The Liver
Biology and Pathobiology

THE LIVER
Biology and Pathobiology

Editors

Irwin M. Arias, M.D.
Professor of Medicine
Director, Liver Research Center
Albert Einstein College of Medicine
Bronx, New York

Hans Popper, M.D., Ph.D.
Gustave L. Levy Distinguished Service
Professor
Mount Sinai School of Medicine
City University of New York
New York, New York

David Schachter, M.D.
Professor of Physiology
Columbia University
College of Physicians and Surgeons
New York, New York

David A. Shafritz, M.D.
Professor of Medicine and Cell Biology
Albert Einstein College of Medicine
Bronx, New York

Raven Press ■ New York

Raven Press, 1140 Avenue of the Americas, New York,
New York 10036

Made in the United States of America

International Standard Book Number 0-89004-575-5
Library of Congress Catalog Number 80-5541

Unbeknown to one of the editors, Hans Popper, his three colleagues have conspired to dedicate this work to him. His intellect has inspired and stimulated at least three generations of hepatologists. His broad range of interest and sustained desire to bridge the gap between advances in basic biology and liver structure, function, and disease exemplify the purpose of this book.

Preface

The roots of contemporary hepatology may be found in the clinical descriptions of the ancients which culminated with the classical writings of the French and German schools in the nineteenth century. Virchow and the generations of morphologists who followed described pathologic processes from gross specimens and light microscopic studies. Their influence dominated studies of the liver until the mid-twentieth century when the influence of post World War II biochemistry and subcellular structure united, and new concepts were introduced into the study of hepatic function, structure, and regulation.

The amazing advances in fundamental biology that have occurred within the past two decades have brought hepatology and other disciplines into new, uncharted and exciting waters. Never before have the opportunities been greater for study of the liver and its diseases than in the era in which we live. Concepts and advances of fundamental biology regarding the structure of cells, how they communicate with each other, how they are assembled and undergo differential turnover without change in morphologic appearance, how they perform their multiple functions under physiologic and pathologic stress, and many other major questions are now being explored using techniques of modern biology.

It is self-evident that dramatic changes in biology will profoundly influence our understanding of liver function and disease, alter our teaching and research, and eventually improve our ability to diagnose, treat, and prevent liver disease. How can a student of the liver and its disease maintain a link to these exciting advances? Most physicians lack the time to take postgraduate courses in basic biology; most basic researchers lack an understanding of liver physiology and disease. For the scientist, the liver is an abundant and easily available source of material for preparation of cells, enzymes, etc. This book is one step in an effort to bridge the ever increasing gap between basic biology and medicine. Numerous excellent volumes exist that describe liver diseases, but none has attempted to bring basic sciences directly into consideration of liver biology and disease processes. We recognize that what was appropriate even as these pages were written will be surpassed in the near future by even more exciting advances.

Toward this end, a group of outstanding basic and clinical investigators have contributed their knowledge in major areas of liver biology and pathobiology. The topics have been integrated to characterize the cells that comprise the liver and their interrelated functions, the function of the liver as an organ in relation to other major organ systems, and a critical analysis of major selected areas of pathobiology.

The authors and editors regard the references to be appropriate for the current state of knowledge and generally reflect the extent of activity in a given area.

The authors and editors will have achieved their goal if the reader finds within these pages exciting glimpses into current state and future directions of our discipline and perspectives that lead to a better understanding of liver function and disease.

Irwin M. Arias
Hans Popper
David Schachter
David A. Shafritz

Contents

Contributors

Philip Aisen, *Departments of Medicine and Physiology, Albert Einstein College of Medicine, Bronx, New York*

Alvito Alvares, *Department of Pharmacology, Uniformed Services School of Medicine, Bethesda, Maryland*

Irwin M. Arias, *Department of Medicine, Director, Liver Research Center, Albert Einstein College of Medicine, Bronx, New York*

Heinz Baumann, *Department of Cell and Tumor Biology, Roswell Park Memorial Institute, Buffalo, New York*

Joseph R. Bloomer, *Department of Medicine, University of Minnesota School of Medicine, Minneapolis, Minnesota*

Harris Busch, *Department of Pharmacology, Baylor College of Medicine, Houston, Texas*

John Caldwell, *Department of Biochemical and Experimental Pharmacology, St. Mary's Hospital Medical School, London, England*

Jose Campra, *Centro Medico De Cordoba, Cordoba, Argentina*

Martin C. Carey, *Gastroenterology Division, Brigham and Women's Hospital, Boston, Massachusetts*

Lawrence Chan, *Departments of Medicine and Cell Biology, Baylor Medical School, Houston, Texas*

Jayanta Roy Chowdhury, *Department of Medicine, Albert Einstein College of Medicine, Bronx, New York*

Robert W. Colman, *Department of Hematology-Oncology, Director, Thrombosis Center, Temple University Health Sciences Center, Philadelphia, Pennsylvania*

Harold O. Conn, *Department of Medicine, Veterans Administration Medical Center, Yale University School of Medicine, New Haven, Connecticut*

Janet Cook, *Department of Cell and Tumor Biology, Roswell Park Memorial Institute, Buffalo, New York*

Gustav Dallner, *Department of Pathology, Karolinska Institute School of Medicine, Stockholm, Sweden*

Darla E. Danford, *Physiological Chemistry Laboratories, Massachusetts Institute of Technology, Cambridge, Massachusetts*

B. deHemptinne, *Catholic University of Louvain, Laboratory of Experimental Surgery, Brussels, Belgium*

Pierre De Meyts, *International Institute of Cellular and Molecular Pathology, Brussels, Belgium*

Helmut Denk, *Department of Pathology, Institute of Pathology, University of Vienna, Vienna, Austria*

Joseph W. DePierre, *Department of Biochemistry, University of Stockholm, Stockholm, Sweden*

Betty Diamond, *Departments of Medicine and Microbiology and Immunology, Albert Einstein College of Medicine, Bronx, New York*

John M. Dietschy, *Department of Medicine, University of Texas Health and Science Center, Dallas, Texas*

Darrell Doyle, *Department of Cell and Tumor Biology, Roswell Park Memorial Institute, Buffalo, New York*

Thomas Duffy, *Department of Biochemistry, Cornell University Medical College, New York, New York*

Sasha Englard, *Department of Biochemistry, Albert Einstein College of Medicine, Bronx, New York*

Murray Epstein, *Department of Medicine, Veterans Administration Medical Center, Miami, Florida*

Serge Erlinger, *Unite de Recherches de Physiopathologie Hepatique, Institut National de la Sante et de la Recherche Medicale, Hôpital Beaujon, Clichy Cedex, France*

H. Dariush Fahimi, *Department of Anatomy, II. Division, Heidelberg, Federal Republic of Germany*

Emmanuel Farber, *Department of Pathology, University of Toronto, Toronto, Ontario, Canada*

Werner W. Franke, *Secretary General, European Cell Biology Organization, Heidelberg, West Germany*

Mark I. Friedman, *Monell Chemical Senses Center, Philadelphia, Pennsylvania*

Paul A. Friedman, *Center for Blood Research, Harvard Medical School, Cambridge, Massachusetts*

Norton B. Gilula, *Department of Cell Biology, Baylor College of Medicine, Houston, Texas*

Robert M. Glickman, *Department of Medicine, Columbia University College of Physicians and Surgeons, New York, New York*

DeWitt S. Goodman, *Department of Medicine, Columbia University College of Physicians and Surgeons, New York, New York*

Carl A. Goresky, *Department of Medicine, Montreal General Hospital, Montreal, Canada*

Roberto J. Groszmann, *Department of Medicine, Veterans Administration Medical Center, Yale University School of Medicine, New Haven, Connecticut*

Jorge J. Gumucio, *Department of Internal Medicine, University of Michigan School of Medicine, Ann Arbor, Michigan*

Jacques Hanoune, *INSERM, Hôpital Henri Mondor, Creteil, France*

Elliot L. Hertzberg, *Department of Biochemistry, Baylor College of Medicine, Houston, Texas*

Peter C. Hinkle, *Department of Biochemistry, Cornell University, Ithaca, New York*

E. Anthony Jones, *Liver Disease Section Digestive Disease Branch, National Institutes of Health, Bethesda, Maryland*

Katherine S. Koch, *Department of Pharmacology, University of California School of Medicine, La Jolla, California*

P. J. Lad, *Department of Pharmacology, University of California School of Medicine, La Jolla, California*

Paul B. Lazarow, *Department of Medicine, Rockefeller University, New York, New York*

Hyman L. Leffert, *Department of Medicine, University of California School of Medicine, La Jolla, California*

Alton Meister, *Department of Biochemistry, Cornell University Medical College, New York, New York*

Deborah L. Miller, *Department of Internal Medicine, The University of Michigan School of Medicine, Ann Arbor, Michigan*

Anatol G. Morell, *Department of Medicine, Albert Einstein College of Medicine, Bronx, New York*

Hamish N. Munro, *Department of Physiological Chemistry, USDA Human Nutrition Research Center on Aging, Tufts University, Boston, Massachusetts*

Alex B. Novikoff, *Department of Pathology, Albert Einstein College of Medicine, Bronx, New York*

Phyllis Marie Novikoff, *Department of Pathology, Albert Einstein College of Medicine, Bronx, New York*

Fred Plum, *Department of Neurology, New York Hospital-Cornell Medical Center, New York, New York*

Hans Popper, *Mount Sinai School of Medicine, City University of New York, New York, New York*

Sue G. Powers, *Department of Biochemistry, Cornell University Medical College, New York, New York*

Juerg Reichen, *Departments of Medicine and Clinical Pharmacology, University of Colorado Medical Center, Denver, Colorado*

Telfer Reynolds, *Department of Medicine, University of Southern California, Los Angeles, California*

Marcos Rojkind, *Department of Biochemistry, Centro de Investigacion Y de Estudios Avanzados del IPN, Mexico, D.F.*

Ronald N. Rubin, *Department of Hematology-Oncology, Temple University Health Sciences Center, Philadelphia, Pennsylvania*

Seymour M. Sabesin, *Department of Medicine, The University of Tennessee Center for the Health Sciences, Memphis, Tennessee*

David Schachter, *Department of Physiology, College of Physicians and Surgeons, New York, New York*

Sam Seifter, *Department of Biochemistry, Albert Einstein College of Medicine, Bronx, New York*

David A. Shafritz, *Departments of Medicine and Cell Biology, Albert Einstein College of Medicine, Bronx, New York*

Dennis Shields, *Department of Anatomy, Albert Einstein College of Medicine, Bronx, New York*

Francis R. Simon, *Department of Medicine, University of Colorado Medical Center, Denver, Colorado*

Harold Skelly, *Department of Pharmacology, University of California School of Medicine, La Jolla, California*

John Edgar Smith, *Department of Medicine, College of Physicians and Surgeons, New York, New York*

Richard J. Stockert, *Department of Medicine, Albert Einstein College of Medicine, Bronx, New York*

Irmin Sternlieb, *Department of Medicine, Albert Einstein College of Medicine, Bronx, New York*

John A. Summerfield, *Department of Medicine, Royal Free Hospital, England*

Stephen D. Turley, *Department of Medicine, University of Texas Health and Science Center, Dallas, Texas*

David H. van Thiel, *Department of Gastroenterology, University of Pittsburgh School of Medicine, Pittsburgh, Pennsylvania*

Allan Wolkoff, *Department of Medicine, Albert Einstein College of Medicine, Bronx, New York*

Stephen P. Young, *Liver Unit, Kings College Hospital, London, England*

Mark A. Zern, *Department of Medicine, Albert Einstein College of Medicine, Bronx, New York*

The Liver
Biology and Pathobiology

SECTION I

Introduction: Organizational Principles

Section I

Introduction: Organizational Principles

The liver in adult man constitutes approximately 2.5% of body weight; at birth, it forms 5%. The structural organization of the parenchymal and vascular elements of the liver is adapted to its special function as a guardian interposed between the digestive tract (and spleen) and the rest of the body. One aspect of this interposition is the handling of large amounts of nutrient amino acids, carbohydrates, lipids, vitamins, and pollutant xenobiotics which enter the body in food and water. A major hepatic function involves effective uptake of substrates from the intestine and their subsequent storage, metabolism, and distribution to blood and bile. Another function of the liver is biotransformation of xenobiotic pollutants, drugs, and endogenous metabolites; these processes occur in the cytosol, endoplasmic reticulum, and nuclear envelope. Monooxygenases utilize atmospheric oxygen to transform exogenous and endogenous substrates and render them susceptible to subsequent biotransformation reactions, such as glucuronidation and sulfation. The major nonoxidative pathway, which requires GSH as substrate, is also most abundant in hepatocytes.

Although the oxidative and nonoxidative biotransformation systems are quantitatively most active and have been best studied in the liver, they are present in other organs, particularly kidney, small intestine, and several endocrine organs. They protect vital systems and, in principle, convert lipid-soluble materials to water-soluble products which can be excreted in bile and urine. Some metabolites formed can be toxic or carcinogenic. Immunologically derived immune complexes enter the liver from the lymphatic system (primarily from the spleen); endotoxins enter from intestinal bacterial flora. Hepatic sinusoidal lining cells have substantial endocytotic and phagocytotic potencies. The liver is quantitatively the most effective site for phagocytosis of solid material, such as bacteria. The formation of bile imposes a need for glandular structure. In addition, the liver accommodates, in sponge-like fashion, at least 300 ml blood in normal adults and thereby participates in the regulation of blood flow and volume.

To meet specific demands, six specific principles govern structure and function: (a) the expression of exocrine and metabolic functions in the same cell; (b) a double blood supply with splanchnic blood from the portal vein exposed to a second interaction with cells in a microvascular system; biliary solutes are reabsorbed in the intestine and undergo enterohepatic circulation, escape from which results from either incomplete reabsorption and loss into the stool or impaired hepatic uptake with entry to the systemic circulation; (c) a specific architectual arrangement of single cells and cell masses to facilitate exchange between blood and hepatocytes; (d) features of perihepatocellular (Disse) spaces, such as the lack of basement membrane, to maximize such exchange; (e) separation of the lumen of biliary from blood spaces compartmentalizing excretory from other hepatocytic functions; and (f) specific biochemical activities of hepatocytic organelles and cell membranes regulating specific functions.

Both structural principles and unique demands made on the liver are reflected in hepatic phylogenesis and ontogenesis. Phylogenetically, the liver first appears in colenterates, such as sea anemones, as a regional thickening of the endodermal primordial gut. This region provides metabolic and storage functions. As a morphologically identified organ develops, specific defense and preservation functions appeared when aquatic animals became terrestrial. For example, overloading by amino acids was associated with development of urea cycle enzymes. The lack of an aquatic milieu, which facilitates exchange, made homeostasis a problem, biotransformation essential, and immunologic reactivity more sophisticated.

In embryonal development, the yolk sac fulfills the early function of the liver. During the fourth week of gestation, an hepatic diverticulum of the endoderm forms in the foregut. The lower part of the diverticulum becomes the anlage of bile duct and gall bladder; the upper part forms epithelial cords, which extend throughout a mesenchymal mass, and the septum transversum, which differentiates into a lacunar blood-filled labyrinth derived from the vitelline veins. The afferent blood vessels eventually become the portal vein. The labyrinth is drained by confluent venous branches which develop into the hepatic veins; the umbilical vein provides an additional source of hepatic blood.

In early embryonal stages, hepatocytes form cords in which (as in a gland) multiple epithelial cells appear on the cut surface to surround the lumen. The epithelial cell masses cluster around a biliary vascular axis to which afferent blood is brought from hepatic arteries and portal veins; bile is secreted in the opposite direction. As metabolic demands rise, the gland-like cords are transformed into a sponge-like wall work, or cellular mass, which is composed of hepatocellular plates meeting at different angles and surrounding the hepatic lacunae. The cell mass is traversed by two tracts of connective tissue which ramify within the liver. The wider one constitutes the portal tracts which carry afferent blood vessels, bile ducts, lymphatics, and nerves; and the narrower one surrounds tributaries of the hepatic veins. The two tracts interdigitate but do not connect. Thus the terminal branches of portal veins and hepatic arteries are separated from hepatic vein tributaries by the hepatic parenchyma. Parenchymal blood flow partly depends on the gradient between pressure in the terminal portal vein, which is estimated at 50 ml water, and in the initial hepatic vein, which is approximately 10 ml water. The more important driving force is hepatic arterial flow, which is regulated by muscular sphincters in arterioles which have a lumen of at least 15 nm in diameter.

Present evidence suggests that sinusoidal flow is continuous and is also modified by local sphincteric action of perisinusoidal cells. The conveyance of the hepatic plates toward the hepatic veins is determined by blood flow, and results in the lobule as the apparent structural unit of the liver. The radius of the lobule is the distance between the terminations of the two connective tissue tracts. Physiologic considerations and histochemical localization of various hepatic functions make the hepatic acinus a more reasonable functional unit than is the lobule. The acinus has the portal tract in its center and consists of parts of several lobules. Since arborization of portal tracts is irregular, hepatic acini assume several shapes. At birth, hepatocytic plates are usually two cells thick; they become one cell thick at the age of 5. This adaptation maximizes contact between blood and hepatocytes.

Hepatocytes surround bile canaliculi which are approximately 1 μm in diameter. Their wall is an adapted part of the hepatocellular plasma membrane and is elongated by formation of finger-like microvilli which often fill the lumen. In the primordial stage, the bile canaliculus appears lined on the cut surface, as in a gland, by several hepatocytes. On subsequent maturation, this is reduced usually to two (or at the most four) hepatocytes. The canaliculi form a chicken-wire-like communicating network in the center of the hepatocytic plates. Approximately 15% of the plasma membrane is formed by bile canaliculi. Even in normal liver, the canaliculi extend as diverticuli into the hepatocytes, but they remain separated from the perihepatocytic spaces by junctional complexes of desmosomes and tight junctions.

Traditionally, the tight junction has been considered to be impermeable; at present, paracellular flow of micromolecular solutes is accepted. The bile canaliculi are the main source of bile released into the duodenum. Through the transitional canals of Herring, they connect to ductules and ducts which form the biliary passages. This system is lined by uniformly shaped epithelial cells, 10 μm in diameter, which have smaller nuclei and mitochondria than the hepatocytes. Biliary epithelial cells lack the characteristic glucose-6-phosphatase reaction of hepatocytes and have a distinct basement membrane on the straight base of the epithelium. Hepatocytes differ from ductal and ductular cells by morphologic and functional criteria, and transformation of one cell type into the other in embryonal development or disease is not established. In contrast, the separation of ductal from ductular cells is less distinct. Although the conduit function of ducts and ductules is prominent, composition of the bile is changed by reabsorption and secretin-dependent secretion. Somatostatin influences canalicular and ductal bile secretion; bicarbonate secretion, which was previously considered specific for the bile ductular system, may also occur in the canaliculi. Approximately one-third of basal human bile secretion (total probably 750 ml/day) seems to be of ductal and ductular origin, to which should be added 20 ml/day mucus, which is formed by glands adnexal to large extrahepatic bile ducts.

The plasma membrane of hepatocytes includes a straight lateral domain (Fig. 1) in which plasma membrane bilayers of contiguous hepatocytes form an intercellular cleft (20 nm in width). Gap junctions provide for communication between neighboring hepatocytes. The hepatocytic plasma membrane which lines the perisinusoidal space has numerous irregular microvilli which protrude into the space. Extensions of the perisinusoidal space between neighboring hepatocytes form a paracellular space which retains a few microvilli; their disappearance indicates the transition to the intercellular cleft. The plasma membrane of the hepatocytes, which is directed toward the perisinusoidal and paracellular spaces, is called the basolateral surface, in analogy to other epithelial cells, and differs chemically and histochemically from the canalicular and straight contiguous surfaces. However, the borders between microvilli-endowed and straight hepatocytic domains are movable, depending on functional demands. In regeneration or in cholestasis, the straight domain is greatly reduced.

The perisinusoidal space is separated from the sinusoid by a layer of sinusoidal cells, of which the endothelial cells are most effective in forming a bar-

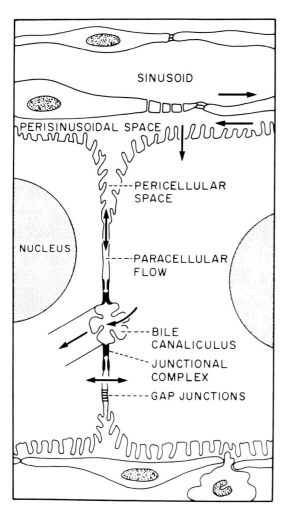

FIG. 1. Principal surfaces (domains) of hepatocytes in relation to the perihepatocellular spaces. Arrows, directions of fluid flow.

rier; other sinusoidal cells have a lesser contribution. The barrier is less tight than that in other organs because the endothelial cells have sieve-like plates which permit fluid, solutes, and even corpuscular elements up to the size of a chylomicron to pass from blood into the perisinusoidal space. In contrast to portal capillaries and gland-like structures, such as the bile ducts, a continuous basement membrane cannot be demonstrated in the perisinusoidal space by electron microscopy. Immunofluorescence studies suggest the presence of basement membrane-like material. The absence of a structurally defined basement membrane facilitates exchange between blood and hepatocytes. Plasticity of the liver is maintained by an ectoskeleton of discontinuous collagen fibrils and a matrix of glycosaminoglycans and glycoproteins, such as laminin and fibronectin. Despite the demonstrable apertures in the endothelial cells, the protein content in perisinusoidal tissue fluid is at least 30% lower than in plasma and increases after cellular injury. This fluid is drained in lymphatics, which begin in the portal spaces and account for the direction of the tissue fluid flow, which parallels that of bile and is opposite to that of blood flow.

Flow of the three fluids is regulated by different factors which, together with chemical mediators (e.g., hormones), determine the functional efficiency of the liver. Innervation of the hepatic parenchyma requires further study. Nervous influence on hepatic function depends greatly on regulation of parenchymal blood flow, which is accomplished by various sphincters, including those of the arterioles and inlet sphincters in the terminal portal veins. In man, hepatic outlet control is not accomplished by muscular sphincters but by the entrance of small hepatic venous tributaries into large ones; contraction of the large veins by a few muscles has a throttle effect.

Various diseases, hepatic and otherwise, not only vary functional demands on the liver but also alter its structure to reflect violations of the structural principles. For example, tissue repair by regeneration or tumorous transformation follow oncogenetic development in that hepatocellular plates again become several cells wide, thus interfering with hepatocyte/blood exchange, which is only partly compensated for by extension of the perisinusoidal space. Abnormal communications between afferent and efferent blood supply characterize cirrhosis; they deprive the body of the function of hepatocytes independently of their structural integrity. Cholestasis alters the relationship between canaliculi and perisinusoidal spaces, thereby modifying bile flow. Therefore, functional and structural alterations in disease assist, as experiments of nature, in the exploration and recognition of basic physiologic and biologic phenomena.

REFERENCES

1. Bolck, F., and Machnik, G. (1978): *Leber and Gallenwege,* Springer-Verlag, Berlin.
2. Elias, H., and Sherrick, J. C. (1969): *Morphology of the Liver.* Academic Press, New York.
3. Popper, H., and Schaffner, F. (1957): *Liver: Structure and Function.* McGraw-Hill, New York.
4. Rappaport, A. M. (1980): Hepatic blood flow: Morphologic aspects and physiologic regulation. In: *Liver and Biliary Tract Physiology, International Review of Physiology, Vol. 21,* edited by N. B. Javitt. University Park Press, Baltimore.

SECTION II

The Cells

Section II

The Cells

A. The Hepatocyte

The parenchymal liver cells, or hepatocytes, are the main functional units of the liver, numbering about 250 billion in the normal adult organ. Although their function, structure, and shape depend on their specific position in the liver cell plate, particularly in the various zones of the acinus, each individual hepatocyte probably has the potential for all functions. The factors that regulate expression of individual hepatocyte functions are poorly understood but are partially determined by hepatic microcirculatory dynamics.

The hepatocyte is a polyhedral multifaceted cell with eight or more surfaces. Its diameter varies between 13 and 30 μm, with the average of 25 μm; its shape resembles that of a small liver. Several structural surface components participate in two or three major domains of the hepatocyte: (a) the basolateral surface (perisinusoidal and paracellular), which has many microvilli, (b) the straight or contiguous domain, and (c) the bile canalicular surface. Hepatocytes represent about 60% of cells in the liver. Because they are larger than the other cells in the liver, they occupy almost 80% of parenchymal volume. In contrast, the sinusoidal cells account for about 6.5% of hepatic volume, and extracellular spaces account for 16 to 20%, of which about two-thirds represent the sinusoidal lumen and one-third the perisinusoidal tissue space of Disse (1). Recent stereologic measurements (2,3), based on morphometric techniques introduced by Weidel (4), indicate that the single mononuclear hepatocyte has an average volume of 11,000 μm³. The cytoplasm contains glycogen granules of 12 nm diameter and occupies one-half the cell; the nucleus occupies a little more than 7% of cell volume. In normal mice, the diploid nucleus has a dry mass of 45 pg, which increases to 190 pg in octoploid hepatocytes (5).

The structure and function of the plasma membrane of the hepatocyte and of organelle membranes are, in principle, the same as in other cells. Most of the specificity of hepatic function results from quantitative variations in the potentials which are expressed in other cells. Relatively few metabolic pathways are specific for hepatocytes. The most important are (a) the urea cycle (ornithine-citrulline-arginine-ornithine), which metabolically regulates the excess of amino acids and ammonia derived from the intestine and its bacterial flora, (b) specific regulations of lipid metabolism related to the massive intestinal absorption of lipids, and (c) formation of bilirubin and bile acids in relation to bile secretion. Details of the structural responses of organelles to specific demands and concomitant biochemical adaptations are discussed in subsequent chapters.

Several quantitative data may aid the reader in appreciating the nature and extent of hepatocyte structure in relation to organelle functions and disease. Quantitation of hepatocyte organelles has been accomplished in human needle biopsy specimens. In principle, the results resemble those found in rodent liver; however, the average size of the hepatocyte may be only half. There are approximately 2,000 mitochondria per hepatocyte, which account for 18% of the total cellular volume. Their average size is 0.8 μm³. Mitochondria are more numerous, larger, and longer in hepatocytes around portal tracts, and are closely related to the rough endoplasmic reticulum, which comprises approximately 7% of cellular space. The smooth endoplasmic reticulum and the Golgi apparatus constitute 12% of cellular volume. The number and size (1 to 6 μm in diameter) of lysosomes vary greatly, even in normal hepatocytes. There are about 1,000 peroxisomes, which average 0.13 μm³ in each hepatocyte. The hepatocyte plasma membrane is 7 nm thick and is a bilayer characteristically found in all cellular membranes. Biochemically, hepatocyte plasma membranes have a relatively high amount of glycosylated protein and lipids and a complex pattern of polypeptides, which is reflected in numerous enzymes that differ in various domains. All plasma membrane domains have a high cholesterol/phospholipid ratio and sphingomyelin content (6). The sinusoidal surface has phagocytotic and endocytotic properties, which are reflected in formation of coated and noncoated vesicles, approximately 100 nm in diameter. The coated pits in the plasma membrane of hepatocytes are less numerous than in fibroblasts. Galactose, glucose, and fucose oligosaccharide extensions of receptors are present in mammalian liver; the most specific for hepatocytes are galactose terminated. Following endocytosis, material is transferred within minutes to lysosomes and to the Golgi zone (7); the ligand is metabolized, and some receptors and other plasma membrane constituents recycle. This general concept applies to materials, such as peptide hormones, which are endocytosed, whereas other proteins, such as immunoglobulin A, are transferred in coated or noncoated vesicles to the bile canaliculi (8). Transcytoplasmic transport is facilitated by the cytoskeleton, the distribution of which has been better visualized since the introduction of glutaraldehyde fixation into electron microscopy and decoration by specific fluorescent antibodies. Quick freeze-deep etching techniques (9) will further improve visualization; present descriptions of the cytoskeleton, therefore, constitute a progress report in this rapidly developing field.

REFERENCES

1. Blouin, A. (1977): Morphometry of liver sinusoidal cells. In: *Kupffer Cells and Other Liver Sinusoidal Cells,* edited by E. Wisse and K. L. Knook, pp. 61–71. Elsevier/Amsterdam.
2. Rohr, H. P., Lüthy, J., Gudat, F., Oberholzer, M., Gysin, C., Stalder, G., and Bianchi, L. (1976): Stereology: A new supplement to the study of human liver biopsy specimens. In: *Progress in Liver Diseases, Vol. V,* edited by H. Popper and F. Schaffner, pp. 24–34. Grune & Stratton, New York.
3. Loud, A. V. (1968): A quantitative stereological description of the ultrastructure of normal rat liver parenchymal cells. *J. Cell Biol.,* 37:27–46.
4. Weidel, E. R. (1969): Stereological principles for morphometry in electron microscopic cytology. *Int. Rev. Cytol.,* 26:235–302.
5. Davies, H. G. et al. (1957): Attempts at measurement of lipid, nucleic acid, and protein content of cell nuclei by microscope-interferometry. *Exp. Cell Res.,* 4:136–149.
6. Evans, W. H. (1970): A biomedical dissection of the functional polarity of the plasma membrane of the hepatocyte. *Biochim. Biophys. Acta,* 604:27–64.
7. Wall, D. A., Wilson, G., and Hubbard, A. L. (1980): The galactose-specific recognition system of mammalian liver: The route of ligand internalization in rat hepatocytes. *Cell,* 21:79–93.
8. Renston, R. H., Maloney, D. G., Jones, A. L., Hradek, G. T., Wong, K. Y., and Goldfine, I. D. (1980): Bile secretory apparatus: Evidence for a vesicular transport mechanism for proteins in the rat, using horseradish peroxidase and ^{125}I insulin. *Gastroenterology,* 78:1373–1388.
9. Heuser, J. (1980): Three-dimensional visualization of coated vesicle formation in fibroblasts. *J. Cell Biol.,* 84:560–583.

The Liver: Biology and Pathobiology, edited by
I. Arias, H. Popper, D. Schachter, and D. A. Shafritz.
Raven Press, New York © 1982.

Chapter 1

Mitochondria

Peter C. Hinkle

Mitochondria are respiratory organelles that constitute about 20% of the cytoplasmic volume of liver cells. Their primary function is to conserve the energy from oxidation of substrates by oxygen as the high-energy phosphate anhydride bonds of ATP. Other functions in liver cells, include citrulline synthesis and regulation of intracellular calcium ion concentration. They are an excellent example of the role of membranes and compartmentation in cellular metabolism. The concentration of tricarboxylic acid cycle intermediates inside mitochondria is important for the rate and regulation of this major pathway. The location of the enzymes of oxidative phosphorylation in the mitochondrial inner membrane not only allows them to interact more rapidly but is crucial for the basic coupling mechanism, which involves the formation and utilization of an electrochemical proton gradient across the membrane.

This chapter outlines the structure and function of liver mitochondria and summarizes the relationship of mitochondria and substrate transport pathways to the major metabolic pathways in liver cells. For a more detailed discussion, the reader is referred to several recent reviews (1–5).

STRUCTURE

The electron micrograph (Fig. 1) shows a typical rat liver mitochondrion. All mitochondria have a basic two-membrane structure: an outer membrane enclosing an inner membrane, which is highly folded. The folds, called cristae, greatly increase the area of the inner membrane. Various lines of evidence

point to a prokaryotic origin of mitochondria, although DNA sequence indicates a complex evolution (6). Liver mitochondria vary in size and shape, depending on their relationship to the blood supply. For a discussion of mitochondrial shape during developmental and other states, see the recent review by Pollak and Sutton (7). The traditional mitochondrial vital stain for light microscopy is Janus green, which is oxidized by mitochondria, resulting in their staining. Fluorescent dyes specific for mitochondria have been found (8), which are lipid-soluble cations accumulated in mitochondria by the large interior negative membrane potential created by respiration. The fluorescence microscope allows excellent visualization of the shape and location of mitochondria in living cells and indicates that some of them are extremely long.

The mitochondrial matrix is a concentrated protein solution of the enzymes of the tricarboxylic acid cycle, fatty acid oxidation, and urea synthesis, as outlined in Table 1. The fact that the protein concentration is unusually high may lead to "microcompartmentation" of intermediates of various pathways (10).

The inner and outer mitochondrial membranes may be separated by density gradient centrifugation after breaking the outer membrane by an osmotic shock (11,12). The enzyme composition of the membranes is also listed in Table 1. The outer membrane functions as a corset to hold the highly folded inner membrane together. It is permeable to molecules less than ~2,000 daltons because of special pores. These pores have been isolated and reconstituted into planar bilayer membranes (13) and liposomes (14). Strangely, when studied in the planar bilayers where electrical mea-

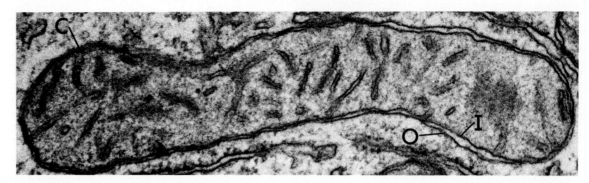

FIG. 1. Mitochondrion of rat liver. O, outer mitochondrial membrane; I, inner mitochondrial membrane; C, crista. ×61,000. (Provided by A. B. Novikoff.)

TABLE 1. *Location of liver mitochondrial enzymes*[a]

Outer Membrane
  Monoamine oxidase
  Cytochrome b_5 reductase
  Cytochrome b_5
  Kynurenine hydroxylase
  Pore protein
  Phospholipase A_2
  Lysophosphatidate acyltransferase
  Glycerophosphate acyltransferase
  Acyl CoA synthetase

Intermembrane Space
  Adenylate kinase
  Nucleosidediphosphate kinase
  DNAse I
  Sulfite-cytochrome c reductase
  D-Xylulose reductase
  Cytochrome c

Inner Membrane
  *F_1-F_0 ATPase (ATP synthase)
  NADH- CoQ reductase (complex I)
  Succinate-CoQ reductase (complex II)
  Glycerol-3-phosphate-CoQ reductase
  Electron-transferring-flavoprotein CoQ reductase
  Choline-CoQ reductase
  Proline-CoQ reductase
  *$CoQH_2$-cytochrome c reductase (complex III)
  Cytochrome c
  *Cytochrome c oxidase
  3-Hydroxybutyrate dehydrogenase (NAD)
  NAD(P) Transhydrogenase
  Inorganic pyrophosphatase
  Carnitine palmitoyltransferase
  Transporters for the following substrates
    *ATP-ADP antiport
    *Phosphate-OH antiport
    Dicarboxylate-P_i antiport
    Tricarboxylate-malate antiport
    Pyruvate-OH antiport
    Glutamate-OH antiport
    Glutamate-aspartate antiport
    α-Ketoglutarate-malate antiport
    L-Ornithine-proton antiport
    Citrulline uniport
    Acryl carnitine-carnitine antiport
    Calcium ion uniport
    Calcium-proton antiport
    Sodium, potassium-proton antiport

Matrix
  Tricarboxylic acid cycle
    Pyruvate dehydrogenase
    Citrate synthase
    Aconitate hydratase
    Isocitrate dehydrogenase (NAD and NADP)
    α-Ketoglutarate dehydrogenase
    Succinyl-CoA synthetase (GTP)
    Fumarate hydratase
    Malate dehydrogenase
  Urea cycle enzymes
    Carbamoyl-phosphate synthase (ammonia)
    Ornithine carbamoyltransferase
  Fatty acid oxidation
    Acetyl-CoA synthetase
    Acyl-CoA synthetase (GTP)
    Acyl-CoA dehydrogenase (ETF)
    Enoyl-CoA hydratase
    Enoyl-CoA isomerase
    3-Hydroxyacyl-CoA dehydrogenase (NAD)
    Acetyl-CoA acetyl transferase
    Acetyl-CoA acyl transferase
    Electron-transferring flavoprotein (ETF)
  Other matrix enzymes
    Fatty acid elongation system
    Aspartate aminotransferase
    Aldehyde dehydrogenase
    Dimethylglycine dehydrogenase (ETF)
    Sarcosine dehydrogenase (ETF)
    Glutamate dehydrogenase (NAD(P))
    Hydroxymethylglutaryl-CoA lyase
    Hydroxymethylglutaryl-CoA synthase
    Nucleosidediphosphate kinase
    Phosphoenolpyruvate carboxykinase (GTP)
    Pyruvate carboxylase
    Aminoacyl-tRNA synthetases
    DNA polymerase
    Elongation factors
    Polyriboadenylate polymerase
    RNA polymerase
    Ribosomes
    Propionyl-CoA carboxylase (ATP)
    Methylmalonyl-CoA mutase
    Methylmalonyl-CoA racemase

[a] For a more complete list and details, see ref. 9. The starred components each constitute about 10% of the membrane.

surements are possible, the protein functions as a voltage-dependent anion channel, which is open only at low voltages. There is presumably little if any membrane potential across the mitochondrial outer membrane, and the voltage dependence of the channel has no known function. The pores are analogous to pores in the outer membrane of bacteria.

The inner membrane has only 20% lipid and contains no cholesterol. It is a fluid membrane and has negative surface potential. This potential holds the majority of the cytochrome c, which is a soluble cationic protein, bound on the outer surface of the inner membrane.

The inner membrane from rat liver mitochondria can also be separated from the outer membrane by treatment with digitonin, which breaks up the latter because it contains cholesterol. The resulting intact inner membrane, called a mitoplast (15), retains oxidative phosphorylation. Liposomes can be fused with mitoplasts to deliver their contents inside and add phospholipid to the membrane (16).

Sonication fragments mitochondria to smaller, sealed vesicles called "submitochondrial particles" (for liver submitochondrial particles, see ref. 17). These vesicles are predominantly inside-out. Electron microscopy, using phosphotungstate negative stain of submitochondrial particles, reveals 90 Å diameter knobs attached to the outside surface. Originally discovered by Fernandez-Moran (18), these were thought to be the respiratory chain and thus were called "elementary particles." Racker and Horstman (19) later showed that they were the ATPase-coupling factor F_1, and that inner membranes stripped of F_1 had a normal respiratory chain but no knobs. Adding back F_1 restored the knobs and oxidative phosphorylation.

OXIDATIVE PHOSPHORYLATION

The Respiratory Chain

The components of the respiratory chain, shown in Fig. 2, have been elucidated during the last 40 years. The iron-sulfur centers (Fe-s) and the hemes of cytochromes are electron carriers, the flavins and coenzyme Q are hydrogen carriers. A possible exception is cytochrome b, which appears to be a hydrogen carrier, probably by a Bohr effect mechanism, which causes dissociation of protons from the protein when the heme is oxidized. Other possible complexities are illustrated by the fact that cytochrome c, the best studied cytochrome, has several anion binding sites in the oxidized state and several cation binding sites in the reduced state (20), which could make the ionic aspects of electron transfer down the chain very complex. These effects may be control mechanisms regulating the midpoint potentials of the electron carriers rather than part of the mechanisms of ion transport across the membrane.

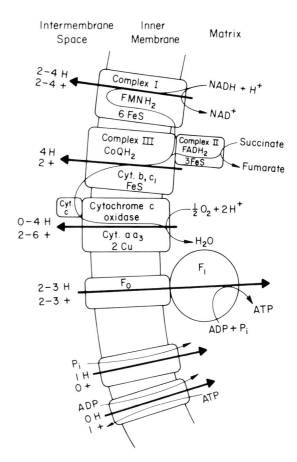

FIG. 2. Diagram of proton transport reactions of the mitochondrial inner membrane. Proton efflux driven by electron transfer down the respiratory chain from NADH or succinate to oxygen and the influx of protons driving ATP synthesis by F_1 and uptake of phosphate and ADP are shown. Thin arrows show electron movement through the complexes (without detail), thick arrows show proton transport. Numbers on the left describe the range of proposals for the stoichiometry of hydrogen (H) and charge (+) transport.

The function of the respiratory chain is to transport protons out of mitochondria, forming an electrochemical proton gradient. This gradient consists of a membrane potential, positive outside, and pH gradient acid outside. Exactly how it does this is still uncertain. Proton transport is a property of the chain itself, since each isolated segment can be incorporated into phospholipid vesicles, which then show the appropriate proton transport process (21–23). The first fact to establish in studies of proton transport is the stoichiometry, currently a subject of much debate. A summary of proposals for the number of protons pumped out of mitochondria for each electron pair transferred from NADH or succinate to oxygen is shown in Table 2. Mitchell (24) proposed and defends (1) the scheme shown in column 1. His proposal is based on studies of rat liver mitochondria, where oxygen pulses were given to anaerobic suspensions of mitochondria in the presence of β-hydroxybutyrate or succinate plus rotenone. The pH of the medium was recorded with a glass electrode. The burst of acid following an oxygen pulse indicated the stoichiometry shown. These values led to Mitchell's "loop" mechanism of proton transport, in which hydrogen and electron carriers alternate in carrying reducing equivalents back and forth across the membrane. This scheme includes the "Q cycle" mechanism for electron transport through the cytochrome b region of the chain (25). More recently, Wikstrom et al. (5) presented evidence that cytochrome oxidase pumps two protons outward across the membrane, in addition to the movement of two electrons inward proposed by Mitchell (4), or moves four positive charges and two protons outward for each electron pair going to oxygen. The groups of Azzone and Lehninger have proposed even higher stoichiometries of proton transport by the respiratory chain (26–28) as listed in column 3 of Table 2. Lehninger (28) has used initial rates of proton transport and oxygen uptake measured with a pH electrode and oxygen electrode to obtain such high ratios and has added N-ethylmaleimide to inhibit phosphate transport, which he claims interferes with measurement of the proton stoichiometry.

The stoichiometries of proton transport by the respiratory chain and by the F_1-F_0 ATPase determine the P/O ratio for synthesis of ATP inside mitochondria. There is an additional complication for the P/O ratio for synthesis of external ATP from external ADP and P_i, as pointed out by Klingenberg (29). The exchange of internal ATP for external ADP catalyzed by the ATP/ADP antiporter is electrogenic and actively exports ATP driven by the membrane potential. One negative electric charge leaves the mitochondrion for each ATP transported to the external medium. The transport of phosphate into mitochondria is an electroneutral process, in exchange for an hydroxide ion or with a proton (30). These two transport systems make the overall transport of ADP and P_i in and ATP out of mitochondria coupled to the influx of one proton, electrically with the ADP and chemically with the P_i. The result is that one more proton is used for the synthesis and transport of ATP out of mitochondria than is used for the actual synthesis on F_1. Mitchell (1) has not accepted the evidence that ATP efflux is electrogenic and proposed that the P/O ratios are the classic values of 2 with succinate- and 3 with NADH-linked substrates (see Table 2). Lehninger (28), Azzone (26,27), and Wikstrom (5) have separately proposed that the H/O ratios are high enough to compensate for the extra proton involved in ATP and P_i transport, so that the P/O ratios for synthesis of external ATP by mitochondria are also the classic values. I recently described measurements of P/O ratios in rat liver mitochondria (31) which were about 1.4 with succinate and 2.2 with β-hydroxybutyrate. These values

TABLE 2. *Proposed coupling ratios of mitochondria*

Ratio	A	B	C	D	E
H/O (succinate)	4	8	6	4	6
H/O (NADH)	6	12	—	6	10
H/ATP (F_1-F_0)	2	3	2	2	3
H/ATP (transport)	0	1	1	1	1
P/O (succinate)	2	2	2	1.3	1.5
P/O (NADH)	3	3	—	2	2.5

A: refs. 1,24; B: refs. 26–28; C: ref. 5; D,E: ref. 31.

are consistent with either of the last two schemes shown in Table 2.

MEASUREMENT OF $\Delta\bar{\mu}_{H^+}$

The value of the electrochemical potential difference (or gradient) of protons across the mitochondrial inner membrane was first measured by Mitchell and Moyle (32) and has been reported many times since, using the same principles for measurement but several different methods (33–35). The principles used are to calculate the membrane potential ($\Delta\psi$) from the distribution of a permeant cation. The potential may be calculated from the Nernst equation,

$$\Delta\psi = \frac{RT}{nF} \ln \frac{C_{in}}{C_{out}}$$

$$= 59 \log \frac{C_{in}}{C_{out}} \text{ (in mV, at T = 25°, n = 1)}$$

Mitchell and Moyle (32) used K^+ ions and valinomycin as the permeant cation, measured uptake with a glass K^+-sensitive electrode, and assumed an internal volume of 0.4 μl/mg to calculate the internal K^+ concentration. Values ranged from 85 to 200 mV in rat liver mitochondria, depending on the external K^+ concentration. The authors also measured the pH gradient from the internal buffering power and the amount of acid appearing outside following a large oxygen pulse. The values for ΔpH ranged from 0.5 to 2.5 pH units. The overall electrochemical proton gradient, $\Delta\bar{\mu}_{H^+}$, was the sum of $\Delta\psi$ and ΔpH, or about 230 mV, positive outside. This is the thermodynamic driving force for proton influx during ATP synthesis, regardless of the detailed mechanism. More recent determinations have given a range of values. Nicholls (34) used radioactively labeled rubidium ions plus valinomycin as the permeant cation and acetate as a permeant acid which distributes across the membrane according to ΔpH and found a $\Delta\bar{\mu}_{H^+}$ essentially identical to that of Mitchell and Moyle (32). He used filtration without washing to separate the mitochondria from the medium for counting the internal isotopes. Others (33–36) have obtained lower values of $\Delta\bar{\mu}_{H^+}$ of 160 to 180 mV using the same or similar isotopic probes and centrifugation to separate the mitochondria from the medium. The value of $\Delta\bar{\mu}_{H^+}$ is relevant to the coupling ratio problem because the thermodynamic energy available can set limits on the possible coupling stoichiometry. When $\Delta\bar{\mu}_{H^+}$ and ΔG_{ATP} formed by mitochondria are compared, for example, a limit for the H/ATP ratio for synthesis and transport can be calculated. The values in rat liver mitochondria range from 2.5 (30) to 8 (36), reflecting the large range in measured values of $\Delta\bar{\mu}_{H^+}$.

Despite the uncertainty about the coupling ratios, there is some knowledge of the mechanism of proton transport by the respiratory chain and through the F_1 ATPase during ATP synthesis. Isotope exchange studies indicate that two or more alternating sites may be involved and that formation of bound ATP from ADP and P_i is a rapidly reversed step (37,38). During ATP hydrolysis, this step reverses, even when there is no electrochemical proton gradient across the membrane. The sequence of the small hydrophobic polypeptide, which forms a proton channel across the membrane leading to F_1, has been determined (39). The subunit structure of F_1 is uncertain; several lines of evidence indicate three copies of each of the large subunits (40), but the more definitive X-ray crystallography indicates two of each (41).

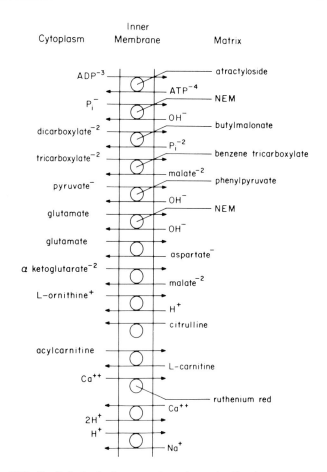

FIG. 3. Substrate transport systems in the inner membrane of mitochondria. (See text for further details.)

SUBSTRATE TRANSPORT

The mitochondrial inner membrane is impermeable to ions in general. Specific transporters are present to allow entry of substrates. There are three types of coupling for the anion transporters: (a) electroneutral proton (or hydroxide) compensated, (b) electroneutral exchange, and (c) electrogenic (2,42). Figure 3 illustrates these transport systems. The adenine nucleotide transporter is electrogenic and exchanges ATP^{-4} for ADP^{-3} (26); it does not transport other nucleotides. The protein has been isolated and reconstituted into liposomes, where it catalyzes the same electrogenic exchange (43,44). It constitutes about 10% of the inner membrane protein. Bongkrekate and atractyloside are potent inhibitors which bind at the inner or outer surfaces of the membrane, respectively. As discussed previously, the electrogenic nature of the exchange causes ATP to be transported out against a gradient, driven by the membrane potential. This raises the Gibbs free energy of ATP outside and uses one-third or one-forth the energy available for ATP synthesis.

Phosphate transport is an electroneutral exchange of the monoanion for hydroxyl ions (30). The transporter has been identified and reconstituted (45). It is inhibited by NEM and mercurials. The fact that phosphate uptake occurs as though with a proton means that the pH gradient drives phosphate uptake and also contributes to the lower Gibbs free energy of ATP inside.

The dicarboxylic acids malate, succinate, and oxaloacetate enter mitochondria by a single transporter, which exchanges them for phosphate. The reaction is only slightly affected by a pH gradient and is presumably the exchange of the dianionic species. Thus phosphate and the phosphate transporter are required for net uptake of malate, the phosphate cycling in with two protons and out as the dianion. This is equivalent to the uptake of malate with two protons and means that a pH gradient drives the uptake of these acids to a maximum of 100-fold when there is a difference of 1 pH unit more basic inside. This serves to keep these intermediates in the matrix, although the exact value of the mitochondrial pH gradient *in vivo* is not known.

The tricarboxylic acids citrate, isocitrate, and *cis*-aconitate, as well as phosphoenolpyruvate, are transported in exchange for malate in an electroneutral, proton-compensated reaction. The transporter is inhibited by benzene-1,2,3-tricarboxylic acid. Pyruvate is transported electroneutrally in exchange for hydroxide in a reaction that shows saturation kinetics and is inhibited by phenylpyruvate or α-cyano-4-hydroxycinnamate. This and other observations indicate that pyruvate enters by its own transporter.

Glutamate has two transporters: (a) an electroneutral exchange for hydroxyl, and (b) an electrogenic exchange for aspartate. The electroneutral glutamate transporter, but not the electrogenic transporter, is inhibited by NEM. Glutamate is concentrated inside mitochondria by the electrogenic transporter driven by the membrane potential. The two glutamate systems together create an electrogenic pathway for asparate efflux, which is driven by the membrane potential.

α-Ketoglutarate is transported by an electroneutral exchange for malate, succinate, or malonate. The α-ketoglutarate-malate exchange and the glutamate-aspartate exchange constitute the transport reactions of the malate-aspartate shuttle for transport of electrons from cytoplasmic to mitochondrial NADH. Since the glutamate-aspartate exchange is electrogenic, this pathway uses one proton per electron pair transported. The alternative pathway for oxidation of cytoplasmic NADH, the glycerol phosphate shuttle, bypasses the first coupling region of the respiratory chain. Thus neither pathway is without energetic cost.

Transporters also play a role in gluconeogenesis. The carboxylation of pyruvate by pyruvate carboxylase occurs inside the mitochondria. Formation of phosphoenolpyruvate from oxaloacetate by phosphoenolpyruvate carboxykinase probably occurs in the cytoplasm (46). Thus the overall pathway uses one matrix ATP, one cytoplasmic GTP, and one electrogenic proton equivalent from utilization of matrix NADH and formation of cytoplasmic NADH. If phosphoenolpyruvate is formed in the matrix, then less energy would be used in the overall pathway (two matrix ATPs).

During urea synthesis, ornithine must enter the mitochondrial matrix and be converted to citrulline, which then returns to the cytoplasm. Studies of these transporters, which occur only in liver mitochondria, have indicated that L-ornithine is taken up as the cation in exchange for a proton (47). Citrulline probably is transported out as the neutral species. Thus the transport reactions do not contribute to the energetics of urea synthesis, except that the equivalent of two protons is saved because two ATP molecules are used inside the mitochondrion instead of in the cytoplasm.

The oxidation of fatty acids requires uptake of acyl-carnitine into the mitochondrion. This occurs by a transporter in exchange for carnitine, an electroneutral exchange. This was originally difficult to demonstrate in liver mitochondria because they lost internal carnitine on isolation. The transporter also catalyzes the net transport of carnitine at about 0.5% the rate of the exchange rate.

The remaining ion transport systems shown in Fig. 3 are for inorganic cations. Liver mitochondria have an active calcium ion uptake system, which has been studied extensively (48–50). This transporter allows calcium ions to permeate with two positive charges, driven by the membrane potential. Attention has been directed at the process by which calcium ions are released by mitochondria. In heart mitochondria, this appears to be a calcium-sodium exchange. In liver mitochondria, however, it is probably a calcium-hydrogen exchange. The efflux pathway may be regulated by the redox state of NADH (51). These two systems serve to buffer the external calcium ion activity at about 10^{-6} M.

The final transporter shown in Fig. 3, hydrogen-sodium (or potassium) exchange, prevents formation of a large pH gradient in mitochondria and slow swelling due to ion leakage by allowing electroneutral sodium and potassium efflux.

BIOSYNTHESIS OF MITOCHONDRIA

Mitochondria contain a small circular DNA which codes for the more hydrophobic subunits of the ATPase, and cytochrome oxidase, and for mitochondrial ribosomal RNA and tRNA. These components are synthesized as in bacteria. A majority of the mitochondrial proteins, however, both soluble and membrane bound, are synthesized in the cytoplasm. They are taken up by mitochondria and clipped to final size by an ATP-requiring protease activity (51–53).

The 16,569 base pairs of human mitochondrial DNA have been sequenced (6). The sequence shows extreme economy in that the genes have none or only a few noncoding bases between them; in many cases, the termination codons are not coded in the DNA but are created posttranscriptionally by polyadenylation of the mRNAs. In addition, there are only 22 tRNA species, and the genetic code differs from the universal code. UGA codes for tryptophan and not termination; UAU codes for methionine not isoleucine; and AGA and AGG code for termination rather than arginine. The sequence probably codes for 13 polypeptides, eight of which are unknown at this time.

REFERENCES

1. Boyer, P. D., Chance, B., Ernster, L., Mitchell, P., Racker, E., and Slater, E. C. (1977): Oxidative phosphorylation and photophosphorylation. *Ann. Rev. Biochem.*, 46:955–1026.
2. Williamson, J. R. (1979): Mitochondrial function in the heart. *Ann. Rev. Physiol.*, 41:486–506.

3. Fillingame, R. H. (1980): The proton-translocating pumps of oxidative phosphorylation. *Ann. Rev. Biochem.*, 49:1079−1114.

4. Mitchell, P. (1979): Compartmentation and communication in living systems. Ligand conduction: A general catalytic principle in chemical, osmotic and chemiosmotic reaction systems. *Eur. J. Biochem*, 95:1−20.

5. Wikstrom, M., Krab, K., and Saraste, M. (1981): Proton-translocating cytochrome complexes. *Ann. Rev. Biochem.*, 50:623−655.

6. Anderson, S., Bankier, A. T., Barrell, B. G., deBruijn, M. H. L., Coulson, A. R., Drouin, J., Eperon, I. C., Nierlich, D. P., Roe, B. A., Sanger, F., Schreier, P. H., Smith, A. J. H., Staden, R., and Young, I. G. (1981): Sequence and organization of the human mitochondrial genome. *Nature*, 290:457−465.

7. Pollak, J. K., and Sutton, R. (1980): The differentiation of animal mitochondria during development. *Trends Biochem. Sci.*, 5:23−27.

8. Johnson, L. V., Walsh, M. L., and Chen, L. B. (1980): Localization of mitochondria in living cells with rhodamine 123. *Proc. Natl. Acad. Sci. USA*, 77:990−994.

9. Ontko, J. A., and Dashti, N. (1976): Enzymes of mitochondria. In: *Cell Biology*, edited by P. I. Altman and D. D. Katz, pp. 161−180. Fed. Am. Soc. Exp. Biol., Bethesda.

10. Sreve, P. A. (1980): The infrastructure of the mitochondrial matrix. *Trends Biochem. Sci.*, 5:120−121.

11. Ernster, L., and Kuylenstierna, B. (1970): Outer membrane of mitochondria. In: *Membranes of Mitochondria and Chloroplasts*, edited by E. Racker, pp. 172−212, Van Nostrand Reinhold, New York.

12. Greenawalt, J. W. (1979): Survery and update of outer and inner mitochondrial membrane separation. *Methods Enzymol.*, 55:88−98.

13. Schein, S. J., Colombini, M., and Finkelstein, A. (1976): Reconstitution in planar lipid bilayers of a voltage-dependent anion-selective channel obtained from paramecium mitochondria. *J. Membr. Biol.*, 30:99−120.

14. Zalman, L. S., Mikaido, H., and Kagawa, Y. (1980): Mitochondrial outer membrane contains protein producing nonspecific diffusion channels. *J. Biol. Chem.*, 255:1771−1774.

15. Schnaitman, C., and Greenawalt, J. S. (1968): Enzymatic properties of the inner and outer membranes of rat liver mitochondria. *J. Cell Biol.*, 38:158−175.

16. Schneider, H., Lemasters, J. J., Hochli, M., and Hackenbrock, C. R. (1980): Fusion of liposomes with mitochondrial inner membranes. *Proc. Natl. Acad. Sci. USA*, 77:442−446.

17. Thayer, W. S., and Rubin, E. (1979): Effects of chronic ethanol intoxication on oxidative phosphorylation in rat liver submitochondrial particles. *J. Biol. Chem.*, 254:7717−7723.

18. Fernandez-Moran, H. (1962): Cell-membrane ultrastructure low-temperature electron microscopy and X-ray diffraction studies of lipoprotein components in lamellar systems. *Circulation*, 26:1039.

19. Racker, E., and Horstman, L. L. (1967): Partial resolution of the enzymes catalyzing oxidative phosphorylation. XIII. Structure and function of submitochondrial particles completely resolved with respect to coupling factor. *J. Biol. Chem.*, 242:2547−2551.

20. Margalit, R., and Schejter, A. (1973): Cytochrome c: A thermodynamic study of relationships among oxidation state, ion-binding and structural parameters. 2. Ion-binding linked to oxidation state. *Eur. J. Biochem.*, 32:500−505.

21. Hinkle, P. C., Kim, J. J., and Racker, R. (1972): Ion transport and respiratory control in vesicles formed from cytochrome oxidase and phospholipids. *J. Biol. Chem.*, 247:1338−1339.

22. Leung, K. H., and Hinkle, P. C. (1975): Reconstitution of ion transport and respiratory control in vesicles formed from reduced coenzyme Q-cytochrome c reductase and phospholipids. *J. Biol. Chem.*, 250:8467−8471.

23. Ragan, C. I., and Hinkle, P. C. (1975): Ion transport and respiratory control in vesicles formed from reduced nicotinamide adenine dinucleotide coenzyme Q reductase and phospholipids. *J. Biol. Chem.*, 250:8472−8476.

24. Mitchell, P. (1966): Chemiosmotic coupling in oxidative and photosynthetic phosphorylation. *Biol. Rev.*, 41:445−502.

25. Mitchell, P. (1976): Possible molecular mechanisms of the protonmotive function of cytochrome systems. *J. Theor. Biol.*, 62:327−367.

26. Pozzan, T., Miconi, V., DiVirgilio, F., and Azzone, G. F. (1979): H+/site, charge/site and ATP/site ratios at coupling sites I and II in mitochondrial e− transport. *J. Biol. Chem.*, 254:10200−10205.

27. Azzone, G. F., Pozzan, T., and DiVirgilio, F. (1979): H+/site, charge/site, and ATP/site ratios at coupling site III in mitochondrial electron transport. *J. Biol. Chem.*, 254:10206−10212.

28. Reynafarje, B., Brand, M. D., and Lehninger, A. L. (1976): Evaluation of the H+/site ratio of mitochondrial electron transport from rate measurements. *J. Biol. Chem.*, 251:7442−7451.

29. Klingenberg, M. (1980): The ADP-ATP translocation in mitochondria, a membrane potential controlled transport. *J. Membr. Biol.*, 56:97−105.

30. Coty, W. A., and Pederson, P. L. (1974): Phosphate transport in rat liver mitochondria. *J. Biol. Chem.*, 249:2593−2598.

31. Hinkle, P. C., and Yu, M. L. (1979): The phosphorus/oxygen ratio of mitochondrial oxidative phosphorylation. *J. Biol. Chem.*, 254:2450−2455.

32. Mitchell, P., and Moyle, J. (1969): Estimation of membrane potential and pH difference across the cristae membrane of rat liver mitochondria. *Eur. J. Biochem.*, 7:471−484.

33. Padan, E., and Rottenberg, H. (1973): Respiratory control and the proton electrochemical gradient in mitochondria. *Eur. J. Biochem.*, 40:431−437.

34. Nicholls, D. E. (1974): The influence of respiration and ATP hydrolysis on the proton-electrochemical gradient across the inner membrane of rat-liver mitochondria as determined by ion distribution. *Eur. J. Biochem.*, 50:305−315.

35. Azzone, G. F., Pozzan, T., Massari, S., and Bragadin, M. (1978): Proton electrochemical gradient and rate of controlled respiration in mitochondria. *Biochim. Biophys. Acta*, 501:296−306.

36. Holian, A., and Wilson, D. F. (1980): Relationship of transmembrane pH and electrical gradients with respiration and adenosine 5′-triphosphate synthesis in mitochondria. *Biochemistry*, 19:4213−4221.

37. Boyer, P. D. (1979): The binding-change mechanism of ATP synthesis. In: *Mechanisms in Bioenergetics*, edited by C. P., Lee, G. Schatz, and L. Ernster, L. pp. 461−479. Addison-Wesley, Reading, Massachusetts.

38. Grubmeyer, C., and Penefsky, H. S. (1981): The presence of two hydrolytic sites on beef heart mitochondrial adenosine triphosphatase. *J. Biol. Chem.*, 256:3718−3727.

39. Sebald, W., Hoppe, J., and Wachter, E. (1979): Amino acid sequence of the ATPase proteolipid from mitochondria chloroplasts and bacteria (wild type and mutants). In: *Function and Molecular Aspects of Biomembrane Transport*, edited by E. Quagliariello, F. Palmieri, S. Papa, and M. Klingenberg, pp. 63−74. Elsevier, New York.

40. Catterall, W. A., Coty, W. A., and Pederson, P. L. (1973): Adenosine triphosphatase from rat liver mitochondria. III. Subunit composition. *J. Biol. Chem.*, 248:7427−7431.

41. Amzel, L. M., and Pederson, P. L. (1978): Adenosine triphosphatase from rat liver mitochondria. Crystallization and X-ray diffraction studies of the F_1-component of the enzyme. *J. Biol. Chem.*, 253:2067−2069.

42. LaNoue, K. P., and Schoolwerth, A. C. (1979): Metabolite transport in mitochondria. *Ann. Rev. Biochem.*, 48:871.

43. Shertzer, H., and Racker, E. (1976): Reconstitution and characterization of the adenine nucleotide transporter derived from bovine heart mitochondria. *J. Biol. Chem.*, 251:2446−2456.

44. Kramer, R., and Klingenberg, M. (1980): Enhancement of reconstituted ADP, ATP exchange activity by phosphatidylethanolamine and by anionic phospholipids. *FEBS Lett.*, 119:257−260.

45. Wohlrab, H. (1980): Purification of a reconstitutively active

mitochondrial phosphate transport protein. *J. Biol. Chem.*, 255:8170–8173.

46. Bentle, L. A., and Lardy, H. A. (1977): P-enolpyruvate carboxykinase ferroactivator. *J. Biol. Chem.*, 252:1431–1440.

47. McGivan, J. D., Bradford, N. M., and Beavis, A. D. (1977): Factors influencing the activity of ornithine aminotransferase in isolated rat liver mitochondria. *Biochem. J.*, 162:147–156.

48. Saris, N., and Akerman, K. E. O. (1980): Uptake and release of bivalent cations in mitochondria. *Curr. Top. Bioenerget.*, 10:103–179.

49. Carafoli, E., and Crompton, M. (1977): The regulation of intracellular calcium. *Curr. Top. Membr. Trans. M.*, 10:151–216.

50. Nicholls, D. (1981): Some recent advances in mitochondrial calcium transport. *TIBS*, 6:36–38.

51. Lehninger, A. L., Vercesi, A., and Bababunmi, E. A. (1978): Regulation of Ca^{2+} release from mitochondria by the oxidation reduction state of pyridine nucleotides. *Proc. Natl. Acad. Sci. USA*, 75:1690–1694.

52. Nelson, N., and Schatz, G. (1979): Energy-dependent processing of cytoplasmically made precursors to mitochondrial proteins. *Proc. Natl. Acad. Sci. USA*, 76:4365–4369.

53. Lewin, A. S., Gregor, I., Mason, T. L., Nelson, N., and Schatz, G. (1980): Cytoplasmically made subunits of yeast mitochondrial F_1-ATPase and cytochrome c oxidase are synthesized as individual precursors, not as polyproteins. *Proc. Natl. Acad. Sci. USA*, 77:3998–4002.

54. Mihara, K., and Blobel, G. (1980): The four cytoplasmically made subunits of yeast mitochondrial cytochrome c oxidase are synthesized individually and not as a polyprotein. *Proc. Natl. Acad. Sci. USA*, 77:4160–4164.

The Liver: Biology and Pathobiology, edited by
I. Arias, H. Popper, D. Schachter, and D. A. Shafritz.
Raven Press, New York © 1982.

Chapter 2

Lysosomes

Alex B. Novikoff

GENERAL CONSIDERATIONS

It is now more than 25 years since de Duve and his colleagues postulated the existence of lysosomes (1,2). An essential aspect was a different scheme of fractionating rat liver homogenates (Fig. 1). Together with Beaufay (3), we tentatively identified the cytochemical entity in rat liver (Fig. 2).

de Duve and his collaborators, at l'Université Catholique de Louvain, postulated the existence of an outer membrane; among the agents that made acid phosphatase (AcPase) lose its "latency" (i.e., inaccessibility of substrate and enzyme) were lipases and proteases. Examination with the electron microscope (Fig. 2) showed the presence of the membranes. On the basis of sedimentation characteristics, the Louvain investigators calculated that the diameters of hepatic lysosomes "must range mostly between 0.25 and 0.8 μ if their density is low (1.10) or between 1.13 and 0.4 μ if their density is high (1.30)." They soon concluded that their density was high. If we assume that the "dense bodies" are spherical *in vivo,* their diameters (Fig. 2) are close to the postulated 0.4 μm. The electron-opaque particles inside the "dense body" (Fig. 2) measured 55 to 77 Å or less, as previously shown by Farrant (4) to be the diameter of isolated ferritin molecules. The presence of these electron-opaque particles helped us draw the tentative conclusion that the "dense bodies" corresponded to the "pericanalicular dense bodies" *in situ* (3).

Although I knew of the heterogeneity of cell types in the liver (Fig. 3) and had popularized such heteroge-

neity in a review, *The Liver Cell: Some New Approaches to Its Study,* written with Essner (7), in my work with de Duve in the 1950s, I treated the rat liver as if it were a tissue consisting only of hepatocytes.

Elsewhere (8) I have considered the effects on the historic development of the lysosome (and peroxisome) fields had there been valid cytochemical procedures available for these two organelles in the early 1950s. Figure 4 shows lysosomes and peroxisomes visualized cytochemically in sections of rat liver. Lysosomes are visualized by their AcPase activity and peroxisomes by their catalase activity. We could have described some of the heterogeneity of lysosomes; however, reliable cytochemical methods at the electron microscope level were not then available. Had they been, they could not yield quantitative data; nor could cytochemical observations establish the concepts of lysosome and peroxisome. These concepts involve ensembles of enzymes within distinctive cytoplasmic particles, the lysosome-containing hydrolases, and the peroxisome enzymes that either produce or destroy hydrogen peroxide.

DEFINITIONS

Biochemically defined, lysosomes are cytoplasmic particles containing a variety of hydrolases, most of which have maximal activities at acid pHs and display latency if the particles are properly isolated. Figure 5 is from de Duve's Nobel Lecture (2). The latency reflects the impermeability of the membranes delimiting the lysosomes to enzymes and substrates. The first iso-

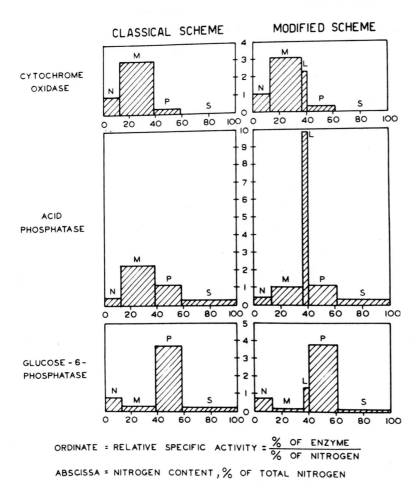

FIG. 1. Change in procedure of fractionation of rat liver homogenates. (From ref. 2, with permission.) Histograms showing distributions of three marker enzymes: glucose-6-phosphatase for microsomes (P), cytochrome oxidase for mitochondria (M), and AcPase for lysosomes. In the modified scheme, M refers to the heavy mitochondrial fraction and L to the light mitochondrial fraction. The nuclear (N) and supernatant (S) fractions are the same in both procedures.

ORDINATE = RELATIVE SPECIFIC ACTIVITY = $\dfrac{\text{\% OF ENZYME}}{\text{\% OF NITROGEN}}$

ABSCISSA = NITROGEN CONTENT, % OF TOTAL NITROGEN

lated lysosomes came from rat liver homogenates. Initially, five such hydrolases were described; at present, far more than 40 are known to reside in hepatic lysosomes. All classes of molecules found in cells may be hydrolyzed by lysosomal enzymes: proteins, nucleic acids, polysaccharides, and lipids (for a 1976 listing, see ref. 10).

As defined morphologically, a lysosome is a cytoplasmic organelle that is surrounded by a membrane and that, under appropriate cytochemical conditions, displays one or more hydrolase activities known to be present in isolated lysosomes. The membrane usually is tripartite but occasionally may be different. In cells endowed with sufficient endoplasmic reticulum (ER), it is likely that lysosomal hydrolases are synthesized on membrane-associated polysomes and gain access to the ER cisternae, through which they are transported to other areas of the cell. Figure 6 indicates that lysosomal hydrolases may go directly from the ER to autophagic vacuoles of two kinds: type 1 (AV₁) and type 2 (AV₂). The characteristic feature of autophagy is that it is endogenous material (organelles or molecules) that is degraded by the lysosomal hydrolases. Exogenous materials may enter cells in "gulps," either by phagocytosis or pinocytosis; endocytosis is the term that encompasses both phagocytosis and

pinocytosis. Endocytic vacuoles become digestive vacuoles, often referred to as phagolysosomes, when they receive lysosomal hydrolases. This involves merger with either primary or secondary lysosomes. Primary lysosomes are vesicles or granules that contain acid hydrolases that have not yet been active in molecular degradation (intracellular digestion). When such degradation begins, the lysosome becomes a secondary lysosome. The most common secondary lysosome is the residual body. The undigestible materials

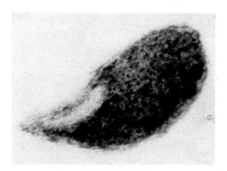

FIG. 2. "Dense body" (which I would now call "residual body") in the L fraction isolated from a rat liver homogenate. Note the external membrane (best seen at left) and the electron-opaque particles inside.

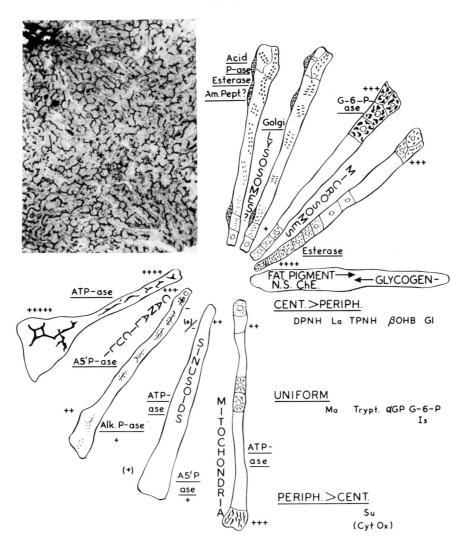

FIG. 3. Diagrammatic representation of a hepatic lobule of the rat. (From ref. 5, with permission.) In the upper left quadrant, a photograph shows a portion of the hepatic lobule stained to demonstrate ATPase activity in the bile canaliculi (6). The quantitative differences between centrolobular and peripheral cells are indicated by plus marks (+) and by schematic representation of the cytologic structures. In the lower right corner, the substrates are arranged, from left to right, in decreasing order of staining produced with tetrazolium (nitro BT). Kupffer cells are indicated where they contain high levels of enzyme activities or large numbers of cytologic structures. The diffuse cytoplasmic staining obtained with unfixed frozen sections when 5'-nucleotidase activity is visualized is more intense (+ +) in the centrolobular area than peripherally (+). It has not been included in the diagram since we have not established whether this represents cytoplasmic (microsomal?) activity or diffusion (enzyme?) from the sinusoidal aspects of the cell. ATPase, adenosinetriphosphatase; A5'P-ase, 5'-nucleotidase; Alk. P'ase, alkaline phosphatase; Am. Pept., aminopeptidase; Acid P-ase, acid phosphatase; G-6-P-ase, glucose-6-phosphatase; cent., centrolobular cells; periph., peripheral cells; DPNH, reduced diphosphopyridine nucleotide; TPNH, reduced triphosphopyridine nucleotide. *Diphosphopyridine nucleotide-linked oxidations:* La, *lactate;* βOHB, betahydroxybutyrate; Gl, glutamate; Ma, malate; αGP, alpha-glycerophosphate. *Triphosphopyridine nucleotide-linked oxidations:* G-6-P, glucose-6-phosphate; Is, isocitrate; Su, succinate; Cyst Ox, cytochrome oxidase.

within the residual bodies take the form of electron-opaque grains, membraneous whorls, and other material. As these residues accumulate, the residual bodies enlarge. Residual bodies may also result from accumulation of materials that cannot be further degraded because of an inherited lack of a specific lysosomal enzyme. These are the ''inclusions'' of storage diseases (considered under ''Pathologies'').

Pinocytosed material is sometimes transported to

ill-defined digestive vacuoles characterized by internal vesicles and called multivesicular bodies (MVB). The term crinophagy was introduced by de Duve (1) to describe an interesting role of lysosomes in the disposal of secretory granules. This was described by Smith and Farquhar (11) in the mammatrophs of anterior pituitary gland of the rat and for other types of secretory cells in the pituitary by Farquhar (12). These authors describe secretory granules as arising from the

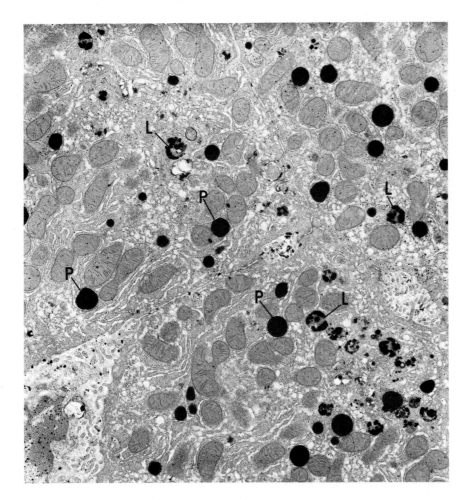

FIG. 4. Lysosomes (L) and peroxisomes (P) visualized cytochemically. (From ref. 9, with permission.)

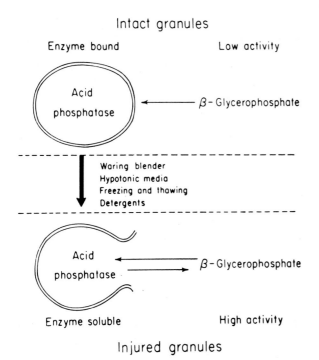

Intact granules

Enzyme bound   Low activity

Acid phosphatase ←———— β-Glycerophosphate

Waring blender
Hypotonic media
Freezing and thawing
Detergents

Acid phosphatase ←———— β-Glycerophosphate
            ————→

Enzyme soluble   High activity

Injured granules

FIG. 5. Diagram of latency of rat liver AcPase, as proposed in 1951. (From ref. 2, with permission.)

innermost element of the Golgi apparatus [element 4 in Fig. 6, where the Golgi apparatus is arbitrarily drawn as having four elements, as in the neurons of dorsal root ganglia (13)].

Figure 6 shows primary lysosomes arising from both the Golgi apparatus and GERL, as coated vesicles. GERL is a specialized region of smooth ER found in some cell types. It is situated at the inner aspect of the Golgi stack and is depicted as forming three kinds of lysosomes: primary lysosomes (coated vesicles), residual bodies, and AV_2.

Microperoxisomes are ubiquitous in animal cells and are also present in some plant cells. They appear to be dilatations of smooth ER, with which they retain multiple attachments. They lack the cores of hepatic peroxisomes (cores are also present in peroxisomal renal tubules) and urate oxidase activity. They contain catalase and probably D-amino acid oxidase and other H_2O_2-producing oxidases.

The work of Friend and Farquhar (14) remains the outstanding study on both the nature of the MVB and the functional role of coated vesicles in any cell type (in this case, the cells in the vas deferens). Coated vesicles transport intravenously injected horseradish

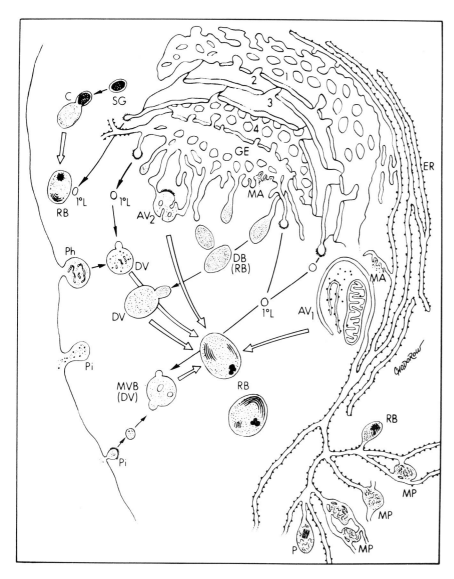

FIG. 6. 1–4, Successive elements of the Golgi stack; 1° L, primary lysosomes; AV₁, type 1 autophagic vacuole; AV₂, type 2 autophagic vacuole; C, crinophagy; DB, dense body; DV, digestive vacuole; ER, endoplasmic reticulum; GE, GERL; MA, microautophagy; MP, micro-peroxisome; MVB, multivesicular body; P, peroxisome; Ph, phago-cytic vacuole; Pi, pinocytic vacuole; RB, residual body; SG, secretory granule. (From ref. 8, with per-mission.)

peroxidase from the cell surface to the MVB; smaller coated vesicles, probably derived from GERL, bring AcPase to the MVB. A recent study from our laboratory (15) on cultured 3T3-L1 cells confirmed these findings. Our study is discussed in the modern framework, beginning with the studies of Pearse (16,17).

GERL

The views of our laboratory concerning the organelle given this irreverent acronym in 1964 (18) were summarized in 1977 (19) and 1979 (20). In 1971, P. M. Novikoff et al. (13) reported cytochemical studies on "thick" sections (0.5 to 1.0 μm) and thin sections (up to 500 Å) of rat dorsal root ganglia. Figure 8 shows a small portion of GERL in a thick section; Fig. 9 shows portions of GERL in thin sections. [See Fig. 40 in ref. 13 for a diagram based on thick and thin sections of

tissues previously incubated for AcPase or nucleoside diphosphatase (NDPase) or thiamine pyrophosphatase (TPPase) (see footnote 1, p. 102, ref. 20).]

Consistent with our cytochemical findings in other cell types are the cytochemical findings in the cell studied by Palade and co-workers (21) for secretory events in the guinea pig exocrine pancreas. These studies are almost universally considered as the paradigm for secretion (see our observations in ref. 22; those on the guinea pig exocrine pancreas are seen in Fig. 10). Our interpretation is that the Golgi apparatus per se is not involved (at least from observations in fixed tissue). In contrast, the condensing vacuoles and related structures (Fig. 10) have cytochemically demonstrable AcPase activity. Fawcett, in his second edition of *The Cell* (23), appears to accept our interpretation but overlooks the evidence in Fig. 10A.

Strong support for our findings in the pancreas exocrine cells comes from the work of Hand and Oliver (24–26) on the exocrine cells of five different salivary

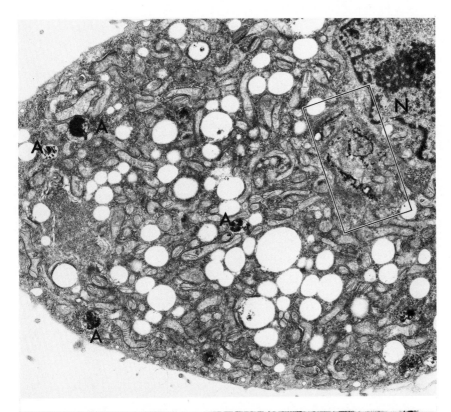

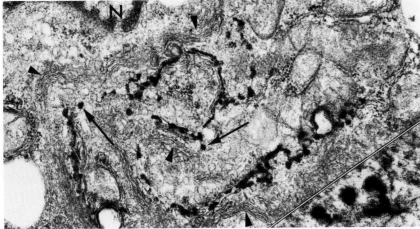

FIG. 7. Differentiating 3T3-L1 cells. (From ref. 15, with permission.) **Upper:** After incubation in AcPase medium. Reaction product makes the numerous autophagic vacuoles (A) and GERL (*boxed area*) visible. ×9,000. **Lower:** Boxed area of upper, enlarged. AcPase reaction product is seen in GERL (unlabeled), the anastomosing nature of which is evident. *Arrowheads,* plane of section passes through the Golgi apparatus, revealing the so-called Golgi stacks. When GERL and adjacent Golgi stacks are seen, it is evident that GERL is always *trans* to the stack (see Fig. 6). Two arrows indicate vesicles that have probably separated from GERL. Three AcPase-positive, apparently coated vesicles appear to be separating from GERL. ×33,000. **Inset,** from another cell. ×65,250.

glands in three species. They considered "immature secretory granules" (i.e., the condensing vacuoles) to be part of GERL. In their studies, condensing vacuoles and tubular elements displayed AcPase but not TPPase activity; the *trans* Golgi element showed TPPase but not AcPase activity, and mature zymogen granules showed neither phosphatase activity. Like us, Hand and Oliver found no structural connections between Golgi elements and GERL.

In reference 20, Fig. 1 schematically depicts GERL in a wide variety of cell types, as interpreted by us and, in some cases, by others. In retrospect, the clear membrane continuities and cytochemically demonstrable AcPase of the MBs described by Robbins et al.

(27) in their classic paper on mitosis are readily interpretable as GERL.

Rome et al. (28) have described properties of a subcellular fraction obtained from cultured human fibroblasts enriched in GERL fragments, the first such fraction to be analyzed. It is not a pure fraction, but it is sufficiently enriched to demonstrate that the same 11 lysosomal hydrolases are present in it and in the lysosome fraction containing residual bodies. The peak buoyant density of the fraction with GERL fragments is 1.085, in contrast to 1.11 for the residual body-containing fraction.

Garvin et al. (29) have recently published interesting cytochemical observations on GERL in cultured hu-

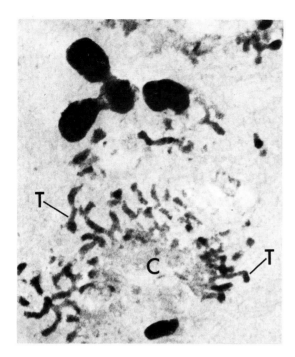

FIG. 8. Small portion of a neuron in fetal rat spinal ganglion, 0.5 μm, incubated for AcPase activity. (From ref. 13, with permission.) A cisternal portion (C) and connecting tubules (T) of GERL are seen. The continuities among the bodies at the top of the figure are interpreted as residual bodies in formation, perhaps from a cisternal portion. ×41,000.

man fibroblasts, including its disruption by addition to the medium of 50 μM chloroquine. Some of the "membranes" described in the initial studies by Fedorko et al. (30,31) may have belonged to GERL.

Finally, it should be noted that GERL (and sometimes other organelles) have cytochemically demonstrable phosphatases capable of hydrolyzing physiologically important substrates, such as pyridoxal-5'-phosphate (32) and analogs of nicotinamide adenine dinucleotide phosphate (33).

FROM GERL TO COMPARTMENT

The view of our laboratory of GERL was extended when P. M. Novikoff et al. (34) studied the Kupffer cells and the phagocytes in spleen of obese Zucker rats fed a cholesterol-enriched diet. We had earlier described (8,35) the continuities, via smooth ER of AV_1, AV_2, and residual bodies (Figs. 11 and 12). Following the description of the lysosomal compartment in phagocytes (34), we found a similar compartment in hepatocytes (Figs. 13–16).

Wall et al. (37) used lactosaminated ferritin to follow its distribution in rat hepatocytes. Indeed, they showed images such as seen in Fig. 13 (secretory vac-

uole, SV) but did not recognize either the lipoprotein particles or the secretory nature of the vacuoles. These authors spoke of a "mottled" appearance in "larger vesicles." Of greater significance, the authors failed to realize that negative findings in cytochemistry, particularly with aryl sulfatase activity (arrow in their Fig. 5B), cannot justifiably be equated with the absence of such activity *in vivo*. Especially is this true if, as the authors write, "in our hands" AcPase cytochemistry gave more "background precipitation." Crisp localizations without background stained are readily obtained (see Figs. 4,7–10,16,18–21, and 23; also see refs. 38 and 39).

There is little question that the AcPase-positive structures in regenerating rat liver described by Jaeken et al. (40) constitute the lysosomal compartment of rat hepatocytes. Similarly, the AcPase system described by Pino et al. (41) in fetal rat liver of Kupffer cells probably constitutes the compartment described by P. M. Novikoff et al. (34).

Hints of similar compartments are to be found in: (a) rat neurohypophysis (42), (b) the salivary glands of *Onychophora*, invertebrates that combine features of annelids and arthropods (43), (c) the human parathyroid gland (44), (d) the system that takes up horseradish peroxidase by endocytosis, following the action of ADH, in toad bladders (45), and (e) the basal lysosomal system described in exocrine acinar cells (46).

PATHOLOGIES

Storage Diseases of Human Liver

Shortly after de Duve and his group had postulated the existence of lysosomes, they began the study of storage diseases of man. This study was under the leadership of Hers, who had collaborated with de Duve since the earlier studies of insulin and glucagon. The book *Lysosome and Storage Diseases* (47) describes approximately 30 diseases characterized by deficiencies of single lysosomal enzymes. Figure 17 is a photograph included in the chapter by Hers and de Barsy (48). A recent discussion of lysosomal storage diseases, with an emphasis on cultural human fibroblasts, is to be found in a book entitled *Lysosomes and Lysosomal Storage Diseases* (49).

Hepatocytes of Rats Injected with Triton WR-1339

Injection of rats with Triton WR-1339 induces the marked formation of AV_1. Figure 18 is interpreted as demonstrating the formation of such autophagic vacuoles by the sequestration of bits of cytoplasm by

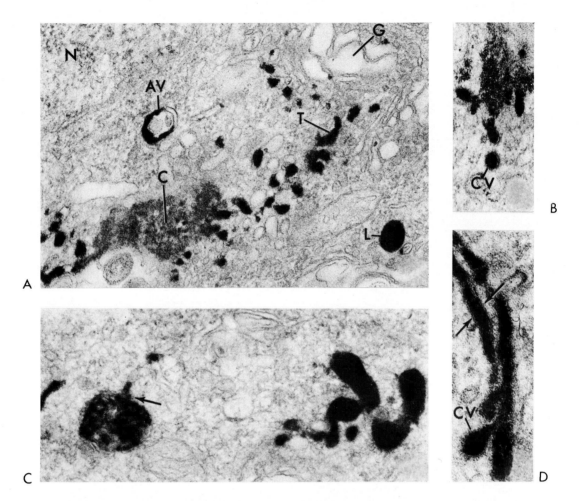

FIG. 9. Portions of neurons in fetal rat spinal ganglia, thin sections, incubated for AcPase activity. (From ref. 13, with permission.) **A:** Both cisternal (C) and tubular (T) portions of GERL are seen. An AV_1 is indicated by AV. A lysosome is indicated by L; it is either a residual body (if sectioned through its interior) or an AV_1 (if sectioned peripherally). The Golgi stack (G) shows no reaction product. N, part of the nucleus. ×41,000. **B:** Small portion of GERL, with some of its tubular and cisternal structures evident. CV, a coated vesicle; AcPase reaction product fills its interior. ×42,000. **C:** The AcPase-positive structures at the right of this micrograph are interpreted as residual bodies in formation, from swellings of GERL. To the left is an AcPase-positive structure, probably an AV_2, with a connection (*arrow*) to a positive tubular structure, probably part of GERL. ×44,000. **D:** A coated vesicle (CV) in continuity with a tubule of GERL. *Arrows,* regions where the delimiting membrane of a GERL tubule is evident. ×80,000.

smooth ER. This mode of autophagy is shown diagrammatically in Fig. 6. Of interest is the accumulation of cytochemically demonstrable AcPase activity (see discussion in ref. 8).

Regenerating Liver of Rat

Normal rat liver shows very few mitotic divisions. Following partial hepatectomy, the number of mitoses increases dramatically, until the liver mass returns to normal.

Prior to the onset of mitosis, dramatic changes occur in the lysosomes. Huge vacuoles appear that are known by a variety of terms; we refer to them as pro-

tein droplets. Mori and I (50) have described these early changes.

The Beige Mouse: The Homolog of the Chédiak-Higashi Disease

Hepatocytes and other cell types have been studied in the beige mutant because light is shed thereby on the origin of the so-called anomalous granules characterizing the human disease and mouse mutant. With AcPase cytochemistry, it was possible to demonstrate, in most cell types, that the granules are enlarged lysosomes (53,54) (Fig. 21). The evidence suggests that these lysosomes arise from GERL (19,53,54) or, in some rare instances, from smooth ER continuous with GERL (Fig. 21).

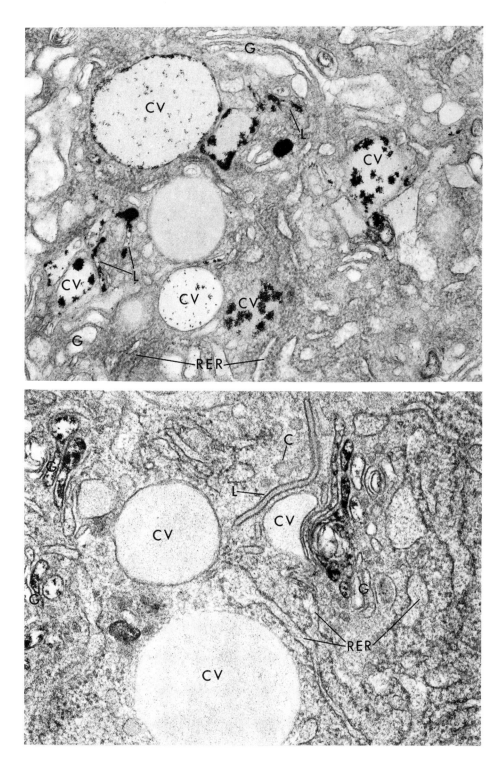

FIG. 10. Portions of pancreatic exocrine cells of the guinea pig. (From ref. 22, with permission.) **Top:** AcPase medium, thin section unstained. AcPase activity is shown by components of GERL: condensing vacuoles (CV), rigid lamellae (L), and coated vesicles (not seen in this section). ×43,200. **Bottom:** NDPase, medium, thin section stained with lead. No portion of the Golgi stack (G) shows AcPase activity. The innermost (*trans*) Golgi element shows NDPase activity. Such activity is not shown by any components of GERL. ×45,000. The rough ER (RER) shows neither AcPase nor NDPase activity. Note the extent of ER directed toward the *trans* aspect of the Golgi stack, probably in a large interruption in the stack (see ref. 22).

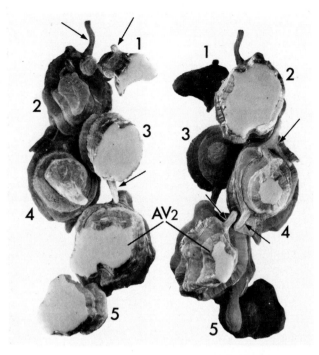

FIG. 11. Two surfaces of a plastic model, reconstructed from 12 consecutive sections of a hepatocyte with hyperplasia of smooth ER. *Arrows,* extensions of smooth ER that interconnect five residual bodies (numbered 1–5) and an AV₂ (see ref. 8). The cut surfaces of the autophagic vacuole and the residual bodies are lighter in the photograph because light-colored rubber was used to fill their interiors. (From ref. 35, with permission.)

Figures 21 and 22 show the accumulations of electron-lucent lipid in the beige lysosomes. When Essner and Oliver (54) described the lysosomes of the hepatocytes in the beige mouse, they wrote: "The accumulation of lipid-like material in GERL and anomalous lysosomes suggests that a disturbance in lipid or lipoprotein synthesis or metabolism may be involved in the pathogenesis of Chédiak-Higashi syndrome."

Cholesterol-Fed Syrian Golden Hamster

Another situation in which GERL appears to be involved in lipid transformations is the one seen in Syrian golden hamsters fed a high cholesterol diet (55). In these hamsters, unlike other mammals we have studied, lipid accumulates within residual bodies. Such lysosomes filled with lipid have been named lipolysosomes (Fig. 23). Hayashi and colleagues (56,57) have described lipolysosomes in human hepatocytes.

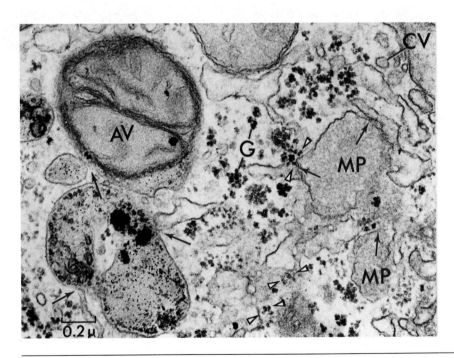

FIG. 12. Portion of a hepatocyte in normal liver, one of 10 consecutive serial sections. Much glycogen (G) is present in the cytoplasm. Three pairs of arrowheads indicate areas in which, as suggested in ref. 8, "microautophagy" of glycogen by smooth ER is occurring. Glycogen, amorphous electron-dense material, and ferritin-like grains are seen in the residual body at bottom left. The two arrows at the left indicate continuities of the residual body with smooth ER. An AV₁ that encloses one or more mitochondria is seen at AV. Dilated smooth ER, with ferritin-like grains, is present at the bottom and to the left of the autophagic vacuole, in a manner suggesting that the vacuole is surrounded by smooth ER (*two arrows*). Smooth ER is continuous with two peroxisomes, possibly microperoxisomes (MP), at the arrows to the right. The continuity of the two peroxisomes is seen in Fig. 2, ref. 35, another of the 10 sections. CV, a coated vesicle. ×44,000. (From ref. 8, with permission.)

FIG. 13 (top left). Portion of a rat hepatocyte 2 min after injection of lactosaminated ferritin. A coated pit at the cell surface displays lactosaminated ferritin (*arrows*). In the secretory vacuole (SV) containing lipoprotein-like particles, the lactosaminated ferritin molecules are barely evident. Note the tubular extensions of SV; they are probably smooth ER. Another portion of the lysosomal compartment is seen beneath the cell surface. ×40,000. (From ref. 36.)

FIG. 14 (top right). Portion of a rat hepatocyte 15 min after injection of lactosaminated ferritin molecules. *Arrows,* lactosaminated ferritin molecules within an autophagic vacuole that contains remnants of a mitochondrion and within a residual body. *Arrowhead,* two morphologic hallmarks of the lysosomal compartment, a thickened membrane and a "halo" beneath it (see ref. 34). ×55,000. (From ref. 36.)

FIG. 15 (bottom). Portion of a rat hepatocyte 15 min after injection of lactosaminated ferritin. *Arrows,* lactosaminated ferritin molecules in a coated vesicle at the upper left, a dilated region of GERL in the center, and another portion of the lysosomal compartment at the right. *Arrowheads,* continuity of the compartment with the ER. ×41,000. (From ref. 36.)

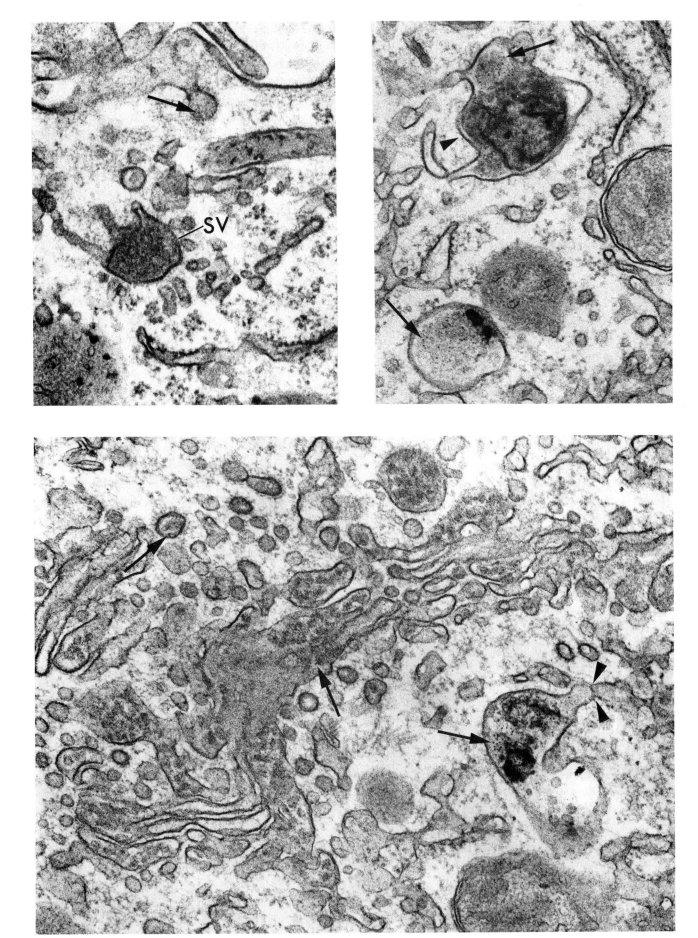

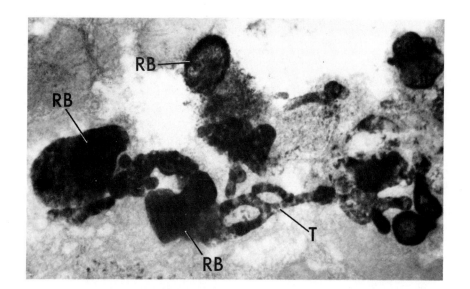

FIG. 16. Portion of a hepatocyte in normal rat liver following incubation for AcPase activity; section approximately 0.25 μm in thickness. ×27,900. (Courtesy P. M. Novikoff, *unpublished.*)

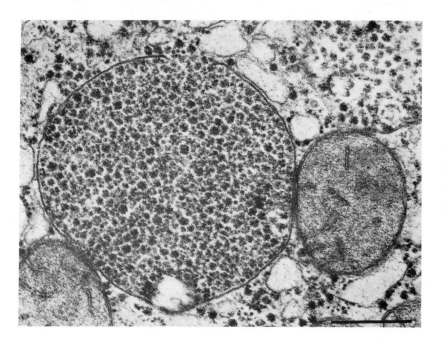

FIG. 17. Portion of a hepatocyte from a patient with type 2 glycogenosis (acid maltase deficiency). Most of the field is occupied by a vacuole filled with α-particulate glycogen. Bar, 0.5 μm. (From ref. 48, with permission.)

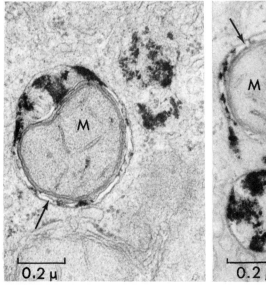
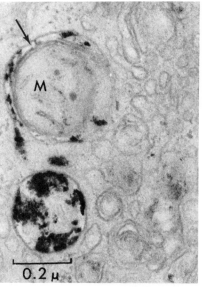

FIG. 18. Portions of hepatocytes in the livers of rats 60 min following intravenous injection of Triton WR-1339 incubated for AcPase activity. Initial events in the formation of AV₁ are seen. The reaction product is seen inside the smooth ER (*arrows*) surrounding mitochondria (M). **Left:** ×64,000. **Right:** ×75,000. (From ref. 8, with permission.)

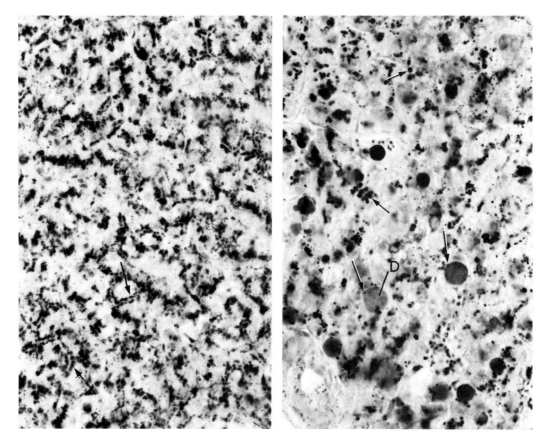

FIG. 19. Left: (From ref. 50, with permission.) Frozen section of liver of control (sham-operated) rat, incubated in CMP medium for 30 min at 37°C. In this relatively thick section (~10 μm), there is considerable overlap of the stained lysosomes. *Arrows,* regions where the pericanalicular distribution of the lysosomes is more evident. ×430. **Right:** Frozen section of regenerating liver 4 hr after partial hepatectomy, processed as in **A.** The largest intracellular structures evident in the section are the protein droplets. The one indicated by *D* shows little reaction product resulting from AcPase activity, whereas the other large droplets show much reaction product. *Long arrows,* lysosomes near the surfaces of protein droplets; *small arrows,* lysosomes which, judging by their size, are probably autophagic vacuoles or residual bodies resulting from them (see Fig. 20). The pericanalicular lysosome distribution **(A)** is no longer evident. This field, like that of **A,** is from the periportal region of the lobule; a bile ductule, with small lysosomes, is at the lower left of the micrograph. ×580.

"Leaky" Lysosomes

Figure 5 is also related to the term "suicide sac," coined by de Duve. In 1973 (8), I contested the generally understood definition of the "suicide sac," namely, that the lysosomes become "leaky" and injure or kill the cells. All of us agree that evidence from homogenized tissue cannot provide unequivocal evidence for *in vivo* effects on the lysosome membranes of "labilizers" and "stabilizers." My position relates to the effects on lysosomal permeability postulated from cytochemistry and electron microscopy. Unequivocal evidence for effects on the membranes of lysosomes is still lacking.

Impaired Ability of Lysosomes to Fuse with Phagocytic Vacuoles

A survey of this vast field is beyond the scope of this chapter. I refer to two recent publications. The first deals with *Mycobacterium tuberculosis* by D'Arcy Hart and Young (58), who first made us aware of the existence of bacteria that escape death because the usual fusion of lysosomes with phagocytic vacuoles does not occur. The second deals with the interesting Legionnaires' disease (59). In the laboratory of Silverstein (60), it has been shown that *Legionella neumophilia* will rapidly multiply inside cultured human monocytes. Again, this results from the im-

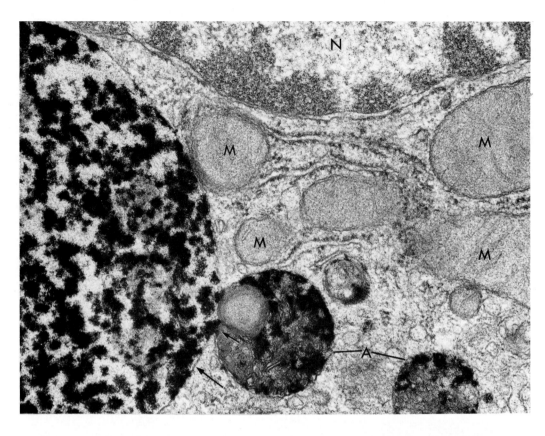

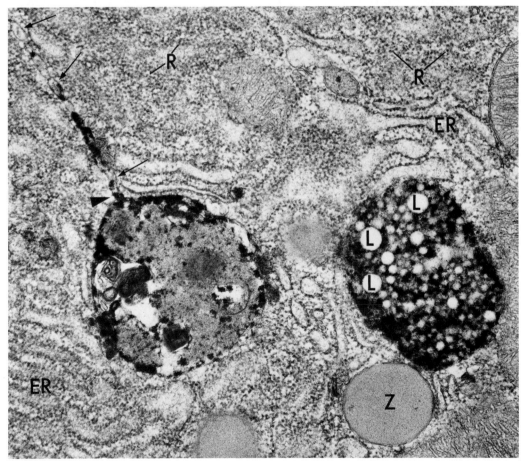

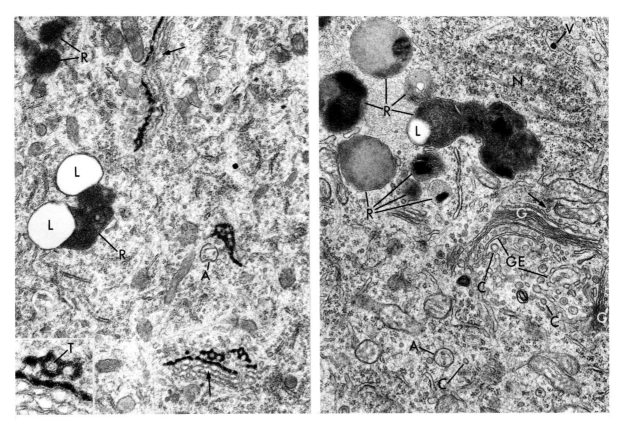

FIG. 22. Portions of two neurons in the dorsal root ganglia of the beige mouse. (From ref. 52, with permission.) **Left:** Micrograph from a ganglion incubated for 30 min for TPPase activity. Reaction product is seen in the *trans*-most element of the Golgi stack (*arrow*). ×16,200. **Inset:** Enlargement in which a tubule (T) is seen enclosed by a polygonal area of this element (see ref. 13). Enlarged lysosomes are labeled R (residual bodies). L, electron-lucent lipid; A, autophagic vacuole. ×36,900. **Right:** Micrograph from a ganglion of unincubated material. A large part of the micrograph is occupied by enlarged lysosomes, labeled residual bodies (R). Only a small part of the electron-lucent lipid (L) shows in this section. *Arrow,* transitional element from ER to Golgi stack; A, autophagic vacuole; C, coated vesicles in formation; G, Golgi stack; GE, GERL; N, nucleus; V, virus. ×19,800.

paired ability of lysosomes to fuse with phagocytic vacuoles.

ACKNOWLEDGMENTS

The work from this laboratory was supported in part by grants to the author from the National Cancer Institute, National Institutes of Health, CA06576 and CA14923, and the American Cancer Society, E32 and CD-125B.

I am indebted to the many colleagues who have contributed to the work and concepts described in this chapter. However, any errors of fact or interpretation are mine alone.

FIG. 20 (top). Portion of hepatocyte from regenerating liver 4 hr after partial hepatectomy incubated in AcPase medium for 30 min at 37°C. Unreactive structures include ER (unlabeled), nucleus (N), and mitochondria (M). Reaction product is seen in the protein droplet at the left and in the autophagic vacuole with which it is apparently fusing. The *short arrow* is directed to reaction product extending from the autophagic vacuole to the droplet, thus indicating the continuity of the droplet and autophagic vacuole. The *long arrow* is directed to a region of the droplet where its tripartite membrane is evident. The continuity of this membrane with the membrane at the bottom of the autophagic vacuole is indistinct, either because of accumulated reaction product or because it is improperly oriented in relation to the electron beam. The body indicated by A, at the right, is either an autophagic vacuole or residual body. ×49,000. (From ref. 50, with permission.)
FIG. 21 (bottom). Portion of a pancreatic acinar cell from a beige mouse, incubated for AcPase. Note the absence of reaction product in rough ER (ER) and zymogen granule (Z). Reaction product is seen within a roughly circular area (at right), which contains lipid-like spheres (L) and within another roughly circular area continuous (*arrowhead*) with a long extension of smooth ER with spotty reaction product. *Arrows,* areas of the extension where the tripartite nature of its delimiting membrane is evident. Higher magnification shows more clearly that the membrane delimiting this extension is thicker than in the ER generally, as at ER in the field, and is like that delimiting the residual body with which it is continuous. R, ribosomes, most of which are probably on rough ER. ×36,000. (From ref. 51, with permission.)

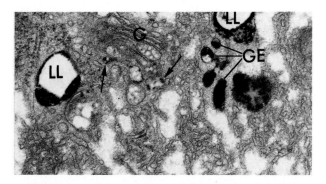

FIG. 23. Portion of a hepatocyte in a male hamster on cholesterol diet, 2 days. Tissue incubated in CMP medium for 30 min. Reaction product is seen in lipolysosomes (LL) and GERL (GE and two arrows). Electron-lucent lipid material is seen in lipolysosomes, GERL, and Golgi apparatus (G). ×27,550. (From ref 55, with permission.)

I am grateful to Dr. Phyllis M. Novikoff for providing Fig. 16. I acknowledge with thanks the patient skill of Mr. George Dominguez in preparing the final photographs, and the devotion of Ms. Brenda Zamboni and Ms. Fay Grad who typed the manuscript.

REFERENCES

1. de Duve, C. (1969): The lysosome in retrospect. In: *Lysosomes in Biology and Pathology,* edited by J. T. Dingle and Honor B. Fell, Vol. 2, pp. 3–40. North-Holland, Amsterdam.
2. de Duve, C. (1975): Exploring cells with a centrifuge. *Science,* 189:186–194.
3. Novikoff, A. B., Beaufay, H., and de Duve, C. (1956): Electron microscopy of lysosome-rich fractions from rat liver. *J. Biophys. Biochem. Cytol.,* 2:179–184.
4. Farrant, J. L. (1954): An electron microscopic study of ferritin. *Biochim. Biophys. Acta,* 13:569–576.
5. Novikoff, A. B. (1959): Cell heterogeneity within the hepatic lobule of the rat (staining reactions). *J. Histochem. Cytochem.,* 7:240–244.
6. Novikoff, A. B., Hausman, D. H., and Podber, E. (1958): The localization of adenosine triphosphatase in liver: *In situ* staining and cell fractionation studies. *J. Histochem. Cytochem.,* 6:61–71.
7. Novikoff, A. B., and Essner, E. (1960): The liver cell: Some new approaches to its study. *Am. J. Med.,* 29:102–131.
8. Novikoff, A. B. (1973): Lysosomes, a personal account. In: *Lysosomes and Storage Diseases,* edited by G. Hers and F. Van Hoof, pp. 1–41. Academic Press, New York.
9. Novikoff, A. B., and Goldfischer, S. (1969): Visualization of peroxisomes (microbodies) and mitochondria with diaminobenzidine. *J. Histochem. Cytochem.,* 17:675–680.
10. Barrett, A. J., and Dean, R. J. (1976): Enzymes of lysosomes. In: *Cell Biology I,* compiled and edited by P. L. Altman and D. D. Katz, pp. 317–324. *Fed. Am. Soc. Exp. Biol.,* Bethesda.
11. Smith, R. E., and Farquhar, M. G. (1966): Lysosome function in the regulation of the secretory process in cells of the anterior pituitary gland. *J. Cell Biol.,* 31:319–347.
12. Farquhar, M. G. (1969): Lysosome function in regulating secretion: Disposal of secretory granules in cells of the anterior pituitary gland. In: *Lysosomes in Biology and Pathology,* edited by J. T. Dingle and H. B. Fell, vol. 2, pp. 462–482. North-Holland, Amsterdam.
13. Novikoff, P. M., Novikoff, A. B., Quintana, N., and Hauw, J.-J. (1971): Golgi apparatus, GERL and lysosomes of neurons in rat dorsal root ganglia, studied by thick section and thin section cytochemistry. *J. Cell Biol.,* 50:859–886.
14. Friend, D. S., and Farquhar, M. G. (1967): Functions of coated vesicles during protein absorption in the rat vas deferens. *J. Cell Biol.,* 35:357–376.
15. Novikoff, A. B., Novikoff, P. M., Rosen, O. M., and Rubin, C. S. (1980): Organelle relationships in the cultured 3T3-L1 preadipocytes. *J. Cell Biol.,* 87:180–196.
16. Pearse, B. M. F. (1975): Coated vesicles from pig brain: Purification and biochemical characterization. *J. Mol. Biol.,* 97:93–98.
17. Pearse, B. M. F. (1976): Clathrin, a unique protein associated with intracellular transfer of membrane by coated vesicles. *Proc. Natl. Acad. Sci. USA,* 73:1254–1255.
18. Novikoff, A. B. (1964): GERL, its form and function in neurons of rat spinal ganglia. *Biol. Bull.,* 127:358.
19. Novikoff, A. B., and Novikoff, P. M. (1977): Cytochemical contributions to differentiating GERL from the Golgi apparatus. *Histochem. J.,* 9:525–551.
20. Novikoff, A. B., and Novikoff, P. M. (1979): Cell organelles and production of secretory products: Hormone action upon cell organelles. *Biol. Cell.* 36:101–110.
21. Palade, G. (1975): Intracellular aspects of the process of protein synthesis. *Science,* 189:71–112.
22. Novikoff, A. B., Mori, M., Quintana, N., and Yam, A. (1977): Studies of the secretory process in the mammalian exocrine pancreas. I. The condensing vacuoles. *J. Cell Biol.,* 75:148–165.
23. Fawcett, D. W. (1981): *The Cell,* second edition. Saunders, Philadelphia.
24. Hand, A. R., and Oliver, C. (1975): Secretory granule formation by the Golgi apparatus and GERL in rat exorbital lacrimal gland acinar cells. *J. Cell Biol.,* 67:154a.
25. Hand, A. R., and Oliver, C. (1977): The relationship between the Golgi apparatus, GERL and secretory granules in acinar cells of the rat exorbital lacrimal gland. *J. Cell Biol.,* 74:399–413.
26. Hand, A. R., and Oliver, C. (1977): Cytochemical studies of GERL and its role in secretory granule formation in exocrine cells. *Histochem. J.,* 9:375–392.
27. Robbins, E., Marcus, P. I., and Gonatas, N. K. (1964): Dynamics of acridine orange-cell interaction. II. Dye-induced ultrastructural changes in multivesicular bodies (acridine orange particles). *J. Cell Biol.,* 21:49–62.
28. Rome, L. H., Garvin, A. J., Allietta, M. M., and Neufeld, E. F. (1979): Two species of lysosomal organelles in cultured human fibroblasts. *Cell,* 17:143–153.
29. Garvin, A. J., Lyubsky, S., and Poore, C. M. (1981): A cytochemical study of GERL in cultured human fibroblasts. *Exp. Cell Res.,* 133:297–307.
30. Fedorko, M. E., Hirsch, J. G., and Cohn, Z. A. (1968): Autophagic vacuoles produced *in vitro.* I. Studies on cultured macrophages exposed to chloroquine. *J. Cell Biol.,* 38:377–391.
31. Fedorko, M. E., Hirsch, J. G., and Cohn, Z. A. (1968): Autophagic vacuoles produced *in vitro.* II. Studies on the mechanism of formation of autophagic vacuoles produced by chloroquine. *J. Cell Biol.,* 38:392–402.
32. Spater, H. W., Novikoff, A. B., Spater, S. H., and Quintana, N. (1978): Pyridoxal phosphatase: Cytochemical localization in GERL and other organelles of rat neurons. *J. Histochem. Cytochem.,* 26:809–821.
33. Smith, C. E. (1981): Correlated biochemical and cytochemical studies of nicotinamide adenine dinucleotide phosphatase (NADPase) activity in ameloblasts using structural analogues of NADP. *J. Histochem. Cytochem.,* 29:822–836.
34. Novikoff, P. M., Yam, A., and Novikoff, A. B. (1981): The lysosomal compartment of macrophages: extending the definition of GERL. *Proc. Natl. Acad. Sci. USA,* 78:5699–5703.
35. Novikoff, A. B., and Shin, W.-Y. (1978): Endoplasmic reticulum and autophagy in rat hepatocytes. *Proc. Natl. Acad. Sci. USA,* 75:5039–5042.
36. Haimes, H. B., Stockert, R. J., Morell, A. G., and Novikoff, A. B. (1981): Carbohydrate-specified endocytosis: localization of ligand in the lysosomal compartment. *Proc. Natl. Acad. Sci. USA,* 78:6936–6939.

37. Wall, D. A., Wilson, G., and Hubbard, A. L. (1980): The galactose-specific recognition system of mammalian liver: The route of ligand internalization in rat hepatocytes. *Cell*, 21:79–93.

38. Novikoff, P. M., and Yam, A. (1978): The cytochemical demonstration of GERL in rat hepatocytes during lipoprotein mobilization. *J. Histochem. Cytochem.*, 26:1–13.

39. Novikoff, P. M., and Yam, A. (1978): Sites of lipoprotein particles in normal rat hepatocytes. *J. Cell Biol.*, 76:1–11.

40. Jaeken, L., Thines-Sempoux, D., and Verheyen, F. (1978): A three-dimensional study of organelle interrelationships in regenerating rat liver. I. The GERL-system. *Cell Biol. Int. Rep.*, 2:501–513.

41. Pino, R. M., Pino, L. C., and Bankston, P. W. (1981): The relationships between the Golgi apparatus, GERL and lysosomes of fetal rat liver Kupffer cells examined by ultrastructural phosphatase cytochemistry. *J. Histochem. Cytochem.*, 29:1061–1070.

42. Boudier, J-A., Marchi, D., Cataldo, C., Massacrier, A., and Cau, P. (1981): Origin and fate of autophagic vacuoles in axons and nerve-endings of the rat neurohypophysis. II. Relationships with axoplasmic reticulum and three dimensional aspects. *Biol. Cell.*, 40:33–40.

43. Nelson, L., Van der Lande, V., and Robson, E. A. (1980): Fine structural and histochemical studies on salivary glands of *Peripatoides Novae-Zealandiae* (Onychophora) with special reference to acid phosphatase distribution. *Tissue Cell*, 2:405–418.

44. Thiele, J. (1977): Human parathyroid gland: A freeze fracture and thin section study. In: *Current Topics in Pathology*, edited by E. Grundmann, and W. H. Kirsten, pp. 31–80. Springer-Verlag, Berlin.

45. Masur, S. K., Rose, T., and Schulman, I. (1981): Ruthenium red and horseradish peroxidase localization in ADH-treated toad bladders. *J. Histochem. Cytochem.*, 29:902 (*Abstr.*).

46. Oliver, C. (1981): Enzyme cytochemical studies of basal lysosomes in exocrine acinar cells. *J. Histochem. Cytochem.*, 29:898 (*Abstr.*).

47. Hers, H. G., and Van Hoof, F. (editors) (1973): *Lysosomes and Storage Diseases*. Academic Press, New York.

48. Hers, H. G., and de Barsy, T. (1973): Type II glycogenesis (acid maltase deficiency). In: *Lysosomes and Storage Diseases*, edited by H. G. Hers and F. Van Hoof, pp. 197–216. Academic Press, New York.

49. Callahan, J. W., and Lowden, J. A. (editors) (1981): *Lysosomes and Lysosomal Storage Diseases*. Raven Press, New York.

50. Mori, M., and Novikoff, A. B. (1977): Induction of pinocytosis in rat hepatocytes by partial hepatectomy. *J. Cell Biol.*, 72: 695–706.

51. Novikoff, A. B., Quintana, N., and Mori, M. (1977): Studies on the secretory process in exocrine pancreas cells. II. C57 black and beige mice. *J. Histochem. Cytochem.*, 62:83–93.

52. Boutry, J.-M., and Novikoff, A. B. (1975): Cytochemical studies on Golgi apparatus, GERL and lysosomes in neurons of dorsal root ganglia in mice. *Proc. Natl. Acad. Sci. USA*, 72:508–512.

53. Oliver, C., and Essner, E. (1973): Distribution of anomalous lysosomes in the beige mouse: A homologue of Chediak-Higashi syndrome. *J. Histochem. Cytochem.*, 21:218–228.

54. Essner, E., and Oliver, C. (1974): Lysosome formation in hepatocytes of mice with Chédiak-Higashi syndrome. *Lab. Invest.*, 30:596–607.

55. Nehemiah, J. L., and Novikoff, A. B. (1974): Unusual lysosomes in hamster hepatocytes. *Exp. Mol. Pathol.*, 21:398–423.

56. Hayashi, H., and Sternlieb, I. (1975): Lipolysosomes in human hepatocytes: Ultrastructural and cytochemical studies of patients with Wilson's disease. *Lab. Invest.*, 33:1–7.

57. Hayashi, H., Winship, D. H., and Sternlieb, I. (1977): Lipolysosomes in human liver: Distribution in livers with fatty infiltration. *Gastroenterology*, 73:651–654.

58. D'Arcy Hart, P., and Young, M. R. (1980): Manipulations of phagosome-lysosome fusion in cultured macrophages: Potentialities and limitations. In: *Mononuclear Phagocytes, Functional Aspects*, edited by Ralph van Furth, pp. 1039–1055. Martinus Nyhoff, Boston.

59. Fraser, W., and McDade, J. E. (1979): Legionellosis. *Sci. Am.*, 241:82–98.

60. Horwitz, M. A., and Silverstein, S. C. (1980): Legionnaires' disease bacterium (*Legionella pneumophila*) multiplies intracellularly in human monocytes. *Am. Soc. Clin. Invest.*, 66:441–450.

The Liver: Biology and Pathobiology, edited by
I. Arias, H. Popper, D. Schachter, and D. A. Shafritz.
Raven Press, New York © 1982.

Chapter 3

Peroxisomes

Paul B. Lazarow

The peroxisome is a subcellular organelle present in many tissues and cells of animals and plants, including unicellular eukaryotes. This chapter deals exclusively with the properties of peroxisomes in liver, specifically with those in parenchymal cells. The bulk of our information comes from studies in rats. The chapter begins with the functions and morphology of peroxisomes, considers their isolation, properties, biogenesis, and turnover, and concludes by describing their possible role in pathology.

FUNCTIONS

Many of the biochemical reactions of peroxisomes are oxidative, functioning in catabolic pathways. Some however, are anabolic reactions, and some end products of peroxisomal reactions serve as building blocks for anabolic reactions elsewhere in the cell.

Respiration

The respiratory pathway of peroxisomes, discovered and characterized by de Duve and his collaborators (1–3), is illustrated in Fig. 1. It consists of a group of oxidases that utilize molecular oxygen to directly oxidize a variety of substrates and produce hydrogen peroxide (H_2O_2), together with catalase, which decomposes the H_2O_2. The substrates for the oxidases (RH_2 in Fig. 1) include lactate, glycolate, and other α-hydroxy acids, urate, D-amino acids, acyl-CoAs, and polyamines, such as spermine (4). The decomposition of H_2O_2 by catalase can occur by two mechanisms: the catalatic reaction shown on top in Fig. 1, or the peroxidatic reaction shown below it. Substrates for peroxidation ($R'H_2$ in Fig. 1) include alcohols, formate, nitrite, and quinones. The peroxidatic reaction is favored by the conditions existing inside peroxisomes, namely, a high catalase concentration and a low and steady formation of H_2O_2. H_2O_2 is probably destroyed peroxidatically to the extent that suitable peroxidatic substrates are available; excess H_2O_2 would be destroyed catalatically. In addition to these direct oxidations, peroxisomes may also participate in the reoxidation of cytoplasmic NADH through coupled reactions (3). One possible scheme is shown in Fig. 2. The extent to which this occurs *in vivo* is unknown.

Peroxisomal respiration differs from mitochondrial respiration in several respects. The energy of the peroxisomal oxidations is not conserved by the formation of ATP but instead is dissipated as heat. These reactions contribute to thermogenesis. Peroxisomal O_2 consumption is not blocked by cyanide and is insensitive to respiratory control. The physiological activity of peroxisomal respiration has been estimated to account for roughly 20% of the oxygen consumption of liver (3,5).

The peroxisome is named for its metabolism of H_2O_2

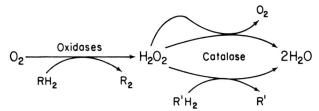

FIG. 1. Respiratory pathway of peroxisomes. (From ref. 3.)

(3). The properties and physiological significance of peroxisomal respiration have been reviewed in detail by de Duve and Baudhin (3) (see ref. 6 for a recent general review of H_2O_2 metabolism).

Lipid Metabolism

β-Oxidation of Fatty Acids

Peroxisomes catalyze the β-oxidation of fatty acids by the reaction sequence illustrated in Fig. 3 (7,8). Long chain acyl-CoAs are the substrates, and acetyl-CoA is formed as an end product. H_2O_2 is formed in the first reaction of this β-oxidation spiral. This differs from the corresponding reaction in mitochondria, where electrons are transferred from an acyl-CoA to the electron transport chain via electron transfer flavoprotein. The oxidase catalyzing this initial peroxisomal reaction appears to be rate limiting and to determine the chain length specificity for the entire reaction sequence. Peroxisomes oxidize saturated acyl-CoAs with chain lengths from seven to 18 or more carbons (8), and long chain unsaturated acyl-CoAs (9).

The subsequent three reactions of the peroxisomal β-oxidation spiral are the same as in the mitochondrial β-oxidation system but are catalyzed by enzymes with different physical properties and substrate specificities. Interestingly, the second and third enzymes, the crotonase and hydroxyacyl-CoA dehydrogenase, together form a bifunctional protein (10).

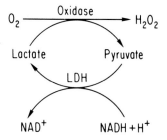

FIG. 2. Hypothetical peroxisomal oxidation of cytosolic NADH by means of coupled reactions. NADH is oxidized by lactate dehydrogenase (LDH) in the cytosol. The lactate diffuses into the peroxisomes, where it is oxidized to pyruvate by L-α-hydroxy acid oxidase. The pyruvate diffuses into the cytosol to complete the cycle. (After ref. 3.)

The capacity of the peroxisomal β-oxidation system in normal rats is approximately of the same order of magnitude as the activity of the mitochondrial β-oxidation system. It is unusual to find an entire reaction sequence duplicated in two organelles, and the physiological roles of peroxisomal and mitochondrial β-oxidation have not yet been elucidated. The properties of the two systems suggest that one mitochondrial function is to oxidize fatty acids to meet the energy needs of the liver, and one peroxisome function is to supply acetyl-CoA for anabolic reactions (e.g., synthesis of cholesterol and bile acids). Peroxisomal β-oxidation in the liver is increased from three- to 10-fold in rats fed a high rat diet (11,12), in genetically obese mice (13), and in rats fed hypolipidemic drugs (14,15).

Fatty Acid Activation

Peroxisomes activate fatty acids to the corresponding acyl-CoAs according to the following reaction:

$$palmitate + CoA + ATP \rightleftharpoons$$
$$palmitoyl\text{-}CoA + AMP + PP_i$$

The peroxisomal acyl-CoA synthetase acts on palmitate and laurate but not on octanoate; its activity is sufficient to keep the peroxisomal β-oxidation system supplied with substrates (16). These results do not

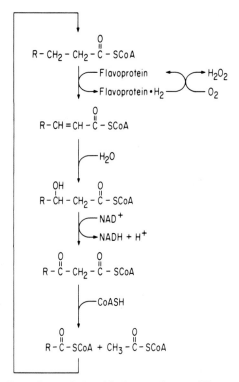

FIG. 3. Peroxisomal β-oxidation pathway. (From ref. 7.)

exclude the possibility that acyl-CoAs formed elsewhere in the cell might also enter peroxisomes for oxidation.

Carnitine Acyltransferase

Peroxisomes catalyze the exchange of short acyl groups (acetyl-, butyryl-, hexanoyl-, and octanoyl-) between CoA and carnitine as follows (17):

$$\text{acyl-CoA} + \text{carnitine} \rightleftharpoons \text{acylcarnitine} + \text{CoA}$$

This provides a mechanism whereby the end products of peroxisomal β-oxidation can be transferred to the mitochondria as carnitine esters for further oxidation.

Ether Glycerolipid Biosynthesis

The enzyme that catalyzes the first reaction of ether glycerolipid biosynthesis (namely, dihydroxyacetone phosphate acyltransferase) has been localized in peroxisomes (18). In addition, some of the enzyme catalyzing the second reaction, dihydroxyacetone phosphate:NADPH oxidoreductase, also appears to be peroxisomal. This is the first instance in which liver peroxisomes have been found to catalyze biosynthetic reactions.

Purine Catabolism

As illustrated in Fig. 4, animals excrete various metabolites as the primary end products of purine catabolism. This is due to the progressive loss of enzymes catalyzing the reactions of purine catabolism during evolution. Four of these enzymes (xanthine dehydrogenase, urate oxidase, allantoinase, and allantoicase) are present in liver peroxisomes in various species; some, however, are found in the cytosol in other species.

Amphibia (frogs), fish (mackerel), and crustaceans (prawns) can catabolize purines all the way to urea and glyoxalate (Fig. 4). The fish liver and crustacean hepatopancreas peroxisomes contain urate oxidase, allantoinase, and allantoicase but not xanthine oxidase, which is found in the cytosol (19). In frog liver, urate oxidase and allantoinase, but not allantoicase, are peroxisomal (20). Rats excrete allantoin; their urate oxidase is located exclusively within peroxisomes. Humans excrete uric acid as the end product of purine catabolism because they lack urate oxidase (and thus are susceptible to gout). Chicken liver has an active xanthine dehydrogenase and low levels of urate oxidase, both of which are located in their peroxisomes. It is clear that peroxisomes play an important role in purine catabolism. On the other

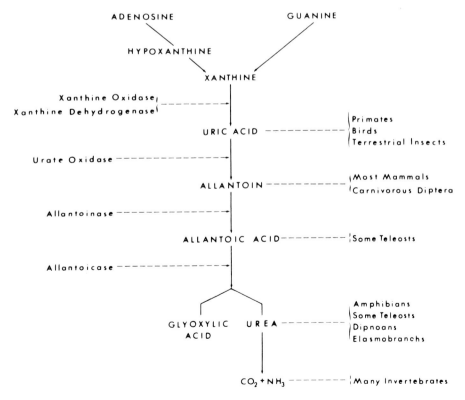

FIG. 4. Reactions of purine catabolism. *Left*, enzymes; *right*, animals using the various metabolites as their end products of purine catabolism. (From ref. 20.)

hand, no species has yet been investigated in which all four enzymes are located together in peroxisomes.

Alcohol Metabolism

Ethanol is a substrate for the peroxidatic reaction of catalase (Fig. 5). This reaction is favored by a high catalase concentration (as occurs in peroxisomes) and by high concentrations of ethanol; it is limited to the rate of H_2O_2 formation. The physiological contribution of peroxisomes to alcohol clearance in ethanol-fed rats or in man has been the subject of some discussion. Alcohol dehydrogenase is found in the cytosol and is responsible for the bulk of alcohol metabolism; from 5 to 25% of ethanol clearance, however, is insensitive to inhibitors of this enzyme (21). Peroxisomes possess the enzymatic capability to oxidize the balance of the ethanol (and in fact considerably more), but only if they are adequately supplied with substrates for H_2O_2 formation. Experiments measuring peroxisomal ethanol oxidation in perfused liver or isolated hepatocytes are not physiologically relevant because under these experimental conditions, the liver cells are deprived of the rich mixture of nutrients normally arriving in the portal blood, including substrates for the oxidases. Oshino et al. (5) applied an elegant spectroscopic method to estimate H_2O_2 formation in the liver of anesthetized rats and calculated that peroxisomes were responsible for about 10% of ethanol clearance.

Several studies (5,22,23) have demonstrated that ethanol peroxidation can be strikingly increased by supplying living rats or perfused livers with substrates (e.g., urate or glycolate) for the peroxisomal oxidases. A possible practical application to inebriety has been discussed (23).

Other Reactions

Rat liver peroxisomes contain an aminotransferase capable of irreversibly transferring amino groups from leucine, phenylalanine, or several other amino acids to glyoxalate, yielding glycine (24).

Since peroxisomes are larger and more abundant in the gluconeogenic tissues, liver and kidney, than in most other mammalian tissues, and since peroxisomes play an important role in gluconeogenesis in plants (25) and unicellular organisms (26), it has long been suspected that liver peroxisomes contribute to gluconeogenesis. They may do so by the exergonic for-

mation of α-keto acids (3) catalyzed by L-α-hydroxy acid oxidase, D-amino acid oxidase, or the aminotransferase mentioned above; the α-keto acids are substrates for gluconeogenesis.

MORPHOLOGY

Peroxisomes are more numerous and larger in size in liver parenchymal cells than in most other mammalian cells. They are usually spherical or slightly elliptical and have one unit membrane, a finely granular matrix, and in some species a dense, paracrystalline core (Fig. 6). In rat liver, peroxisomes have a mean diameter of 0.6 to 0.7 μm, although they range in size from 0.2 to 1.0 μm. According to morphometric analysis (27,28), there are between 370 and 620 peroxisomes per parenchymal cell, and together they take up about 1.5 to 2% of the parenchymal cell volume. The average peroxisome has one-fourth to one-sixth the volume of the average mitochondrion, and peroxisomes are four to two times less numerous than mitochondria.

There is a core in many liver peroxisomes. In rat liver, the core consists of urate oxidase in a cylindrical paracrystalline array of hollow tubules. Longitudinal sections show a striated appearance, whereas perfect cross sections show an array of circles. Human hepatic peroxisomes lack both urate oxidase and cores. In general, there is a good correlation between the presence of urate oxidase in peroxisomes and the presence of a core, but the converse is not necessarily true. The structure of the core varies considerably among species and may be worm-shaped or branched instead of cylindrical; it may lack the internal paracrystallinity (29). When present, cores facilitate the identification of peroxisomes in electron micrographs, but their presence is not essential.

In some species, peroxisomes contain a marginal plate, which is a flat, electron-dense structure located in the periphery of the organelle, almost adjacent to the membrane. The thickness of the marginal plate ranges from 8 to 15 nm. These structures are common in insectivores and nonhuman primates; they are absent in human and rat liver peroxisomes. Nothing is known of their biochemical composition. (See ref. 29 for a comparative review of peroxisome ultrastructure.)

The disposition of peroxisomes throughout the hepatocyte and among cells in different regions of the liver lobule is fairly uniform. There are no great concentrations of peroxisomes in any one region of the cell or in one part of the lobule, except that peroxisomes are somewhat more abundant in cells near the central vein (27).

Peroxisomes tend to occur in clusters within the cell (Fig. 7A) (30–33). Occasionally, they appear to be interconnected (Fig. 7B) (31,33–35); such images are more

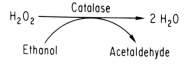

FIG. 5. Peroxidatic oxidation of ethanol by catalase.

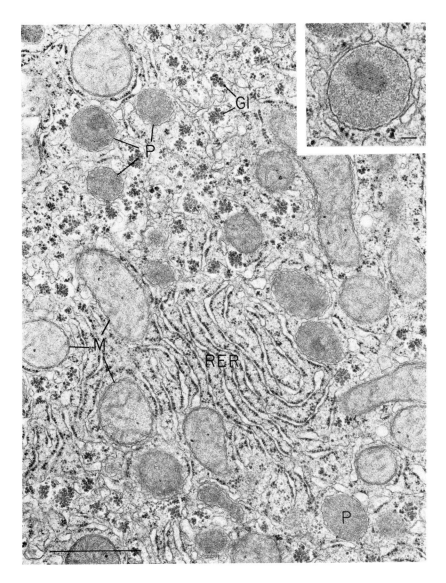

FIG. 6. Electron micrograph of rat liver. P, peroxisomes; M, mitrochondria; RER, rough endoplasmic reticulum, Gl glycogen in region of smooth ER. *Bar* = 1 μm. **Inset:** Peroxisome showing striated core. *Bar* = 100 nm.

common at times of peroxisome proliferation. The total volume of peroxisomes in a cell may be more constant than the size of individual peroxisomes. Two morphometric analyses (27,28) agree closely on the total peroxisome volume but differ by almost a factor of two on the total number and individual volume of peroxisomes. Administration of triiodothyronine increased the number of peroxisomes fivefold, but the average volume decreased threefold; thus total peroxisome volume was less than doubled (36). These facts suggest that peroxisomes may constitute a single mass that can be variously subdivided.

Peroxisomes often occur in close association with elements of the endoplasmic reticulum (ER) (Figs. 6 and 7). Whether or not there are luminal connections between these two types of organelles is a matter of controversy. Some investigators claim that there are many such continuities (37), while others disagree (34,38). In any case, the physical proximity of per-

oxisomes and ER may facilitate biochemical cooperation.

"Tails" are observed occasionally on peroxisomes (Fig. 7C) (29,30,32,39). They sometimes have been interpreted as connections to the ER but may be connections to other peroxisomes. Some tails with loops or other unusual structures have been described as "gastruloid cisternae" (40).

It has been suggested (41) that peroxisomes may be interconnected in space and time to form a "peroxisome reticulum" entirely distinct from the ER. The contents of the peroxisomes would form one pool within the cell, kept in continuity by fission and fusion and/or by interconnections. New peroxisomes could form by fission from preexisting ones. This concept would explain most of the available data on the biogenesis and turnover of peroxisomes discussed below.

The shape of peroxisomes is altered by the adminis-

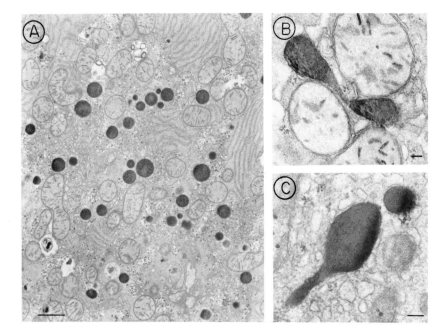

FIG. 7. Electron micrographs of rat liver in which the peroxisomes have been stained with the diaminobenzidine cytochemical staining reaction for catalase (107). **A:** Clustering of peroxisomes. **B:** Dumbbell-shaped peroxisome. **C:** Peroxisome with a "tail." *Bar* = 1 μm in **A** and 250 nm in **B** and **C**.

tration of a number of unrelated compounds that may produce highly elongated or oddly shaped particles (40,42). The abundance and total volume of peroxisomes may be strikingly increased by a variety of hypolipidemic drugs (see below). This increase in peroxisome mass is a separate phenomenon from the proliferation of ER produced by phenobarbital (28,43).

Liver peroxisomes were first observed under the electron microscope by Rouiller and Bernhard (44), who described them by the name "microbody," a term that had previously been applied to a similar structure in rat kidney by Rhodin (45). The term is still in use in the electron microscopic literature to describe a structure with a single membrane, a diameter of roughly 0.2 to 1 μm, and often a core. However, because some such structures in various cell types are biochemically unrelated to peroxisomes, the more specific biochemical name "peroxisome" is preferred. The terminology of these organelles is discussed in more detail by de Duve (46).

ISOLATION AND PHYSICAL PROPERTIES

Peroxisomes, mitochondria, and lysosomes in liver have roughly similar sizes. Therefore, a mitochondrial fraction prepared by classic differential centrifugation procedures contains all three organelles. Peroxisomes may be separated from the other particles by equilibrium density centrifugation, as shown in Fig. 8 (2,47). This figure illustrates the application of the method of analytical cell fractionation (48) to the elucidation of cell structure.

Certain properties of peroxisomes have been de-

duced from their sedimentation behavior under a variety of conditions. The average peroxisome has a dry weight of 24 fg (24×10^{-15} g), a dry density of 1.32 g/cm³, and a sedimentation coefficient in 0.25 M sucrose of 4,400 S (3). Peroxisomes are permeable to sucrose; therefore, unlike lysosomes and mitochondria, they are osmotically inactive in sucrose gradients, where they have an equilibrium density of 1.32, equal to their dry density. Peroxisomes can be purified almost 40-fold starting from a rat liver homogenate. They constitute 2.5% of total liver protein or about 6.5 mg protein per gram liver (47).

Catalase is the most abundant protein of rat liver peroxisomes, contributing 16% to the total peroxisomal protein. The core contributes 10% of the peroxisomal protein and is mostly, if not exclusively, urate oxidase. All other proteins are present in smaller amounts, according to analysis by sodium dodecyl sulfate polyacrylamide gel electrophoresis.

The polypeptide composition of the peroxisome membrane is simple and unique (49); it contains only a few major proteins, which are not found in the membranes of the ER or the mitochondria. The phospholipids of the peroxisome membrane are the same as those found in the ER, but the proportions are different. The peroxisome membrane is permeable to such molecules as sucrose, lactate, urate, and D-amino acids.

BIOGENESIS

Most of the experimental information on peroxisome biogenesis comes from studies on catalase, the

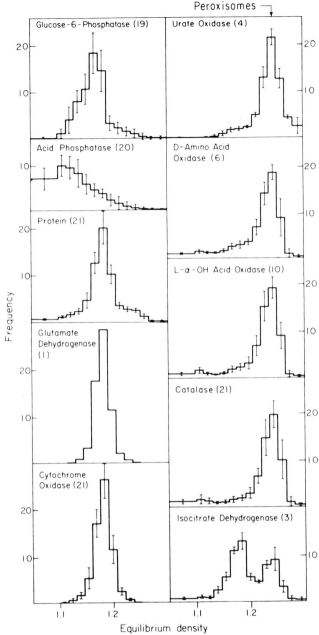

FIG. 8. Purification of peroxisomes. A small mitochondrial fraction was prepared by differential centrifugation and then subfractionated by equilibrium density centrifugation in a linear sucrose gradient. The positions of the organelles in the gradient at the end of the centrifugation were determined by assaying their marker enzymes: glucose-6-phosphatase (microsomes), acid phosphatase (lysosomes), glutamate dehydrogenase and cytochrome oxidase (mitochondria). Isocitrate dehydrogenase is located partly in mitochondria and partly in peroxisomes. Numbers of experiments in parentheses. (From ref. 47.)

principal enzyme of the organelle. As illustrated in Fig. 9, catalase is synthesized *in vivo* in rat liver as an apomonomer (50) that appears to be located in the cell sap (51,52). It enters peroxisomes posttranslationally,

with a half life of 14 min (52), without undergoing detectable proteolytic processing (53). Inside the organelle, it acquires heme and aggregates to form the active tetrameric enzyme.

When catalase mRNA is translated *in vitro* in the wheat germ or the reticulocyte lysate cell-free protein synthesizing system, the product has the same molecular mass as the subunit of the mature enzyme (53). Catalase mRNA is found in a free but not a bound polysome fraction (54). There is no evidence for any role of the ER in the biogenesis of catalase.

The simplest hypothesis for peroxisome biogenesis is that newly synthesized peroxisomal proteins are added to preexisting peroxisomes by posttranslational uptake (52). These would potentially include soluble, core, and membrane proteins. New peroxisomes could form by fission from old peroxisomes or from the suggested peroxisome reticulum (41).

A previous hypothesis for peroxisome biogenesis suggested that catalase and other soluble peroxisome proteins are segregated cotranslationally into the ER (like secretory proteins) and find their way through the ER cisternae to outpouchings which accumulate peroxisome proteins and eventually bud off to form peroxisomes (3). This attractive hypothesis engendered fruitful experiments, which have served to disprove the hypothesis.

Many unanswered questions remain concerning peroxisome biogenesis, including the site of synthesis and assembly of the membrane proteins and the mechanism of entry of the soluble proteins (see ref. 41 for a recent review).

TURNOVER

It is thought that peroxisomes are destroyed randomly by autophagy (3). Peroxisomes have been observed within autophagic vacuoles by several investigators (cited in ref. 29).

Rat liver peroxisomal proteins appear to have approximately the same half-life (55). The observed value, obtained by labeling proteins *in vivo* with [³H]-leucine, is 3.5 days. When these data are corrected for the reutilization of the isotope, however, the half-life decreases to 1.5 days (56), which agrees with the half-life determined for catalase by two other independent methods (57). There is one apparent case of asynchronous turnover of peroxisome proteins. In a mutant strain of mice, the half-life of catalase is 50% of normal, resulting in a doubling of the steady-state amount of catalase (58). The activity of urate oxidase is also increased but only by 20%, not by the 100% expected if the mutation affected the half-life of all peroxisome proteins equally.

No hint has been found for the maturation and aging of peroxisomes as individual particles. For example,

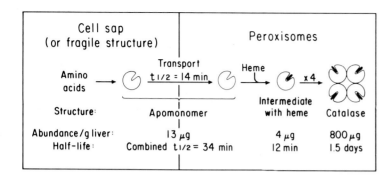

FIG. 9. Catalase biogenesis *in vivo* in rat liver. (From ref. 41.)

small peroxisomes do not grow gradually to become large peroxisomes (59). The turnover of catalase is independent of particle size. These facts are consistent with the idea that peroxisomes exchange their contents with one another and are destroyed randomly.

PATHOLOGY

Hypolipidemic Drugs and Atherosclerosis

Peroxisomes are greatly affected by hypolipidemic drugs. The activity of the peroxisomal β-oxidation system is increased eightfold in the livers of rats treated with clofibrate for 1 week (Fig. 10) (7). Some analogs of clofibrate produce similar effects but at much lower doses (15,60). Other hypolipidemic drugs with different structures (tibric acid and Wy-14,643) increase the peroxisomal β-oxidation capacity of the whole liver as much as 18-fold (14). Two chemically different compounds not usually considered to be hypolipidemic—di-(2-ethylhexyl)phthalate and acetylsalicylic acid—have been shown to both lower serum triglycerides and increase hepatic peroxisomal β-ox-

idation (61,62). Taken together, these results suggest that the peroxisomes play an important role in the lowering of serum triglycerides caused by these drugs.

The first evidence of an effect of clofibrate on peroxisomes was the discovery that the drug caused a striking proliferation of the organelle as well as an increase in catalase activity (63). Other hypolipidemic drugs have similar effects (64,65). These proliferated peroxisomes do not have the same biochemical composition as normal peroxisomes. β-Oxidation increases by an order of magnitude, while catalase (which in normal liver is the most abundant peroxisomal enzyme) increases by only 50 to 100%. Urate oxidase, D-amino acid oxidase, and L-α-hydroxy acid oxidase all decrease in activity (63,66).

Hypolipidemic drugs also elevate other enzymes of lipid metabolism in several liver organelles. Carnitine acyltransferase, which is located in peroxisomes, mitochondria, and ER (17), is increased by an order of magnitude (67,68). The longer chain length carnitine acyltransferases are also elevated but to a lesser extent (69).

Clofibrate causes a two- to threefold increase in the activity of fatty acid-activating enzymes in liver (70). These enzymes are located in the ER, mitochondria, and peroxisomes, and the activity in the three organelles is increased approximately in parallel by the drug treatment (16).

The modest increase in catalase activity caused by clofibrate has no obvious connection to the hypolipidemic properties of the drug. Several reports in the literature, however, link catalase activity to atherosclerosis. A lyophilized preparation of bovine liver catalase was reported to lower serum cholesterol levels when injected into guinea pigs, dogs, humans (71), and rabbits (72). A purified, dialyzed peroxidatic subunit of catalase (prepared by alkaline-treatment of bovine liver catalase) partially protected rabbits against atherosclerosis induced by a high cholesterol diet (73).

Feinstein (74) and his colleagues selected and bred a strain of "acatalasemic" mice. These mice have normal amounts of an abnormal catalase. The liver

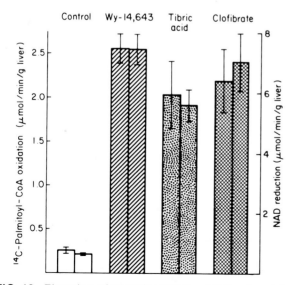

FIG. 10. Elevation of peroxisomal β-oxidation in rat liver by administration of hypolipidemic drugs. (From ref. 14.)

enzyme is unstable and easily loses its catalatic activity; in so doing, it acquires (or reveals) a large peroxidatic activity (75,76). Goldfischer et al. (77) found that in these acatalasemic mice, the serum cholesterol and triglyceride concentrations are significantly lower than in control mice. The mutant mice also have impaired synthesis of cholesterol and fatty acids (78). Thus, as pointed out by Goldfischer et al. (77), mice with a genetically altered catalase and rabbits injected with catalase or peroxidase share the property of having decreased serum lipid levels. It must be emphasized that no causal explanation or connection of these observations is known, but the coincidence is curious.

Takahara et al. (79) have investigated a rare, recessive acatalasemia among Japanese. The only clinical symptom noted was occasional ulceration or gangrenous degeneration around the teeth. Aebi and Suter (80) have reviewed later studies of acatalasemic individuals of other nationalities who are asymptomatic.

Infection and Inflammation

Acute bacterial infection (elicited by subcutaneous administration of pneumococci to rats) produces a 50% decrease in the number and total volume of peroxisomes in 24 hr, accompanied by significant decreases in catalase and urate oxidase activities (81). In contrast, mitochondrial, soluble, and lysosomal enzymes were unaffected.

Turpentine-induced inflammation in rats causes decreases of catalase and three peroxisomal oxidases ranging from 33 to 60% (82). Hepatocytes isolated from these rats had only half the normal capability to oxidize oleic acid; the activity of peroxisomal β-oxidation was not determined. Canonico et al. (81,82) note that the effects of septic and aseptic stress on peroxisomes and on lipid metabolism in liver appear in several respects to be opposite to the effects of hypolipidemic drugs.

Acute viral hepatitis with jaundice may affect peroxisomes differently from bacterial infection or inflammation. Numerous peroxisomes were noted in the livers of mice infected with ectromelia virus (mouse pox) and showing jaundice (83) and in biopsy specimens of patients with acute viral hepatitis and jaundice (84). No systematic investigations yet have been performed.

Tumors

Liver of Tumor-Bearing Animals

The catalase activity of the liver is depressed to as little as 5% of the control value in rats bearing hepatomas, lymphomas, sarcomas, and carcinomas (85). Among the remarkable features of this effect is that the catalase depression increases with tumor mass and is completely reversible by removing the tumor. Liver catalase activity also returns to normal values in a strain of mice in which an implanted sarcoma grows for 3 weeks and then regresses spontaneously (85). In contrast, kidney catalase is depressed only modestly, and blood catalase is unaffected. (See ref. 86 for a review of the literature on the possible mechanisms whereby liver catalase is decreased by a tumor elsewhere in the body.) Hepatic catalase decreases in humans with liver metastases and increases again in individuals who respond to chemotherapy (87).

Tumors affect peroxisome abundance and catalase activity. A combined morphological and biochemical study of rats bearing Ehrlich ascites tumors found that the number of hepatic peroxisomes decreased by 40%, hepatic catalase activity dropped 50%, and urate oxidase lost not more than 15 to 17% of its activity (88). Thus tumors do not decrease all peroxisomal enzymes in parallel, just as hypolipidemic drugs do not increase all peroxisomal enzymes in parallel.

Hepatomas

The degree of morphological differentiation of Morris hepatomas is inversely correlated with their growth rate (89). Among various alterations that occur are striking changes in the peroxisomes, ranging from a decrease in size (in hepatomas with intermediate growth rates) to complete absence (in rapidly growing hepatomas). This inverse correlation extends as well to the Novikoff and Reuber hepatomas (90).

The changes in abundance of peroxisomes are accompanied by equally striking changes in the activities of peroxisomal enzymes (91). The activity of catalase in general follows the abundance of peroxisomes, although there are some notable exceptions. Urate oxidase and D-amino acid oxidase activities correlate with catalase to the extent that both are very low or absent in the rapidly growing hepatomas (with a single exception). However, the two oxidases vary considerably in their activity among the intermediate and slow-growing hepatomas. In some cases, they are more than twice the normal values. The extremes in the individual enzyme activities occur in different rather than in the same hepatomas.

The subcellular compartmentation of catalase, urate oxidase, and D-amino acid oxidase varies among hepatomas (92). In several Morris hepatomas with moderate growth rates, all three enzymes are located exclusively in peroxisomes, but the peroxisomes have somewhat altered physical properties. In a rapidly growing HC hepatoma, peroxisomes are absent, catalase is entirely in the cytosol (although abundant), and the oxidases are absent altogether.

Alcoholism

An increase in peroxisome abundance has been reported in the livers of alcohol-consuming men (93) and rats (94), but this was not confirmed in a later morphometric study (95). Ethanol peroxidation by catalase is increased in rats receiving ethanol chronically, but this accounts for only a small part of the observed increase in ethanol clearance (21). As discussed above, H_2O_2 formation is the rate-limiting step in peroxisomal ethanol metabolism. Unfortunately, there is no direct spectroscopic measurement of H_2O_2 formation *in vivo* in ethanol-treated rats as there is in normal rats (5).

Clofibrate administration increases the rate of ethanol clearance in rats (96,97) and prevents the formation of fatty liver during both acute (98) and chronic (99) ethanol feeding. Some of the increase in ethanol clearance is due to hepatomegaly caused by the drug. Prevention of fatty liver may be attributable to the induction by clofibrate of peroxisomal β-oxidation. Increased H_2O_2 formation during peroxisomal fatty acid oxidation probably contributes to the more rapid ethanol clearance (97).

Zellweger's Cerebrohepatorenal Syndrome

Babies with this rare familial disease show multiple complex symptoms, as the name implies. They have no detectable peroxisomes in their hepatocytes and renal proximal tubules, although liver catalase activity is normal (100). Mitochondria also appear to be defective, ultrastructurally and functionally, in liver and brain. Other cellular changes include a deficiency of smooth ER and an excess of glycogen in the hepatocytes. The primary defect in this disease is not known.

In a similar syndrome (101), peroxisomes are absent, catalase is absent (as determined spectroscopically), and mitochondria are altered (although differently). Smooth ER is normal.

Other Diseases

Liver peroxisomes occasionally appear to proliferate in patients with Wilson's disease, in which copper accumulates in the liver (102). However, this is not a consistent occurrence; pathological alteration of mitochondria is more common.

A greater than normal abundance of peroxisomes has also been described in Reye syndrome (103,104). On the other hand, Svoboda and Reddy (105) found that the number of peroxisomes was normal in Reye syndrome patients, but they often contained cores which normal human liver peroxisomes do not. Sternlieb and Quintana (106) described the altered

appearance of peroxisomes in liver biopsies of patients with a number of different diseases.

In view of the fact that peroxisomes tend to occur in clusters in normal liver, anecdotal mention of proliferated peroxisomes in disease states should be considered cautiously. Different electron microscopic sections may contain different numbers of peroxisomes, making morphometric analysis essential for the reliable evaluation of possible changes.

SUMMARY

At present, there are no known "peroxisomal diseases," in the sense that we know of no primary enzymatic defect in the peroxisomes that is responsible for illness. One biochemical alteration of peroxisomes that is clearly related to health is the elevation of the peroxisomal β-oxidation system by hypolipidemic drugs. This increase in peroxisomal enzymes appears to play an important role in the hypotriglyceridemic action of these drugs. Peroxisomes are also altered, sometimes strikingly, in a variety of other disease states. From the biochemical point of view, we know too little about the reasons for these changes. Further research is required to evaluate their significance.

ACKNOWLEDGMENTS

The work of the author was supported by NIH grants AM-19394 and HL-20909 and NSF grant PCM77-11151.

I thank Karrie Polowetzky and Martha Morse for their expert typing of the manuscript, Helen Shio for the preparation of Figs. 6 and 7, and Miklos Muller for his critical reading of the manuscript. Figures 1, 4, 8, and 9 are reprinted with the permission of Physiological Reviews, The New York Academy of Sciences, The Journal of Cell Biology, and Springer, Inc., respectively.

REFERENCES

1. de Duve, C., Beaufay, H., Jacques, P., Rahman-Li, Y., Sellinger, O. Z., Wattiaux, R., and de Coninck, S. (1960): Intracellular localization of catalase and of some oxidases in rat liver. *Biochim. Biophys. Acta*, 40:186–187.
2. Beaufay, H., Jacques, P., Baudhuin, P., Sellinger, O Z., Berthet, J., and de Duve, C. (1964): Tissue fractionation studies. 18. Resolution of mitochondrial fractions from rat liver into three distinct populations of cytoplasmic particles by means of density equilibration in various gradients. *Biochem. J.*, 92:184–205.
3. de Duve, C., and Baudhuin, P. (1966): Peroxisomes (microbodies and related particles). *Physiol. Rev.*, 46:323–357.
4. Holtta, E. (1977): Oxidation of spermidine and spermine in rat liver: Purification and properties of polyamine oxidase. *Biochemistry*, 16:91–100.
5. Oshino, N., Jamieson, D., Sugano, T., and Chance, B. (1975):

Optical measurement of the catalase-hydrogen peroxide intermediate (compound I) in the liver of anaesthetized rats and its implication to hydrogen peroxide production in situ. *Biochem. J.,* 146:67−77.

6. Chance, B., Sies, H., and Boveris, A. (1979): Hydroperoxide metabolism in mammalian organs. *Physiol. Rev.,* 59:527−605.

7. Lazarow, P. B., and de Duve, C. (1976): A fatty acyl-CoA oxidizing system in rat liver peroxisomes; enhancement by clofibrate, a hypolipidemic drug. *Proc. Natl. Acad. Sci. USA,* 73:2043−2046.

8. Lazarow, P. B. (1978): Rat liver peroxisomes catalyze the β-oxidation of fatty acids. *J. Biol. Chem.,* 253:1522−1528.

9. Osmundsen, H., Neat, C. E., and Norum, K. R. (1979): Peroxisomal oxidation of long chain fatty acids. *FEBS Lett.,* 99:292−296.

10. Osumi, T., and Hashimoto, T. (1979): Peroxisomal β-oxidation system of rat liver. Copurification of enoyl-CoA hydratase and 3-hydroxyacyl-CoA dehydrogenase. *Biochem. Biophys. Res. Commun.,* 89:580−584.

11. Neat, C. E., Thomassen, M. S., and Osmundsen, H. (1980): Induction of peroxisomal β-oxidation in rat liver by high-fat diets. *Biochem. J.,* 186:369−371.

12. Ishii, H., Fukumori, N., Horie, S., and Suga, T. (1980): Effects of fat content in the diet on hepatic peroxisomes of the rat. *Biochem. Biophys. Acta,* 617:1−11.

13. Murphy, P. A., Krahling, J. B., Gee, R., Kirk, J. R., and Tolbert, N. E. (1979): Enzyme activities of isolated hepatic peroxisomes from genetically lean and obese male mice. *Arch. Biochem. Biophys.,* 193:179−185.

14. Lazarow, P. B. (1977): Three hypolipidemic drugs increase hepatic palmitoyl-coenzyme A oxidation in the rat. *Science,* 197:580−581.

15. Inestrosa, N. C., Bronfman, M., and Leighton, F. (1979): Detection of peroxisomal fatty acyl-coenzyme A oxidase activity. *Biochem. J.,* 182:779−788.

16. Krisans, S., Mortensen, R. M., and Lazarow, P. B. (1980): Acyl-CoA synthetase in rat liver peroxisomes. Computer-assisted analysis of cell fractionation experiments. *J. Biol. Chem.,* 255:9599−9607.

17. Markwell, M. A. K., McGroarty, E. J., Bieber, L. L., and Tolbert, N. E. (1973): The subcellular distribution of carnitine acyltransferases in mammalian liver and kidney. A new peroxisomal enzyme. *J. Biol. Chem.,* 248:3426−3432.

18. Hajra, A. K., Burke, C. L., and Jones, C. L. (1979): Subcellular localization of acyl coenzyme A:dihydroxyacetone phosphate acyltransferase in rat liver peroxisomes (microbodies). *J. Biol. Chem.,* 254:10896−10900.

19. Noguchi, T., Takada, Y., and Fujiwara, S. (1979): Degradation of uric acid to urea and glyoxylate in peroxisomes. *J. Biol. Chem.,* 254:5272−5275.

20. Scott, P. J., Visentin, L. P., and Allen, J. M. (1969): Enzymatic characteristics of peroxisomes of amphibian and avian liver and kidney. *Ann. NY Acad. Sci.,* 168:244−264.

21. Khanna, J. M., and Israel, Y. (1980): Ethanol metabolism. In: *Liver and Biliary Tract Physiology I,* edited by N. B. Javitt, pp. 275−315. University Park Press, Baltimore.

22. Oshino, N., Chance, B., Sies, H., and Bucher, T. (1973): The role of generation in perfused rat liver and the reaction of catalase compound I and hydrogen donors. *Arch. Biochem. Biophys.,* 154:117−131.

23. Thurman, R. G., and McKenna, W. (1974): Activation of ethanol utilization in perfused liver from normal and ethanol-pretreated rats. The effect of hydrogen peroxide generating substrates. *Hoppe Seylers Z. Physiol. Chem.,* 355:336−340.

24. Hsieh, B., and Tolbert, N. E. (1976): Glyoxylate aminotransferase in peroxisomes from rat liver and kidney. *J. Biol. Chem.,* 251:4408−4415.

25. Beevers, H. (1969): Glyoxysomes of castor bean endosperm and their relation to gluconeogenesis. *Ann. NY Acad. Sci.,* 168:313−324.

26. Blum, J. J., and Connett, R. J. (1972): Analysis of metabolism in tetrahymena. In: *Proceedings of the International Symposium on Environmental Physiology,* edited by R. Em. Smith,

J. P. Hannon, J. L. Shields, B. A. Horwitz, pp. 59−66. Federation of American Societies for Experimental Biology.

27. Loud, A. V. (1968): A quantitative stereological description of the ultrastructure of normal rat liver parenchymal cells. *J. Cell Biol.,* 37:27−46.

28. Weibel, E. R., Staubli, W., Gnagi, H. R., and Hess, F. A. (1969): Correlated morphometric and biochemical studies on the liver cell. I. Morphometric model, stereologic methods, and normal morphometric data for rat liver. *J. Cell Biol.,* 42:68−91.

29. Hruban, Z., and Rechcigl, M. (1969): *Microbodies and Related Particles.* Academic Press, New York.

30. Novikoff, A. B., and Shin, W. Y. (1964): The endoplasmic reticulum in the Golgi zone and its relationship to microbodies, Golgi apparatus and autophagic vacuoles in rat liver cells. *J. Microsc.* 3:187−206.

31. Legg, P. G., and Wood, R. L. (1970): New observations on microbodies: A cytochemical study on CPIB-treated rat liver. *J. Cell Biol.,* 45:118−129.

32. Essner, E. (1970): Observations on hepatic and renal peroxisomes (microbodies) in the developing chick. *J. Histochem. Cytochem.,* 18:80−92.

33. Reddy, J., and Svoboda, D. (1971): Microbodies in experimentally altered cells. VIII. Continuities between microbodies and their possible biologic significance. *Lab. Invest.,* 24:74−81.

34. Rigatuso, J. L., Legg, P. G., and Wood, R. L. (1970): Microbody formation in regenerating rat liver. *J. Histochem. Cytochem.,* 18:893−900.

35. Reddy, J. K., and Svoboda, D. (1973): Further evidence to suggest that microbodies do not exist as individual entities. *Am. J. Pathol.,* 70:421−432.

36. Fringes, B., and Reith, A. (1980): The formation of microbodies (Mb) under triiodothyronine (T3) influence in rat liver. A stereological study by electron microscopy. *Eur. J. Cell Biol.,* 22:166.

37. Novikoff, P. M., Novikoff, A. B., Quintana, N., and Davis, C. (1973): Studies on microperoxisomes. III. Observations on human and rat hepatocytes. *J. Histochem. Cytochem.,* 21:540−558.

38. Fahimi, H. D., Gray, B. A., and Herzog, V. K. (1976): Cytochemical localization of catalase and peroxidase in sinusoidal cells of rat liver. *Lab. Invest.,* 34:192−201.

39. Tsukada, H., Mochizuki, Y., and Konishi, T. (1968): Morphogenesis and development of microbodies of hepatocytes of rats during pre- and postnatal growth. *J. Cell Biol.,* 37:231−243.

40. Hruban, Z., Gotoh, M., Slesers, A., and Chou, S. F. (1974): Structure of hepatic microbodies in rats treated with acetylsalicylic acid, clofibrate, and dimethrin. *Lab. Invest.,* 30:64−75.

41. Lazarow, P. B., Shio, H., and Robbi, M. (1981): Biogenesis of peroxisomes and the peroxisome reticulum hypothesis. In: *Biological Chemistry of Organelle Formation,* edited by T. Bucher, W. Sebald, and H. Weiss, pp. 187−206. Springer-Verlag, New York.

42. Hruban, Z., Swift, H., and Slesers, A. (1966): Ultrastructural alterations of hepatic microbodies. *Lab. Invest.,* 15:1884−1901.

43. Staubli, W., Hess, R., and Weibel, E. R. (1969): Correlated morphometric and biochemical studies on the liver cell. II. Effects of phenobarbital on rat hepatocytes. *J. Cell Biol.,* 42:92−112.

44. Rouiller, C., and Bernhard, W. (1956): "Microbodies" and the problem of mitochondrial regeneration in liver cells. *J. Biophys. Biochem. Cytol. [Suppl.],* 2:355−359.

45. Rhodin, J. (1954): Correlation of ultrastructural organization and function in normal and experimentally changed proximal convoluted tubule cells of the mouse kidney. *Doctoral dissertation,* Karolinska Institute.

46. de Duve, C. (1969): Evolution of the peroxisome. *Ann. NY Acad. Sci.,* 168:369−381.

47. Leighton, F., Poole, B., Beaufay, H., Baudhuin, P., Coffey, J. W., Fowler, S., and de Duve, C. (1968): The large scale

separation of peroxisomes, mitochondria and lysosomes from the livers of rats injected with Triton WR-1339. *J. Cell Biol.,* 37:482–512.

48. de Duve, C. (1975): Exploring cells with a centrifuge. *Science,* 189:186–194.

49. Fujiki, Y., Fowler, S., Hubbard, A. L., and Lazarow, P. B. (1981): Comparison of rat liver peroxisome membranes with endoplasmic reticulum and mitochondrial membranes. *Fed. Proc.,* 40:1616.

50. Lazarow, P. B., and de Duve, C. (1973): The synthesis and turnover of rat liver peroxisomes IV. Biochemical pathway of catalase synthesis. *J. Cell Biol.,* 59:491–506.

51. Redman, C. M., Grab, D. J., and Irukulla, R. (1972): The intracellular pathway of newly formed rat liver catalase. *Arch. Biochem. Biophys.,* 152:496–501.

52. Lazarow, P. B., and de Duve, C. (1973): The synthesis and turnover of rat liver peroxisomes. V. Intracellular pathway of catalase synthesis. *J. Cell Biol.,* 59:507–524.

53. Robbi, M., and Lazarow, P. B. (1978): Synthesis of catalase in two cell-free protein-synthesizing systems and in rat liver. *Proc. Natl. Acad. Sci. USA,* 75:4344–4348.

54. Goldman, B. M., and Blobel, G. (1978): Biogenesis of peroxisomes: Intracellular site of synthesis of catalase and uricase. *Proc. Natl. Acad. Sci. USA,* 75:5066–5070.

55. Poole, B., Leighton, F., and de Duve, C. (1969): The synthesis and turnover of rat liver peroxisomes. II. Turnover of peroxisome proteins. *J. Cell Biol.,* 41:536–546.

56. Poole, B. (1971): The kinetics of disappearance of labeled leucine from the free leucine pool of rat liver and its effect on the apparent turnover of catalase and other hepatic proteins. *J. Cell Biol.,* 246:6587–6591.

57. Price, V. E., Sterling, W. R., Tarantola V. A., Hartley, R. W., Jr., and Rechcigl, M., Jr. (1962): The kinetics of catalase synthesis and destruction in vivo. *J. Biol. Chem.,* 237:3468–3475.

58. Ganschow R. E., and Schimke R. T. (1969): Independent genetic control of the catalytic activity and the rate of degradation of catalase in mice. *J. Biol. Chem.,* 244:4649–4658.

59. Poole, B., Higashi, T., and de Duve, C. (1970): The synthesis and turnover of rat liver peroxisomes. III. The size distribution of peroxisomes and the incorporation of new catalase. *J. Cell Biol.,* 45:408–415.

60. Lazarow, P. B. (1980): Elevation of peroxisomal β-oxidation by bezafibrate. In: *Lipoproteins and Coronary Heart Disease: New Aspects in the Diagnosis and Therapy of Disorders of Lipid Metabolism,* edited by H. Greten, P. D. Lang, and G. Schettler, pp. 96–100. Gerhard Witzstrock, New York.

61. Osumi, T., and Hashimoto, T. (1978): Enhancement of fatty acyl-CoA oxidizing activity in rat liver peroxisomes by di-(2-ethylhexyl)phthalate. *J. Biochem.,* 83:1361–1365.

62. Ishii, H., and Suga, T. (1979): Clofibrate-like effects of acetyl-salicylic acid on peroxisomes and on hepatic and serum triglyceride levels. *Biochem. Pharmacol.,* 28:2829–2833.

63. Hess, R., Staubli, W., and Reiss, W. (1965): Nature of the hepatomegalic effect produced by ethyl-chlorophenoxyisobutyrate in the rat. *Nature,* 208:856–858.

64. Reddy, J. K., Azarnoff, D. L., Svoboda, D. J., and Prasad, J. D. (1974): Nafenopin-induced hepatic microbody (peroxisome) proliferation and catalase synthesis in rats and mice: Absence of sex difference in response. *J. Cell Biol.,* 61:344–358.

65. Reddy, J. K., and Krishnakantha, T. P. (1975): Hepatic peroxisome proliferation: Induction by two novel compounds structurally unrelated to clofibrate. *Science,* 190:787–789.

66. Leighton, F., Coloma, L., and Koenig, C. (1975): Structure, composition, physical properties, and turnover of proliferated peroxisomes. A study of the trophic effects of Su-13437 on rat liver. *J. Cell Biol.,* 67:281–309.

67. Solberg, H. E., Aas, M., and Daae, L. N. W. (1972): The activity of the different carnitine acyltransferases in the liver of clofibrate-fed rats. *Biochem. Biophys. Acta,* 280:434–439.

68. Moody, D. E., and Reddy, J. K. (1974): Increase in hepatic carnitine acetyltransferase activity associated with peroxisomal (microbody) proliferation induced by the hypolididemic drugs clofibrate, nafenopin and methyl clofenapate. *Res. Commun. Pathol. Pharmacol.,* 9:501–510.

69. Moody, D. E., and Reddy, J. K. (1978): The hepatic effects of hypolipidemic drugs (clofibrate, nafenopin, tibric acid and Wy-14,643) on hepatic peroxisomes and peroxisomal-associated enzymes. *Am. J. Pathol.,* 90:435–445.

70. Daae, L. N. W., and Aas, M. (1973): Fatty acid activation and acyl transfer in rat liver during clofibrate feeding. *Atherosclerosis,* 17:389–400.

71. Barcelo, P., Muset, P. P., Sola, L. S., Laporte, J., and Valdecasas, F. G. (1960): Premieres etudes pharmacologiques sur l'hepatocatalase et son emploi therapeutique. In: *First European Symposium on Medical Enzymology,* edited by N. Dioguardi, pp. 342–349. Karger, Basel.

72. Caravaca, J., May, M. D., and Dimond, E. G. (1963): Inhibition of squalene and cholesterol biosynthesis by hepatocatalase (caperase). *Biochem. Biophys. Res. Commun.,* 10:189–194.

73. Caravaca, J., Dimond, E. G., Sommers, S. C., and Wenk, R. (1967): Prevention of induced atherosclerosis by peroxidase. *Science,* 155:1284–1287.

74. Feinstein, R. N. (1970): Acatalasemia in the mouse and other species. *Biochem. Genet.,* 4:135–155.

75. Goldfischer, S., and Essner, E. (1970): Peroxidase activity in peroxisomes (microbodies) of acatalasemic mice. *J. Histochem. Cytochem.,* 18:482–489.

76. Feinstein, R. N., Savol, R., and Howard, J. B. (1971): Conversion of catalatic to peroxidatic activity in livers of normal and acatalasemic mice. *Enzymologia,* 41:345–358.

77. Goldfischer, S., Roheim, P. S., Edelstein, D., and Essner, E. (1971): Hypolipidemia in a mutant strain of "acatalasemic" mice. *Science,* 173:65–66.

78. Cuadrado, R. R., and Bricker, L. A. (1973): An abnormality of hepatic lipogenesis in a mutant strain of acatalasemic mice. *Biochem. Biophys. Acta,* 306:168–172.

79. Takahara, S., Hamilton, H. B., Neel, J. V., Kobara, T. Y., Ogura, Y., and Nishimura, E. T. (1960): Hypocatalasemia: A new genetic carrier state. *J. Clin. Invest.,* 39:610–619.

80. Aebi, H., and Suter, H. (1971): Acatalasemia. *Adv. Hum. Genet.,* 2:143–199.

81. Canonico, P. G., White, J. D., and Powanda, M. C. (1975): Peroxisome depletion in rat liver during pneumococcal sepsis. *Lab. Invest.,* 33:147–150.

82. Canonico, P. G., Rill, W., and Ayala, E. (1977): Effects of inflammation on peroxisomal enzyme activities, catalase synthesis and lipid metabolism. *Lab. Invest.,* 37:479–486.

83. Leduc, E. H. (1960): Changes in fine structure of the mouse liver induced by the ectromelia virus. *Anat. Rec.,* 136:230.

84. Schaffner, F. (1966): Intralobular changes in hepatocytes and the electron microscopic mesenchymal response in acute viral hepatitis. *Medicine,* 45:547–552.

85. Greenstein, J. P. (1947): *Biochemistry of Cancer.* Academic Press, New York.

86. Kampschmidt, R. F. (1965): Mechanism of liver catalase depression in tumor-bearing animals: a review. *Cancer Res.,* 25:34–45.

87. Ohnuma, T., Maldia, G., and Holland, J. F. (1966): Hepatic catalase activity in advanced human cancer. *Cancer Res.,* 26:1806–1818.

88. Mochizuki, Y. (1968): An electron microscope study on hepatocyte microbodies of mice bearing Ehrlich ascites tumor. *Tumor Res.,* 3:1–33.

89. Dalton, A. J. (1964): An electron microscopical study of a series of chemically induced hepatomas. In: *Cellular Control Mechanisms and Cancer,* edited by P. Emmelot and O. Muhlbock, pp. 211–225. Elsevier, New York.

90. Hruban, Z., Swift, H., and Rechcigl, M., Jr. (1965): Fine structure of transplantable hepatomas of the rat. *J. Natl. Cancer Inst.,* 35:459–473.

91. Mochizuki, Y., Hruban, Z., Morris, H. P., Slesers, A., and Vigil, E. L. (1971): Microbodies of Morris hepatomas. *Cancer Res.,* 31:763–773.

92. Wattiaux, R., Wattiaux-De Conninck, S., Van Dijck, J. M., and Morris, H. P. (1970): Subcellular particles in tumors—III. Peroxisomal enzymes in hepatoma HO and Morris hepatomas 7794A, 7794B, 5123A and 7316A. *Eur. J. Cancer,* 6:261–268.

93. Rubin, E., and Lieber, C. S. (1967): Early fine structural

changes in the human liver induced by alcohol. *Gastroenterology,* 52:1–13.

94. Porta, E. A., Hartroft, W. S., and de la Iglesia, F. A. (1965): Hepatic changes associated with chronic alcoholism in rats. *Lab. Invest.,* 14:1437–1455.

95. Dobbins, W. O., Rollins, E. L., Brooks, S. G., and Fallon, H. J. (1972): A quantitative morphological analysis of ethanol effect upon rat liver. *Gastroenterology,* 62:1020–1033.

96. Kahonen, M. T., Ylikahri, R. H., and Hassinen, I. (1971): Ethanol metabolism in rats treated with ethyl-α-p-chlorophenoxyisobutyrate (clofibrate). *Life Sci.,* 10:661–670.

97. Carter, E. A., and Isselbacher, K. J. (1973): The effect of ethyl-α-p-chlorophenoxyisobutyrate (clofibrate) on alcohol metabolism. *Life Sci.,* 13:907–917.

98. Brown, D. F. (1966): The effect of ethyl α-p-chlorophenoxyisobutyrate on ethanol-induced hepatic steatosis in the rat. *Metabolism,* 15:868–873.

99. Spritz, N., and Lieber, C. S. (1966): Decrease of ethanol-induced fatty liver by ethyl α-p-chlorophenoxyisobutyrate. *Proc. Soc. Exp. Biol. Med.,* 121:147–149.

100. Goldfisher, S., Moore, C. L., Johnson, A. B., Spiro, A. J., Valsamis, M. P., Wisniewski, H. K., Ritch, R. H., Norton, W. T., Rapin, I., and Gartner, L. M. (1973): Peroxisomal and mitochondrial defects in the cerebro-hepato-renal syndrome. *Science,* 182:62–64.

101. Versmold, H. T., Bremer, H. J., Herzog, V., Siegel, G., Bassewitz, D. B. von, Irle, U., Voss, H. V., Lombeck, I., and Brauser, B. (1977): A metabolic disorder similar to Zellweger syndrome with hepatic acatalasia and absence of peroxisomes, altered content and redox state of cytochromes, and infantile cirrhosis with hemosiderosis. *Eur. J. Pediatr.,* 124:261–275.

102. Sternlieb, I. (1972): Evolution of the hepatic lesion in Wilson's disease (hepatolenticular degeneration). In: *Progress in Liver Diseases, Vol. IV,* edited by H. Popper and F. Schaffner, pp. 511–525. Grune & Stratton, New York.

103. Thaler, M. M., Bruhn, F. W., Applebaum, M. N., and Goodman, J. (1970): Reye's syndrome in twins. *J. Pediatr.,* 77:638–646.

104. Partin, J. C., Schubert, W. K., and Partin, J. S. (1971): Mitochondrial ultrastructure in Reye's syndrome (encephalopathy and fatty degeneration of the viscera). *N. Engl. J. Med.,* 285:1339–1343.

105. Svoboda, D. J., and Reddy, J. K. (1975): Pathology of the liver in Reye's syndrome. *Lab. Invest.,* 32:571–579.

106. Sternlieb, I., and Quintana, N. (1977): The peroxisomes of human hepatocytes. *Lab. Invest.,* 36:140–149.

107. Novikoff, A. B., Novikoff, P. M., Davis, C., and Quintana, N. (1972): Studies on microperoxisomes. II. A cytochemical method for light and electron microscopy. *J. Histochem. Cytochem.,* 20:1006–1023.

The Liver: Biology and Pathobiology, edited by
I. Arias, H. Popper, D. Schachter, and D. A. Shafritz.
Raven Press, New York © 1982.

Chapter 4

Endoplasmic Reticulum

Gustav Dallner and Joseph W. DePierre

GENERAL CONSIDERATIONS

Three-Dimensional Structure

Electron micrographs of the rat hepatocyte show the endoplasmic reticulum (ER) to be present throughout the cytoplasm as an extensive network of tubules, vesicles, and lamellae. The reconstructed three-dimensional structure represented in Fig. 1 gives an idea of the complexity of this network (see ref. 1). The cytoplasmic surface of 60% of the ER is normally dotted with ribosomes; these regions, called the rough endoplasmic reticulum (RER), are generally arranged in parallel arrays of broad flattened bags (cisternae). The smooth endoplasmic reticulum (SER), which is often found in the region of the Golgi apparatus, consists of widely dispersed tubules and vesicles not infrequently associated with glycogen deposits. The membranes of the ER as seen in the electron microscope are 50 to 80 Å thick. The lumen of the RER is 200 to 300 Å wide (mean width, 260 Å), and the lumen of the SER is 300 to 600 Å wide (mean width, 430 Å). The morphological and morphometric characteristics of the ER vary from region to region (peripheral, midzonal, central) of the liver lobe.

A number of morphometric investigations of the rat hepatocyte ER have been performed. On the average, this organelle occupies 15.3% of the total cell volume; the volume of the ER of 756 μm^3 per hepatocyte is 2.5 times that of the nucleus and 65% of the mitochondrial volume. The surface area of the ER (approximately 63,000 μm^2 per hepatocyte) is about 37.5 times the surface area of the plasma membrane and 8.5 times the surface area of the outer mitochondrial membrane. On another scale, the surface area of the ER has been estimated to be between 7.3 and 11 m^2/g liver, with 2.8 mg phospholipid and 4.7 mg protein per m^2. The ER network of an individual hepatocyte has about 12.7 million attached ribosomes.

Molecular Composition

Morphological observations suggest that the ER is a major cell constituent, a suggestion borne out by biochemical studies (for detailed references, see ref. 1). The ER of 1 g (wet weight) liver contains 40 to 50 mg protein and about 15 mg phospholipid. Using values for the recovery of enzymatic markers and chemical constituents in the microsomal fraction as well as estimates of the purity of this fraction, it can be calculated that the ER contains 19% of total protein, 48% of total phospholipid, and 58% of total RNA of the rat

The Cisternal Systems

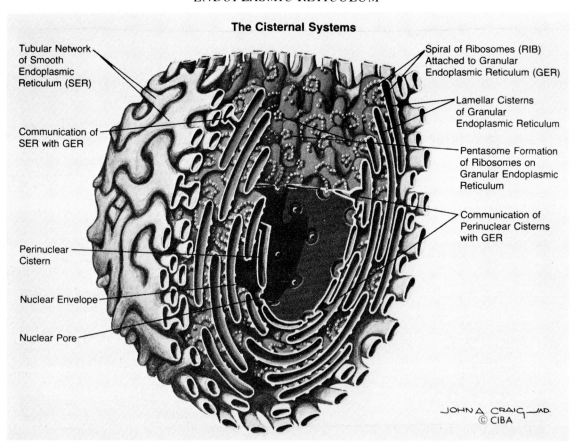

Tubular Network
of Smooth
Endoplasmic
Reticulum (SER)

Communication of
SER with GER

Perinuclear
Cistern

Nuclear Envelope

Nuclear Pore

Spiral of Ribosomes (RIB)
Attached to Granular
Endoplasmic Reticulum (GER)

Lamellar Cisterns
of Granular
Endoplasmic Reticulum

Pentasome Formation
of Ribosomes on
Granular Endoplasmic
Reticulum

Communication of
Perinuclear Cisterns
with GER

JOHN A CRAIG AD.
© CIBA

FIG. 1. Three-dimensional structure of the ER in the hepatocyte. (From Clinical Symposia 25/4. Reproduced by courtesy of CIBA-GEIGY Ltd., Basel, Switzerland. All rights reserved.)

hepatocyte. Uncertainties are involved in such a calculation, but the quantitative importance of the ER as a cellular organelle is apparent.

Compositional studies of isolated rat liver microsomes reveal that the membrane of the ER is about 70% protein and 30% lipid (of which 85% is phospholipid) by weight. One can estimate, using 800 as the molecular weight of a "typical" phospholipid and 50,000 as the molecular weight of an "average" microsomal protein, that there are approximately 23 molecules of phospholipid per protein molecule in the ER membrane. The quantitative relationship of phospholipids to membrane proteins in microsomes is strikingly constant in developing and adult rat liver and is not greatly changed by various treatments.

Microsomal phospholipids consist of about 55% phosphatidylcholine, 20 to 25% phosphatidylethanolamine, 5 to 10% phosphatidylserine, 5 to 10% phosphatidylinositol, and 4 to 7% sphingomyelin. The fatty acid moieties of these phospholipids are chiefly the 16:0, 16:1, 18:0, 18:1, 18:2, 20:4, and 22:6 species; the relative amounts of these species present are dependent on the diets of the animals. Microsomes also contain cholesterol (0.6 mg/g liver), triglycerides (0.5 mg/g liver), small amounts of cholesterol esters and free fatty acids, and vitamin K.

In addition, microsomal membranes contain proteins that are about 2% carbohydrate by weight. These glycoproteins contain the neutral sugars mannose and galactose, the former in two- to fourfold higher amounts than the latter. The main hexosamine in ER glycoproteins is glucosamine; only minute quantities of galactosamine can be detected. It is well established that sialic acid is the terminal sugar of some of the oligosaccharide chains on these glycoproteins. The structure of practically all membrane glycoproteins, including those of the ER, seems to involve N-glycosidic linkage between asparagine and N-acetylglucosamine as the only type of bond between protein and carbohydrate moieties.

Relevance of *In Vitro* Studies to *In Vivo* Structure

Structural and functional studies of the ER are performed with isolated microsomal fractions whose morphology is vastly different from that of the intact organelle *in vivo* (see ref. 1). Unlike other organelles, such as mitochondria and lysosomes, the ER is extensively disrupted even by gentle homogenization of the liver. This breakage does not seem to be purely mechanical but involves an active "pinching off" (Fig. 2).

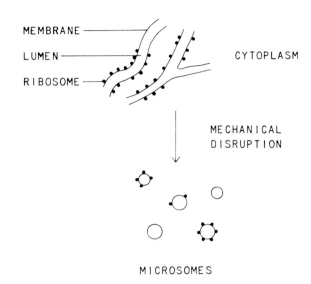

FIG. 2. Schematic representation of the morphology of the ER.

Thus fragments of the ER that can be isolated from a tissue homogenate are in the form of closed vesicles, the so-called microsomes. Several criteria indicate that the outer surface of these vesicles corresponds to the cytoplasmic surface of the ER; consequently, the inside of the vesicle corresponds to the luminal surface of the intact organelle: (a) ribosomes, which are always found on the cytoplasmic surface of the ER, occur on the outer surface of microsomal vesicles; (b) albumin, which is always found in the lumen of the ER, is always found inside microsomal vesicles; (c) histochemical studies demonstrate that the active site of glucose-6-phosphatase is present on the luminal surface of the ER and on the inner surface of microsomal vesicles; (d) ferritin-labeled antibodies have been used to demonstrate that cytochrome b_5 is localized on the cytoplasmic surface of the ER and on the outer surface of microsomal vesicles; (e) freeze-fracture studies also support this relationship between the structures of the intact organelle and microsomal vesicles.

Unfortunately, it has not yet been possible to obtain microsomal vesicles with the opposite orientation, similar to the inside-out vesicles that can be prepared from the erythrocyte membrane or from the mitochondrial inner membranes. Other techniques for getting at the inside surface of microsomal vesicles have been developed (see below).

It should be remembered that fragmentation of the ER during homogenization or some aspect of the procedure used to isolate microsomes may cause subtle changes in the structure of the membrane. Nevertheless, on the basis of our present knowledge, it is reasonable to assume that structural information obtained from studies on isolated microsomes accurately reflects the situation *in vivo*.

STRUCTURAL ASPECTS

Lateral Heterogeneity

At present, the most widely used techniques for investigation of enzyme topology in the lateral plane of membranes are subfractionation (including disruption of the membrane into smaller pieces), normal and freeze-fracture electron microscopy, and reconstitution of membranes from isolated components (for details, see refs. 2 and 3). Other techniques have been developed, e.g., cross-linking of membrane proteins to one another and photolysis-induced cross-linking of the fatty acid moiety of phospholipids to proteins in their immediate vicinity, and should find broader application.

Since breakage of the ER during homogenization occurs transversely, subfractionation of microsomes might reveal heterogeneities in the lateral plane of this organelle. Microsomal vesicles are heterogeneous with respect to size, density, and surface charge; these differences can be used to subfractionate them. There is no known relationship between such properties and the levels of different enzymes present; thus there is no reason to believe that separation of microsomal vesicles on the basis of physicochemical characteristics will reveal lateral enzymatic heterogeneities, even if these exist. In addition, the number of ribosomes and the types of proteins present on microsomal vesicles have also been used as bases for subfractionation.

Histochemical, immunochemical, and other investigations suggest that it will not be possible to find qualitative differences between microsomal vesicles, i.e., to isolate vesicles that contain certain enzymes of the ER but not others. Glucose-6-phosphatase, cytochrome b_5, and NADPH-cytochrome c reductase are present in essentially all vesicles derived from the ER by homogenization.

A variety of enzymes have been found by subfractionation studies to be distributed heterogeneously along the lateral plane of the ER. These enzymes include NADPH-cytochrome c reductase, cytochrome P-450, NADH-cytochrome c reductase, cytochrome b_5, glucose-6-phosphatase, nucleoside diphosphatase, and ATPase. Virtually all the enzymes that have been carefully examined using this approach have shown such a heterogeneous distribution. This is also true for microsomal glycoproteins. An example of microsomal heterogeneity is given in Fig. 3. After rate differential centrifugation, the smaller vesicles in the upper part of the gradient are enriched in electron transport enzymes, while the larger vesicles in the lower part are enriched in ATPase.

Three additional conclusions may be drawn from studies on the subfractionation of rat liver micro-

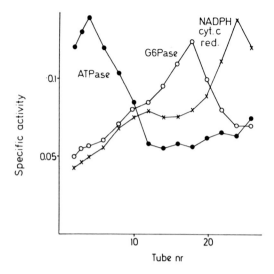

FIG. 3. Distribution of some enzymes of rough microsomal subfractions after rate differential centrifugation on a stabilizing gradient. Tube no. 1 represents the bottom of the gradient.

TABLE 1. *Some widely used approaches to investigate the transverse distribution of membrane proteins*

Accessibility to
Proteases
Lactoperoxidase-catalyzed iodination
Antibodies, lectins, and other macromolecules with specific binding sites
Nonpenetrating substrates and effectors of enzyme activity
Other nonpenetrating reagents
Involvement in vectorial processes, e.g., vectorial release of product, H^+ translocation
Reconstitution of membranes from isolated components

somes. First, in agreement with histochemical and immunological studies, the differences in the enzyme activities of different vesicles are quantitative, not qualitative. Second, the smaller the size of the vesicles, the more clearly heterogeneities can be revealed by subfractionation. Finally, the larger the number of subfractionation steps employed, the more clearly microsomal heterogeneities can be revealed. Thus the best approach is analogous to the one used in protein purification, in which one chromatographic separation is followed by another based on the same or a different principle.

It is possible, although unlikely, that microsomal heterogeneities revealed by subfractionation reflect differences between the ER systems of different hepatocytes or of different parts of the same hepatocyte, rather than a heterogeneous lateral distribution of enzymes in a single, continuous system. If, however, the heterogeneity is within a single continuous membrane system, this would mean that the enzymes involved do not all "float" around freely in the membrane, as proposed for certain membrane proteins in the fluid mosaic model of membrane structure.

Transverse Asymmetry

Some of the most widely used approaches for determining the transverse distribution of membrane proteins are listed in Table 1 (see ref. 2). Rat liver microsomes are freely permeable to uncharged molecules with molecular weights up to at least 600, whereas charged substances with a molecular weight as low as 90, as well as macromolecules, do not cross the vesicle membrane. In addition, treatment of micro-

somes with proteases does not destroy their permeability barrier to macromolecules. Thus only the outer surface of intact microsomal vesicles is susceptible to proteolytic attack. These properties have allowed the approaches given above to be used in investigation of the transverse topology of the membrane proteins of the ER.

Table 2 gives this topology for various enzymes. It can be seen that all enzymes that have been studied are asymmetrically localized. In the erythrocyte membrane, more proteins are localized at the cytoplasmic surface than at the outer surface; this also is true for the ER. In the present case, it is not yet certain that some of the enzymes listed as being on the luminal surface are not simply soluble enzymes trapped inside the vesicles.

Binding of Membrane Proteins

Cytochrome b_5 is an integral membrane protein of the ER (for detailed references, see refs. 2 and 3). It apparently plays a role in fatty acid desaturation. Evidence shows that it can provide an electron required for drug metabolism by the cytochrome P-450 system. Studies on cytochrome b_5 have resulted in a relatively detailed picture of how this integral protein is bound to the microsomal membrane. Most of this work has been carried out in the laboratories of Strittmatter and Sato.

Cytochrome b_5 has been solubilized in an active form from microsomes both with detergents and by hydrolysis with proteases. The cytochrome purified after solubilization with proteases has a molecular weight of about 11,000, is soluble in neutral aqueous buffers, does not bind phospholipid or detergent molecules, and cannot be reincorporated into microsomal or other membranes. The detergent-solubilized cytochrome has a molecular weight of 16,700, is highly aggregated in neutral aqueous buffers, binds phospholipid and detergent molecules, and can be reincorporated into microsomal membranes in a functional state. These and other observations led to the conclu-

TABLE 2. *Transverse distribution of various enzymes of the ER*

Enzyme	Localization	Criteria
Cytochrome b_5	Cytoplasmic surface	Release with protease Inhibition with antibodies Electron microscopy (EM) 　of ferritin-labeled 　antibody Lack of latency
NADH-cytochrome b_5 reductase	Cytoplasmic surface	Release with protease Inhibition with antibodies Lack of latency Nonpenetrating reagents
NADPH-cytochrome c reductase	Cytoplasmic surface	Release with protease Inhibition with antibodies Lack of latency Localization of products EM of ferritin-labeled 　antibody
Cytochrome P-450	Cytoplasmic surface	Denaturation with 　protease ^{125}I-labeling Localization of 　products Nonpenetrating reagents
ATPase	Cytoplasmic surface	Denaturation with 　protease Localization of 　products
5'-Nucleotidase	Cytoplasmic surface	Inhibition with 　antibodies and 　concanavalin A Lack of latency Localization of 　product
Nucleoside pyrophosphatase	Cytoplasmic surface	Release with protease
GDP-mannosyl, UDP-glucos- 　aminyl, UDP-glucosyl- 　transferases	Cytoplasmic surface	Denaturation with 　protease Nonpenetrating reagents
Nucleoside diphosphatase	Luminal surface	Lack of protease 　effect Lack of antibody 　inhibition Latency
Glucose-6-phosphatase	Luminal surface	Protease denaturation 　only in presence of 　deoxycholate Localization of 　products
Acetanilide-hydrolyzing 　esterase	Luminal surface	Lack of effect of 　various proteases No absorption of 　specific antibodies
β-Glucuronidase	Luminal surface	Lack of protease 　effect Release with low 　concentrations of 　deoxycholate Latency

sion that cytochrome b_5 has a catalytically active, hydrophilic head and a noncatalytically active, hydrophobic tail. The extra 44 amino acid residues present in the detergent-solubilized cytochrome, but not in the protease-solubilized cytochrome, are about 60% hydrophobic.

Further details concerning the amino acid sequence of cytochrome b_5 and the relationship between this sequence and its topology in the membrane have been obtained (Fig. 4). Both the amino and carboxyl terminals of the polypeptide extend into the cytoplasm, while a stretch of 17 amino acids near the C-terminal is buried in the membrane; this part is obviously anchoring the molecule to the ER. Proteases cleave this cytochrome beside arg-88 and lys-90 in the primary sequence. Asparagine in the 20 and 105 positions in the sequence of Asn-X-Thr (or Ser) gives two possibilities for attachment of an oligosaccharide chain by an N-glycosidic binding.

There is strong evidence that NADH-cytochrome b_5 reductase binds to the membrane of the ER in the same manner as does cytochrome b_5. Microsomal NADPH-cytochrome c reductase seems also to bind in this manner. Finally, the microsomal enzymes stearyl-CoA desaturase and nucleoside pyrophosphatase and intestinal aminopeptidase may also be amphipathic proteins that are bound to their membranes by a hydrophobic tail.

It is important to ask how general this type of model may be for the binding of integral proteins to membranes. Not all integral membrane proteins fit this model; strictly hydrophobic membrane proteins have already been recognized and isolated. In addition, the activities of a large number of membrane enzymes are dependent on the type of phospholipids immediately surrounding them as well as on the physical state of these phospholipids. Many membrane proteins, such as transport and receptor proteins, have functions that are more basically connected with the membrane than is the function of cytochrome b_5. These considerations suggest that many membrane proteins need more intimate contact with the hydrophobic region of their membranes than do cytochrome b_5 and its reductase.

Investigations with microsomes may also show how certain peripheral proteins are bound to their membranes. Murine microsomal β-glucuronidase consists of two different kinds of polypeptide chains: one is the catalytic subunit, and the other has properties that would be predicted for a protein designed to anchor the active subunit to the membrane of the ER. The suggestion that the anchor protein, called egasyn, serves essentially as a receptor for the active β-glucuronidase is similar to the model for the binding of peripheral proteins to membranes proposed by Singer.

Complexes

At least two electron-transport chains are localized in the membrane of the ER (see refs. 1 and 2). The first system is composed of at least two protein components, cytochrome P-450 and NADPH-cytochrome P-450 reductase. It uses electrons from NADPH in the oxidation of xenobiotics, steroids, and fatty acids. Microsomes contain a single reductase molecule for every 20 to 30 molecules of cytochrome P-450. In addition, there are a number of "accessory enzymes," such as epoxide hydrase and UDP-glucuronyl transferase, which are also localized on the ER and whose functions are closely linked to that of the cytochrome P-450 system.

The second microsomal electron-transport chain is composed of at least three protein components: cytochrome b_5, NADH-cytochrome b_5 reductase, and fatty acyl-CoA desaturase. It uses electrons from NADH in the desaturation of fatty acids. Microsomes contain a single reductase molecule for approximately every 30 molecules of cytochrome b_5. In addition, there is ample evidence that the cytochrome b_5 system and the cytochrome P-450 system interact. The interaction of so many different components, most of which apparently interact directly without mobile, low molecular weight intermediates, might be facilitated by the formation of complexes similar to those found in the inner mitochondrial membrane.

Studies involving subfractionation of microsomes have demonstrated that the cytochrome P-450 and the

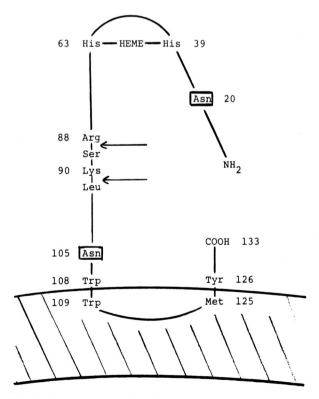

FIG. 4. Molecular relationship of cytochrome b_5 to the ER membrane. (Data from ref. 5.)

cytochrome b_5 systems can be partially separated from one another and from other microsomal enzymes, such as phosphatases. However, the components of a given chain are generally distributed in a similar manner. Such findings are consistent with the organization of the cytochrome P-450 system into one complex and the organization of the cytochrome b_5 system into another, but not with the existence of a single complex containing both chains.

Other evidence concerning the possible organization of microsomal electron-transport chains into complexes comes from reincorporation studies. Both cytochrome b_5 and cytochrome P-450 can be reincorporated into microsomes such that they can be reduced enzymatically and function normally. This would seem to rule out the possibility that all cytochrome and reductase molecules sit together in tight complexes where no components can enter or leave.

Finally, when NADH-cytochrome b_5 reductase and cytochrome b_5 are incorporated into liposomes, NADH-cytochrome c reductase activity (which involves both of these components) shows breaks in its Arrhenius plot at the transition temperatures of the lipids, whereas NADH-ferricyanide reductase activity (which only involves the reductase molecule) does not. This observation suggests that translational diffusion is important in the interaction of these two proteins in a membrane.

Relationship of Proteins to Lipids

Several investigations have been concerned with the relationship of microsomal membrane proteins to the phospholipid molecules of the membrane bilayer (for details, see refs. 1 and 2). It was suggested that cytochrome P-450 is enclosed in a phospholipid halo, which is more rigid than the bulk of microsomal lipids and undergoes crystalline-liquid-crystalline phase change at about 32°C. It was estimated that about 20% of the microsomal phospholipids are located in this halo, which may affect the diffusion of lipid-soluble substrates to and of lipid-soluble products away from the cytochrome P-450 molecule.

Demonstration that detergent-solubilized cytochrome b_5 immobilizes spin-labeled stearic acid and phosphatidylcholine led to the estimate that this protein immobilizes 2 to 4 molecules of phospholipid in its immediate vicinity in the microsomal membrane. Cytochrome b_5 is being used in many model systems to investigate the interaction between proteins and lipids in membranes. For instance, the effect of cytochrome b_5 incorporation on the size, density, permeability, strength, and melting temperature of phosphatidylcholine vesicles is being determined.

The functional properties of many proteins in different biological membranes are intimately related to the microenvironment provided by membrane lipids; the proteins of the membrane of the ER are no exception. The cytochrome P-450 system has been shown by treatment with agents that disrupt protein-lipid interactions, reconstitution experiments, and Arrhenius plots to be functionally dependent on the nature and state of neighboring phospholipid molecules. Similar types of experiments have demonstrated the functional relationship of microsomal glucose-6-phosphatase to phospholipids. Cytochrome b_5 also shows such a relationship. Finally, the exact relationship of microsomal UDP-glucuronyltransferase to membrane phospholipids is still controversial.

FUNCTIONAL AND DYNAMIC ASPECTS

Metabolism of Xenobiotics

One of the most important cellular functions localized on the ER is the metabolism of xenobiotics (see ref. 4). The cytochrome P-450 system (including NADPH-cytochrome P-450 reductase and the many different isozymes of the cytochrome itself), the cytochrome b_5 system, epoxide hydrolase, an activatable glutathione S-transferase, and UDP-glucuronosyl-transferase activities are all localized on this organelle. Many of these detoxifying systems are found in other compartments of the cell as well. In the same way that the liver is the organ for detoxication, the ER is the organelle of the cell for detoxication.

The majority of xenobiotics to which we are exposed are hydrophobic and poorly soluble in water. Since the system of the body for excreting undesirable substances and waste products is based on aqueous solutions (ie., blood, urine, and bile), most xenobiotics cannot be excreted in unchanged form. The major goal of cellular detoxication systems is simply to convert hydrophobic xenobiotics to water-soluble products. Unfortunately, the cytochrome P-450 system, which catalyzes the first step in the metabolism of many xenobiotics, often produces metabolites (e.g., epoxides, radicals, carbonium ions) that are capable of reacting with cellular proteins, RNA, and DNA and thereby giving rise to toxic effects and even cancer. Epoxide hydrolase and glutathione S-transferases metabolize these reactive intermediates further to more inert products.

The properties of many of the enzyme systems involved in detoxication are described in detail elsewhere in this volume. Here we discuss briefly the topology of various xenobiotic metabolizing systems in the ER and possible functional consequences of these structural features.

Why are drug-metabolizing systems localized in a membrane? This is not absolutely necessary, since a number of bacteria have functional, soluble cytochrome P-450 systems. One speculation is that since the xenobiotics, which are substrates for these enzyme systems, are hydrophobic and therefore concentrated in membranes, placing these enzymes in a membrane gives them access to higher concentrations of their substrates. Another possibility is that the effectiveness of detoxication is increased by assembling the systems involved into multienzyme complexes resembling those present in the inner mitochondrial membrane. Indeed, there is some evidence that cytochrome P-450 and its reductase form such a complex to some extent; the same may be true for cytochrome b_5 and its reductase (see above).

The lateral and transverse topology of different xenobiotic-metabolizing enzymes is discussed above. The finding that certain microsomal vesicles are enriched in the cytochrome P-450 system, the cytochrome b_5 system, or epoxide hydrolase suggests that certain regions of the ER may exist which are specialized for detoxication. On the other hand, certain hepatocytes may be specialized for detoxication, and the ER in these cells may be richer in xenobiotic-metabolizing enzymes.

The localization of NADPH-cytochrome P-450 reductase at the cytoplasmic surface of the ER is not difficult to explain. Since its cofactor NADPH is produced in the cytoplasm, positioning this enzyme at the luminal surface would require a special system for transporting NADPH across the bilayer or for producing NADPH in the lumen itself. It is consequently not surprising that at least a portion of the cytochrome P-450 molecule is localized at the cytoplasmic surface as well. This molecule must presumably interact with the portion of its reductase that contains flavoprotein and extends into the cytoplasm. Similar reasoning can be employed in search of an explanation for the localization of NADH-cytochrome b_5 reductase and cytochrome b_5 at the cytoplasmic surface of the ER.

An additional consequence of the localization of xenobiotic-metabolizing systems on the ER should be mentioned. Many of these systems, including the cytochrome P-450 system, the cytochrome b_5 system, epoxide hydrolase, and UDP-glucuronosyltransferase can be induced; i.e., when animals are exposed to large amounts of certain xenobiotics, the activities of these systems in the liver can be increased. In all cases that have been studied in detail, this increase in activity reflects an increased amount of enzyme protein. Induction of xenobiotic-metabolizing systems also occurs in humans. For instance, the activity of benzpyrene monooxygenase (a reaction catalyzed by the cytochrome P-450 system) is 13 times higher in cells from the lungs of smokers than in corresponding cells from nonsmokers.

When the amounts of different xenobiotic-metabolizing systems present on the ER increase in response to inducers, other components of the ER are also affected. After administration of phenobarbital to rats, not only are the microsomal levels of the cytochrome P-450 system and of epoxide hydrolase dramatically increased, but the amount of phospholipid present in the ER per gram liver increases to between 2 and 2.5 times the control level. Most other inducers cause a much less extensive hypertrophy of this organelle; e.g., *trans*-stilbene oxide increases the phospholipid content of the microsomal fraction no more than 28%. Certain inducers, such as 3-methylcholanthrene, cause no hypertrophy. Why this hypertrophy occurs in response to certain inducers is not clear. Perhaps more "room" in the lipid bilayer is required to accommodate the increased levels of xenobiotic-metabolizing enzymes. In any case, the hypertrophy of the ER, especially after administration of phenobarbital, and the return of this organelle to control levels after cessation of treatment, offer interesting systems for the investigation of membrane biogenesis and degradation.

Synthesis and Transport of Proteins

Principally three types of proteins are produced by ribosomes bound to the ER of the liver (see ref. 6): (a) The most intensive synthesis is devoted to secretory proteins, since the majority of the blood proteins originates from the liver. (b) All membrane proteins of the ER, with few exceptions, are produced by bound ribosomes and inserted directly into the membrane. It appears that the newly synthesized membrane proteins are placed at once with the correct topology in the transverse plane and that their mobility is subsequently restricted to the lateral plane. (c) A sizeable portion of the protein of intracellular organelles other than ER originates from the ER. These may be transported in membrane-bound form or as soluble protein in the lumen. After arrival at their final destination, these proteins can either be incorporated into membrane or become a soluble component in the luminal compartment of the organelle.

The biosynthetic pathways and the processing of newly synthesized proteins is a large chapter in cell biology and is discussed in detail elsewhere in this book. With respect to transport, there are two main groups: proteins translocated either in the membrane or in the lumen. Knowledge about protein movement within the membrane is limited. It is not easy to visualize how a large number of proteins on the outer and the inner surface and, in certain cases, even as transmembrane proteins, move along the lateral plane at different speeds. Obviously, a number of specific signals are built into the molecules directing their movement within the membrane.

Schematic pictures of secretion often show nascent proteins appearing free in the lumen after transport through the membrane. This occurs commonly, but not always. Those proteins which are completed, for example, by glycosylation, are tightly attached to the inner side of the membrane at certain phases of the completion process, obviously as a part of the substrate-enzyme-acceptor complex. Thus a portion of the secretory proteins may not be extractable from the luminal compartment. On the other hand, certain microsomal enzymes are loosely attached to the inner surface (e.g., nucleoside diphosphatase, β-glucuronidase), are liberated easily, and appear as soluble proteins even after a mild extraction procedure. It has been established that the secretory process is independent of continuous protein synthesis. Inhibition of the biosynthetic and completion processes does not influence transport in the ER system. The transport process should require energy, but the exact details involved have not yet been elucidated. In the case of the pancreas, the first "ATP-lock" is localized in the terminal portion of the RER.

Glycosylation in the ER

The ER of the liver contains a complete glycosylation system able to synthesize branching oligosaccharide chains (see refs. 7 and 8). Glycosyl transferases are also present in other intracellular membranes, but it is not yet clear whether these enzymes can synthesize a complete chain or if they are devoted to the completion of chains assembled elsewhere. In any case, most glycosylation in the hepatocyte takes place in the endoplasmic membrane system. It appears that all glycoproteins produced in the liver have a single type of protein-sugar interaction, namely, an N-glycosidic binding between asparagine and N-acetylglucosamine.

Two types of glycoproteins are synthesized in the liver ER: membrane constituents and secretory proteins. Secretory proteins may be divided into two groups: (a) blood proteins, which leave the cell, and (b) proteins that remain within the cell but leave the ER, such as viral proteins or plasma membrane constituents. The core of the carbohydrate moieties of secretory proteins is thought to be assembled on a dolichol pyrophosphate molecule; no sequential assembly occurs on the polypeptide itself (Fig. 5). In the first step, GlcNAc-1-P is transferred from UDP-GlcNAc to Dol-P, and the accumulation of additional sugars occurs on this dolichol-pyrophosphate molecule. The next GlcNAc and the following five mannoses are transferred directly from the nucleotide-activated form; for the following four mannoses and three glucoses, the sugar is transferred first to dolichol monophosphate and subsequently to the growing oligosaccharide chain.

Transfer of the core portion to the protein takes place while the nascent chain is still attached to the ribosomes (Fig. 6). This fact is a general finding, but it is possible that glycosylation of some proteins may even occur at a later stage. Glycosylation of the asparagine residue occurs only if the tripeptide Asn-X(any amino acid)-Thr(or Ser) is present, but it is not known why some of these sequences are glycosylated and others are not.

The secretory glycoproteins so far investigated exhibit a processing of the core part in the protein-bound form involving specific glycosidases distributed along the endoplasmic channels and Golgi vesicles. Two glucosidases are involved in the hydrolysis of the three glucoses, after which an α-1,2-mannosidase liberates four mannoses. Removal of two additional mannoses requires a signal, which is the transfer of glucosamine by the UDP-GlcNAc transferase type 1. Addition of terminal GlcNAc, galactose, sialic acid, or fucose takes place in the Golgi system.

Two types of carriers capable of functioning in sugar transfer reactions have so far been identified: (a) dolichol phosphate (Fig. 7), which is able to react with GlcNAc, mannose, and glucose; and (b) retinol phosphate, which accepts only mannose. Dolichol occurs in liver mainly in a nonphosphorylated form and consists of several components (Fig. 7). The number of isoprene residues may vary between 16 and 23, and the α-isoprene is saturated, which stabilizes this lipid to such an extent that it survives heating in alkaline solution. The amount and composition of dolichol depends on the type of liver investigated (Table 3). Human liver contains more than 1 mg dolichol/g wet weight; the amount is much less in the liver of various animals. Comparing dolichols of human liver to rat liver, it is apparent that human dolichols are generally longer polyprenols than those in rat liver. The extreme size of the dolichol molecule raises the question of how this molecule is located in the membrane and how it functions. The size of dolichol in fully extended form exceeds considerably the width of the membrane. It will be a task for the future to find suitable methods to establish the three-dimensional arrangement of this lipid in the membrane.

Regulation of Amount of Lipid Intermediate

Several mechanisms for the regulation of glycoprotein synthesis exist. All sugars can be transferred by several glycosyl transferases, depending on the type of the glycosidic bond established and the nature of the acceptor used. Consequently, it is difficult to speak about glycosyl transferase activity if one is not using a

UDP-GlcNAc

P-Dolichol

GlcNAc-PP-Dolichol
$\downarrow \leftarrow$ UDP-GlcNAc
(GlcNAc)$_2$-PP-Dolichol
$\downarrow \leftarrow$ (GDP-Man)$_5$
Man$_5$-(GlcNAc)$_2$-PP-Dolichol
$\downarrow \leftarrow$ (Man-P-Dolichol)$_4$
Man$_9$-(GlcNAc)$_2$-PP-Dolichol
$\downarrow \leftarrow$ (Glc-P-Dolichol)$_3$
Glc$_3$-Man$_9$-(GlcNAc)$_2$-PP-Dolichol

FIG. 5. Assembly of core oligosaccharide on dolichol-PP.

specific acceptor and if the product is not identified chemically. Under certain conditions, however, such as acute alcohol intoxication, certain glycosyltransferase activities may be greatly increased. Thus both the amount of available protein acceptor and the level of glycosyltransferase activity influence the amount and type of oligosaccharide produced.

An additional important regulation of N-glycosylation in the liver occurs through dolichol biosynthesis and production of the active carrier, dolichol monophosphate. The early steps in dolichol biosynthesis are identical with those of cholesterol. Farnesylpyrophosphate acts as a precursor for both dolichol and ubiquinone, and the enzymic steps for the production of this compound are localized in the mitochondria. Several investigations indicate that the amount

$$CH_3 \qquad\qquad CH_3$$
$$| \qquad\qquad\qquad |$$
$$PO_4\text{-}CH_2\text{-}CH_2\text{-}CH\text{-}CH_2\text{-}(CH_2\text{-}CH=C\text{-}CH_2)_n$$

FIG. 7. Structure of the dolichol phosphates.

of dolichol may regulate protein glycosylation. HMG-CoA-reductase is inhibited in different systems by 25-hydroxycholesterol or compaction. These inhibitors decrease the biosynthesis of dolichol phosphate and the N-glycosylation of proteins in parallel. On the other hand, the amount of dolichol increases in hypercholesterolemia, and N-glycosylation increases simultaneously.

At the end of its biosynthesis, dolichol is present in the pyrophosphate form. The same compound is liberated when the core oligosaccharide is transferred to protein. Dolichol pyrophosphate is dephosphorylated to monophosphate in the liver through the action of a bacitracin-sensitive phosphatase present mainly in lysosomes and plasma membranes. Also, an active fluoride-sensitive monophosphatase produces the free alcohol. The majority of the liver dolichol is present as the free alcohol or the alcohol esterified with a fatty acid. On the outer surface of the microsomes is a CTP-mediated kinase which phosphorylates dolichol and which may be an important regulatory factor in the production of the active lipid intermediate, dolichol

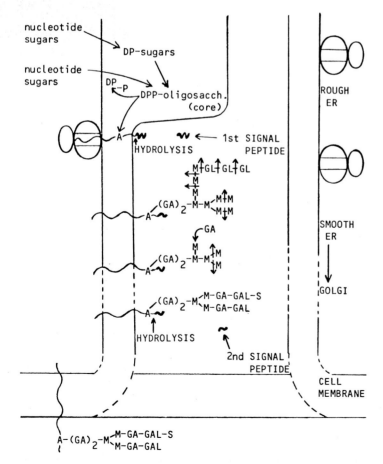

FIG. 6. Processing and completion of the protein-bound oligosaccharide in the ER-Golgi system. DP, dolichol-P; DPP, dolichol-PP; A, asparagine; GA, N-acetylglucosamine; M, mannose; GL, glucose; GAL, galactose; S, siliac acid.

TABLE 3. *Distribution of dolichol in liver from different origins*

Origin	Concentration (μg/g wet weight)	Main components[a]
Chicken	182	
Human	1,226	*20*, 21, 19
Pig	69–129	*19*, 20, 18
Rabbit	10–40	*18*, 19, 17, 20
Rat	23–50	*18*, 19, 17

[a] Value of N in Fig. 7, main component italicized.

monophosphate. Dolichols and dolichol phosphates are present in all intracellular membranes, which indicates an active transport in the soluble cytoplasm. Consequently, a protein carrier for these compounds should exist.

Dolichol is present in various amounts in all organs, but it is questionable whether polyprenol synthesis occurs in all these organs. Therefore, one cannot exclude the possibility that a portion of the dolichol synthesized in the liver is transported in the blood bound to a carrier and taken up by different cells by a mechanism similar to that described for the uptake of dolichol-containing liposomes by isolated hepatocytes.

Membrane Glycoproteins

Oligosaccharide chains covalently bound to protein are present on both the outer and inner surfaces of ER membranes. Various investigations indicate that a number of enzymes in the ER, such as cytochromes P-450 and b_5, β-glucuronidase, AMPase, nucleotide pyrophosphatase, and NADH-ferricyanide reductase, are glycoproteins. It is probable that a number of other enzymes are also glycoproteins, but it is difficult to study this possibility for several reasons. In contrast to secretory proteins, membrane proteins of the ER seem to possess a single, short oligosaccharide chain. In the case of cytochrome P-450, for example, this consists of two mannoses and one glucosamine per protein molecule. Since most of the enzymes occur in small amounts, direct measurement of the amount of sugar present is difficult.

Secretory proteins, which are produced in large amounts, have short half-lives in the liver (15 to 30 min). On the other hand, membrane proteins, which are produced in relatively small amounts, have half-lives of several days. The functional importance of oligosaccharides on ER membrane proteins is unknown. Blood proteins require for normal function (e.g., ability to function as coagulation factor) the presence of a complete oligosaccharide chain; however, it is not required for transport of the protein itself in the ER and for its release from the Golgi system to the blood. Similarly, the antigenicity and receptor ca-

pacity of many plasma membrane proteins require an intact sugar chain.

In the case of lysosomal enzymes, the terminal mannose of the core oligosaccharide is phosphorylated in the rough microsomes by a transfer of glucosamine-1-P. The subsequent removal of glucosamine leaves mannose-6-P as a signal for transport to the lysosomes. This terminal phosphate is hydrolyzed upon arrival of the enzyme at its final destination; completion of the oligosaccharide chain can then take place.

Short oligosaccharide chains are probably necessary to fix enzymes at certain positions in the membrane and direct them into close proximity to neighboring enzymes for interaction, e.g., in consecutive electron transport. If cytochrome b_5 is glycosylated on the asparagine in position 105 (Fig. 4), which seems likely, the above hypothesis would gain some support.

Intramembranous Distribution of Glycosyl Transferases

Activated sugars are synthesized in the cytoplasm. Therefore, some enzymes of the transferase complex should be present on the cytoplasmic surface of the ER. Dolichol-mediated protein glycosylation is the dominating pathway in rough microsomes but is less prominent in smooth microsomes. Experiments with surface probes indicate that many of the glycosyltransferase activities are present on the outer surface of rough microsomal membranes and that, at least in these membranes, several glycosylating systems involving or lacking dolichol phosphate are present in different compartments. The dolichol pathway, described in Fig. 5, is probably not involved in glycosylation of several membrane proteins, which necessitates the existence of other glycosylating systems in the ER. Cytochrome P-450 does not contain the characteristic diacetylchitobiose residue; this does not exclude the possibility that synthesis occurs along the lines described for secretory proteins but suggests the possibility of another pathway. Such a pathway might involve glucosamine transfer without dolichol involvement, as described for ribonuclease A or O-glycosylation through dolichol phosphate-mannose, known to occur in yeast.

Phospholipid Synthesis and Movement

Phospholipids produced in the ER have several different functions. (a) Phospholipids and cholesterol form the basic bilayer construction of all membranes; (b) lipids are produced for secretion and are components of various lipoproteins; and (c) most phospholipids are produced exclusively in the ER and there is extensive and continuous transport to other intracellular membranes.

Because most steps involved in phospholipid synthesis appear to be localized on the cytoplasmic surface of the ER, and because of the various functions of phospholipids, a considerable movement of these molecules in ER membranes must occur. Physical studies suggest isotropic motion in microsomal membranes. Also, at least a part of phospholipids is in a nonbilayer form, such as inverted micelles; the exchange between these different forms is rapid. Experiments with exchange proteins suggest a completely free exchange of the total phosphatidylcholine pool between liposomes and microsomes; i.e., flip-flop motion involving all the lipids seems to occur within minutes.

Despite these findings, one wonders whether such an unlimited free movement of phospholipid molecules in the ER is compatible with normal function. Biosynthesis on one side of the membrane may involve an active transfer to the opposite side, which does not necessarily imply free transmembrane movement. Such a transfer is well investigated in the case of proteins, which undergo an active, vectorial transfer not involving flip-flop. Enzymes may require a specific type of lipid for catalysis and may immobilize a fraction of these lipids.

Considerable transverse asymmetry in the distribution of microsomal phospholipids has been questioned but not disproved. In the presence of exchange proteins, microsomal phosphatidylcholine exchanges with liposomes within a few minutes, a finding that does not necessarily reflect the *in vivo* situation. In fact, pulse labeling with glycerol-^{3}H suggests that the transfer of phosphatidylcholine and phosphatidylethanolamine from rough microsomes to inner mitochondrial membranes requires several hours; it is a relatively slow process.

Nearest neighbor analysis of phosphatidylethanolamine with difluorodinitrobenzene indicates compartmentalization of this lipid in microsomes rather than random distribution (Table 4). The biological validity of these findings is strengthened by comparison to corresponding data for inner mitochondrial membranes and erythrocytes, where there is also a compartmentalization, but with quite a different pattern. Pulse labeling with radioactive glycerol-^{3}H also

indicates that the exchange between the monomer and the protein-bound form is a time-requiring process. Obviously, the results obtained for lipid arrangement and movement within the ER depend on the methods used and may not mirror events taking place in the living cell.

Turnover of Proteins and Phospholipids in the ER Membranes

The membranes of the ER represent the most dynamic portion of the intracellular membrane system (see ref. 10). The average half-life of ER proteins in rat liver is 60 to 70 hr, considerably shorter than the mean half-life of proteins in other organelles. Investigation of individual proteins demonstrates that their turnovers differ and range between a few hours and several days (Table 5). It is clear that individual enzymes are synthesized and degraded independently, indicating that membrane formation and degradation are complex processes that involve many synthetic and degradation reactions that occur simultaneously at different rates. Newly synthesized membrane proteins must be placed into an already existing membrane as single components and must also be removed by single reactions. Even enzymes that interact functionally and lie close to one another in the membrane, such as the electron transport enzymes, exhibit different turnovers. Characteristically, even different parts of the same enzyme—such as the apoprotein and the heme-prosthetic group of cytochromes b_5 and P-450—exhibit different turnover rates. Since membrane composition is stable and displays relatively limited changes even under pathological conditions, the insertion and removal of individual proteins must be strictly coordinated.

The different turnovers of membrane proteins may involve specific proteases; if so, a number of proteolytic reactions occur simultaneously. Therefore, under normal conditions, degradation is a heterogenous event, as is the biosynthetic process; the ER membrane cannot be engulfed as a whole for degradation in autophagosomes. Endogenous proteases demonstrate specificity with respect to the charge, hydrophobicity, and size of the protein substrate, which also indicates that the initial steps in degradation are probably not

TABLE 4. *Cross-linking of phosphatidylethanolamine with 1,5-difluoro-2,4-dinitrobenzene*

PE	Microsomes	Inner mitochondrial membranes (% total)	Erythrocytes
FDNP-PE	26	39	22
PE-DNP-PE	9	32	49
PE-DNP-PS	2	1	25
PE-DNP-protein	63	28	4

TABLE 5. *Turnover rates of microsomal enzymes in rat liver*

Enzymes	Half-lives (hr)
Stearyl CoA desaturase	4
HMG-CoA reductase	4
Nucleoside diphosphatase	30
Cytochrome P-450 (protein)	40
Cytochrome P-450 (heme)	22
NADPH-cytochrome P-450 reductase	70
Arylacylamidase	100
Cytochrome b_5 (protein)	100
Cytochrome b_5 (heme)	45
NADH-cytochrome b_5 reductase	140
Total microsomal membrane protein	70

lysosomal. The partially degraded protein molecule may enter the lysosomes, where complete hydrolysis to amino acids takes place. Turnover rates may be affected by several factors, which may be the mechanism for selected changes in enzyme composition. Several drugs increase the amounts of certain enzymes, not only by increasing their synthetic rates but also to a greater or lesser degree by decreasing their turnover rate.

The turnover rates of phospholipids are even more rapid than are those of enzymes. Phospholipid turnover may involve several phases, where the initial rapid phase is followed by a somewhat slower phase. During the first rapid phase, the half-life of microsomal phosphatidylcholine is 14 hr, phosphatidylethanolamine 16 hr, phosphatidylserine 23 hr, and sphingomyelin 38 hr. Drugs influence the synthesis and degradation of phospholipids, just as they do in the case of proteins.

Despite the highly individual rates of turnover of practically all proteins and lipids in the ER, the basic composition, that is, the ratio between phospholipids and proteins, never changes significantly. Obviously, the dynamic nature is restricted to individual molecules and does not affect the overall structural make-up of the membrane. This indicates that normal functions of the ER, which are necessary for maintenance of the cell, require a basic membrane structure that cannot be abolished or even changed significantly.

Involvement in Carbohydrate Metabolism: Glucose-6-Phosphatase

Glucose-6-phosphatase hydrolyzes glucose-6-phosphate to release free glucose and inorganic phosphate (see ref. 1). The substrate is provided by the breakdown of glycogen and by the process of gluconeogenesis. The freed glucose subsequently can be transported from the cytoplasm of the hepatocyte into the blood. This process is central in maintaining the concentration of glucose in the blood within normal physiological limits.

Glucose-6-phosphatase is localized on the ER in hepatocytes. Evidence indicates that the active site of this enzyme is located at the luminal surface of the ER. Since glucose-6-phosphate is produced in the cytoplasm, there may be a transport protein in the membrane of the ER which carries glucose-6-phosphate across this membrane. Strong indications for the existence of such a transport protein have been reported. Glucose-6-phosphatase seems to be a relatively nonspecific enzyme, hydrolyzing a large number of different hexose phosphates. The specificity in the system is provided by the transport protein, which is highly selective for glucose-6-phosphate.

The functional consequences of this arrangement of the glucose-6-phosphatase system in the membrane of the ER are still a mystery. Arion, who has done much of the important work in this area, suggests that this topology may provide the cell with subtle mechanisms for regulating the conversion of glucose-6-phosphate to glucose. Considering the importance of this conversion, this hypothesis is attractive; however, it remains to be tested.

REFERENCES

1. DePierre, J. W., and Dallner, G. (1975): Structural aspects of the membrane of the endoplasmic reticulum. *Biochim. Biophys. Acta*, 415:411–472.
2. DePierre, J. W., and Ernster, L. (1977): Enzyme topology of intracellular membranes. *Annu. Rev. Biochem.*, 46:201–262.
3. DePierre, J. W., and Dallner, G. (1976): Isolation, subfractionation and characterization of the endoplasmic reticulum. In: *Biochemical Analysis of Membranes*, edited by A. H. Maddy, pp. 79–131. Chapman and Hall, London.
4. DePierre, J. W., Seidegard, J., Morgenstern, R., Balk, L., Meijer, J., and Astrom, A. (1981): In: *Mitochondria and Microsomes*, edited by C. P. Lee, G. Schatz, and G. Dallner, Addison-Wesley, Boston pp. 585–610.
5. Tajima, S., Enomoto, K., and Sato, R. (1978): Nature of tryptic attack on cytochrome b_5 and further evidence for the two-domain structure of the cytochrome molecule. *J. Biochem.*, 84:1573–1586.
6. Palade, G. E. (1975): Intracellular aspects of the process of protein synthesis. *Science*, 189:347–358.
7. Kornfeld, R., and Kornfeld, S. (1980): Structure of glycoproteins and their oligosaccharide units. In: *The Biochemistry of Glycoproteins and Proteoglycans*, edited by W. J. Lennarz, pp. 1–34. Plenum, New York.
8. Dallner, G., and Hemming, F. W. (1981). In: *Mitochondria and Microsomes*, edited by C. P. Lee, G. Schatz, and G. Dallner, pp. 655–681. Addison-Wesley, Boston.
9. van Deenen, L. L. M. (1981): Topology and dynamics of phospholipids in membranes. *FEBS Lett.*, 123:3–15.
10. Omura, T. (1980): Cytochrome P-450 linked mixed function oxidase. Turnover of microsomal components and effects of inducers on the turnover. Phospholipids, proteins and specific enzymes. *Pharmacol. Ther.*, 8: 489–499.

The Liver: Biology and Pathobiology, edited by
I. Arias, H. Popper, D. Schachter, and D. A. Shafritz.
Raven Press, New York © 1982.

Chapter 5

Cytoskeletal Filaments

Helmut Denk and Werner W. Franke

The cytoplasm contains two major components, which are distinguished by their solubility properties: (a) solid and/or gelled structures, and (b) cytosol. The cytosol constitutes the internal milieu of the cell and is the site of many fundamental cell functions. It contains soluble proteins, RNA, and enzymes, which constitute about 25% of total cell protein. The existence of intracellular "skeletal" structures was postulated as early as 1928 but was later regarded as fixation artifact. Biochemical techniques and localization at the light and electron microscopic level, however, have clearly established the existence and significance of an elaborate system of cytoskeletal structures in most, if not all, eukaryotic cells. Prominent components of this system are several classes of distinct filaments, notably microfilaments, intermediate-sized filaments, and microtubules. These filaments form with membranous structures a mutually interacting complex system which, among other functions yet to be elucidated, plays a major role in the regulation of shape and mobility, intracellular movements, including contractile and secretory processes, mitosis, and cell cleavage. The organization of these filaments and their association with nonfilamentous components depends on cell differentiation and environmental factors. Various pathologic conditions affect these cytoskeletal structures (for further information, see refs. 1–6).

THE MICROFILAMENT (ACTOMYOSIN) SYSTEM

Properties and Functions

Nonmuscle cells contain an actomyosin system, which is often associated with actin-containing microfilaments. Microfilaments measure 4 to 7 nm in diameter and are composed of globular (G) actin molecules, which form filamentous (F) actin. Each filament consists of two strands of F-actin coiled around each other. F-actin microfilaments are often densely fasciated into bundles of variable thickness. An assembly-disassembly equilibrium exists between F- and G-actin subunits which are free or bound to certain proteins (actin-binding proteins). Under physiologic conditions, specific mechanisms involving actin-associated proteins maintain actin in an unpolymerized, nonfilamentous state at concentrations that exceed the critical concentration for aggregation. Intracellular calcium is also involved in maintenance of F-actin filaments (for further details, see refs. 1,3, and 7–8).

The equilibrium of assembly and disassembly can be disturbed by many chemicals and drugs. For example, the fungal metabolite cytochalasin B binds, at substoichiometric concentrations relative to actin, to high affinity binding sites on the ends of F-actin filaments,

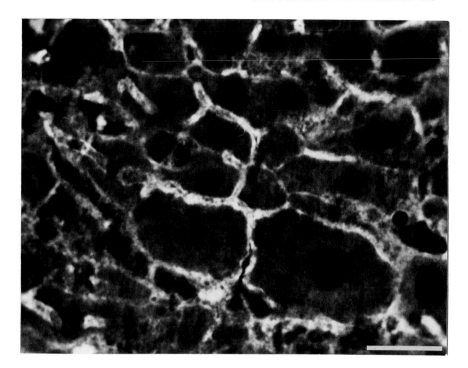

FIG. 1. Actin-specific staining of hepatocytes and bile canaliculi (mouse liver) revealed by indirect immunofluorescence using antibodies to actin. Bar, 20 μm).

inhibits filament elongation, and disrupts the regular arrangements of microfilaments (10–12). Phalloidin, one of the toxic principles of the mushroom *Amanita phalloides*, stabilizes F-actin and promotes or induces polymerization of G-actin, resulting in accumulation of microfilaments (13,14). In contrast to muscle cells, only low concentrations of myosin are present in nonmuscle cells. As in muscle cells, myosin molecules in nonmuscle cells also contain a Ca^{2+}-activated ATPase, which is located in the globular heads of the molecule. The less ordered distribution of the actomyosin filament system in nonmuscle cells, in comparison with muscle cells, and the lower concentration of myosin may account for less efficient contractile activity in this system (1,4).

Presence and Distribution in Hepatocytes

Actin comprises about 1 to 2% of the protein of mammalian liver (4,16–18). Hepatocyte actin is normal β- and γ-nonmuscle actin (K. Weber and J. Vandenkerckhove, *personal communication*). Hepatocyte-associated myosin is similar in amino acid composition to skeletal and cardiac muscle myosin. The actin-myosin ratio in hepatocytes is considerably greater than in skeletal muscle (4,16). Actin-containing microfilaments form a three-dimensional meshwork, which extends throughout the cytoplasm and is concentrated in the subcortical cytoplasm of hepatocytes, particularly around bile canaliculi as a pericanalicular web (4,19–22). (Fig. 1; see also Fig. 10). They may be associated with cell organelles, except mitochondria (4), and have been found in isolated hepatocyte nuclei.

The significance of intranuclear actin is controver-

sial (23). In contrast, nuclei usually are not stained by actin antibodies in immunofluorescence microscopy of liver sections or cultured hepatocytes (19). Actin is also associated with isolated plasma membrane preparations, but the mode of its anchorage to the plasma membrane is unclear (21). The actin content of hepatocyte microfilaments has been demonstrated by their affinity to heavy meromyosin, which results in formation of typical arrowhead-like complexes (20), and by immunomorphologic localization at the light and electron microscopic levels. Immunofluorescence microscopy reveals actin- and myosin-specific immunostaining at the periphery of hepatocytes and encircling bile canaliculi (polygonal staining pattern), which results from the high density of microfilaments in this location (22) (Fig. 1). Actin and myosin antibodies usually do not show conspicuous fibril staining within the cytoplasm of hepatocytes *in situ*, possibly because of the paucity of microfilaments traversing this cytoplasmic region (19,22). As shown by electron microscopy, actin microfilaments are present in parallel arrays in the cores of intracanalicular microvilli, similar to what has been described in greater detail in the microvilli of the intestinal brush border (10,19–21). In isolated and cultured hepatocytes, relatively thick and extended cables of microfilaments are visualized by indirect immunofluorescence microscopy, either as pole-oriented "stress" fibers or as concentric arrays, depending on the cellular growth state, and are similar to the cables found in other cell types in culture (19).

Currently available data are compatible with a function of the microfilament system in motile phenomena of the hepatocyte. The concentration of this filament system around bile canaliculi suggests a specific relationship to bile secretion. The filaments may provide tone to the canalicular system by maintaining canaliculi in a contracted state. They may also regulate bile flow through cycles of contractions and relaxations (active contractions of bile canaliculi have recently been demonstrated by time-lapse kinephotomicrography) and microvillar core contractions (4,14,17,20,24–27). Actin filaments are also probably involved in shaping the sinusoidal cell cortex of the hepatocyte, as suggested by formation of zeiotic blebs in these regions after application of phalloidin or cytochalasin B (14,25,27). Details of biologic functions of the hepatocyte which involve actin remain to be elucidated.

Pathology of the Hepatic Microfilament System

Phalloidin-induced hyperplasia of actin filaments in rat hepatocytes is a striking example of toxic damage to the microfilament system. Bile canaliculi become progressively dilated, with partial swelling and bleb-like transformation of microvilli (14). Under the influence of cytochalasin B *in vivo* and *in vitro,* microfilaments appear to be detached from the canalicular membrane and are transformed to heap-like aggregates of nonordered filaments together with amorphous and granular material. The canaliculi are dilated, and microvilli are reduced in number (25). In addition to these morphologic effects, cytochalasin B inhibits several enzyme activities and may also have other effects on membranes (17).

In the liver of griseofulvin-poisoned mice, the microfilament system, particularly around bile canaliculi, becomes progressively deranged. This alteration is accompanied by canalicular alterations (e.g., dilatation and microvillar abnormalities) (19). Intoxications of this type are associated with decreased (bile salt-dependent and -independent) bile flow, suggesting that an intact microfilament system is involved in bile secretion (14,17,24,25,27,28). Moreover, the canalicular and pericanalicular changes are ultrastructural features which also occur in various cholestatic conditions in animals and man (25,29–31). In the course of liver regeneration after partial hepatectomy and in experimental and human cirrhosis, microfilaments are rearranged and increase in amount, as shown by immunofluorescence and electron microscopy (32–34). As a consequence of parenchymal damage, fibroblasts (myofibroblasts), which contain abundant microfilaments, appear and may be related to an increased contractility of the cirrhotic organ (35).

INTERMEDIATE-SIZED FILAMENT SYSTEM

Properties and Functions

Intermediate-sized filaments are a family of morphologically similar, unbranched, tubular structures with diameters of 6 to 11 nm. They are characterized by insolubility in nondenaturing buffers over a broad range of high and low ionic strengths and in nondenaturing detergents at neutral and alkaline pH. Their structural rigidity suggests that they serve cytoskeletal functions, such as maintenance of cell shape and stability, integration and compartmental organization of the cytoplasmic space, support of the contractile filament systems and microtubules, and guidance to organelle movements (36).

Despite common morphologic features, intermediate-sized filaments are heterogeneous with respect to subunit composition and antigenicity. Filaments of the cytokeratin type are present in epidermal cells (prekeratin filaments). Structures which are closely related by immunologic criteria are also found in most, if not all, nonkeratinizing epithelial cells of diverse vertebrate organs either attached to desmosomes (tonofilaments) or free; their constituent proteins, therefore, have been termed cytokeratins (37). They are easily identified by immunologic cross-reactivity with authentic epidermal prekeratin polypeptides isolated from different species. They are insoluble in neutral buffers but are dissolved at acidic or alkaline pH and by denaturing solvents (e.g., 8 M urea). Filaments readily reform after dissolution of their subunits after removal of the denaturing solvent by dialysis. Electrophoretic separation of the purified material on polyacrylamide gels performed under denaturing and reducing conditions reveals a complex but characteristic composition with a set of polypeptides, usually two or more, ranging in molecular weight from 40,000 to 68,000 (see also Fig. 2).

At present, it cannot be excluded that individual intracellular filaments are slightly heterogeneous in regard to their cytokeratin polypeptide composition (36). Moreover, cytokeratin filaments in different types of epithelial cells show considerable differences in polypeptide composition. It is not clear whether these compositional differences represent precursor-product relationships or reflect different lines of cell differentiation (9,36–39). At least in the skin, no relationship exists between the polypeptides of various sizes; different keratin polypeptides are translated from different mRNA molecules (40). Intermediate-sized filaments from cells in culture differ in their polypeptide composition from those of cells grown in the body, indicating that regulatory processes of an undetermined nature influence the pattern of keratin expression (41).

In a variety of mesenchymal cells grown in the body and in culture, but also in cultured cells of epithelial origin, including hepatocytes, bundles of intermediate-sized filaments occur in conspicuous arrays in the perinuclear cytoplasm. In contrast to the cytokeratin filaments described above, the chemical composition of these filaments is simple; they contain only one major subunit protein with a molecular weight of 57,000, termed vimentin. In cultured cells, phosphorylated

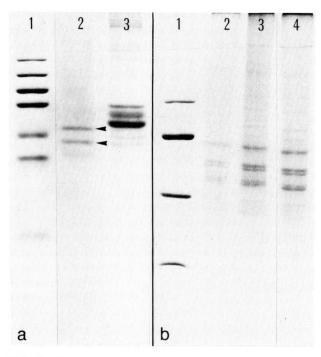

FIG. 2. Electrophoretic separation on SDS-polyacrylamide gels (10% polyacrylamide) of cytokeratin material from mouse liver (**a,** slot 2) and epidermis (**a,** slot 3) and Mallory body material isolated from liver of griseofulvin-fed mice (**b,** slots 2 to 4). Standard proteins are coelectrophoresed in slot **a**(1) (*from top to bottom:* β-galactosidase, phosphorylase a, transferrin, bovine serum albumin, glutamate dehydrogenase, actin) and in slot **b**(1) (*from top to bottom:* phosphorylase a, bovine serum albumin, actin, chymotrypsinogen). Bands indicated by arrowheads in slot **a**(2) are the major cytokeratin components of mouse liver (upper band, with relative molecular weight of 55,000, is termed A; lower band, with relative molecular weight of 48,000, is termed D).

and unphosphorylated forms of vimentin occur. In a variety of cells, vimentin filaments coexist with other types of intermediate-sized filaments. For example, vimentin and cytokeratin filaments occur in diverse epithelial cells in culture, and vimentin and desmin filaments occur in myogenic and muscle cells in culture and in several types of muscles grown in the body (19,36,42,43).

Desmin filaments are composed of a subunit protein of ~53,000 molecular weight (desmin). They are abundant in various forms of smooth muscle tissue and in myoblasts of skeletal and cardiac muscle. Phosphorylated variants have also been described. In mature cardiac and skeletal muscle, desmin has been visualized by immunofluorescence microscopy within Z-lines and at cell-to-cell junctions, notably intercalated disks. In this location, it is likely that the protein is organized in a mode different from that present in intermediate-sized filaments, which traverse the cytoplasm (43; see ref. 36 for review and further references).

Neurofilaments are major filamentous components of neurons, in addition to microtubules. Their chemical composition varies in different animal species. In rodents, they consist of three major polypeptides with molecular weights of 210,000, 160,000, and 68,000. In some lower animals, neurofilaments consist of only two major polypeptides. The high molecular weight polypeptide is susceptible to proteolytic degradation, resulting in formation of smaller polypeptides. The significance of the two smaller polypeptides present as native molecules in rodent neurofilaments has been established by *in vitro* translation assays using mRNA preparations from brain (see ref. 36 for further information and references).

Glial filaments contain the "glial fibrillary acidic protein" (GFA protein), which has a molecular weight of 50,000 to 55,000 as major, if not exclusive, subunit protein. They occur in the cytoplasm of astrocytes growing in the body or in culture. In both situations, they can coexist with vimentin filaments (36).

Intermediate-Sized Filaments in Normal Liver

Distribution in Different Cell Types

Hepatocytes of several animal species, including man, contain tufts of intermediate-sized filaments of the cytokeratin type, which are often closely associated with desmosomes (19; see also Fig. 10). Demonstration of these filaments is sometimes facilitated if glutaraldehyde-fixed tissue is extracted with detergents, such as deoxycholate or Triton X-100 (44). Such bundles of cytokeratin filaments are particularly prominent in the pericanalicular region, where they are often interwoven with microfilaments, and close to the nucleus. Occasionally, bundles of intermediate-sized filaments span the distance between canaliculus and sinusoidal liver cell surface, suggesting that they form an elaborate cytoplasmic meshwork, as in other cell types (see also 45–47).

In bile duct epithelial cells, desmosomes with attached intermediate-sized filaments of the cytokeratin type are more frequent and prominent than in hepatocytes (29; see ref 19 for further information). Desmosomes and tonofilaments are absent from mesenchymal cells in the liver, including endothelial and Kupffer cells (19). In contrast, these cells contain loosely arranged intermediate-sized filaments of the vimentin type, which are especially frequent in Kupffer cells (19; and Fig. 3). Desmin filaments are not present in hepatocytes or bile duct epithelial cells. In liver, desmin filaments are restricted to certain smooth muscle cells of larger blood vessels (Fig. 4). Neurofilaments occur in liver tissue and are specific for adrenergic nerve axons, which are present in some mammalian species (Fig. 5) (for references on liver innervation, see ref. 48).

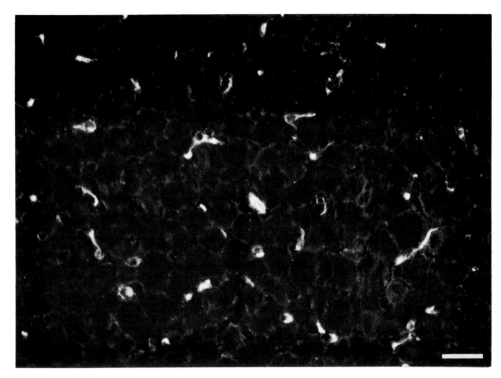

FIG. 3. Kupffer cells in rat liver are specifically decorated by indirect immunofluorescence by antibodies to vimentin. Hepatocytes remain unstained. Bar, 30 μm.

Chemical Composition of Cytoskeletal Filaments of Hepatocytes

As in other epithelial cells, intermediate-sized filaments associated with hepatocytes are highly resistant to extraction in various buffers, a feature which facilitates isolation and purification (see refs. 45,49, and 50 for further details). Upon dissolution of cytoskeletal proteins under denaturing conditions, intermediate-sized filaments spontaneously reform following removal of the denaturing solvent. The cytoskeletal material of mouse, rat, and human hepatocytes, which is resistant to extraction in high salt buffers and Triton X-100, is characterized by several polypeptide bands with molecular weights of 40,000 to 55,000 (45,49; H. Denk, R. Krepler, and W. W. Franke, *unpublished observations*). As shown in Fig. 2 for mouse liver cytoskeleton proteins, two major polypeptides, one (polypeptide A) with an apparent molecular weight of ~55,000 and the other (polypeptide D) with an apparent molecular weight of ~48,000, are prominent. If liver cytoskeleton polypeptides are separated accord-

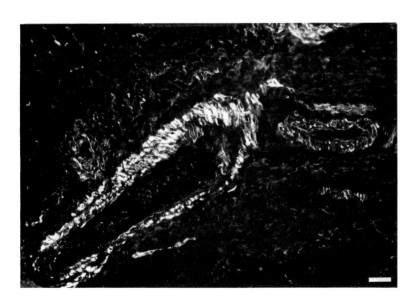

FIG. 4. Specific decoration by indirect immunofluorescence microscopy of smooth muscle cells of the arterial wall in bovine liver with antibodies to desmin. Bar, 30 μm.

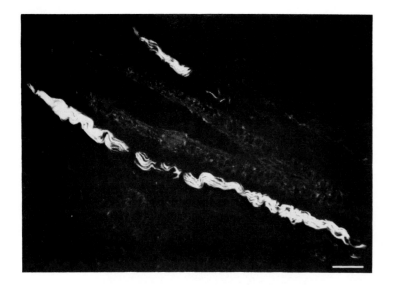

FIG. 5. Specific decoration by indirect immunofluorescence microscopy of nerve axons in bovine liver with antibodies to neurofilament protein. Bar, 30 μm. (Courtesy of Dr. J. Kartenbeck, Heidelberg.)

ing to their isoelectric points and then according to their molecular weights, the individual polypeptides focus between pH 5.2 and 6.5, and the major components appear as a typical series of isoelectric variants differing in isoelectric points by 0.05 to 0.08 pH, probably reflecting different degrees of phosphorylation (49) (Fig. 6). The less acidic, unphosphorylated component is usually the predominant isoelectric variant in each polypeptide species. Similar "pairs of isoelectric variants" have been described for various other protein constituents of intermediate-sized filaments and, in the case of vimentin and desmin, represent different degrees of phosphorylation (see ref. 49 for references and ref. 36 for review).

Immunologic Relationship

Broad immunologic cross-species and cross-organ reactivity is characteristic of the cytokeratin protein family (36,51). However, several antisera to epidermal prekeratin do not react in immunofluorescence and immunoperoxidase microscopy with the cytoskeleton meshwork in epithelial cells of certain parenchymal organs, including hepatocytes and acinar cells of pancreas. Tonofilaments are revealed in these cells by electron microscopy (19,39,46,47). This suggests that cytokeratin filaments are either immunologically heterogeneous or differ in the accessibility of their antigenic determinants.

The possibility of inaccessible antigenic determinants *in situ* is suggested by immunolocalization studies using antibodies to the isolated cytoskeleton polypeptides A and D from mouse liver. Both antibody preparations precipitate cytoskeleton proteins A and D in double immunodiffusion tests. By immunofluorescence microscopy on frozen tissue sections, however, only antibodies to component D reveal an elaborate,

three-dimensional cytoplasmic fibril meshwork in hepatocytes, with concentration of fluorescence around bile canaliculi and other subcortical areas (Fig. 7). Those findings agree with the increased density of tonofilaments in the hepatocyte cortex (45). In accordance with the wide immunologic cross-species and cross-organ reactivity of cytokeratins is the finding that antibody to polypeptide D reacts with hepatocytes and bile duct epithelial cells in other animals and with a variety of epithelial cells from different organs and species *in situ* and in culture (49) (Fig. 8). Antibody preparations to liver cytoskeleton component A do not effectively stain hepatocytes *in situ* but strongly stain fibrils in epidermal, myoepithelial, and bile duct epithelial cells. These observations support the con-

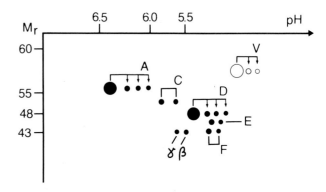

FIG. 6. Schematic presentation of mouse liver cytokeratin components (A to F) separated by two-dimensional gel electrophoresis according to molecular weight and isoelectric point (*solid circles*). Liver cytokeratin polypeptides consist of several isoelectric variants. The least acidic component is the predominant isoelectric variant and is unphosphorylated, whereas the more acidic variants are phosphorylated. Residual actin is present as β- and γ-actin. *Open circles*, isoelectric variants of vimentin (V). Vimentin is absent from hepatocytes in situ and is included only for comparison.

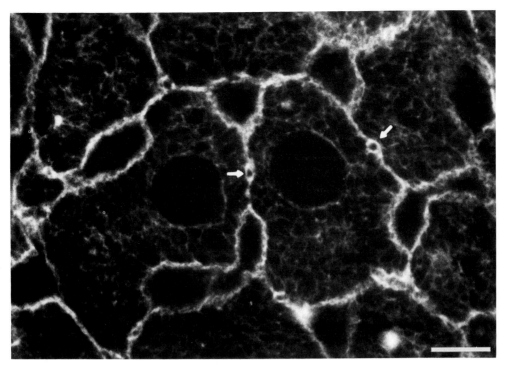

FIG. 7. Specific decoration of a distinct cytoplasmic meshwork in hepatocytes of mouse liver by indirect immunofluorescence microscopy using antibodies to mouse liver cytokeratin polypeptide component D. Fluorescence intensity is concentrated at the periphery of the hepatocytes and around bile canaliculi (*arrows*). Bar, 10 μm.

cept of differences of accessibility of cytokeratin antigens (45,49). Immunoreactivity of cytokeratin present in bile duct epithelia differs from that of hepatocytes. A strongly fluorescent dense filamentous meshwork is revealed with antibodies to liver cytokeratins A and D and with antibodies to various epidermal preparations (19,52).

Cytokeratins are restricted to epithelial elements in the liver as revealed by immunofluorescence microscopy. Intermediate-sized filaments of cells of mesenchymal origin, including endothelial and Kupffer cells, are decorated only by antibodies against vimentin (19) (Fig. 3).

Intermediate-Sized Filaments in Isolated and Cultured Hepatocytes

Cells cultured *in vitro* are widely used as model systems to study cell functions under defined experimental conditions. Work with hepatocytes and hepatoma cell lines has been particularly helpful in elucidating various metabolic and secretory processes. The major problem of directly transferring results obtained from cultured cells to an explanation of organ functions *in situ* is the deviation of cultured cells from their precursors *in situ*. This is also pertinent to cytoskeleton components, since isolated and cultured hepatocytes and hepatoma cells show considerable deviations from liver-specific patterns. Whereas the

pattern of major cytoskeletal proteins of freshly isolated hepatocytes is identical to that of hepatocytes grown *in situ*, the cytoskeleton of hepatocytes grown *in vitro*, even for periods as short as 24 to 36 hr, contain additional major polypeptides. Components of these polypeptides have molecular weights ranging from 59,000 to 69,000. In their position after two-dimensional gel electrophoresis (separation according to molecular weights combined with isoelectric focusing), some polypeptides resemble cytokeratins from epidermal cells. This may explain why cultured hepatocytes, in contrast to hepatocytes grown *in situ*, often do not stain with antibodies to epidermal prekeratin. Vimentin can appear *de novo* in cultured hepatocytes, and newly formed vimentin filaments aggregate into juxtanuclear whorls in response to colcemide treatment (19; see ref. 50 for further details).

The results suggest that the expression of different cytoskeletal proteins is subject to environmental influences, particularly to cell-to-cell interactions and changes in growth conditions.

Pathology of the Intermediate-Sized Filament Cytoskeleton in Liver Cells

Since studies of the cytokeratin system of the liver have only recently begun, relatively few pathologic conditions related to the intermediate-sized filament system of the hepatocytes are described.

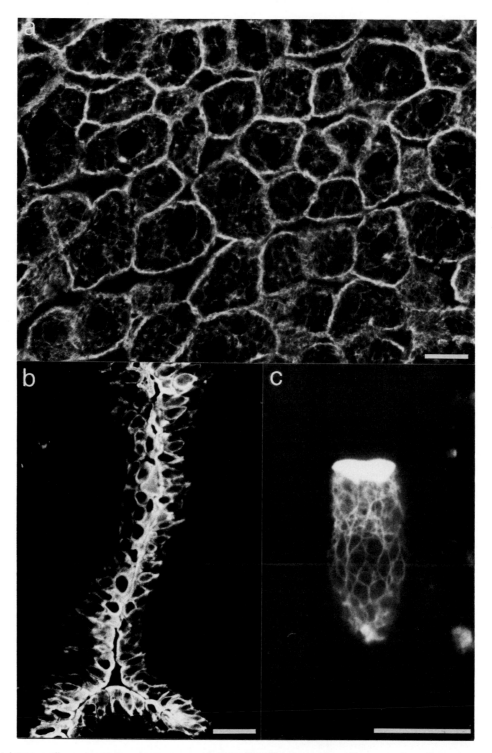

FIG. 8. Indirect immunofluorescence microscopy using antibodies to mouse liver cytokeratin component D demonstrating lack of species- and organ-specificity of these antibodies. **a:** Specific decoration of a filamentous cytoplasmic meshwork and staining of hepatocytes in rat liver. Bar, 20 μm. **b:** Specific decoration of mouse urothelium. Bar, 20 μm. **c:** Specific decoration of a filamentous cytoskeleton meshwork in epithelial cell isolated from mouse small intestine Bar, 20 μm.

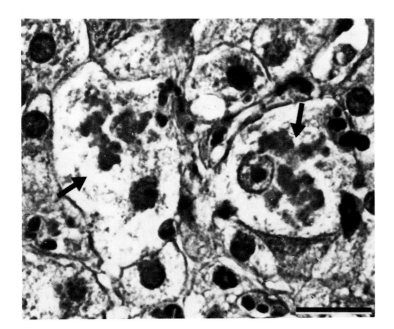

FIG. 9. Hepatocytes containing irregular Mallory body inclusions (*arrows*) in a liver biopsy from a patient with alcoholic hepatitis. Chromotrope aniline blue stain. Bar, 20 μm.

Mallory Bodies

Mallory bodies (Fig. 9) are cytoplasmic inclusions usually associated with liver cell damage in chronic alcoholics (53; see refs. 54–56 for reveiw and further details). Mallory bodies, however, are neither alcohol- nor liver-specific lesions. They are associated, although less frequently, with chronic cholestatic conditions, Wilson disease, Indian childhood cirrhosis, and other types of cirrhoses, hepatocellular tumors, and several metabolic disturbances involving the liver. They are experimentally produced in mice by chronic intoxication with griseofulvin. Mallory body-like lesions have also been observed in pneumocytes in patients with asbestosis.

Mallory bodies consist of tubular, unbranched filaments with diameters of 10 to 20 nm, arranged either in bundles or distributed in a random fashion (Fig. 10). Occasionally, particularly in the center of Mallory bodies and in older lesions, the filamentous ultrastructure is replaced by granular and amorphous material, which usually stains intensely with heavy metal ions (Fig. 11). Transmission electron microscopy, particularly of negatively stained material, shows a fuzzy and apparently stain-repellent surface coat. When this coat is penetrated by staining material, a central core cylinder, 7 nm in diameter, is contoured, which is similar in size to intermediate-sized filaments (Fig. 12).

Mallory body filaments are related to cytokeratin filaments, as judged from immunofluorescence microscopy using antibodies to cytokeratin and cytokeratin components from various sources, including bovine epidermis (52,57). These antibodies specifically react with Mallory bodies in human and murine hepatocytes

(57) (Fig. 13). The close relationship of Mallory body filaments to hepatocyte cytokeratins is further substantiated by the specific reaction of antibodies to major liver cytokeratin components with Mallory bodies (45) (Figs. 14 and 15). Antibodies to component A of liver cytokeratin strongly decorate Mallory bodies in all stages of their development. This clearly indicates that the development of Mallory bodies is accompanied by changes in antigenicity or in accessibility of antigenic determinants to antibodies. Diminution and severe derangement of the cytoskeletal meshwork accompany the evolution of Mallory bodies, suggesting that synthesis or assembly of normal cytokeratin is altered in these pathologic conditions, and that cytokeratin material eventually is incorporated into Mallory bodies (Fig. 15).

The isolated Mallory body material is highly resistant to nondenaturing solvents. It can be partially dissolved in high concentrations (8 M) of urea and SDS under reducing conditions. Electrophoresis of denatured Mallory body material in polyacrylamide gels shows a set of three polypeptide doublets ranging in molecular weight from 48,000 to 66,000 (50) (Fig. 2). Thus the major polypeptides from isolated Mallory bodies resemble hepatocytic cytokeratins but show additional major polypeptides of molecular weights larger than 55,000.

Based on these results, it seems clear that polypeptides of the cytokeratin type are major filament constituents of Mallory body material and that inclusion of other cell proteins in Mallory bodies is not excluded. Localization of antigenic components other than prekeratin in Mallory bodies has been reported (58). Phospholipid and carbohydrate materials may also be included in Mallory bodies (see ref. 54 for further

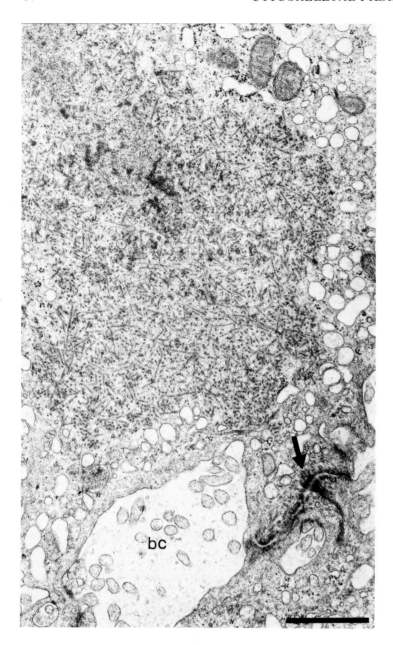

FIG. 10. Accumulation of Mallory body filaments in a hepatocyte in close vicinity to a distended bile canaliculus (bc). Pericanalicular area and microvilli contain microfilaments. *Arrow,* desmosome with attached tonofilaments. Bar, 1 μm.

information on chemical composition of Mallory bodies). Elucidation of the chemical nature of the insoluble portion of Mallory bodies is particularly needed.

The metabolic background of Mallory body formation is unclear. It is noteworthy that conditions which lead to Mallory body development (chronic alcoholism, griseofulvin intoxication) often are associated with an increased density of bundles of intermediate-sized filaments in their early stages, particularly in Mallory body-free hepatocytes. These changes suggest that accumulation of intermediate-sized filament material, either by increased production or decreased degradation, could be a precursor anomaly (19,59). Although the detailed function of the intermediate-sized filament cytoskeleton remains to be clarified, it is likely that dis-

turbance of the cytoskeleton architecture deprives the liver cell of its internal support and contributes to cell swelling, a phenomenon well known to pathologists since Mallory's first description in 1911 (53). Mallory body formation is reversible. During recovery from intoxication, Mallory bodies disperse into smaller granular units at the cell periphery, as revealed by immunofluorescence and electron microscopy (57,60) (Fig. 16), which suggest that Mallory body material may be used for reformation of normal cytoskeleton structures.

Intermediate-Sized Filaments in Liver Tumors

Morphology and antigenicity of intermediate-sized filaments appear to be highly conserved during neo-

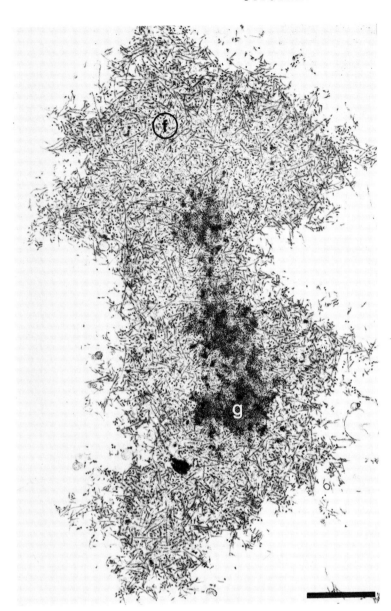

FIG. 11. Electron micrograph of Mallory body material isolated from the liver of a griseofulvin mouse; note the filamentous (f) and granular-amorphous (g) portions. Bar, 1 μm.

plastic transformation (61). Hepatocellular adenomas and carcinomas contain intermediate-sized filaments, which closely resemble those described in nonneoplastic hepatocytes by immunofluorescence and electron microscopy. The tumor cells are strongly stained by antibodies to liver cytokeratins and certain epidermal prekeratins from desmosome-attached tonofilaments. Cytokeratin filaments also occur in cholangiocellular carcinomas, which retain their broad immunoreactivity with several types of cytokeratin antibodies, including those to epidermal prekeratin. In contrast, mesenchymal neoplasms of the liver (angiosarcomas and other types of sarcomas) react with vimentin antibodies like the nonneoplastic cells from which they are derived. Because of maintenance of the specificity of intermediate-sized filaments in liver neoplasms, immunofluorescence microscopy using appropriate antibodies is a valuable method to identify and characterize various types of tumors. As in nonneoplastic hepatocytes grown *in vitro*, intermediate-sized filaments in cultured cells derived from liver tumors show considerable aberrations in their polypeptide composition and frequently contain vimentin and cytokeratin filaments (50). In some cultured hepatoma cells, cytokeratin and vimentin filaments are both included in large juxtanuclear aggregates reminiscent of, but not identical to, Mallory bodies (62).

Intermediate-Sized Filaments in Other Types of Liver Cell Injury

In fatty liver, fibrils of the intermediate-sized filament cytoskeleton are pushed to the cell periphery by masses of lipid accumulating in the cytoplasm but

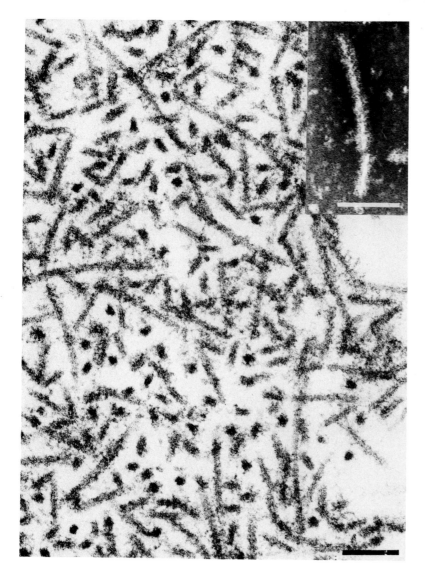

FIG. 12. Electron micrograph of Mallory body filaments isolated and purified from griseofulvin mouse liver. Filaments represent rigid, unbranched rods with outer diameters of 14 to 20 nm. Note the irregular fuzzy outline of the filaments. Bar, 0.1 μm. *Inset:* Details of the ultrastructure of a Mallory body filament in a negatively stained preparation. The fuzzy coat material and a core filament 6 to 7 nm in diameter are visible. Bar, 0.1 μm.

otherwise are not significantly altered, at least as revealed by immunofluorescence microscopy (45). In liver cirrhosis, the cytoskeleton is not conspicuously altered (H. Denk, R. Krepler, and W. W. Franke, *unpublished observations*). No studies exist on the behavior of intermediate-sized filaments in other liver diseases, including cholestasis and viral hepatitis.

MICROTUBULES

Properties and Functions

Microtubules are present in the cytoplasm of almost all eukaryotic cells. Fairly uniform in size, they are straight and hollow structures, several micrometers long, with an outer diameter of 20 to 26 nm. In contrast to microtubules of cilia and flagella, most cytoplasmic microtubules are relatively labile structures, particularly when cells are treated with drugs, such as colchicine, colcemid, griseofulvin, vinca alkaloids, and

others, or are exposed to high calcium concentrations. Microtubules are composed of tubulin which is a dimer consisting of either identical (α- or β-tubulin) or different (α- and β-tubulin) monomers with similar molecular weights (values range from 50,000 to 56,000). A dynamic equilibrium exists between free dimers and polymerized tubulin. Nucleotides are involved in controlling the rates of nucleation and elongation of microtubules. Several microtubule-associated proteins are regular components of microtubular structures. Microtubules are involved in the maintenance of cell shape, polarity of movement, distribution and movements of cell organelles, secretory processes, and complex particle movements during mitotic and meiotic divisions (see refs. 1,3,8,15, and 63 for further information).

Microtubular System in Hepatocytes

Tubulin comprises about 1% of the soluble protein in hepatocytes, but only about 40% of tubulin is assem-

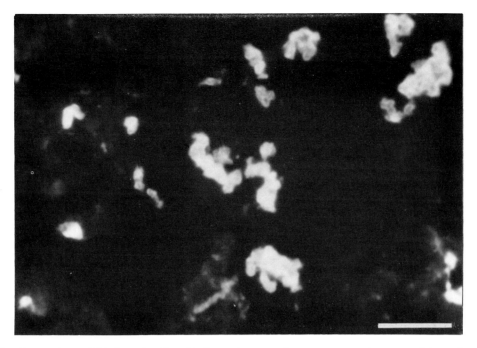

FIG. 13. Specific decoration of Mallory bodies (indirect immunofluorescence microscopy) in a liver biopsy from a patient with alcoholic hepatitis using antibodies to a prekeratin polypeptide component (molecular weight, 58,000) derived from desmosome-attached tonofilaments of bovine muzzle epidermis. Bar, 20 μm.

bled in microtubules (64). Liver cell regeneration increases hepatocellular tubulin content, as determined by the colchicine binding assay (65). Microtubules traverse the cytoplasm of hepatocytes for long distances. Disturbance of the microtubular system by antitubulin drugs and ethanol profoundly influences intracellular translocation of proteins, phospholipids, and triglycerides and several secretory processes, such as the secretion of albumin, other plasma proteins, and lipoproteins (66–68). Swelling of hepatocytes concomitant with accumulation of the Golgi apparatus and secretory vesicles often occurs after acute and chronic exposure to ethanol and at least partly results from retention of substances normally exported

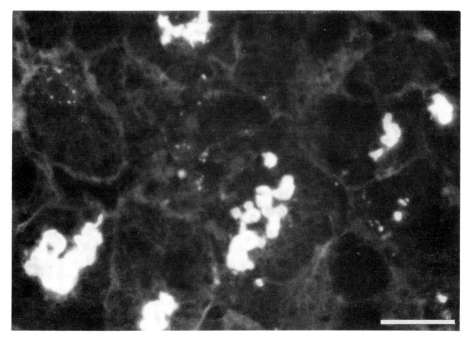

FIG. 14. Specific decoration of Mallory body inclusions (indirect immunofluorescence microscopy) in griseofulvin mouse liver by antibodies to mouse liver cytokeratin component A. Only Mallory bodies are specifically stained. Bar, 20 μm.

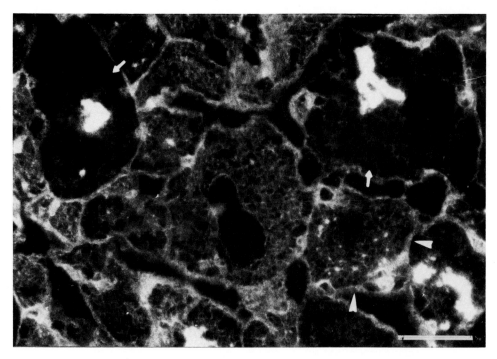

FIG. 15. Indirect immunofluorescence microscopy using antibodies to mouse liver cytokeratin component D performed on a frozen section of liver from a mouse that received griseofulvin for 3 months. The hepatocyte in the center displays a regular cytoplasmic filament meshwork resembling the intact cytoskeleton. In an adjacent hepatocyte (*arrowheads*), tiny Mallory body granules are visible. Two additional hepatocytes (*arrows*) contain larger Mallory body inclusions and have a diminished and severely deranged cytoplasmic filament meshwork. Bar, 20 μm.

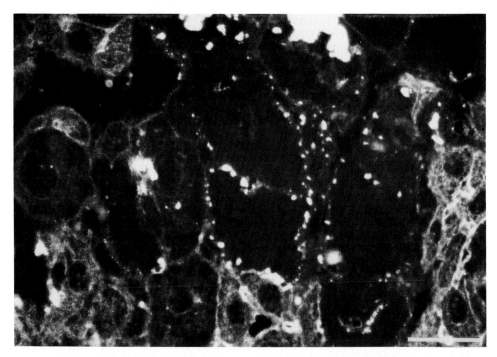

FIG. 16. Hepatocytes with small Mallory body granules arranged at the periphery of the cells in a liver from a mouse that was treated with griseofulvin in high concentrations for 3 months and allowed to recover on a griseofulvin-free diet for 1 month. Indirect immunofluorescence microscopy using antibodies to mouse liver cytokeratin component D. Bar, 20 μm.

from the liver cell (56,69). Colchicine also inhibits the biliary secretion of phospholipid, cholesterol, and bile salts, which suggests an effect of the microtubular system on bile secretion (70); however, this is controversial (71), particularly since some effects of colchicine do not involve microtubules (72–74).

AUTOANTIBODIES TO CYTOSKELETAL PROTEINS IN LIVER DISEASES

Antibodies that react with smooth muscle-associated antigens, i.e., smooth muscle antibodies, have diagnostic significance in clinical hepatology (see ref. 75 for review). Since the initial reports emphasizing the association of smooth muscle antibodies with chronic active hepatitis, antibodies of this type have been found in alcoholic liver disorders, primary biliary cirrhosis, and acute viral hepatitis and in nonhepatic disorders. The antibodies are heterogeneous with respect to the antigens which they recognize. Consequently, smooth muscle antibodies have been divided into those directed against actin and those of nonactin types (76). Actin antibodies are predominant in chronic active hepatitis, whereas nonactin antibodies (including antibodies to components of intermediate-sized filaments, such as desmin and vimentin) occur in alcoholic liver disease, viral infections, and in cancer patients (76). Antibodies to tubulin occur in infectious mononucleosis (75).

The biologic significance of these autoantibodies is unclear, but it is likely that they indicate cell damage. However, filaments of the vimentin type can activate complement in an antibody-independent manner which may aggravate tissue damage (77).

REFERENCES

1. Adelstein, R. S., Scordilis S. P., and Trotter, J. A. (1979): The cytoskeleton and cell movement: General considerations. *Methods Achiev. Exp. Pathol.*, 8:1–41.
2. Clarke, M., and Spudich, J. A. (1977). Nonmuscle contractile proteins: The role of actin and myosin in cell motility and shape determination. *Annu. Rev. Biochem.* 46:797–822.
3. DeRobertis, E. D. P., and DeRobertis, E. M. F. (1980): *Cell and Molecular Biology*, pp. 179–205. Saunders, Philadelphia.
4. Fisher, M. M., and Phillips, M. J. (1979). Cytoskeleton of the hepatocyte. In: *Progress in Liver Diseases, Vol. VI*, edited by H. Popper and F. Schaffner, pp. 105–121. Grune & Stratton, New York.
5. Pollard, T. D. (1977): Cytoplasmic contractile proteins. In: *International Cell Biology* edited by B. R. Brinkley and K. R. Porter pp. 378–387. Rockefeller University Press, New York.
6. Stossel, T. P. (1978) Contractile proteins in cell structure and function. *Annu. Rev. Med.*, 29:427–457.
7. Gordon, D. J., Boyer, J. L., and Korn, E. D. (1977): Comparative biochemistry of nonmuscle actins. *J. Biol. Chem.*, 252: 8300–8309.
8. Henderson, D., and Weber. K. (1979). Three-dimensional organization of microfilaments and microtubules in the cyto-

skeleton. Immunoperoxidase labelling and stereo-electron microscopy of detergent extracted cells. *Exp. Cell Res.*, 124:301–316.
9. Jackson, B. W., Grund, C., Schmid, E. Bürki, K., Franke, W. W., and Illmensee, K. (1980): Formation of cytoskeletal elements during mouse embryogenesis: Intermediate filaments of the cytokeratin type and desmosomes in preimplantation embryos. *Differentiation*, 17:161–179.
10. Flanagan, M. D., and Lin, S. (1980): Cytochalasins block actin filament elongation by binding to high affinity sites associated with F-actin. *J. Biol. Chem.*, 255, 835–838.
11. Lindberg, U., Carlsson, L., Markey, F., and Nystrom, L. E. (1979): The unpolymerized form of actin in non-muscle cells. *Methods Achiev. Exp. Pathol.*, 8:143–170.
12. MacLean-Fletcher, S., and Pollard, T. D. (1980): Mechanism of action of cytochalasin B on actin. *Cell*, 20:329-341.
13. Dancker, P., Löw, I., Hasselbach, W., and Wieland, T. (1975): Interaction of actin with phalloidin: Polymerization and stabilization of F-actin. *Biochem. Biophys. Acta*, 400:407–414.
14. Gabbiani, G., Montesano, R., Tuchweber, B., Salas, M., and Orci, L. (1975): Phalloidin induced hyperplasia of actin filaments in rat hepatocytes. *Lab. Invest.*, 33:562–569.
15. Luduena, R. F. (1979): Biochemistry of tubulin. In: *Microtubules*, edited by K. Roberts and J. S. Hyams, pp. 65–116. Academic Press, London.
16. Brandon, D. L. (1976): The identification of myosin in rabbit hepatocytes. *Eur. J. Biochem*, 65:139–146.
17. Elias, E., and Boyer, J. L. (1979): Mechanism of intrahepatic cholestasis. In: *Progress in Liver Diseases, Vol. VI*, edited by H. Popper and F. Schaffner, pp. 457–470 Grune & Stratton, New York.
18. Gordon, D. J., Boyer, J. L., and Korn, E. D. (1977): Comparative biochemistry of nonmuscle actins. *J. Biol. Chem.*, 252:8300–8309.
19. Franke, W. W., Schmid, E., Kartenbeck, J., Mayer, D., Hacker, H. J., Bannasch, P., Osborn, M., Weber, K., Denk, H., Wanson, J. C., and Drochmans, P. (1979): Characterization of the intermediate-sized filaments in liver cells by immunofluorescence and electron microscopy. *Biol. Cell.*, 34:99–110.
20. French, S. W., and Davies, P. L. (1975): Ultrastructural localization of actin-like filaments in rat hepatocytes. *Gastroenterology*, 68:765–774.
21. Oda, M., Price, V. M., Fisher, M. M., and Phillips, M. J. (1974): Ultrastructure of bile canaliculi with special reference to the surface coat and the pericanalicular web. *Lab. Invest.*, 31:314–323.
22. Trenchev, P., Sneyd, P., and Holborow, E. J. (1974): Immunofluorescent tracing of smooth muscle contractile protein antigens in tissues other than smooth muscle. *Clin. Exp. Immunol.*, 16:125–136.
23. LeStourgeon, W. M. (1978): The occurrence of contractile proteins in nuclei and their possible functions. In: *The Cell Nucleus, Vol. VI., Chromatin*, edited by H. Busch, pp. 305–326 Academic Press, New York.
24. French, S. W. (1976): Is cholestasis due to microfilament failure? *Hum. Pathol.*, 7:243–244.
25. Oda, M., and Phillips, M. J. (1977): Bile canalicular membrane pathology in cytochalasin B-induced cholestasis. *Lab. Invest.*, 37:350–356.
26. Oshio, C., and Phillips, M. J. (1980): Contraction of bile canaliculi as evidenced by time-lapse cinephotomicrography. *Gastroenterology*, 79:1043(*Abstr.*).
27. Phillips, M. J., Oda, M., Mak, E., Fisher, M. M., and Jeejeebhoy, K. N. (1975): Microfilament dysfunction as a possible cause of intrahepatic cholestasis. *Gastroenterology*, 69:48–58.
28. Dubin, M., Maurice, M., Feldman, G., and Erlinger, S. (1978): Phalloidin-induced cholestasis in the rat: Relation to changes in microfilaments. *Gastroenterology*, 75:450–455.
29. Biava, C. G. (1964): Studies on cholestasis. A reevaluation of the fine structure of normal human bile canaliculi. *Lab. Invest.*, 13:840–864.
30. DeVos, R., DeWolf-Peeters, C., Desmet, V., Eggermont, E.,

and VanAcker, K. (1975): Progressive intrahepatic cholestasis (Beyler's disease): Case report. *Gut*, 16:943–950.

31. Steiner, J. W., and Carruthers, J. S. (1961): Studies on the fine structure of the terminal branches of the biliary tree. II. Observations of pathologically altered bile canaliculi. *Am. J. Pathol.*, 39:41–63.

32. Gabbiani, G., and Ryan, G. B. (1974): Development of a contractile apparatus in epithelial cells during epidermal and liver regeneration. *J. Submicr. Cytol.*, 6:143-157.

33. Lampert, I. A., Trenchev, P., and Holborow, E. J. (1974): Contractile protein changes in regenerating rat liver. *Virchows Archiv. [Cell Pathol.]*, 15:351–355.

34. Toh, B. H., Cauchi, M. N., and Muller, H. K. (1977): Actin-like contractile protein in carbon tetrachloride-induced cirrhosis in the rat. *Pathology*, 9:187–194.

35. Irle, C., Kocher, O., and Gabbiani, G. (1980): Contractility of myofibroblasts during experimental liver cirrhosis. *J. Submicr. Cytol.*, 12:209–217.

36. Lazarides, E. (1980): Intermediate filaments as mechanical integrators of cellular space. *Nature*, 283:249–256.

37. Franke, W. W., Weber, K., Osborn, M., Schmid, E., and Freudenstein, C. Antibody to prekeratin: Decoration of tonofilament-like arrays in various cells of epitheloid character. *Exp. Cell Res.*, 116:429–445.

38. Milstone, L. M., and McGuire, J. (1981): Different polypeptides form the intermediate filaments in bovine hoof and esophageal epithelium and in aortic endothelium. *J. Cell Biol*, 88:312–316.

39. Sun, T. T., Shih, C., and Green, H. (1979): Keratin cytoskeletons in epithelial cells of internal organs. *Proc. Natl. Acad. Sci. USA*, 76:2813–2817.

40. Fuchs, E., and Green, H. (1979): Multiple keratins of cultured human epidermal cells are translated from different mRNA molecules. *Cell*, 17:573–582.

41. Fuchs, E., and Green, H. (1978): The expression of keratin genes in epidermis and cultured epidermal cells. *Cell*, 15:887–897.

42. Franke, W. W., Schmid, E., Winter, S., Osborn, M., and Weber, K. (1979): Widespread occurrence of intermediate-sized filaments of the vimentin-type in cultured cells from diverse vertebrates. *Exp. Cell Res.*, 123:25–46.

43. Gard, D. L., Bell, P. B., and Lazarides, E. (1979): Coexistence of desmin and the fibroblastic intermediate filament subunit in muscle and nonmuscle cells: Identification and comparative peptide analysis. *Proc. Natl. Acad. Sci. USA*, 76:3894–3898.

44. Yokoda, S., and Fahimi, H. D. (1979): Filament bundles of prekeratin type in hepatocytes: Revealed by detergent extraction after glutaraldehyde fixation. *Biol. Cell.* 34:119-126.

45. Denk, H., Franke, W. W., Dragosics, B., and Zeiler, I. (1981): Pathology of cytoskeleton of liver cells. Demonstration of Mallory bodies (alcoholic hyalin) in murine and human hepatocytes by immunofluorescence microscopy using antibodies to cytokeratin polypeptides from hepatocytes. *Hepatology* 1:9–20.

46. Jahn, W. (1980): The cytoskeleton of rat liver parenchymal cells. *Naturwissenschaften*, 67:568.

47. Jahn, W. (1980): Visualization of a filamentous network in cryosections of liver tissue. *Eur. J. Cell Biol.*, 20:301–304.

48. Forssmann, W. G., and Ito, S (1977): Hepatocyte innervation in primates. *J. Cell Biol.*, 74:299–313.

49. Franke, W. W., Denk, H., Kalt, R., and Schmid, E. (1981): Biochemical and immunological identification of cytokeratin proteins present in hepatocytes of mammalian liver tissue. *Exp. Cell Res.*, 131:299–318.

50. Franke, W. W., Mayer, D., Schmid, E., Denk, H., and Borenfreund, E. (1982): Differences of expression of cytoskeletal proteins in cultured rat hepatocytes and hepatoma cells. *Exp. Cell Res.*, 131:299–318.

51. Franke, W. W., Weber, K., Osborn, M., Schmid, E., and Freudenstein, C. (1978): Antibody to prekeratin: Decoration of tonofilament-like arrays in various cells of epitheloid character. *Exp. Cell Res.*, 134:345–365.

52. Franke, W. W., Denk, H., Schmid, E., Osborn, M., and Weber, K. (1979): Ultrastructural, biochemical, and immunologic characterization of Mallory bodies in livers of griseofulvin-treated mice. Fimbriated rods of filaments containing prekeratin-like polypeptides. *Lab. Invest.*, 40:207–220.

53. Mallory, F. B. (1911): Cirrhosis of the liver. Five different types of lesions from which it may arise. *Bull. Johns Hopkins Hosp.*, 22:69–75.

54. Denk, H., Franke, W. W., Kerjaschki, D., and Eckerstorfer, R. (1979): Mallory bodies in experimental animals and man. *Int. Rev. Exp. Pathol.* 20:77–121.

55. French, S. W., and Burbige, E. J. (1979): Alcoholic hepatitis: Clinical, morphologic, pathogenic, and therapeutic aspects. In: *Progress in Liver Diseases, Vol. VI*, edited by H. Popper and F. Schaffner, pp. 557–579. Grune & Stratton, New York.

56. French, S. W., and Davies, P. L. (1975): The Mallory body in the pathogenesis of alcoholic liver disease. In: *Alcoholic Liver Pathology*, edited by J. M. Khanna, Y. Israel, and H. Kalant, pp. 113–170. Addiction Research Foundation of Ontario, Toronto.

57. Denk, H., Franke, W. W., Eckerstorfer, R., Schmid, E., and Kerjaschki, D. (1979): Formation and involution of Mallory bodies ("alcoholic hyalin") in murine and human liver revealed by immunofluorescence microscopy using antibodies to prekeratin. *Proc. Natl. Acad. Sci. USA*, 76:4112–4116.

58. Morton, J. A., Fleming, K. A., Trowell, J. M., and McGee, J. O'D. (1980): Mallory bodies—immunohistochemical detection by antisera to unique nonprekeratin components. *Gut*, 21:727–733.

59. Petersen, P. (1977): Alcoholic hyalin, microfilaments and microtubules in alcoholic hepatitis. *Acta Pathol. Microbiol. Scand.*, 85:384–394.

60. Denk, H., and Franke W. W. (1981): Rearrangement of the hepatocyte cytoskeleton after toxic damage: Involution, dispersal and peripheral accumulation of Mallory body material after drug withdrawal. *Eur. J. Cell Biol.*, 23:241–249.

61. Bannasch, P., Zerban, H., Schmid, E., and Franke, W. W. (1980): Liver tumors distinguished by immunofluorescence microscopy with antibodies to proteins of intermediate-sized filaments. *Proc. Natl. Acad. Sci. USA*, 77:4948–4952.

62. Borenfreund, E., Schmid, E., Bendich, A., and Franke, W. W. (1980): Constitutive aggregates of intermediate-sized filaments of the vimentin and cytokeratin type in cultured hepatoma cells and their dispersal by butyrate. *Exp. Cell Res.*, 127:215–235.

63. Weber, K., and Osborn, M. (1979): Intracellular display of microtubular structures revealed by indirect immunofluorescence microscopy. In: *Microtubules*, edited by K. Roberts and J. S. Hyams, pp. 279–313. Academic Press, London.

64. Patzelt, C., Singh, A., LeMarchand, Y., Orci, L., and Jeanrenaud, B. (1974): Colchicine binding protein of the liver. Its characterization and relation to microtubules. *J. Cell Biol.* 66:609–620.

65. Lawrence, J. H., and Wheatby, D. N. (1974): Microtubule protein in normal and regenerating liver. *Cytobios*, 10:111–122.

66. Gregory, D. H., Vlahcevic, Z. R., Prugh, M. F., and Swell, L. (1978): Mechanism of secretion of biliary lipids: Role of a microtubular system in hepatocellular transport of biliary lipids in the rat. *Gastroenterology*, 74:93–100.

67. Redman, C. M., Banerjee, D., Howell, K., and Palade, G. E. (1975): Colchicine inhibition of plasma protein release from rat hepatocytes. *J. Cell Biol.*, 66:42–59.

68. Redman, C. M., Banerjee, D., Manning, C., Huang, C. Y., and Green, K. (1978): In vivo effect of colchicine on hepatic protein synthesis and on the conversion of proalbumin to serum albumin. *J. Cell Biol.*, 77:400–416.

69. Baraona, E., Leo, M. A., Borowsky, S. A., and Lieber, C. S. (1975): Alcoholic hepatomegaly: Accumulation of protein in the liver. *Science*, 190:794–795.

70. Olinger, E. J., and Malham, L. (1978): Correlation of the effects of colchicine on bile acid secretion and microtubule depolymerization in isolated rat hepatocytes. *Gastroenterology*, 79:1041 (*Abstr.*).

71. Stein, O., Sanger, L., and Stein, Y. (1974): Colchicine-induced inhibition of lipoprotein and protein secretion into the serum and lack of interference with secretion of biliary phospholipids and cholesterol by rat liver in vivo. *J. Cell Biol.*, 62:90–103.

72. Scott, T., Brady, S. D., Crother, C., Nosal, C., and McClure,

W. O. (1980): Fast axonal transport in the presence of high Ca^{++}: Evidence that microtubules are not required. *Proc. Natl. Acad. Sci. USA,* 77:5909–5913.

73. Stadler, J., and Franke, W. W. (1974): Characterization of the colchicine binding of membrane fractions from rat and mouse liver. *J. Cell Biol.,* 60:297–303.

74. Tauber, R., and Reutter, W. (1980): A colchicine-sensitive uptake system in Morris hepatomas. *Proc. Natl. Acad. Sci. USA,* 77:5282–5286.

75. Toh, B. H. (1979): Smooth muscle autoantibodies and autoantigens. *Clin. Exp. Immunol.,* 38:621–628.

76. Kurki, P., Virtanen, I., Stenman, S., and Linder, E. (1978): Characterization of human smooth muscle autoantibodies reacting with cytoplasmic intermediate filaments. *Clin. Immunol. Immunopathol.,* 11:379–387.

77. Linder, E., Lehto, V. P., and Stenman, S. (1979): Activation of complement by cytoskeletal intermediate filaments. *Nature,* 278:176–177.

The Liver: Biology and Pathobiology, edited by
I. Arias, H. Popper, D. Schachter, and D. A. Shafritz.
Raven Press, New York © 1982.

Chapter 6

Nucleus, DNA, and Chromatin

Harris Busch

The nucleus, the major repository of genetic information in the cell, contains DNA and its associated proteins. Small amounts of DNA are also present in mitochondria; little if any is found in the cell membrane or the endoplasmic reticulum. The genetic information of the cell nucleus becomes operational in the cytoplasm in the form of polysomes, which contain messenger RNA (template RNA), ribosomes, and associated biosynthetic elements.

Whether the nucleus represents a small structure in a large cell or a giant structure in a relatively small cell, a layer of cytoplasm always separates it from the plasma membrane of the cell. The cytoplasm plays an important role in the feedback interactions of the nucleus with an array of stimuli. The nucleus is part of an integrated system by which cells respond to extracellular and intracellular stimuli. These stimuli interact with the nuclear informational system to produce specific products (Table 1) that permit responses to the environment and its functional demands. The cell nucleus has a huge variety of potential products that alter cellular function remarkably from organ to organ.

A major question in cell and molecular biology regards the nature of control systems that regulate the genome. Since DNA content and composition are the same in virtually all cells of an individual (except red blood cells and haploid cells), it remains totipotent throughout the life of the cell. The substances that govern gene expression, therefore, must be derived from the cytoplasm or external cellular milieu directly or by interaction with appropriate "receptor" or "carrier" molecules interacting with specific genetic loci.

So much new information has accumulated on the structures (Fig. 1) and products (Table 1) of the cell nucleus that the subject has been the topic of symposia, reviews, and multivolume treatises (1–6). Important aspects of DNA subelements in the cell nucleus are rapidly coming into sharp focus.

One fundamental question is how the nucleus offers significant chemical or physical advantages over the random distribution of DNA in juxtaposition to cytoplasmic elements found in microorganisms. The nucleus segregates the genetic information in a compact state distant from the major sites of phenotypic function. It has a continuing, moment-to-moment interaction with cytoplasmic events and replenishes the special polysomes destroyed or metabolized in normal cell function. It reacts quantitatively and qualitatively to an altered cell environment, but the advantages of such specialization are not obvious. Among the possi-

Table 1. *Nuclear products*

DNA
  Complete DNA replication during cell division
  Gene amplification or repetition
RNA
  Messenger RNA
    mRNA sequences
    poly(A) 3′ termini
    The 5′ cap (? nucleus)
  rRNA
    28 S
    18 S
    5.8 S
    5 S
  tRNA
    tRNA nucleotide sequence
    Many modified tRNA nucleotides
  LMWN RNA
    Uridine-rich nuclear RNA U1, U2, U3
    Other species including 4.5 S RNA_{I-III}, 5 S RNA_{III},
    8 S RNA
  Precursor processing reactions for each RNA species
Ribonucleoprotein particles
  mRNP particles
    Informosomes
    Polysomes
  rRNA particles
    Granular nucleolar elements
    Completed ribosomes

ble reasons for segregation of genetic material into the cell nucleus are: (a) protection of genetic elements from cleavage of other degradative reactions resulting from release or hyperactivity of cytoplasmic hydrolytic enzymes, or (b) separation of the "storage elements" from the main sites of synthesis and metabolic activity of specialized cytoplasmic enzymes and complex structures. The large numbers and types of products present in the cell nucleus may be well separated from unrelated elements to increase efficient functioning.

Differences in the substances and enzymes present in specialized cell nuclei have been reported. For example, thymus nuclei contain most of the enzymes of glycolysis and oxidative phosphorylation. On the other hand, highly purified nuclei, such as the commonly studied liver nucleus, contain few if any such enzymes or corresponding structures.

In cells in which the nuclei have been lost, such as reticulocytes, cell function continues for long periods of time. The red cell is a useful oxygen carrier up to 120 days, even though it is totally lacking in nuclear elements. In the enucleated reticulocyte, polysomes continue to function for the synthesis of hemoglobin. Globin mRNA has a long half-life (7). Thus nuclear functions are not absolutely necessary for the useful life of such cells.

In cells that are either slowly or never reproduced, such as nerve cells of the cerebrum, cerebellum, and other components of the central nervous system, the nucleus and auxiliary structures may be extremely active in replacement processes. Such processes include ribosome synthesis and synthesis of Nissl substance (8).

The cytoplasm influences nuclear function through either specific products or feedback loops. The experiments on nuclear transplantation by Briggs and King (9), which demonstrated the totipotency of the nuclei of the frog egg, and the subsequent experiments of Gurdon (10), which demonstrated totipotency of nuclei in highly differentiated tissues, have established that the cell nucleus is responsive to cytoplasmic stimuli. We have suggested that the nucleus serves a role like that of a musical instrument, with specific capacities responsive to a series of specific manipulations.

NUCLEAR STRUCTURES

Many light microscopic studies have been performed on nuclei and nucleoli (8,11). Recent elegant advances in scanning and electron microscopy have provided improved two- and three-dimensional analyses of the nuclear structures as well as their spatial interrelationships (Table 2).

The fundamental structure of the cell nucleus is rather simple. As seen in Fig. 2, isolated nuclei are circumscribed by a refractile, highly permeable, double-layered envelope. The basic nuclear framework is the "nuclear ribonucleoprotein network" ("nuclear matrix"), of which the hub is the nucleolus (Fig. 3). The nuclear envelope and the nuclear matrix provide both the basic elements of nuclear structure and the sites of attachment of critical nuclear elements (Table 2). In general, the nucleus may be considered to be a unit structure containing an internal matrix surrounded by a double-layered envelope of high porosity. Although at one time the nucleus was thought to be an amorphous structure (with the exception of the nucleoli), improved methods have shown that it contains a series of particulate structures that serve special and important roles in its function. For example, specific elements involved in "RNA splicing" are now being clarified and represent important areas of future research.

The Nuclear Envelope

The nuclear envelope (Figs. 2–5) consists of two portions: an outer layer, which is frequently covered by ribosomes and is in contact with the cytoplasm and endoplasmic reticulum, and an inner layer, which is composed of "membrane." The inner layer is in contact with chromatin and the nuclear elements. The two layers join at the nuclear pores, which are shown in cross section (Fig. 5A) and on end (Fig. 5B). These

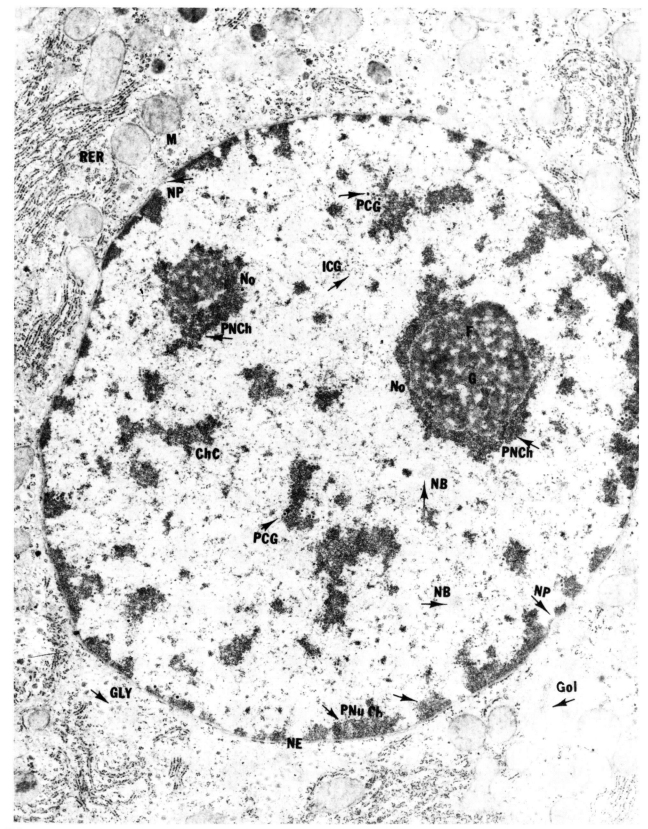

FIG. 1. Electron micrograph of a rat liver cell nucleus. Within the nucleus, nucleoli (No) are surrounded by perinucleolar chromatin (PNCh). The nucleoli consist of granular (G) and fibrillar (F) elements. Chromocenters (ChC) are distributed randomly with the nucleoplasm. Frequently, perichromatin granules (PCG) are associated with these chromocenters. Within the nucleus, occasional nuclear bodies (NB) and interchromatin granules (ICG) are seen, which are apparently cross sections of the nuclear ribonucleoprotein network. The inner layer of the nuclear envelope (NE) surrounds a conspicuous layer of dense chromatin (PNuCh). The clear areas within this heterochromatin layer usually mark the location of the nuclear pores (NP). Glycogen elements (GLY) are present in the cytoplasm. Mitochondria (M) and rough endoplasmic reticulum (RER) are distributed throughout the cytoplasm. Occasional Golgi (Gol) complexes are seen around the nuclear periphery. Lead citrate-uranyl acetate staining (× 16,200). (Courtesy of T. Unuma and Y. Daskal.)

Table 2. *Nuclear structures*

Nuclear envelope
  Outer layer—continuation of the endoplasmic reticulum
  Inner layer
  Nuclear pores
  Juxtaenvelope chromatin
Chromatin—chromosomes
  Interphase chromatin
    "Euchromatin"—dispersed chromatin
    Heterochromatin—condensed chromatin
  Meiotic chromatin
    Chromatin in various states of condensation
    Defined metaphase chromosomes
Nucleolus
  Nucleoli in various stages of cell function
  "Nucleolar chromosomes"
  rDNA and its controls
  Preribosomal RNA
  Interlocks of rRNA and ribosomal protein synthesis
  The nucleolar channel system
Nuclear ribonucleoprotein network
Nuclear particles
  Perichromatin granules
  Interchromatin granules
  Nuclear bodies
  Nuclear rodlets
  Nuclear inclusions
  mRNP precursor particles (informosomes)

structures are not simply holes in the nuclear wall but contain a number of elements arranged in a highly ordered form. A schematic diagram of these structures (Fig. 6) was presented by Franke and Scheer (12). Studies in progress on the nuclear envelope are aimed at discerning more about its semipermeability and the mechanism of penetration of the large particles and other elements from the nucleus into the cytoplasm. The nucleus is continuously "sensing" the cytoplasmic function; its response is in the form of large particles that must pass through the nuclear envelope. Presumably, nuclear pores serve to permit large "packages" to migrate from the nucleus into the cytoplasm. Some electron micrographs support this suggestion (Fig. 7).

The Nuclear Ribonucleoprotein Network

Studies in our laboratory demonstrated the presence of a network of ribonucleoproteins within the nucleus that has subsequently become of considerable interest (13). As shown in Fig. 3, dense strands emerge from the nucleolus, spreading throughout the nuclear matrix and terminating in the inner layer of the nuclear envelope. These dense strands were studied with respect to their RNA content and were shown to contain AU-rich RNA in addition to the GC-rich RNA of the nucleolar products (14,15). This network not only contains unusual elements that might represent elementary nuclear structures but also serves as a pathway for com-

pletion and packaging of nuclear products on their way to the cytoplasm. The nuclear ribonucleoprotein elements might be the "interchromatinic granules" in thin sections of transmission microscopy (Fig. 1).

Recent expansions of these studies by Berezney and Coffey (13) and Comings and Okada (16) have strengthened the idea that this network is a specialized nuclear component. It contains three major proteins which are distinct from other nuclear proteins; in addition, it contains some DNA which may be different from the remainder of the nuclear DNA.

Nuclear Particulate Structure

Of the nuclear particulate structures, the nucleolus is the largest and most important in terms of synthesis of ribosomal elements. The largest and most important functional "structure" of the nucleus is the chromatin, within which are a number of important granular elements (Figs. 1,4), referred to as the interchromatinic dense granules. These are readily visible in most electron micrographs that are fixed and stained by conventional standards (8). The possibility that dense granules are the strands of the nuclear ribonucleoprotein network is noted above. Their arrangement in large and small bundles agrees with this possibility.

Perichromatin Granules

Of the dense elements in the nucleus, the most interesting are the perichromatin granules (Figs. 1,8) best seen in some states when cellular function is inhibited. Recent studies from our laboratory showed that large numbers of these granular elements accumulated in regions adjacent to the chromatin masses. Among the most interesting features of these granules are the halos that surround them, producing a "bulls-eye" appearance. These granules contain low molecular weight (U6) nuclear RNA, mRNA, and "informosomal proteins." Clearly, further morphological and biochemical analyses of their functional roles are necessary.

Among the larger elements in the cell nucleus are the nuclear bodies, which are distributed throughout the nucleoplasm. Such bodies are composed primarily of fibrillar elements, either densely or rather loosely packed (Fig. 9). These bodies have been classified as granular, simple, and coiled bodies, but the distinctions are at present unclear. Whether they represent "inclusion bodies" related to viral or other infections or sites of degradation of various nuclear elements is not yet known.

Juxtanucleolar Bodies

Of particular interest to morphologists are the juxtanucleolar bodies originally described by Terzakis

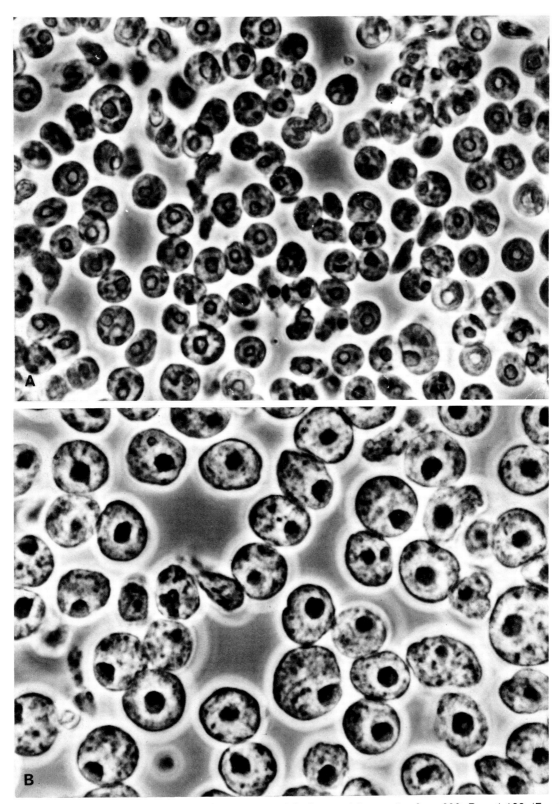

FIG. 2. Phase microscopy of a preparation of isolated nuclei of normal liver cells. **A:** × 600; B: × 1,100. (From ref. 8.)

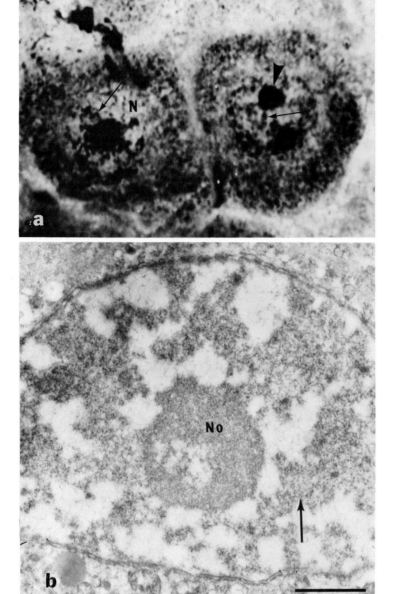

FIG. 3. a: Smear of liver cells extracted with 0.14 M NaCl stained with toluidine blue without previous fixation. The nuclear RNP network (*arrow*) seems to radiate from the nucleolus (*arrowhead*). × 2,200. **b:** Nuclear residue from Walker tumor after treatment with dilute (0.14 M) and concentrated (2 M) saline solutions. The nucleolus (No) is attached to a network (*arrow*) composed of particles and filaments. × 14,000. (From ref. 8.)

(17) in human uterine tissues. These bodies are generally believed to be formed by cytoplasmic invaginations that form a honey-combed mass (when viewed in cross section) apparently next to or within the nucleolar structures (Fig. 10). On longitudinal section, these structures appear to be channels composed primarily of unit membrane; in some areas, the membrane appears to be doubled (Fig. 11). Their function is completely unknown.

Statellite Bodies

Among the other nuclear bodies described in specific tissues are the "statellite bodies" found in neurons in the cerebral cortex (Fig. 12). They appear in close proximity to the nucleolus but are definitely not related to cytoplasmic invaginations because they lack peripheral membrane. Apparently, they represent specialized localizations of chromatin masses. One suggestion is that they represent amplified gene segments but proof for this has not been presented.

Other Types of Nuclear Elements

Bouteille et al. (17a) illustrated the many types of structures seen in the cell nucleus (Fig. 4). They noted the presence of intranuclear rodlets (INR) and certain coiled bodies (CB), which represent unique nuclear structures. Many of these structures are present in

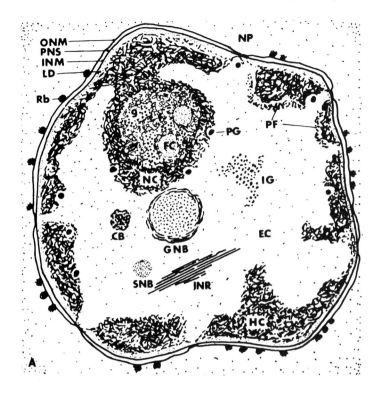

FIG. 4A. Ideal section of a nucleus, showing all major components. The nucleus is surrounded by outer (ONM) and inner (INM) nuclear membranes, which enclose the perinuclear space (PNS), which is a part of the rough endoplasmic reticulum and has ribosomes (Rb) attached. Between the chromatin and the inner membrane lies the lamina densa (LD), which is thinner in front of the nuclear pores (NP). The chromatin is found as heterochromatin (HC), nucleolus-associated chromatin (NC), and euchromatin (EC). The nucleolus shows granular (g) components and fibrillar centers (FC). In the borderline of the chromatin, many perichromatin granules (PG) and a layer of perichromatin fibrils (PF) (of which only a portion has been drawn) are present. In the interchromatin space, a cluster of interchromatin granules (IG), granular nuclear body (GNB), simple nuclear body (SNB), coiled body (CB), and an intranuclear rodlet (INR) have been drawn. (From ref. 17a.)

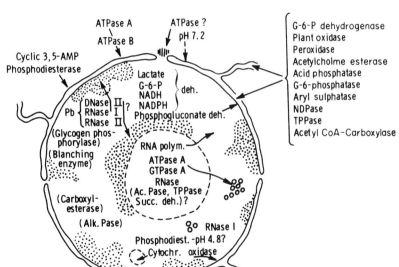

FIG. 4B. Diagram illustrating localization of cytochemically detectable enzymes in different components of the cell nucleus. *Dotted areas;* condensed chromatin; *small circles,* interchromatinic granules; *interrupted line,* and the nucleolus. The enzymes in brackets were observed only in isolated cases. The question mark indicates that the presence of the enzyme is uncertain. Alk. Pase, alkaline phosphatase; Ac. Pase, acid phosphatase; TPPase, thiamine pyrophosphatase; Succ. deh., succinic dehydrogenase. (From ref. 34.)

such small amounts that no specific biochemical studies have been made.

CHROMATIN

As noted above, the main constituent of the nucleus is chromatin, which is a complex of nuclear DNA, its associated proteins, RNA, and small molecules (18). Chromatin is the interphase state of the chromosomes and has been the object of intensive investigations, which are now improving in precision despite the enormous complexity and unusual properties of chromatin.

The basic problems in manipulation of chromatin relate to the difficulties in handling of chemical evaluations of molecules of such enormous size as DNA, which is now generally believed to be as long as the chromatids. The former concept that each chromosome contained hundreds of thousands of individual DNA molecules has now been largely discarded in favor of the idea that the DNA is essentially continuous in these giant structures.

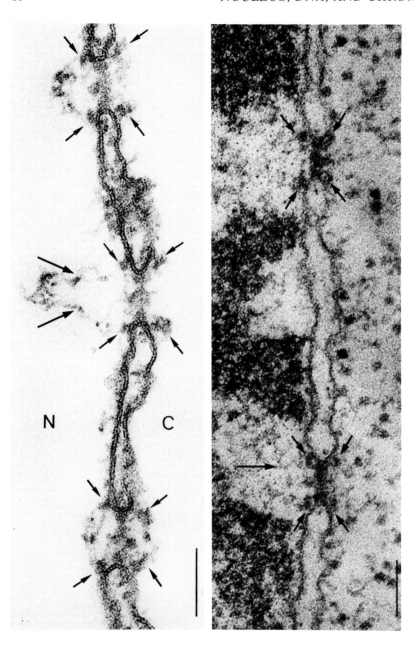

FIG. 5A. Section through the nuclear envelope showing the continuous nature of the membrane and discontinuities at nuclear pores. Pores are not empty but contain stainable hazy components (*arrows*). C, cytoplasm; N, nucleus. (From ref. 12.)

The task of sorting out a specific DNA cistron in an intact form from such structures has challenged many investigators. Except for rare cases, such as the "amplified" and segregated rDNA found in some "statellites," individual DNA species had not been isolated from chromatin until recently. With cloning and restriction endonucleases, much information is accumulating.

NUCLEAR PROTEINS-HISTONES

DNA-associated proteins have added to the complexity of the problem. It has long been known (19) that the histones in chromatin are approximately equal in weight to the DNA; furthermore, DNA is closely associated with histones in somatic cells. Accordingly

it appeared that the histones had some critical structural or stabilizing role, particularly since the number of charges that were positive on the histones were roughly equal to the number of negative charges on the DNA.

There are significant interactions between histones, which are sufficient in themselves to produce small nuclear bodies (Fig. 13), referred to as "nu bodies" (20). These nu bodies are apparently composed of histone subunits, i.e., one molecule each of histone 2A, 2B, 3, and 4. They may be related to structures containing only histone 1. The role of nu bodies is undefined. They are randomly distributed in both transcribed and untranscribed chromatin. Moreover, virtually all the liver sequences transcribed into mRNA are present in "nu body-associated DNA." Accord-

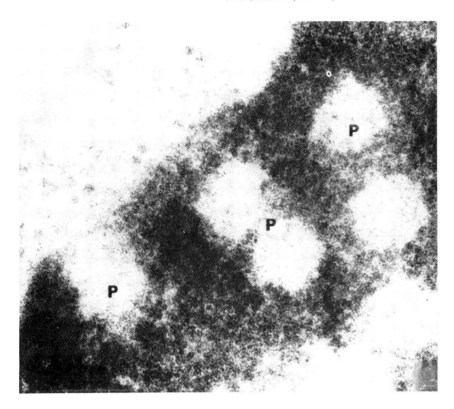

FIG. 5B. Vertical section through the nuclear envelope at the nuclear pores (P). (From ref. 12.)

ingly, nu body formation is random with respect to DNA sequence, and the presence of nu bodies in a specific DNA region is not sufficient to restrict transcription.

Histones contain a variety of modified structures, including phosphoserine, acetylserine, mono- and dimethyllysine, methylarginine, and other phosphorylated derivatives, including phosphohistidine. The extent of phosphorylation of specific histones varies with the stages of the cell cycle. During cell division, phosphorylation of many histones has been demonstrated (21).

One specific phosphorylation, i.e., that of histone 1, the lysine-rich histone group, has been studied by Langan (22,23) in relation to the hormonal effects of glucagon. The specificity of the phosphorylation suggests that there may be a specific interaction between this histone and the genome. No precise interaction between the phosphorylated histone and DNA or other nonhistone or histone proteins has been found (24).

Histone metabolism is of interest primarily because the major synthetic reactions involved in histone formation occur during or shortly prior to the synthesis of DNA. Some evidence exists for histone turnover

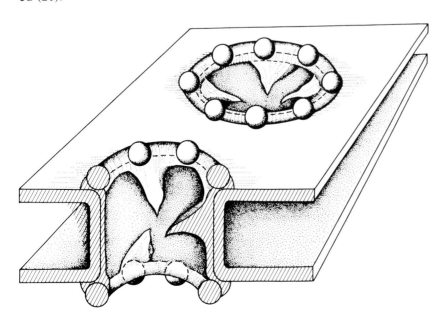

FIG. 6. Model of the pore complex (12). The pore center is frequently occupied by a dense element of variable shape and size. The massive projecting tips contain fibrils, which can be directly visualized in certain cells and preparations. Such internal fibrils can be radially arranged (often connecting the central granule with the pore wall and the annular granules, respectively) and may constitute a so-called inner ring structure. Fibrillar threads are also seen frequently in continuity with the central and annular granules, especially at the inner (nucleus-oriented) annulus.

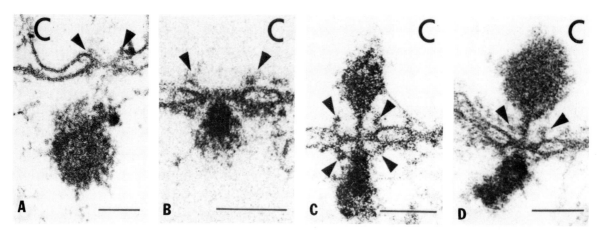

FIG. 7. Possible sequence of events for penetration of the pore complexes (*arrowheads,* some annular granules). The large globule approaches the pore complex and becomes connected to it by thin filaments **(A)**; it reaches the pore center **(B)** and elongates into a 100 to 150 Å broad rod. The material passes the pore center in this rod-like form, transitorily assuming a typical dumbbell-shaped configuration **(C)**. The material rounds into a spheroid particle **(D)** is deposited on the cytoplasmic side (C). **A,** × 83,000; **B,** × 135,000; **C,** × 110,000; **D,** × 100,000. Bars, 0.1 μm. (From ref. 12.)

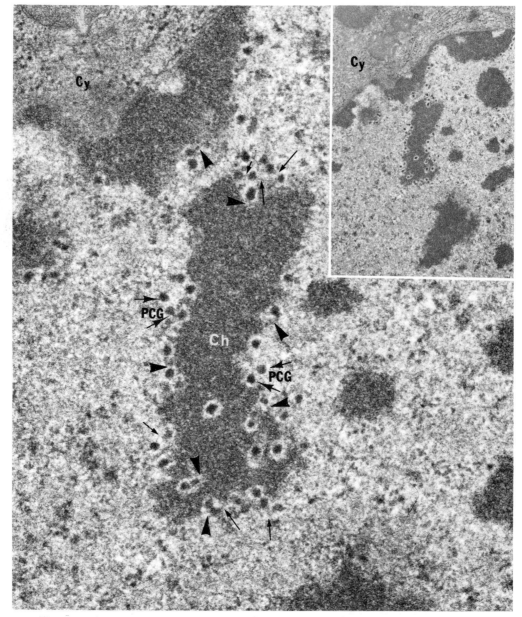

FIG. 8. High magnification of perichromatin granule (PCG) complex in rat liver nucleus treated with 200 mg/kg cycloheximide. Perichromatin fibrils (*arrowheads*) connect the PCG to the chromocenter (Ch). Finer filaments (*arrows*) interconnect the PCG proper. Cy, cytoplasm (× 62,000). **Inset,** × 15,750.

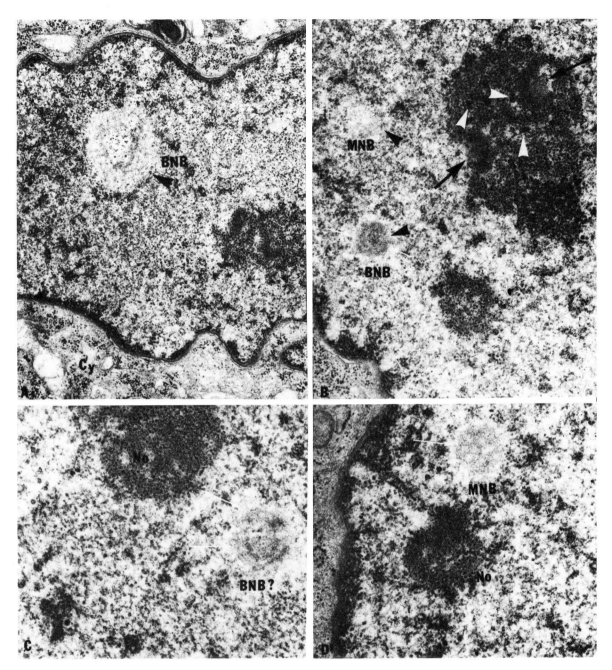

FIG. 9. Type 1 alveolar epithelial cells from a patient. **A:** Beaded nuclear body (BNB) (*black arrowheads*) may be differentiated into a membranous cortex and a granular core. × 127,000. **B:** Nucleoli contain fibrillar centers (*arrows*), condensed fibrillar components, and microspherules (*white arrowheads*). × 31,500. At higher magnifications, **(C)** nuclear bodies are surrounded by a halo of low electron density (*white arrows*). In this halo, fine filaments interconnect the nuclear body and nucleoplasmic components. This particular nuclear body appears to be intermediate between the membranous and beaded variety. × 40,500. **D:** Alveolar interstitial fibroblast with a characteristic membranous nuclear body (MNB). Lead citrate-uranyl acetate staining. × 41,000.

throughout the cell cycle, but there is little information on the rates and extent of these synthetic events.

Recently, much attention has been directed to the genes coding for histones. Poly(A−) histone mRNA is produced in high concentration prior to synthesis of histones, and following the S phase of the cell cycle, its concentration diminishes rapidly. There has been considerable interest in the mechanisms of histone synthe-

sis, particularly with respect to the role of nonhistone proteins in stimulating synthesis of histone mRNA by specific interaction with the genome (6). In the case of histone mRNA synthesis, it appears that a specific nonhistone protein plays a special role in initiating these synthetic reactions.

Another facet of histone synthesis that has become of great interest is the arrangement of histone mes-

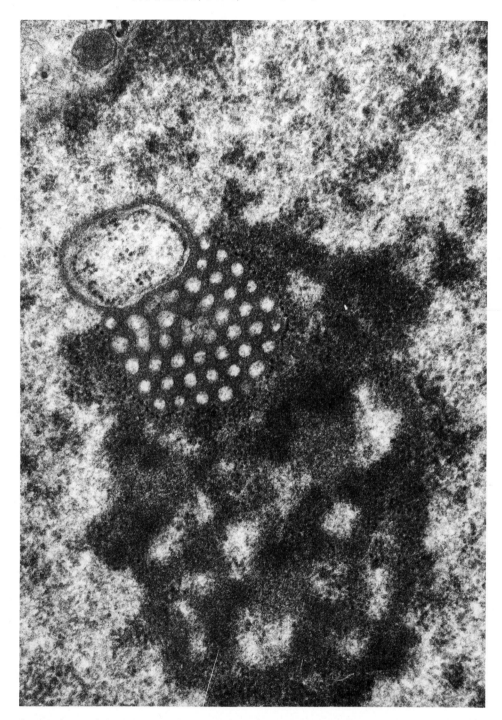

FIG. 10. Portion of an endometrial secretory cell nucleolus showing the nucleolar channel system at the periphery. The system appears to have a honeycomb-like structure in a circular profile about 500 to 600 Å in diameter. The channels contain amorphous material of low density and small granules and are embedded in a rather dense, amorphous matrix material. Peripheral to the matrix is a row of densely staining 150 Å granules which are denser than the nucleolar granular elements. An apparent invagination of cytoplasm is present in the region just above and to the left of the nucleolar channel system. × 47,700. (Courtesy of Dr. John A. Terzakis, Columbia University.)

sages on the DNA sequences, i.e., the precise positioning of the histone genes, coding for specific histone fractions. At present, this area is being explored by several investigators.

Nonhistone Nuclear Proteins

It is well recognized that most (if not all) nuclear proteins are synthesized in the cytoplasm and must be

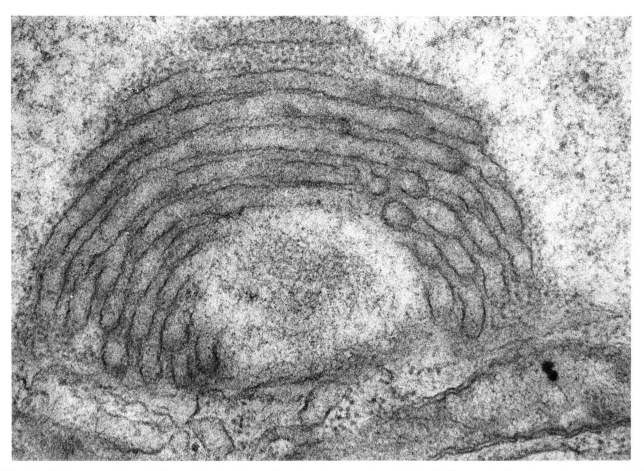

FIG. 11. High-power view of the nucleolar channel system in an endometrial cell. The nucleolar channels are bounded by a well-defined, triple-layered membrane. Within a channel, long fibrils are present. × 85,000. (Courtesy John A. Terzakis, Columbia University.)

present there in small amounts (25). Procedures for nuclear isolation (8) result in preparations that will simplify the already complex problems of nuclear protein chemistry (26).

It has become clear (27) that the nonhistone proteins are a heterogeneous series of molecular species, including proteins of the nuclear envelope, the nuclear sap, chromatin mRNP, and those of the nucleolus (Table 3). Each of these groups contains important subgroups that include various enzymes, phosphoproteins, processing enzymes, and transport elements (18).

In recent years, great interest has centered on proteins that are "chromatin associated," largely because "gene control proteins" are present in these fractions (Table 4). The evidence that gene control proteins are in chromatin was obtained by preextraction of citric acid nuclei with dilute salt solution (0.15 M NaCl, 0.1 M Tris) followed by distilled water to swell the chromatin. Following these extractions, the residue, called "chromatin," was demonstrated to exhibit "fidelity" of transcription by analysis of products generated after incubation with RNA polymerase and appropriately

labeled nucleoside triphosphates. The products produced were then hybridized in competition studies with RNA of specific tissues (28–30). A key finding was that on reconstitution of the chromatin initially dissociated with high salt (2 M NaCl, 5 M urea, 0.01 M Tris, pH 8.3), the RNA transcripts were characteristic of the tissue or origin of the nonhistone proteins and not the DNA or the histones. Subsequent findings have supported these conclusions (Table 4).

A crucial unanswered question is whether nonhistone proteins specifically bind to DNA or to other types of proteins. Many DNA-binding proteins have been found in eukaryotic cells. Although their interaction with DNA may account for their activity, a clearcut demonstration of "1 protein:1 mRNA" has not yet been established.

Studies on binding of hormones to nonhistone proteins (Table 4) have been interesting. The studies of Jensen and DeSombre (31) on estrogen receptor interaction initiated much work in this field (Table 4). Studies of O'Malley and Means (32) have shown a clearcut relationship between the steroid hormone-receptor complex and the production of special mRNA

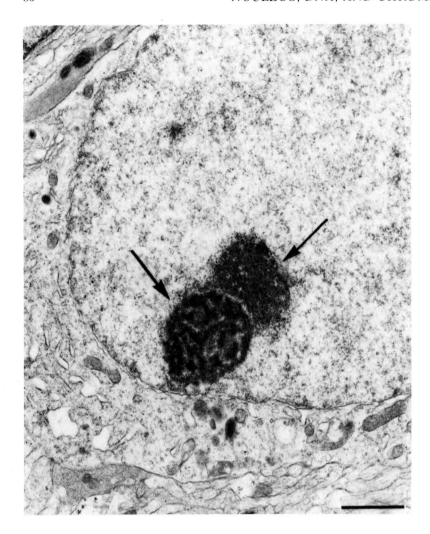

FIG. 12. Nucleolus (*left arrow*) with satellite body (*right arrow*) in a pyramidal neuron in the cerebral cortex of a rat. Specimens were postfixed in osmium tetroxide after perfusion of the rat with 2% formaldehyde and glutaraldehyde. × 15,300. (Courtesy W. Caley, Department of Anatomy, Baylor College of Medicine.)

related to oviduct proteins. A diagram of these interactions was developed by Higgins and associates (33) (Fig. 14).

The nonhistone proteins serve important enzymatic functions (Table 5) and have interesting nuclear localizations (34) (Fig. 4). Some of these proteins bind to mRNA in complex systems for processing and splicing reactions.

Links Between the Nonhistone Proteins and the Histones

Two-dimensional gel electrophoresis has shown that there are many nuclear protein molecules (Fig. 15), in excess of 1,000 types (1,35–39). Continuing efforts to isolate and identify individual nuclear proteins led to the demonstration of new HMG molecules (high mobility proteins) by Goodwin et al. (40). A particularly interesting protein, A24, so named because of its migration on 2-D gel electrophoresis, appears to be a conjugated form of histone 2A and ubiquitin, a polypeptide bound to histone 2A, apparently in an isopeptide linkage (41). The ubiquitin can be cleaved

off physiologically. Although the functional role of this protein is not yet known, the nonhistone "arm" of the protein may be a lever by which the 2A histone may be a site for HMG and other protein associated with DNA. This possibility was suggested by the changes observed in nucleolar content of protein A24 during activation of nucleolar function (Fig. 16).

Of the other proteins currently identified, the silver-staining phosphoprotein C23 (42) appears to have some derepressor function or enhancement of RNA polymerase activity. The possibility that some of these proteins serve as specific derepressors remains to be evaluated. Moreover, the possibility that specific proteins interact with "receptor-protein complexes" is under study with respect to hormonal systems and undoubtedly will be studied for other types of systems as well.

Goldstein (43) has suggested that there is a class of "nucleocytoplasmic" or "cytonucleoprotein" proteins or nucleic acids which are in relatively constant communication between the nucleus and the cytoplasm. Such proteins might serve to carry information into the nucleus and thereby provide one arm of the feedback loop that affects overall cellular function. Such

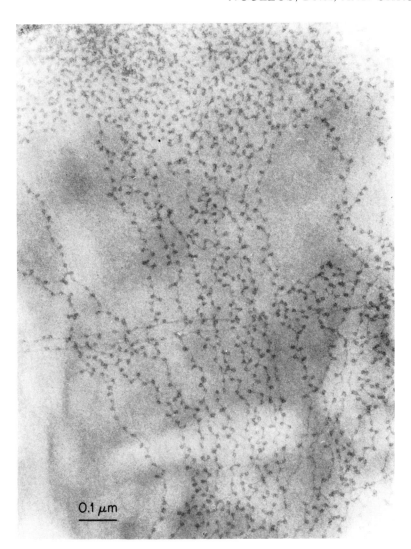

FIG. 13. Nu bodies. Chromatin fibers streaming out of a rat thymus nucleus. Spheroid chromatin units (nu bodies) exhibit local variations in arrangement and separation, possibly due to differential stretching of the fibers. Negative stain 0.5% ammonium molybdate, pH 7.4. ×293,000. (From ref. 18.)

0.1 μm

"informational proteins" or "receptor proteins" that are present in the cytoplasm for longer periods of time may be in rapid equilibrium with the cell nucleus. Their entry into the nucleus may be related to conformational changes or to other changes, such as binding to specific elements or interaction with other polypeptide molecules. It has been suggested that such proteins may be in the nucleoplasm or in the group of readily extractable nuclear proteins (0.15 M NaCl, 0.35 M NaCl). It will be necessary in future years to clarify the roles of the various proteins in these extracts so that more meaningful information can be derived regarding their nuclear distribution and function.

Metaphase Chromosomes

Although the functional state of the chromatin is largely represented by the interphase amorphous nucleus, the most dramatic changes in the chromosomes occur during mitosis. These chromosomes are identified by their sizes and shapes as well as their banding patterns when stained with special stains. The complexity of the chromosomes has only recently become visualizable by scanning electron microscopic techniques, which permit a clearer appreciation of the detailed ultrastructure of chromosomes (Fig. 17). The chromosomes per se offer a particularly interesting opportunity for studies of genetic aberrations as well as their relationships to human clinical disorders. Once the chromosomes enter metaphase, the synthetic reactions involving their template function cease, and no new RNA is made. As pointed out by Hodge et al. (44), protein synthesis does continue during metaphase and the polysomes carry over into the next generation of daughter cells (Fig. 18). The ramifications of these events for the transmission of genetic information are indeed important.

During the last decade, there has been remarkable evolution of new information on chromosomes of eukaryotic cells, their underlying structure, and important aspects of gene localization. For many years, the localization of nucleolus organizer regions (NORs) was identified by means of secondary constrictions

Table 3. *Nuclear nonhistone proteins*

Nuclear membrane proteins
    Structural proteins
    Transport proteins
    Processing enzymes
    Nuclear pore proteins
Nuclear sap proteins
    Cytonucleoproteins
      Receptors, normal and modified
      RNP particle proteins
        Small U1 and U2 RNA
        Samarina particles
      Informosomes
    Phosphoproteins
    Enzymes
Chromatin-bound proteins
    Solubility classification
      Acid soluble
        Acid soluble
        Acid insoluble
          Solubilized by DNase
          DNase residue
      Soluble in dilute NaCl
      Solubility in concentrated NaCl
        Soluble in 2 M NaCl
        Soluble in 3 M NaCl 7 M urea
      Soluble in phenol
      Soluble in sodium dodecyl sulfate
    Structural proteins
    Gene control proteins
    Phosphoproteins
    Enzymes
Nucleolar proteins
    Ribosomal precursor proteins
    Structural proteins
    rDNA control proteins
    Phosphoproteins
    Enzymes

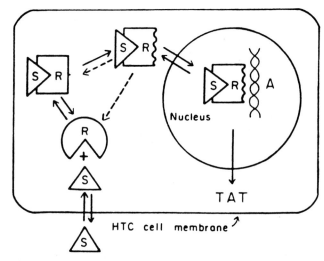

FIG. 14. Early steps in glucocorticoid action. The steroid (S) enters the cell and binds to the cytoplasmic receptor protein (R). In the case of inducer steroids, the receptor-steroid complex has a different conformation from the unbound receptor. Further changes, "activation," occur in the R-S complex, exposing a nuclear binding site. The active complex binds to the nuclear acceptor site (A), and tyrosine aminotransferase (TAT) is eventually induced. (From ref. 33.)

Table 4. *Evidence for specificity of nonhistone proteins (NHP)*[a]

Test system
Organ-specific transcription of chromatin
Tissue-specific restriction of DNA
Tissue-specific binding of progesterone receptor
Mechanism of action of female sex hormones
NHP in chromatin—organ specificity
Tumor transcriptional specificity; regenerating liver specificity
Tissue specificity of NHP
Antigenic specificity of chromatin
Specificity of mitotic proteins
Phosphoproteins in gene regulation
Stimulation of synthesis by phytohemagglutinin

[a] From ref. 18.

seen in various types of chromosomes. Special techniques, such as those employed by Ruddle and colleagues have permitted mapping of specific markers on special chromosomes.

To detail the progress of chromosomology would necessitate an extensive review of both markers and ultrastructural analysis, which are beyond the scope of this chapter (1,45,45a). It should be noted, however, that despite the extensive progress that has been made in this complex and important field, an enormous amount of information is yet to be obtained, particularly because the structures present in the metaphase chromosomes are so complex. At least two of the chromosome components that are particularly relevant to nuclear elements are well identified, i.e., the gene segments coding for histones (46), and for rRNA (8). In both instances, the information obtained is fragmentary but offers a basis for intensive studies on other gene segments.

RNA

In a sense, mRNA synthesis is the most specific nuclear function. The biosynthetic reactions involve complex events in enzymatic and structural chemistry. Through interaction of specific nonhistone proteins with the genome, specific mRNA species are produced and transported to the cytoplasm (Fig. 18). Recently, specific individual mRNA species have been isolated, including mRNA for hemoglobin, histones, globin, albumin and ovalbumin. The polysomes, which ultimately translate mRNA into proteins, are associated with a host of initiation and elongation factors.

Synthesis of mRNA

The processes involved in RNA synthesis are apparently similar to those for rRNA synthesis. The en-

Table 5. *Nuclear enzymes*

RNA synthesis and processing
RNA polymerases A, B, etc.
RNA modification enzymes; methylases, formation of modified bases
RNA trimming or special cleavage enzymes
RNases; exo- and endonucleolytic

DNA synthesis
  "True" synthetases
  Ligases
  Excision enzymes
  Terminal addition enzymes
  DNases
  Modification enzymes; methylases, etc.

Other modification and synthetic enzymes
Histone phosphokinases, methylases acetylases, de-acetylases, proteases
  Nonhistone protein kinases and methylases
  Nucleoside kinases
  NAD pyrophosphorylase

Dehydrogenases
  Steroid dehydrogenase
  Cytochrome oxidase
  Glycerol-3-phosphate dehydrogenases
  Glyceraldehyde-3-phosphate dehydrogenase
  Succinate, malate, isocitrate, lactate, NADH. NADPH. glucose 6-phosphate, phosphogluconate
Transferases: glycosyl for glycogen phosphorylases and branching enzymes
Enzymes of uncertain function
  ATPases
  Carboxylesterases
  Phosphatases
  5'-Nucleotidases
  Phosphodiesterase

zyme RNA polymerase II catalyzes transcription of mRNA as a consequence of the availability of "open gene complexes." This enzyme and associated factors link nucleoside triphosphates covalently into 3',5'-phosphodiester bonds of mRNA. There are critical elements of the "initiation reactions" involved in starting these gene readouts, as well as termination factors that are still only incompletely understood. Although mRNA is linearly synthesized in the nucleus, critical modification reactions are known to occur at each end of mRNA (Fig. 19). A large portion of the mRNA molecules become polyadenylated; i.e., an oligomer of approximately 200 adenylic residues is added to the 3' end by a poly(A) polymerase reaction (47).

Virtually all functional mRNA contains "5' cap" structures essential for activity in protein synthesis (Fig. 19). The 5' cap is added by a series of reactions involving guanylyl transferases and methylating enzymes that form the $m^7G(5')ppp(5')Y^mpZ^mp$ "cap." The formation of this cap probably occurs partly in the nucleus and partly in the cytoplasm. The 5' cap appears to serve as an allosteric binding site for proteins involved in the initiation of protein synthesis or for mRNA binding directly to special ribosomal proteins (19,47).

Studies of specialized mRNA species, such as globin mRNA, ovalbumin mRNA, and others, have been successful. Although the specific enzyme RNA polymerase II is involved in transcription of the DNA, it must be closely associated in these transcriptional events with the methylases, pyrophosphorylases, and poly(A) polymerases that are responsible for the synthesis of the completed mRNA. In addition, important

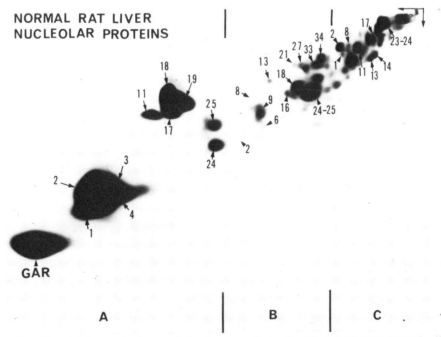

NORMAL RAT LIVER
NUCLEOLAR PROTEINS

GAR

A   B   C

FIG. 15. Separation of acid soluble nucleolar proteins by two-dimensional gel electrophoresis (35), 10% acid-urea horizontal dimension, 12% SDS vertical dimension.

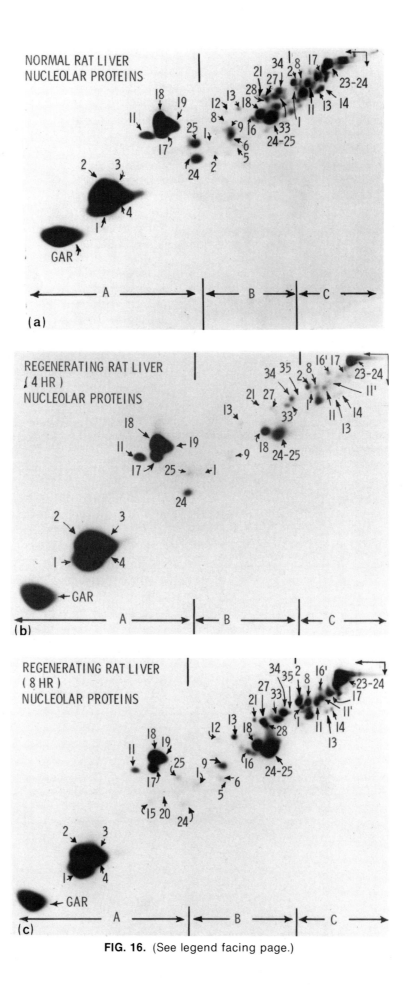

FIG. 16. (See legend facing page.)

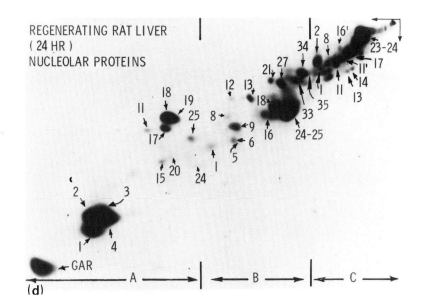

FIG. 16. A–D. Two-dimensional gel electrophoretic patterns of normal and regenerating liver nucleolar proteins (35). Marked changes were found in the concentration of proteins A11, A24, C13, and C14 from the normal levels **(a)**, 4-hr **(b)**, 8-hr **(c)**, and 24-hr **(d)** of regenerating liver.

initiation and termination factors have been identified in both bacterial and eukaryotic systems. For detailed studies on transcription of a specific mRNA, more sharply defined systems must be developed. Among the more satisfactory studies thus far are those on transcription of globin mRNA sequences from bone marrow chromatin (48,49). DNA-dependent RNA polymerase II has been shown to transcribe globin gene sequences under appropriate conditions.

Timing of mRNA Synthesis

The synthesis of mRNA occurs in individual cells and in specialized tissues in an ordered time frame, which is essential for production of products initially in the fetus and later in specific adult tissues. One of the most important types of timing for mRNA synthesis is that occurring during the cell cycle, particularly in the G_1, S, and G_2 phases. There is greater interest in this subject because of the "cycle-specific proteins" present in growing and dividing tissues which have been shown to have high antigenic activities (50).

Processing of Newly Synthesized mRNA

Initially, it was thought that the primary transcript of mRNA is in fact the cytoplasmic mRNA, which must be appropriately methylated and processed on the 5' and 3' ends for its completion. More recently, it has been discovered that mRNA is read as a long precursor molecule (HnRNA, dRNA) that undergoes a series of cleavage reactions to form the specific mRNA product.

Another type of processing that occurs for newly synthesized mRNA is its combination with proteins, particularly the protein in mRNP particles believed to be involved in mRNA transport. Such particles are similar to the RNP particles observed in the nuclear ribonucleoprotein network (8) and the perichromatin granules (Figs. 1,3,4).

Controls of mRNA Production

With respect to DNA of the cell nucleus, most genes that could produce messenger RNA are silent. It is logical that common repressor mechanisms exist, and that only a few "depressor mechanisms" are active; thus reading of 2 to 5% of the total genes occurs. Despite recent suggestions that DNA methylation is involved in gene shut-off, the molecules currently assigned the role of depressors are the nonhistone proteins.

The concept that nonhistone proteins control specific mRNA transcripts implies that there are specific control proteins for many kinds of mRNA molecules. Critical elements may be linked; i.e., one nonhistone protein may regulate the synthesis of several products. Such "coupled synthesis" may be exemplified by rRNA synthesis and the many proteins involved in ribosome formation. Similar kinds of controls may exist for other products, including plasma proteins and clotting factors synthesized by the liver. It is inconceivable, however, that individual nonhistone proteins control each of the reactions of the corresponding messenger RNA species, otherwise there would be an endless cascade of controls.

The question of interlocking controls has been suggested recently (51) to involve self-feedback controls for individual protein species; i.e., regulators, such as "receptor proteins," may regulate their own synthesis. In addition, a single receptor-protein complex may not only stimulate production of several messages but may also activate gene segments for both rRNA and ribosomal protein synthesis (Fig. 20).

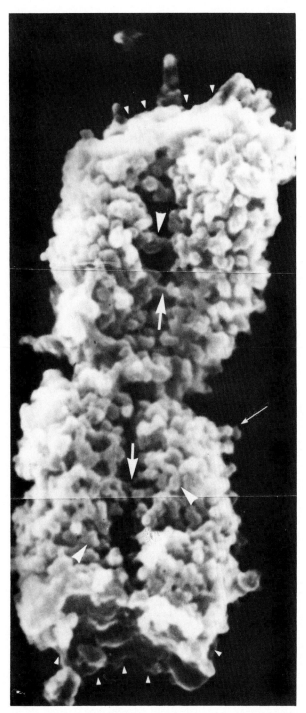

FIG. 17. Scanning electron micrograph of whole-mount isolated CHO metaphase chromosome 2. Membranous plate-like structures (*small arrowheads*) connects both chromatids only at their distal ends. Multiple inter-chromatidal connections (*large arrows*) are seen in the interchromatidal furrow. Highly coiled topical "micro-convules" (*large arrowheads*) and axial coiling (*small arrows*) are present. × 65,000. (From ref. 70.)

Chromosomal RNA

Specific "chromosomal RNA species" have been reported to exert significant roles in effecting the syn-

thesis of mRNA. One of the suggested functions for the low molecular weight nuclear RNA (LMWN RNA) is that they function as "gene gates" or to maintain "stable open complexes" in the genome (52,53). At present, little evidence exists for a specifying role for low molecular weight RNA for control or derepression of the genes. Rather, there appear to be more satisfactory lines of evidence for a special role of these molecules, particularly in "splicing" of pre-mRNA. The older results on 3.3 S chromosomal RNAs are no longer considered to be valid, inasmuch as they may be degradation artifacts.

THE NUCLEOLUS

The nucleolus (Fig. 1) synthesizes about 85% of all cellular RNA and plays an essential role in production of new ribosomes (8). It is the product of NORs of chromatin, which apparently contain the rDNA and the specific sites of structural organization for interlocking nucleolar proteins and RNA products. The nucleolus is the sole cellular location of specific cellular and nuclear components (Table 6). One remarkable facet of nucleolar function is the production of the enormous chains of nucleotides (12,000) of 45 S pre-rRNA synthesized by RNA polymerase I (54–56) with great rapidity on repetitive genes. These are methylated, cleaved, and modified as the molecules are being formed. In addition, the nucleolus is a site of protein binding to the newly synthesized RNA to form the nucleolar granular elements (Fig. 21). These granular elements are the RNP products of the nucleolus (Fig. 20); after isolation by various procedures, they have been shown to contain the modified long preribosomal RNA chains and, in addition, some proteins that migrate to cytoplasmic ribosomes and others that do not.

Further maturation of nucleolar products occurs in the nuclear ribonucleoprotein network (8), which may provide the locus for joining additional ribosomal and polysomal proteins to these preribosomal elements to complete the fully matured polysomes. The fibrillar elements of the nucleolus apparently provide the matrix composed of rDNA, the RNA polymerase, and juxtaposed enzymes. These elements are involved in the earliest stages of preribosomal RNA synthesis.

Light Spaces

"Light spaces" are visible in many nucleoli between the fibrillar and granular masses (Fig. 21). These spaces are probably the nucleololini reported by Love and Soriano (57) to contain important nucleolar elements, including perhaps some important nucleolar enzymes. Unfortunately, no satisfactory methods have been developed to isolate or identify the compo-

NUCLEUS **CYTOPLASM**

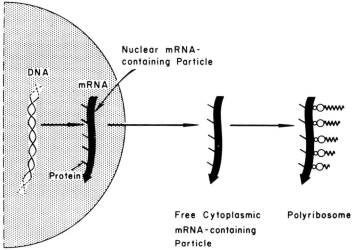

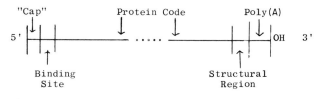

FIG. 18. Scheme of synthesis and transport of mRNA from the nucleus to cytoplasm where it functions as part of the polyribosome complex. (Courtesy of Dr. Edgar C. Henshaw, Harvard University Medical School.)

nents of the light spaces or to evaluate their structural and functional roles. The soluble elements of these structures likely are extracted by a variety of nucleolar fractionation procedures.

rDNA

Beginning with the demonstration of the NOR by Heitz (58) and the studies of McClintock (59,60), extensive studies have been made on nucleolar DNA in a wide variety of species (8). The "secondary constrictions" or NOR in chromosomes have been described earlier. The presence in the nucleolus of several classes of DNA has been demonstrated by light and electron microscopic techniques, including special stains, i.e., acridine orange, coriphosphine O, Feulgen stain, and methyl green. Some DNA regions can be "geographically" segregated into perinucleolar chromatin and intranucleolar chromatin. rDNA can also be subfractioned into condensed and dispersed nucleolar chromatin. The precise coding chromatin for nucleolar rDNA has not yet been defined in geographical entities. Accordingly, it is still unknown whether pre-rRNA migrates centrifugally from within the nucleolar matrix.

Aside from the localization of DNA within the nucleolus by staining techniques, splendid electron microscopic analysis has been made of DNA within the nucleoli after specific types of digestion (8). These microscopic studies have supported the concept that the genes for production of rRNA are localized to specific chromosomal regions and are not randomly dispersed. With the spreading technique developed by Kleinschmidt (61), Miller and Beatty (62) made excellent studies on "Christmas tree" patterns for synthesis of rRNA in the nucleolar cores of Xenopus (Fig. 22). The results support the reported tandem redundant

RNA genes simultaneously transcribed along the nucleolar matrix. Although these products have still not been related to chemical entities, the concept of progressive growth of chains fits well to the concept of long final products of pre-RNA and the associated RNP.

With the development of improved hybridization techniques, attempts have been made to establish specific information on the localization of rDNA genes. The concentration of rDNA in the nucleolus is 10 times that of rDNA throughout the remainder of the nucleus (Fig. 23). Accordingly, the nucleoli contain 90% or more of total rDNA, at least in Novikoff hepatoma ascites cells (63,64).

Products of Nucleolar RNA

The original RNA product of the nucleolus consists of 45 S pre-RNA and oligomers of sedimentation coefficients up to 85 S. By a series of unique and specific endonucleolytic cleavages, these giant nucleolar RNAs are cleaved to three major ribosome species: 28 S, 18 S, and 5.8 S rRNA (Fig. 24). The presence of both rRNA species in 45 S nRNA was proved by hybridization competition studies (64). Both 18 S and 28 S rRNA compete with the hybridization of 45 S RNA; when combined, they compete independently. These data indicate that each 45 S nRNA molecule contains one molecule of the two rRNA species.

FIG. 19. Structure of mRNA.

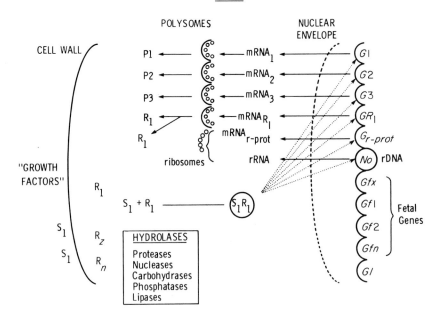

FIG. 20. Response of cells to stimulus (S_1) with formation of stimulus-receptor complex (S_1R_1), which impinges upon a group of genes (G1-GR_1, G_{r-prot}, and $G_{No-rDNA}$), to produce a series of mRNAs, ribosomes, and polysomes, which synthesize specific products, including R_1. The "battery" of fetal genes is not involved in these normal responses. P1-P3, protein readouts.

Ribosomal and Preribosomal RNA

Ribosomal RNA consists of four major types: 28 S, 18 S, and 5.8 S, and 5 S RNA, with approximate molecular weights of 1.7 million, 0.6 million, 50,000, and 40,000, respectively. Each ribosome contains one each of these molecules in its total structure, which has a sedimentation coefficient of approximately 80 S. The 18 S and 28 S rRNA molecules are the backbones of the 40 S and 60 S subunits of the ribosomes. The 5 S RNA molecule apparently is part of a small ribonucleoprotein particle in the 60 S ribosomal subunit. It is essential for the function of the ribosome, but a definitive function has not yet been defined. Unequivocal evidence has now been provided that the source of ribosomal 5.8 and 28 S RNA is the nucleolus, but the source of the 5 S RNA is extranucleolar. It is apparently synthesized on a one-to-one basis with the other ribosomal RNA species. The sequence of 5.8 S rRNA has recently been defined.

Table 6. *Specific nucleolar components*

rDNA
U3 low molecular weight RNA
Specific elements
Fibrillar elements
Granular elements
Interelement "spaces"
Proteins
RNA polymerase I
Silver staining proteins B23, C23

Spacers

As shown in Fig. 24, there are several products, P1, P2, and P3, referred to as spacers, i.e., segments of 45 S RNA readouts, that do not appear in the final ribosome products. These spacers are currently under study; spacer regions may contain U-rich segments. Studies are necessary to position the loci of the U-rich segments in the overall 45 S RNA sequences. Brown and his colleagues (64a) made extensive studies on the regions between the rDNA gene loci, i.e., the "gene spacers." Their impression is that the spacer regions are specific species. On the other hand, the coding regions for rRNA are constant from species to species.

Nucleolar Proteins and Control of Nucleolar Function

Nucleolar proteins can be divided as follows: (a) structural elements, including (i) the histones, (ii) special proteins of the preribosomal particles, and (iii) ribosomal proteins; (b) enzymes of RNA synthesis (RNA polymerase I) and processing (exonucleases and endonucleases); and (c) gene control proteins. Although there is much information on proteins of the first group, gene control proteins are least well understood and perhaps the most important. Control of nucleolar function in gene expression may reside in specific elements that are either phosphoproteins (see below) or other specific types of nonhistone proteins. Moreover, the important participation of the nucleolus

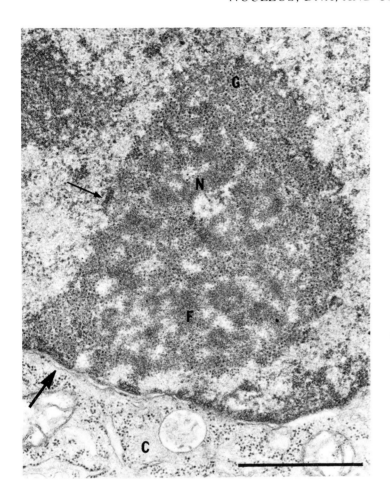

FIG. 21. Electron micrograph of a nucleolus (N) *in situ* showing the fibrillar elements (F) and the granular elements (G). *Heavy arrow,* outer layer of the nuclear envelope; *thin arrow,* nuclear rodlet. Between the fibrillar elements of the nucleolus are the light spaces, which undoubtedly are filled with enzymes and other functional elements of the nucleolus. C, cytoplasm. Bar = 1 nm.

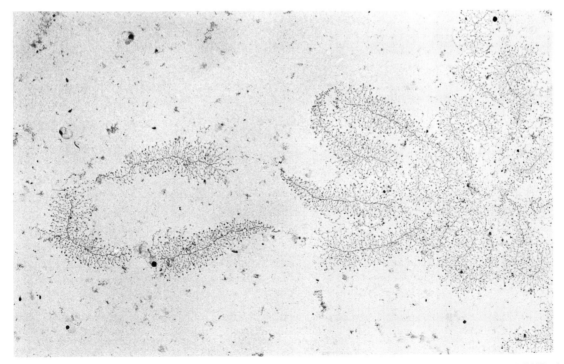

FIG. 22. "Miller" picture of "Christmas trees" of nucleolar rRNA readouts, synthesized preribosomal RNP elements. (Courtesy of Dr. O. L. Miller.)

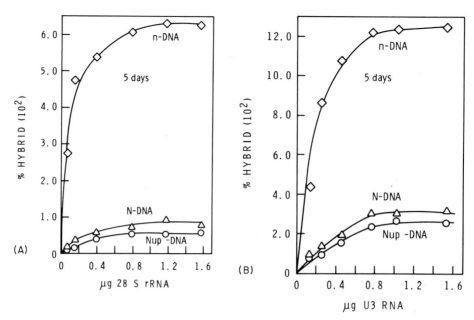

FIG. 23. (A) Hybridization plateau (5 days) of 28S rRNA with nucleolar DNA (n-DNA), whole nuclear DNA (N-DNA), and extranucleolar DNA (Nup-DNA). **(B)** Similar hybridization plateaus (5 days) for U3 low molecular weight RNA which is limited in localization to the nucleolus.

in many regulatory and phase-specific events indicates that such proteins must be commonly involved in increased gene activity.

With improved methods for isolation of rDNA and various binding proteins, it is now possible to achieve a more satisfactory approach to isolation and analysis of proteins involved in promotion or derepression of rDNA and DNA_{r-prot}. Such studies are important in understanding production of most cellular RNA and specific controls on this major gene set.

At one time, the nucleolus was considered a simple structure with a small number of elements. The development of technology for determination of the numbers and types of those constituents has led to the view

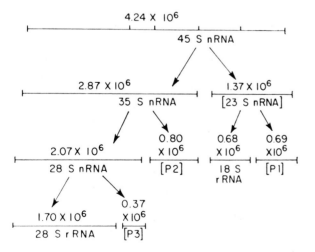

FIG. 24. Cleavage reactions of nucleolar 45S RNA. n, Nucleolar; r, ribosomal; P1, P2, and P3, postulated polynucleotide intermediates, which have not yet been defined.

that the nucleolus contains more than 200 species of proteins (35). Two-dimensional polyacrylamide gel electrophoresis (Fig. 15) has established that in addition to all the varieties of histones, approximately 90 nonhistone proteins are extractable from nucleoli with 0.4 N H_2SO_4. Another group of proteins is acid-insoluble but is extractable under conditions that require solvents that dissociate hydrogen bonds and destroy hydrophobic molecular reactions. RNA polymerase I that is uniquely localized to the nucleolus accounts for several polypeptides, which are presumably enzyme subunits. Also, many proteins are elements of the nucleolar ribonucleoproteins of the granular elements (Fig. 21) and the ribosomes. Presumably, control elements in the nucleolus require much more careful identification and analysis.

Of the nuclear phosphoproteins, one is specifically localized to the nucleolus, i.e., protein C23, a recently described nucleolus-specific phosphoprotein that apparently accounts for the bulk of ^{32}P incorporated into nucleolar proteins (65). This silver staining protein (42) contains highly acidic phosphopeptides (66).

MORPHOLOGICAL CORRELATES OF ALTERED rRNA PRODUCTION

Almost all cell growth or cell enlargement is intimately correlated with the synthesis of new ribosomes. In this process, the nucleolus plays a major role, exemplified by its enlargement and the corresponding increase in the number of granular elements. The synthetic reactions of the nucleolus are catalyzed by RNA polymerase I, a specific polymerase localized to the nucleolus. The activity in synthesis of pre-rRNA varies greatly with the state of the nucleolus and the cell. In cells, such as the circulating lymphocyte, there is a small nucleolus, and the amount of rRNA produced is correspondingly very limited. The ultrastructure of these nucleoli was extensively studied by Busch and Smetana (8), who referred to them as "ring-shaped" nucleoli, although in three dimensions they are "shell-like." The amount of granular elements produced by these nucleoli is very small, and the rate of ribosome replacement is correspondingly limited. The nucleolus of the normal liver is also a rather small structure; it contains relatively large amounts of fibrillar elements and relatively small amounts of granular elements.

The nucleoli with the highest rates of production of ribosomes are those of rapidly growing tissues, including malignant tumors, regenerating liver, "activated" lymphocytes, and nucleoli of some drug-treated tissues (i.e., nucleoli of thioacetamide-treated cells). In the normal liver, the rate of production of 45 S pre-rRNA is approximately 3 to 5 fg/min/nucleolus. In thioacetamide-treated cells and in some malignant tumors, the rate of 45 S pre-rRNA biosynthesis is 40 to 45 fg/min/nucleolus.

CONTROL OF NUCLEOLAR RNA SYNTHESIS

In the nucleolus, a series of "triggering events" apparently precedes the synthetic reactions involved in rRNA synthesis. Such reactions are presumably related to gene derepression, i.e., either more rDNA cistrons become available for rRNA synthesis or the activity of the polymerase is increased. A search is in progress in this and other laboratories for specific gene derepressors associated with the activation of these systems. Several different kinds of activation reactions may have a final common pathway of increased rRNA production (Fig. 20).

ENHANCED PRODUCTION OF RIBOSOMES

Although the synthesis of rRNA is essential for production of ribosomes, other kinds of events must occur simultaneously. Included in this category are synthetic reactions for 5 S rRNA, which occurs at extranucleolar loci, and synthesis of ribosomal proteins (r proteins). Although neither of these is as well understood as the synthesis of the rRNA, the mechanism for synthesis of r proteins is somewhat clearer.

There were two possible explanations for increased synthesis of r proteins: (a) increased rates of synthesis on existing $mRNA_{r-prot}$, or (b) increased production of $mRNA_{r-prot}$. These possibilities have been resolved by analysis of the two-dimensional gel products produced

from mRNA of normal liver, regenerating liver, and the Novikoff hepatoma. Evidence is reported for an increase in the amount of mRNA for ribosomal proteins in growing tissues. This increased synthesis is quantitatively similar to the increase in rRNA synthesis; i.e., a five- to sixfold increase in $mRNA_{r-prot}$ has been determined.

COUPLED SYNTHESIS OF rRNA and $mRNA_{prot}$

In a variety of bacterial systems, evidence has been presented for coassociated ribosomal protein and ribosomal RNA synthesis (67–69). This coupling has been based in part on gene proximity, as well as on the obvious need for correlated or simultaneous synthesis. In eukaryotic cells, the synthesis of rRNA and r proteins is only under limited study with respect to its temporal similarity; the likelihood that the two are made together has now been supported by evidence for increases in both products during liver regeneration. Kinetic studies on the relationships of synthesis of r proteins and rRNA (70) have shown a close temporal proximity.

Although the genes for rRNA are clustered and tandemly related, the r protein genes are not identified. The suggestion has been made that the corresponding mRNAs are derived from a broad group of genes in various chromosomes. The "triggers" for their synthesis must be capable of affecting many genes. To establish the mechanisms for these activations will require extensive study because of the numbers and types of genes that must be involved.

HORMONE INDUCTION OF COUPLED SYNTHESIS OF mRNA AND RIBOSOMES

The synthesis of ribosomes, their products, and associated cofactors, which are the elementary cellular machinery for protein synthesis, is closely related to the synthesis of mRNA. In the feedback circuitry of the cell is an overall coupled synthesis of ribosomes, mRNA, and thus the polysomes. Studies of DeSombre et al. (71) and Cohen and Hamilton (51) have established synthesis of a variety of products following administration of estrogens. These products include specific mRNA for the new estrogen-stimulated transcripts as well as the corresponding products related to new ribosome synthesis.

These results establish an unequivocal role for the nucleolus as a responsive gene segment essential to the biosynthesis of new ribosomes for polysomes, either for altered directions of cell function or for replacement of metabolically unstable structures that are necessary for maintenance homeostasis.

LMWN RNA

Special interest from both structural and functional points of view has been recently directly to special LMWN RNA, which differs markedly in structure from other types of cellular RNA. Studies on these molecules showed the remarkable 5' cap of RNA species, which is different from the 5' cap of mRNA by virtue of the presence of the base $m^{2,2,7}$ trimethylguanosine, rather than the m^7G of mRNA in the 5'-terminal nucleotide. The presence of this base apparently eliminates the possibility that translational systems in the cytoplasm can utilize these low molecular weight RNA species.

Of the major U-rich species of the LMWN RNA, only U3 RNA is specifically localized to the nucleolus; it does not appear to be present in any other site in the cell. This RNA must serve an important role in rRNA synthesis. The number of U3 RNA molecules in the nucleolus is approximately 200,000 (0.3 attamoles or 0.2 pg/nucleolus), which is a large excess over the rDNA genes or the numbers of polymerase molecules. These may be regulatory, since many kinds of control elements exceed the number of genes with which they interact; i.e., the estrogen receptors in the cell nucleus exceed (100,000-fold) the number of gene sites available for specific transcripts.

Among the suggestions for the function of the U3 RNA and other LMWN RNA are the following: (a) they maintain "open" gene complexes; (b) they may form a critical component of the nucleolar fibrillar elements, which are the presumed sites of transcription of the rDNA; and (c) they may form an RNP complex with subunits of RNA polymerases which transcribe the RNA.

U1 and U3 SnRNA

The U1, U2, and U3 RNA, for which the sequences are defined, contain the 5' cap structure. Other RNAs for which the structures are known include 4.5 S, U4, and U6 RNA. The 4.5 S RNA structure contains no modified nucleotides and no 5' cap. Little is known about the other molecules in the nucleoplasmic fractions, i.e., 4.5 S RNA_{II}, 4.5 S RNA_{III}, and 5 S RNA. The nucleoplasm contains a minimum of six special RNA species, whereas the nucleolus contains only one. These low molecular weight RNA species are unique molecules and not degradation products of higher molecular weight RNA. However, it is not yet clear whether they have precursors that are high molecular weight (HMW) RNA species. The function of these RNA species is difficult to analyze because the systems involved in their functional role are undefined. They are probably functional as ribonucleoprotein complexes and not as free RNA molecules. Recently, RNP complexes that contain U1 and U2 RNA were extracted from chromatin of Novikoff hepatoma ascites cells with 0.01 M Tris-HCl, pH 8. This same extract contains most of the RNA polymerase activity. These RNP complexes were purified; approximately 10 proteins were associated with U1 and U2 RNA in these fractions (72).

CYTOPLASMIC COMMUNICATION

The nucleus communicates with the cytoplasm by means of polysomes, the ribonucleoprotein particles whose constituents are mRNP particles, and the ribosomal rRNP particles. The mRNP particles contain both the mRNA and special proteins associated with mRNA. The rRNP particles contain a multiplicity of proteins and four major species of RNA: 28 S, 18 S, 5.8 S, and 5 S rRNA. Although these are major products, the nucleus also produces a variety of other RNA species that never pass out into the cytoplasm. The functions of the latter species are unknown at present, although they have been suggested to relate specifically to control mechanisms that affect gene function.

On the other hand, how does the cytoplasm communicate with the nucleus? This subject is one of special interest at present (43). It is generally considered that nuclear proteins of the nonhistone type may have those special functions. Nuclear proteins with communicative functions are thought to carry information related to hormone responses into the nucleus; furthermore, there is increasing evidence that they con-

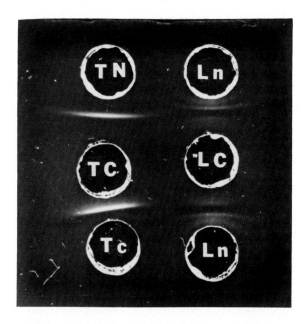

FIG. 25A. Immunoprecipitin bands showing that antibodies to tumor chromatin (TC) and liver chromatin (LC) formed specific immunoprecipitates with liver (Ln) and tumor (TN) nucleolar extracts. Only one dense band was found in the tumor, whereas three (or four) were found for the liver. No cross immunoreactivity was found in these preparations.

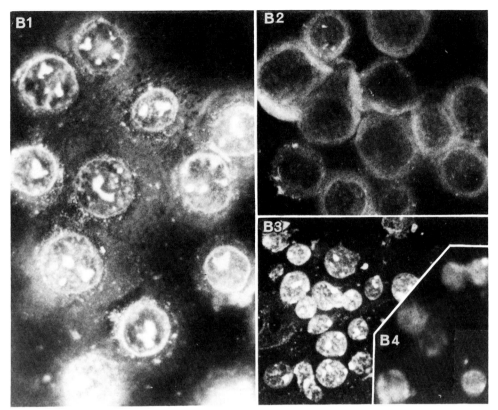

FIG. 25B. Immunofluorescence of cells reacted with preabsorbed antinucleolar antisera; preabsorbed antitumor nucleolar antiserum and Novikoff hepatoma cells **(B1)** or normal liver cells **(B4)**, preabsorbed antiliver nucleolar antiserum with Novikoff hepatoma cells **(B2)** or normal liver cells **(B3)**. All photomicrographs ×1,800.

trol synthesis of globin, histones, and other special proteins. Thus one form of communication depends on movement of molecules from the cytoplasm to the nucleus, where they serve as triggers or specific binding elements for special gene function.

Although the moment-to-moment functioning of the nucleus is becoming better understood, the most dramatic events that occur with respect to the cell nucleus occur during cell division, at which time, great changes take place. The nuclear envelope with its many important structures undergoes virtually complete dissolution; the nuclear chromatin becomes condensed into metaphase chromosomes, and, through a combination of highly specific interactions with tubulin and spindles, the chromosomes segregate into maternal and daughter units. These events terminate with cellular reconstitution and reformation of the stable structures of normal nuclei in new cells. Interestingly, in the course of mitosis, a temporary but total interspersion of nuclear and cytoplasmic elements occurs, which ends abruptly with the reestablishment of a new nuclear envelope in the daughter cells.

Recently, in a search for nuclear elements that may be involved in gene controls, we have been conducting studies on nucleolar antigens (Fig. 25). Differences in antigens of normal liver and tumors have been demonstrable. This approach may be useful in answering

questions about mechanisms of cytoplasmic communication and orderly progress of cell function.

REFERENCES

1. Busch, H. (editor) (1974): Part I. General aspects of molecular biology of cancer. I. Introduction. In: *The Molecular Biology of Cancer*, pp. 1–39. Academic Press, New York.
2. Busch, H. (editor) (1978): *The Cell Nucleus, Chromatin A, Vol. 4.* Academic Press, New York.
3. Busch, H. (editor) (1978): *The Cell Nucleus, Chromatin B, Vol. 5.* Academic Press, New York.
4. Busch, H. (editor) (1978): *The Cell Nucleus, Chromatin C, Vol. 6.* Academic Press, New York.
5. Elgin, S. C. R., and Weintraub, H. (1975): Chromosomal proteins and chromatin structure. *Annu. Rev. Biochem.,* 44:725–774.
6. Stein, G. S., and Kleinsmith, L. J. (editors) (1975): *Chromosomal Proteins and Their Role in the Regulation of Gene Expression.* Academic Press, New York.
7. Greenberg, J. R. (1975): Messenger RNA metabolism of animal cells. *J. Cell Biol.,* 64:269–288
8. Busch, H., and Smetana, K. (1970): *The Nucleolus.* Academic Press, New York.
9. Briggs, R., and King, J. J. (1952): Transplantation of living nuclei from blastula cells into enucleated frogs eggs. *Proc. Natl. Acad. Sci. USA,* 38:455–463.
10. Gurdon, J. B. (1974): The genome in specialized cells, as revealed by nuclear transplantation in amphibia. In: *The Cell Nucleus, Vol. 1,* edited by H. Busch, pp. 471–489. Academic Press, New York.
11. Montgomery, T. H. (1898): Comparative cytological studies with special regard to the nucleus. *J. Morphol.,* 15:265–564.
12. Franke, W. W., and Scheer, U. (1974): Structures and functions

of the nuclear envelope. In: *The Cell Nucleus, Vol. 1*, edited by H. Busch, pp. 220–347. Academic Press, New York.

13. Berezney, R., and Coffey, D. S. (1976): The nuclear protein matrix: Isolation, structure and functions. *Adv. Enzyme Regul.*, 14:63–100.

14. Steele, W. J., and Busch, H. (1966): Increased content of high molecular weight RNA fractions in nuclei and nucleoli of livers of thioacetamide-treated rats. *Biochim. Biophys. Acta*, 119: 501–509.

15. Steele, J. W., and Busch, H. (1966): Studies on the ribonucleic acid components of the nuclear ribonucleoprotein network. *Biochim. Biophys. Acta*, 129:54–67.

16. Comings, D. E., and Okada, T. A. (1976): *Exp. Cell. Res.*, 103:341–360.

17. Terzakis, J. A. (1965): The nucleolar channel system of human endometrium. *J. Cell Biol.*, 27:293–304.

17a. Bouteille, M., Laval, M., and Dupuy-Coin, A. M. (1974): Localization of nuclear functions is revealed by ultrastructural autoradiography and cytochemistry. In: *The Cell Nucleus*, edited by H. Busch, pp. 5–74. Academic Press, New York.

18. Busch, H., Ballal, N. R., Olson, M. O. J., and Yeoman, L. C. (1975): Chromatin and its nonhistone proteins. *Methods Cancer Res.*, 11:43–121.

19. Busch, H. (1965): *Histones and Other Nuclear Proteins.* Academic Press, New York.

20. Olins, A. L., and Olins, D. E. (1974): Spheroid chromatin units (v bodies). *Science*, 183:330–332.

21. Olson, M. O. J., and Busch, H. (1974): Nuclear proteins. In: *The Cell Nucleus, Vol. 3*, edited by H. Busch, pp. 212–269. Academic Press, New York.

22. Langan, T. A. (1969): Phosphorylation of liver histone following the administration of glucagon and insulin. *Proc. Natl. Acad. Sci. USA*, 64:1276–1283.

23. Langan, T. A. (1969): Action of adenosine 3′,5′-monophosphate-dependent histone kinase in vivo. *J. Biol. Chem.*, 224: 5763–5765.

24. Kleinsmith, L. J., Stein, J., and Stein, G. (1975): Direct evidence for a functional relationship between nonhistone chromosomal protein phosphorylation and gene transcription. In: *Chromosomal Proteins and Their Role in the Regulation of Gene Expression*, edited by G. S. Stein and L. J. Kleinsmith, pp. 59–56. Academic Press, New York.

25. Comings, D. E., and Tack, L. O. (1973): Non-histone proteins—The effect of nuclear washes and comparison of metaphase and interphase chromatin. *Exp. Cell. Res.*, 82:175–191.

26. Comings, D. E., and Harris, D. C. (1975): Nuclear proteins. I. Electrophoretic comparison of mouse nucleoli, heterochromatin, euchromatin and contractile proteins. *Exp. Cell. Res.*, 96:161–179.

27. Steele, W. J., and Busch, H. (1963): Studies on acidic nuclear proteins of the walker tumor and liver. *Cancer Res.*, 23: 1153–1163.

28. Paul, J., and Gilmour, R. S. (1966): Template activity of DNA is restricted in chromatin. *J. Mol. Biol.*, 16:242–244.

29. Paul, J., and Gilmour, R. S. (1966): Restriction of deoxyribonucleic acid template activity in chromatin is organspecific. *Nature*, 210:992–993.

30. Paul, J., and Gilmour, R. S. (1968): Organ-specific restriction of transcription in mammalian chromatin. *J. Mol. Biol.*, 34: 305–316.

31. Jensen, E. V., and DeSombre, E. R. (1972): Mechanism of action of the female sex hormones. *Annu. Rev. Biochem.*, 41:203–230.

32. O'Malley, B. W., and Means, A. R. (1974): Effects of female steroid hormones on target cell nuclei. In: *The Cell Nucleus, Vol. 3*, edited by H. Busch, pp. 380–416. Academic Press, New York.

33. Higgins, S. J., Rousseau, G. G., Baxter, J. D., and Tomkins, G. M. (1973): Early events in glucocorticoid action. Activation of the steroid receptor and its subsequent specific nuclear binding studied in a cell-free system. *J. Biol. Chem.*, 248: 5866–5872.

34. Vorbrodt, A. (1974): Cytochemistry of nuclear enzymes. In:

The Cell Nucleus, Vol. 3, edited by H. Busch, pp. 309–344. Academic Press, New York.

35. Orrick, L. R., Olson, M. O. J., and Busch, H. (1973): Early events in glucocorticoid action. Activation of the steroid receptor and its subsequent specific nuclear binding studied in a cell-free system. *Proc. Natl. Acad. Sci. USA*, 70:1316–1320.

36. Peterson, J. L., and McConkely, E. H. (1967): Non-histone chromosomal proteins from HeLa cells. *J. Biol. Chem.*, 251:548–554.

37. Peterson, J. L., and McConkey, E. H. (1967): Proteins of friend leukemia cells. *J. Biol. Chem.*, 251:555–558.

38. Yeoman, L. C., Taylor, C. W., and Busch, H. (1973): Two-dimensional polyacrylamide gel electrophoresis of acid extractable nuclear proteins of normal rat liver and Novikoff hepatoma ascites cells. *Biochem. Biophys. Res. Commun.*, 51:956–966.

39. Yeoman, L. C., Taylor, C. W., Jordan, J. J., and Busch, H. (1973): Two-dimensional polyacrylamide gel electrophoresis of chromatin proteins of normal rat liver and Novikoff hepatoma ascites cells. *Biochem. Biophys. Res. Commun.*, 53:1067–1076.

40. Goodwin, G. H., Nicolas, R. H., and Johns, E. W. (1975): An improved large scale fractionation of high mobility group nonhistone chromatin proteins. *Biochim. Biophys. Acta*, 405: 280–291.

41. Goldknopf, I. L., French, M. F., Musso, R., and Busch, H. (1977): Presence of protein A24 in rat liver nucleosomes. *Proc. Natl. Acad. Sci. USA*, 74:5492–5495.

42. Lischwe, M. A., Smetana, K., Olson, M. O. J., and Busch, H. (1979): Proteins C23 and B23 are the major nucleolar silver staining proteins. *Life Sci.*, 25:701–708.

43. Goldstein, L. (1974): Movement of molecules between nucleus and cytoplasm. In: *The Cell Nucleus, Vol. 1*, edited by H. Busch, pp. 388–438. Academic Press, New York.

44. Hodge, L. D., Robbins, E., and Scharff, M. D. (1969): Persistence of messenger RNA through mitosis in HeLa cells. *J. Cell Biol.*, 40:497–507.

45. Arrighi, F. E. (1974): Mammalian chromosomes. In: *The Cell Nucleus, Vol. 2*, edited by H. Busch, pp. 1–32. Academic Press, New York.

45a. Kucherlapti, R. S., Creagen, R. P., and Ruddle, F. H. (1974): Progress in human gene mapping by somatic cell hybridization. In: *The Cell Nucleus, Vol. 2*, edited by H. Busch, pp. 209–222. Academic Press, New York.

46. Birnstiel, M. (1975): Anatomy of gene-cluster coding for 5 histone proteins of sea-urchin, a progress report. In: *Molecular Biology of the Mammalian Genetic Apparatus, Vol. 1*, edited by P. O. T'so, pp. 87–89. Elsevier, Amsterdam.

47. Busch, H., Choi, Y. C., Daskal, Y., Liarakos, C. D., Rao, M. R. S., Ro-Choi, T. S., and Wu, B. C. (1976): *Methods of Cancer Res.*, 8:101–197.

48. Steggles, A. W., Wilson, G. N., Kantor, J. A., Picciano, D. J., Falvey, A. K., and Anderson, W. F. (1974): *Proc. Natl. Acad. Sci. USA*, 71:1219–1223.

49. Wilson, G. N., Steggles, A. W., and Neinhuis, A. W. (1975): Strand-selective transcription of globin genes in rabbit erythroid cells and chromatin. *Proc. Natl. Acad. Sci. USA*, 72:4835–4839.

50. Rule, A. H., and Goleski-Reilly, C. (1974): Phase-specific oncocolar antigens: A theoretical framework for "carcinoembryonic antigen' specificities. *Cancer Res.*, 34:2083–2087.

51. Cohen, M. E., and Hamilton, T. H. (1975): Effects of estradiol 73β on the synthesis of specific uterine nonhistone chromosomal proteins. *Proc. Natl. Acad. Sci. USA*, 72:4346–4350.

52. Ro-Choi, T. S., and Busch, H. (1974): Low molecular weight nuclear RNA. In: *The Molecular Biology of Cancer*, edited by H. Busch, pp. 241–276. Academic Press, New York.

53. Ro-Choi, T. S., and Busch, H. (1974): Low molecular weight nuclear RNAs. In: *The Cell Nucleus, Vol. 3*, edited by H. Busch, pp. 152–211. Academic Press, New York.

54. Chambon, P., Gissenger, F., Kedinger, C., Mandel, J. L., and Meilhac, M. (1974): Animal nuclear DNA-dependent RNA polymerases. In: *The Cell Nucleus, Vol. 3*, edited by H. Busch, pp. 270–308. Academic Press, New York.

55. Roeder, R. G., and Rutter, W. J. (1969): Multiple forms of DNA-dependent RNA polymerase in eukaryotic organisms. *Nature*, 224:234–237.

56. Roeder, R. G., and Rutter, W. J. (1970): Multiple ribonucleic acid polymerase and ribonucleic acid synthesis during sea urchin development. *Biochemistry,* 9:2543–2553.

57. Love, R., and Soriano, R. Z. (1971): Correlation of nucleolini with fine structural nucleolar constituents of cultured normal and Neoplastic cells. *Cancer Res.,* 31:1030–1037.

58. Heitz, E. (1933): Über Total Und Partielle Somatische Heteropyknose Sowie Strukturelle Geschlechtschromosomen Bei Drosophila Funebris. *Z. Zellforsch. Mikrosk. Anat.,* 19:720–742.

59. McClintock, B. (1934): The relation of a particular chromosomal element to the development of the nucleoli in Zea Mays. *Z. Zellforsch. Mikrosk. Anat.,* 21:294–328.

60. McClintock, B. (1961): Some parallels between gene control systems in maize and in bacteria. *American Naturalist,* 95:265–328.

61. Kleinschmidt, A. K. (1968): Monolayer techniques in electron microscopy of nucleic acid molecules. In: *Methods in Enzymology, Vol. 12, Nucleic Acids,* edited by L. Grossman and K. Moldave, pp. 361–377. Academic Press, New York.

62. Miller, O. L., Jr., and Beatty, B. R. (1969): Visualization of nucleolar genes. *Science,* 164:955–957.

63. Sitz, T. O., Nazar, R. N., Spohn, W. H., and Busch, H. (1973): Similarity of ribosomal and ribosomal precursor RNAs from rat liver and the Novikoff ascites hepatoma. *Cancer Res.,* 33:3318–3321.

64. Quagliarotti, G., Hidvegi, E., Wikman, J., and Busch, H. (1970): Structural analysis of nucleolar precursors of ribosomal ribonucleic acid. Comparative hybridizations of nucleolar and ribosomal ribonucleic acid with nucleolar deoxyribonucleic acid. *J. Biol. Chem.,* 245:1962–1969.

64a. Brown, P. D., Wensink, P. C., and Jordan, E. (1972): A comparison of the ribosomal DNA of Xenopus laevis and Xenopus niederi. *J. Mol. Biol.,* 63:57–73.

65. Olson, M. O. J., Ezrailson, E. G., Guetzow, K., and Busch, H. (1975): Localization and phosphorylation of nuclear, nucleolar and extranucleolar non-histone proteins of Novikoff hepatoma ascites cells. *J. Mol. Biol.,* 97:611–619.

66. Mamrack, M. D., Olson, M. O. J., and Busch, H. (1979): Amino acid sequence and sites of phosphorylation in a highly acidic region of nucleolar nonhistone protein C23. *Biochemistry,* 18:3381–3386.

67. Jaskunas, S. R., Burgess, R., Lindahl, L., and Nomura, M. (1975): Identification of two copies of the gene for the elongation factor EF-Tu in E. coli. *Nature,* 257:458–462.

68. Lindahl, L., Jaskunas, S. R, Dennis, P., and Nomura, M. (1975): Clusters of genes in Escherichia coli for ribosomal proteins, ribosomal RNA, and RNA polymerase subunits. *Proc. Natl. Acad. Sci. USA,* 72:2743–2747.

69. Watson, R. J., Parker, J., Fiil, N. P., Flaks, J. G., and Friesen, J. D. (1975): New chromosomal location for structural genes of ribosomal proteins. *Proc. Natl. Acad. Sci. USA,* 72:2765–2769.

70. Busch, H., Hirsch, F., Gupta, K. K., Rao, M., Spohn, W., and Wu, B. (1976): Structural and functional studies on the "5'-cap": A. Survey method for mRNA. *Prog. Nucleic Acid Res.,* 19:39–61.

71. DeSombre, E. R., Mohla, S., and Jensen, E. V. (1972): Estrogen-independent activation of the receptor protein of calf uterine Cytosol. *Biochem. Biophys. Res. Commun.,* 48:1601–1608.

72. Raj, N. B. K., Ro-Choi, T. S., and Busch, H. (1975): Nuclear ribonucleoprotein complexes containing U1 and U2 RNA. *Biochemistry,* 14:4380–4385.

The Liver: Biology and Pathobiology, edited by
I. Arias, H. Popper, D. Schachter, and D. A. Schafritz.
Raven Press, New York © 1982.

Chapter 7

Hepatic Protein Synthesis and its Regulation

Mark A. Zern, David A. Shafritz, and Dennis Shields

The purpose of this chapter is to review the basic mechanism for hepatic protein synthesis, the factors that regulate synthesis of specialized proteins in the liver, in particular albumin, and the influence of altered physiologic states and pathologic conditions on hepatic protein synthesis.

MECHANISM FOR HEPATIC PROTEIN SYNTHESIS

With few exceptions, eukaryotic cells contain a complex network of subcellular structures devoted to specific metabolic processes. The basic subcellular structure on which protein synthesis occurs is the polyribosome. This macromolecular aggregate is composed of multiple ribosomes held together by a linear messenger RNA (mRNA) molecule (containing the genetic signal), which has been transcribed in the nucleus and transferred to the cytoplasm. Detailed analysis of the protein synthesis mechanism is beyond the scope of this discussion, and only an abbreviated view is presented. As shown schematically in Fig. 1, the protein synthesis mechanism can be separated into three major steps: (a) initiation, (b) elongation, and (c) termination. Amino acids, ATP, GTP, monovalent

(K^+) and divalent (Mg^{2+}) cations, transfer RNAs (tRNAs), mRNA, ribosomal subunits, and many protein factors interact in a precise fashion to complete these various steps.

Initiation is the most complex step and has received the most attention (for reviews, see refs. 1–3). It requires a special initiator tRNA ($tRNA_f^{Met}$), which, when activated (acylated) with methionine (Met-tRNA$_f$), can interact with initiation factor eIF-2 and GTP to form a ternary complex (Met-tRNA$_f$·eIF-2·GTP); this starts the initiation process. eIF-2 has three polypeptide subunits; phosphorylation of the small subunit (38,000 daltons) inhibits formation of the ternary complex, thereby inhibiting initiation. Inhibition of protein synthesis by a hemin-controlled inhibitor (HCI) or 2′-3′ oligo A (mediated by interferon) is thought to occur through inactivation of eIF-2 (2,3). Inhibition of protein synthesis by oxidized glutathione also may occur through inactivation of eIF-2. Methionyl tRNA$_f$ responds to the code word AUG, but it has been found that the Met-tRNA$_f$·eIF-2·GTP complex can join to the 40 S ribosomal subunit in the absence of exogenous template. Another methionyl-tRNA species, Met-tRNA$_m$, responds to the codon AUG. $tRNA_m^{Met}$ is acylated by a synthetase separate from

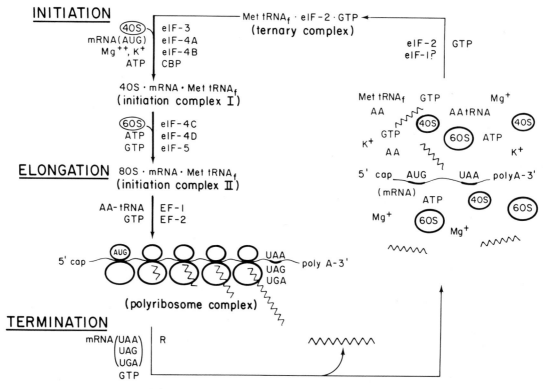

FIG. 1. Steps in eukaryotic protein synthesis.

that activating $tRNA_f^{Met}$ (4). It does not form a complex with eIF-2 and GTP but adds methionine to internal positions of the growing peptide chain; i.e., it is not involved in the initiation mechanism but is utilized during elongation.

RNA is synthesized in the nucleus and is released into the cytoplasm in protein complexes referred to as messenger ribonucleoprotein particles (mRNPs). mRNPs range in size from 30,000 to >100,000 daltons (5). Their specific function(s) has not been identified. Some are similar in size to specific initiation factors or subunits of initiation factors, but additional characterization studies are needed (5). The 5′ end of mRNA has a unique structure, 7-N methyl guanosine in a 5′ to 5′ triphosphate linkage to the penultimate nucleotide, which is usually 6-0 methyl adenosine or 6-0 methyl guanosine (for review, see ref. 6). The exact function of this structure (referred to as the mRNA 5′ cap) has not been defined, but a 24,000 dalton polypeptide has been identified which binds to the cap (cap binding protein or CBP) and is required for initiation of protein synthesis (7). The initiation codon (AUG) is separated from the cap by an oligonucleotide sequence of variable length, ranging from 50 to 200 nucleotides and referred to as the mRNA leader region (8). Initiation factor eIF-4B, which also binds to mRNA, appears to have a function together with CBP in bringing mRNA to the ribosome (9) or in orienting mRNA on the ribosome to permit protein synthesis to begin (phasing). A series of eIF-4B components with unique properties

for translating specific mRNAs has been reported (10), but this area has been the subject of much controversy (1).

Four or five other initiation factors have been identified (2); the specific function of only one has been clearly described. In the presence of ATP (and GTP), eIF-5 causes joining of the 60 S subunit to the initiation complex (2). During this process, ATP and GTP are hydrolyzed. A second AA-tRNA joins the initiated 80 S ribosome under the influence of elongation factor EF-1 and the second triplet codon of the mRNA. The first peptide bond is formed by a catalytic reaction involving peptidyl transferase, an integral ribosomal protein residing on the 60 S subunit. This completes initiation.

Peptide bond formation is repeated sequentially under the direction of subsequent triplet codons, which are specific for given amino acids in a 5′ to 3′ reading direction of the mRNA (elongation). Elongation factor EF-1 brings successive AA-tRNAs to the ribosome through intermediate formation of an AA-tRNA·EF-1·GTP complex, similar to the ternary complex for initiation. Elongation factor EF-2 (translocase) provides energy for movement of the ribosome down the mRNA through a GTP-dependent hydrolytic reaction. Formation of each peptide bond also requires energy provided by GTP hydrolysis. As the ribosome moves approximately 30 codon units, a second initiation event can occur at the initial AUG codon. The polyribosome complex is formed as successive ribosome units are added to mRNA during the translation process.

Polypeptide chain elongation is a self-perpetuating event until a termination signal is reached. Termination signals are nonsense codons, i.e., triplet code words that do not code for any amino acyl tRNA. In both prokaryotic and eukaryotic cells, three termination signals have been discovered: UAA, UAG, and UGA. When such a signal is reached, polypeptide chain elongation ceases (termination). In conjunction with a protein complex, R (11), the polypeptide chain is separated from its 3' terminal AA-tRNA (GTP hydrolysis is again required); the protein and deacylated tRNA are released from the mRNA; and the various components reenter the cytosol pool.

Unless one or more of the above steps is interrupted, protein synthesis continues in a cyclic process. Under normal circumstances in biologically active cells, initiation represents the rate-limiting step in eukaryotic protein synthesis and is most readily subject to modulation or regulation (1). Therefore, physiologic or other factors that alter either the cellular composition of mRNA or the initiation mechanism have the greatest influence on protein synthesis. Later portions of this chapter deal with derangements in hepatic protein synthesis produced by alterations in amino acid supply, hepatotoxins (alcohol and carbon tetrachloride), hormonal changes, and certain pathologic states, including diabetes, thyroid dysfunction, and chronic renal failure.

Role of the Rough Endoplasmic Reticulum and Free Polyribosomes

Ultrastructural studies performed in the 1950s and 1960s showed that parenchymal cells of certain tissues, such as pancreas, mammary gland, and liver, possess a rich network of endoplasmic reticulum (ER) related to the secretory function of these organs. A large portion of the ribosomal complement in these cells is attached to membranous structures comprising the rough endoplasmic reticulum (RER). In rapidly dividing, germinal, or neoplastic cells (such as the intestinal crypt cell, HeLa cells, or fibroblasts in tissue culture) and in nonsecretory cells (such as reticulocytes or striated muscle), the ER is poorly developed. Most of the ribosomes in these cells are present in free cytoplasmic polyribosomes.

It was subsequently discovered that newly synthesized, secretory proteins accumulate on or within the RER, and it was proposed that secretory proteins are synthesized selectively in the RER, whereas intracellular proteins are synthesized on free polyribosomes (12–14). Numerous theories were developed to explain the preferential synthesis of certain proteins on membrane-bound polyribosomes. These included

separate classes of ribosomes for the free versus membrane-bound fraction, special ribosomal proteins that anchored membrane-bound ribosomes to the ER, preferential affinity of certain classes of mRNA for membranous structures through mRNA-protein interaction (specific membrane mRNP proteins), and direct anchorage of polysomes containing nascent polypeptide chains to the membrane. A variant of the latter theory has been confirmed and is described in detail.

The Signal Sequence Hypothesis for Synthesis of Secretory Proteins

Various *in vitro* studies have shown that secretory proteins are synthesized as precursor molecules. These precursors contain 15 to 30 extra amino acids in the N-terminal segment which are usually quite hydrophobic. Blobel and Dobberstein (15,16) showed that the N-terminal hydrophobic sequence serves as a signal for polyribosomes synthesizing secretory proteins to associate with the RER. Using isolated mRNAs in a reconstituted cell-free system devoid of membranes, these investigators demonstrated that immunoglobin L-chain (a secreted protein) was synthesized as a precursor containing an extra N-terminal amino acid sequence of ~3,000 daltons. Globin (a nonsecreted protein) was not synthesized as a precursor. When a pancreatic membrane fraction was added to the reconstituted system, newly synthesized immunoglobulin L-chain was internalized into membrane vesicles and was no longer present as a precursor; globin was not internalized. Amino acid sequencing data showed that the "pre" immunoglobulin L-chain polypeptide contained 24 extra N-terminal amino acids, beginning with the usual initiating amino acid methionine (coded by AUG) and was strongly hydrophobic in its amino acid composition (between amino acids 11 and 18).

From these and similar studies with pancreatic tissue (22), Blobel and co-workers (15–17) proposed a model for synthesis of secretory proteins called the "signal sequence" hypothesis (Fig. 2). In this model, translation of all mRNA begins on free ribosomes in the cytoplasm. The initial N-terminal peptide region for secretory proteins is hydrophobic (with a similar amino acid sequence). As this peptide region emerges through the ribosome surface during protein synthesis, it serves as a signal for attachment of the ribosome to the membrane structure. The N-terminal peptide is cleaved by a specific enzyme residing on the internal surface of the ER, so that it does not appear in the final product (Fig. 2A). Once the protein has entered the ER, synthesis continues vectorially through the membrane structure, and the completed product is released into the intracisternal space. Although details concerning specific steps in this mechanism are not well established, this basic model has attractive features

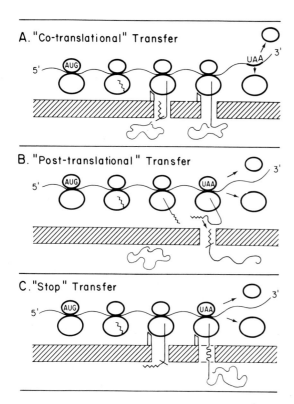

FIG. 2. Signal sequence hypothesis for synthesis of secretory and membrane-associated proteins.

and has been confirmed in many systems (18). In the case of chicken ovalbumin, a secretory product of the oviduct, the N-terminal sequence is hydrophobic but is not cleaved (19). Since ovalbumin was shown to have the functional equivalent of a signal sequence (19), this finding is not inconsistent with the basic premise of the "signal sequence" hypothesis; namely, that the hydrophobic nature of the N-terminal segment of the nascent polypeptide chain, rather than the primary sequence of the mRNA, serves as the signal for polysomes synthesizing secretory proteins to attach to the RER. This model does not exclude other mechanisms for synthesis of membrane-constituent proteins and other intracellular or cytosolic proteins.

Synthesis of Integral Membrane Proteins

The previously described mechanism for translocation or vectorial synthesis of secreted proteins has been termed cotranslational transfer (Fig. 2A). Variants of this mechanism are utilized for synthesis of membrane proteins of subcellular organelles and for synthesis of cell surface membrane proteins. For certain proteins of subcellular organelles, protein synthesis begins and is completed on free polyribosomes. The resultant protein is later incorporated into membranous structures by interactions between a hydrophobic peptide segment and specific receptors within the membrane. This mechanism has been termed posttranslational transfer (Fig. 2B). Examples include uricase and cat-

alse, both of which are peroxisomal proteins (20). It should be emphasized that in posttranslational transfer, hydrophobic domains are still thought to be responsible for interaction of newly synthesized protein with membrane constituents. The precise position of the hydrophobic signal and the mechanism for processing have not been clarified.

Another mechanism has been identified for synthesis of several cell surface membrane proteins (for review, see ref. 21). In these cases, protein synthesis begins on free polyribosomes, the nascent chain becomes attached to membranous structures through hydrophobic interactions of a precursor signal sequence, and vectorial synthesis continues as for a secreted protein (Fig. 2C). As the carboxy terminus is approached, however, a special event occurs which stops translocation and freezes the protein within the membrane (stoptransfer). A hydrophilic domain is reached, which is preceded by a hydrophobic domain. This in turn, is preceded by another hydrophilic region, so that the hydrophobic domain is sandwiched between two highly polar regions. Protein synthesis is completed beyond this region on the cytoplasmic face of the ER; thus a transmembrane protein is generated. Examples of stoptransfer have been described for specific viral proteins and for cell surface immunoglobulins. In the case of Semliki-forest virus, hydrophobic peptide regions for two integral viral membrane proteins, E1 and E2, have been identified and sequenced near the carboxy terminal region (22). These hydrophobic regions are of sufficient length to span the lipid bilayer in the form of an α-helix (22). Interesting features of mRNAs and genes for membrane-associated versus secreted immunoglobulins are discussed below.

ALBUMIN SYNTHESIS AS A PRECURSOR MOLECULE

The signal sequence hypothesis predicted that serum albumin would be synthesized in the liver as a precursor molecule. Early evidence for a precursor was obtained by several investigators, but this precursor (termed proalbumin) contained only five to six extra N-terminal amino acids (23–25). Subsequently, Strauss et al. (26) proved that rat albumin is indeed synthesized as a precursor molecule (preproalbumin) with an extra hydrophobic N-terminal sequence of 24 amino acids (the last six amino acids were identical to those found in proalbumin). As with other secretory proteins, the "pre" portion is cleaved before polypeptide chain synthesis is completed, so that it has not been possible to identify preproalbumin directly in liver tissue.

SUBCELLULAR DISTRIBUTION OF ALBUMIN mRNA

If the signal sequence hypothesis were correct, it should be possible to demonstrate specific association of albumin mRNA with membrane-bound polyribosomes in the liver. This has been accomplished by subcellular fractionation of membrane-bound and free polysomes and quantitation of albumin mRNA in various subcellular fractions by molecular hybridization with purified albumin DNA probes. Determination of cell-free albumin synthesis with membrane-bound versus free polysomes can be used as a preliminary index of albumin mRNA segregation. Such measurements may not be accurate, however, because many factors alter relative and absolute rates of synthesis of specific proteins in cell-free systems (27).

The impetus for using molecular hybridization to study metabolism of specific mRNAs in animal cells came from the discovery in the early 1970s of an enzyme capable of synthesizing DNA *in vitro* from an RNA template (i.e., an RNA-dependent DNA polymerase). This enzyme, referred to as "reverse transcriptase," requires, in addition to an RNA template, a double-stranded primer region. In eukaryotic cells, most mRNAs and their precursors (but not other types of RNA) contain a 3' noncoding sequence of poly (A). By adding synthetic oligo (dT) to the reaction mixture, a double-stranded region is formed at the 3' end of the mRNA, leaving the remaining sequence as a primed template for reverse transcriptase. The reaction (Fig. 3) also requires a divalent cation (Mg^{2+}) and all four deoxyribonucleoside triphosphates (dXTPs); actinomycin D is added to prevent self-copying of newly synthesized DNA. Due to Watson-Crick base pairing, DNA synthesized from mRNA, referred to as cDNA, is precisely complementary in base sequence to the mRNA from which it was generated. Using radioactive dXTP substrates, cDNA can be prepared at very high specific activity (10^6 to 10^8 cpm/µg). Under appropriate conditions, this material can be used as an accurate and highly sensitive probe for detecting RNA

sequences to which the cDNA is specifically complementary. As ordinarily employed, this assay is 1,000 times more sensitive for detecting mRNA than the most sensitive protein-synthesizing system. A potential limitation is that the mRNA need not be intact or biologically active to hybridize with cDNA. This property may also be of advantage, however, since only a slight alteration of mRNA during metabolism or isolation may render it biologically inactive but still capable of detection by molecular hybridization.

Quantitation of Albumin mRNA Sequences by Molecular Hybridization

If a labeled cDNA probe is prepared from a purified specific mRNA, hybridization to any RNA fraction measures precisely the number of sequences present in the RNA that are complementary to the DNA. Critical factors are purity of the mRNA from which the DNA has been prepared and conditions under which hybridization is performed. Once it is established that the materials and hybridization conditions are specific, a simple titration curve can be performed by using a fixed amount of [^{3}H]cDNA and increasing amounts of RNA (saturation hybridization). The amount of mRNA required to protect a given cpm of labeled cDNA is a constant for each preparation of cDNA, as long as hybridization is performed to completion. If the specific activity (cpm/µg) of the cDNA is known and a purified mRNA standard is available, the amount of mRNA necessary to protect a given cpm of cDNA can be determined.

To obtain quantitative information on the amount and subcellular distribution of albumin mRNA in liver, it is essential to use cellular fractionation and isolation procedures which provide uniformly high yields of undegraded polyribosomes. Ramsey and Steele developed such techniques (28). Using these methods in conjunction with molecular hybridization, Yap et al. (27) determined that 97% of total albumin mRNA sequences in normal rat liver cytosol are in membrane-bound polysomes, 2% are in free polysomes, and 1% are in the postribosomal fraction. These findings, which confirmed and extended earlier studies by cell-free protein synthesis (29), are consistent with expectations of the signal sequence hypothesis.

Studies in Hepatomas, Cell Lines, and Other Model Systems

Studies of albumin mRNA metabolism and function in hepatoma cell lines in tissue culture have recently come under scrutiny. Peterson (30) reported three clonal derivatives of rat hepatoma cells which synthesize and secrete albumin at different levels (high, medium, and low). The level of albumin mRNA in these cell lines correlated directly with the level of

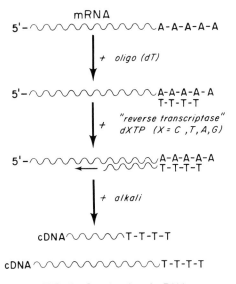

FIG. 3. Synthesis of cDNA.

albumin synthesis. A similar result has been obtained by Sell et al. (31), using molecular hybridization technology. Synthesis of albumin, a constitutive process, occurs at three different levels in these hepatoma cell lines, depending on the level of cytoplasmic albumin mRNA. Examining factors that control albumin gene transcription and albumin mRNA processing and metabolism in these cells would be instructive.

Specific Morris hepatomas do or do not synthesize albumin (32−34). Albumin synthesis is present in two lines (#5123tc or D and #9121), and secretion is either markedly depressed or absent (33,34). In Morris hepatoma #5123D, RER is sparse, disorganized, and vacuolated. In one study, albumin was reported to be synthesized on free polyribosomes but not secreted from the cell (35). These results could be explained by deletion of all or part of the mRNA region coding for the N-terminal hydrophobic peptide of albumin, by an abnormality in the properties of the membrane, or by absence of a specific protein(s) involved in association of albumin mRNA or albumin synthesizing polysomes with the ER. Strauss et al. (36) reported synthesis of normal preproalbumin with an mRNA extract from Morris hepatoma #5123tc, suggesting that the coding portion of the mRNA is intact.

ALBUMIN GENE ORGANIZATION AND TRANSCRIPTION

Although expression of the albumin gene appears relatively fixed in adult life, understanding its expression at the molecular level is important: (a) albumin synthesis represents a major liver cell differentiated function; (b) albumin mRNA is the most abundant mRNA species in normal adult liver; and (c) relatively little is known about the mechanism for activation of the albumin gene (i.e., induction during embryonal development). Until recently, it had been assumed that functional cytoplasmic mRNAs represent direct co-linear transcripts of a continuous sequence of DNA in the genome. Data from prokaryotic systems supported this view. This dogma of one gene−one mRNA−one polypeptide chain has been revised on the basis of recent studies. The impetus for much of this work has come from advances in recombinant DNA technology during the last 5 years.

Basically, it has been found that specific eukaryotic genes are mosaics: sequences that are expressed in the final polypeptide product ("exons") are held in an alternating matrix with unexpressed sequences ("introns" or "intervening sequences"). The general methodology used to establish the discontinuous nature of eukaryotic genes is relatively straightforward and conceptually similar to peptide mapping. Purified cellular DNA is cleaved with various restriction endonucleases (enzymes that recognize 4 to 6 base pair regions in double-stranded DNA and cleave both strands at

these sites). The resulting fragments are separated by gel electrophoresis and transferred onto a nitrocellulose filter using the method of Southern (38). The filter is hybridized with a radioactively labeled unique species of cDNA prepared from the specific mRNA under investigation. This cDNA is usually prepared in large quantity in highly purified form by cloning in a bacterial plasmid. Using this cDNA as a hybridization probe, it is possible to construct a physical map of restriction endonuclease cleavage sites in DNA regions surrounding the coding sequences in the structural gene. It is also possible to determine the orientation of the gene and the direction of transcription within this map. Restriction endonuclease cleavage maps also can be used to locate various classes of sequences that might neighbor the gene, for example, repetitive DNA, palindromes, oligo dA:dT clusters. Such sequences are suspected to impart regulatory actions in gene expression.

SYNTHESIS, PROCESSING, AND METABOLISM OF EUKARYOTIC mRNAs

The discovery of intervening sequences within eukaryotic genes has introduced a new level of complexity in mRNA synthesis and metabolism. Intervening sequences have been found in the α- and β-globin genes of rabbit and mouse (39,40), the immunoglobulin gene of mouse (41,42), the ovalbumin gene of chicken (43,44), and many other genes (45). Coding sequences (exons) and intervening sequences (introns) are transcribed continuously in the nucleus, resulting in an mRNA precursor of high molecular weight (HnRNA), which is subsequently processed to mRNA and released into the cytoplasm (see Fig. 4). The mechanism for mRNA processing has not been fully elucidated; but during this process, introns are excised in a precise fashion, and exons are ligated in a head-to-tail fashion to form functional mRNAs (46).

In the case of the rabbit β-globin gene, there is an intervening sequence of 600 base pairs at the 3′ end of the gene (39). A similar sized intron is also found at the 3′ end of the mouse β-globin gene (40). In addition, a smaller intervening sequence is located close to the 5′ end of the mouse β-globin gene. These inserts appear to represent a general property of the β-globin gene, even in tissues in which this gene is inactive. This suggests that the inserts are not involved in gene activation or deactivation. The similar position and size of the 3′ insert in the β-globin gene of two species widely separated in evolution suggests that this insert has a conserved role in the function of this gene.

In the chicken, ovomucoid and ovalbumin gene coding sequences are split by at least six to seven intervening sequences (44). The total length of ovalbumin introns is at least three times that of the exons.

Generally, introns are longer than exons and are widely separated. Administration of estrogen to immature chicks results in cytodifferentiation of tubular gland cells and increased steady-state levels of ovalbumin and ovomucoid mRNAs. In the case of ovalbumin, gene organization in both oviduct cells (highly specialized in ovalbumin synthesis) and erythrocytes (not expressing ovalbumin) is similar. In other words, exon rearrangement in the ovalbumin gene does not take place during cytodifferentiation, at least with ovalbumin in the avian species. Similar conclusions have been reached with the β-globin gene (39). Studies with immunoglobulin genes in mammals have shown that, in the germ line (embryonic tissue), sequences coding for the variable region and those coding for the constant region of immunoglobulin L-chain lie separate from each other. These two genetic regions move from distant to close but not contiguous positions during differentiation of lymphocyte precursors. This type of rearrangement, however, may be unique to the immunoglobulin system (41,42).

Sala-Trepat et al. (47), using full-length, radiolabeled albumin cDNA, reported that the albumin gene is transcribed from a nonrepetitive fraction of the rat genome. They estimated that there are about 1.5 albumin genes per haploid genome and determined that the EcoR1 restriction enzyme maps for albumin genes are similar in rat liver and rat hepatoma DNA. Using albumin cDNA probes, restriction enzyme mapping, and DNA R-looping, these investigators determined that the rat albumin gene coding sequence is distributed over at least 14.5 kilobases of continuous cellular DNA, and that the albumin gene contains 13 intervening sequences (48). Figure 4 is a schematic diagram illustrating the salient features in albumin synthesis, beginning with transcription of the albumin gene and concluding with secretion of the albumin protein molecule.

During processing of mRNA precursors, deletion of noncoding or intervening sequences is a precise event. It is reasonable to expect that certain mutations at the boundaries of regions to be spliced out may affect mRNA maturation or function. It has been found in certain α- and β-thalassemias that globin genes are altered in a silent intervening or precursor sequence (49–52). It has also been suggested that Lepore-like crossovers, which produce decreased amounts of defective globin chains, may be defective in the same way (53). Therefore, the presence of intervening sequences in genes poses new and unexpected questions relevant to gene organization and protein synthesis which can be applied to the albumin system. Such abnormalities may account for the lack of albumin mRNA in the liver of an analbuminemic rat strain identified in Japan (54) and in analbuminemic humans (59). These defects could be related to abnormalities in

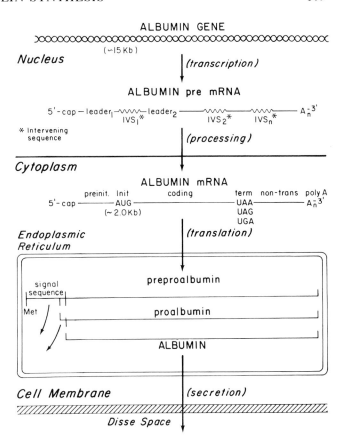

FIG. 4. Steps in albumin synthesis.

albumin gene organization, gene transcription, or processing of the albumin mRNA precursor (see Fig. 4).

In the case of mouse immunoglobulin μH-chain mRNA, a unique observation has been made regarding mRNA processing. A single gene codes for two distinct μH-chain mRNAs, which differ only in their 3' sequence past the fourth constant region domain (56). Depending on whether IgM is to be secreted or cell-surface bound, the amount of these two mRNAs varies in the cytoplasm. This alteration in mRNA structure is caused by variation in mRNA processing, which produces two distinct mRNAs. This leads to synthesis of different carboxy terminal regions for these two proteins, which are otherwise identical. The membrane-associated form of μH-chain contains a stop-transfer sequence, which is not present in the secreted form of this protein (56,57).

In adenovirus (Ad)-infected HeLa cells, a single primary RNA transcript (synthesized in the nucleus) can give rise to a whole series of distinct mRNA products depending on how processing events proceed (46). Thus a single mRNA precursor may give rise to different specific mRNAs at different times or under different cellular conditions. Swaneck et al. (58) identified ovalbumin mRNA precursors in chick oviduct nuclei. The authors used cloned cDNA to ovalbumin mRNA and prepared a DNA fragment that contains only ovalbumin cDNA sequences. Utilizing recombinant cloned cDNA to ovalbumin mRNA, they analyzed the distribution of nuclear ovalbumin mRNA sequences, which were fractionated by agarose gel electrophoresis under denaturing conditions. The results suggested transcription of the entire ovalbumin gene into a large precursor molecule, followed by excision of intervening sequences to form mature ovalbumin mRNA. Similar studies should determine events in synthesis and metabolism of nuclear precursors to albumin mRNA in liver and various hepatoma cell lines, as well as in various pathophysiologic states. In preliminary studies, Strair et al. (59) identified a presumptive nuclear precursor to albumin mRNA in rat liver and in cultured hepatoma cells. It will be interesting to determine whether nuclear albumin mRNA-processing events are modified under different cellular conditions or stresses.

The concentration of a specific mRNA in a cell is a function of both its rate of synthesis and its rate of destruction. Most studies on mRNA stability have been performed with total poly A-containing message. By utilizing a probe for a specific message, it is possible to examine the fate of that particular mRNA. Wilson et al. (60) used this technique to study Ad-2-specific mRNAs in transformed cells. They found that discrete mRNAs appear to turn over randomly, and that while bulk mRNA appears to have an average half-life of 4 to 5 hr, individual mRNAs can have much shorter half-lives. This study dealt with two Ad-2-mRNAs only in logarithmically growing rat cells. These same mRNAs are also produced early in virus infection of HeLa cells (60). Preliminary results with a pulse label and actinomycin D chase showed that the half-lives of the two Ad-2-mRNAs are greatly lengthened during lytic infection of HeLa cells as compared to the same mRNAs under different physiologic conditions. The question of whether specific mRNAs have fixed intrinsic half-lives or half-lives that can vary could be of great importance in understanding the regulation of protein synthesis.

On the basis of theoretical calculations, Bastos et al. (61) concluded that high accumulation of globin mRNA in terminally differentiated erythrocytes cannot be accounted for simply by synthesis rates or mRNA processing. Lodish and Small (62) reported a differential destruction of mRNA for a 64,000 dalton polypeptide (polypeptide I) compared to globin mRNA during maturation of erythrocytes. Lowenhaupt and Lingrel (63) have shown in murine erythroleukemic cells that the half-life of globin mRNA is 50 hr early after induction, whereas it is 17 hr late in induction; i.e., the stability of globin mRNA changes during the induction process. Other investigators (45,64–66) report that the half-life of specific mRNAs may vary during specific induction or differentiation, but results in these systems are somewhat less firm.

Studies of albumin mRNA function in acute amino acid deprivation suggest that modulation or regulation of albumin synthesis may occur at the level of initiation or mRNA-ribosome-membrane association (27). It is not surprising that mRNA for a "luxury function" protein, such as albumin, would be amenable to storage in a nonfunctional state. This does not imply that cytoplasmic albumin mRNA has an increased half-life when albumin synthesis is suppressed and albumin mRNA accumulates in mRNPs. Molecular hybridization studies will provide answers to some of these questions.

NUTRITIONAL EFFECTS ON PROTEIN METABOLISM

The molecular basis for the role of nutritional factors in regulating protein synthesis is not well understood. Studies have concentrated on three areas: (a) fasting and the effect of refeeding, (b) force-feeding of diets deficient in a specific amino acid, such as threonine, and (c) use of protein-calorie-deficient diets.

Fasting and Refeeding

There is general agreement that fasting causes a decrease in hepatic protein synthesis (67–69). This finding occurs in all animal models (rat, mouse, or rabbit), regardless of whether intact tissue (perfused liver), liver slices, or cell-free systems are utilized. In most studies, all proteins are affected. In fasted rats, however, Peters and Peters (67) found a disproportionate reduction in albumin synthesis compared to intracellular proteins. Others have suggested that synthesis of all hepatic proteins decreases at the same rate (70), and Wilson et al. (71) reported that albumin synthesis is more refractory than other hepatic proteins to conditions that limit protein synthesis.

As indicated previously, differences in mRNA affinity for the initiation complex may explain variations in translation rates for specific mRNAs (2,72–75). Controversy exists, however, as to whether the relative affinity of mRNAs is secondary to innate qualities of the mRNAs (74) or to initiation factors that favor specific groups of mRNAs (3). Sonenshein and Braverman reported a preferential affinity of immunoglobulin L-chain mRNA for polyribosomes in mouse myeloma cells (73). When myeloma cells are starved, the proportion of immunoglobulin to total protein increases because starvation limits the ability of cells to initiate, thereby favoring synthesis of proteins from high affinity mRNAs (73). When cyclohexamide is added to the medium (leading to a relative increase in initiation capacity compared to polypeptide chain elongation), the proportion of immunoglobulin/total protein decreases because initiation affinity is no longer the rate-limiting step controlling protein synthesis (73).

The best studied example demonstrating differential initiation rates for specific mRNAs is the globin system (2,72,74). In crude reticulocyte lysate, α-globin mRNA initiates protein synthesis only 60% as frequently as β-globin mRNA (74). In another cell-free reticulocyte system, translation of β-chains is 50 times more efficient than that of α-chains. When excess initiation factors are present, however, binding of α- and β-globin mRNAs to the ribosome and subsequent translation are essentially equal (76). It has been proposed that starvation for certain amino acids may act by influencing initiation of protein synthesis (77). Under adverse cellular conditions, such as starvation or amino acid deprivation, competition of various mRNA species for existing ribosomes may favor initiation and translation of more efficient mRNAs. This has not been demonstrated directly in liver.

Alterations in RNA content, polyribosome aggregation, and mRNA subcellular distribution are other mechanisms proposed to explain variations in protein synthesis caused by fasting (27,68,69,78). According to McNurlan et al. (68), decreased RNA content upon fasting of rats for 48 hr exceeds the diminution of protein synthesis; i.e., the amount of protein synthesis per gram RNA was essentially unchanged. Therefore, the decrease in protein synthesis was secondary to the decrease in RNA content. In perfused fasted rabbit liver, Rothschild et al. (69) demonstrated a marked disaggregation in polysomes of the RER, where albumin synthesis occurs. Free cytoplasmic polyribosomes were not disaggregated (69). Whether the disaggregation of membrane-bound polyribosomes resulted from a decreased initiation rate compared to elongation was not determined (69). Another possible explanation for the decrease in RNA content and polysome disaggregation in fasting could be activation or release of ribonucleases. Increased ribonuclease activity has been reported in protein-calorie malnutrition (79) and in hypophysectomized rats (80).

The influence of fasting on the subcellular distribution of albumin mRNA has been studied directly by Yap et al. (27,78). These investigators employed RNA-cDNA hybridization techniques to determine the absolute content of albumin mRNA in various subcellular fractions of rat liver. Total cytoplasmic albumin mRNA was decreased 40% by an 18-hr fast, and the ratio of albumin mRNA/unit of polyribosomal RNA was also diminished. Although the proportions of free and membrane-bound polysomes were unchanged, there was significant disaggregation of membrane-bound polysomes with little effect on free polysomes (78). While fasting led to a decrease in albumin mRNA associated with membrane-bound polysomes and an increase in albumin messenger in free polysomes, the greatest change was a 25-fold increase in albumin

mRNA in the postribosomal supernatant fraction. This albumin mRNA was complexed to protein as mRNPs (78). Similar complexes have been found in other systems associated with limitation of translation (81); it has been proposed that mRNPs may serve as a cytoplasmic storage pool for mRNAs (27).

Another possible mechanism for decreased protein synthesis in fasting is the loss of high-energy phosphate compounds. Both ATP and GTP are required at many steps in the protein synthesis mechanism. GDP inhibits formation of the ternary aminoacyl tRNA-elongation factor complex by competing with GTP (82). Conditions that alter the energy level of the cell may regulate protein biosynthesis at the level of initiation (82). Gilch and Mager (83) have shown that glucose starvation can lead to ATP and GTP depletion, which can result in translational inhibition.

The effect of refeeding fasted animals has been evaluated to determine whether abnormalities of the protein synthesis machinery are rapidly reversible. Feeding a diet complete in amino acids results in prompt improvement in protein synthesis (69,84–88). Controversy exists, however, as to which nutrients are essential in refeeding experiments. Much of the evidence supports the theory that tryptophan is a crucial amino acid in the refeeding diet. Tryptophan alone may be sufficient to correct many of the abnormalities in hepatic protein synthesis in fasted animals (84–86, 88,89), although this observation has been the subject of long-term controversy (79,90).

Several mechanisms may be involved in correction of hepatic protein synthesis by refeeding of tryptophan or complete amino acid mixtures. Studies demonstrate an increase in polysome aggregation and RNA content toward normal (69,84,88). Although there is evidence that trytophan increases cytoplasmic RNA levels by increasing transcription (89), Murty et al. (85) suggest at least one other mechanism. Rats were pretreated with cordycepin (2-deoxyadenosine), which inhibits nuclear RNA synthesis. When these animals were given tryptophan, there was an increase in the cytoplasmic poly (A^+) RNA and a decrease in the nuclear poly (A^+) RNA compared to control animals given cordycepin but not tryptophan. The authors concluded that tryptophan effects a posttranscriptional or translational step and that transport of mRNA from the nucleus to the cytoplasm is the most likely site of tryptophan action (84,85). The specific importance of tryptophan in albumin synthesis has not been explained and is surprising considering its limited representation in the albumin molecule. The N-terminal sequence of rat preproalbumin (the signal sequence), however, contains tryptophan (91). Perhaps it is this characteristic that makes tryptophan especially important in albumin synthesis.

Yap et al. (78) suggested another mechanism for the rapid effect of refeeding on protein synthesis. Within 1 hr after refeeding a complete amino acid mixture, but not tryptophan alone, cytoplasmic albumin mRNA re-shifted from the mRNP pool to membrane-bound polysomes (78). The investigators proposed that albumin mRNA, which is not required for cell survival, is stored as mRNPs under adverse conditions for protein synthesis and can be quickly reutilized when conditions become more favorable (78). Therefore, the polysome-mRNP equilibrium for a specific mRNA may be an important variable in determining the level of synthesis for a specific protein.

Force-Feeding of a Threonine-Deficient Diet

Sidransky and co-workers (92,93) employed an unusual diet to evaluate nutritional factors influencing hepatic protein synthesis. By forcefeeding rats with a threonine-deficient diet for 1 to 10 days, these investigators observed morphologic and biochemical changes similar to Kwashiorkor in humans. Pathologic alterations included hepatomegaly associated with increased fat, glycogen, and free polyribosomes. There was a small increase in hepatic protein synthesis compared to control animals (rats force-fed a complete amino acid diet). The increase occurred in both serum proteins and intracellular proteins. Increased hepatic protein synthesis was associated with an increase in total RNA content (93), average size of mRNA (93), polysome aggregation (92), and activity of initiation factors (94). Increased hepatic protein synthesis was explained on the basis of increased availability of amino acids secondary to increased muscle catabolism and diminished muscle protein synthesis (93); however, albumin synthesis was decreased in this system (rats force-fed a tryptophan-deficient diet).

Protein-Calorie-Deficient Diet

Although various authors consider their experimental diets to be strictly protein-deficient, experimental animals generally weigh less than controls, which suggests both protein and caloric deficiency (95–97). Most reports indicate that protein-calorie deficiency decreases hepatic protein synthesis (79,95–101), but some studies report an increase in synthesis of intrahepatic proteins (102,103). In protein-calorie malnutrition, the mechanism considered responsible for decreased hepatic protein synthesis is disaggregation of polysomes (79,87,95,98,100). Some studies also demonstrate diminished RNA content (79,101,104). One study indicated a decrease in RNA synthesis (101). Enwonwu and Munro (104) attributed the decrease in RNA content to be secondary to an increase of ribonuclease activity, which is probably caused by lysosomal activation or depression of ribonuclease inhibitor activity (79). The precise role of ribonuclease

inhibitor in protein synthesis in vivo has not been elucidated.

Sato et al. (98) evaluated the effect of protein depletion on the average polypeptide chain assembly time, which was prolonged in protein-deficient animals, suggesting an effect at the elongation step. There was no difference in poly (A$^+$) mRNA content between fed and deficient animals, and polysome disaggregation in the fasted state returned to normal following administration of cyclohexamide (98). Correction of polysome disaggregation by cyclohexamide (which inhibits polysome elongation and causes a shift to heavier polysomes) suggests that a defect in the initiation rate is more significant than perturbation of elongation (98). In addition, Sato and others have found that refeeding with a total amino acid mixture corrects polysome disaggregation and augments protein synthesis (79,87, 98,99).

Another mechanism that may influence protein synthesis in nutritionally deprived cells is the availability of activated amino acids (105–111). Using both artificial and natural mRNA templates in cell-free systems, Anderson and Gilbert (105,106) showed that variations in specific aminoacyl tRNAs could influence the rate of protein synthesis. Ogilvie et al. (109) evaluated the influence of limiting one essential amino acid in the medium on protein synthesis by Ehrlich ascites tumor cells. Moderate limitation of an aminoacylated species primarily influenced the rate of elongation, while effects on polysome aggregation or initiation steps required a diminution to less than 50% of control values (109). Other investigators found that aminoacylated tRNAs provide stability to the polyribosome (110).

Osterman (108) suggested that changes in the physiologic state of the cell alter the composition of isoaccepting tRNA species. When there is marked limitation in certain isoaccepting species, translation of mRNAs that employ these tRNAs will be hampered in comparison to other mRNAs that employ other isoaccepting species (2). Support for this mechanism is provided by the finding that the composition of the tRNA pool is noticeably different when a tissue hyperproduces a specific protein (112). Sharma et al. (113) reported that tRNA from chicken oviducts stimulates production of ovalbumin by chicken oviduct cells, whereas tRNA from rooster and rat liver has no effect. In addition, tRNA from rat hepatoma cells decreases ovalbumin synthesis in oviduct cells and induces synthesis of faulty ovalbumin (113). For a summary of the various mechanisms proposed for inhibition of hepatic protein synthesis by fasting or protein-calorie malnutrition, see Table 1.

The role of protein degradation in regulation of hepatic protein synthesis is unclear. Goldberg and St. John (114) reported that in vivo protein degradation rates are initially high in fasting or amino acid depriva-

TABLE 1. *Mechanisms proposed for inhibition of hepatic protein synthesis by fasting or protein-calorie malnutrition*

Mechanism	References
Inhibition of initiation	77,98,150
Decreased RNA content	68,79,101,104
Disaggregation of membrane-bound polyribosomes	69,79,89,95,98,100
Decreased availability of amino-acyl tRNAs	109
Shifting of mRNA from poly-somes to mRNPs	27,78
ATP and GTP depletion	83
Increased ribonuclease activity	79,104

tion and then decrease. This fall does not occur in studies utilizing isolated cells (114). Under normal cellular conditions, there is a marked variation in degradation rates of different proteins in rat liver, ranging from 12 min to 25 days (115). The half-life of the average hepatic protein is between two and three days and may vary with the size of the protein, subcellular location, hormonal factors, and nutritional state of the animal (114).

EFFECT OF ETHANOL ON HEPATIC PROTEIN SYNTHESIS

Serum albumin levels frequently are depressed in cirrhotic patients. Alcohol abuse contributes significantly to this problem; three reviews have evaluated the influence of ethanol on hepatic protein synthesis (116–118). It is assumed that ethanol has a toxic effect on protein synthesis in cirrhotic liver, but results of various studies are conflicting (69,119–137). Differences in experimental design may account for some of these differences: acute versus chronic ethanol exposure; oral versus parenteral administration of ethanol, variations in other nutrients; use of intact animals versus perfusion of isolated rabbit or rat liver; liver slices versus intact livers; isolated hepatocytes versus cell-free ribosomal preparations. Differences in ethanol levels achieved in animals, or in ethanol concentrations in perfusates or culture medium, as well as specific types of proteins studied, also may account for different results. A summary of the basic findings in various systems, with appropriate references, is given in Table 2.

There is general agreement that *in vitro* protein synthesis in liver from animals acutely treated with ethanol is decreased. Table 3 presents a summary of the proposed mechanisms. Rothschild et al. (69,122–124) have shown this in the isolated perfused rabbit liver. Kirsch et al. (125) demonstrated diminished albumin synthesis under the influence of ethanol in the isolated perfused rat liver. Liver slices also show diminished protein synthesis when incubated with

TABLE 2. *Effects of ethanol on hepatic protein synthesis*

Ethanol administration	References
Acute	
In vitro	
Inhibition of intracellular and export protein synthesis	69,121–126,131–133,137
Depressed glycoprotein synthesis	120
In vivo	
No change or decreased protein synthesis	127,133–135
Chronic	
In vitro	
Increased synthesis of export proteins	128,131,135
In vivo	
Conflicting results	119,130,135,136

ethanol (126). According to Kuriyama et al. (131), acute administration of ethanol diminishes protein synthesis by mouse liver ribosomes. Inhibition of protein synthesis by ethanol also occurs in isolated hepatocytes (121,132,133,137). Tuma and Sorrell (120) demonstrated that glycoprotein synthesis is affected adversely by ethanol. Controversy exists, however, regarding the effect of acute ethanol administration on protein synthesis *in vivo*. Some authors suggest a diminution in protein synthesis under such conditions (135); others report no effect on general protein or albumin synthesis (127,133,134). Baraona and co-workers (133) postulate inhibition of protein secretion to explain the apparent inconsistencies.

Conflicting results have been reported on the effect of chronic ethanol administration *in vivo*. There was a decrease in hepatic protein synthesis in rats, according to Nadkarni et al. (136) and Banks et al. (130). In other studies of rats with chronic low serum ethanol levels, however, Renis et al. (135) found no change in hepatic protein synthesis. In contrast, Baraona et al. (119) reported increased liver protein and proalbumin synthesis in rats after chronic ethanol administration.

When chronic ethanol administration is evaluated *in vitro*, a more consistent picture emerges. Isolated microsomes from ethanol-treated rats showed increased protein synthesis when compared to control animals (135). Kuriyama et al. (131) also demonstrated an in-

TABLE 3. *Mechanisms proposed for diminished protein synthesis after acute ethanol administration*

Mechanism	References
Decreased RNA/DNA ratio	122
Polysome disaggregation	69
Production of acetaldehyde	125,126
Generation of excess reducing equivalents	116,117,125,133,138

crease in protein synthesis with polysomes extracted from mice fed ethanol chronically. Zern and Shafritz (128) found that membrane-bound polysomes, but not free polysomes, from ethanol-treated rats incorporate more [^{3}H]leucine in cell-free protein synthesis than control animals. These results suggest that any decrease in protein or albumin synthesis after chronic ethanol administration *in vivo* probably results from posttranslational changes or other mechanisms.

Tables 1 and 3 show some similar changes which are similar in the effects of nutrient deprivation and acute ethanol administration on the hepatic protein synthesis machinery. Acute ethanol administration causes polysome disaggregation (69) and a decrease in the RNA/DNA ratio (122) in a manner similar to fasting. Fasting augments the acute effects of ethanol administration on protein synthesis (122,123,134). After ETOH administration, addition of tryptophan or a combination of amino acids leads to a reaggregation of polysomes and a return of the RNA/DNA ratio toward normal (69,122). In addition, Oratz et al. (123) have reported that spermine and arginine work synergistically to correct the disaggregation of polysomes and decrease in albumin synthesis caused by ethanol administration. Finally, amino acid supplementation corrects the depression in protein synthesis caused by acute ethanol administration (69,122,125,134). Therefore, acute ethanol administration and nutritional deficiency may operate through interference of a common molecular mechanism (121).

Certain effects of ethanol administration related to its subsequent oxidation are not produced by nutritional deficiency, namely, production of acetaldehyde and generation of excess reducing equivalents. Which of these factors is more significant in the toxic effect of ethanol on protein synthesis is not known. Acetaldehyde produces a concentration-dependent inhibition of protein synthesis in rat liver slices and in perfused rabbit liver (124,126). Addition of acetaldehyde directly to the culture medium, however, does not suppress protein synthesis in isolated hepatocytes (133). Oratz et al. (124) suggest that acetaldehyde may depress protein synthesis in a manner distinct from ethanol; the influence of acetaldehyde was not increased in fasted animals, nor did it cause polysome disaggregation.

Both oxidation of ethanol to acetaldehyde (by alcohol dehydrogenase) and subsequent oxidation of acetaldehyde to acetate generate excess reducing equivalents. This leads to an increase in the NADH:NAD ratio, which has several metabolic consequences, including inhibition of galactose elimination, fatty acid oxidation, and tricarboxylic acid cycle activity. In addition, the lactate/pyruvate ratio is increased (138). This change in redox levels in the cytosol and mitochondria is significant in the toxic effect of

ethanol on hepatic protein synthesis (116,117,126, 133,138). The proponents of this theory cite the following evidence to support their claims:

1. Oxidation of ethanol is required for its negative effect on protein synthesis. Perin et al. (126,129) and Baraona and co-workers (133) have demonstrated that pyrazole, an inhibitor of alcohol dehydrogenase, abolishes the inhibition of protein synthesis by ethanol in rat liver slices and in isolated hepatocytes. Also ethanol does not inhibit protein synthesis in tissues or cells which are low in alcohol dehydrogenase activity (126,129,137).

2. Sorbitol and other substances that elevate the NADH:NAD ratio depress protein synthesis in liver (126), while substances that scavenge reducing equivalents, such as methylene blue, reduce or prevent ethanol-induced inhibition of hepatic protein synthesis (129,133). Kirsch et al. (125), however, observed that although methylene blue corrects the lactate/pyruvate level, it does not attenuate the effect of ethanol on protein synthesis (125).

3. There is good evidence for attenuation or absence of ethanol-induced redox changes after chronic alcohol ingestion (138). Most studies do not demonstrate a reduction in protein synthesis following chronic ethanol administration (see above). Acute ethanol creates a high NADH:NAD ratio and inhibits protein synthesis, whereas chronic ethanol administration neither elevates the NADH:NAD ratio nor inhibits protein synthesis. Diminished generation of reducing equivalents in the chronic state may result from other pathways of ethanol metabolism which create acetaldehyde but do not generate NADH (117,138). Whatever the cause, changes in the redox state, as measured by elevated lactate/pyruvate levels or inhibition of galactose inhibition, are not found in animals fed ethanol chronically (138). When liver slices from these animals are compared to controls, inhibition of the tricarboxylic acid cycle and fatty acid oxidation by ETOH was attenuated (138).

Still unanswered is how a rise in the NADH:NAD ratio might affect the protein synthesis machinery at the molecular level. One possibility involves the equilibrium between nicotinamide and adenine nucleotides in the cytosol, such that an increase in the NADH:NAD ratio produces a decrease in the ATP/ADP ratio (139). Both ATP and GTP are involved in the initiation and elongation steps of protein synthesis (88,140), and adenine and guanine nucleotides are in equilibrium. GDP inhibits formation of the elongation factor EF-1 ternary complex by competing with GTP (82). Therefore, conditions that alter the energy level of the cell can affect protein biosynthesis. Depletion of ATP as a result of the altered redox state may be a significant mechanism for the effect of ethanol on protein synthesis. This mechanism has been postulated to explain suppression of protein synthesis by glucagon. Requero et al. (140) found that when an isolated liver is perfused with glucagon, the lactate/pyruvate ratio is elevated. Concurrently, the ATP/ADP ratio decreases; the pattern of ATP decrease corresponds to the pattern of decrease in hepatic protein synthesis (140).

Altered energy levels may affect protein synthesis, which may explain the reversal of alcohol-induced inhibition of protein synthesis by propylthiouracil (PTU) (136). Israel et al. (141) proposed that chronic ethanol ingestion results in a hypermetabolic state, which involves increased utilization of ATP via stimulation of the Na^+-K^+-dependent ATPase system. PTU may act by attenuating this hypermetabolic state and inhibiting the use of ATP. This could return the ATP/ADP ratio to normal and alleviate the block in protein synthesis.

PROTEIN SECRETION BY THE HEPATOCYTE

The effect of ethanol on hepatic protein secretion is disputed. Baraona and co-workers (119,133) found a decrease in secretion of hepatic proteins *in vivo* after ethanol administration. Tuma and Sorrell (120) reported that ethanol decreases glycoprotein secretion in rat liver slices. Therefore, some of the changes in overall protein synthesis in liver after ethanol administration may be secondary to effects on protein secretion. Unless intracellular degradation also increases, a combination of increased synthesis with diminished secretion should increase the protein content in the liver cell. Lieber (116) suggests that an increased osmotic load from cellular sequestration of normally secreted protein draws water into the cell and may account for hepatomegaly in alcoholic fatty liver.

Mørland and co-workers (118,121), however, observed no significant change in protein secretion after ethanol administration to isolated rat hepatocytes. They separated synthesis from secretion by giving a short pulse of [^{3}H]valine before measuring the effect of ethanol on protein secretion. In contrast to the effect of ethanol, colchicine decreased protein secretion in their system (118,121). Rothschild and co-workers (118) suggest that secretion plays a significant role in serum protein levels in cirrhosis. In cirrhosis, collagen accumulation alters the normal pathway of protein secretion into plasma; proteins that are normally secreted, enter the ascitic fluid rather than the serum. This may explain hypoalbuminemia in alcohol-induced cirrhosis, despite increased hepatic protein synthesis; another explanation may be a decrease in functioning hepatocyte mass. This was suggested by Yap et al. (142), who observed no change in cell-free protein synthesis activity or albumin mRNA content per mi-

crogram liver RNA in CCl_4-induced cirrhosis in rats. Alternatively, chronic ethanol administration may affect protein synthesis in cirrhotic liver differently from its effect on the fatty liver. Decreased nutrition may also reduce albumin synthesis in the cirrhotic patient.

HORMONAL EFFECTS ON PROTEIN SYNTHESIS

Hormones are thought to exert their effect by inducing biosynthesis of specific proteins, depending on the genetic structure of the cell. Estimates have put the number of inducible proteins at 1% or less of expressed protein (143). The influence of a particular hormone on hepatic protein synthesis *in vivo* is difficult to delineate. (For a capsule summary, see Table 4.) One complicating factor is that several hormones often interact to produce a given effect; e.g., $\alpha_2\mu$-globulin synthesis in liver is stimulated by androgens, thyroxine, glucocorticoids, and growth hormone (144). The nutritional status of the animal also may influence hormonal effects or induce other hormones. For example, glucose starvation leads to ATP deprivation, which subsequently leads to translational inhibition similar to the effect of hemin on initiation factor eIF-2 (83). The question is whether inhibition of protein synthesis is secondary to diminished insulin, increased glucagon, or an unrelated phenomenon. Evidence suggests that a specific hormone may affect protein biosynthesis at several levels (143), making evaluation of its influence on a particular mechanism more difficult.

Glucagon and cAMP

Although some specific proteins are induced by glucagon, e.g., tyrosine aminotransferase (145), glucagon has generally been associated with diminished hepatic protein synthesis (3,140,146,147). *In vivo* studies reveal an increase in polypeptide chain completion

TABLE 4. *Effects of hormones and endocrinopathies on hepatic protein synthesis*

Hormone or endocrine abnormality	References
Glucagon depresses protein synthesis (mediated via cAMP)	3,140,146,147
Diabetes has no effect or decreases protein synthesis; insulin corrects abnormalities in protein synthesis in diabetic rats	151–155
Hypophysectomy has no effect or decreases protein synthesis	80,158–160
Thyroid hormone increases protein synthesis in hypothyroid or euthyroid animals and in humans	118,162–165

time with glucagon (147). Glucagon decreases protein synthesis in isolated hepatocytes and in liver slices (3). One recently proposed mechanism involves an increase in the NADH:NAD ratio and subsequent diminution of ATP levels (140). A more established mechanism involves elevation of cAMP levels by glucagon (3). Cyclic AMP has an antianabolic effect, presumably on translation (146). Major actions of cAMP include stimulating gluconeogenesis and glycogenolysis. This antianabolic effect would permit amino acid utilization for gluconeogenesis (146). cAMP is thought to act on the initiation process by means of a cAMP-dependent protein kinase (146). Protein kinases that inhibit translation act in a manner similar to the cAMP-independent protein kinase, the hemin-controlled inhibitor (HCI) (148).

HCI and other cAMP-dependent protein kinases in rat liver, rabbit reticulocyte, and Krebs ascites cells all phosphorylate the smallest subunit of eIF-2, which limits initiation (3,139). The action of these inhibitors is overcome by adding excess eIF-2 (149). Phosphorylation-dephosphorylation of eIF-2 by cAMP-dependent protein kinase may be a major means for regulating initiation of protein synthesis (148). This is significant because the overall rate of protein synthesis is roughly proportional to the initiation rate constant (150).

Diabetes and Insulin

The influence of experimentally induced diabetes on protein synthesis is unclear. *In vivo* studies by Pain and Garlick (151) suggest no change in protein synthesis; Ingebretson and co-workers (152), however, demonstrated impaired synthesis of secreted proteins in isolated hepatocytes of diabetic rats. Jefferson et al. (153–155) studied diabetic perfused rat liver and observed that secretory protein synthesis was reduced to a much greater extent than intracellular protein synthesis. Albumin was the most significantly affected protein. The authors proposed that the diminution in albumin synthesis is secondary to disorganization of the RER (156). The polysome size was unchanged (154), but the total number of polysomes was diminished in the membrane-bound fraction (153). Both cell-free protein synthesis and recombinant DNA techniques were employed to determine that albumin mRNA content was decreased in diabetic animals (155). Insulin injection restored albumin synthesis and albumin mRNA levels to normal (155). Unfortunately, the results are problematic, because induction of diabetes led to weight loss in experimental rats and possibly to protein-calorie malnutrition. Insulin led to subsequent weight gain and correction of protein synthesis. Although these findings may explain the mechanism for insulin action in protein synthesis, nutritional factors may be a critical variable in their system. Other authors (157) suggest that diminished specific amino-

acyl tRNA synthetases may regulate hepatic protein synthesis in diabetes. These studies require further documentation.

Hypophysectomy and Growth Hormone

Hypophysectomy has been used as a model to determine the effect of growth hormone on hepatic protein synthesis. Most (80,158,159) but not all (80,160) studies indicate that hypophysectomy decreases protein synthesis. Taylor et al. (158,159) found diminished protein and albumin synthesis in perfused liver *in vivo* and in isolated hepatocytes from hypophysectomized animals when compared to controls. They also found a 50% reduction in albumin mRNA content in experimental animals (158); growth hormone replacement returned albumin mRNA levels to normal. However, hypophysectomized animals experienced a 20% weight loss from the time of operation to the time of the experiment (3 to 5 months later). Hypophysectomized animals gained considerable weight during growth hormone treatment. Since previous studies had shown that growth hormone alone was incapable of restoring levels of mRNA (161), improved nutrition may explain the increase in albumin mRNA levels. These studies indicated that administration of corticosteroids, dihydrotestosterone, and thyroxine, as well as growth hormone, was necessary for significant repletion of mRNA (161). In other studies, Brewer et al. (80) found that protein synthesis was only occasionally decreased in hypophysectomized animals. When this occurred, there was disaggregation of polysomes associated with a corresponding increase in RNAse activity. When growth hormone was given, RNAse activity, the polysome profile, and *in vitro* protein synthesis returned to normal (80).

Thyroid Hormone

Thyroid hormone increases protein synthesis in healthy humans and in laboratory animals *in vivo* and *in vitro* (118,162–165). mRNA and rRNA levels in thyroidectomized animals are reduced, and triiodothyronine administration leads to a rise in nuclear RNA synthesis. Carter and Faas (162) recently observed an early increase in protein synthesis after thyroid hormone administration that was blocked by α-amanitin. This suggested that the effect was dependent on RNA synthesis, in contrast to earlier reports that thyroxine stimulated the elongation step of polypeptide synthesis (164).

Other Hormones

Transcriptional and posttranscriptional control studies in systems other than liver have shown marked changes in the half-life of specific messenger RNAs with induction by hormones (63,167,168). The importance of transcription and mRNA processing is stressed in the work of Tsai et al. (169), who found less than one molecule of ovalbumin nuclear RNA per cell in uninduced oviduct cells. After induction, there were hundreds of molecules of ovalbumin nuclear RNA per cell, and thousands of molecules per cell in the cytoplasm (169). Future studies will be necessary to determine whether albumin mRNA transcription, processing, or half-life is influenced by hormonal or other physiologic or pathologic parameters. Although no known hormone is involved, albumin is induced from a low level of synthesis in fetal life to become the major adult serum protein (170). Albumin mRNA levels in the rat range from 2,000 copies per cell at 16 days gestation to 60,000 copies per cell 2 weeks after birth and throughout adult life.

In addition to transcriptional regulation, there is evidence for significant posttranscriptional control of specific albumin mRNA content. A recent report by Hofer et al. (171) indicates that while 0.4% of nuclear poly (A+) molecules are homologous to albumin cDNA, 10% of cytoplasmic poly (A+) molecules react with this probe (i.e., represent albumin mRNA). Evidence that RNA processing or transport from nucleus to the cytoplasm may in fact alter the relative mRNA content in a cell has been presented by Harpold and co-workers (172). These investigators cloned DNA sequences to unselected mRNAs from Chinese hamster ovary cells and found that the relative cytoplasmic content of poly (A+) RNA for at least one-third of the clones was considerably different from the relative nuclear content (172). This indicates that posttranscriptional events may play a significant role in determining the cytoplasmic concentration of many mRNA species.

EFFECT OF CHRONIC RENAL FAILURE

Few studies have evaluated the effect of chronic renal failure (uremia) on hepatic protein synthesis separate from the influence of nutritional factors. In pair-fed animals of essentially similar age and weight, Grossman et al. (173) found decreases in the serum albumin level, in cell-free albumin synthesis, and in average polysome size (especially membrane-bound polyribosomes). There was no change in protein synthesis with free polysomes but a reduction in synthesis of secreted proteins by membrane-bound polysomes and a marked decrease in albumin synthesis (173). Diminished synthesis of albumin (*in vitro*) plus increased intracellular accumulation of albumin suggested a block in secretion. Using hybridization studies, Zern et al. (174) demonstrated an increased amount of albumin mRNA sequences per gram liver and an increase in total polysomes in the cells of uremic animals, but a diminution of full-sized albumin mRNA and decreased albumin synthesis when compared to controls. Therefore, both synthesis and secretion of albumin from the hepatocyte may be influenced in separate ways by uremia in rats.

CONCLUSION

It is difficult to evaluate the influence of variations in physiologic state on the complex functions of hepatic protein synthesis. Each system has its advantages and disadvantages. Ideally, one wishes to understand the effect of the perturbation on the intact animal. Interrupting homeostatic mechanisms with one intrusion, however, often influences other regulators of protein synthesis. This may yield a change in protein biosynthesis, as demonstrated by an *in vivo* effect, but obscures the true mechanisms of action of the substance studied. Studies that attempt to avoid this difficulty by employing *in vitro* systems run the risk of evaluating a mechanism that may have no physiologic importance. For example, the use of a messenger-dependent rabbit-reticulocyte lysate system to evaluate rat liver mRNA content was an advance over previous systems in that it permitted unequivocal demonstration of liver-specific proteins in a heterologous system. Use of protein synthesis machinery from reticulocytes, however, exhibited properties that are not present in liver. In addition, the reticulocyte system quantifies translatable mRNA, not total mRNA content, a problem that can be rectified by concurrent use of cDNA hybridization. However, combining protein synthesis with hybridization measurements may not necessarily delineate all the factors that may influence synthesis of a specific protein.

This leads to a basic problem in elucidating mechanisms involved in changes in protein synthesis caused by changes in the physiologic state, i.e., the multiplicity of regulation. There is evidence for regulation at the following levels: gene rearrangement, transcription, processing, and transport of mRNA from nucleus to cytoplasm; translation of mRNA; turnover or degradation of mRNA (in the cytoplasm); and protein turnover directly. Although these multilayered levels of regulation [originally proposed by Scherrer and Marcaud (175)] make analysis complex, these factors and steps must be considered. When vast differences in protein synthesis exist during various physiologic states, major changes in specific mRNA content may be occurring. Minor or temporary perturbations in hepatic protein biosynthesis may be caused by changes in physiologic states without alteration in total mRNA content of the cell. The task, therefore, is to understand the complex function of protein synthesis while maintaining awareness of the limitations placed on us by the complexity of the system with which we are dealing.

REFERENCES

1. Lodish, H. (1976): Translational control of protein synthesis. *Ann. Rev. Biochem.*, 45:39–72.

2. Revel, M., and Groner, Y. (1978): Post-transcriptional and translational controls of gene expression in eukaryotes. *Ann. Rev. Biochem.*, 47:1079–1126.

3. Ochoa, S., and de Haro, C. (1979): Regulation of protein synthesis in eukaryotes. *Ann. Rev. Biochem.*, 48:549–580.

4. Shafritz, D. A., and Anderson, W. F. (1970): Factor dependent binding of methionyl-tRNA's to reticulocyte ribosome. *Nature*, 227:918–920.

5. Shafritz, D. A. (1977): Messenger RNA and its translation. In: *Molecular Mechanisms of Protein Biosynthesis*, edited by H. Weissbach and S. Pestka, pp. 555–601. Academic Press, New York.

6. Shatkin, A. J. (1976): Capping of eucaryotic mRNAs. *Cell*, 9:645–653.

7. Chang, A. C., Erlich, H. A., Gunsalus, R. P., Nunberg, J. H., Kaufman, R. J., Schimke, R. T., and Cohen, S. N. (1980): Initiation of protein synthesis in bacteria at a translational start codon of mammalian cDNA. *Proc. Natl. Acad. Sci. USA*, 77:1442–1446.

8. Berk, A. J., and Sharp, P. A. (1977): Ultraviolet mapping of the adenovirus 2 early promoters. *Cell*, 12:45–55.

9. Padilla, M., Canaani, D., Groner, Y., Weinstein, J., Bar-Joseph, M., Merrick, W., and Shafritz, D. A. (1978): Initiation factor eIF-4B (IF-M₃)-dependent recognition and translation of capped versus uncapped eukaryotic mRNAs. *J. Biol. Chem.*, 253:5939–5945.

10. Heywood, S. M., Kennedy, D. S., and Bester, A. J. (1974): Separation of specific initiation factors involved in the translation of myosin and myoglobin messenger RNAs and the isolation of a new RNA involved in translation. *Proc. Natl. Acad. Sci. USA*, 71:2428–2434.

11. Caskey, T. (1977): Peptide chain termination. In: *Molecular Mechanisms of Protein Biosynthesis*, edited by H. Weissbach and S. Pestka, pp. 413–467. Academic Press, New York.

12. Siekevitz, P., and Palade, G. E. (1960): A cytochemical study on the pancreas of the guinea pig. V. *In vivo* incorporation of leucine-1-C¹⁴ into the chymotrypsinogen of various cell fractions. *J. Biophys. Biochem. Cytol.*, 7:619–630.

13. Peters, T., Jr. (1962): The biosynthesis of rat serum albumin. Properties of rat albumin and its occurrence in liver cell fractions. *J. Biol. Chem.*, 237:1181–1185.

14. Peters, T., Jr. (1962): The biosynthesis of rat serum albumin. II. Intracellular phenomena in the secretion of newly formed albumin. *J. Biol. Chem.*, 237:1186–1189.

15. Blobel, G., and Dobberstein, B. (1975): Transfer of proteins across membranes. I. Presence of proteolytically processed and unprocessed nascent immunoglobulin light chains on membrane-bound ribosomes of murine myeloma. *J. Cell Biol.*, 67:835–851.

16. Blobel, G., and Dobberstein, B. (1975): Transfer of proteins across membranes. II. Reconstitution of functional rough microsomes from heterologous components. *J. Cell Biol.*, 67:852–862.

17. Devillers-Thiery, A., Kindt, T., Scheele, G., and Blobel, G. (1975): Homology in amino-terminal sequence of precursors to pancreatic secretory proteins. *Proc. Natl. Acad. Sci. USA*, 72:5016–5020.

18. Blobel, G. (1977): Mechanisms for the intracellular compartmentation of newly synthesized proteins. In: *Gene Expression, Proceedings* of the 11th FEBS Meetings, Copenhagen, edited by P. Schambye, vol. 43, pp. 99–108. Pergamon, Oxford.

19. Palmiter, R. D., Gagnon, J., and Walsh, K. A. (1978): Ovalbumin: A secreted protein without a transient hydrophobic leader sequence. *Proc. Natl. Acad. Sci. USA*, 75:94–98.

20. Goldman, B. M., and Blobel, G. (1978): Biogenesis of peroxisomes: Intracellular site of synthesis of catalase and uricase. *Proc. Natl. Acad. Sci. USA*, 75:5066–5070.

21. Blobel, G., Walter, P., Chang, C. N., Goldman, B. M., Erickson, A. H., and Lingappa, V. R. (1979): Translocation of proteins across membranes: The signal hypothesis and beyond. In: *Secretory Mechanisms*, etited by C. R. Hopkins and C. J. Duncan, pp. 9–36. Cambridge University Press, London.

22. Garaff, H., Frischauf, A. M., Simons, K., Lehrach, H., and Delius, H. (1980): Nucleotide sequence of cDNA coding for semliki forest virus membrane glycoproteins. *Nature*, 288:236–241.

23. Judah, J. D., Gamble, M., and Steadman, J. H. (1973): Biosynthesis of serum albumin in rat liver. *Biochem. J.*, 134:1083–1091.

24. Russel, J. H., and Geller, D. M. (1975): The structure of rat proalbumin. *J. Biol. Chem.*, 250:3409–3413.

25. Urban, J., Inglis, A. S., Edwards, K., and Schreiber, G. (1974): Chemical evidence for the difference between albumin from microsomes and serum and a possible precursor product relationship. *Biochem. Biophys. Res. Commun.*, 61:494–501.

26. Strauss, A. W., Donahue, A. M., Bennett, C. D., Rodkey, J. A., and Alberts, A. W. (1977): Rat liver preproalbumin. *In vitro* synthesis and partial amino acid sequence. *Proc. Natl. Acad. Sci. USA*, 74:1358–1362.

27. Yap, S. H., Strair, R. K., and Shafritz, D. A. (1978): Effect of short-term fast on the distribution of albumin messenger RNA in rat liver. *J. Biol. Chem.*, 253:4944–4950.

28. Ramsey, J. C., and Steele, W. J. (1976): A procedure for the quantitative recovery of homogeneous populations of undegraded free and bound polysomes from rat liver. *Biochemistry*, 15:1704–1712.

29. Shafritz, D. A. (1974): Evidence for non-translated messenger RNA in membrane-bound and free polysomes of rabbit liver. *J. Biol. Chem.*, 249:89–93.

30. Peterson, J. A. (1976): Clonal variation in albumin messenger RNA activity in hepatoma cells. *Proc. Natl. Acad. Sci. USA*, 73:2056–2060.

31. Sell, S., Thomas, K., Michaelson, M., Sala-Trepat, J., and Bonner, J. (1979): Control of albumin and α-fetoprotein expression in rat liver and in some transplantable hepatocellular carcinoma. *Biochem. Biophys. Acta*, 564:173–178.

32. Richardson, U. I., Tashjian, A. H., Jr., and Levine, L. (1969): Establishment of a clonal strain of hepatoma cells which secrete albumin. *J. Cell Biol.*, 40:236–247.

33. Schreiber, G., Boutwell, R. K., Potter, V. R., and Morris, H. P. (1966): Lack of secretion of serum protein by transplanted rat hepatomas. *Cancer Res.*, 26:2357–2361.

34. Urban, J., Kartenbeck, J., Zimber, P. I., Timko, J., Lesch, R., and Schreiber, G. (1972): Increase of extravascular albumin pool and intracellular accumulation of vesicles in transplanted Morris hepatoma 9121. *Cancer Res.*, 32:1971–1975.

35. Uenoyama, K., and Ono, T. (1972): Synthesis of albumin by the free polyribosomes in 5123 hepatoma. *Biochim. Biophys. Acta*, 281:124–129.

36. Strauss, A., Bennett, C., Donohue, A. M., Rodkey, J., and Alberts, A. W. (1977): Rat hepatoma 5123TC albumin mRNA directs the synthesis of pre-proalbumin identical to rat liver pre-proalbumin. *Biochem. Biophys. Res. Commun.*, 77:1224–1230.

37. Kreibich, G., Ulrich, B. L., and Sabatini, D. D. (1978): Proteins of rough microsomal membranes related to ribosome binding. I. Identification of ribophorins I and II, membrane proteins characteristic of rough microsomes. *J. Cell Biol.*, 77:464–486.

38. Southern, E. M. (1975): Detection of specific sequences among DNA fragments separated by gel electrophoresis. *J. Mol. Biol.*, 98:503–517.

39. Jeffreys, A. J., and Flavell, R. A. (1977): The rabbit B-globin gene contains a large insert in the coding sequence. *Cell*, 12:1097–1108.

40. Tilghman, S. M., Tiemeier, D. C., Seidman, J. G., Peterlin, B. M., Sullivan, M., Maizel, J., and Leder, P. (1978): Intervening sequences of DNA identified in the structural portion of mouse B-globin gene. *Proc. Natl. Acad. Sci. USA*, 75:725–729.

41. Brack, C., Hirama, M., Lenhard-Schuller, R., and Tonegawa, S. (1978): A complete immunoglobulin gene is created by somatic recombination. *Cell*, 15:1–14.

42. Seidman, J. G., and Leder, P. (1978): The arrangement and rearrangement of antibody genes. *Nature*, 276:790–795.

43. Breathnach, R., Mandel, J. L., and Chambon, P. (1977): Ovalbumin gene is split in chicken DNA. *Nature,* 270:314–319.

44. Lai, E. C., Woo, S. L. C., Dugaiczyk, A., Catterall, J. F., and O'Malley, B. W. (1978): The ovalbumin gene: Structural sequences in native chicken DNA are not contiguous. *Proc. Natl. Acad. Sci. USA,* 75:2205–2209.

45. Dawid, I., and Wahli, W. (1979): Application of recombinant DNA technology to question of development biology: A review. *Dev. Biol.,* 69:305–328.

46. Darnell, J. E., Jr. (1979): Transcription units for mRNA production in eukaryotic cells and their DNA viruses. In: *Progress in Nucleic Acid Research and Molecular Biology, Vol. 22,* edited by W. E. Cohn, pp. 327–353. Academic Press, New York.

47. Sala-Trepat, J. M., Sargent, T., Sell, S., and Bonner, J. (1979): α-Fetoprotein and albumin genes of rats. No evidence for amplification-deletion or rearrangment in rat liver carcinogenesis. *Proc. Natl. Acad. Sci. USA,* 76:695–699.

48. Sargent, T. D., Wu, J. R., Sala-Trepat, J., Wallace, R. B., Reyes, A. A., and Bonner, J. (1979): The rat serum albumin gene: Analysis of cloned sequences. *Proc. Natl. Acad. Sci. USA,* 76:3256–3260.

49. Mears, J. G., Ramirez, F., Leibowitz, D., and Bank, A. (1978): Organization of human α- and β-globin genes in cellular DNA and the presence of intragenic insets. *Cell,* 15:15–23.

50. Orkin, S. H., Alter, B. P., and Altay, C. (1978): Application of endonuclease mapping to the analysis and prenatal diagnosis of thalassemia caused by globin gene detection. *N. Engl. J. Med.,* 297:166–172.

51. Fritsch, E. F., Lawn, R. M., and Maniatis, T. (1979): Characterization of deletions which affect the expression of fetal globin genes in man. *Nature,* 279:598–603.

52. Liebhaber, S. A., Goosens, M. J., and Kan, Y. W. (1981): Differences in the structure and expression of the two α-globin genes. *Clin. Res.,* 29:513A.

53. Ramirez, F., Mears, G., Nudel, U., Bank, A., Luzzatto, L., Gambino, R., Cimino, R., and Quattrin, N. (1979): Defects in DNA and globin messenger RNA in homozygotes for hemoglobin lepore. *J. Clin. Invest.,* 63:736–742.

54. Nagase, S., Shimamune, K., and Shumiya, S. (1979): Albumin-deficient rat mutant. *Science,* 205:590–591.

55. Cormode, E. J., Lyster, D. M., and Israels, S. (1975): Analbuminemia in a neonate. *J. Pediatr.,* 86:862–867.

56. Rogers, J., Early, P., Carter, C., Calame, K., Bond, M., Hood, L., and Wall, R. (1980): Two mRNAs with different 3' ends encode membrane-bound and secreted forms of immunoglobulin μ chain. *Cell,* 20:303–312.

57. Early, P., Rogers, J., Davis, M., Calame, K., Bond, M., Wall, R., and Hood, L. (1980): Two mRNAs can be produced from a single immunoglobulin μ gene by alternative RNA processing pathways. *Cell,* 20:313–319.

58. Swaneck, G. E., Nordstrom, J. L., Kreuzalev, F., Tsai, M. J., and O'Malley, B. W. (1979): Effect of estrogen on gene expression in chicken oviducts: Evidence for transcriptional control of ovalbumin gene. *Proc. Natl. Acad. Sci. USA,* 76:1049–1053.

59. Strair, R. K., Yap, S. H., Nadal-Ginard, B., and Shafritz, D. A. (1978): Identification of a high molecular weight putative precursor to albumin mRNA in the nucleus of rat liver. *J. Biol. Chem.,* 253:1328–1331.

60. Wilson, M. C., Sawicki, S. G., White, P. A., and Darnell, J. E., Jr. (1978): A correlation between the rate of poly (A) shortening and half-life of messenger RNA in adenovirus transformed cells. *J. Mol. Biol.,* 126:23–36.

61. Bastos, R. N., Volloch, Z., and Aviv, H. (1977): Messenger RNA population analysis during erythroid differentiation: A kinetical approach. *J. Mol. Biol.,* 110:191–203.

62. Lodish, H. F., and Small, B. (1976): Different lifetimes of reticulocyte messenger RNA. *Cell,* 7:59–65.

63. Lowenhaupt, K., and Lingrel, J. B. (1978): A change in the stability of globin mRNA during the induction of murine erythroleukemia cells. *Cell,* 14:337–344.

64. Buckingham, M. E., Cohen, A., and Gros, F. (1976): Cytoplasmic distribution of pulse-labelled poly (A) containing RNA, particularly 26S RNA, during myoblast growth and differentiation. *J. Mol. Biol.,* 103:611–626.

65. Cox, R. F., Haines, M. E., and Emtage, J. S. (1974): Quantitation of ovalbumin mRNA in hen and chick oviduct by hybridization to complementary DNA. *Eur. J. Biochem.,* 49:225–236.

66. Farmer, S. R., Henshaw, E. C., Berridge, M. V., and Tata, J. R. (1978): Translation of *xenopus* vitellogenin mRNA during primary and secondary induction. *Nature,* 273:401–403.

67. Peters, T., Jr., and Peters, J. C. (1972): The biosynthesis of rat serum albumin. VI. Intracellular transport of albumin and rates of albumin and liver protein synthesis *in vitro* under various physiological conditions. *J. Biol. Chem.,* 247:3858–3863.

68. McNurlan, M. A., Tomkins, A. M., and Garlick, P. J. (1979): The effect of starvation on the rate of protein synthesis in rat liver and small intestine. *Biochem. J.,* 178:373–379.

69. Rothschild, M., Oratz, M., and Schreiber, S. S. (1974): Alcohol, amino acids and albumin synthesis. *Gastroenterology,* 67:1200–1213.

70. Pain, V. M., Garlick, P., J., and McNurlan, M. A. (1978): Synthesis of albumin and of total plasma proteins by liver of fed and starved rats. *Proc. Nutr. Soc.,* 37:29A.

71. Wilson, S. H., Hill, H. Z., and Hoagland, M. B. (1967): Physiology of rat liver polysomes. *Biochem. J.,* 103:567–572.

72. Beuzrad, Y., and London, I. (1974): The effects of hemin and double stranded RNA on α and β-globin synthesis in reticulocyte and Krebs II ascites cell-free systems and the relationship of these effects to an initiation factor preparation. *Proc. Natl. Acad. Sci. USA,* 71:2863–2866.

73. Sonenshein, G. E., and Braverman, G. (1976): Regulation of immunoglobulin synthesis in mouse myeloma cells. *Biochemistry,* 15:5497–5500.

74. Lodish, H. F. (1974): Model for the regulation of mRNA translation applied to haemoglobin synthesis. *Nature,* 251:385–388.

75. Lodish, H. F. (1976): Translational control of protein synthesis. *Ann. Rev. Biochem.,* 45:39–72.

76. Kabat, D., and Chappell, M. R. (1977): Competition between globin messenger ribonucleic acids for a discriminating initiation factor. *J. Biol. Chem.,* 252:2684–2690.

77. Von Heyne, G., Nilsson, L., and Blomberg, C. (1977): Translation and messenger RNA secondary structure. *J. Theor. Biol.,* 68:321–329.

78. Yap, S. H., Strair, R. K., and Shafritz, D. A. (1978): Identification of albumin mRNPs in the cytosol of fasting rat liver and influence of tryptophan or a mixture of amino acids. *Biochem. Biophys. Res. Commun.,* 83:427–433.

79. Enwonwu, C. O., and Sreebny, L. M. (1971): Studies of hepatic lesions of experimental protein-calorie malnutrition in rats and immediate effects of refeeding an adequate protein diet. *J. Nutr.,* 101:501–514.

80. Brewer, E. N., Foster, L. B., and Sells, B. H. (1969): A possible role for ribonuclease in the regulation of protein synthesis in normal and hypoplysectomized rats. *J. Biol. Chem.,* 244:1389–1392.

81. Schochetman, G., and Perry, R. P. (1972): Characterization of the messenger RNA released from L cell polyribosomes as a result of temperature shock. *J. Mol. Biol.,* 63:577–590.

82. Walton, G. M., and Gill, G. N. (1975): Nucleotide regulation of a eukaryotic protein synthesis initiation couplex. *Biochim. Biophys. Acta,* 390:231–245.

83. Gilch, H., and Mager, J. (1975): Inhibition of peptide chain initiation in lysates from ATP-depleted cells. *Biochim. Biophys. Acta,* 414:293–308.

84. Murty, C. N., Verney, E., and Sidransky, H. (1976): Effect of tryptophan on RNA transport from nucleus to cytoplasm in rat liver. *Fed. Proc.,* 35:498.

85. Murty, C. N., Verney, E., and Sidransky, H. (1976): Effect of tryptophan on polyriboadenylic acid and polyadenylic acid-messenger ribonucleic acid in rat liver. *Lab. Invest.,* 34:77–85.

86. Wunner, W. H., Bell, J., and Munro, H. N. (1966): The effect of feeding with a tryptophan-free amino acid mixture on rat liver polysomes and ribosomal ribonucleic acid. *Biochem. J.,* 101:417–423.

87. Fleck, A., Shepherd, J., and Munro, H. N. (1965): Protein synthesis in rat liver: Influence of amino acids in diet on microsomes and polysomes. *Science*, 150:628–630.

88. Sidransky, H., Sarma, D. S. R., Bongiorno, M., and Verney, E. (1968): Effect of dietary tryptophan on hepatic polyribosomes and protein synthesis in fasted mice. *J. Biol. Chem.*, 243:1123–1132.

89. Oravec, M., and Korner, A. (1971): Stimulation of ribosomal and DNA-like RNA synthesis by tryptophan. *Biochim. Biophys. Acta*, 247:404–407.

90. Kelman, L., Saunders, S. J., Wicht, S., Firth, L., Corrigall, A., Kirsch, R. E., and Terblanche, J. (1972): The effects of amino acids on albumin synthesis by the isolated perfused rat liver. *Biochem. J.*, 129:805–809.

91. Strauss, A. W., Bennett, C. D., Donohue, A. M., Rodkey, J. A., and Alberts, A. W. (1977): Rat liver pre-proalbumin: Complete amino acid sequence of the pre-piece. *J. Biol. Chem.*, 252:4846–4855.

92. Sidransky, H., Staehelin, T., and Verney, E. (1964): Protein synthesis enhanced in the liver of rats force-fed a threonine-devoid diet. *Science*, 146:766–768.

93. Sidransky, H. (1976): Nutritional disturbances of protein metabolism in the liver. *Am. J. Pathol.*, 84:649–667.

94. Murty, C. N., Verney, E., and Sidransky, H. (1974): Initiation factors in protein synthesis of liver and skeletal muscle of rats force-fed a threonine-devoid diet. *Proc. Soc. Exp. Biol. Med.*, 145:74–79.

95. Pain, V. M., Clemens, M. J., and Garlick, P. J. (1978): The effect of dietary protein deficiency on albumin synthesis and on the concentration of active albumin messenger ribonucleic acid in rat liver. *Biochem. J.*, 172:129–135.

96. Quartey-Papafio, P., Garlick, P. J., and Pain, V. M. (1980): Effect of dietary protein on liver protein synthesis. *Biochem. Soc. Trans.*, 15:357.

97. Peters, T., Jr. (1973): Biosynthesis of rat serum albumin. VII. Effects observed in liver slices. *Am. J. Physiol.*, 224:1363–1368.

98. Sato, K., Noda, K., and Natori, Y. (1979): The effect of protein depletion on the rate of protein synthesis in rat liver. *Biochim. Biophys. Acta*, 561:475–483.

99. Morgan, E. H., and Peters, T., Jr. (1971): The biosynthesis of rat serum albumin. V. Effect of protein depletion and refeeding on albumin and transferrin synthesis. *J. Biol. Chem.*, 246:3500–3507.

100. Tavill, A. S., East, A. G., Black, E. G., Nadharni, D., and Hoffenberg, R. (1973): Regulatory factors in the synthesis of plasma proteins by the isolated perfused rat liver. In: *Protein Turnover, Ciba Foundation Symposium*, vol. 9, edited by G. E. W. Wolstenholme and M. O'Connor, pp. 155–173. Elsevier Excerpta Medica, Amsterdam.

101. Wannemacher, R. W., Wannemacher, C. F., and Yatvin, M. B. (1971): Amino acid regulation of ribonucleic acid and protein in the liver of rats. *Biochem. J.*, 124:385–397.

102. Haider, M., and Tarver, H. (1969): Effect of diet on protein synthesis and nucleic acid levels in rat liver. *J. Nutr.*, 99:433–445.

103. Garlick, P. J., Millward, D. J., James, W. P. T., and Waterlow, J. C. (1975): The effect of protein deprivation and starvation on the rate of protein synthesis in tissues of the rat. *Biochem. Biophys. Acta*, 414:71–84.

104. Enwonwu, C. O., and Munro, H. N., (1970): Rate of RNA turnover in rat liver in relation to intake of protein. *Arch. Biochem. Biophys.* 138:532–539.

105. Anderson, W. F., and Gilbert, J. M. (1969): tRNA-dependent translational control of *in vitro* hemoglobin synthesis. *Biochem. Biophys. Res. Commun.*, 36:456–462.

106. Anderson, W. F. (1969): The effect of tRNA concentration on the rate of protein synthesis. *Proc. Natl. Acad. Sci. USA*, 62:566–573.

107. Pain, V. M., and Clemens, M. J. (1973): The role of soluble protein factors in the translational control of protein synthesis in eukaryotic cells. *FEBS Lett.*, 32:205–212.

108. Osterman, R. A. (1979): Participation of tRNA in regulation of protein biosynthesis at the translational level in eukaryotes. *Biochimie*, 61:323–342.

109. Ogilvie, A., Huschka, V., and Kersten, W. (1979): Control of protein synthesis in mammalian cells by aminoacylation of

110. Warrington, R. C., Wratten, N., and Hechtman, R. (1977): L-histidinol inhibits specifically and reversibly protein and ribosomal RNA synthesis in mouse L cells. *J. Biol. Chem.*, 252:5251–5257.

111. Vaughan, M. H., and Hansen, B. S. (1973): Control initiation of protein synthesis in human cells. Evidence for a role on uncharged transfer ribonucleic acid. *J. Biol. Chem.*, 248:7087–7091.

112. Chavancy, G., Garel, J. P., and Daillie, J. (1975): Functional adaptation of aminoacyl tRNA synthetases to fibroin biosynthesis in the silkgland of BOMBYX MORI L. *FEBS Lett.*, 49:380–384.

113. Sharma, O. K., Mays, L. L., and Borek, E. (1975): Functional differences in protein synthesis between rat liver tRNA and tRNA from Novikoff hepatoma. *Biochemistry*, 14:509–514.

114. Goldberg, A. L., and St. John, A. C. (1976): Intracellular protein degradation in mammalian and bacterial cells. Part 2. *Ann. Rev. Biochem.*, 45:747–803.

115. Wang, C., and Towster, O. (1975): Turnover studies on proteins of rat liver lysosomes. *J. Biol. Chem.*, 250:4896–4902.

116. Lieber, C. S. (1980): Alcohol, protein metabolism and liver injury. *Gastroenterology*, 79:373–390.

117. Sorrell, M. F., and Tuma, D. J. (1979): Effects of alcohol on hepatic metabolism: Selected aspects. *Clin. Sci.*, 57:481–489.

118. Rothschild, M. A., Oratz, M., and Schreiber, S. S. (1980): In: *Albumin Synthesis in Liver and Biliary Tract Physiology*. I. *International Review of Physiology*, edited by N. B. Javitt, vol. 21, pp. 249–274. University Park Press, Baltimore.

119. Baraona, E., Leo, M. A., Borowsky, S. A., and Lieber, C. S. (1977): Pathogenesis of alcohol-induced accumulation of protein in the liver. *J. Clin. Invest.*, 60:546–554.

120. Tuma, D. J., and Sorrell, M. E. (1981): Effects of ethanol on the secretion of glycoproteins by rat liver slices. *Gastroenterology*, 80:273–278.

121. Mørland, J., Rothschild, M. A., Oratz, M., Mongelli, J., Donor, D., and Schreiber, S. S. (1981): Protein secretion in suspensions of isolated rat hepatocytes: No influence of acute ethanol administration. *Gastroenterology*, 80:159–165.

122. Rothschild, M. A., Oratz, M., Mongelli, J., and Schreiber, S. S. (1971): Alcohol-induced depression of albumin synthesis: Reversal by tryptophan. *J. Clin. Invest.*, 50:1812–1818.

123. Oratz, M., Rothschild, M. A., and Schreiber, S. S. (1976): Alcohol, amino acids and albumin synthesis. II. Alcohol inhibition of albumin synthesis reversed by arginine and spermine. *Gastroenterology*, 71:123–127.

124. Oratz, M., Rothschild, M. A., and Schreiber, S. S. (1978): Alcohol, amino acid and albumin synthesis. III. Effects of ethanol, acetaldehyde and 4-methylpyrazole. *Gastroenterology*, 74:672–676.

125. Kirsch, R. E., Frith, L., Stead, R. H., and Saunders, S. J. (1973): Effect of alcohol on albumin synthesis by the isolated perfused rat liver. *Am. J. Clin. Nutr.*, 26:1191–1194.

126. Perin, A., Scalabrino, G., Sessa, A., and Arnaboldi, A. (1974): *In vitro* inhibition of protein synthesis in rat liver as a sequence of ethanol metabolism. *Biochim. Biophys. Acta*, 366:101–108.

127. Mørland, J. (1975): Incorporation of labelled amino acids into liver protein after acute ethanol administration. *Biochem. Pharmacol.*, 24:439–442.

128. Zern, M. A., and Shafritz, D. A. (1980): The effect of chronic ethanol administration on the hepatic polysome population and protein synthesis. *Gastroenterology*, 79:1070.

129. Perin, A., Sessa, A., and Desideri, M. A. (1979): Ethanol and liver protein synthesis. In: *Metabolic Effects of Alcohol*, edited by P. Avogaro, C. R. Sirton, and E. Tremoli, pp. 273–289. Elsevier, Amsterdam.

130. Banks, W. L., Kline, E. S., and Higgins, E. S. (1970): Hepatic composition and metabolism after ethanol consumption in rats fed liquid purified diets. *J. Nutr.*, 100:581–593.

131. Kuriyama, K., Sze, P. Y., and Rauscher, G. E. (1971): Effects of acute and chronic ethanol administration on ribosomal protein synthesis in mouse brain and liver. *Life Sci.*, 10:181–189.

132. Mørland, J., and Bessesen, A. (1977): Inhibition of protein synthesis by ethanol in isolated rat liver parenchymal cells. *Biochim. Biophys. Acta*, 474:312–320.

133. Baraona, E., Pikkarainen, P., Salaspuro, M., Finkelman, F.,

and Lieber, C. S. (1980): Acute effects of ethanol on hepatic protein synthesis and secretion in the rat. *Gastroenterology,* 79:104–111.

134. Jeejeebhoy, K. N., Phillips, M. J., Bruce-Robertson, A., Ho, J., and Sodtke, V. (1972): The acute effect of ethanol on albumin, fibrinogen and transferin synthesis in the rat. *Biochem. J.,* 126:1111–1126.

135. Renis, M., Giovine, A., and Bertolino, A. (1975): Protein synthesis in mitochondrial and microsomal fractions from rat brain and liver after acute or chronic ethanol administration. *Life Sci.,* 16:1447–1458.

136. Nadkarni, G. D., Deshpande, V. R., and Pahuya, D. N. (1979): Reversal of alcohol-induced inhibition of plasma protein synthesis by propylthiouracil. *Biochem. Med.,* 22:64–69.

137. Mørland, J., Bessesen, A., and Svendsen, L. (1979): Incorporation of labelled amino acids into proteins of isolated parenchymal and nonparenchymal rat liver cells in the absence and presence of ethanol. *Biochim. Biophys. Acta,* 561:464–474.

138. Salaspuro, M. P., Shaw, S., Jaytilleke, E., Ross, W. A., and Lieber, C. S. (1981): Attenuation of the ethanol-induced hepatic redox change after chronic alcohol consumption in baboons: Metabolic consequences *in vivo* and *in vitro. Hepatology,* 1:33–38.

139. Krebs, H. A. (1971): Glucogenesis and redox state. In: *Regulation of Gluconeogenesis,* edited by H. D. Soling and B. Willms, pp. 114–117. Academic Press, New York.

140. Requero, A. M., Diaz, J. P., Ayuso-Parrilla, M. S., and Parrilla, R. (1979): On the mechanism of glucagon-induced inhibition of hepatic protein synthesis. *Arch. Biochem. Biophys.* 195:223–234.

141. Israel, Y., Kalant, H., Orrego, H., Khanna, J. M., Videla, L., and Phillips, J. M. (1975): Experimental alcohol-reduced hepatic necrosis: Suppression by propylthiouracil. *Proc. Natl. Acad. Sci. USA,* 72:1137–1141.

142. Yap, S. H., Strair, R. K., and Shafritz, D. A. (1978): Albumin mRNA distribution and changes in experimental metabolic disease. In: *Albumin Metabolism Function and Clinical Use,* edited by S. H. Yap, C. L. H. Majoor, and J. H. M. van Tongeren, pp. 49–66. Martinus Nijhoff BV, The Hague, The Netherlands.

143. Rosenfeld, M. G., and Barrieux, A. (1979): Regulation of protein synthesis by polypeptide hormones and cyclic AMP. In: *Advances in Cyclic Nucleotide Research, Vol. 11,* edited by P. Greengard and G. A. Robison, pp. 205–264. Raven Press, New York.

144. Kurtz, D. T., Sippel, A. E., Ansah-Yiadon, R., and Feigelson, P. (1976): Effects of sex hormones on the level of messenger RNA for the rat hepatic protein $\alpha_2\mu$ globulin. *J. Biol. Chem.,* 251:3594–3598.

145. Wicks, W. D. (1974): Regulation of protein synthesis by cAMP. *Adv. Cyclic Nucleotide Res.,* 4:335–438.

146. Bloxham, D. P., and Klaopongpan, A. (1979): The involvement of adenosine 3'5' cyclic monophosphate in the translational control of protein synthesis. *Int. J. Biochem.,* 10:1–5.

147. Ayuso-Parrilla, M. S., Martin-Requero, A., Diaz, J. P., and Parrilla, R. (1976): Role of glucagon on the control of hepatic protein synthesis and degradation in the rat *in vivo. J. Biol. Chem.,* 251:7785–7790.

148. Ranu, R. S. (1980): Regulation of protein synthesis in eukaryotes by the protein kinases that phosphorylate initiation factor eIF-2. *FEBS Lett.,* 112:211–215.

149. Cherbas, L., and London, I. M. (1976): On the mechanism of delayed inhibition of protein synthesis in heme-deficient rabbit reticulocyte lysates. *Proc. Natl. Acad. Sci. USA,* 73:3506–3510.

150. Bergman, J. E., and Lodish, H. (1979): A kinetic model of protein synthesis application to hemoglobin synthesis and translational control. *J. Biol. Chem.,* 254:11927–11937.

151. Pain, V. M., and Garlick, P. J. (1974): Effect of streptozotocin diabetes and insulin treatment on the rate of protein synthesis in tissues of the rat *in vivo. J. Biol. Chem.,* 249:4510–4514.

152. Ingebretson, W. R., Moxley, M. A., Allen, D. O., and Wagle, S. R. (1972): Studies in gluconeogenesis, protein synthesis and cyclic AMP levels in isolated parenchymal cells following insulin withdrawal from alloxan diabetic rats. *Biochem. Biophys. Res. Commun.,* 49:601–607.

153. Jefferson, L. S. (1980): Role of insulin in the regulation of protein synthesis. *Diabetes,* 29:487–496.

154. Peavy, D. E., Taylor, J. M., and Jefferson, L. S. (1979): Regulation of hepatic albumin and total protein synthesis in normal and diabetic rats. *Diabetes,* 28:390–394.

155. Peavy, D. E., Taylor, J. M., and Jefferson, L. S. (1978): Correlation of albumin production rates and albumin mRNA levels in livers of normal, diabetic and insulin-treated diabetic rats. *Proc. Natl. Acad. Sci. USA,* 75:5879–5883.

156. Pain, V. M., Lamoix, J., Bergeron, J. J. M., and Clemens, M. J. (1974): The effect of diabetes on the ultrastructure of the hepatocyte and on the distribution and activity of ribosomes in the free and membrane-bound populations. *Biochem. Biophys. Acta,* 353:487–498.

157. Germanyuk, Y. L., and Mironenko, V. I. (1969): Insulin and the attachment of amino acids to the liver transfer RNAs. *Nature,* 222:486–487.

158. Keller, G. H., and Taylor, J. M. (1978): Effect of hypophysectomy and growth hormone treatment on albumin mRNA levels in the rat liver. *J. Biol. Chem.,* 254:276–278.

159. Feldhoff, R. C., Taylor, J. M., and Jefferson, L. S. (1977): Synthesis and secretion of rat albumin *in vivo* in perfused liver, and in isolated hepatocytes. *J. Biol. Chem.,* 252:3611–3616.

160. Korner, A. (1964): Regulation of the rate of synthesis of messenger ribonucleic acid by growth hormone. *Biochem. J.,* 92:449–456.

161. Roy, A. K., and Dowbenko, D. J. (1977): Role of growth hormone in the multihormonal regulation of messenger RNA for a $\alpha_2\mu$ globulin in the liver of hypophysectomized rats. *Biochemistry,* 16:3918–3922.

162. Carter, W. J., and Faas, F. H. (1979): Early stimulation of rat liver microsomal protein synthesis after tri-iodothyronine injection *in vivo. Biochem. J.,* 182:651–654.

163. Tata, J. R., and Widnell, C. C. (1966): Ribonucleic acid synthesis during the early action of thyroid hormones. *Biochem. J.,* 98:604–620.

164. Carter, W. J., Faas, F. H., and Wynn, J. O. (1976): Stimulation of peptide elongation by thyroxine. *Biochem. J.,* 156:713–717.

165. Mathews, R. W., Oronsky, W. A., and Haschemeyer, A. E. V. (1973): Effect of thyroid hormone on polypeptide chain assembly kinetics in liver protein synthesis *in vivo. J. Biol. Chem.,* 248:1329–1333.

166. Guyette, W. A., Matusik, R. J., and Rosen, J. M. (1979): Prolactin-mediated transcriptional and post-transcriptional control of casein gene expression. *Cell,* 17:1013–1023.

167. Palmiter, R. D. (1975): Quantitation of parameters that determine the rate of ovalbumin synthesis. *Cell,* 4:189–197.

168. Puckett, L., Chambers, S., and Darnell, J. E. (1975): Short-lived messenger RNA in HeLa cells and its impact on the kinetics of accumulation of cytoplasmic polyadenylate. *Proc. Natl. Acad. Sci. USA,* 72:389–393.

169. Tsai, S. Y., Tsai, M. J., Lin, C. T., and O'Malley, B. W. (1979): Effect of estrogen on ovalbumin gene expression in differentiated nontarget tissues. *Biochemistry,* 18:5726–5731.

170. Sell, S., Sala-Trepat, J. M., Sargent, T. D., Thomas, K., Nahon, J. L., Goodman, T. A., and Bonner, J. (1980): Molecular mechanisms of control of albumin and alphafetoprotein production: A system to study the early effects of chemical hepatocarcinogens. *Cell Biol. Int. Rep.,* 4:235–254.

171. Hofer, E., Alonso, A., Krieg, L., Schatzl, U., and Sekeris, C. E. (1979): Purification of albumin mRNA from rat liver content of albumin-specific sequences in cytoplasmic and nuclear RNA. *Eur. J. Biochem.,* 97:455–462.

172. Harpold, M. M., Evans, R. M., Salditt-Georgieff, M., and Darnell, J. E. (1979): Production of mRNA in Chinese hamster cells: Relationship of the rate of synthesis to the cytoplasmic concentration of nine specific mRNA sequences. *Cell,* 17:1025–1035.

173. Grossman, S. B., Yap, S. H., and Shafritz, D. A. (1977): Influence of chronic renal failure on protein synthesis and albumin metabolism in rat liver. *J. Clin. Invest.,* 59:869–878.

174. Zern, M. A., Yap, S. H., Strair, R. K., Kaysen, G. A., and Shafritz, D. A. (1981): The effects of chronic renal failure on hepatic protein synthesis and albumin mRNA in rats. *Hepatology* (abstr.), 1:561.

175. Scherrer, K., and Marcaud, L. (1968): Messenger RNA in avian erythroblasts at the transcriptional and translational levels and the problem of regulation in animal cells. *J. Cell. Physiol.* 72:(*Suppl. 1*), 1:181.

The Liver: Biology and Pathobiology, edited by
I. Arias, H. Popper, D. Schachter, and D. A. Shafritz.
Raven Press, New York © 1982.

Chapter 8

Lipoprotein Metabolism

Robert M. Glickman and Seymour M. Sabesin

When one considers the large flux of lipid that passes through the liver each day, it is not surprising that this organ subserves central metabolic functions in various aspects of lipid and lipoprotein metabolism (Table 1). These functions include uptake, oxidation, or metabolic conversion of free fatty acids; synthesis of cholesterol and phospholipids, and formation and secretion of specific classes of plasma lipoproteins. In the fasting state, a large proportion of the lipid that circulates as plasma lipoproteins originates in the liver through the biosynthesis of specific lipoproteins. In addition to lipoprotein synthesis, the liver participates in other essential aspects of plasma lipoprotein metabolism, including metabolic transformations of lipoproteins in the plasma and catabolism of low density lipoproteins (LDL), high density lipoproteins (HDL), and chylomicron remnants. Recognition of the functions and importance of the liver in lipid and lipoprotein metabolism makes it easy to appreciate that alterations in hepatic structure and function associated with hepatocellular injury or cholestasis result in profound abnormalities in the concentration and composition of lipids and lipoproteins within the liver and plasma. These abnormalities directly reflect alterations in hepatic lipoprotein formation and/or secretion, as well as derangements in liver-regulated meta-bolic and catabolic processes. The major objective of this chaper is to review the biochemical and physiological aspects of hepatic lipoprotein formation and metabolism and to discuss mechanisms by which impairment of these processes results in abnormalities of hepatic and plasma lipoprotein metabolism.

OVERVIEW OF LIPOPROTEIN METABOLISM

A brief overview is presented to facilitate an understanding of the role of the liver in lipoprotein metabolism. Plasma lipoprotein formation, structure, and metabolism have been reviewed extensively; recent articles should be consulted for comprehensive discussions (1–11).

The plasma lipoproteins are molecular complexes of lipids and specific proteins called apoproteins. These complexes have been defined by their chemical and physical properties after isolation by sequential ultracentrifugation. Table 2 summarizes the chemical and physical characteristics of human plasma lipoproteins, their sources, and major functions. As isolated from plasma, lipoproteins can be visualized electron microscopically using negative staining techniques (Fig. 1). They appear as spherical particles of rather characteristic size range in each density class, al-

TABLE 1. *Role of liver in lipid and lipoprotein metabolism*

Synthesis	
Lipids	Triglyceride, cholesterol, phospholipid
Apoproteins	A−I, A−II, B, C−I, C−II, C−III, E
Lipoproteins	VLDL, nascent HDL
Enzymes	LCAT, hepatic triglyceride lipase
Catabolism	Chylomicron and VLDL remnants, LDL, HDL[a]
Biliary excretion	Cholesterol, phospholipids

[a] VLDL remnants in man are catabolized to LDL in the plasma but are taken up by the liver and catabolized by hepatocytes in rats.

though there is considerable heterogeneity in the size of triglyceride-rich lipoproteins of intestinal origin (chylomicrons) isolated from plasma after ingestion of a fatty meal.

Figure 2 is a simplified scheme of plasma lipoprotein metabolism which serves to emphasize several major points: (a) intestinal and hepatic synthesis of certain lipoprotein classes; (b) formation of lipoprotein remnants secondary to triglyceride hydrolysis by lipoprotein lipase; (c) formation and addition of cholesteryl esters to nascent HDL via lecithin cholesterol acyltransferase (LCAT); (d) transfer of cholesteryl esters from HDL to the pathway leading to LDL formation; and (e) uptake of chylomicron remnants and HDL by the liver and catabolism of LDL by peripheral cells and the liver. LCAT deficiency results in plasma accumulation of nascent discoidal HDL. Since cholesteryl esters cannot be formed, LCAT deficiency prevents conversion of HDL discs to spherical particles.

Lipoproteins are dynamic particles which are in a constant state of synthesis, degradation, and removal from the plasma compartment. During the process of lipoprotein catabolism, nascent secretory particles of intestinal or hepatic origin undergo triglyceride hydrolysis, acquire new apoproteins by exchange with other lipoproteins, lose apoproteins of endogenous origin, and thus become altered drastically in size and composition. The lipoprotein end-products of these complex transformations are important in many ways. Thus LDL is a major source of cholesterol for peripheral cells, and HDL provides a reservoir for cholesterol, accepting "excess" cholesterol from peripheral cells and transporting it to the liver for excretion (in bile), degradation, or reutilization.

As recent studies have shown, receptor-mediated processses are important for uptake and clearance by the liver of certain lipoproteins following their initial catabolism in the plasma compartment. Mechanisms involved in hepatic lipoprotein clearance and the resultant effects on hepatic cholesterol and bile acid metabolism are discussed elsewhere in this volume.

HEPATIC SYNTHESIS OF LIPOPROTEINS

Very Low Density Lipoproteins

The major triglyceride-rich lipoproteins secreted by the liver are very low density lipoproteins (VLDL). When isolated from plasma by ultracentrifugation and visualized by electron microscopy, VLDL appear as spherical particles with a diameter of 280 to 800 Å (Fig. 1). Their composition is shown in Table 2. When recovered from isolated hepatic perfusates, their lipid composition is essentially similar to plasma VLDL; however, nascent VLDL from liver acquire additional protein (apoproteins) on exposure to plasma, giving

TABLE 2. *Characterization of plasma lipoproteins[a]*

Parameter	Chylomicrons	VLDL	LDL	HDL
Source	Intestine	Liver	Plasma	Intestine, liver
Size (Å)	800−5,000	280−800	≈200	50−150
Density (g/ml)	<0.95	0.95−1.006	1.006−1.063	1.063−1.210
Electrophoretic mobility	Origin	Pre-β	β	α
Lipid content (%)	≈98	≈90	≈75	≈50
Lipid classes (% of total lipid)[b]	≈90 TG	≈60 TG	≈60 CH	≈50 PL
	≈8 PL	≈20 PL	≈30 PL	≈32 CH
	≈5 CH	≈17 CH	≈10 TG	≈10 TG
Protein (%)	0.5−2.5	10−13	20−25	45−55
Major apoproteins	B, C−I, C−II, C−III	B, C−III, E	B	A−I, A−II
Minor apoproteins	A−I, A−II, E	A−I, A−II, C−I, C−II	C−I, C−II, C−III, E	B, C−I, C−II, C−III, E
Functions/metabolism	Dietary TG transport; peripheral lipolysis to form chylomicron remnants	Endogenous TG transport; peripheral lipolysis to form LDL	CE transport; uptake by cells and regulation of cholesterol biosynthesis	LCAT substrate; transfer and exchanges of apoproteins (apo C, E) and lipids (PL, CE); CH removal from cells

[a] Data derived from many published sources.
[b] TG, triglyceride; PL, phospholipid; CH, cholesterol; CE, cholesteryl ester.

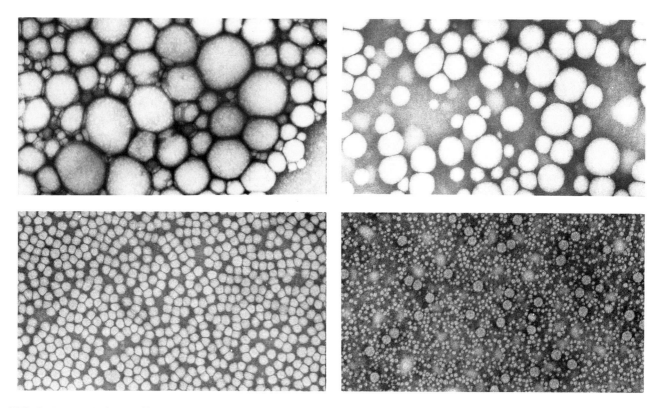

FIG. 1. Isolated plasma lipoproteins visualized by electron microscopy of negatively stained preparations. **A:** Chylomicrons (×51,300); **B:** VLDL; **C:** LDL; **D:** HDL (B,C,D: ×11,400).

them a characteristic pre-β mobility on lipoprotein electrophoresis. Considerable insight into VLDL formation and secretion has been provided by ultrastructural studies.

Ultrastructural Aspects of Hepatic Lipoprotein

Formation and secretion

Morphological aspects of the assembly, intracellular transport, and secretion of lipoproteins have been investigated by electron microscopy in the intact or isolated perfused rat liver (12–15). Ultrastructural studies have defined the subcellular pathways of hepatic VLDL formation under varying physiological conditions. Since VLDL are readily observed within hepatocyte subcellular organelles, electron microscopy has been useful elucidating certain aspects of VLDL assembly and intracellular transport.

The formation of VLDL begins with triglyceride and apoprotein synthesis. After uptake by the hepatocyte, fatty acids may be esterified to form triglycerides. The initial step in apoprotein formation involves genetic transcription of the mRNA coding for apoprotein synthesis. Specific genes probably exist for each individual apoprotein, but relatively little is known regarding these genes or their regulation (16). After their formation on polyribosomes of the rough endoplasmic

reticulum (RER), nascent apoproteins are translocated into the RER cisternae, where they commence a vectorical transport through the ER channels toward their assembly with the lipid moieties.

The enzymes involved in triglyceride, cholesterol, and phospholipid synthesis are located in the smooth ER (SER), and presumably the newly formed lipids are also directed into the SER cisternae. Because of their electron density, after fixation, the lipid portion of the VLDL particle is visualized easily. Thus particles of VLDL size and morphology can be observed within channels of the ER and in the Golgi complex. Since apoproteins cannot be seen directly, however, immunohistochemical techniques are required to reveal their localization. Recent studies using ferritin-conjugated antibodies directed against rat apoprotein of B (the major apoprotein of nascent VLDL) suggest that assembly of the lipid and apoprotein B of VLDL occurs at the transition zone between SER and RER (17). Nascent VLDL are then transported to the Golgi apparatus, where their synthesis is completed. This process may involve glycosylation of lipoproteins prior to their sequestration in secretory vesicles.

The exact mechanism by which nascent lipoproteins are transported from the ER into the Golgi apparatus is not known. One proposed mechanism suggests structural continuity between the ER reticulum and Golgi complex with transport of nascent VLDL through

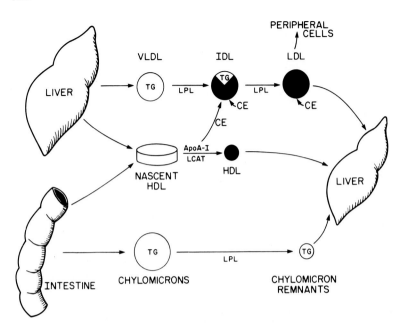

FIG. 2. Simplified scheme of plasma lipoprotein metabolism. Key events are the hydrolysis of triglyceride-rich lipoproteins by lipoprotein lipase (LPL), the conversion of VLDL to IDL, the progressive enrichment of IDL and LDL with cholesteryl esters (CE) transferred from HDL as a result of the LCAT reaction, and the removal of LDL and chylomicron remnants by peripheral cells and the liver.

tubular extensions of the ER directly into Golgi cisterna (15). It was suggested by Claude (15) that VLDL within the SER were transported directly into the Golgi, since the SER membranes appeared to extend into the Golgi complex. The coalescence of SER tubular extensions into the Golgi resulted in formation of sacs filled with 400 Å lipoprotein particles. Since lipoprotein particles were not seen within the RER, it was concluded that the RER synthesized the apoproteins, whereas the SER was involved in lipid synthesis. The specific function of the Golgi in lipoprotein synthesis was not determined, except that the Golgi zones became filled with secretory vesicles which segregated particles of VLDL size. Figure 3 is an electron micrograph of rat liver, showing VLDL within Golgi cisternae and in secretory vesicles derived from the Golgi complex.

Alternatively, it has been suggested that nascent lipoproteins and other secretory proteins are brought to the Golgi by transport in vesicles derived by "budding off" from transitional elements of the smooth-surfaced extentions of the ER (18,19). These vesicles, containing single VLDL particles, migrate from the ER to the Golgi complex and deliver nascent VLDL into the Golgi cisternae by merging with the cisternal membranes.

Current evidence suggests that transport of nascent lipoproteins into the Golgi apparatus is obligatory for their final assembly and secretion; however, the exact function of the Golgi apparatus in this regard has not been established (12,15). The Golgi may serve to complete the assembly of nascent proteins, perhaps by addition of sugar moieties catalyzed by glycosyltransferases located in Golgi membranes (20). Biochemical evidence supporting this sequence of assembly and transport to the Golgi complex has been obtained by

subcellular fractionation studies in which purified lipoprotein particles similar to VLDL in size and composition have been prepared from isolated Golgi vesicles (21,22). Thus studies of lipoprotein synthesis and transport in the isolated rat liver, perfused with free fatty acids, have shown an increase in the number of particles of VLDL size in the Golgi complex within 5 min of perfusion; particles of similar size and appearance can be recovered from the d < 1.006 fraction of the perfusate (13). Particles of VLDL size have been localized in the Golgi zone following intravenous injection of ^{3}H-palmitate (23).

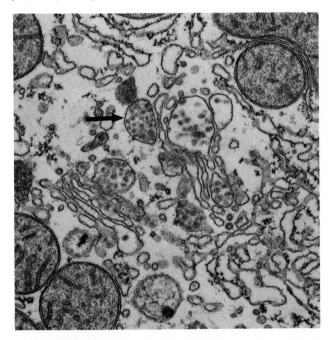

FIG. 3. Electron microscopic appearance of a rat hepatocyte showing VLDL particles in the Golgi complex and in a secretory vesicle (*arrow*). ×28,500.

Cortisone increases hepatic VLDL production in the rabbit. After 6 days of administration, the Golgi complex becomes prominent and contains large secretory vesicles containing clusters of VLDL particles (22). Marked accumulation of secretory vesicles in the Golgi, concomitant with enhanced VLDL formation and increased plasma lipids, suggests a prominent role for the Golgi apparatus in VLDL assembly and secretion.

Characterization of the lipoproteins obtained from purified rat liver Golgi fractions and recovered by ultracentrifugation at d < 1.006 revealed a lipid composition similar to plasma VLDL (21). Electron microscopy showed the Golgi-derived particles to be similar in size to circulating VLDL. Immunochemical studies, using antisera specific for plasma VLDL revealed antigenic similarities. This provided further evidence that these lipoproteins are precursors of plasma VLDL (21). In another characterization of purified hepatic Golgi VLDL, Mahley and co-workers (24) used specific antisera and polyacrylamide gel electrophoresis to compare Golgi with plasma VLDL and with VLDL derived from isolated hepatic perfusates. Since the Golgi VLDL contained the same major apoproteins as VLDL obtained from rat plasma or hepatic perfusates, there was additional evidence that Golgi-derived VLDL are the precursors of plasma VLDL.

In a correlative biochemical and morphological study of the synthesis and intracellular transport of lipoproteins by the liver, Glaumann et al. (25) investigated the incorporation of radioactive glycerol into triglyceride and phospholipids of isolated lipoproteins in various subcellular compartments. After pulse-labeling, triglyceride obtained from rough and smooth microsomal fractions showed a high rate of labeling with a peak at 6 min followed by a quick fall-off. Golgi lipoproteins were labeled maximally at 10 to 20 min; there was a 10 to 15 min interval before labeled VLDL appeared in the serum. Lipoprotein particles obtained from the RER contained phospholipids and triglycerides in relatively small amounts but were rich in protein. In contrast, particles from the SER and particularly from the Golgi apparatus were enriched in triglyceride and phospholipid and thus resembled plasma VLDL. It was concluded that assembly of the apoprotein and lipid moieties into lipoprotein particles begins in the RER and continues in the SER. There is a change in the chemical composition and size of the particles as they traverse the ER, with the final remodeling in the Golgi apparatus prior to secretion (25).

The smooth-surfaced secretory vesicles, containing nascent VLDL, leave the Golgi zones, migrate through the cytoplasm, and merge with the lateral plasmalemma of the hepatocyte, thereby secreting VLDL into the space of Disse by a process called exocytosis. Relatively little information is available concerning the mechanism by which secretory vesicles are directed toward the space of Disse. Recent studies (26,27) have demonstrated that colchicine and other related alkaloids can inhibit VLDL secretion. The inhibitory effects of colchicine may result from interference in formation of microtubules. Although microtubules probably subserve several functions, it has been postulated that they direct vectorial movement of secretory vesicles toward the cell membrane, thereby controlling the secretory process.

Novikoff (28–30) has described a specialized subcellular component [Golgi, ER, lysosomes (GERL)], which is located in proximity to the Golgi apparatus. GERL can be distinguished cytochemically from the ER and the innermost elements of the Golgi apparatus by the specificity of its staining for acid phosphatase (28,29). VLDL-size particles have been demonstrated in the smooth-surfaced cisternae and tubules of GERL (31), suggesting direct entry of VLDL from the ER into GERL, thereby "bypassing" the Golgi apparatus. Metabolic transformation of VLDL within GERL has been suggested by the irregular size and shape of VLDL in GERL and the appearance of so-called "residual bodies" containing homogeneous electron-dense material. VLDL catabolism, perhaps related to apoprotein degradation and partial triglyceride lipolysis is thought to occur in "residual bodies" (31). Thus ultrastructural differences between VLDL morphology in GERL and Golgi suggest a degradative function for GERL, perhaps related to lipoprotein catabolism. There is good evidence for such a function, since GERL contains lysosomal enzyme activity, and there is a striking accumulation of VLDL in GERL during reversal of experimental fatty liver (32).

Biochemical Features of VLDL Synthesis

As shown in Table 2, the major lipids comprising VLDL are triglycerides (60%), phospholipids (20%), and cholesterol (17%). The esterified:unesterified cholesterol ratio in VLDL is 1.0; the predominant phospholipids are lecithin and sphingomyelin. Protein comprises about 10 to 13% of the particle by weight. The liver is capable of synthesizing all the various components of the VLDL particle.

VLDL secretion by the liver is directly coupled to the intracellular concentration of fatty acids within the hepatocyte and the metabolic state of the liver. Free fatty acids (FFA) available to the liver may be derived from endogenous or exogenous sources. During fasting or conditions of low fat diet, most FFA are probably derived from lipolysis of adipose tissue triglycerides through the action of hormone sensitive lipases. After eating a fatty meal, plasma FFA and, subsequently, hepatic VLDL become enriched in dietary fatty acids. FFA are transported in the circulation almost entirely complexed to albumin in a molar ratio of 0.5 to 2. Uptake of FFA by the liver is essentially proportional to the concentration of FFA in plasma (or in the medium used in hepatic studies). Thus uptake of FFA is not a rate-limiting factor in the subsequent metabolism of fatty acids. The process is thought to be passive and is not influenced by various hormones. The fate of the fatty acids within the hepatocyte is influenced primarily by the existing nutritional and hormonal state. In general, fatty acids can be reesterified to triglyceride or oxidized to CO_2 and ketone bodies. Whether triglycerides or ketones are formed appears to be regulated in a reciprocal manner in various nutritional or hormonal states. Fasting, insulin lack, glucagon, cylic AMP, and cyclic GMP accelerate ketogenesis. Conversely, feeding, insulin replacement, and estrogens enhance triglyceride formation and VLDL secretion (33).

A cytosolic protein, fatty acid binding protein (FABP), has been purified by Ockner et al. (34) from many tissues, including liver. FABP has a molecular weight of 12,000 daltons. Its affinity is higher for unsaturated than for saturated fatty acids. FABP may be responsible for transport of fatty acids to the SER, the site of triglyceride resynthesis (35). Recent studies have shown that the level of FABP may be under hormonal control (36). It is increased by estrogens and is present in higher concentrations in liver from female as compared to male rats. Hepatic VLDL secretion is greater in female than male rats, and VLDL secretion is enhanced by estrogen treatment. FABP probably functions to reduce the intracellular content of FFA and to provide directed intracellular movement of fatty acids within the hepatocyte.

Triglyceride synthesis from fatty acids occurs in the SER, where microsomal enzymes catalyze the esterification of glycerol by fatty acid CoA derivatives to form triglycerides. Studies in the isolated perfused liver by Heimberg and Wilcox (37) demonstrated that 50% more VLDL triglyceride is secreted when the liver is perfused with oleic acid compared to palmitic acid. Similar results have been obtained in the intestine by Ockner et al. (38), suggesting that the physical properties of secreted VLDL are affected by the type of fatty acid incorporated into triglyceride. Phospholipids required for lipoprotein formation also are synthesized in the SER (39). In the rats, cholesterol is synthesized in the SER, as are some cholesteryl esters, whereas in man, cholesteryl esters are formed in the plasma by the LCAT reaction. Hepatic cholesterol metabolism and the rate-limiting enzymes involved in this process (3-hydroxyl-3-methylglutaryl-CoA reductase and acyl-CoA cholesterol acyltransferase) are reviewed elsewhere in this volume. While the precise interrelationships between hepatic cholesterol synthesis and VLDL formation and secretion are largely unknown, these components may be a source for lipoprotein cholesterol and cholesterol esters.

The major remaining component of hepatic VLDL, i.e., specific apoprotein constituents, are actively synthesized by the liver during VLDL formation. Studies with the isolated perfused liver have confirmed that radioactive amino acids are actively incorporated into apo B, apo E, and to a lesser extent, apo C proteins.

Apo B comprises approximately 30% of VLDL protein. New data in the rat and in man indicate that distinctive forms of apo B are present. These may be characteristic of the tissue apoprotein origin, namely, liver or intestine (40–43). The intestinal form is characteristic of mesenteric lymph triglyceride-rich lipoproteins (chylomicrons) and appears in the plasma of rats after cholesterol feeding. It has a molecular weight in the rat of 240,000 versus 350,000 for plasma LDL, which is known to be derived primarily from the catabolism of hepatic VLDL. Recent studies (41,43) in the rat suggest that the liver may produce both forms of apo B. In man, the studies of Kane et al. (42) demonstrated an intestinal apo B of 264,000 molecular weight, while plasma LDL contained apo B of 459,000 or two smaller subunits (407,000 and 144,500). These findings strongly indicate that in man, the liver and intestine produce characteristic forms of apo B.

The importance of apo B in triglyceride transport is underscored by the human disease abetalipoproteinemia, in which there is a characteristic absence of triglyceride-containing lipoproteins in plasma and an absence of immunochemically detectable apo B. Both the liver and intestine contain increased amounts of triglyceride, an expression of the total inability to secrete triglyceride-rich lipoproteins. The intestine of patients with abetalipoproteinemia contains no immunochemically detectable apo B. Direct studies have not been performed on liver from such patients, but a similar defect undoubtedly is present. Thus apo B synthesis appears to be an absolute requirement for VLDL and chylomicron synthesis and secretion. Evidence that apo B synthesis occurs early in VLDL formation is suggested by immunochemical localization studies of Alexander and co-workers (17). Apo B was visualized in RER and appeared associated with triglyceride droplets in interconnecting profiles of RER and SER. In abetalipoproteinemia, hepatocytes contain large triglyceride droplets, and Golgi vacuoles contain no VLDL, further indicating that apo B is added to the lipids at an early stage in VLDL formation. Additional evidence for the importance of apoprotein synthesis in VLDL secretion is provided by experimental studies using protein synthesis inhibitors. Bar-on et al. (44) administered cyclohexamide to rats and found that VLDL secretion by the perfused liver continues for up to 60 min and then decreases sharply. The studies demonstrate the requirement for active protein synthesis in VLDL secretion and also suggest the presence of a limited preformed pool of apoproteins.

Recent studies using isolated hepatocytes in monolayer culture have demonstrated VLDL secretion and apoprotein synthesis (45,46). Newly secreted VLDL contain two major apoproteins, apo B and apo E. Small amounts of radioactivity are incorporated into apo C and apo A-I. It should be noted that hepatic VLDL differ markedly in their apoprotein composition when compared to VLDL-sized particles, as isolated from mesenteric lymph of rat or man. Intestinal VLDL contain the intestinal form of apo B and have as their major apoproteins apo A-IV and apo A-I. The intestine does not appear to synthesize apo E, a major apoprotein of hepatic VLDL. Newly secreted VLDL, whether from the perfused liver or from isolated hepatocytes, contain less of the C apoproteins than plasma VLDL. It is known that C apoproteins can transfer from plasma HDL to triglyceride-rich particles (i.e., VLDL and chylomicrons). These apoproteins have a relatively long half-life in plasma. The apparent low synthetic rates of C apoproteins by the liver, therefore, may be sufficient to maintain plasma levels. In addition, the C apoproteins appear to be secreted on hepatic HDL (see below). Studies with isolated cultured rat hepatocytes indicate that VLDL secretion is modulated in a manner similar to *in vivo* stimuli. Thus sucrose feeding, fatty acids, and cyclic nucleotides all increase VLDL secretion, while protein synthesis inhibitors block VLDL secretion, despite active triglyceride synthesis.

While many physiological stimuli can affect the synthesis of VLDL and its components, less is known about the molecular mechanisms of apoprotein synthesis and how a given stimulus operates to influence VLDL formation. Significant progress has been made in elucidating the regulation of VLDL formation and secretion by estrogens. In a series of elegant studies, Chan and co-workers (47,48) explored estrogenic effects on VLDL synthesis in the cockerel. The studies show that synthesis of apo A-II, a major apoprotein of cockeral VLDL, is increased 10-fold by estrogen administration. Estrogen binds to specific receptors in the liver cell nucleus, resulting in enhancement of RNA polymerase activity and synthesis of VLDL mRNA. This mRNA is transported to the cytoplasm, where it is translated into pre-apo-VLDL. The pre-apo-VLDL (MW 11,000), containing a signal sequence, is cleaved by a protease yielding apo A-II (MW 9,400). This apoprotein is then released and binds phospholipids and triglycerides in the SER; however, the details of this process are not known. Thus the synthetic sequence for this apoprotein appears to conform to the hypothesis of Blobel and Dob-

berstein (49) for secretory protein biosynthesis. Other stimuli that influence VLDL secretion probably will share features in common with the above model. Such information is essential to enable an understanding of human lipoprotein disorders.

LDL Secretion

Current concepts of LDL formation indicate that LDL are formed in the plasma from the catabolism of hepatic VLDL (5). Perfused livers of the monkey (50) and swine (51) secrete some particles in the LDL range; however, the quantitative importance of this source of LDL is unknown. Isolated cultured hepatocytes do not secrete LDL. As discussed below, the liver may synthesize LDL particles under conditions of high cholesterol feeding (52); an analogous situation has been suggested in human familial hypercholesterolemia. In the absence of VLDL secretion, there is no formation of LDL; this is a characteristic finding in abetalipoproteinemia. The catabolism of intestinal trigylceride-rich particles (i.e., chylomicrons) does not result in LDL formation but rather in formation of so-called chylomicron remnant particles, which are rapidly taken up and catabolized by the liver. Therefore, although the liver does not directly synthesize LDL under most circumstances, formation of LDL is totally dependent on hepatic VLDL secretion.

HDL Secretion

The liver shares with the intestine a central role in HDL formation. Current concepts of HDL formation indicate that these particles can be formed by two processes: lipolytic or secretory (53). Substantial evidence exists that triglyceride-rich particles (derived from either liver or intestine) can generate HDL as a result of lipolysis. Lipoprotein lipase, present in capillary endothelial cells of many tissues (e.g., skeletal muscle, heart, adipose tissue), rapidly hydrolyzes the core triglyceride of chylomicrons or VLDL reducing the size of the apolar lipid core. This results in redundant surface material which is composed primarily of phospholipid and apoprotein. This surface material dissociates from the remnant particle and distributes into the HDL fraction of plasma, where it may interact with the preexisting pool, thereby increasing its mass. Some material may dissociate from the chylomicron surface as discoidal or vesicular particles (11). Remodeling of these particles takes place with the formation of cholesteryl esters, which distribute to form the core of a particle. This converts the discoidal structure into a spherical HDL particle. As mentioned previously, formation of cholesteryl esters results from activity of LCAT, an enzyme synthesized in the liver but acting in plasma (54).

In addition to formation of HDL through lipolysis of triglyceride-rich lipoproteins, there is evidence that HDL particles may be directly secreted by both intestine and liver (55,56). Studies using isolated perfused rat liver have demonstrated particles in the HDL density range containing the major apoproteins of circulating HDL (55). Evidence for *de novo* synthesis of HDL apoproteins is provided by the incorporation of radioactive amino acids by the perfused liver into these apoproteins. Additional evidence that the perfusate HDL are not filtered from plasma comes from an analysis of their composition and morphology. Whereas plasma HDL are spherical particles with a phospholipid:cholesterol ester (PL/CE) ratio of ≈ 1, HDL from hepatic perfusates have a PL/CE ratio greater than 1 and contain much less cholesterol ester. In addition, the apoprotein pattern of perfusate HDL differs from plasma in that the particles are apo E rich (apo $E/_{A-I} \approx 10$), whereas plasma HDL contain predominantly apo A-I with little apo-E. Morphologically, perfusate HDL are discoidal particles reflecting their phospholipid-rich, cholesterol ester-poor composition. These bilamellar discoidal particles form rouleaux when examined by negative staining (55). Similar particles have been isolated from rat mesenteric lymph but contain apo A-I as their major apoprotein in contrast to hepatic HDL (56,57). Discoidal HDL have been isolated from single pass as well as recirculating hepatic perfusions and are abundant when an LCAT inhibitor is added to the perfusate to prevent cholesterol esterification after secretion (55).

Discoidal HDL particles, newly secreted by the liver or intestine, probably undergo extensive modifications when entering plasma. Various *in vitro* studies with cultured cells indicate that discoidal HDL are excellent acceptors for unesterified cholesterol. Subsequently, LCAT, acting on discoidal HDL as substrate, synthesizes cholesteryl esters and converts the discs to spherical particles. Apo E-rich discoidal HDL from the liver must also acquire additional apoproteins, such as apo E and apo A-I, which are present on circulating plasma lipoproteins. It is currently not known what proportion of circulating HDL derives from lipolysis of triglyceride-rich lipoproteins or are directly secreted by liver and intestine.

Less is known concerning metabolic factors within the liver that control the secretion of HDL. Available evidence suggests that HDL secretion is somewhat independent of hepatic VLDL secretion. Orotic acid, which specifically inhibits hepatic VLDL secretion, had little effect on HDL secretion by the perfused liver (58). In addition, experimental nephrosis in the rat is associated with a marked increase in HDL secretion by the perfused rat liver without a proportional increase in VLDL secretion (59). The increased HDL

secretion in nephrosis was associated with a change in apoprotein content of perfusate HDL. The particles become greatly enriched in apo A-I at the expense of their normal apo E content. The mechanisms responsible for these changes are unknown but suggest that formation of HDL and synthesis of HDL apoproteins have been altered dramatically. Further studies are required to determine additional metabolic factors which influence the synthesis and secretion of HDL by the liver.

The intracellular events in HDL formation are largely unknown. Particles of the density and electrophoretic mobility of HDL containing HDL apoproteins have been isolated from Golgi preparations (60,61). Discoidal HDL have not been visualized by electron microscopy within hepatocytes, undoubtedly because of their small size (190 × 45 Å) and the lack of rouleaux formation in fixed sections. In contrast to VLDL, no information is available concerning the subcellular pathway of HDL assembly and secretion.

HEPATIC CATABOLISM OF LIPOPROTEINS

In addition to its major biosynthetic role, the liver is important in several other aspects of plasma lipoprotein metabolism (62−64). Most important is the removal from plasma of remnant particles resulting from the partial catabolism of triglyceride-rich lipoproteins (65,66).

Chylomicrons and VLDL

Newly synthesized (nascent) VLDL and chylomicrons contain triglyceride as the principal component of the particle core. Before the triglyceride in these lipoproteins can be used as an energy source, it must by hydrolyzed by lipoprotein lipase (LPL). The nascent particles acquire the activator of LPL, apo C-II, by rapid transfer from HDL. Triglyceride hydrolysis ensues in relation to vascular endothelial cells, where LPL is localized (67). This enzymatic process is repeated numerous times with gradual depletion of core triglyceride and, in the case of VLDL, replacement of core lipids by cholesteryl esers transferred from HDL (Fig. 2). Chylomicrons apparently obtain most of their complement of cholesteryl esters within the intestinal absorptive cell.

As triglyceride lipolysis proceeds, the particles become smaller, more dense, and poorer substrates for LPL, particularly as apo C-II is depleted. During lipolysis, the surface lipids, phospholipids, unesterified cholesterol, and C apoproteins are removed and contribute to the formation of additional nascent HDL (see above). Eventually, a lipoprotein particle results, which is relatively refractory to further LPL action because of substrate (triglyceride) or activator (apo C-II) depletion or accumulation of inhibitors. At this point, at least in man, the metabolic pathways of VLDL and chylomicrons diverge. The VLDL, having been catabolized to intermediate density particles, become further enriched with cholesteryl esters by transfer from HDL. As triglyceride and residual C-apoproteins are removed, the particles are quantitatively transformed into LDL. In contrast, the remnants of chylomicron metabolism, still containing some triglyceride, are cleared by the liver (Fig. 2).

The exact mechanism of remnant clearance is not known. It is dependent on the presence of apoprotein E and C apoproteins in the remnant particles and on receptors for apo E located on hepatocyte surface membranes (68–74). On the basis of recent reports, a clear role of apo E in the hepatic clearance of triglyceride-rich lipoproteins has been established. Shelburne et al. (72) have demonstrated that addition of apo E to either rat lymph chylomicrons or triglyceride emulsions increased their uptake by nonrecirculating perfused livers. When lymph chylomicrons were exposed to plasma and became enriched in both apo E and C apoproteins, however, uptake was inhibited (72), an effect attributed primarily to apo C-III-I. Windler et al. (75) showed that incubation of either VLDL or small lymph chylomicrons with C apoproteins inhibited their uptake by perfused liver. Addition of apo E to small chylomicrons increased hepatic uptake. They concluded that apo E and apo C have opposing but independent effects on hepatic uptake of triglyceride-rich lipoproteins but did not conclude that a specific ratio of apo E:apo C-III-I was regulatory.

Havel et al. (76) studied hepatic remnant removal further utilizing ^{125}I-labeled apo E complexed with egg lecithin in lamellar form. These investigators have observed that uptake is dependent on the presence of specific isoforms of human apo E. Thus when all the isoforms of human apo E (from normals) were present, uptake was similar to rat apo E. When apo E from dysbetalipoproteinemia patients was used (deficient in E3 and E4), however, uptake was greatly reduced (76). The authors concluded that apo E3 and E4 are essential for recognition by the hepatic receptor of triglyceride-rich lipoproteins and that lack of these isoforms is the underlying defect in dysbetalipoproteinemia. In animal studies, the cholesteryl esters in chylomicron remnants have been shown to regulate the activity of hepatic 3-hydroxymethylglutaryl coenzyme-A reductase (HMG Co-A reductase), the rate-controlling enzyme of cholesterol synthesis (77). This is discussed more fully elsewhere in this volume.

LDL

No clear consensus exists as to the major site of LDL catabolism. The important studies of Brown and Goldstein (78,79) have demonstrated in *in vitro* ca-

tabolism by LDL by cultured skin fibroblasts and a variety of other peripheral cells. These cells possess specific receptors for apo B, which permit binding, internalization, and subsequent degradation of the LDL particle. It has been demonstrated that the perfused rat liver can take up and degrade LDL. Receptors on liver cell membranes have been found for apo B and apo E and are markedly increased by treatment with pharmacological doses of estrogens (73,75,76,80). Estrogen treatment also enhances catabolism by the liver of lipoproteins, including LDL (80). Therefore, while the liver undoubtedly can catabolize LDL, the magnitude is unknown. Further studies are needed to determine whether hepatic LDL receptors on hepatocytes are identical to those on peripheral cells. Available data suggest that they are quite similar (78).

HDL

The catabolism of HDL is complex; it is clear that a number of HDL components may be catabolized independently of the removal of the intact particle from the circulation. For example, cholesterol esters transfer from HDL to other lipoproteins, which are subsequently degraded. Similarly, unesterified cholesterol may rapidly equilibrate and leave the HDL particle. It is difficult to be confident about the catabolic fate of HDL. Studies on the fate of radioiodinated HDL have shown that the liver can take up HDL, and that labeled HDL apoproteins are sequestered by hepatocyte lysosomes (81,82). HDL binding and uptake have been demonstrated by isolated rat hepatocytes. This process can be inhibited by chloroquine, supporting the importance of lysosomes in HDL catabolism after binding and internalization by the hepatocyte membrane (83–85). In general, the results of *in vitro* uptake studies have not agreed with the observed rates of uptake by isolated hepatocytes. Peripheral cells (i.e., fibroblasts, vascular smooth muscle cells, vascular endothelial cells also can catabolize HDL. This uptake does not involve the LDL receptor, although a subfraction of HDL (containing apo E) competes with LDL for cell surface receptors (86). Thus, although it is clear that the liver can degrade HDL, the quantitative importance of this organ in HDL catabolism is not known.

ROLE OF LCAT IN LIPOPROTEIN METABOLISM

Because esterification of cholesterol in plasma by LCAT is a key reaction in lipoprotein metabolism, it is pertinent to emphasize salient features of the LCAT reaction. Cholesterol esterification occurs in the plasma and is attributable to LCAT, which is synthesized by the liver and is secreted into plasma. Recognition that most of the plasma-esterifying activity is due to an acyltransferase, and not to a combination of a cholesterol esterase and a lecithinase or to a reversible cholesterol ester hydrolase, was of major significance.

The basic function of LCAT is in the transfer of a fatty acyl group, usually polyunsaturated, from the 2-position of lecithin to unesterified cholesterol to form cholesteryl esters. Evidence for the LCAT reaction is as follows: (a) Incubation of radioactive cholesterol or radioactive lecithin with plasma results in the formation of labeled cholesterol ester, but incubation with radioactive FFA does not; (b) unesterified cholesterol and lecithin decrease at nearly equimolar rates during incubation of plasma, suggesting that lecithin is the principal acyl donor and that one fatty acyl group per molecule lecithin is transferred; and (c) more than 80% of the fatty acid transferred is unsaturated. This provides evidence that essentially one fatty acid is transferred per lecithin molecule and indicates that most of the fatty acids originate from the 2-position.

As indicated earlier, LCAT utilizing nascent HDL as substrate causes the transformation of the discoidal into spherical particles. This occurs as cholesteryl esters are synthesized and form the core of the HDL particle. The LCAT reaction is crucial to formation of plasma HDL, since the cholesteryl esters produced by LCAT are strongly hydrophobic and will thermodynamically seek a position between the lamellae of the discoidal nascent HDL. With repeated acquisition of free cholesterol and conversion into cholesteryl esters by the LCAT reaction, the HDL particles assume a spherical configuration with an oily, hydrophobic core of cholesteryl esters (11).

Subsequent sections dealing with lipoprotein changes in liver disease emphasize the striking abnormalities in lipoprotein metabolism that occur in liver disease can be largely attributed to LCAT deficiency.

EXPERIMENTAL CONDITIONS OF ALTERED HEPATIC VLDL SYNTHESIS

The liver can respond to an increased supply of FFA by enhanced triglyceride synthesis and a subsequent increase in VLDL formation and secretion. In most circumstances, the ability of the liver to rapidly synthesize and secrete VLDL and their efficient plasma catabolism does not result in an accumulation of triglycerides in either the hepatocyte or in plasma. However, there are clinical and experimental conditions in which an imbalance occurs between hepatic triglyceride formation and the synthesis and/or secretion of VLDL; this leads to fatty liver. Human diseases associated with fatty liver include certain forms of toxic hepatitis, uncontrolled diabetes, and excessive ethanol ingestion. Experimental models have been developed in an effort to understand the pathogenesis of fatty liver and the mechanism of VLDL synthesis and secretion (12). Certain drugs or toxins appear to affect specific steps in the pathway leading to VLDL formation or secretion (87,88). Other drugs are associated with concomitant hepatocellular injury, thereby producing derangements in plasma lipoprotein metabolism strikingly similar to human alcoholic hepatitis (89–92).

Numerous theories proposed for the pathogenesis of fatty liver are based on derangements of hepatic triglyceride synthesis and secretion (12,93). These include not only abnormalities of physiological and biochemical regulation, but also derangements in the steps by which VLDL lipid and lipoproteins are synthesized and assembled into nascent lipoprotein particles. These particles are transported sequentially through subcellular compartments and are secreted from the hepatocyte into the bloodstream.

Derangements of these events, singly or in combination, can be involved in the pathogenesis of fatty liver (93). Thus an increased supply of fatty acids, leading to an imbalance between triglyceride synthesis and secretion, could result from enhanced fatty acid mobilization from adipose tissue, increased hepatic fatty acid synthesis, or decreased fatty acid oxidation by hepatocyte mitochondria. Assembly of triglycerides into VLDL might be impaired as a consequence of inhibited apoprotein synthesis or inadequate apoprotein formation, which might occur when an excessive triglyceride load is available for lipoprotein formation. Defects in one or more of the steps involved in the intracellular transport or secretion of VLDL also can lead to fatty liver. These defects include interference with VLDL transport from the ER to the Golgi complex, impaired Golgi function which prevents the final glycosylation of VLDL apoproteins, decreased secretory vesicle formation, and impaired movement of secretory vesicles to the cell membrane.

Electron microscopic studies of human or experimental fatty liver reveal a monotonous engorgement of the cytoplasm with triglyceride droplets. Since triglycerides and apoproteins are synthesized in relation to the membranes of SER and RER, and the secretory particle is transported within the channels formed by these tubular organelles, an accumulation of triglyceride results in vesiculation of the ER. Vesiculation is caused by coalescence of triglyceride molecules into larger lipid droplets, which remain confined by the distended ER (88). With prolonged steatosis, there is progressive aggregation of triglyceride into very large droplets, which eventually assume enormous proportions and impinge upon the barriers imposed by ER membranes, resulting in formation of massive lipid aggregates.

Effects of Alcohol on Hepatic VLDL

Experimentally, the administration of ethanol to rats causes a rapid enhancement of VLDL synthesis and secretion (94). This effect results in a marked proliferation of VLDL in rat hepatocyte Golgi and active secretory vesicle formation within 90 min of intragastric administration of ethanol. These acute effects of ethanol are multifactorial, reflecting enhanced mobilization of fatty acids from adipose tissue and increased hepatic fatty acid synthesis from acetate, a major metabolite of alcohol. Baraona and Lieber (94) have comprehensively reviewed many aspects of the effects of ethanol on peripheral and hepatic lipid and lipoprotein metabolism.

As mentioned previously, fatty liver can develop if there is an imbalance between the extent of triglyceride formation and the ability of the liver to assemble and/or secrete triglycerides as VLDL. Ethanol may affect this process by increasing the supply of fatty acids brought to the liver. This is accomplished in part by increasing the mobilization of fatty acids from adipose tissue, possibly by release of norepinephrine and other hormones that promote adipose tissue triglyceride lipolysis. The supply of fatty acids is also increased by the availability of acetate, a product of ethanol metabolism. If ethanol has caused hepatocyte injury, the mitochondrial oxidation of fatty acids may be impaired. This results in an excess of fatty acids which could then be used for triglyceride synthesis. Hepatocyte injury induced by ethanol also can result in impaired protein synthesis, thereby interfering with the availability of apo B required for VLDL formation. At the subcellular level, alcohol can affect one or more of the steps in intracellular transport, packaging, or secretion of nascent VLDL. These include the movement of vesicles containing nascent VLDL from the ER to the Golgi complex, glycosylation of nascent VLDL in the Golgi, and formation of secretory vesicles. Movement of secretory vesicles containing nascent VLDL to the cell membrane for secretion may be regulated by microtubules. Ethanol has been shown to interfere with the export of several hepatic secretory proteins, and there is evidence that it interferes with microtubule formation (94).

Orotic Acid-Induced Defect in VLDL Secretion

Feeding 1% orotic acid in a semisynthetic diet produces a profound accumulation of triglycerides in rat liver, associated with a specific defect in VLDL secretion (87,88). Since orotic acid does not interfere specifically with protein or lipoprotein synthesis, it has been suggested that it may prevent assembly and/or secretion of lipoproteins (58). Apparently, hepatic synthesis of apoproteins involved in VLDL formation is not prevented following orotic acid feeding; however, there is a marked decrease in plasma triglyceride, cholesterol, and apo-B concentration. The isolated perfused rat liver obtained from orotic acid-treated animals cannot release VLDL but can secrete albumin and other plasma proteins (87).

Ultrastructural analysis of the alterations in rat hepatic subcellular organelles following orotic acid feeding suggests that orotic acid induces a defect in either the intracellular transport of nascent VLDL from the ER to the Golgi or in the final formation of VLDL within the Golgi complex (88,95,96). This interpretation is based on the distention of Golgi cisternae and vesicles with lipid droplets within the first few days of orotic acid feeding (when plasma triglyceride levels are decreasing rapidly) and the absence of VLDL in Golgi cisternae when fatty liver is well developed (95). With orotic acid feeding, there is a progressive distention of the ER, causing vesiculation of the cisternae as small lipid droplets aggregate into large triglyceride-rich droplets (88,97). Orotic acid may produce an interference with normal Golgi function. In the early phases of orotic acid-induced fatty liver, the Golgi cisternae are distended with lipid, secretory vesicles do not form, and there is no evidence of VLDL exocytosis. After 10 or more days of orotic acid feeding, however, the Golgi complexes are flattened and devoid of lipoprotein particles, suggesting a defect in the entrance of nascent VLDL into the Golgi complex (95).

The plasma lipoproteins are actually glycolipoproteins; however, the role of glycosyl moieties in determining the structure, secretion, and metabolism of lipoproteins is not known. Since there is evidence that the final assembly of lipoproteins occurs within the Golgi apparatus, and this subcellular organelle is thought to be the site of important terminal glycosylations in glycoprotein synthesis, secretion of lipoproteins by hepatic Golgi may depend on the addition of a carbohydrate moiety (98,99). The orotic acid-induced secretory block may be related to a defect in the glycosylation of certain VLDL apoproteins within the Golgi. Orotic acid is known to produce an imbalance in hepatic nucleotide levels, causing an increase in uridine and a decrease in adenine and cytidine nucleotides (100). The decreased availability of specific sugars for transfer to completely glycosylated apoproteins within the Golgi might cause the secretory block. In this regard, there is some evidence that a defect in glycoprotein formation can occur after orotic acid feeding (98,99).

The decrease in cytidine nucleotides may have important implications for the pathogenesis of fatty liver, since the hepatic Golgi contain a sialytransferase which catalyzes the incorporation of sialic acid from CMP-N-acetylneuraminic acid into a sialidase-treated apo C peptide isolated from VLDL (101). A decrease in the availability of this sugar nucleotide might prevent adequate sialylation of C-peptides in the Golgi and could explain the observations discussed above. If VLDL secretion is dependent on the presence of the sugar moieties of the VLDL apoproteins, then defective sialylation of the C-peptides could cause the secretory block. In this regard it is of interest that addition of adenine to the orotic acid diet not only reverses the hepatic triglyceride accumulation but also specifically restores to normal the balance of uridine and adenine nucleotides in the liver.

Effects of Galactosamine on Plasma Lipoproteins

In rats, intraperitoneal injection of galactosamine (GalN) produces hepatocellular injury secondary to uridylate trapping in the form of uridine disphosphate hexosamines (102–104). A decrease in rat plasma LCAT activity following GalN injection has been reported (91). Compositional studies of plasma lipoproteins after GalN have shown that the plasma lipoproteins are deficient in cholesteryl esters and enriched in unesterified cholesterol and phospholipid (91,92). These compositional alterations are associated with changes in lipoprotein ultrastructure characterized by the formation of bilamellar discoidal lipoproteins in both the LDL and HDL fractions. In addition to the alterations in lipid composition. GalN produces striking abnormalities in apoprotein composition, particularly in VLDL and HDL. Thus the VLDL are characterized by a decreased content of apo E and C-apoproteins, while the discoidal HDL are enriched in apo E and deficient in apo A-I, A-II, and A-IV. These findings are similar to some of the alterations in lipoprotein composition and ultrastructure reported in human alcoholic hepatitis with secondary LCAT deficiency and in familial LCAT deficiency. They reflect the importance of cholesterol esterification in nascent HDL and the subsequent transfer of cholesteryl esters to other lipoproteins for the normal pathways of lipoprotein metabolism to occur.

The remarkable alteration in plasma lipoprotein composition associated with GalN-induced hepatitis may reflect the central role of LCAT in lipoprotein metabolism. Since GalN produces direct hepatocellular injury causing pathological changes similar to viral or toxic agents which produce hepatocellular injury and necrosis, the LCAT deficiency may be secondary to loss of the enzyme from the damaged hepatocytes. The accumulation in plasma of abnormal lipoproteins is apparently not due to impaired hepatic VLDL secretion, since ultrastructural studies of GalN hepatitis have shown distention of hepatocyte Golgi zones with lipoprotein droplets and secretion of these lipoproteins into the perisinusoidal space of Disse (105).

Effects of 4-Aminopyrazolopyrimidine on Hepatic VLDL Formation and Secretion

4-Aminopyrazolopyrimidine (APP), an adenine analog, rapidly produces a selective defect in VLDL secretion and fatty liver in the rat (106). Thus 18 hr after APP, plasma triglycerides are greatly reduced, and lipoprotein electrophoresis shows absent pre-beta (VLDL) and only traces of beta (LDL) bands (106). By electron microscopy, alterations in Golgi and ER are evident within a few hours. Golgi cisternae become distended with VLDL-size particles; however, secretory vesicles do not form (107). Although the SER becomes dilated by an accumulation of lipid, VLDL-size particles are present in smooth-surfaced extensions of the ER; there is evidence of vesicular transport of lipoprotein particles into the Golgi. By 18 hr, the Golgi cisternae are markedly distended with lipid, and the ER assumes various configurations of distention and vesiculation; other subcellular organelles are normal, however, and hepatocyte necrosis is not observed (107). Thus VLDL-size particles accumulate in the Golgi even when plasma triglycerides and VLDL are markedly decreased. These findings suggest that the VLDL secretory block induced by APP occurs within the Golgi, leading to a secondary accumulation of triglycerides within the ER.

Effects of Hypercholesterolemic Diets on Hepatic Golgi Lipoprotein Formation

Experimentally, hypercholesterolemia and alterations in the composition and electrophoretic properties of plasma lipoproteins can be induced in certain animal species by feeding diets containing high concentrations of cholesterol (108). Induction of these changes is enhanced by supplementing the diets with saturated fats and by making the animals hypothyroid. Changes in plasma lipoproteins include the appearance of a beta-migrating VLDL (β-VLDL), which are cholesterol-enriched compared to normal VLDL, an increase in the concentration of intermediate density lipoproteins (IDL) and LDL, and the formation of an unusual HDL termed HDL_c (108). HDL_c are uniquely related to feeding a high cholesterol diet. They are quite similar to LDL in lipid composition but differ in that they contain apo E and A-I and do not contain apo B, the characteristic apoprotein of LDL. After cholesterol feeding, all the unusual lipoproteins are characterized by their enrichment in cholesteryl esters and apo E.

These unusual lipoproteins may represent either a direct hepatic secretory product or result from the accumulation of chylomicron remnants. Earlier studies in the cholesterol-fed rabbit suggested that the cholesteryl ester-enriched LDL actually represented chylomicron remnants which could not be cleared readily by the liver (109). Some years ago, however, Roheim and co-workers (110) showed that the liver of cholesterol-fed rats could secrete 50% more lipoprotein cholesterol than controls. There is also evidence that cholesterol feeding increases apoprotein synthesis by the liver, particularly apo E (111,112).

Two excellent studies have attempted to specifically determine what type of lipoproteins the hypercholesterolemic rat liver can synthesize and secrete (85,113). Using isolated hepatic perfusion, Noel and co-workers (113) have shown that the liver from hypercholesterolemic rats can secrete cholesterol-ester and apo E-rich lipoproteins similar to those isolated from plasma. Thus the hypercholesterolemic liver secretes apo E at a high rate and synthesizes cholesterol ester-rich, apo C-deficient VLDL. The LDL was enriched in cholesterol and contained apo E as well as apo B. Radioisotopic studies showed incorporation of ^{3}H-leucine into apo-VLDL and apo-LDL secreted by the livers of hypercholesterolemic animals. An analysis of the apoproteins by polyacrylamide gel electrophoresis suggested hepatic synthesis of the apoprotein constituents of the hypercholesterolemic lipoproteins.

In an elegant study, Swift and co-workers recently approached the question of formation of hypercholesterolemic lipoproteins more directly by determining the composition of lipoproteins purified from hepatic Golgi preparations (52). They showed that Golgi VLDL from hypercholesterolemic rats contained four times the total cholesterol mass found in controls. The VLDL were devoid of apo C and migrated electrophoretically between beta and pre-beta. The authors isolated an LDL fraction from the Golgi which were smaller than VLDL, displayed beta-electrophoretic mobility, were enriched in cholesteryl esters, and contained apo E as well as apo B. Each of these studies indicates that cholesteryl ester-rich, apo C-deficient VLDL and the apo E-containing LDL found in the plasma of hypercholesterolemic rats are not merely VLDL and chylomicron remnants but are synthesized and secreted by the liver.

These observations are important, since they demonstrate that the liver can respond to dietary influences by synthesizing lipoproteins of novel composition and thus contribute to dietary-induced hypercholesterolemia. Moreover, they provide evidence that, under certain conditions, the liver can synthesize a type of LDL particle. This finding is of considerable interest in view of prevailing concepts that LDL is formed exclusively in plasma as a direct product of VLDL catabolism.

LIPOPROTEIN AND LIPID ABNORMALITIES IN HUMAN LIVER DISEASE

Having considered the importance of the liver in the normal synthesis and metabolism of plasma lipoproteins, it is appropriate to briefly discuss the lipid and lipoprotein abnormalities that occur in liver diseases characterized by hepatocellular injury or cholestasis. This is particularly pertinent since alterations in the concentration and composition of plasma lipids and lipoproteins occur invariably in liver disease. These changes can be attributed to abnormalities in lipoprotein synthesis, LCAT deficiency, lipolytic defects, and abnormalities in the hepatic recognition and uptake of remnant lipoprotein particles, as well as regurgitation into plasma of biliary lipids. These derangements reflect the central role of the liver in lipoprotein metabolism and are expressed by hypercholesterolemia, decreased percent cholesteryl esters, hypertriglyceridemia, and complex abnormalities in the structure and lipid and apoprotein composition of the plasma lipoproteins.

This complex subject has been discussed extensively in several recent reviews (62–64) and is considered here only briefly, emphasizing the major abnormalities in lipid and lipoprotein metabolism that characteristically occur in liver disease.

Lipoprotein Changes in Hepatocellular Disease

Alterations in Plasma Lipids

Modest hypertriglyceridemia (250 to 500 mg/dl) occurs frequently in association with hepatocellular disease, as described in alcoholic, viral, and drug-induced hepatitis. In some patients with severe alcoholic fatty liver, massive hypertriglyceridemia is attributable to specific effects of alcohol on lipid metabolism and may not reflect alcohol-induced derangements in hepatocellular function. Hypertriglyceridemia in liver disease is transient, with plasma triglyceride levels returning to normal with resolution of the disease. The triglycerides usually are recovered in an abnormal LDL fraction, which may represent the accumulation of remnant lipoproteins because of impaired lipolysis or ineffective remnant clearance by the injured liver. Remnant accumulation in liver disease could be explained by defective hepatocyte receptors, alterations in the apo E and C-apoprotein content of remnants, or by a decrease in the activity of hepatic triglyceride lipase. Hepatic triglyceride lipase is located on the surface of hepatocyte and is thought to function in the hydrolysis of residual triglycerides in remnant particles. There is evidence for hepatic triglyceride lipase deficiency in liver disease, but the other possible explanations for remnant accumulation have yet to be proved.

Perhaps the most characteristic alteration in plasma lipids in hepatocellular disease is a decrease in the percent cholesteryl esters which occurs almost invariably. The importance of the liver in the synthesis and secretion of LCAT provides the most likely explanation for the cholesteryl ester deficiency. In addition to decreased cholesteryl esters, patients with liver disease may have increased lecithin and unesterified cholesterol and decreased lysolecithin. These changes in cholesterol and phospholipids are similar to those described in familial LCAT deficiency. It is well documented that plasma LCAT activity is decreased in hepatocellular disease and that LCAT deficiency is the principal explanation for the decreased cholesteryl esters (114–121). Thus the decrease in LCAT activity and the parallel depression in cholesteryl ester concentration are related to the extent of liver damage and increase concomitantly with clinical recovery (116, 117,119,120,122,123).

There are several possible explanations for LCAT deficiency in hepatocellular disease; perhaps most likely is inadequate synthesis or loss of the enzyme secondary to hepatocyte necrosis. There is no evidence that LCAT inhibitors occur in plasma in liver disease. Although a striking deficiency of apo A-I frequently occurs, which is required for LCAT activation, the minute quantity of activator required tends to exclude apo A-I deficiency as a plausible explanation. Decreased plasma cholesterol esterification could result from the release of cholesteryl ester hydrolase from damaged hepatocytes (124,125). The net cholesterol-esterifying activity of plasma may be the result of a balance between LCAT and cholesteryl ester hydrolase activity (126). This activity, however, has not been demonstrated in the plasma of patients with liver disease, and cholesterol-esterifying ability has been closely correlated with independent assays of LCAT activity in patients with liver disease. This suggests that net cholesterol esterification can be best equated with LCAT activity (127). Furthermore, LCAT deficiency is found in hepatectomized animals (128), and decreased LCAT activity and lipoprotein abnormalities similar to those of patients with hepatocellular injury have been described in ethionine (129), carbon tetrachloride (130), and galactosamine (91,92) hepatitis. These results suggest that defective cholesterol esterification reflects decreased LCAT availability. Until sufficient purification of human LCAT is achieved to permit actual quantitation of enzyme protein, however, a primary LCAT deficiency cannot be proved.

Lipoprotein Electrophoretic Abnormalities

Lipoprotein electrophoretic patterns are consistently abnormal in hepatocellular disease. Characteristically, the α-lipoprotein band is absent or greatly reduced, and the pre-β and β-lipoprotein bands are replaced by a single band migrating between the β and pre-β position. These rather characteristic changes occur in all types of hepatocellular disease, with similar patterns described in patients with alcoholic, viral, and drug-induced hepatitis. With clinical improvement, there is a gradual reappearance of the α band and the resolution of the single abnormally migrating band into β and pre-β components. The electrophoretic abnormalities reflect alterations in the concentration and composition of the plasma lipoproteins. These are described more fully below but basically consist of (a) a greatly decreased concentration of normal HDL, which is replaced by a discoidal particle enriched in apo E and deficient in apo A-I and C-peptides, (b) a triglyceride-rich LDL fraction, which is depleted in cholesteryl esters, and (c) the accumulation of VLDL, which are deficient in C-apoproteins and apo E. The lipoprotein electrophoretic changes probably reflect the abnormal electrophoretic mobility of these unusual lipoproteins.

Lipoprotein Composition in Hepatocellular Disease

On the basis of the uniformity of plasma lipid and lipoprotein electrophoretic abnormalities in various types of liver disease, there is good reason to expect that the apoprotein and lipid composition of the plasma lipoproteins would also be similar, despite the etiology of the hepatocellular injury. Relatively few detailed analytical studies of lipoprotein composition in hepatocellular disease have been performed. These have been confined essentially to alcoholic hepatitis, probably because of the infectious hazard of purifying lipoproteins from patients with viral hepatitis.

Detailed compositional studies of lipoprotein fractions isolated by ultracentrifugation, performed at various intervals throughout the course of illness in patients with alcoholic hepatitis, have revealed compositional abnormalities in each of the fractions (115,131). Most prominent are profound depressions in the percent cholesteryl esters, which can remain reduced for many weeks before gradually returning towards normal. In VLDL, the decrease in cholesteryl esters is accompanied by moderate increase in phospholipids. In addition to a striking decrease in the percent cholesteryl esters in LDL, this fraction is characterized by an enrichment in triglycerides and phospholipids. The HDL fraction is remarkable for the decrease in percent cholesteryl esters which, in very sick patients, can persist at low levels for several months. These compositional abnormalities are associated with ultrastructural changes that can be observed by electron microscopy of negatively stained lipoproteins isolated by sequential ultracentrifugation from plasma.

In alcoholic hepatitis, the VLDL contain particles similar in structure and size to normal VLDL. The LDL contain a mixture of spherical particles similar in appearance and size to normal LDL and others which are much larger (500 nm). In some patients, the LDL fraction contains lipoproteins that appear as bilamellar vesicles or chains of discoidal particles. The HDL fractions contain some spherical particles of approximately normal HDL size, but most of the lipoproteins appear as long chains of stacked bilamellar discs measuring 150 to 240 nm in diameter and 30 to 50 nm in thickness (132) (Fig. 4).

An analysis of the specific apoprotein composition and concentration in the VLDL, LDL, HDL of patients with alcoholic hepatitis shows remarkable abnormalities, probably attributable to defective lipoprotein metabolism (132). Characteristically, the VLDL are enriched in apo B, but the C peptides and apo E may be nearly absent. The LDL fraction contains apo B similar to normal LDL; the apoprotein content of HDL, however, is strikingly abnormal. Normal HDL contain apo A-I, apo A-II, the apo C peptides, and a trace of apo E. In contrast, the predominant apoprotein in alcoholic hepatitis is apo E, and apo A-I is severely deficient.

With recovery from alcoholic hepatitis, there is a gradual return toward normal of the apoprotein composition of the VLDL and HDL. This is associated with an increase in plasma LCAT activity and a corresponding increase in the percent cholesteryl esters in plasma (133). The return toward normal of the apoproteins in the isolated lipoprotein fractions is characterized by a decrease in apo E in HDL and an increase

in apo A-I. The relative proportion of apo B in VLDL gradually decreases, while apo C and apo E content increases.

Thus it is evident that alcoholic hepatitis is associated with many abnormalities in the concentration and composition of blood lipids and lipoproteins. The cause of these changes is multifactorial, reflecting complex biosynthetic, enzymatic, and catabolic derangements in lipoprotein catabolism (62–64). An interpretation of the compositional abnormalities in alcoholic hepatitis is compatible with the concept that the liver secretes primarily two lipoprotein types: nascent HDL, whose major apoprotein is apo E, and nascent VLDL, containing only apo B. Normally, nascent HDL is acted upon by LCAT, and resulting cholesteryl esters are transferred to nascent VLDL along with apo E and apo C. Therefore, HDL containing primarily apo A-I is the major component of the HDL fraction. In alcoholic hepatitis, because of LCAT deficiency, cholesteryl esters are not formed, and nascent HDL accumulates. As a result of the cholesteryl ester deficiency, there is no transfer of lipids or apoproteins to nascent VLDL. Thus nascent VLDL containing primarily apo B accumulates. Partial hydrolysis of the triglyceride in nascent VLDL results in accumulation of a triglyceride-rich fraction floating in the LDL density range. Complete triglyceride hydrolysis may be limited by the C-apoprotein deficiency, since apo C-II is required for lipoprotein lipase activation. This fraction contains primarily apo B, but its further metabolism to LDL is impaired, probably because of the cholesteryl ester deficiency.

Alterations of plasma lipoproteins in chronic parenchymal liver disease are similar to those of acute liver injury but usually are less striking. Electrophoretic patterns may be normal in chronic liver disease but frequently show a decrease in the α band and an absent pre-β. This probably reflects on-going hepatocellular injury and impaired triglyceride and cholesterol synthesis. The cholesteryl esters have been reported as normal (122) to slightly decreased (114,117,120) in chronic liver disease; LCAT is depressed (114,117, 118,120,122), indicating the activity of the injurious process.

Lipid and Lipoprotein Abnormalities in Cholestatic Liver Disease

Lipid and lipoprotein abnormalities similar to those in parenchymal liver injury are found in cholestatic liver disease, even in the virtual absence of hepatocellular injury. These changes include abnormal lipoprotein electrophoretic patterns identical to those in patients with hepatitis, elevated plasma lipids, and abnormalities in the lipid and apoprotein composition

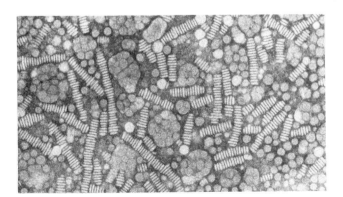

FIG. 4. Negatively stained preparation of nascent HDL which appear as chains of bilamellar discs from a patient with alcoholic hepatitis. ×114,000.

of lipoprotein fractions (62–64). There are differences, however, in some of the lipid and lipoprotein changes. This is particularly true in regard to the extraordinary elevation of plasma cholesterol and phospholipid and the appearance in cholestatic plasma of a variety of unusual lipoproteins, including the classic cholestatic lipoprotein, lipoprotein-X (Lp-X) (Fig. 5). Furthermore, although decreased LCAT activity does occur in cholestasis, it is not found invariably as in the case of hepatocellular disease. Since elevated plasma cholesterol is characteristic of cholestasis, in some patients whose LCAT activity is normal, the absolute concentration of cholesteryl esters is normal, but the percent cholesteryl esters is decreased relative to the enormous increase in plasma unesterified cholesterol.

The increased phospholipid and free cholesterol are complexed in an equimolar ratio with albumin and some C-apoproteins (134–137). The lipids form a bilamellar vesicular structure Lp-X, which traps albumin in the aqueous core and adsorbs C-apoproteins on the surface. Although Lp-X floats at the density of LDL (138,139), only traces of cholesteryl ester and triglyceride are present, and apo B, the main component of normal LDL, is absent (135,138). Initially, the C-apoprotein component was mistakenly believed to be a unique new apoprotein, designated apo X; therefore, the total complex was designated Lp-X. Lp-X appears as 400 to 600 nm diameter, 100 nm thick discs with a tendency to form rouleaux (140) (Fig. 5). It has the peculiar property of cathodal migration on agar gel electrophoresis, permitting its semiquantitative determination in whole plasma.

The two most likely explanations for the origin of Lp-X are the regurgitation of biliary lipids and substrate accumulation secondary to LCAT deficiency. Proponents of the latter hypothesis emphasize the presence of an Lp-X-like lipoprotein in sera from patients with familial LCAT deficiency and the fact that the composition of Lp-X from patients with liver disease could represent the accumulation of an LCAT

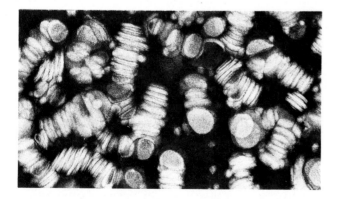

FIG. 5. Negatively stained preparations of the cholestatic lipoprotein Lp-X. ×114,000.

substrate. Cholestatic plasma may enhance LCAT activity (117), suggesting that Lp-X, directly or indirectly, can serve as an LCAT substrate. LCAT activity is decreased in many patients with biliary obstruction (116,117,140), and an inverse relationship has been observed between Lp-X concentration and LCAT activity, suggesting that LCAT deficiency causes an accumulation of excess substrate, which aggregates as Lp-X (140). However, the concept that cholestatic plasma, containing Lp-X, is a superior LCAT substrate has been challenged. One study showed that LCAT activity was decreased in cholestatic plasma (117), while another showed that Lp-X can inhibit LCAT (137). In the latter case, Lp-X concentration remained constant, even upon prolonged incubation with an LCAT source (137).

The decrease in LCAT activity is variable in obstructive jaundice. LCAT activity may be normal or even increased in some patients (122). Normal LCAT activity in cholestasis has been documented, particularly when it is of short duration, as in acute cholelithiasis (122). It appears that decreased LCAT activity is associated with a longer duration of cholestasis than when LCAT activity is normal. Lp-X is consistently detected in patients with primary biliary cirrhosis who have severe intrahepatic cholestasis, but LCAT activity is usually normal. This finding suggests that LCAT deficiency and Lp-X formation are independent events, and that Lp-X results from biliary stasis, whereas LCAT deficiency reflects hepatocellular injury, which is usually a late finding in primary biliary cirrhosis.

The results of recent experiments designed to investigate the source of Lp-X indicate that Lp-X may be derived from a precursor lipoprotein complex which is normally excreted by the liver into the bile but which is converted into Lp-X when it is regurgitated into the plasma during cholestasis (141). The concentration of phospholipids and free cholesterol in bile are similar to those of Lp-X, but bile does not contain any apoproteins; nor does it form bilamellar vesicles when visualized by electron microscopy. A lipid-protein complex similar in lipid composition to native bile and Lp-X can be isolated from bile by ultracentrifugation. This lipoprotein differs from Lp-X in electrophoretic mobility and immunochemical reactivity (141). The addition of bile salts produces some changes in the properties of the bile lipoprotein, causing it to migrate anodally and to react with antialbumin antibodies in a manner similar to that of native bile. When native or water-dialyzed bile is incubated *in vitro* with albumin or serum, a lipoprotein is formed which is remarkably similar to Lp-X in such characteristics as lipid composition and cathodal migration on agarose electrophoresis. The amount of Lp-X formed after the addition of albumin or serum depends on the concentration of bile salts and the bile lipoprotein. By electron microscopy, Lp-X formed *in vitro* appears as bilamellar vesicles and stacked discs, structures similar to Lp-X.

These experiments point to the possibility that Lp-X is formed as a consequence of the interaction of bile and serum constituents, particularly albumin. Thus it has been suggested that during cholestasis, Lp-X is formed when biliary constituents reflux into the blood (141).

It is not certain, however, that all the lipid abnormalities of cholestasis are due to Lp-X, since compositional abnormalities of all classes of plasma lipoproteins occur, and the quantity of Lp-X in the blood may not account for the entire elevation of free cholesterol and phospholipids. Although Lp-X represents one specific abnormal lipoprotein in cholestasis, it is evident that complex abnormalities in the metabolic interconversions of plasma lipoproteins occur in cholestatic liver disease and that these cannot be explained merely by the reflux of biliary constituents into plasma. For example, cholestatic and hepatic liver diseases are often accompanied by defective cholesterol esterification related to a decreased LCAT activity; many of the lipoprotein compositional abnormalities can be explained by LCAT deficiency.

SUMMARY

This chapter summarizes current information on the mechanisms involved in hepatic lipoprotein formation, secretion, and catabolism. Many questions remain unanswered concerning the molecular events in lipoprotein formation. Specifically, the control mechanisms involved in lipoprotein secretion need further delineation. What factors influence the synthesis of specific apoproteins? Can these rates of synthesis be altered? Are there interrelationships between the intestinal and hepatic synthesis of lipoproteins? Similarly, more information is needed concerning events involved in the catabolism of lipoproteins by the liver. Of great importance is new information on specific hepatic recognition and transport systems for lipoprotein catabolism. Little is known concerning the linkage of lipoprotein catabolism and biliary excretion of bile salts and cholesterol, an essential process for cholesterol homeostasis. A full understanding of these mechanisms will permit therapeutic modulations of lipoprotein metabolism. Such drug or dietary therapies are likely to be of great value in the treatment of hyperlipidemias and in our understanding and therapy of atherosclerosis. Based on recent progress in elucidating many areas of lipoprotein metabolism, we can confidently look forward to major advances in our further understanding of this area.

ACKNOWLEDGMENTS

This research was supported by grant HL-27369-01 from the National Institutes of Health, General Clinical Research Center grant RR 00211 (Dr. Sabesin), and by National Institutes of Health grants AM 21367, HL 21006, and AM 07330 (Dr. Glickman).

REFERENCES

1. Eisenberg, S., and Levy, R. I. (1975): Lipoprotein metabolism. *Adv. Lipid Res.*, 13:1–89.
2. Eisenberg, S. (1976) Lipoprotein metabolism and hyperlipidemia. In: *Atherosclerosis Reviews*, edited by R. Paoletti and A. M. Gotto, pp. 23–60. Raven Press, New York.
3. Morrisett, J. D., Jackson, R. L., and Gotto, A. M. (1975): Lipoproteins: Structure and function. *Ann. Rev. Biochem.*, 44:183–207.
4. Jackson, R. L., Morriset, J. D., and Gotto, A. M. Jr. (1976): Lipoprotein structure and metabolism. *Physiol. Rev.*, 56:259.
5. Schaefer, E. J., Eisenberg, S., and Levy, R. I. (1978): Lipoprotein apoprotein metabolism. *J. Lipid Res.*, 19:667.
6. Smith, L. C., Pownall, H. J., and Gotto, A. M., Jr. (1978): The plasma lipoproteins: Structure and metabolism. *Ann. Rev. Biochem.*, 47:751–777.
7. Havel, R. J. (1975): Lipoprotein and lipid transport. *Adv. Exp. Med. Biol.*, 63:37–59.
8. Kane, J. P. (1977): Plasma lipoproteins: Structure and metabolism. In: *Lipid Metabolism in Mammals*, edited by F. Snyder, pp. 209–957. Plenum, New York.
9. Morrisett, J. D., Jackson, R. L., and Gotto, A. M., Jr. (1977): Lipid-protein interactions in the plasma lipoproteins. *Biochim. Biophys. Acta*, 472:93–133.
10. Osborne, J. C., Jr., and Brewer, H. B., Jr. (1977): The plasma lipoproteins. *Adv. Protein Chem.*, 31:253–337.
11. Tall, A. R., and Small, D. M. (1978): Plasma high-density lipoproteins. *N. Engl. J. Med.*, 299:1232–1236.
12. Stein, O., Bar-on, H., and Stein, Y. (1972): Lipoproteins and the liver. In: *Progress in Liver Disease, Vol. IV*, edited by H. Popper and F. Schaffner, pp. 45–62. Grune & Stratton, New York.
13. Hamilton, R. L., Regen, D. M., Gray, M. E., and LeQuire, V. S. (1967): Lipid transport in liver. I. Electron microscopic identification of very low density lipoproteins in perfused rat liver. *Lab. Invest.*, 16: 305–319.
14. Jones, A. L., Ruderman, N. B., and Herrera, M. G. (1967): Electron microscopic and biochemical study of lipoprotein synthesis in the isolated perfused rat liver. *J. Lipid Res.*, 8:429–446.
15. Claude, A. (1970): Growth and differentiation of cytoplasmic membranes in the course of lipoprotein granule synthesis in the hepatic cell. I. Elaboration of elements of the Golgi complex. *J. Cell Biol.*, 47:745–766.
16. Hay, R., and Getz, G. S. (1979): Translation in vivo and in vitro of proteins resembling apoproteins of rat plasma very low density lipoprotein. *J. Lipid Res.*, 20:334–348.
17. Alexander, C. A., Hamilton, R. L., and Havel, R. J. (1976): Subcellular localization of B apoprotein of plasma lipoproteins in rat liver. *J. Cell Biol.*, 69:241–263.
18. Sabesin, S. M., Frase, S., and Finberg, R. P. (1978): Biogenesis of rat hepatocyte Golgi during the induction of lipoprotein secretion by sucrose feeding. *Gastroenterology (Abstr.)*, 75:963.
19. Palade, G. E. (1975): Intracellular aspects of the process of protein secretion. *Science*, 189:347–358.
20. Mahley, R. W., Brown, W. V., and Schachter, H. (1974): Incorporation of sialic acid into sialidase-treated apolipoprotein of human, very low density lipoprotein by a pork liver siayltransferase. *Can. J. Biochem.*, 52:655–664.
21. Mahley, R. W., Hamilton, R. L., and LeQuire, V. S. (1969): Characterization of lipoprotein particles isolated from the Golgi apparatus of rat liver. *J. Lipid Res.*, 10:433–439.

22. Mahley, R. W., Gray, M. E., Hamilton, R. L., and LeQuire, V. S. (1968): Lipid transport in liver. II. Electron microscopic and biochemical studies of alterations in lipoprotein transport induced by cortisone in the rabbit. *Lab. Invest.,* 19:358.

23. Stein, O., and Stein, Y. (1966): Visualization of intravenously injected 9, 10-^{3}H$_2$-palmitic acid in rat liver by electron microscopic autoradiography. *Isr. J. Med. Sci.,* 2:239–242.

24. Mahley, R. W., Bersot, T. P., and LeQuire, V. S. (1970): Identity of very low density lipoprotein apoproteins of plasma and liver Golgi apparatus. *Science,* 168:380–382.

25. Glaumann, H., Bergstrand, H., and Erickson, J. L. E. (1975): Studies on the synthesis and intracellular transport of lipoprotein particles in rat liver. *J. Cell Biol.,* 64:356–377.

26. Le Marchand, Y., Singh, A., Assimacopoulos-Jeannet, F., Orci, L., Rouiller, C., and Jeanrenaud, B. (1973): A role for the mictotubule system in the release of very low density lipoproteins by perfused mouse liver. *J. Biol. Chem.,* 248:6862-6870.

27. Reaven, E., and Reaven, G. M. (1978): Dissociation between rate of hepatic lipoprotein secretion and hepatocyte microtubule content. *J. Cell Biol.,* 77:735–742.

28. Novikoff, A. B. (1976): The endoplasmic reticulum: A cytochemist's view (A review). *Proc. Natl. Acad. Sci. USA,* 73:2781–2787.

29. Novikoff, A. B., and Novikoff, P. M. (1977): Cytochemical studies on Golgi apparatus and GERL. *Histochem. J.,* 9:525–551.

30. Novikoff, P. M., Novikoff, A. B., Quintana, N., and Hauw, J. J. (1971): Golgi apparatus, GERL and lysosomes of neurons in rat dorsal root ganglia, studied by thick section and thin section cytochemistry. *J. Cell Biol.,* 50:850–886.

31. Novikoff, P. M., and Yam, A. (1978): Sites of lipoprotein particles in normal rat hepatocytes. *J. Cell Biol.,* 76:1–11.

32. Novikoff, P. M., and Edelstein, D. (1977): Reversal of orotic acid-induced fatty liver in rats by clofibrate. *Lab. Invest.,* 36:215–231.

33. Heimberg, M., Gohn, E. H., Klausner, H. A., Soler-Argilaga, C., Weinstein, I., and Wilcox, H. G. (1978): Regulation of hepatic metabolism of free fatty acids. Interrelationships among secretion of very low density lipoproteins, ketogenesis and cholesterogenesis. In: *Disturbances in Lipid and Lipoprotein Metabolism,* edited by J. M. Dietschy, A. M. Gotto, Jr., and J. A. Ontko, pp. 251–284. Clinical Physiology Series, American Physiologic Society, Washington, D.C.

34. Ockner, R. K., Manning, J. M., Pappenhausen, R. B., and Ho, W. K. L. (1972): A binding protein for fatty acids in cytosol of intestinal mucosa, liver, myocardium and other tissues. *Science,* 177:56–58.

35. Ockner, R. K., and Manning, J. M. (1976): Fatty acid binding protein. Role in esterification of absorbed long chain fatty acid in rat intestine. *J. Clin. Invest.,* 58:632–641.

36. Ockner, R. K., Burnett, D. A., Lysenko, N., and Manning, J. A. (1979): Sex differences in long chain fatty acid utilization and fatty acid binding protein concentration in rat liver. *J. Clin. Invest.,* 64:172–181.

37. Heimberg, M., and Wilcox, H. G. (1972): The effects of palmitic and oleic acid on the properties and composition of the very low density lipoproteins secreted by the liver. *J. Biol. Chem.,* 247:875–880.

38. Ockner, R. K., Hughes, F. B., and Isselbacher, K. J. (1969): Very low density lipoproteins in intestinal lymph: Role in triglyceride and cholesterol transport during fat absorption. *J. Clin. Invest.,* 48:2367–2373.

39. Van Golde, L. M., Raben, G. J., Batenburg, J. J., Fleischer, B., Zambrano, F., and Fleischer, S. (1974): Biosynthesis of lipids in Golgi complex and other subcellular fractions from rat liver. *Biochim. Biophys. Acta,* 360:179–192.

40. Krishnaiah, K. V., Walker, L. F., Borensztajn, J., Schonfeld, G., and Getz, G. S. (1980): Apolipoprotein B variant derived from rat intestine. *Proc. Natl. Acad. Sci. USA,* 77:3806–3810.

41. Wu, A. L., and Windmueller, H. G. (1981): Variant forms of plasma apolipoprotein B. Hepatic and intestinal biosynthesis and heterogenous metabolism in the rat. *J. Biol. Chem.,* 256:3615–3618.

42. Kane, J. P., Hardman, D. A., and Paulus, H. E. (1980): Heterogeneity of apolipoprotein B: Isolation of a new species from human chylomicrons. *Proc. Natl. Acad. Sci. USA,* 77:2465–2469.

43. Elovson, J., Huang, Y. O., Baker, N., and Kannan, R. (1981): Apolipoprotein B is structurally and metabolically heterogenous in the rat. *Proc. Natl. Acad. Sci. USA,* 78:157–161.

44. Bar-on, H., Kook, A. I., Stein, O., and Stein, Y. (1973): Assembly and secretion of very low density lipoproteins by rat liver following inhibition of protein synthesis with cycloheximide. *Biochim. Biophys. Acta,* 306:106–114.

45. Kempen, H. J. M. (1980): Lipoprotein secretion by isolated rat hepatocytes: Characterization of the lipid carrying particles and modulation of their release. *J. Lipid Res.,* 21:671–680.

46. Davis, R. A., Englehorn, S. C., Pangburn, S. H. Weinstein, D. B., and Steinberg, D. (1979): Very low density lipoprotein synthesis and secretion by cultured rat hepatocytes. *J. Biol. Chem.,* 254:2010–2016.

47. Chan, L., Jackson, R. L., O'Malley, B. W. and Means, A. R. (1976): Synthesis of very low density lipoproteins in the cockerel. Effects of estrogen. *J. Clin. Invest.,* 58:368–379.

48. Chan, L., Snow, L. D., Jackson, R. L., and Means, A. R. (1979): Hormonal regulation of lipoprotein synthesis in the cockerel. In: *Ontogeny of Receptors and Reproductive Hormone Action,* edited by T. H. Hamilton, J. H. Clark, and W. A. Sadler, pp. 331–351. Raven Press, New York.

49. Blobel, G., and Dobberstein, B. (1975): Transfer of proteins across membranes. Presence of proteolytically processed and unprocessed nascent immunoglobulin light chain on membrane-bound ribosomes of murine myeloma. *J. Cell Biol.,* 67:835.

50. Illingworth, D. R. (1975): Metabolism of lipoproteins in nonhuman primates. Studies on the origin of low density lipoprotein apoprotein in the plasma of the squirrel monkey. *Biochim. Biophys. Acta,* 388:38–51.

51. Nayaka, N., Chung, B. K., Patsch, J. R., and Taunton, D. O. (1977): Synthesis and release of low density lipoproteins by the isolated perfused pig liver. *J. Biol. Chem.,* 252:7530–7533.

52. Swift, L. L., Manowitz, N. R., Dunn, G. D., and LeQuire, V. S. (1980): Isolation and characterization of hepatic Golgi lipoproteins from hypercholesterolemic rats. *J. Clin. Invest.,* 66:415–425.

53. Nicoli, A., Miller, N. E., and Lewis, B. (1980): High density lipoprotein metabolism. *Adv. Lipid Res.,* 17:53–106.

54. Glomset, J. A. (1968): The plasma lecithin: cholesterol acyltransferase reaction. *J. Lipid Res.* 9:155–167.

55. Hamilton, R. L., Williams, M. C., Fielding, C. J., and Havel, R. J. (1976): Discoidal bilayer structure of nascent high density lipoproteins from perfused rat liver. *J. Clin. Invest.,* 58:667–680.

56. Green, P. H. R., Tall, A. R., and Glickman, R. M. (1978): Rat intestine secretes discoid high density lipoprotein. *J. Clin. Invest.,* 61:528–534.

57. Glickman, R. M., and Green, P. H. R. (1977): The intestine as a source of apolipoprotein A-I. *Proc. Natl. Acad. Sci. USA,* 74:2569–2573.

58. Marsh, J. B. (1976): Apoproteins of the lipoproteins in a non-recirculating perfusate of rat liver. *J. Lipid. Res.,* 17:85–90.

59. Marsh, J. B., and Sparks, C. E. (1979): Hepatic secretion of lipoproteins in the rat and the effect of experimental nephrosis. *J. Clin. Invest.,* 64:1229–1237.

60. Mahley, R. W., Bersot, T. P., Levy, R. K., Windmueller, H. G., and LeQuire, V. S. (1970): Identity of lipoprotein apoproteins of plasma and liver Golgi apparatus in the rat. *Fed. Proc. (Abstr.),* 29:629.

61. Hamilton, R. L. (1972): Synthesis and secretion of plasma lipoproteins. Pharmacologic control of lipid metabolism. *Adv. Exp. Med. Biol.,* 26:7–24.

62. Sabesin, S. M. (1979): Role of the liver and intestine in lipoprotein metabolism. *Viewpoints Dig. Dis.,* II (5)(*Suppl.*).

63. Sabesin, S. M., Ragland, J. B., and Freeman, M. R. (1979): Lipoprotein disturbances in liver disease. In: *Progress in Liver Diseases, Vol. VI,* edited by H. Popper and F. Schaffner, pp. 243–262. Grune & Stratton, New York.

64. Sabesin, S. M., Bertram, P. D., and Freeman, M. R. (1980): Lipoprotein metabolism in liver disease. In: *Advances in*

Internal Medicine, Vol. 25, edited by G. H. Stollerman, pp. 117–141. Year Book, New York.

65. Redgrave, T. C. (1970): Formation of cholesterol ester-rich particulate lipid during metabolism of chylomicrons. *J. Clin. Invest.,* 49:465–471.

66. Mjos, O. D., Faergeman, O., Hamilton, R. L., and Havel, R. J. (1974): Characterization of remnants of lymph chylomicrons and lymph and plasma very low density lipoproteins in "supradiaphragmatic" rats. *Eur. J. Clin. Invest.,* 4:382–383.

67. Fielding, C. J., and Havel, R. J. (1977): Lipoprotein lipase. *Arch. Pathol. Lab. Med.,* 101:225–299.

68. Cooper, A. D. (1977): The metabolism of chylomicron remnants by isolated perfused rat liver. *Biochim. Biophys. Acta,* 488:464–474.

69. Cooper, A. D., and Yu, P. Y. S. (1978): Rates of removal and degradation of chylomicron remnants by isolated perfused rat liver. *J. Lipid Res.,* 19:635–643.

70. Carrella, M., and Cooper, A. D. (1979): High affinity binding of chylomicron remnants to rat liver plasma membranes. *Proc. Natl. Acad. Sci. USA,* 76:338–342.

71. Sherrill, B. C., and Dietschy, J. M. (1977): Characterization of the sinusoidal transport process responsible for uptake of chylomicrons by the liver. *J. Biol. Chem.,* 253:1859–1867.

72. Shelburne, F., Hanks, J., Meyers, W., and Quarfordt, S. (1980): Effect of apoproteins on hepatic uptake of triglyceride emulsions in the rat. *J. Clin. Invest.,* 65:652–658.

73. Windler, E. E., Chao, Y. S., and Havel, R. J. (1980): Determinants of hepatic uptake of triglyceride-rich lipoproteins and their remnants in the rat. *J. Biol. Chem.,* 255:5475–5478.

74. Sherrill, B. C., Innerarity, T. L., and Mahley, R.W. (1980): Rapid hepatic clearance of the canine lipoproteins containing only the E apoproteins by a high affinity receptor. *J. Biol. Chem.,* 255:1804–1807.

75. Windler, E. E., Kovanen, P. T., Chao, Y. S., Brown, M. S., Havel, R. J., and Goldstein, J. L. (1980): The estradiol-stimulated lipoprotein receptor of rat liver. *J. Biol. Chem.,* 255:10464–10471.

76. Havel, R. J., Chao, Y. S., Windler, E. E., Kotite, L., and Guo, L. S. S. (1980): Isoprotein specificity in the hepatic uptake of apolipoprotein E and the pathogenesis of familial dysbetalipoproteinemia. *Proc. Natl. Acad. Sci. USA,* 77:4349–4353.

77. Cooper, A. D. (1976): The regulation of 3-hydroxy-3-methylglutaryl coenzyme A reductase in the isolated perfused rat liver. *J. Clin. Invest.,* 57:1461–1470.

78. Brown, M. S., and Goldstein, J. L. (1976): Receptor mediated control of cholesterol metabolism. *Science,* 191:150–154.

79. Brown, M. S., Kovanen, P. T., and Goldstein, J. L. (1981): Regulation of plasma cholesterol by lipoprotein receptors. *Science,* 212:628–635.

80. Kovanen, P. T., Brown, M. S., and Goldstein, J. L. (1979): Increased binding of low density lipoprotein to liver membranes from rats treated with 17 α-ethinyl estradiol. *J. Biol Chem.,* 254:11367–11373.

81. Roheim, P. S., Rachmilewitz, D., Stein, O., and Stein, Y. (1971): Metabolism of iodinated high density lipoproteins in the rat. *Biochim. Biophys. Acta,* 248:315–329.

82. Rachmilewitz, D., Stein, O., Roheim, P. S., and Stein, Y. (1972): Metabolism of iodinated high density lipoproteins in the rat: Autoradiographic localization in the liver. *Biochim. Biophys. Acta,* 270:414–425.

83. Nakai, T., and Whayne, T. F., Jr. (1976): Catabolism of canine apolipoprotein A-I: Purification, catabolic rate, organs of catabolism, and the liver subcellular catabolic site. *J. Lab. Clin. Med.,* 88:6380.

84. VanBerkel, T. J., Koster, J. F., and Hulsmann, W. C. (1977): High density lipoprotein and low density lipoprotein catabolism by human liver and parenchymal and non-parenchymal cells from rat liver. *Biochim. Biophys. Acta,* 486:586–589.

85. Stein, Y., Ebin, V., Bar-On, H., and Stein, O. (1977): Chloroquin-induced interference with degradation of serum lipoproteins in rat liver studied in vivo and in vitro. *Biochim. Biophys. Acta,* 486:286–297.

86. Mahley, R. W., Innerarity, T. L., Pitas, R. E., Weisgraber,

K. H., Browen, J. H., and Gross, E. (1977): Inhibition of lipoprotein binding to cell surface receptors of fibroblasts following selective modification of arginyl residues in arginine-rich and B apoproteins. *J. Biol. Chem.,* 252:7279–7287.

87. Windmueller, H. G. (1964): An orotic acid-induced, adenine-reversed inhibition of hepatic lipoprotein secretion in the rat. *J. Biol. Chem.,* 239:530.

88. Sabesin, S. M., Frase, S., and Ragland, J. B. (1977): Accumulation of nascent lipoproteins in rat hepatic Golgi during induction of fatty liver by orotic acid. *Lab. Invest.,* 37:127–135.

89. Koff, R., Gordon, G., and Sabesin, S. M. (1971): D-Galactosamine hepatitis. I. Hepatocellular injury and fatty liver following a single dose. *Proc. Soc. Exp. Biol. Med.,* 137:696.

90. Koff, R., Fitts, J. J., and Sabesin, S. M. (1971): D-Galactosamine hepatotoxicity. II. Mechanism of fatty liver production. *Proc. Soc. Exp. Biol. Med.,* 138:89.

91. Sabesin, S. M., Kuiken, L. B., and Ragland, J. B. (1975): Lipoprotein and lecithin:cholesterol acyltransferase changes in galactosamine-induced rat liver injury. *Science,* 190:1302–1304.

92. Sabesin, S. M., Kuiken, L. B., and Ragland, J. B. (1975): Lipoprotein abnormalities in galactosamine hepatitis: A model of experimental lecithin:cholesterol acyltransferase deficiency. *Scand. J. Clin. Lab. Invest.,* 38:187–193.

93. Lombardi, B. (1966): Considerations on the pathogenesis of fatty liver. *Lab. Invest.,* 15:1.

94. Baraona, E., and Lieber, C. S. (1979): Effects of ethanol on lipid metabolism. *J. Lipid Res.,* 20:289–315.

95. Novikoff, P. M., Roheim, P. S., Novikoff, A. B., and Edelstein, B. S. (1974): Production and prevention of fatty liver in rats fed clofibrate and orotic acid diets containing sucrose. *Lab. Invest.,* 30:732.

96. Novikoff, P. M., and Edelstein, D. (1977): Reversal of orotic acid-induced fatty liver in fats by clofibrate. *Lab. Invest.,* 36:215–231.

97. Rajalakshmi, S., Adams, W. R., and Handschumacher, R. E. (1969): Isolation and characterization of low density structures from orotic acid-induced fatty livers. *J. Cell Biol.,* 41:625–636.

98. Pottenger, L. A., Frazier, L. E., DuBien, H. L., Getz, G. S., and Wissler, R. W. (1973): Carbohydrate composition of lipoprotein apoproteins isolated from rat plasma and from livers of rats fed orotic acid. *Biochim. Biophys. Res. Commun.,* 54:770.

99. Pottenger, L. A., and Getz, G. S. (1971): Serum lipoprotein accumulation in the liver of orotic acid-fed rats. *J. Lipid Res.,* 12:450.

100. Marchetti, M., Puddu, P., and Caldarera, C. M. (1964): Metabolic aspects of orotic acid fatty liver: Nucleotide control mechanisms of lipid metabolism. *Biochem. J.,* 92:46.

101. Wetmore, S., Mahley, R. W., Brown, W. V., and Schachter, H. (1974): Incorporation of sialic acid into sialidase-treated apolipoprotein of human, very low density lipoprotein by pork liver sialyltransferase. *Can. J. Biochem.,* 52:655.

102. Decker, K., and Keppler, D. (1974): Galactosamine hepatitis: Key role of the nucleotide deficiency period in the pathogenesis of cell injury and cell death. *Rev. Physiol. Biochem. Pharmacol.,* 71:78–106.

103. Decker, K., Keppler, D., Rudigier, J., and Domischke, W. (1971): Cell damage by trapping of biosynthetic intermediates. The role of uracil nucleotides in experimental hepatitis. *Hoppe Seylers Z. Physiol. Chem.,* 352:412–418.

104. Keppler, D., Rudigier, J., Bischoff, E., and Decker, K. (1970): The trapping of uridine phosphates by D-galactosamine, D-glucosamine and 2-deoxy-d-galactose. A study on the mechanism of galactosamine hepatitis. *Eur. J. Biochem.,* 17:246–253.

105. Sabesin, S. M., and Koff, R. S. (1976): D-Galactosamine hepatotoxicity IV. Further studies of the pathogenesis of fatty liver. *Exp. Mol. Pathol.* 24:424–434.

106. Shiff, T. S., Roheim, P. S., and Eder, H. A. (1971): Effects of high sucrose diets and 4-aminopyrazolopyrimidine on serum lipids and lipoproteins in the rat. *J. Lipid Res.,* 12:596–603.

107. Freeman, M. R., Frase, S., and Sabesin, S. M. (1978): Hepatocyte Golgi alterations in the selective inhibition of very

low density lipoprotein secretion produced by 4-aminopyrazolopyrimidine. *Gastroenterology*, 74:1036 (*Abstr.*).

108. Mahley, R. W. (1978): Alterations in plasma lipoproteins induced by cholesterol feeding in animals including man. In: *Disturbances in Lipid and Lipoprotein Metabolism*, edited by J. M. Dietschy, A. M. Gotto, Jr., and J. A. Ontko, pp. 181–197. American Physiological Society, Washington, D.C.

109. Ross, A. C., and Zilversmit, D. B. (1977): Chylomicron remnant cholesteryl esters as the major constituent of very low density lipoproteins in plasma of cholesterol fed rabbits. *J. Lipid Res.*, 18:169–181.

110. Roheim, P. S., Haft, D. E., Gidez, L. I., White, A., and Eder, H. A. (1963): Plasma lipoprotein metabolism in perfused rat livers. II. Transfer of free and esterified cholesterol into the plasma. *J. Clin. Invest.*, 42:1277–1285.

111. Frnka, J., and Resier, R. (1974). The effects of diet cholesterol on the synthesis of rat serum apolipoproteins. *Biochim. Biophys. Acta*, 360:322–338.

112. Roth, R. I., and Patsch, J. R.(1978): Metabolism of the "arginine-rich" protein in the rabbit. *Fed. Proc.*, 37:1322.

113. Noel, S. P., Wong, L., Dolphin, P. J., Dory, L., and Rubinstein, D. (1979): Secretion of cholesterol-rich lipoproteins by perfused livers of hypercholesterolemic rats. *J. Clin Invest.*, 64:674–683.

114. Turner, K. B., McCormach, G. H., Jr., and Richards, A. (1953): The cholesterol esterifying enzyme of human serum. I. In liver disease. *J. Clin. Invest.*, 32:801–806.

115. Sabesin, S. M., Hawkins, H. L., Kuiken, L., and Ragland, J. B. (1977): Abnormal plasma lipoproteins and lecithin: cholesterol acyltransferase deficiency in alcoholic liver disease. *Gastroenterology*, 72:510–518.

116. Wengeler, H., Greten, H., and Seidel, D. (1972): Serum cholesterol esterification in liver disease. Combined determinations of lecthin: cholesterol acyltransferase and lipoprotein-X. *Eur. J. Clin. Invest.*, 2:372–378.

117. Calandra, S., Martin, M. J., and McIntyre, N. (1971): Plasma lecithin:cholesterol acyltransferase activity in liver disease. *Eur. J. Clin. Invest.*, 1:352–360.

118. Simon, J. B., and Scheig, R. (1970): Serum cholesterol esterification in liver disease. Importance of lecithin:cholesterol acyltransferase. *N. Engl. J. Med.*, 283:841–846.

119. Gjone, E., and Blomhoff, I. P. (1970): Plasma lecithin:cholesteryl acyltransferase in obstructive jaundice. *Scand. J. Gastroenterol.*, 5:305–308.

120. Gjone, E., Blomhoff, I. P., and Wienecke, I. (1971): Plasma lecithin:cholesterol acyltransferase activity in acute hepatitis. *Scand. J. Gastroenterol.*, 6:161–168.

121. Gjone, E., and Norum, K. R. (1970): Plasma lecithin:cholesterol acyltransferase and erythrocyte lipids in liver disease. *Acta Med. Scand.*, 187:153–161.

122. Ritland, S., Blomhoff, J. P., and Gjone, E. (1973): Lecithin:cholesterol acyltransferase and lipoprotein-X in liver disease. *Clin. Chim. Acta*, 49:251–259.

123. Blomhoff, J. P., Skrede, S., and Ritland, S. (1974): Lecithin:cholesterol acyltransferase and plasma proteins in liver disease. *Clin. Chim. Acta*, 53:197–207.

124. Simon, J. B., Kepkay, D. L., and Poon, R. (1974): Serum cholesterol esterification in human liver disease: Role of lecithin:cholesterol acyltransferase and cholesterol ester hydrolase. *Gastroenterology*, 66:539–547.

125. Stokke, K. T. (1972): The existence of an acid cholesterol esterase in human liver. *Biochim. Biophys. Acta*, 270:156–166.

126. Jones, D. P., Sosa, F. R., Shartsis, J., Shah, P. T., Shromack, E., and Beher, W. T. (1971): Serum cholesterol esterifying and cholesterol ester hydrolyzing activity in liver diseases: Relationships to cholesterol, bilirubin, and bile salt concentration. *J. Clin. Invest.*, 50:259–265.

127. Simon, J. B. (1974): Lecithin:cholesterol acyltransferase in human liver disease. *Scand. J. Clin. Lab. Invest.*, 33(137):107–113.

128. Fex, G., and Wallinder, L. (1970): Decreased esterification of (^{3}H) cholesterol by serum from partially hepatectomized rats in vitro. *Biochim. Biophys. Acta*, 210:341–343.

129. Lossow, W. J., Shah, S. N., Brot, N., and Chaikoff, I. L. (1963): Effect of ethionine treatment on esterification in vitro of free (4-^{14}C) cholesterol by rat plasma. *Biochim. Biophys. Acta*, 70:593–595.

130. Sugano, M., Hori, K., and Wada, M. (1969): Hepatotoxicity and plasma cholesterol esterification by rats. *Arch. Biochim. Biophys.*, 129:588-596.

131. Ragland, J. B., Heppner, C., and Sabesin, S. M. (1978): The role of lecithin:cholesterol acyltransferase deficiency in the apoprotein metabolism of alcoholic hepatitis. *Scand. J. Clin. Lab. Invest.* [Suppl. 150], 38:208–213.

132. Ragland, J. B., Bertram, P. D., and Sabesin, S. M. (1978): Identification of nascent high density lipoproteins containing arginine-rich protein in human plasma. *Biochim. Biophys. Res. Commun.*, 80:81–88.

133. Sabesin, S. M., Hawkins, H. L., Bertram, P. D., Mann, J. A. and Peace, R. J. (1978): Alcoholic hepatitis. *Gastroenterology*, 74:276–286.

134. Switzer, S. (1967): Plasma lipoproteins in liver disease. I. Immunologically distinct low density lipoproteins in patients with biliary obstruction. *J. Clin. Invest.*, 46:1855–1866.

135. Seidel, D., Alaupovic, P., and Furman, R. H. (1969): A lipoprotein characterizing obstructive jaundice. I. Method for qualitative separation and identification of lipoproteins in jaundiced subjects. *J. Clin. Invest.* 48:1211–1223.

136. Magnani, H. N. (1976): The influence of Lp-X and other lipoproteins associated with hepatic dysfunction of the activity of lecithin:cholesterol acyltransferase. *Biochim. Biophys. Acta*, 450:390–401.

137. Ritland, S., and Gjone, E. (1975): Quantitative studies of lipoprotein-X in familial lecithin:cholesterol acyltransferase deficiency and during cholesterol esterification. *Clin. Chim. Acta*, 59:109–119.

138. Seidel, D., Alaupovic, P., Furman, R. H., and McConathy, W. J. (1970): A lipoprotein characterizing obstructive jaundice. II. Isolation and partial characterization of the protein moieties of low density lipoproteins. *J. Clin. Invest.*, 49:2396–2407.

139. Hamilton, R. L., Havel, R. J., Kane, J. P., Blaurock, S. E., and Sata, T. (1971): Cholestasis: Lamellar structure of the abnormal human serum lipoprotein. *Science*, 172:475–478.

140. Gjone, E., Javitt, N. B., Blomhoff, J. P., and Fausa, O. (1973): Studies of lipoprotein-X (Lp-X) and bile acids in familial LCAT deficiency. *Acta Med. Scand.*, 194:377–378.

141. Manzato, E., Fellin, R., Baggio, G., Walch, S., Neubeck, W., and Seiden, D. (1976): Formation of lipoprotein-X. Its relationship to bile compounds. *J. Clin. Invest.*, 57:1248–1260.

The Liver: Biology and Pathobiology, edited by
I. Arias, H. Popper, D. Schachter, and D. A. Shafritz.
Raven Press, New York © 1982.

Chapter 9

Intracellular Organelles and Lipoprotein Metabolism in Normal and Fatty Livers

Phyllis Marie Novikoff

One of the prominent functions of the hepatocytes, which are the main cell type found in mammalian liver, is the metabolism of lipids and lipoproteins. The hepatocyte is a polarized cell with extensive surfaces exposed to the spaces of Disse, where lipid interchanges with plasma occur. Free fatty acids and glycerol are removed by the hepatocytes and are combined within the hepatocytes to form triacylglycerols (TG). The release of lipids from the hepatocytes to the plasma occurs after TG, along with cholesterol and phospholipids, have combined with proteins and carbohydrate moieties to form lipoglycoproteins (LP). LP are found in blood plasma and lymph and serve in the transport of lipids. In addition to the hepatocytes, the absorptive cells of the small intestine participate in the metabolism of lipids and LP.

This chapter focuses on the intracellular organelles involved in lipid and LP metabolism in normal rat hepatocytes and the modulation of these organelles in hepatocytes from a variety of experimentally induced fatty livers. The essence of modulation is the capacity of an organism to change or adapt to new or altered circumstances. Modulations that occur in hepatocytes center primarily on changes in organelle structure and how these structural changes can be correlated with altered functions. Paralleling these changes are a myriad of other changes, such as those in enzyme activities (see ref. 1 for a review of enzymes involved in lipid metabolism). This topic and the biochemical and biophysical properties of the blood and lymph LP and the properties of plasma membranes and other cytomembranes are outside the scope of this chapter. (For a review of plasma LP, see ref. 2 and chapter by Glickman and Sabesin; for a review of membranes, see ref. 3 and chapter by Dallner.)

ORGANELLES AND LIPOPROTEIN METABOLISM

Some general comments on the structure and participation of organelles in lipid and LP metabolism are briefly presented. The organelles presently known to be involved in lipid and LP metabolism are the plasma membrane and its modification, microvilli, endoplasmic reticulum (ER), Golgi apparatus, GERL, lysosomes, peroxisomes (including microperoxisomes), mitochondria, and storage or "cytosolic"[1] lipid spheres.

---

[1] The nature of what constitutes cytosol (hyaloplasm, ground substance, cell matrix, or cell sap) is presently undergoing investigation. Is it composed of soluble and structureless components, or is it a highly organized and complex structural entity (cytoskeleton), or a combination of both? (See refs. 4 and 5 for discussions.)

Plasma Membrane

The plasma membranes of the apical surfaces of the hepatocyte have numerous microvilli which project into the spaces of Disse. This specialization of the plasma membrane greatly amplifies the surface area of the hepatocyte. It is at these apical surfaces that lipids, after being hydrolyzed to free fatty acids and glycerol by the activity of lipases, enter the hepatocytes. The mechanism (or mechanisms) of how these molecular forms permeate the apical plasma membranes is unknown. It is also at these apical surfaces that lipid exits the hepatocyte as LP particles after undergoing numerous modifications within the intracellular compartments of the hepatocyte. The lateral plasma membranes lack microvilli; however, it has not been determined if lipids enter the hepatocytes along the lateral plasma membranes. Microvilli are present on plasma membranes that face the bile canalicular and function in the secretion of bile.

Endoplasmic Reticulum

The ER, an extensive membraneous system that courses through the cytoplasm, is composed of flattened cisternal elements, often in parallel arrays or configurations, and anastomosing tubules. In 1945, Porter et al. (6), after examining cultured fibroblast cells with the electron microscope, were the first to describe and name this organelle. The earliest descriptions of the ER in hepatocytes were those of Dalton et al. (7), Bernhard et al. (8), and Fawcett (9). The rough ER, studded with ribosomes, many in the form of polysomes (10), and the smooth ER comprise one interconnected system. Enzymes synthesizing TG and phospholipids are considered to be located within the rough ER, whereas cholesterol synthesis is thought to be a function of the smooth ER. Some of these enzymes are located within the membrane of the ER, while others are found within the cisternal space (11).

The synthesis of the apoproteins of the LP and the partial glycosylation of the LP is a function of the ER. The linking of the proteins and carbohydrate moieties to the lipid components to form the LP particles that are ultimately secreted also occurs in the ER. It is not known, however, whether this takes place in the rough or the smooth ER. The ER also functions in transporting lipids and LP to other parts of the hepatocytes, where they can be stored as cytosolic lipid spheres, packaged for secretion by the Golgi apparatus, and degraded by GERL and lysosomes.

Storage Lipid Spheres

Relatively few lipid spheres accumulate within the cytoplasm in untreated hepatocytes. These structures are generally spherical in shape, are not bounded by a tripartite membrane, and vary in size from 0.5 to 2.0 μm in diameter. When present, they are usually located near the sinusoidal aspect of the hepatocyte. In untreated hepatocytes, they are composed predominantly of TG. They also contain cholesterol, phospholipids, protein, and carbohydrates (12). These spheres are stainable by lipid stains (Oil red O, Sudan black B) and are often referred to as lipids, even though they may contain proteins and carbohydrates. The appearance of these lipid spheres in the electron microscope varies with fixation and other preparative procedures. They can appear electron opaque or electron lucent. With our procedures, the lipid spheres and also the lipoprotein particles are generally electron lucent, with an electron-opaque limit that appears as a fine line; this fine line is not a membrane.

Intimately associated with the surface of the lipid spheres are cisternae of smooth ER. The extent of the surface that is encased by smooth ER probably reflects the physiologic state of the hepatocyte. Since the ER is involved in lipid metabolism, this intimate relationship of the ER to the spheres probably has functional significance. Other organelles closely associated with the spheres are the mitochondria and peroxisomes.

Golgi Apparatus

The Golgi apparatus consists of four to five smooth membrane-enclosed cisternae or elements. The elements are parallel to each other, separated by a relatively constant distance of about 20 nm. They are kept in a relatively fixed position by unknown mechanisms. The apparatus is an extensive organelle which undulates and twists through much of the cytoplasm. Its three-dimensional appearance is difficult to appreciate in ultrathin sections, where only portions of the elements are seen; this portion is referred to as a Golgi stack. Because of the plane of sectioning, the Golgi stacks may appear as several separate units; in reality, however, they are continuous and form one Golgi apparatus. Often, the stacks exhibit a curved or crescent shape, resulting in a concavity on one aspect and a convexity on the other.

Several descriptive terms in the literature refer to this observed morphologic polarity. Ehrenreich et al. (13) introduced the term *cis* to refer to the outer, convex, or forming aspect, and *trans* to refer to the inner, concave, or maturing aspect. This morphologic polarity of the Golgi apparatus may be a reflection of its functions, the *cis* aspect receiving materials from the ER, and the *trans* aspect producing secretory vacuoles.

In hepatocytes, the nascent LP particles, which are incompletely glycosylated, are transported by the ER to the *cis* aspect of the Golgi apparatus within ER-derived, smooth-surfaced vesicles or cisternae, often referred to as transitional vesicles. Direct continuities of the ER with the *cis* face of the Golgi apparatus have not been found. The lipoprotein particles within these transitional vesicles are large enough to be visible by electron microscopic procedures. These particles, called liposomes, measure approximately 40 nm. They become incorporated into the elements of the Golgi apparatus, in which they undergo additional glycosylation and possibly other modifications, forming a class of LP particles known as very low density lipoprotein (VLDL) particles.

Vacuoles containing the VLDL particles emerge from the elements and transport the VLDL for ultimate secretion. Which elements and where in the elements these Golgi-derived vacuoles originate has not been determined. Each element shows LP particles within dilations; the extent of the dilations within the elements varies with the physiologic state of the hepatocyte. Images showing lateral dilations of the elements and vacuoles at the *trans* face of the Golgi apparatus suggest that these are the sites of origin of the VLDL-containing vacuoles. Because of the twisting nature of the apparatus, the *cis* and *trans* aspects may be difficult to distinguish by morphologic criteria alone; by combining cytochemistry with morphology, this difficulty can be overcome. The most *cis* element can be identified by a prolonged staining with osmium. Only this element shows a deposition with the reduced osmium (14). The most *trans* element possesses the enzymes nucleoside diphosphatase and thiamine pyrophosphatase (15). Only this element is visualized using a lead capture method in which either inosine, uridine, quanidine diphosphate, or thiamine pyrophosphate acts as substrate (16,17). The intervening elements in the Golgi stack do not display the osmium-reducing property or the enzyme activities. The elements of the Golgi apparatus in hepatocytes and in many other cell types display this specificity of staining.

Biochemical analysis of fractions considered enriched in the Golgi apparatus show an association of several glycosyl transferases involved in glycoprotein synthesis (18). Morphologic assessment of these fractions shows other membraneous structures, including GERL, as well as recognizable Golgi stacks. The precise localizations of the transferases in intact hepatocytes and isolated fractions await the development of an *in situ* method.

GERL and Related Lysosomes

GERL is a hydrolase-rich region of smooth ER, initially described in the small neurons of the rat dorsal root ganglia (19). (Direct continuities with the ribosome-studded ER and the cytochemical demonstration of several hydrolases have established this organelle as a specialized area of the ER.) This region of smooth ER is generally but not exclusively found spatially related to the *trans* element of the Golgi apparatus. Although morphologic continuities between the *trans* element and GERL have not been demonstrated, this does not rule out possible functional relationships between these structures. In rat hepatocytes, GERL consists of interconnected cisternae and tubules, including flattened tubules referred to as rigid lamellae (20). LP particles and a finely granular material are present within GERL. Often a clear zone, or "halo," about 10 nm wide is evident between its contents and the delimiting membrane.

The delimiting membrane of portions of GERL appear thicker than other areas of ER and may exhibit spikes or coated regions on its exoplasmic surface. A variety of lysosomes (residual bodies, coated vesicles, and autophagic vacuoles) arise from this structure. Residual bodies, containing LP particles and particulate matter of a heterogeneous nature, probably arise from dilations of the cisternal portions of GERL; they frequently possess a "halo" beneath its membrane. Coated vesicles probably derive from the coated areas of GERL. In hepatocytes, the hydrolase-rich nature of GERL, residual bodies, autophagic vacuoles, and coated vesicles has been demonstrated *in situ* and in homogenates with a cytochemical procedure which showed the presence of one acid hydrolase, namely, acid phosphatase. Presumably other hydrolases, including lipases, are present in GERL and its derivatives. The hydrolases aryl sulfatase and E600-resistant esterase have been cytochemically demonstrated in other cell types (21–23). (For an extensive discussion of the history, origins, diversity of forms and functions of lysosomes, and the contributions of biochemistry and cytochemistry, see refs. 24–26 and Chapter 2.

The presence of LP particles of various sizes (20 to 40 nm), shapes, and densities in the acid hydrolase milieu of GERL and residual bodies suggests that these particles may undergo partial or complete catabolism. The origins and biochemical composition of the LP particles within GERL and the functions of GERL in LP metabolism are under study. The involvement of this organelle in lipid and LP metabolism is discussed in subsequent sections in this chapter.

Peroxisomes and Microperoxisomes

Peroxisomes were defined biochemically by de Duve and Baudhuin in 1966 (27) as cytoplasmic particles that contain both catalase, a H_2O_2-destroying enzyme, and at least one H_2O_2-generating enzyme. In rat hepatocytes, peroxisomes are approximately 0.5 μm, are membrane delimited, show a granular appearance in their matrix, and contain a crystalline core or nucleoid, which is believed to be urate oxidase. Broad continuities between the membrane of the ER and the membrane of the peroxisomes have been frequently observed in rat hepatocytes (28–30).

These observations suggest that peroxisomes arise as dilations or expansions of the ER. Peroxisomes from rat liver have been isolated and shown to contain fatty acid oxidases and ligases, thus suggesting their possible role in the β-oxidation of fatty acids and in the biosynthesis of lipids (31–33). In hepatocytes from untreated rat livers and from rat livers with experimentally induced lipid deposition or removal, peroxisomes are intimately associated with the surfaces of the cytosolic or storage lipid spheres (34–35). This close spatial relationship, in conjunction with the presence of lipid-metabolizing enzymes, supports their role in lipid metabolism.

The term microperoxisome was introduced by Novikoff and Novikoff in 1972 (36) to distinguish these structures from the peroxisomes of rat liver and kidney. Microperoxisomes are membrane-delimited particles, smaller in size (their diameters range from 0.15 to 0.25 μm), lack nucleoids, often appear in clusters, and have numerous slender continuities with the ER. Elongate forms of these structures are commonly encountered. They arise as dilations of the ER and retain some continuity with it. Microperoxisomes are considered to be the progenitors of rat hepatocyte peroxisomes. Like the peroxisomes, they contain catalase and are spatially related to lipid spheres. Microperoxisomes are numerous in cell types engaged in lipid metabolism, e.g., epithelial cells of the small intestine (36), interstitial cells of the testis (37), adrenocortical cells (38), and cultured 3T3L-1 preadipocyte cells (39) (for a listing of other cell types, see refs. 40 and 41).

Peroxisomes can be easily identified morphologically by the presence of a nucleoid. To aid in the identification of microperoxisomes, the enzyme catalase can be cytochemically demonstrated. Modifications of a diaminobenzidine procedure, originally introduced by Graham and Karnovsky (42) to stain exogenously injected horseradish peroxidase (HRP), permit the identity of these structures with certainty at both the light and electron microscope level (43,44).

Rat hepatocyte peroxisomes have been shown to increase in size and number with the administration of hypolipidemic drugs (45–47). Clofibrate (CPIB, ethyl-p-cholorphenoxyisobutyrate) and nafenopin (2-methyl-2 [p-(1,2,3,4 tetrahydro-1-naphthyl)phenoxy]-propionic acid) are among the drugs that have been commonly employed as peroxisomal proliferators. Concomitant with the increase in numbers of peroxisomes is an increase in enzyme catalase synthesis (48,49).

Mitochondria

In 1949, Kennedy and Lehningner (50) showed in studies of rat liver that oxidation of fatty acids occurs in mitochondria, and that adenosine triphosphate (ATP) is required to enzymatically activate the oxidation of fatty acids. In 1952, Palade (51) observed in the pancreas the close proximity of mitochondria to the surface of storage lipid spheres and related this structural apposition to their functional role in lipid metabolism. In hepatocytes and other cell types that contain storage lipid spheres, mitochondria are always intimately associated with the surfaces of the lipid spheres. This structural association probably correlates with their functional relationship in lipid metabolism.

An important phenomenon was described by Hackenbrock et al. (52) regarding mitochondria in intact and isolated hepatocytes from rat liver. The ultrastructural appearance of mitochondria in the presence or absence of adenosine diphosphate (ADP) (i.e., when phosphorylation and respiration were or were not occurring) showed two different configurations, either orthodox or condensed. In the condensed configuration, the matrix is more electron dense, and the spaces within the cristae are enlarged when compared to the orthodox configuration. These conformational changes may be important in the formation of ATP. The relationship of these changes to lipid metabolism remains to be explored.

OVERVIEW OF MORPHOLOGIC EVENTS IN LIPOPROTEIN METABOLISM

Figure 1 is a schematic representation of the morphologic sequence of events in the uptake, transport, secretion, storage, and degradation of lipids and lipoproteins in normal hepatocytes and in hepatocytes in which the sequence has been experimentally altered. Numerous investigators have contributed to the understanding of the structure-function interrelationships of the organelles involved in lipid and lipoprotein metabolism (for a partial list, see ref. 35).

There is considerable agreement on the following events in normal rat hepatocytes. Hepatocytes can make lipids *de novo* from carbohydrates and other substances. They can absorb lipids from the circulation, which enter hepatocytes at the space of Disse in the form of free fatty acids and glycerol. The fatty acids and glycerol traverse the plasma membrane and the membrane of the ER, which are in close proximity to each other (Fig. 1.1), and are reesterified to TG within the ER (Fig. 1.2). The ER contains enzymes for reesterification and synthesis of other lipids.

Processing of lipids continues in the ER with the addition of specific proteins (apoproteins) and carbo-

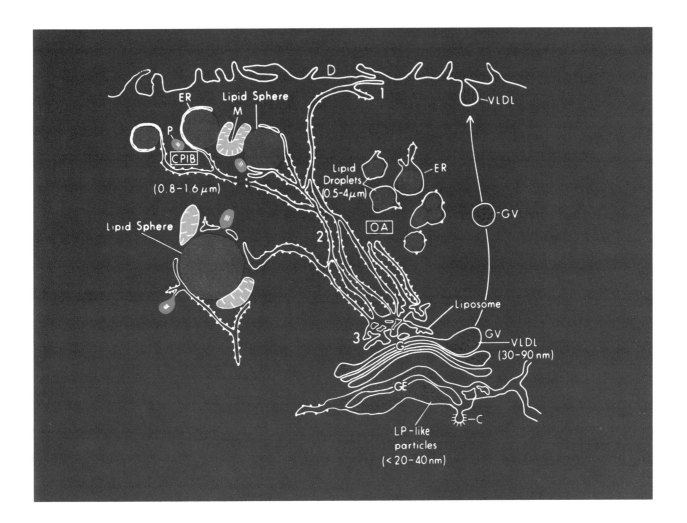

FIG. 1. Schematic representation of the organelles involved in various aspects of lipid and lipoprotein metabolism in rat hepatocytes. The sequence of morphologic events in the uptake, transport, secretion, storage, and degradation of lipids and lipoproteins is illustrated. The structural changes in the ER induced with OA, that is, vesiculation, and by CPIB, that is, proliferation of smooth ER, and the relationship of the ER to lipid deposition are also illustrated. See text for details. Lipid spheres, lipid droplets, liposomes, and lipoprotein particles (LP) are colored red; peroxisomes (P), green; mitochondria (M), yellow. The membranes of the ER (including ribosomes), of the Golgi apparatus (G) and Golgi-derived vacuoles (GV), and of GERL (GE) are white. The constellation of organelles, that is, the relationship of the ER, P, and M to the surface of the cytosolic lipid spheres, is shown for normal rat hepatocytes (*lower left*) and for hepatocytes from CPIB-treated rats (*upper left*). Within the elements of the Golgi apparatus and GV are the VLDL particles ranging in size from 30 to 90 nm. Within the cisternae of GE are LP-like particles ranging in size from 20 to 40 nm. One type of lysosome, a coated vesicle, is shown forming from GE.

hydrate moieties (mannose and glucosamine), forming nascent LP complexes. These complexes, which are not visible by electron microscopic procedures, may follow several pathways; one results in secretion, one in degradation, and one in storage.

The complexes that enter the secretory pathway are transported within transitional vesicles or cisternae derived from the ER (Fig. 1.3) to the *cis* aspect of the Golgi apparatus. The complexes within the transitional structures are visible by electron microscopic procedures and are called liposomes. The isolation and biochemical characterization of liposomes have not been achieved. These liposomes enter the elements of the Golgi apparatus, where further glycosylation (addition of glucosamine, galactose, fucose?, and sialic acid?) transforms liposomes into VLDL particles. The VLDL particles are packaged into vacuoles that are derived from dilations in the elements of the Golgi apparatus. These Golgi-derived vacuoles detach from the elements and move to the sinusoidal surface of the hepatocyte, where vacuole and plasma membrane fuse; VLDL particles are released into the space of Disse by exocytosis.

Via direct continuities with the ER, LP particles are transported to GERL, an acid hydrolase-rich area of smooth ER located at the *trans* aspect of the Golgi apparatus. GERL gives rise to a variety of lysosomes, including residual bodies. One type of lysosome illustrated is the coated vesicle. GERL and residual bodies (not illustrated) contain LP particles of various sizes. In the presence of hydrolases, transformations of the protein, carbohydrate, and lipid moieties of the particles may occur in GERL and residual bodies, possibly leading to partial or complete catabolism or to conversion of LP particles for secretion.

Lipids and LP are transported by the ER for storage and are deposited in the cytosol in the form of spheres, known as "cytosolic" or "storage" lipid spheres. In normal hepatocytes, their numbers are few, and they are situated at the sinusoidal pole of the hepatocyte. Smooth ER, peroxisomes, and mitochondria are intimately associated with the surfaces of the lipid spheres. This constellation of organelles is illustrated in the lower left of Fig. 1.

In hepatocytes from rats treated with CPIB, the number of lipid spheres increases, and the smooth ER covers a greater surface of the lipid spheres. Peroxisomes, which also increase in number, and mitochondria retain their association with the spheres as described for untreated hepatocytes. The ER associated with the lipid surface is flattened; its membrane appears thicker, and it wraps incompletely in a ribbon-like fashion around a more extensive area of the lipid surface. Elsewhere, the ER appears to be normal. Also as in untreated hepatocytes, the secretory pathway and acid hydrolase-rich structures remain normal.

In hepatocytes from rats treated with orotic acid (OA), the ER undergoes a dramatic morphologic change. The entire ER breaks into vesicles, and one or more lipid droplets are deposited within each one. These lipid-containing ER vesicles are present throughout the cytoplasm of the hepatocyte. With OA, the pathway for the secretion of VLDL is interrupted: transitional vescicles and liposomes at the *cis* face of the Golgi apparatus disappear; Golgi elements are flattened and show no VLDL; Golgi vacuoles are absent; and VLDL particles are no longer secreted. GERL is reduced in size and lacks LP particles.

The effects of OA can be reversed by treating rats with CPIB. This results in the return of the ER to its usual morphologic configuration and reestablishment of the secretory pathway for VLDL GERL is enlarged in the reversed hepatocytes when compared to untreated hepatocytes and is distended with numerous LP particles.

EXPERIMENTALLY INDUCED FATTY LIVERS IN RATS

Several unrelated agents cause accumulation of lipid within mammalian hepatocytes producing fatty liver. Among them are ethionine, OA, alcohol, carbon tetrachloride, galactosamine, choline deficiency, cholesterol, CPIB, and sucrose. The pathogenic mechanisms leading to induction of fatty livers are not completely understood for any agent and most likely are different with each. When examined grossly, fatty livers have similar appearances; their size and weight are increased, and they are pale beige or white. Although fatty livers may show uniformity when examined by the unaided eye in the intact animal, remarkable diversities are seen when studied by microscopy. Light and electron microscopy, alone or in combination with histo- and cytochemistry, have permitted the study of aspects of lipid metabolism not possible by other approaches. Knowledge of these morphologic observations and correlation with biochemical studies of fatty livers may provide clues for formulating pathogenic mechanisms. Only fatty livers induced by OA, CPIB, sucrose, and cholesterol are discussed in this chapter.

OA-Induced Fatty Livers

Although OA is an intermediate in pyrimidine nucleotide synthesis in microorganisms and higher animals, rats fed a purine-free diet containing 1% OA develop a fatty liver, in which most of the lipid accumulated is newly synthesized TG. Concomitant with the decrease in plasma levels of TG and cholesterol is the disappearance of VLDL and apo B, its major apoprotein. These effects can be prevented and reversed by adding adenine to the diet.

Light microscopic observations of oil red O-stained frozen sections of these fatty livers show numerous spherical lipid droplets filling the cytoplasm of all hepatocytes from the sinusoidal to the bile canicular aspects. The hepatocytes are enlarged and rounder than normal. Initially, the droplets appear in hepatocytes close to the portal triad. Subsequently, all hepatocytes show lipid droplets throughout the cytoplasm. Lipid deposition in hepatocytes near the portal triad occurs in the liver of rats after 4 days on the diet; by 8 days, deposition has progressed to hepatocytes in the central vein area. Paralleling this is reduction in plasma apo B level to half that in normal plasma by the fourth day, with a virtual absence of apo B by the eighth day.

The asynchronous response of hepatocytes to the OA diet (revealed by light microscopy) offers the advantage of studying the morphologic sequence of changes in many hepatocytes from the same animal as lipid deposition proceeds. Before lipid is evident in hepatocytes, nucleoside diphosphatase (NDP) activity, a "marker" enzyme of the basophilic clumps (which consist of parallel arrays of rough ER), is diminished or lost (53).

Ultrastructural studies show dramatic changes in the structural appearance of the intracellular organelles within these hepatocytes (34,35,53). The most striking alterations occur in the ER system, which undergoes extensive vesiculation (Fig. 2). It is completely transformed from parallel arrays of cisternae and anastomosing tubules into rounded vesicles. The lipid droplets that accumulate in these hepatocytes are located within the cisternae of ER vesicles. Ribosomes are attached to many but not all ER vesicles.

The ER appears to be the first organelle effected by the OA diet. Electron microscopic studies of the ER in hepatocytes from rats fed the OA diet for 1 to 3 days (at this time lipid droplets are not evident) show images that are interpreted as early stages in vesicular formation. This is consistent with the light microscopic observation of the changes in NDP activity. As a consequence of the vesiculation of the ER, profound changes ensue in structurally and functionally related structures, namely, transitional vesicles, Golgi apparatus, GERL, and peroxisomes.

Figure 3 shows the appearance of the Golgi apparatus and GERL in untreated hepatocytes. These structures are drastically altered in hepatocytes of rats fed OA. Transitional vesicles, which transport nascent LP particles from the ER to the Golgi apparatus, are not formed. Because of morphologic interruption at this step in the secretory pathway, the elements of the Golgi apparatus lack VLDL particles, are flattened, and do not produce VLDL-containing vacuoles (Fig. 4a; compare with Fig. 4b). Microsomes isolated from livers of OA-fed rats showed an increase in the apoproteins characteristic of VLDL (54,55); the carbohydrate composition of these apoproteins is deficient in N-acetylglucosamine, galactose, fucose, and sialic acid (56). These carbohydrate moieties are considered to be added to LP particles as they move through the smooth ER and the Golgi apparatus. Other plasma proteins, including albumin, continue to be secreted, suggesting the existence of a secretory pathway that does not involve VLDL-containing, Golgi-derived vacuoles. Continuities between the ER and GERL, which is reduced in size and devoid of LP particles, disappear. It is not known if any part of GERL vesiculates along with the rest of the ER. Decreased catabolism

of lipid in GERL may in part contribute to the accumulation of lipid within the ER.

In the course of ER vesiculation, peroxisomes are reduced in number, and microperoxisomes are rarely present. The peroxisomes, with eccentric nucleoids, are found near the lipid-containing vesicles (Fig. 2). Many mitochondria are found in the condensed configuration closely apposed to the lipid-filled vesicles. Since peroxisomes and mitochondria possess lipid-metabolizing enzymes, reduction in the peroxisome population and the presence of condensed mitochondria may have functional significance in the pathogenesis of OA-induced fatty liver.

Reversal of the OA-Induced Fatty Liver by CPIB

The structural and functional modulations in organelles involved in lipoprotein metabolism are most dramatically demonstrated in the induction and subsequent reversal of the OA fatty liver (35). This reversal can be achieved by a hypolipidemic drug, CPIB, which can also produce a mild fatty liver in rats. Interestingly, an established fatty liver is completely reversed with CPIB, even while OA feeding continues. When examined grossly, the liver has regained its normal red-brown color. Liver weights, however, remained essentially unchanged. This is explained by the hepatomegalia caused by CPIB. Light microscopic examination of frozen sections of the reversed livers shows a paucity of lipid spheres. As in hepatocytes from untreated rats, these spheres are located near the sinusoidal aspect of the hepatocyte. The removal of lipid follows a similar progression in the liver lobule as the deposition. The lipid diminishes initially in hepatocytes near the portal triad, and clearing proceeds progressively toward the central vein. This permitted a reasonable reconstruction of the morphologic events involved in the removal of lipid from hepatocytes. (For a detailed description of the intermediate stages in this reversal process, especially changes of the ER, see ref. 35.)

The ultrastructure of the hepatocyte after reversal by CPIB shows a remarkable restoration of the ER to its normal configuration (Fig. 5). The parallel arrays of rough ER and the anastomosing network of smooth ER tubules, characteristic of normal hepatocytes, have reappeared. Lipid droplets have been completely removed from the cisternae of the ER. The structural and functional relationship of the ER to the Golgi apparatus is restored with the reappearance of liposomes within transitional vesicles. The Golgi apparatus contains VLDL in the dilations of its elements (Fig. 4b). VLDL-containing vacuoles, apparently Golgi derived, are present in the Golgi zone and near the apical

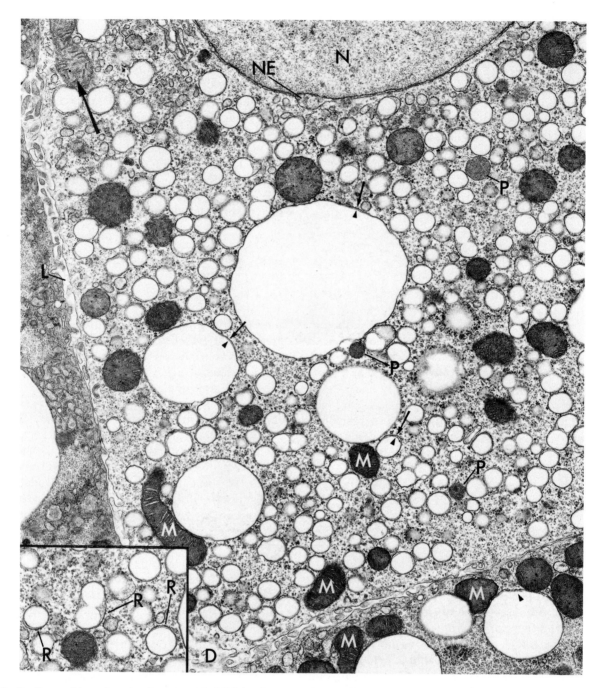

FIG. 2. Portions of hepatocytes from a rat fed OA for 2 weeks. One or more lipid droplets is present within the vesicles of ER; a finely granular material is also present and is most evident in the inset. *Arrowheads,* limits of the lipid droplets; *arrows,* ER of the vesicles. Ribosomes (R) are present on some of the ER vesicles membranes **(inset).** Numerous free ribosomes and glycogen particles are seen in the cytosol. The distinction between the two structures is not clear because of the similarity in size range and density. The lipid droplets vary in size; the largest in the field measures 4.5 μm. Some of the mitochondria that are closely applied to the droplet-containing vesicles are indicated by M. Most of the mitochondria have the condensed configuration; one of the few with the orthodox configuration is indicated by an arrow. Few peroxisomes (P) are present. At NE, an area of nuclear envelope is indicated in which the two ER membranes are separated by a material like that found in the ER vesicles. Also labeled are lateral plasma membrane (L) and space of Disse (D). ×11,250. (From ref. 35, with permission.)

plasma membrane that faces the space of Disse. Thus the entire morphologic pathway involved in synthesis, transport, and secretion of VLDL has been reestablished. Correlating with this morphologic restoration is the return of apo B to the plasma.

A striking finding is enlargement of GERL. Its cisternal and tubular portions are more extensive and are distended by numerous LP particles (57). These LP particles are more closely packed, electron opaque, and smaller when compared with particles within the

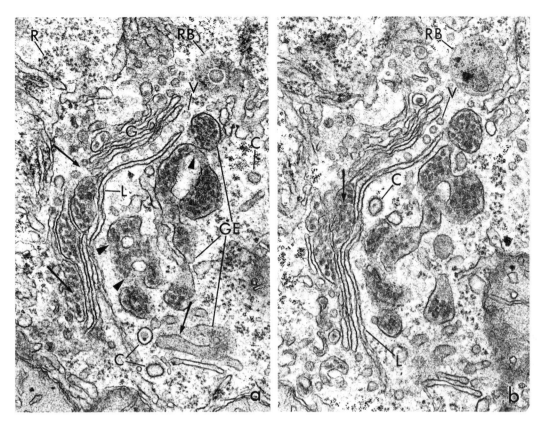

FIG. 3. Golgi zones of hepatocytes from the portal triad area of unincubated material from an untreated rat liver. These figures represent serial sections. *Long arrows,* VLDL particles in a dilation of a Golgi element. The particles are electron-opaque in this preparation. The anastomosing nature of GERL (GE) is seen in both sections but is more apparent in **a** (*arrowheads*). Within its cisternae are electron-opaque LP particles and a finely granular material (*arrowheads* and *short arrow*). Numerous small vesicles (V) are seen between the Golgi stack and a portion of GE. A portion of GE labeled (L) is a rigid lamella. Three coated vesicles (C) are seen in **a** and another in **b**. A residual body (RB) is cut tangentially in **a** and slightly more transversely in **b**, thereby revealing a part of its delimiting tripartite membrane. These serial sections also show that the elements of the Golgi apparatus are continuous; compare area near the long arrow in **a** with same area in **b**. The elements appear discontinuous in one plane of section. This apparent discontinuity may result from the undulating nature of the Golgi apparatus. ×43,000. (From ref. 20, with permission.)

Golgi apparatus (Fig. 4b; also see Fig. 1 in ref. 57). Associated with enlargement of GERL is the presence of numerous residual bodies; some are filled with LP particles and others with matrixes containing electron-lucent and electron-opaque areas (Figs. 6c, d).

The extensive nature of GERL, although recognizable by its ultrastructural features, and its distinction from the Golgi apparatus were confirmed by cytochemistry with two different procedures. The anastomosing cisternae and tubules of GERL, residual bodies, and coated vesicles show acid phosphatase but not NDP activity (Figs. 6a, b, 7), whereas the inner element of the Golgi apparatus displays NDP but not acid phosphatase activity (Figs. 6a, b). In the reversal experiment, GERL most likely functions in the removal of the lipid from the ER and in the transformations, including degradation of LP particles.

Peroxisomes increase in number and size and show eccentric nucleoids (Fig. 5). Broad continuities between their membrane and the membrane of the ER, similar to those seen in nafenopin-treated rats (58)

(Figs. 8a, b), are frequently encountered. Their role in lipid removal is suggested by close proximity to the surface of large storage lipid spheres that appear in the early stages of the reversal process. The biochemical or molecular mechanisms by which CPIB reverses the OA fatty liver are unknown.

Morphologic Differences Between OA- and CPIB-Induced Fatty Livers

CPIB produces a mild fatty liver in rats that have a diet-induced hyperlipemia (34,59), which results from a diet containing 60% sucrose (60). This CPIB effect does not occur in chow-fed rats (34,59). The nature of the deposition of lipid spheres in hepatocytes and the relationship of the ER to the lipid spheres differs completely from that of OA (34). After 1 day on the CPIB diet, numerous lipid spheres appear and are concentrated and restricted to the region of the hepatocytes close to the sinusoids. All hepatocytes show this pattern of lipid accumulation, which is sustained for 30

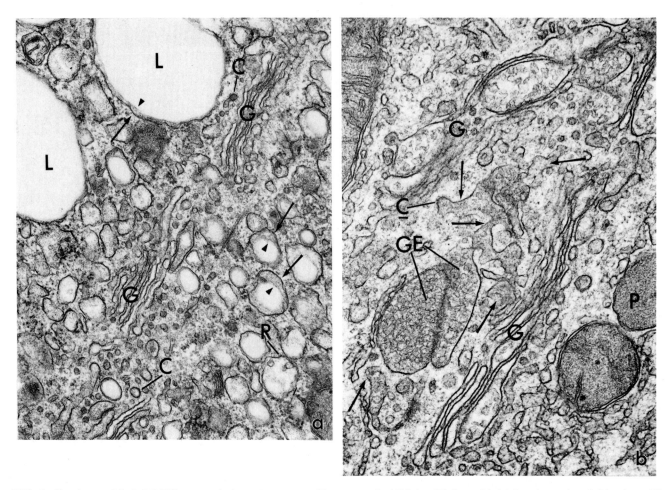

FIG. 4. Portions of Golgi-GERL zones in hepatocytes. **a:** From a rat fed OA for 15 days. Lipid droplets of variable sizes fill the vesicles of ER (*arrows*). A granular material between the limit of the lipid (*arrowheads*) and the ER membranes is evident. The elements of the Golgi stack are flattened and do not contain VLDL or lipid particles. VLDL containing secretory vacuoles are also absent. GERL is much reduced in size. A coated vesicle (C) (lower left) and one still attached to a small tubule of GERL (upper right) are the only distinguishing morphologic entities observed of this organelle. Ribosomes (R) are still attached to the ER membranes. ×31,500. **b:** From a rat fed the same diet as in Fig. 5. The elements of a portion of the Golgi apparatus (G) are distended with VLDL particles. GERL (GE) is much enlarged and contains LP particles within its tubular and expanded cisternal portions. The particles appear smaller, more densely packed, and more electron-opaque than the particles in the elements of the Golgi apparatus. Tubular portions of GERL are indicated by arrows and the cisternal portions are indicated by GE. A coated area is seen on a tubular portion of GERL. ×43,000. (From ref. 35, with permission.)

days, the longest time studied. Rarely do lipid spheres extend to the region of the bile canaliculus.

Ultrastructural observations show numerous electron-lucent lipid spheres with a peripheral dense thin line as its boundary (Fig. 9). The nature of this line is not known; however, it does not have the appearance of a tripartite membrane. The "cytosolic" lipid spheres lie free in the cytoplasm; i.e., they are not surrounded by a tripartite membrane. Smooth ER, which proliferates, spirals around each of the spheres in a sheet or ribbon-like fashion and is often found in continuity with rough ER. The cisternae of the smooth ER, enwrapping the spheres, flatten; the membrane of the smooth ER becomes thicker and more darkly stained than the rough ER with which it is continuous or the ER elsewhere in the hepatocyte (Fig. 9).

In contrast with OA-fed rats, in which all lipid droplets are within the cisternae of the ER vesicles, these lipid spheres are never found in the cisternae of the ER. Serial sectioning reveals some aspects of the geometric arrangements of the ER-lipid sphere relationship. The ER does not completely encircle the lipid sphere. However, more of the lipid surface is covered by the ER than is exposed to the cytosol. Peroxisomes and mitochondria are either in direct contact with the lipid surface or close to the enveloping ER. The constellation of lipid spheres-smooth ER-peroxisomes or microperoxisomes-mitochondria differs from untreated hepatocytes in the extent of the area of contact between the lipid surface and the smooth ER and the increased numbers of peroxisomes or microperoxisomes on the lipid surfaces.

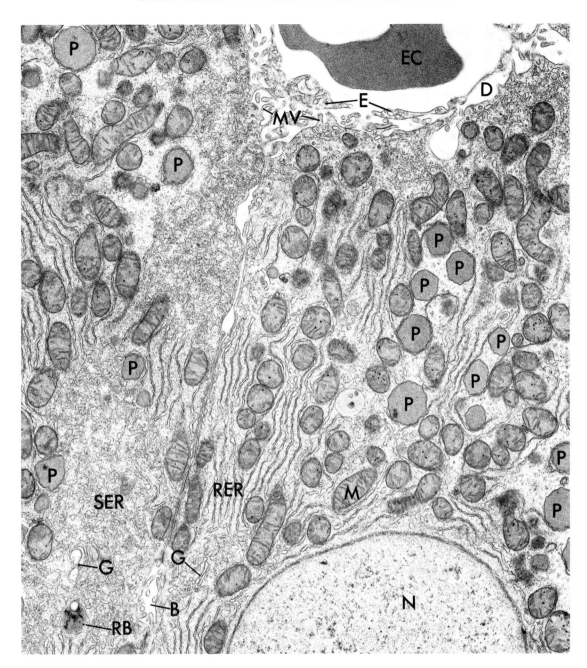

FIG. 5. Portions of two hepatocytes from a rat fed OA for 7 days and then CPIB plus OA for 15 days. The parallel arrays of rough ER (RER) and the anastomosing smooth ER (SER) are restored to their normal configuration. Lipid droplets are not evident within the cisternae of ER. Numerous peroxisomes (P) are present, some of which contain eccentric nucleoids. It has not been ascertained if those peroxisomes without nucleoids are microperoxisomes which may develop into peroxisomes, because serial sections on these hepatocytes were not performed. Even at this magnification (×11,250), the proximity of the ER to the peroxisomes is evident. This section is cut to reveal only a small area of the Golgi apparatus (G) and GERL (not labeled). A residual body (RB), containing an electron-lucent area, probably lipid, is present. All the mitochondria (M) show the orthodox configuration. Also labeled are the microvilli (MV), which project into the space of Disse (D), a portion of the nucleus (N), and a portion of the bile caniliculus (B). Outside the hepatocyte, portions of an endothelial cell (E) and an erythrocyte (EC) are seen. (From ref. 35, with permission.)

The secretory pathway for lipoproteins is unperturbed. Liposomes are transported via smooth ER to the Golgi apparatus where particles resembling VLDL are formed and packaged into vacuoles; the Golgi-derived vacuoles move to the plasma membrane where the particles are released by exocytosis into the space of Disse. However, GERL is hypertrophied and contains numerous lipoprotein particles. Autophagic vacuoles and residual bodies are numerous; these residual bodies do not contain the large lipid spheres depicted in Figs. 6c and d. Although the mild fatty liver is manifested early (within 24 hr), the hypolipidemic effect of

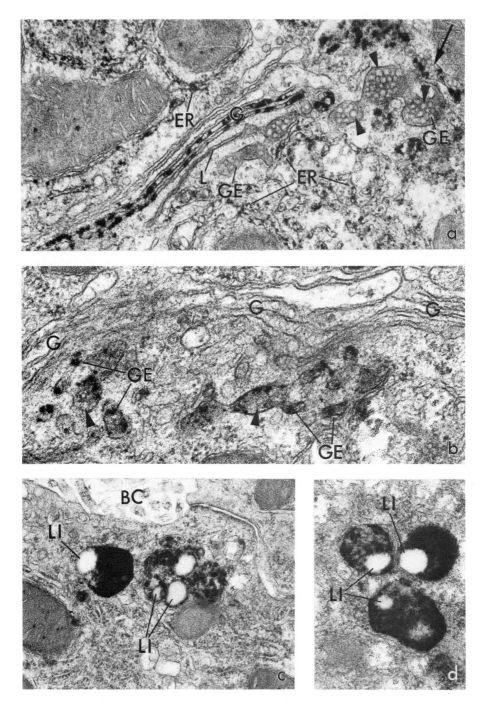

FIG. 6. Portions of hepatocytes from rats fed OA for 7 days, and CPIB plus OA for 8 days **(a, c, d)** and 15 days **(b)**. **a:** Incubated for thiamine pyrophosphatase activity for 90 min at neutral pH. Electron-opaque reaction product is seen in the innermost or *trans* element of the Golgi stack (see refs. 20 and 82 for a discussion of the complex geometric arrangement of the innermost Golgi element of the Golgi apparatus). The rigid lamellae (L), the cisternal and tubular portions of GERL (GE), are devoid of reaction product. Within portions of GE are LP particles (*arrowheads*) and also a finely granular material. Some reaction is also present in the ER. *Arrow upper right,* LP particles, presumably VLDL within a portion of the innermost Golgi element, along with reaction product. The ER is seen in close continuity with portions of GE. ×39,600. **b:** Incubated for acid phosphatase activity at pH 5.0 for 12 min. The Golgi stack (G) lacks reaction product. GE shows reaction product along with LP particles in its anastomosing cisternal and tubular portions. The LP particles are visible in GE (*arrowheads*) because the incubation time was brief, thereby preventing the reaction product from obscuring the particles. Residual bodies (not illustrated) show LP particles with a heterogeneity in size and shape. ×43,200. **c** and **d:** Incubated for acid phosphatase activity for 30 min. Large electron-lucent lipid-like spherical areas are seen in residual bodies (LI). These areas probably formed from the smaller LP particles in residual bodies. Reaction product is present in the residual bodies. ×40,000. (From ref. 57, with permission.)

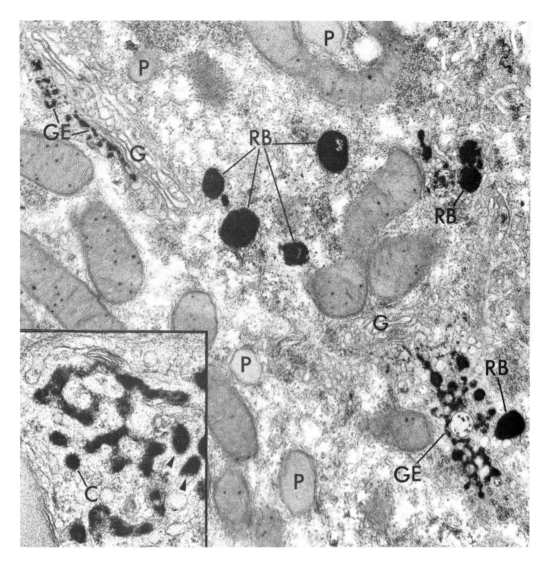

FIG. 7. Portion of hepatocyte from a rat treated as in Fig. 6b. Section incubated for acid phosphatase 30 min. The elements of the Golgi stacks lack reaction product. The extensive nature of GERL (GE) and the numerous residual bodies (RB) are revealed by the intense reaction product. In sections that are perpendicular through the Golgi stack (*upper left*), the anastomosing nature of GE is not evident. When cut tangentially, however, the anastomosing tubular nature of GE is evident. Serial sections are needed to ascertain if the RB are separate from GE or connected to GE. **Inset,** a coated vesicle (C), presumably detached and derived from GE, is positive for acid phosphatase. Coated areas (*arrowheads*) are present on some areas of the anastomosing tubules of GE. ×26,000; **inset,** ×56,000. (From ref. 57, with permission.)

CPIB in hyperlipemic rats occurs much later (after 8 days). The mechanisms of action of CPIB in lowering plasma lipids have not been established. The contributions of the increased degradative capacity of GERL, along with proliferation of the smooth ER and peroxisomes, in reducing plasma lipids must be explored.

FATTY LIVERS IN GENETIC OBESE RATS

The mutant rat, known as the Zucker fatty rat, inherits obesity as an autosomal Mendelian trait (61). These rats are hyperlipemic, hyperinsulinemic, and normoglycemic (62). An extreme fatty liver develops when they are fed a sucrose-enriched diet (63). Hyperlipemia, but not fatty liver, occurs in heterozygous or homozygous lean Zucker rats with this diet, suggesting that heredity plays a major role. This diet also produces hyperlipemia, but not fatty livers, in Sprague-Dawley (60) and Lewis (64) rats.

Observations on Hepatocytes

After 1 week on the sucrose-enriched diet, numerous and large electron-lucent lipid spheres fill the cy-

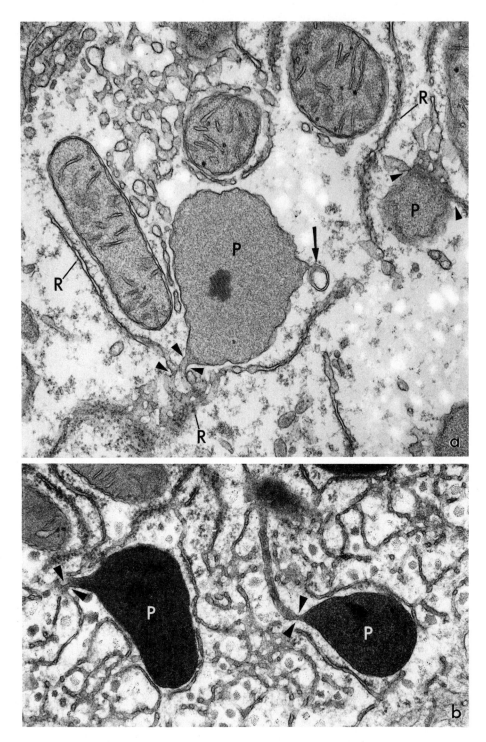

FIG. 8. Portions of hepatocytes from livers of rats administered nafenopin by gavage. **a:** Unincubated material. Two peroxisomes (P), one very large and showing or containing a nucleoid, have several continuities with the smooth ER (*arrowheads*). The smooth ER connected to the peroxisomes is continuous with the rough ER. Ribosomes (R) are evident on the ER membranes. The larger peroxisome also shows a continuity with a small tab of smooth ER (*arrow*) that may have separated from the rough ER. ×36,000. **b:** Incubated for catalase activity in a medium containing diaminobenzidine for 10 min at pH 9.7, 37°C. The two peroxisomes in the field are enlarged, and both show nucleoids that may be somewhat obscured by the electron-opaque reaction product. The upper peroxisome shows a distinct continuity (*arrowheads*) between the delimiting membrane of the peroxisome and the membrane of the smooth ER. Within this extension of smooth ER is electron-opaque reaction product similar to that seen in the matrix of the peroxisome. The lower peroxisome also shows a continuity with the smooth ER (*arrowheads*) which, in turn, is continuous with the RER. ×35,000.

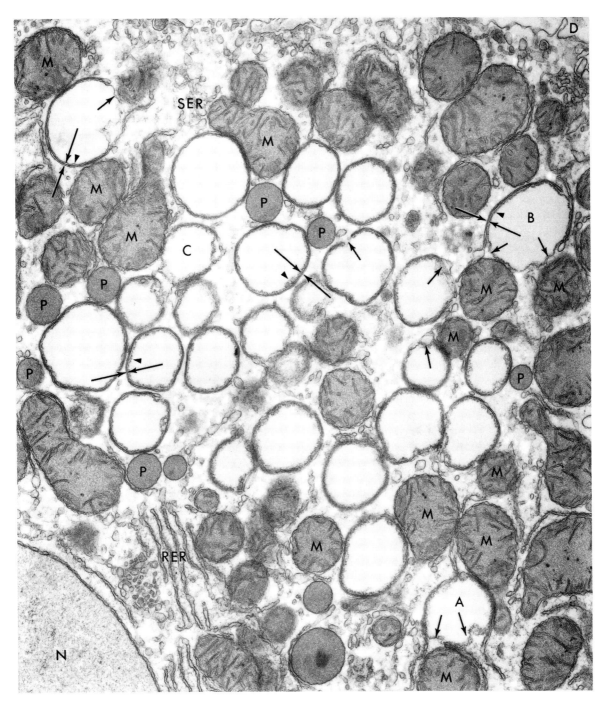

FIG. 9. Portion of a hepatocyte from a rat fed CPIB and sucrose for 8 days. Part of the nucleus is seen at N and some of the space of Disse at D. Little rough ER (RER) and smooth ER (SER) is seen in this field. The numerous storage lipid spheres are electron lucent except for irregular electron-opaque line at their peripheries (*arrowheads*). This line is not a delimiting membrane; the composition or its nature is unknown. It may represent or be of a proteinaceous nature. *Apposing long arrows,* some of the flattened ER surrounding lipid spheres; *short arrows,* regions where SER is not present at this level of sectioning. In contrast to storage lipid spheres in untreated hepatocytes, the ER membranes surround a greater area of the lipid spheres, do not undulate, and appear thicker and more darkly stained, or both. Two separate SER sheets appear to surround spheres A, B, and C. Often these SER are found to be continuous with RER (not illustrated). The possibility that the two sheets or flattened cisternae of SER might join outside the plane of section cannot be ruled out, since serial sections were not made of the tissue used in this figure. Mitochondria are closely associated with the spheres and are often found in areas where the SER is interrupted or absent. Also closely associated with the spheres are numerous peroxisomes. Whether any microperoxisomes are present would require serial sectioning to be sure that a nucleoid is absent. ×18,900. (From ref. 34, with permission.)

toplasm of all the hepatocytes. These spheres are not enclosed within a membrane but have portions of their surfaces intimately associated with the ER, peroxisomes, and mitochondria (Fig. 10). In this respect, they resemble the lipid spheres of untreated rat but differ in their size, number, and location within the hepatocyte. The massive accumulation of lipids, mostly TG, in the fatty liver is not coincident with or accompanied by a decrease in the release of lipids from the liver. Ultrastructural studies show that the morphologic secretory pathway for LP particles is intact. Larger LP particles are produced, however, filling the elements of the Golgi apparatus, GERL, and vacuoles (Fig. 11b) and are secreted into the space of Disse (Figs. 11e, f). These particles are two to three times larger than those produced and secreted by the hepatocytes from chow-fed obese rats (compare Figs. 11a, c, d with 11b, e, f). Results from experiments with injection of Triton WR1339 [which inhibits the activity of plasma lipoprotein lipases (65)] show that LP particles are secreted from the sucrose-induced fatty liver (L. Gidez, *unpublished*). These data correlate with morphologic observations, thereby demonstrating that LP particles are secreted even during massive deposition of lipid in hepatocytes.

Hepatocyte ultrastructural changes identical to those described in the sucrose-induced fatty liver of the genetic obese rat were produced in a nonobese rat with pancreatic hormones and a sucrose diet (64). Lewis rats were made diabetic with streptozoticin injected into the portal vein with pancreatic islet transplants, and fed a sucrose-enriched diet. Fatty liver did

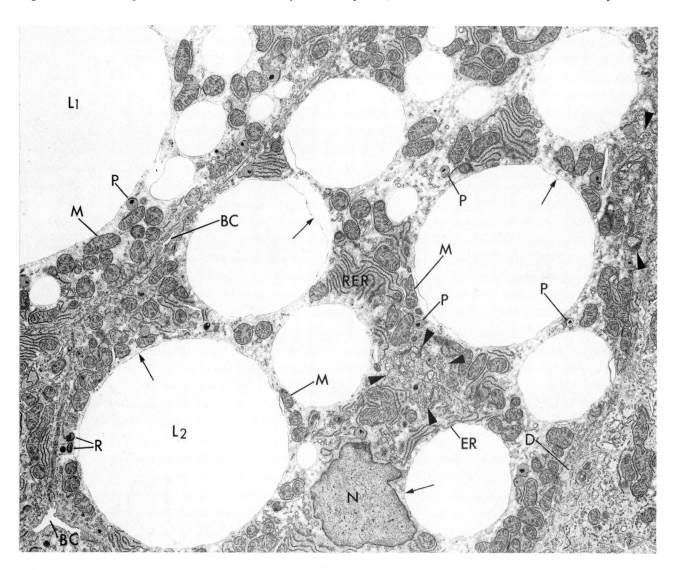

FIG. 10. Portion of a hepatocyte from a Zucker fatty rat fed a 60% sucrose diet for 1 week. Numerous and large electron-lucent lipid spheres fill the cytoplasm. The close proximity of the ER, the peroxisomes (P), and the mitochondria (M) to the surface of the lipid spheres is evident. The diameters of L_1 and L_2 are approximately 14 and 9 μm, respectively. Also labeled are bile caniliculus (BC), space of Disse (D), nucleus (N), residual bodies (R), and rough ER (RER). ×5,500. (From ref. 64, with permission.)

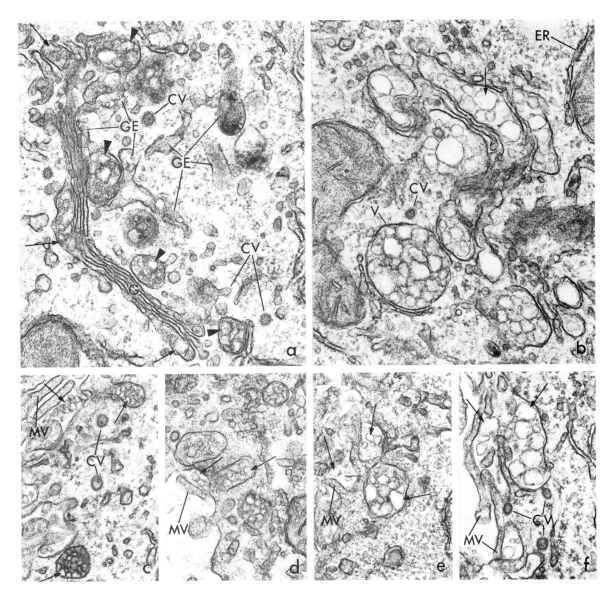

FIG. 11. Portions of Golgi GERL zones. **a:** From a portion of a hepatocyte from a genetically obese (Zucker) rat fed a chow diet. **b:** From a similar rat fed an enriched sucrose diet for 1 week. The elements of the Golgi apparatus (G) show distensions containing VLDL particles (*arrows*). *Arrowheads,* LP particles in portions of GERL (GE). Coated vesicles (CV) are also present in this zone. **b:** Much enlarged LP particles (*arrows*) in distended portions of the Golgi apparatus, in regions of GERL, and in a presumably secretory vacuole. **c–f:** Portions of sinusoidal aspects of genetically obese Zucker rats. **c, d:** From a rat fed chow; **e, f:** from a rat fed as in **b.** Microvilli (MV) project in the space of Disse. **c, d:** *arrows,* LP particles in vacuoles, some of which are in contact with and within the space of Disse. These particles are in the same size range as those in **a. e, f:** Much enlarged LP particles in vacuoles and in the space of Disse. These particles are similar in size to those in **b.** CV, coated vesicles. **a, b,** ×39,000; **c-f,** ×30,000. (From ref. 63, with permission.)

not result, but numerous white spots, consisting of lipid-filled hepatocytes, appeared in all liver lobes. Only hepatocytes surrounding the portal triads, which lodged the pancreatic islets, showed accumulation of cytosolic lipid spheres with intimate associations to the ER, peroxisomes, and mitochondria (Fig. 12) and enlarged LP particles within the Golgi apparatus, GERL, and vacuoles. These changes occurred only in hepatocytes close to the islet cells and may reflect their response to higher levels of hormones together with fructose or another metabolite of sucrose.

Hepatocytes from fatty livers induced in obese rats by a 2% cholesterol diet are qualitatively similar to those in sucrose-induced fatty livers. All hepatocytes show numerous cytosolic lipid spheres within their cytoplasms with the same intimate association with the ER, peroxisomes, and mitochondria.

The extent of the surface of the spheres covered by ER varies among the lipid spheres. Some spheres are enclosed by cisternae of ER; others show none or little at their surfaces (Fig. 13). Peroxisomes appear more numerous, particularly in hepatocytes with cytochemi-

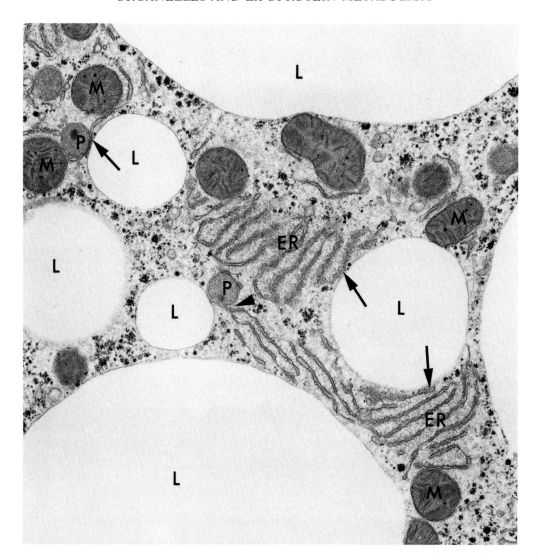

FIG. 12. Portion of a hepatocyte from the portal triad area of the hepatic lobule from the liver of a Lewis rat. The rat was treated as follows: diabetes induced by streptozotozin, followed by intraportal transplant of isolated pancreatic islets, and fed a sucrose diet for 2 weeks. Numerous lipid spheres (L) of various sizes fill the cytoplasm of the hepatocytes near the transplant (see Fig. 2A in ref. 64). The limit of the lipid spheres appears as a fine line (*arrows*). The close proximity of the ER, the peroxisomes (P), and mitochondria (M) to the surface of the lipid spheres is evident. *Arrowhead,* near continuity between the membrane of the ER and the membrane of a nucleoid-containing peroxisome. ×17,000. (Courtesy of Ana Yam.)

cally demonstrable catalase activity (Fig. 13). Relevant to this observation are reports that peroxisomes isolated from livers of rats fed a high fat diet showed increases in catalase and in β-oxidation of fatty acids (66,67). Large LP particles are found in the Golgi apparatus, GERL, vacuoles, and the space of Disse, suggesting that accumulation of cholesterol, like accumulation of TG, does not interfere with the secretion of LP particles. In addition, excessive deposition of cholesterol does not affect the capacity of these hepatocytes to endocytose exogenously administered HRP (68). After 5 and 10 min postinjection of HRP, some portions of GERL and some residual bodies (those generally containing LP particles) show the endocytosed peroxidase; at the same time, peroxi-

dase-negative portions of GERL and residual bodies are also evident (Fig. 14). Observations on Kupffer cells from these HRP injected fatty livers led to reexamination of the concept that GERL and residual bodies may comprise an extensive interconnecting lysosomal compartment in macrophages, hepatocytes, and other cell types (see chapter by A. B. Novikoff). The presence or absence of HRP may reflect heterogeneity in the structure and function of the lysosomal compartment in hepatocytes from the cholesterol-induced fatty liver. HRP is transported to structures morphologically similar to those found in untreated hepatocytes which have endocytosed galactose-terminated glycoproteins (asialoglycoproteins) by a receptor-mediated process (69).

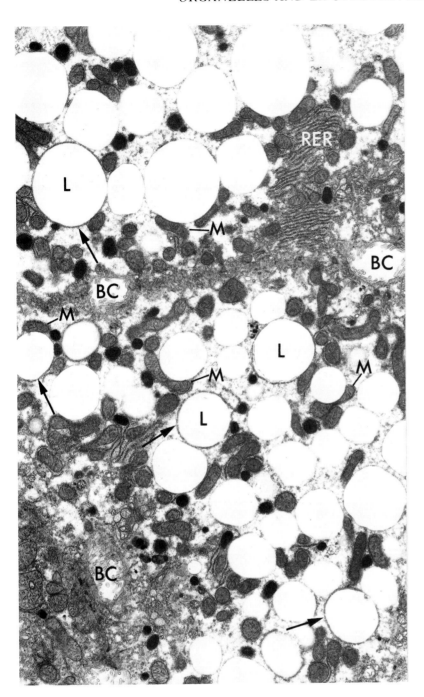

FIG. 13. Portion of two hepatocytes from an obese Zucker rat fed a 2% cholesterol diet for 2 weeks. Numerous electron-lucent storage or "cytosolic" lipid spheres (L) are distributed throughout the cytoplasm. This section of the liver had been incubated in a medium containing diaminobenzidine for 5 min at pH 9.7, 37° C. (44). The close association of the peroxisomes to the surface of the lipid spheres is more striking with the cytochemical visualization of their catalase activity. The relationship of the ER (*arrows*) to the surface of some but not all the lipid spheres (see Figs. 9 and 10 for comparison) is evident. Also evident is the close proximity of the mitochondria to the spheres. BC, bile canaliculi. ×8,000.

Observations on Kupffer Cells

Kupffer cells show dramatic changes in cholesterol-induced fatty livers of obese rats. The cells become enlarged and increase in numbers, particularly in the periportal areas of the hepatic lobule. Lipoprotein particles, similar in morphologic appearance and size to those found in the Golgi apparatus and GERL of hepatocytes, in the space of Disse, and in blood sinusoids, are found within membrane-enclosed structures (Fig. 15). The particles appear to enter Kupffer cells by several endocytic mechanisms: (a) membrane indentations forming endocytic vacuoles, (b) envelopment by microvilli or filapodia, (c) "vermiform invaginations" of the plasma membrane, and (d) coated pits. An extensive lysosomal compartment, which includes a network of interconnected residual bodies and GERL, develops and contains lipoprotein particles and lipid-like inclusions. This system shows cytochemically demonstrable acid phosphatase activity.

Intravenously injected tracer HRP and endogenously produced lipoprotein particles are rapidly taken up by the Kupffer cells and transported to the entire lysosomal system (70). These observations raise the possibility that Kupffer cells, in addition to hepato-

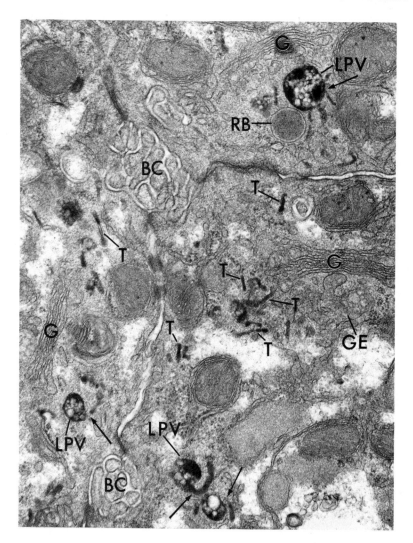

FIG. 14. Portions of three hepatocytes from a centrilobular area in an obese Zucker rat fed a 2% cholesterol diet for 2 weeks. Rat was injected with HRP, 10 mg/100 g weight, into the tail vein and killed after 10 min. Vibratome sections (20 to 30 μm) were incubated for peroxidase by the method of Graham and Karvovsky (42) at pH 7.4 for 10 min. Peroxidase is found in vacuoles (LPV) containing electron-lucent lipoprotein particles. Some of these LPV have smooth surfaced tubular extensions which are also positive for HRP (*arrows*). Several smooth surfaced cisternae or tubules (T), probably portions of GERL, are positive for peroxidase and are located in the Golgi zone. The Golgi apparatus (G) is negative for peroxidase. Also negative at this point are some residual bodies (RB) and a portion of GERL (GE) containing LP particles within its cisternae. BC, bile caniliculi. ×31,500.

cytes, participate in the uptake and degradation of lipoprotein particles. The origin and nature of these particles remains to be established. Relevant to these observations are studies on isolated Kupffer cells, which show uptake of several classes of iodinated lipoprotein particles and degradation of their lipid and apoprotein components. Among the lipoprotein particles metabolized by the Kupffer cells were rat chylomicra and VLDL remnants, rat and human VLDL, low density lipoprotein (LDL), and high density lipoprotein (HDL) (71–74).

RELEVANCE OF CULTURED 3T3-L1 PREADIPOCYTES TO HEPATOCYTES

Green (75) and colleagues established several cloned lines from disaggregated Swiss mouse embryos capable of differentiating into adipocyte-like cells. One of these, designated 3T3-L1, showed a 50- to 100-fold increase in enzymes involved in TG biosynthesis, a massive accumulation of TG, and an increased response to a variety of hormones, including insulin

(76–78). Biochemical studies have contributed significantly to understanding the metabolic events that occur in these cells during lipogenesis and lipolysis. These cells provide not only a unique system to study cellular organelles during differentiation but a useful model system to study lipid metabolism in hepatocytes as well.

Ultrastructural study revealed features of the differentiating 3T3-L1 cells similar to those of hepatocytes (39). These cells showed the ER spatially close to the plasma membrane and lipid deposited as cytosolic spheres with ER, microperoxisomes, and mitochondria intimately associated with the spheres (Fig. 16). These observations suggest that the 3T3-L1 cells may function in a manner similar to hepatocytes in the uptake, synthesis, transport, and accumulation of lipids. Little is known about the deposition of lipid in the form of spheres and the enlargement of the spheres. The differentiating 3T3-L1 are suitable for studying these processes, with an emphasis on the intimate relationships of the ER, microperoxisomes, and mitochondria to the spheres. These cells possess the greatest num-

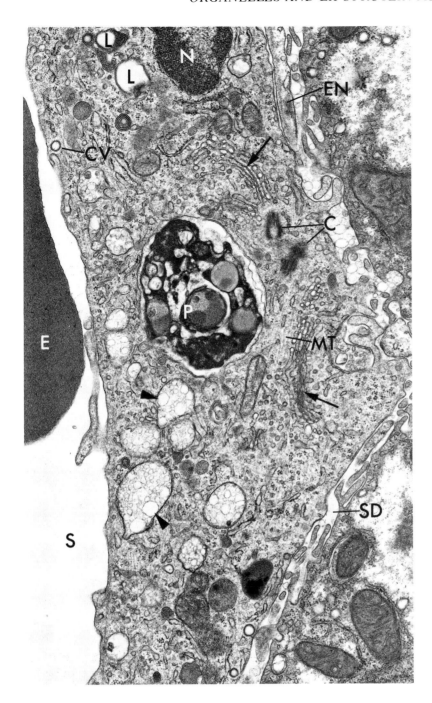

FIG. 15. Portion of a Kupffer cell from a cholesterol-fed obese Zucker rat. Numerous vacuoles containing endocytosed lipoprotein particles (LP) of various sizes are evident. *Arrowheads,* electron-lucent LP in endocytic vacuoles, in a coated vesicle, and in the space of Disse (SD). LP are also found in the blood sinusoids (not present in this liver which was initially fixed by perfusion). Portions of residual bodies contain electron-lucent lipid (L). The Golgi apparatus (*arrows*) lacks LP. Also labeled are: several coated vesicles (CV) near the plasma membrane; a platelet (P) that has been endocytosed by the Kupffer cell; centriole (C); microtubules (M); endothelial cell (EN); nucleus (N); and erythrocyte (E). ×19,000.

ber of microperoxisomes of all cell types thus far studied. This is dramatically shown by the cytochemical presence of the enzyme catalase (Fig. 16). The isolation of microperoxisomes from these cells and biochemical analysis for lipid-metabolizing enzymes might provide evidence that the microperoxisomes participate in the biosynthesis of lipids, as shown in hepatocytes and in brain (79). These cells may also be advantageous in studying the significance of the asymmetrical distribution of biosynthetic enzymes for phospholipids and TG on the cytoplasmic side of microsomal vesicles (80), and the morphologic relation-

ship of the ER to the surface of the cytosolic lipid spheres.

SIGNIFICANCE OF LIPID AND LIPOPROTEIN PARTICLES WITHIN GERL

The existence of a new pathway for the transport of lipids and lipoprotein particles in untreated rat hepatocytes emerged from morphologic and cytochemical studies on hepatocytes in which massive deposition of lipid was followed by subsequent removal of lipids (20,34,35). This new pathway involves direct chan-

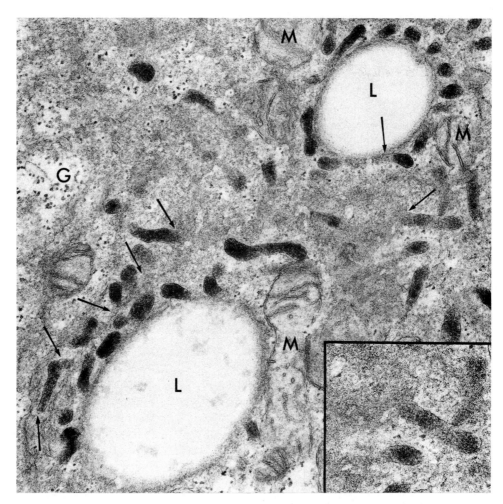

FIG. 16. Differentiating cultured 3T3L-1 cells 4 to 5 days after treatment with dexamethasone and methylisobutylxanthine. This cell was incubated to reveal sites of catalase using a medium containing diaminobenzidine at pH 9.7 for 90 min. Numerous microperoxisomes are present in these cells and contain catalase. These organelles appear electron opaque after incubation for this enzyme. These organelles are found juxtaposed to the surface of the many storage lipid spheres that accumulate in these cells as they continue to differentiate. The lipid spheres are cut somewhat tangentially so that the ER surrounding its surface is not clearly delineated. *Arrows,* regions where contiguities, possibly continuities, between the ER and microperoxisomes are present. **Inset,** higher magnification, showing a glancing view of an elongated microperoxisome continuous with a portion of fenestrated ER. Mitochondria (M) are also seen close to the lipid surfaces. ×29,700; **inset,** ×40,500. (From ref. 39, with permission.)

neling of lipoprotein particles and other materials to GERL from the ER through membrane continuities between ER and GERL. This pathway is distinct from the well-known and studied secretory pathway for the transport of nascent VLDL particles from the ER to the Golgi apparatus via transitional vesicles. Lipoprotein particles and other materials may be transported from the ER to GERL indirectly after passage through the Golgi apparatus. A close structural and possibly functional relationship exists between these two structures; however, direct continuities have not been observed.

Metabolic events that occur within GERL in relation to lipid and lipoprotein metabolism must be explored. The recognition of GERL as a separate organelle and the isolation of this organelle would contribute to our

understanding of these events. The biochemical properties of the lipoprotein particles and the hydrolytic enzymes (except for acid phosphatase) present in GERL (e.g., lipases) or other enzymes (e.g., glycosyl transferases) have not been determined.

The presence of lipoprotein particles within an acid hydrolase environment strongly suggests that catabolic events occur within GERL. The significance of the catabolic events raises innumerable questions as to the functions of this extensive hydrolase-rich system. GERL may play a role in the following: (a) regulating the secretory process of various classes of lipoproteins, analogous to, but not akin to, crinophagy in hormone-secreting cells (81); (b) secretion of lipoproteins by remodeling, altering, or transforming their lipid, protein, and carbohydrate moieties; (c) glycosylation of lipoprotein particles (82,83); (d) interconversions of lipoprotein particles as occur in the plasma (2), and degradation of chylomica remnants, VLDL remnants, LDL, and HDL (84–87); (e) proteolytic cleavage of proalbumin to albumin (88–89) (although not directly related to lipoprotein metabolism); studies to reveal the functions of this organelle in hepatocytes and other cell types offer an exciting area of future research.

ACKNOWLEDGMENTS

These investigations were supported by National Institutes of Health grants CA06576 and AM23078. I am grateful for the encouragement from, the advice of, and the critical discussions with Alex B. Novikoff during the course of these experiments.

REFERENCES

1. Lands, W. E. M., and Crawford, C. G. (1976): Enzymes of membrane phospholipid metabolism in animals. In: *The Enzymes of Biological Membranes*, edited by A. Martonosi, pp. 3–85. Plenum, New York.
2. Havel, R. J., Goldstein, J. C., and Brown, M. S. (1980): Lysoproteins and lysid transport. In: *Metabolic Control and Disease*, edited by P. K. Bondy and L. E. Rosenberg, pp. 393–494. Saunders, Philadelphia.
3. Singer, S. J. (1971): The molecular organization of biological membranes. In: *Structure and Function of Biological Membranes*, edited by L. I. Rothfield, pp. 145–222. Academic Press, New York.
4. Wolosewick, J. J., and Porter, K. R. (1979): Microtrabecular lattice of the cytoplasmic ground substance. *J. Cell Biol.*, 82:114–139.
5. Fulton, A. B., Wan, K. M., and Penman, S. (1980): The spatial distribution of polyribosomes in 3T3 cells and the associated assembly of proteins into the skeletal framework. *Cell*, 20:849–857.
6. Porter, K. R., Claude, A., and Fullam, E. F. (1945): A study of tissue culture cells by electron microscopy. *J. Exp. Med.*, 81:233–247.
7. Dalton, A. J., Kahler, H., Striebick, M. J., and Lloyd, B. (1950): Finer structure of hepatic, intestinal and renal cells of the mouse as revealed by the electron microscope. *J. Natl. Cancer Inst.*, 11:439–461.
8. Bernhard, W., Haguenau, F., Gautier, A., and Oberling, C. (1952): La structure submicroscopique des éléments basophiles cytoplasmiques dans le foie, le pancréas, et les glandes salivaires. *Z. Zellforsch. Mikrosk. Anat.*, 37:281–300.
9. Fawcett, D. W. (1955): Observations on the cytology and electron microscopy of hepatic cells. *J. Natl. Cancer Inst. [Suppl.]*, 15:1475–1502.
10. Palade, G. (1975): Intracellular aspects of the process of protein synthesis. *Science*, 189:347–358.
11. Bell, R. M., and Coleman, R. A. (1980): Enzymes of glycerolipid synthesis in eukaryotes. *Ann. Rev. Biochem.*, 49:459–487.
12. DiAugustine, R. P., Schaefer, J. M., and Founts, J. R. (1973): Hepatic lipid droplets. Isolation, morphology and composition. *Biochem. J.*, 132:323–327.
13. Ehrenreich, J. H., Bergeron, J. J. M., Siekevitz, P., and Palade, G. E. (1973): Golgi fractions prepared from rat liver homogenates I. Isolation procedure and morphological characterization. *J. Cell Biol.*, 59:45–72.
14. Friend, D. S., and Murray, M. (1965): Osmium impregnation of the Golgi apparatus. *Am. J. Anat.*, 17:135–141.
15. Cheetham, D., Morre, J., Pannek, C., and Friend, D. S. (1971): Isolation of a Golgi apparatus-rich fraction from rat liver. IV. Thiamine pyrophosphatase. *J. Cell Biol.*, 49:899–905.
16. Novikoff, A. B., and Goldfischer, S. (1961): Nucleosidediphosphatase activity in the Golgi apparatus and its usefulness for cytological studies. *Proc. Natl. Acad. Sci. USA*, 47:802–810.
17. Novikoff, A. B., and Heus, M. (1963): A microsomal nucleoside diphosphatase. *J. Biol. Chem.*, 238:710–716.
18. Schacter, H., and Roseman S. (1980): Mammalian glycosyltransferases. Their role in the synthesis and function of complex carbohydrates and glycolipids. In: *Biochemistry of Glycoproteins and Proteoglycans*, edited by W. J. Lennarz, pp. 85–160. Plenum, New York.
19. Novikoff, A. B. (1964): GERL, its form and function in neurons of rat spinal ganglia. *Biol. Bull.*, 127:358.
20. Novikoff, P. M., and Yam, A. (1978): Sites of lipoprotein particles in normal rat hepatocytes. *J. Cell Biol.*, 76:1–11.
21. Decker, R. S. (1974): Lysosomal packaging in differentiating and degenerating anuran lateral motor column neurons. *J. Cell Biol.*, 61:599–612.
22. Bentfeld, M. E., and Bainton, D. F. (1975): Cytochemical localization of lysosomal enzymes in rat megakaryocytes and platelets. *J. Clin. Invest.*, 56:1635–1649.
23. Paavola, L. G. (1978): The corpus luteum of the guinea pig II. Cytochemical studies on the Golgi complex, GERL, and lysosomes in luteal cells during maximum progesterone secretion. *J. Cell Biol.*, 79:45–73.
24. de Duve, C., and Wattiaux, R. (1966): Functions of lysosomes. *Ann. Rev. Physiol.*, 28:435–492.
25. de Duve, C. (1975): Exploring cells with a centrifuge. *Science*, 75:186–194.
26. Novikoff, A. B. (1973): Lysosomes, a personal account. In: *Lysosomes and Storage Diseases*, edited by G. Hers and F. Van Hoof, pp. 1–41. Academic Press, New York.
27. de Duve, C., and Baudhuin, P. (1966): Peroxisomes (microbodies and related particles). *Physiol. Rev.*, 46:323–357.
28. Novikoff, A. B., and Shin, W.-Y. (1964): The endoplasmic reticulum in the Golgi zone and its relations to microbodies, Golgi apparatus and autophagic vacuoles in rat liver cells. *J. Microsc.*, 3:187–206.
29. Essner, E. (1967): Endoplasmic reticulum and the origin of microbodies in fetal mouse liver. *Lab. Invest.*, 17:71–87.
30. Reddy, J., and Svoboda, D. (1971): Microbodies in experimentally altered cells. VIII. Continuities between microbodies and their possible biologic significance. *Lab. Invest.*, 24:72–81.
31. Lazarow, P. B., and De Duve C. (1976): A fatty acyl-CoA oxidizing system in rat liver peroxisomes; enhancement by clofibrate, a hypolipidemic drug. *Proc. Natl. Acad. Sci. USA*, 73:2043–2046.
32. Lazarow, P. B. (1978): Rat liver peroxisomes catalyse the β-oxidation of fatty acids. *J. Biol. Chem.*, 253:1522–1528.
33. Krisans, S. K., Mortensen, R. M., and Lazarow, P. B. (1980): Acyl-CoA synthetase in rat liver peroxisomes. *J. Biol. Chem.*, 255:9599–9607.
34. Novikoff, P. M., Roheim, P. S., Novikoff, A. B., and Edelstein, D. (1974): Production and prevention of fatty liver in rats fed clofibrate and orotic acid diets containing sucrose. *Lab. Invest.*, 30:732–750.
35. Novikoff, P. M., and Edelstein, D. (1977): Reversal of orotic acid-induced fatty liver in rats by clofibrate. *Lab. Invest.*, 36:215–231.
36. Novikoff, P. M., and Novikoff, A. B. (1972): Peroxisomes in absorptive cells of mammalian small intestine. *J. Cell. Biol.*, 53:532–560.
37. Reddy, J., and Svoboda, D. (1972): Microbodies (peroxisomes) in the interstitial cells of rodent testes. *Lab. Invest.*, 26:657–665.
38. Black, V. H., and Bogart, B. I. (1973): Peroxisomes in inner adrenal cortical cells of fetal and adult guinea pigs. *J. Cell Biol.*, 57:345–358.
39. Novikoff, A. B., Novikoff, P. M., Rosen, O. M., and Rubin, C. S. (1980): Organelle relationships in cultured 3T3-L1 preadipocytes. *J. Cell Biol.*, 87:180–196.
40. Novikoff, A. B., Novikoff, P. M., Davis, C., and Quintana, N.

(1973): Studies on microperoxisomes. V. Are microperoxisomes ubiquitous in mammalian cells? *J. Histochem. Cytochem.*, 21:737–755.

41. Novikoff, A. B. (1976): Occurrence of peroxisomes based on morphological criteria. In: *Cell Biology,* edited by P. L. Altman and B. D. Katz, pp. 332–334. Federation of the American Society of Experimental Biology, Bethesda.

42. Graham, R. C., Jr., and Karnovsky, M. J. (1966): The early stages of absorption of injected horseradish peroxidase in the proximal tubules of mouse kidney: Ultrastructural cytochemistry by a new technique. *J. Histochem. Cytochem.*, 14:291–302.

43. Novikoff, A. B., and Goldfischer, S. (1969): Visualization of peroxisomes (microbodies) and mitochondria with diaminobenzidine. *J. Histochem. Cytochem.*, 17:675–680.

44. Novikoff, A. B., Novikoff, P. M., Davis, C., and Quintana, N. (1972): Studies on microperoxisomes. II. A cytochemical method for light and electron microscopy. *J. Histochem. Cytochem.*, 20:1006–1022.

45. Svoboda, D. J., and Azarnoff, D. L. (1966): Response of hepatic microbodies to a hypolipidemic agent, ethyl chlorophenoxyisobutyrate (CPIB). *J. Cell Biol.*, 30:422–450.

46. Legg, P. G., and Wood, R. L. (1970): New observations on microbodies. A cytochemical study on CPIB-treated rat liver. *J. Cell Biol.*, 45:118–129.

47. Tolbert, N. E. (1981): Metabolic pathways in peroxisomes and glyoxysomes. *Ann. Rev. Biochem.*, 50:133–157.

48. Reddy, J. K. (1974): Hepatic microbody proliferation and catalase synthesis induced by methyl clofenapate, a hypolipidemic analog of CPIB. *Am. J. Pathol.*, 75:103–114.

49. Reddy, J. K., Azarnoff, D. L., Svoboda, D. J., and Prasad, J. D. (1974): Nafenopin-induced hepatic microbody (peroxisome) proliferation and catalase synthesis in rats and mice. *J. Cell Biol.*, 61:344–358.

50. Kennedy, E. P., and Lehninger, A. L. (1949): Oxidation of fatty acids and tricarboxylic acid cycle intermediates by isolated rat liver mitochondria. *J. Biol. Chem.*, 179:957–972.

51. Palade, G. E. (1952): The fine structure of mitochondria. *Anat. Rec.*, 114:427–451.

52. Hackenbrock, C. R., Rehn, T. G., Weinback, E. C., and Lemasters, J. J. (1971): Oxidative phosphorylation and ultrastructural transformation in mitochondria. *J. Cell Biol.*, 51:123–137.

53. Novikoff, A. B., Roheim, P., and Quintana, N. (1966): Changes in rat liver cells induced by orotic acid feeding. *Lab. Invest.*, 15:27–49.

54. Rajalakshi, S., Adams, W. R., and Handschumacher, R. E. (1969): Isolation and characterization of low density structures from orotic acid-induced fatty livers. *J. Cell Biol.*, 41:625–636.

55. Pottenger, L. A., and Getz, G. S. (1971): Serum lipoprotein accumulation in the livers of orotic acid-fed rats. *J. Lipid Res.*, 12:450–459.

56. Pottenger, L. A., Frazier, L. E., DuBien, L. H., Getz, G. S., and Wissler, R. W. (1973): Carbohydrate composition of lipoprotein apoproteins isolated from rat plasma and from the livers of rats fed orotic acid. *Biochim. Biophys. Res. Commun.*, 54:770–776.

57. Novikoff, P. M., and Yam, A. (1978): The cytochemical demonstration of GERL in rat hepatocytes during lipoprotein mobilization. *J. Histochem. Cytochem.*, 26:1–13.

58. Novikoff, A. B., Novikoff, P. M., Mori, M., and Levine, W. (1975): Cytochemical studies on rat hepatocytes following nafenopin treatment. *J. Histochem. Cytochem.*, 23:314–315.

59. Segal, P., Roheim, P. S., and Eder, H. A. (1972): Effect of clofibrate on lipoprotein metabolism in hyperlipidemic rats. *J. Clin. Invest.*, 51:1632–1638.

60. Shiff, T. S., Roheim, P. S., and Eder, H. A. (1971): Effects of high sucrose diets and 4-aminopyrazolopyrimidine on serum lipids and lipoproteins in the rat. *J. Lipid Res.*, 12:596–603.

61. Zucker, L. M., and Zucker, T. F. (1961): Fatty, a new mutation in a rat. *J. Hered.*, 53:275–278.

62. Bray, G. (1977): The Zucker-fatty rat. *Fed. Proc.*, 36:148–153.

63. Novikoff, P. M. (1977): Fatty liver induced in Zucker "fatty"

(ff) rats by a semisynthetic diet rich in sucrose. *Proc. Natl. Acad. Sci. USA*, 74:3550–3554.

64. Eder, H. A., Novikoff, P. M., Novikoff, A. B., Yam, A., Beyer, M., and Gidez, L. I. (1979): Biochemical and morphologic studies on diabetic rats: Effects of sucrose-enriched diet in rats with pancreatic islet transplants. *Proc. Natl. Acad. Sci. USA*, 76:5905–5909.

65. Schotz, M. C., Scanu, A., and Page, I. H. (1957): Effect of triton on lipoprotein lipase of rat plasma. *Ann. J. Physiol.*, 188:399–402.

66. Ishii, H., Fukumori, N., Hone, S., and Sugar, T. (1980): Effects of fat content in the diet on hepatic peroxisomes of the rat. *Biochim. Biophys. Acta*, 617:1–11.

67. Neat, C. E., Thomassen, M. S., and Osmundsen, H. (1980): Induction of peroximal β-oxidation in rat liver by high-fat diets. *Biochim. J.*, 186:369–371.

68. Novikoff, P. M., and Yam, A. (1981): Uptake of horseradish peroxidase by Kupffer cells and hepatocytes from cholesterol-fed obese rats. *J. Cell. Biol.*, 87:311a.

69. Stockert, R. J., Haimes, H., Morell, A. G., Novikoff, P. M., Novikoff, A. B., and Sternlieb, I. (1980): Endocytosis of asialoglycoprotein-enzyme conjugates by hepatocytes. *Lab. Invest.*, 43:556–563.

70. Novikoff, P. M., Yam, A., and Novikoff, A. B. (1981): The lysosomal compartment of macrophages: Extending the definition of GERL. *Proc. Natl. Acad. Sci. USA*, 78:5699–5703.

71. Van Berkel, T. J. C., and Van Tol, A. (1979): Role of parenchymal and non-parenchymal rat liver cells in the uptake of cholesterol-labelled serum lipoproteins. *Biochem. Biophys. Res. Commun.*, 89:1097–1101.

72. Van Tol, A., and Van Berkel, T. J. C. (1980): Uptake and degradation of rat and human very low density (remnant) apolipoproteins by parenchymal and non-parenchymal rat liver cells. *Biochim. Biophys. Acta*, 619:156–166.

73. Ose, L., Ose, T., Norum, K. R., and Berg, T. (1979): Uptake and degradation of ^{125}I-labelled high density lipoproteins in rat liver cells *in vivo* and *in vitro*. *Biochim. Biophys. Acta*, 574:521–536.

74. Van Berkel, T. J. C., Vaandrager, H., Kruijt, J. K., and Koster, J. F. (1980): Characteristics of acid lipase and acid cholesteryl esterase activity in parenchymal and non-parenchymal rat liver cells. *Biochim. Biophys. Acta*, 617:446–457.

75. Green, H. (1978): Conversion of 3T3 Cells. In: *Miami Winter Symposia. Differentiation and Development*, edited by F. Ahmad, T. R. Russel, J. Schultz, and R. Werner, vol. 15 pp. 12–36. Academic Press, New York.

76. Coleman, R. A., Brent, B. C., Mackall, J. C., Student, A. K., Lane, M. D., and Bell, R. M. (1978): Selective changes in microsomal enzymes of triacylglyceral phosphatidylcholine, and phosphatidylethanoline biosynthesis during differentiation of 3T3-L1 preadipocytes. *J. Biol. Chem.*, 253:7256–7261.

77. Kuri-Harcuch, W., and Green, H. (1977): Increasing activity of enzymes on pathway of triacylglycerol synthesis during adipose conversion of 3T3 cells. *J. Biol. Chem.*, 252:2158–2160.

78. Rubin, C. S., Hirsch, A., Fung, C., and Rosen, O. M. (1978): Development of hormone receptors and hormonal responsiveness *in vitro*. *J. Biol. Chem.*, 253:7570–7578.

79. Hajra, A. K., and Burke, C. (1978): Biosynthesis of phosphatidic acid in rat brain via acyl dihydroxyacetone phosphate. *J. Neurochem.*, 31:125–134.

80. Coleman, R., and Bell, R. M. (1978): Evidence that biosynthesis of phosphateylethanolamine, phosphatidylcholine and triacylglyceral occurs on the cytoplasmic side of microsomal vesicles. *J. Cell Biol.*, 76:245–253.

81. Smith, R. E., and Farquhar, M. G. (1966): Lysosome function in the regulation of the secretory process in cells of the anterior pituitary gland. *J. Cell Biol.*, 31:319–347.

82. Novikoff, P. M., Novikoff, A. B., Quintana, N., and Hauw, J.-J. (1971): Golgi apparatus, GERL and lysosomes of neurons in rat dorsal root ganglia, studied by thick section and thin section cytochemistry. *J. Cell Biol.*, 50:859–886.

83. Bennett, G., and O'Shaughnessy, D. (1981): The site of incorporation of sialic acid residues into glycoproteins and the subsequent fates of these molecules in various rat and mouse cell types as shown by radioautography after injection of [^{3}H] N-acetylmannosamin I. Observations in hepatocytes. *J. Cell Biol.,* 88:1–15.

84. Eisenberg, S. (1979): Lipoprotein metabolism. *Prog. Biochem. Pharmacol.,* 15:1.

85. Scanu, A., and Landsberger, F. R. (1980): Lipoprotein structure. *Ann. N.Y. Acad. Sci.,* 348:1.

86. Chao, Y.-S., Jones, A. L., Hradek, G. T., Windler, E. E. T., and Havel, R. J. (1981): Autoradiographic localization of the sites of uptake, cellular transport and catabolism of low density lipoproteins in the liver of normal and estrogen-treated rats. *Proc. Natl. Acad. Sci. USA,* 78:597–601.

87. Brown, M. S., Kovanen, P. T., and Goldstein, J. L. (1981): Regulation of plasma cholesterol by lipoprotein receptors. *Science,* 212:628–635.

88. Quin, P. S., and Judah, J. D. (1978): Calcium-dependent Golgi-vesicle fusion and cathepsin B in the conversion of proalbumin into albumin in rat liver. *Biochem. J.,* 172:301–309.

89. Yokata, S., and Fahimi, D. (1981): Immunocytochemical localization of albumin in the secretory apparatus of rat liver parenchymal cells. *Proc. Natl. Acad. Sci. USA,* 78:4970–4974.

The Liver: Biology and Pathobiology, edited by
I. Arias, H. Popper, D. Schachter, and D. A. Shafritz.
Raven Press, New York © 1982.

Chapter 10

Hormonal Control of Gene Expression

Lawrence Chan

GENE EXPRESSION

Proteins in living cells serve two primary functions: (a) they are the structural elements upon which cells are built; and (b) they serve as enzyme catalysts for chemical reactions in living systems. Hormones regulate cell function primarily by altering the expression and activity of some of these proteins. This chapter reviews the basic molecular mechanisms by which various hormones modulate expression, or synthesis, of specific proteins in eukaryotic cells.

The structure of a protein is ultimately determined by its gene. A gene may be defined as a sequence of DNA which is responsible for the synthesis of a single polypeptide chain. The transfer of genetic information from gene to protein through messenger RNA can be represented as follows:

$$DNA \rightleftharpoons RNA \rightarrow protein$$

This formula, the "central dogma" proposed by Crick (1,2), implies that genetic information is maintained by replication of DNA, which is then expressed by the synthesis of RNA and protein. Under certain cir-

cumstances (e.g., RNA tumor viruses) RNA molecules can be transcribed into DNA by an RNA-dependent DNA polymerase, reverse transcriptase. In the normal adult organism, however, the usual flow of genetic information is unidirectional, from DNA to RNA to protein. In simplistic terms, gene expression can be modified at either of these two major sites:

$$^3 DNA \overset{1}{\rightleftharpoons} RNA \overset{2}{\rightarrow} protein^4$$

at the transcriptional or the translational level. Because of the complex nature of the informational transfer, the levels of regulation in transcription and translation potentially involve numerous steps. Furthermore, the maintenance of genetic information can also be modulated at the level of DNA replication and posttranslational protein modification and degradation. Since some of these reactions require the participation of new hormone-induced proteins or of altered levels of preexisting proteins, such as specific enzymes, the detailed scheme of the hormonal control of gene expression is extremely complex. Only the earliest and possibly primary action of hormones on cellular function are reviewed. Other aspects of hormonal action in hepatic protein synthesis are discussed elsewhere in this volume.

DEFINITION AND CLASSIFICATION OF HORMONES

A hormone is a chemical messenger secreted by one cell (an "endocrine" cell), which modulates the function and activity of another cell (a "target" cell). Classically, the target cell is at some remote site, and the hormone is carried to this site by the circulatory system. There are many exceptions to this generalization, and hormones often reach their target cells by diffusion through tissue fluid without going through the intravascular compartment. It has also been proposed that some hormones [e.g., somatostatin in the pancreatic islets (3)] might migrate to neighboring target cells within the same organ. Hence the only prerequisite for labeling any molecule a hormone is that it must act specifically on a cell other than the cell that produces it.

Hormones can be classified according to their structure or function. The traditional classification based on hormone structure (e.g., polypeptide hormones, steroid and sterol hormones, and amine hormones) is invaluable in terms of the biosynthesis of these hormones. Even though there is some overlap in the mechanism of action of hormones within each structural group, this classification is largely unsatisfactory from the standpoint of function. The simplest and most general classification of hormones is that which takes into account both the initial site of interaction of the hormone with the target cell and the chemical structure of the hormone molecule (Table 1).

The major membrane receptor-mediated hormones include the polypeptide hormones, catecholamines, and neurotransmitters. The major intracellular receptor-mediated hormones include the steroid and sterol hormones and the thyroid hormones. Apart from differences in the initial steps of action, the two major classes of hormone are distinct in other ways: the membrane receptor-mediated hormones exist largely as free molecules in blood and have evanescent half-lives (minutes), whereas the intracellular receptor-mediated hormones are mostly bound to specific plasma proteins and generally have longer half-lives (hours to days).

HORMONE RECEPTORS IN HORMONE ACTION

General Principles

The fluids bathing various tissues in the body contain a multitude of different chemical molecules, including numerous hormones. For a cell to respond to

TABLE 1. *General classification of hormones*[a]

Membrane receptor-mediated hormones
    Peptide hormones
    Catecholamines
    Neurotransmitters

Intracellular receptor-mediated hormones
    Steroid hormones
    Vitamin D sterols
    Thyroid hormones[b]

---

[a] This is a simplified classification of hormones based on both their site of initial interaction with the target cell and the chemical structure. For most hormones, the two alternative receptor pathways may not be mutually exclusive. However, the major mode of action of these hormones is listed according to our present understanding.

[b] Recently, Cheng et al. (96) presented evidence that tetramethylrhodamine-labeled triiodothyronine appears to be taken up by cultured mouse fibroblasts via membrane receptor-mediated endocytosis. Similar techniques have not been applied to the steroid and sterol hormones. Since intracellular receptors clearly have been well demonstrated for these hormones, the classification remains valid.

some of these hormones, it must possess specific receptors which recognize the hormones and bind them selectively. The presence or absence of specific hormone receptors determines whether a cell is a target for the specific hormones involved.

Hormone Receptors: Basic Criteria

A number of criteria must be satisfied before a cellular component or molecule is labeled a receptor to a specific hormone.

High affinity of binding.

Hormone molecules are bound to receptors and are retained on the surface of or inside the target cell against a concentration gradient; hormones generally circulate at relatively low concentrations (10^{-10} to 10^{-8} M). Furthermore, various plasma proteins bind various hormones with considerable affinity; hence receptor hormone binding is characterized by high affinity. To explore the concept of high affinity more quantitatively, we examine the following equation:

$$R + H \rightleftharpoons RH \rightarrow R^*H \rightarrow Effect \qquad [1]$$

where R is the receptor, H is the hormone molecule, RH is the receptor hormone complex, and R^*H represents a hypothetical transition state required for RH to produce an effect. For simplicity, consider the initial part of the reaction:

$$R + H \underset{k_{-1}}{\overset{k_1}{\rightleftharpoons}} RH \qquad [2]$$

where k_1 and k_{-1} are the association and dissociation rate constants, respectively.

Now

$$k_1 = \frac{[RH]}{[R] \cdot [H]} \qquad [3]$$

and

$$k_{-1} = \frac{[R] \cdot [H]}{[RH]} \qquad [4]$$

At equilibrium, the rate of conversion of R and H into RH (namely, $k_1 [R] \cdot [H]$) is equal to the rate of the dissociation of RH into R and H (namely, $k_{-1} [RH]$). That is,

$$k_1 [R]_e \cdot [H]_e = k_{-1}[RH]_e \qquad [5]$$

hence

$$\frac{k_1}{k_{-1}} = \frac{[RH]_e}{[R]_e \cdot [H]_e} = Ka \qquad [6]$$

where Ka is defined as the equilibrium constant of association. By inverting equation [6], we obtain

$$\frac{k_{-1}}{k_1} = \frac{[R]_e \cdot [H]_e}{[RH]_e} = Kd \qquad [7]$$

where Kd is the equilibrium constant of dissociation, often referred to simply as "dissociation constant."

A simple binding curve for a hormone to its receptor is shown in Fig. 1A. The interrupted lines represent nonspecific and total (specific + nonspecific) binding. Nonspecific binding is measured as the amount of labeled hormone bound in the presence of excess quantities of homologous hormone. The linear increase in nonspecific binding indicates that this component is nonsaturable; i.e., it has unlimited capacity for the hormone (see below). Specific binding, on the other hand, is saturable and takes the form of a rectangular hyperbola. It can be described by a form of the Michaelis-Menton equation, derived from equation [7], as

$$[RH] = \frac{([RH] + [R]) \cdot [H]}{Kd + [H]} \qquad [8]$$

when half of the receptor sites are occupied; i.e., $[RH] = 1/2([RH] + [R])$, then $Kd = [H]$ (Fig. 1A). This is a direct way to determine Kd. Unfortunately, since the total number of binding sites ($[RH] + [R]$) is an asymptotic function, the Kd cannot be accurately estimated from the binding curve shown in Fig. 1A. A popular graphic method for obtaining both ($[RH] + [R]$) and Kd simultaneously is Scatchard analysis (4)

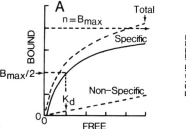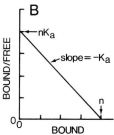

FIG. 1. A: Receptor hormone binding curve. **B:** Scatchard plot of receptor hormone binding.

(Fig. 1B). The derivation of the Scatchard equation is as follows. From equation [6]:

$$\begin{aligned}
\frac{[RH]}{[H]} &= Ka\,[R] \\
&= Ka\,([HR] + [R] - [HR]) \\
&= Ka[HR] - Ka\,([HR] + [R]) \qquad [9]
\end{aligned}$$

Thus a plot of $[RH]/[H]$ versus $[RH]$ will give $-Ka$ as the slope, $Ka\,([HR] + [R])$ as the Y-intercept and ($[HR] + [R]$) as the X-intercept. For simplicity, n, the molarity of total binding sites, is used in Fig. 1B to represent the function ($[HR] + [R]$). Kd can be derived from the relationship $Kd = 1/Ka$.

Since Ka and n can be readily obtained from Scatchard analysis, it is simple to compare these parameters in different experimental situations. For example, the "steeper" the binding curve, the higher the affinity of binding (or Ka which has units of M^{-1}); the X-intercept also can be directly compared for the total number of hormone binding sites (n) in such circumstances.

Although Scatchard plots are popular, there are alternative ways of expressing binding data, each of which offers certain features that render it particularly useful in defined situations. The double reciprocal (Lineweaver-Burk) plot (5) (Fig. 2A) gives an accurate measure of 1/n. However, it gives larger percentage errors at lower free hormone concentrations and hence larger errors in the 1/nKa value. The direct linear plot (Eisenthal-Cornish-Bowden) (6–8) (Fig. 2B) is simple and can be plotted directly ($[HR]$ versus $[H]$) without calculations; Kd and n are obtained directly from the intersection of multiple lines projecting on the X and Y axes, respectively. Hence hormone receptors are characterized by their high affinity as defined by a low Kd, generally ranging from 10^{-8} to 10^{-10} M.

Finite binding capacity.

As discussed above, receptor hormone binding displays saturation kinetics. This property differentiates the "nonspecific" binding sites, which are of "unlimited" capacity. In a binding curve (Fig. 1A) using

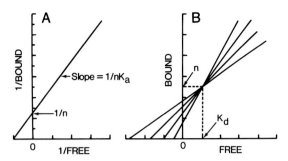

FIG. 2. A: Lineweaver-Burk plot of receptor hormone binding. **B:** Direct linear plot (Eisenthal-Cornish-Bowden) of receptor hormone binding.

radiolabeled hormones, nonspecific binding sites cannot be effectively competed by an excess of unlabeled hormone. Specific saturable binding sites represent from 15 to 30% to >95% of total binding, depending on both the specific hormone and the specific tissue examined. For intracellular receptors, in tissues such as the liver, generally "nonspecific" binding sites constitute a fairly high proportion of the total binding, since the liver contains a multitude of structural and enzymatic proteins that bind various ligands nonspecifically (or, in some cases, such as steroid hormones, specifically).

Hormone specificity.

Cellular receptors (membrane associated or soluble) discriminate between various hormones and "pick them out" by binding to these molecules specifically. Other types of hormones, however, exist in "classes." For example, many steroid hormones can be classified as mineralocorticoids, e.g., aldosterone, 11-deoxycorticosterone, and fludrocortisone. It is now evident that these mineralocorticoids all bind to the same receptors.

The assessment of the "fit" of a particular hormone molecule to a receptor involves competition with an excess of the prototype hormone, which, in the case of mineralocorticoids, would be aldosterone. It should be noted that agonist as well as antagonist hormone analogs bind to specific receptors. For example, spironolactone binds with high affinity to the mineralocorticoid receptor. The analogous situation occurs with other steroid hormone antagonists, e.g., antiestrogens and antiandrogens. This concept is even more important in the case of membrane receptors. Numerous hormone analogs bind to these receptors with high affinity, e.g., anti-α- and β-adrenergic agents, and various polypeptide hormone analogs. Some of these analogs are especially convenient tools to study receptor biochemistry, since they are more easily obtained in a labeled form than the parent hormone, e.g., [3H]dihydroalprenolol binding to the β-adrenergic re-

ceptor. Hence hormone specificity defines whether or not a tissue is a target organ for a class of hormones.

Tissue specificity.

Only certain organs and tissues will respond to a particular hormone at physiologic concentrations. For example, the classic target organs for estrogens include the vagina, uterus, and pituitary, and for parathyroid hormone, the kidney and bone. For a number of hormones, e.g., glucocorticoid and thyroid hormones, however, it is likely that their specific receptors are widely distributed. This is easily appreciated if we realize that these types of hormones exert general effects on many tissues. Even for hormones with more restrictive actions, such as androgens and estrogens, tissues and organs previously not recognized to be targets have now been found to contain specific receptors. For example, estrogen receptors have been found in skin as well as in liver, albeit in low concentrations compared to those in the uterus. Hence, the terms "target" and "nontarget" tissues probably signify a quantitative rather than a qualitative difference between these tissues. This will be important in future investigations.

Biologic response.

Since hormone receptor binding usually is studied under highly artifactual conditions, before any interaction is labeled receptor binding, it must be followed by a biologic response. The latter can be in the form of some physical change (e.g., water imbibition in the uterus in response to estrogen), changes in enzyme activity (e.g., many hormone-induced changes in adenylate cyclase activity or RNA polymerase activities), or growth and cell division. While biologic response ideally is a prerequisite for designating any interaction receptor binding, it is often difficult to establish such a relationship. This is especially true in the case of many noncyclic nucleotide-mediated peptide hormones, e.g., insulin receptors in monocytes. The best examples for correlation of the presence of receptors with biologic responses are (a) in the case of testicular feminization, where the absence of normal androgen receptors results in the expression of the female phenotype in a genetic male (10), and (b) the absence of normal glucocorticoid receptors in steroid-resistant lymphoma cell lines (11).

Receptor-Hormone Interactions

Interpretations of the nonlinear Scatchard plots.

A common observation in hormone receptor binding studies is the nonlinearity of many Scatchard analyses. There are two possible situations (12):

1. A concave-downward Scatchard analysis (Fig.

3A) implies that as the amount of ligand increases (so that the amount bound goes up), the slope becomes steeper; i.e., the apparent affinity constant increases. This can be caused by "cooperativity" or a "homotropic" allosteric effect involving a di- or polyvalent receptor. However, errors in estimation of tracer concentrations or nonspecific counts should be excluded.

2. A concave-upward Scatchard plot (Fig. 3B) is a more common situation in binding experiments. Possibilities include (a) heterogeneity or multiplicity of receptor-binding sites, and (b) presence of negative cooperativity, i.e., a di- or polyvalent receptor, with a reduction of affinity of remaining sites after the first site(s) are filled. Other possible artifactual considerations, such as differences in affinities of the labeled and unlabeled ligand, and errors in separation of bound and free ligand, should also be excluded. Negative cooperativity is dealt with elsewhere in this volume.

The heterogeneity of three classes of binding sites is represented in Fig. 3B: one with "high" affinity, one with "intermediate" affinity, and one with "nonspecific" interactions. The high and intermediate sites are specific, saturable sites; the "nonspecific" sites are nonsaturable and can be identified by competition experiments (Fig. 1A). Data plots for the specific sites can be obtained by vectorial analysis (the sum of the component curves should equal the composite curve) or by a computer program. A common error is direct extrapolation of the curve to the X-axis (interrupted lines in Fig. 3B), which invariably overestimates n. Such an erroneous maneuver also underestimates the affinity for the higher affinity class and overestimates that for the lower affinity class of receptors.

Role of Hormone Receptors in Hormone Action

We examine the role of intracellular hormone receptors in the mode of action of hormones. The steps involved in such a pathway can be divided into the following (13): (a) delivery of hormone to, and its binding by, target tissue; (b) translocation of the hormone receptor complex into the nucleus; (c) hormone receptor interactions with chromatin; and (d) hormone-induced alterations in gene expression.

Delivery of Hormone to, and Its Binding by, Target Tissue

The soluble receptor-mediated hormones are preferentially retained by their target organs. With the exception of thyroid hormones, specific cytoplasmic receptors bind their respective class of hormones as they diffuse through the cell membrane. Since most of the hormones are delivered to the target organ via the bloodstream, they are largely presented to the tissue in the form of noncovalent complexes with proteins (14–17). The affinities of these binding proteins vary considerably, with association constants of 10^6 to 10^9 M^{-1} (Table 2). Their presence in plasma restricts the delivery of free hormone to target cells. Hence they may act as both carrier proteins and modulators of hormone action.

The concentration of these binding proteins in plasma varies considerably under physiologic and pathologic conditions. For example, the concentration of both cortisol binding globulin (CBG) and sex steroid binding globulin (SBG) are regulated by estrogen and testosterone and are markedly elevated during the second and especially the third trimester of pregnancy. Furthermore, both of these proteins are also regulated by other hormones, such as thyroid hormones. It is likely that variations in the concentrations of these binding proteins result in modulations of steroid hormone action. For example, increases in SBG concentrations during pregnancy might offset the possible androgenization resulting from elevated unbound testosterone. The importance of these binders in the

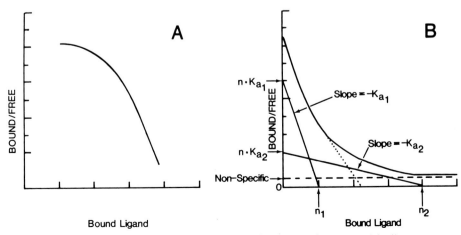

FIG. 3. Nonlinear Scatchard plot of receptor hormone binding.

TABLE 2. *Properties of the major high affinity hormone binders in plasma* [a]

Plasma binder	Molecular weight (daltons)	Plasma concentration (M^{-1})	Approximate affinity constant at 37° C (M^{-1})
CBG	52,000	7×10^7	3×10^7 (to cortisol)
			9×10^7 (to progesterone)
			6×10^6 (to aldosterone)
SBG	98,000	$4-6 \times 10^8$ (nonpregnant women)	1×10^9 (to dihydrotestosterone)
		$2-3 \times 10^7$ (pregnant women)	2×10^7 (to testosterone)
Vitamin D binding protein	55,000	6×10^6	5×10^9 (to estradiol)
			6×10^8 (to 25-hydroxy-vitamin D_3)
Thyroxine-binding globulin (TBG)	63,000	6×10^7	3×10^7 (to 1,25-dihydroxy-vitamin D_3)
			2×10^{10} (to thyroxine)
Thyroxine-binding prealbumin (TBPA)	70,000	$3-5 \times 10^6$	2×10^9 (to triiodothyroxine)
			2×10^8 (to thyroxine)[b]
			1.6×10^7 (to triiodothyronine)

[a] Compiled from data from a number of laboratories.
[b] There appears to be two binding sites with widely different affinities, 2×10^8 and 2×10^6 M^{-1}.

modulation of hormone action has been confirmed by *in vitro* studies, which demonstrate that their presence markedly affects both the uptake and retention of steroids by target cells.

Another protein molecule with high binding affinity for estrogen not listed in Table 2 is α-fetoprotein. This protein binds estradiol with high affinity (Ka, 10^{10} M^{-1}) and probably functions by limiting the delivery of otherwise toxic levels of hormone to peripheral tissues in the human fetus. The concentration of α-fetoprotein gradually declines from high levels in the newborn to very low levels just before puberty. This decline may allow increased delivery of estrogen to the target organs at a critical time of development.

In addition to the high-affinity plasma binders listed in Table 2, other molecules in blood bind steroid hormones with lower affinity. Furthermore, CBG also binds to testosterone and estradiol with low affinity (18). Albumin is probably the most important low-affinity binder for thyroid and steroid hormones because of its high concentration in blood (7×10^{-4} M) and its high capacity for these hormones. There is good evidence *in vitro* that the uptake and retention of steroid hormones is affected by the addition of albumin to the medium. Since plasma concentrations of albumin vary markedly under pathological states such as prematurity, cirrhosis of the liver, nephrotic syndrome, and malnutrition, some of the complications of these disease states might be modulated by changes in albumin concentrations.

Another important effect of plasma binding proteins on intracellular receptor-mediated hormone action is that they might differentially affect the action of one hormone with respect to another. For example, when tested *in vitro* in the absence of plasma, estradiol dem-onstrates a 10-fold greater affinity for receptor than estriol. When administered intravenously *in vivo*, however, both estriol and estradiol stimulate early uterotropic events in a comparable fashion (19,20). This probably is the result of a 10- to 100-fold higher affinity of plasma binding proteins for estradiol than for estriol. This consideration is especially important in the case of synthetic steroids, which generally bind plasma proteins with widely different affinities compared with the natural steroids.

Another important function of the plasma binders is the storage of various hormones. The vascular system is a reservoir for large amounts of steroid hormones, thyroid hormones, and sterol vitamins. This function is especially important for the latter two classes of hormone, since the production of the thyronines and vitamin D is highly dependent on exogenous input in the form of diet (iodides or vitamin D-containing foodstuff) or sunlight. If denied access to these external sources, man becomes deficient in these hormones. For both these two hormone systems, the specific plasma proteins bind the less active prohormones with considerably higher affinity. This suggests that the primary function of these proteins is storage rather than modulation of the action of their specific ligands. The relative importance of these proteins as modulators of hormone action is unknown, since this aspect of their possible function has not been studied as thoroughly as that for the steroid hormone-binding proteins.

Translocation of the Hormone-Receptor Complex to the Cell Nucleus

After a hormone is bound to a cytoplasmic receptor, the next step in its action involves transfer of the hormone-receptor complex into the target cell nucleus. It is within the latter compartment that the hormone exerts its influence on gene activity.

For all the intracellular receptor-mediated hormones, except thyroid hormones, the cytoplasmic hormone receptor complex undergoes a temperature-dependent "activation" step before it is transferred to the nucleus. This "two-step mechanism" was independently proposed by Jensen et al. (21) and Gorski et al. (22) for estrogen action in the uterus. It has been found to be true for other steroid hormones (13), as well as for 1,25-dihydroxyvitamin D (23), in their respective target tissues. The activation step may or may not be accompanied by measurable conformational change in the hormone receptor complex. Furthermore, in some systems, additional factors become associated with the complex before it is translocated to the cell nucleus.

Concomitant with the transfer of the hormone receptor complex into the nucleus, the concentration of cytoplasmic hormone receptor complex is depleted. This provides additional evidence that it is a direct transfer of the hormone receptor complex itself, rather than of the hormone only, into the nuclear compartment. This cytoplasmic depletion of the receptor is followed by its reappearance or "replenishment" hours later. At present, it is not certain how much of this replenishment is mediated by recycling and how much represents *de novo* synthesis of protein receptor.

Evidence suggests that the cellular compartmentalization of receptor molecules is correlated with biologic responses. Clark and Peck (24) suggested that long-term nuclear retention of estrogen receptors is required for true uterine growth. They have shown that treatment of the immature rat with various estrogenic compounds results in altered uterine growth. The nature of these alterations is dependent on the nuclear retention of the estrogen receptor steroid complex. Treatment with estrogenic compounds, such as estradiol, which cause long-term nuclear retention of the receptor, results in true uterine growth. On the other hand, single injections of short-acting estrogens, such as estriol, which are not retained in the nucleus, result in no significant uterine growth. In addition, nuclear retention of receptor steroid complex has been correlated temporarily with RNA polymerase activities and increase in RNA synthesis initiation sites (20). Korach et al. (25) recently found that a variety of analogs of diethylstilbestrol may be ineffective estrogens because they alter the normal rate of receptor clearance from the nucleus. This clearance process may be an essential component in the mechanism of estrogen hormone action. Hence both nuclear retention and replenishment of cytoplasmic receptors are important factors in steroid hormone action.

Thyroid hormones differ from other soluble receptor-mediated hormones in one important way; namely, triiodothyronine and thyroxine seem to bind directly to specific nuclear receptors without a cytoplasmic intermediary (26–28). They are found in the nucleus in equal amounts, whether or not the cell has been previously exposed to the hormone. An excellent correlation also has been observed between the affinity of the binding between the thyroid hormones and various iodothyronine analogs to the receptors, and the biologic potency of the analog (29,30).

Hormone Receptor Interactions with Chromatin

The nuclear receptors of the various hormones interact with the target cell nuclear chromatin. The two major components in the latter with which the receptors interact are nuclear DNA and nuclear proteins.

Receptor-DNA interaction.

Nuclear receptors of steroid and thyroid hormones often can be released partially or almost completely upon treatment with deoxyribonuclease (31,32). This indicates that DNA is an important component of the nuclear acceptor sites for the receptors. Studies of DNA binding of various receptors generally reveal no specificity for the source of DNA; prokaryotic as well as eukaryotic DNA from a wide variety of organisms bind these receptors with equal affinity. Furthermore, denatured (single-stranded) DNA binds receptor more effectively than does native (double-stranded) DNA. The absence of specificity of receptor-DNA binding indicates that other components in chromatin may be important in the interaction of the receptor with target cell genome.

Receptor-chromosomal protein interaction.

Steroid hormone receptors bind to target cell chromatin to a much greater extent than to nontarget cell chromatin. This tissue specificity, which is absent in binding studies on naked DNA, appears to reside in the nonhistone protein fraction of nuclear chromatin. Various partially purified fractions of nonhistone proteins have been described which bind steroid receptors. In the chick oviduct system, two distinct forms of the progesterone receptor have been described. They are the A (MW 79,000) and B (MW 117,000) "subunits" (33–36). Although these two proteins differ significantly in physicochemical characteristics, they are similar in many respects. For example, both display identical hormone-binding kinetics and steroid specificity; both are capable of binding to DNA (DNA-cellulose), although the interaction of A with DNA is much stronger than that of B. On the other hand, the B protein, but not the A protein, binds well to chromatin. These differential binding properties suggest that the A protein might function *in vivo* as the actual gene regulatory protein, whereas the B protein might facilitate the binding of A to the correct region of chromatin.

In the case of thyroid hormone receptors, apart from binding experiments, the receptors can be fixed to chromatin with formaldehyde (37). Formaldehyde treatment of chromatin fixes histones and a small proportion of the nonhistone proteins to DNA. The distribution of histones fixed on chromatin by this technique was nonrandom and did not result from histone exchange during the experiment (14). This provides further evidence for the close association of the receptors to proteins associated with chromatin.

Hormone-Induced Alterations in Gene Expression

Once the hormone receptor complex interacts with chromatin, various alterations in gene expression have been observed. These include changes in RNA polymerase activities (38–40) and in the availability of various DNA regions for transcription. The latter has been revealed by measurement of chromatin template activity *in vitro* (41), by hybridization analyses of RNA sample isolated under various hormonal conditions (42), and by an alteration in the number of RNA synthesis initiation sites (39). Observations on the genomic effects of various hormones have been made on a limited number of systems and are discussed in the following section.

HORMONAL REGULATION OF GENE EXPRESSION

Recent Concepts of Gene Structure

A detailed structure of hormone-regulatable genes forms the basis for any theory about how hormones affect gene expression. The genetic material for a number of hormone-regulatable proteins has been purified and amplified by recombinant DNA techniques. These include ovalbumin, ovomucoid, conalbumin, vitellogenin, apoVLDL-II, growth hormone, and beta-lipotropin or "procorticotropin." Since ovalbumin is the best characterized system, it is presented as a model of a steroid hormone-regulatable gene.

The ovalbumin structural gene was purified and amplified by cloning in the bacterial strain ×1776 using the tetracycline-resistant plasmid pMB9. By this technique, McReynolds et al. (43) cloned a 1,859 base-pair segment corresponding to the entire coding sequence (1,158 nucleotides) plus 64 noncoding nucleotides at the 5′-end and 637 noncoding nucleotides at its 3′-end, excluding the polyadenylate tail. Using the cloned ovalbumin structural gene as a probe, segments of the natural gene were identified in total chick DNA. These segments are amplified by insertion into the bacteriophage lambda systems (λ-gtWES · B and Charon 4A). Detailed analyses of the cloned genomic ovalbumin gene uncovered unexpected findings. These observations, coupled with analogous findings in the structure of other natural genes (44,45), revolutionized our thinking on the structure-organization of eukaryotic genes and the regulation of expression of these genes.

Instead of an exact complimentary replica of the cytoplasmic mRNA, the natural ovalbumin gene was found to be discontinuous (46–50), as shown schematically in Fig. 4. The structural gene sequence is divided into eight portions in genomic chick DNA by seven intervening DNA sequences, or introns. Therefore, the chromosomal ovalbumin gene is not colinear with its mature cytoplasmic mRNA product. The natural gene (>8,000 bases long) is approximately four times longer than the mRNA (1,859 bases long). The distribution of the introns is nonrandom, since all seven introns appear in the 5′-half of the structural gene (with respect to the mRNA).

The presence of intervening sequences has been detected in the genes of numerous other proteins, as well as in the tRNA genes and the cytochrome b gene of yeast mitochondria (44,45). There are a number of exceptions, the most notable of which are the histone genes, which seem not to contain introns (51). The origin and significance of introns in eukaryotic genes are unknown and have been discussed in previous reviews (44,45,52). They are apparently needed for the expression of genomic transcripts as mature cytoplasmic mRNAs (53). Superficially, the inclusion of introns in native DNA appears to be a redundant, wasteful mechanism, since none of the introns is expressed as a protein. However, the additional DNA may allow for a more flexible modulation of protein expression under various selective processes.

Induction of Specific Protein Synthesis by Steroid, Thyroid, and Sterol Hormones

Regulation of protein synthesis in target tissues is undoubtedly a major action of intracellular receptor-mediated hormones. The rate of synthesis of large numbers of proteins is affected by hormones in tissues which respond by growth and differentiation (e.g., chick oviduct in response to estrogen). In differentiated tissues, such as the liver, it is likely that these hormones cause major changes in the rate of synthesis of only a small proportion (probably 1% or less) of proteins expressed. For example, Ivarie and O'Farrell (54) have analyzed the pattern of newly synthesized proteins in cultured hepatoma cells in response to glucocorticoids. The cellular proteins were pulse la-

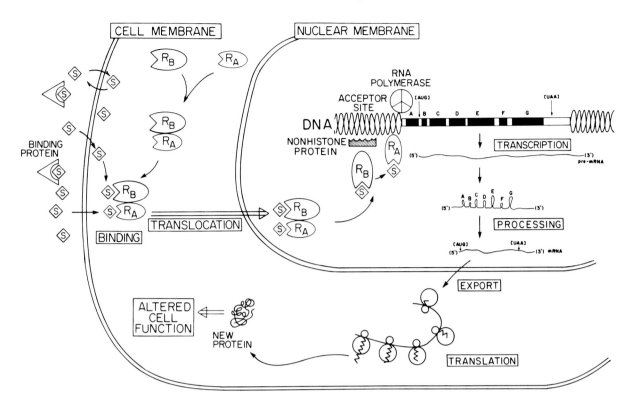

FIG. 4. Control of gene expression by steroid hormones. (Reprinted with permission from ref. 97.) The gene structure shown is that of ovalbumin. Introns are shown in black and labeled alphabetically. The steroid hormone receptor structure is based on information from the progesterone receptor in the chick oviduct; it may or may not hold for other steroid hormones. S, steroid hormone; R_A and R_B, steroid hormone receptor subunits. The steroid receptor dimer (R_A + R_B) enters the nucleus and binds to chromatin "acceptor sites" composed of DNA and nonhistone protein. After this interaction in a manner not yet completely understood, transcription of the ovalbumin gene (and other induced genes) is initiated. The primary transcript is a large RNA molecule that contains a complement of the entire natural gene (structural sequences plus intervening sequences). After transcription, a series of complex processing reactions occurs, such that the intervening sequence RNA segments are specifically excised, and the structural sequences are ligated together to form the mature biologically active mRNA. After export to the cytoplasm and translation of these mRNA molecules on cytoplasmic ribosomes, new hormone-induced proteins appear.

beled by radioactive methionine and were separated into individual spots by the sensitive technique of two-dimensional electrophoresis. Over 1,000 labeled proteins could be resolved by this technique. These workers found that in cultured hepatoma cell lines, glucocorticoid caused a consistent, major increase in the rate of synthesis of about seven proteins, as revealed by the appearance of radioactive spots, and infrequent changes in another 16 proteins (either induced and/or repressed). Since minor (10 to 20%) changes in synthesis are not detected by their technique, many more proteins may be modulated by glucocorticoids. The observation does indicate that in differentiated tissues, hormone-induced changes are highly selective, affecting only about 0.5 to 1% of genes being expressed. Similarly, in pituitary cell lines in culture, dexamethasone and triiodothyronine significantly affect the synthesis of only three identifiable proteins (55): growth hormone [which is stimulated by triiodothyronine (56)], prolactin (which is inhibited by dexamethasone), and p16, a protein of unidentified function

(which is stimulated by triiodothyronine). Inhibition (or repression) of the expression of specific proteins is probably equally important in the mechanism of action of these hormones.

Because of the complexity of hormone-induced responses, important advances in our knowledge of hormonal control of gene expression have been made through studies in model systems. Many of these studies have been reviewed previously (57). They represent important contributions to our understanding of hormone action. Studies of proteins in Table 3 generally indicate that in most of the model systems studied, intracellular receptor-mediated hormones regulate the expression of specific proteins at a pretranslational level. Except for embryonal or dormant cells and altered physiologic states, an alteration in the rate of synthesis of any protein is associated with a similar alteration in the concentration of its specific mRNA. This indicates the mRNA availability is probably more important than efficiency of translation in the action of these hormones, even though translational efficiency

TABLE 3. *Specific proteins induced by intracellular receptor-mediated hormones* [a]

Hormone	Tissue	Protein
Estrogen	Chick oviduct	Ovalbumin
	Chick oviduct	Conalbumin
	Chick oviduct	Lysozyme
	Chick oviduct	Ovomucoid
	Chick liver	apoVLDL-II
	Chick liver	Vitellogenin
	Xenopus liver	Vitellogenin
	Rat pituitary	Prolactin
Progesterone	Chick oviduct	Avidin
	Rabbit uterus	Uteroglobin
Androgen	Rat liver	α-2u-globulin
	Mouse liver	Major urinary protein complex
	Rat prostate	Aldolase
Glucocorticoids	Rat liver	Tyrosine aminotransferase
	Rat liver	Tryptophan oxygenase
	Rat kidney	PEP carboxykinase
	Mouse mammary cells	Mammary tumor virus RNA
	Embryonic chicken retina	Glutamine synthetase
	Rat pituitary cell culture	Growth hormone
	Rat pituitary	Corticotropin [b]
Vitamin D	Chick intestine	Calcium binding protein
Triiodothyronine	Rat pituitary cell culture	Growth hormone

[a] Includes those proteins the mRNAs of which have been demonstrated by translation or nucleic acid hybridization. The level of regulation can be evaluated only in these instances. (See ref. 57 for references to most of these studies.)
[b] Corticotropin mRNA is "turned off" rather than induced by glucocorticoids.

may also be altered in certain situations. The availability of mRNA is controlled by the rate of transcription and posttranscriptional processing of the intranuclear transcripts, as well as the rate of degradation of the mature mRNAs. Presently, there is no evidence that posttranscriptional processing represents a primary hormone-regulatable step in the supply of translatable mRNAs. However, both the rates of transcription and degradation of mRNAs seem to be important in determining the availability of specific mRNAs under the influence of various hormones.

Differential Hormonal Control of Specific Gene Products

Regulation of the expression of specific genes is a major mechanism of action of many hormones. Two different aspects of this process are intriguing in terms of the underlying mechanisms: (a) in the same tissue, different hormone-responsive genes often are regulated at entirely different rates; and (b) in a number of instances, the same gene product is expressed in two

different tissues, and the response of these tissues to a specific hormone is entirely different. In the chick oviduct, estrogen stimulates the synthesis of a number of different egg white proteins. The rate with which these proteins respond to the hormone is unique for each. For example, in response to a single injection of estrogen to hormone-withdrawn chicks, the initial rate of accumulation of conalbumin mRNA in the oviduct is considerably more rapid than that for ovalbumin mRNA (58). However, the maximum response is lower than that for ovalbumin. An even more dramatic example is the effect of estrogen on several different liver proteins in the cockerel. In this animal, apoVLDL-II (59), a major egg yolk protein, seems to accumulate in the liver most rapidly; this is followed closely by the accumulation of vitellogenin, another major yolk protein. ApoA-I, an apoprotein in avian high density lipoproteins, does not show any detectable response to a single dose of the hormone and accumulates only after multiple injections. Ovalbumin, an oviduct protein normally not expressed in the liver, also begins to accumulate, albeit at low levels, in this organ after multiple injections of the hormone (60,61). In the case of apoVLDL-II, vitellogenin and ovalbumin, the specific mRNAs can be shown to respond in a similar fashion after estrogen treatment (62–64).

These observations on the differential responses of different proteins to the same hormone are interesting. Undoubtedly, some of the differences could be accounted for by secondary effects of the hormone on the tissue. However, other factors involving hormone receptor and chromosomal protein ("acceptors") interactions are probably also important.

Another intriguing observation is that the same protein expressed in two different tissues responds differently to the same hormone. Conalbumin in the chick oviduct and transferrin in the avian liver appear to comprise identical polypeptide chains (60). This protein appears also to be produced in a number of other tissues, including spleen, kidney, lung, brain, and bone marrow (65). The regulation of this protein in the chick oviduct and liver was studied by Lee et al. (66), who found that both estrogen and progesterone cause a rapid and marked accumulation of hybridizable mRNA for conalbumin in the oviduct. In the liver, however, there was a significant lag in the response of transferrin mRNA to estrogen, and the degree of stimulation was much less (1.5- to twofold compared to six- to eightfold in the oviduct). Furthermore, progesterone was without effect on transferrin synthesis.

Similarly, uteroglobin appears to be produced in both lung and endometrium. However, only the endometrium responds to progesterone treatment with an accumulation of the mRNA for this protein (67). This failure of the lung to respond to the hormone is probably not due to the lack of progesterone receptors in this tissue, since such specific receptors are demonstrable in pulmonary tissues. However, the possibility remains that uteroglobin mRNA is expressed in some cell types, whereas progesterone receptors are present in other cell types. Future studies on the conalbumin-transferrin and uteroglobin systems will yield clues as to the mechanism by which tissue-specific regulation of genes is established during differentiation and development.

Effects of Steroid Hormones on Specific Gene Transcription

Since the chick oviduct is the best studied of the hormone-inducible systems, investigations carried out in this model system are analyzed in detail. It is likely that similar mechanisms are involved in the regulation of gene expression by other hormones. DNA probes prepared from structural and intervening sequences within the natural ovalbumin gene were used to study the expression of these sequences in estrogen target and nontarget tissues *in vivo* and *in vitro*. Both introns and exons (structural sequences) of the ovalbumin genes are completely transcribed *in vivo* (68). Indeed, Roop et al. (69) have mapped the 5'- and 3'-ends of transcripts of the natural ovalbumin gene and found them to be coincident with the beginning and end of the structural sequence of the natural gene. When oviduct nuclei are incubated *in vitro,* they seem to synthesize RNA complementary to introns and exons at comparable rates (68). This observation again indicates that the ovalbumin gene is expressed in the nuclei in its entirety.

Under steady-state conditions, however, when sequences from total cellular RNA, nuclear RNA, and polysomal RNA of the chick oviduct were quantified, the intervening sequence transcripts were essentially all confined to the nucleus. There was also a substantial difference in the ratio of ovalbumin mRNA (structural sequence) to intervening sequence RNA in the nucleus (10-fold) as compared to the cytoplasm (2,000-fold). This indicates either that the intervening sequence transcripts are rapidly processed (degraded) as soon as they reach the cytoplasm, or, more likely, that they are degraded in the nucleus. Further studies on the processing of primary transcripts indicate that intervening sequences are removed in a nonrandom fashion. The order of removal of the various intervening sequences is not obligatory, however, and follows more than one preferred order (70).

As a direct demonstration of transcriptional regulation of ovalbumin synthesis by estrogen in the chick oviduct, Swaneck et al. (71) isolated nuclei from the oviduct, liver, and spleen of chickens in different states of estrogen stimulation. They were incubated *in vitro* and allowed to synthesize RNA, using radiolabeled ribonucleotides as precursor. The concentration of transcripts of structural and intervening DNA sequences was determined by hybridizing the newly synthesized radiolabeled RNA to filters containing cloned ovalbumin cDNA or fragments of the natural ovalbumin gene containing most of the intervening sequences. Of the RNA synthesized by oviduct nuclei from chickens chronically stimulated with diethylstilbestrol, 0.23% corresponded to ovalbumin mRNA. Transcripts were not detected in radiolabeled RNA synthesized by spleen and liver cell nuclei. After 60 hr of hormone withdrawal, synthesis of ovalbumin mRNA by oviduct nuclei also could not be detected. After readministration of estrogen, a gradual increase in ovalbumin mRNA synthesis was observed which began at 1 hr and reached a plateau by 8 hr. For the intervening sequences, similar kinetics were observed for the initial 4 hr. These studies (71), coupled with those by Roop et al. (68,69), strongly support the concept that estrogen regulates ovalbumin synthesis at the level of ovalbumin gene transcription.

Regulation of Specific Gene Expression by Membrane Receptor-Mediated Hormones

Generally, the mode of action of these hormones is different and often involves the generation of "second messengers" following hormone receptor binding on the cell surface. In a number of such hormones, however, especially those which have trophic effects on the target cell, control of specific gene expression is an important mechanism of action.

Membrane receptor-mediated hormones as primary regulators of specific protein synthesis have been studied at the mRNA level in three systems: the induction of tyrosine aminotransferase mRNA by adenosine 3',5'-monophosphate (cAMP) and glucagon (72), the induction of phosphoenolpyruvate (PEP) carboxykinase by cAMP (73), and the induction of casein mRNA by prolactin (74).

Hepatic tyrosine aminotransferase mRNA and PEP carboxykinase in hepatoma cells are readily induced by glucocorticoids. It has long been known that both these enzymes can be induced by cAMP administration (71). Until recently, the mechanism of action of this cyclic nucleotide in the stimulation of the synthesis of these two enzymes was unclear. It has been proposed that this action of cAMP could be mediated at the translational level (75). However, Iynedjian and Hanson (73) demonstrated that the functional level of hepatic mRNA coding for PEP carboxykinase rapidly increased in concert with enzyme activity during induction by dibutyryl cAMP administration *in vivo*. Similarly, Ernest and Feigelson (72) demonstrated that a single injection of dibutyryl cAMP and theophylline stimulated both hepatic tyrosine aminotransferase enzymic activity and functional activity of its mRNA as assayed in the wheat germ system. The authors further demonstrated that glucagon given *in vivo* also stimulated hepatic tyrosine aminotransferase at the level of its mRNA.

These studies on hepatic enzyme regulation by cAMP and glucagon raise the possibility that these two hormones regulate specific gene expression at a pretranslational level. Since these studies were performed in intact animals, and mRNA activities were examined hours after hormone administration, however, some indirect effects of these hormones on mRNA activity could not be excluded. Similar studies will soon be carried out in tissue-culture systems involving the same enzymes, since all the techniques are presently available. Only then can one conclude whether cAMP and glucagon exert direct effects on the mRNA activity of PEP carboxykinase or tyrosine aminotransferase.

The only system in which *in vitro* studies were performed is the rodent mammary gland organ culture, where casein mRNA is induced by prolactin (74).

Terry (74a) first demonstrated the induction of casein mRNA in a mouse mammary gland culture. The mRNA activity was assayed in a cell-free protein synthesis system, and the induction was carried out over a 6-day period by a combination of insulin + prolactin + cortisol. Matusik and Rosen (74) studied the induction process in a rat mammary gland explant. They detected casein mRNA sequences by molecular hybridization with a specific cDNA probe and observed induction of the mRNA within 1 hr of addition of prolactin to the culture medium. They further demonstrated that hydrocortisone was not necessary for casein mRNA induction by prolactin, but the steroid was required for maximal accumulation of casein mRNA. Furthermore, induction of the mRNA by prolactin was inhibited in a dose-dependent manner by the simultaneous addition of progesterone to the organ culture. The study of Matusik and Rosen (74) appears to be the first demonstration of the rapid induction of a specific mRNA by a peptide hormone. Their system will serve as a valuable model for further studies on the peptide hormone regulation of specific gene expression.

In addition to studying the influence of prolactin on the rate of casein mRNA transcription in mammary gland organ culture, Guyette et al. (76) studied the contribution of posttranscriptional events in prolactin action. They found that within 1 hr, prolactin stimulated the rate of casein mRNA transcription two- to fourfold. This increased rate of transcription, however, was not sufficient to account for the rapid accumulation of casein mRNA. When they measured the half-life of casein mRNA, they found that it was increased 17- to 25-fold in the presence of prolactin. This change in casein mRNA half-life, coupled with a two- to fourfold increase in the rate of transcription, completely accounted for the accumulation of casein mRNA observed after prolactin addition. The observation of Guyette et al. (76) was the first evidence that modulation of the stability of a hormone-induced mRNA is an important action of prolactin in the mammary gland.

Hormonal Regulation of Specific Gene Expression in the Liver

The liver is a metabolically active organ. It contains a multitude of enzymes and secretory proteins and responds to essentially all the hormones listed in Table 1. Since most of the membrane receptor-mediated hormones have generalized actions in multiple target cells, it is expected that the liver contains receptors to these hormones and responds to them. This is also true for the steroid hormone glucocorticoid and thyroid hormones, which have metabolic effects on almost all tissues in the body. The liver is a classic organ in studies carried out on these hormones.

As discussed above, both glucocorticoid and thyroid hormones exert major influences on the expression of a selected number of hepatic proteins. They also probably modulate the concentration of numerous other proteins. For example, the hepatic synthesis of three enzymes involved in amino acid metabolism (tyrosine aminotransferase, tryptophan oxygenase, and PEP carboxykinase) are all stimulated by glucocorticoid treatment. In the first two instances, the stimulation was shown to be a result of a hormone-induced accumulation of the specific mRNAs.

What is generally less well appreciated is that the liver is also a target organ for the sex steroid hormones. It is the source of the major plasma proteins, which include albumin, plasma clotting factors and inhibitors, the acute phase proteins, lipoproteins, renin-substrate, and various hormone-binding proteins. It is known that sex steroid hormone administration is associated with changes in the plasma concentration of some of these hepatic secretory proteins; e.g., estrogen therapy is associated with an increase in clotting factors VII and X (77) and a decrease in the clotting inhibitor antithrombin III (78), an increase in very low density lipoproteins (79), renin-substrate (80), and an increase in the concentration of the plasma hormone binders, thyroxine-binding globulin (TBG) (81) and CBG (Table 2). Androgen therapy often is associated with different effects on these proteins. In addition, estrogen therapy leads to an increased incidence of gallstones (82) and liver tumors (83). What is not clear is which of these sex steroid-induced changes in liver function are mediated directly by estrogen-hepatocyte interaction and which are caused by indirect effects of the hormones on the liver. In at least one instance, the effect of estrogen appears to be direct, namely, stimulation of apolipoprotein synthesis in an animal model (84). In the cockerel, estrogen treatment stimulates the synthesis of a specific apolipoprotein in very low density lipoproteins, apoVLDL-II, by stimulating the accumulation of its specific mRNA. This effect of estrogen temporally follows closely the accumulation of nuclear estrogen receptors in the liver and increase in RNA polymerase activities (85). It should be pointed out that estrogenic modulation of lipoprotein metabolism is complex, since in the rat, estrogen increases the uptake of very low density lipoproteins by the liver (86,87). Similarly, estrogen receptors have been characterized in the rat liver (88) and appear to have the same general properties as the corresponding receptors in the uterus, except that they are present in considerably lower concentrations. Furthermore, androgen receptors have also been demonstrated in the rat liver and are absent in animals with the testicular feminization syndrome (89).

In summary, numerous hormone receptors have been demonstrated in the mammalian liver. This organ is a direct target for the action of many of these hormones, and it responds by modulation of its various metabolic pathways as well as by an alteration of its secretory pattern.

Future Studies

At present, there is little doubt that many intracellular receptor-mediated hormones and some membrane receptor-mediated hormones regulate gene expression by modulating the intracellular concentration of specific mRNAs at a transcriptional level and probably also at the level of mRNA degradation. It is also known that specific hormone receptors are important in this respect (Fig. 4). With the widespread application of molecular cloning and DNA sequencing, our concept of eukaryotic gene structure has undergone tremendous evolution; however, our understanding of specific interactions at potential regulatory regions is quite limited. During the past few years, two major advances in immunologic and biochemical techniques will likely lead to important breakthroughs with respect to hormone action. The development of monoclonal antibodies to estrogen receptors by Greene et al. (90) will prove valuable tools for probing receptor structure, function, and localization. The development of DNA-dependent, cell-free, *in vitro* transcription systems (91–93) will also facilitate the delineation of the steps involved in gene transcription. Recently, Wasylyk et al. (94) and Tsai et al. (95) utilized such techniques to study the structural requirements of the DNA template for specific initiation of RNA synthesis in hormone responsive systems. Using cloned genomic ovalbumin DNA templates of various lengths, Tsai et al. (95) found that sequences upstream from the cap-site (5′-end of the structural gene region) which contain an AT (deoxyadenylate-thymidylate)-rich region known as the Hogness box having the sequence TATATAT were essential for the correct initiation of transcription of the ovalbumin gene. However, natural DNA fragments containing similar AT-rich segments not normally located in the immediate 5′-flanking region of an authentic gene did not serve as promotors for initiation of transcription. Similar observations were made for conalbumin, another estrogen-regulated gene, by Wasylyk et al. (94). These results suggest that the Hogness box is essential but not sufficient for specific initiation of RNA synthesis.

Such studies indicate that advances are being made regarding the mechanism of hormone regulation of specific gene expression. Many unexplored areas remain, however, such as the regulatory roles of the nonhistone and histone proteins, the interaction of nuclear hormone receptors with some of these proteins and with DNA, and the intermediates of membrane receptor-mediated hormone regulation of gene expression. Furthermore, we still know very little about the enzymes involved in posttranscriptional RNA processing, the export of such RNA molecules into the cytoplasm, or the factors regulating the stability of cytoplasmic RNAs. Much experimentation is required before the biochemistry of hormonal control of gene expression will be understood in precise detail.

REFERENCES

1. Crick, F. H. C. (1958): On protein synthesis. *Symp. Soc. Exp. Biol.,* 12:138–163.
2. Crick, F. H. C. (1970): Central dogma of molecular biology. *Nature,* 227:561–562.
3. Unger, R., and Orci, L. (1977): Possible role of pancreatic D-cell in normal and diabetic states. *Diabetes,* 26:241–244.
4. Scatchard, G. (1949): The attractions of proteins for small molecules and ions. *Ann. NY Acad. Sci.,* 51:660–672.
5. Lineweaver, H., and Burk, D. (1934): The determination of enzyme-dissociation constants. *J. Am. Chem. Soc.,* 56:658–666.
6. Cornish-Bowden, A., and Eisenthal, R. (1974): Statistical considerations in the estimation of enzyme kinetic parameters by the direct linear plot and other methods. *Biochem. J.,* 139:721–730.
7. Eisenthal, R., and Cornish-Bowden, A. (1974): The direct linear plot: A new graphical procedure for estimating enzyme kinetic parameters. *Biochem. J.,* 139:715–720.
8. Woosely, J. T., and Muldoon, T. G. (1976): Use of the direct linear plot to estimate binding constants for protein-ligand interactions. *Biochem. Biophys. Res. Commun.,* 71:155–160.
9. Anderson, N. S., III, and Fanestil, D. D. (1978): Biology of mineralocorticoid receptors. In: *Receptors and Hormone Action, Vol. 11,* edited by B. W. O'Malley and L. Birnbaumer, pp. 323–351. Academic Press, New York.
10. Keenan, B. S., Meyer, W. J., III, Hadjian, A. J., and Migeon, C. J. (1974): Syndrome of androgen insensitivity in man: Absence of 5α-dihydrotestosterone binding protein in skin fibroblasts. *J. Clin. Endocrinol. Metab.,* 38:1143–1146.
11. Tosenau, W., Baxter, J. D., Rousseau, G. G., and Tomkins, G. M. (1972): Mechanism of resistance to steroids: Glucocorticoid receptor defect in lymphoma cells. *Nature [New Biol.],* 237:20–24.
12. Rodbard, D. (1973): Mathematics of hormone-receptor interaction. I. Basic principles. In: *Receptors for Reproductive Hormones,* edited by B. W. O'Malley and A. R. Means, pp. 289–326. Plenum, New York.
13. Chan, L., and O'Malley, B. W. (1976): Mechanism of action of the sex steroid hormones. *N. Engl. J. Med.,* 294:1322–1328, 1372–1381, 1430–1437.
14. Doenecke, D., and McCarthy, B. J. (1975): Protein content of chromatin fractions separated by sucrose gradient centrifugation. *Biochemistry,* 14:1366–1372.
15. Westphal, U. (1971): *Steroid-Protein Interactions.* Springer-Verlag, New York.
16. Westphal, U. (1980): Mechanism of steroid binding to transport proteins. In: *Pharmacological Modulation of Steroid Action,* edited by E. Genazzani, pp. 33–47. Raven Press, New York.
17. Woeber, K., and Ingbar, S. H. (1974): Interactions of thyroid hormones with binding proteins. In: *Handbook of Physiology, Vol. III. Thyroid,* edited by M. A. Greer and D. H. Solomon, pp. 187–196. Williams & Wilkins, Baltimore.
18. Stroupe, S. D., Harding, G. B., Forsthoefel, M. W., and Westphal, U. (1978): Kinetic and equilibrium studies on steroid interaction with human corticosteroid-binding globulin. *Biochemistry,* 17:177–182.
19. Anderson, J. N., Peck, E. J., Jr., and Clark, J. H. (1975): Estrogen-induced uterine responses and growth: Relationship to receptor estrogen binding by uterine nuclei. *Endocrinology,* 96:160–167.
20. Harden, J. W., Clark, J. H., Glaser, S. R., and Peck, E. J., Jr. (1976): Estrogen receptor binding by uterine nuclei: Relationship to endogenous nuclear RNA polymerase activity. *Biochemistry,* 15:1370–1374.
21. Jensen, E. V., Suzuki, T., Kawashima, T., Stumpf, W. E., Jungblut, P. W., and DeSombre, E. R. (1968): A two-step mechanism for the interaction of estradiol with rat uterus. *Proc. Natl. Acad. Sci. USA* 59:632–638.
22. Gorski, J., Toft, D., Shyamala, G., Smith, D., and Notides, A. (1968): Hormone receptors: Studies on the interaction of estrogen with the uterus. *Recent Prog. Horm. Res.* 24:45–80.
23. Brumbaugh, P. F., and Haussler, M. R. (1974): 1,25-Dihydroxycholecalciferol receptors in intestine. II. Temperature-dependent transfer of the hormone to chromatin via a specific cytosol receptor. *J. Biol. Chem.,* 249:1258–1262.
24. Clark, J. H., and Peck, E. J., Jr. (1976): Nuclear retention of receptor-oestrogen complex and nuclear acceptor sites. *Nature,* 260:635–637.
25. Korach, K. S., Metzler, M., and McLachlan, J. A. (1979): Diethylstilbestrol metabolites and analogs. New probes for the study of hormone action. *J. Biol. Chem.,* 254:8963–8968.
26. Oppenheimer, J. H., Schwartz, H. L., Surks, M. I., Koerner, D., and Dillman, W. H. (1976): Nuclear receptors and the initiation of thyroid hormone action. *Recent Prog. Horm. Res.,* 32:529–565.
27. Samuels, H. H., and Tsai, J. S. (1973): Thyroid hormone action in cell culture: Demonstration of nuclear receptors in intact cells and isolated nuclei. *Proc. Natl. Acad. Sci. USA,* 70:3488–3492.
28. Spindler, B. J., MacLeod, K. M., Ring, J., and Baxter, J. D. (1975): Thyroid hormone receptors. Binding characteristics and lack of hormonal dependency for nuclear localization. *J. Biol. Chem.,* 250:4113–4119.
29. Dietrich, S. W., Bolger, M. B., Kollman, P. A., and Jorgensen, E. C. (1971): Thyroxine analogues. 23. Quantitative structure-activity correlation studies *in vivo* and *in vitro* thyromimetic activities. *J. Med. Chem.,* 20:863–880.
30. Koerner, D., Schwartz, H. L., Surks, M. I., Oppenheimer, J. H., and Jorgensen, E. C. (1975): Binding of selected iodothyronine analogues to receptor sites of isolated rat hepatic nuclei: High correlation between structural requirements for nuclear binding and biological activity. *J. Biol. Chem.,* 250:6417–6423.
31. Chan, L., and Tindall, D. J. (1981): Steroid hormone action. In: *Pediatric Endocrinology,* edited by R. Collu, J.-R. Ducharme, and H. Guyda, pp. 63–97. Raven Press, New York.
32. MacLeod, K. M., and Baxter, J. D. (1976): Chromatin receptors for thyroid hormones: Interactions of the solubilized proteins with DNA. *J. Biol. Chem.,* 251:7380–7387.
33. Schrader, W. T., and O'Malley, B. W. (1972): Progesterone-binding components of chick oviduct. IV. Characterization of purified subunits. *J. Biol. Chem.,* 247:51–59.
34. Vedeckis, W. V., Freeman, M. R., Schrader, W. T., and O'Malley, B. W. (1980): Progesterone binding components of chick oviduct: Partial purification and characterization of a calcium-activated protease which hydrolyzes the progesterone receptor. *Biochemistry,* 19:335–343.
35. Vedeckis, W. V., Schrader, W. T., and O'Malley, B. W. (1979): Structural relationships between the chick oviduct progesterone receptor A and B proteins. In: *Steroid Hormone Receptor Systems,* edited by W. W. Leavitt and J. H. Clark, pp. 309–327. Plenum, New York.
36. Vedeckis, W. V., Schrader, W. T., and O'Malley, B. W. (1980): Progesterone-binding components of chick oviduct: Analysis of receptor structure by limited proteolysis. *Biochemistry,* 19:343–349.
37. Charles, M. A., Ryffel, G. U., Obinata, M., McCarthy, B. J., and Baxter, J. D. (1975): Nuclear receptors for thyroid hormone: Evidence for nonrandom distribution with chromatin. *Proc. Natl. Acad. Sci. USA,* 72:1787–1791.
38. Glasser, S. R., Chytil, F., and Spelsberg, T. C. (1972): Early effects of oestradiol-17 on the chromatin and activity of the deoxyribonucleic acid-dependent ribonucleic acid polymerases (I and II) of the rat uterus. *Biochem. J.,* 130:947–957.
39. Snow, L. D., Eriksson, H., Hardin, J. W., Chan, L., Jackson,

R. L., Clark, J. H., and Means, A. R. (1978): Nuclear estrogen receptor in the avian liver: Correlation with biologic response. *J. Steroid Biochem.*, 9:1017–1026.

40. Widnell, C. C., and Tata, J. R. (1966): Additive effects of thyroid hormone, growth hormone and testosterone on deoxyribonucleic acid-dependent ribonucleic acid polymerase in rat liver nuclei. *Biochem. J.*, 98:621–629.

41. Church, B. R., and McCarthy, B. J. (1970): Unstable nuclear synthesis following estrogen stimulation. *Biochim. Biophys. Acta*, 199:103–114.

42. Liarakos, C. D., Rosen, J. M., and O'Malley, B. W. (1973): Effect of estrogen on gene expression in the chick oviduct. II. Transcription of chick tritiated unique deoxyribonucleic acid as measured by hybridization in ribonucleic acid excess. *Biochemistry*, 12:2809–2816.

43. McReynolds, L. A., Catterall, J. F., and O'Malley, B. W. (1977): The ovalbumin gene: Cloning of a complete ds-cDNA in a bacterial plasmid. *Gene*, 2:217–231.

44. Gilbert, W. (1979): Introns and exons: Playgrounds of evolution. In: *Eucaryotic Gene Regulation*, edited by R. Axel, T. Maniatis, and C. F. Fox, pp. 1–12. Academic Press, New York.

45. Leder, P. (1978): Discontinuous genes. *N. Engl. J. Med.*, 298:1079–1081.

46. Breathnach, R., Mandel, J. L., and Chambon, P. (1977): Ovalbumin gene is split in chicken DNA. *Nature*, 270:314–319.

47. Doel, M. T., Houghton, M., Cook, E. A., and Carey, N. H. (1977): The presence of ovalbumin mRNA coding sequences in multiple restriction fragments of chicken DNA. *Nucleic Acids Res.*, 4:3701–3713.

48. Lai, E. C., Woo, S. L. C., Dugaiczyk, A., Catterall, J. F., and O'Malley, B. W. (1978): The ovalbumin gene: Structural sequences in native chicken DNA are not contiguous. *Proc. Natl. Acad. Sci. USA*, 75:2205–2209.

49. Mandel, J. L., Breathnach, R., Gerlinger, P., LeMur, M., Gannon, F., and Chambon, P. (1978): Organization of coding and intervening sequences in the chicken ovalbumin split gene. *Cell*, 14:641–653.

50. Weinstock, R., Sweet, R., Weiss, M., Cedar, H., and Axel, R. (1978): Intragenic DNA spacers interrupt the ovalbumin gene. *Proc. Natl. Acad. Sci. USA*, 75:1299–1303.

51. Schaffner, W., Junz, G., Daetwyler, H., Telford, J., Smith, H. O., and Birnsteil, M. L. (1978): Genes and spacers of cloned sea urchin histone DNA analyzed by sequencing. *Cell*, 14:655–671.

52. O'Malley, B. W., Roop, D. R., Lai, E. C., Nordstrom, J. L., Catterall, J. F., Swaneck, G. E., Colbert, D. A., Tsai, M.-J., Dugaiczyk, A., and Woo, S. L. C. (1979): The ovalbumin gene: Organization, structure, transcription and regulation. *Recent Prog. Horm. Res.*, 35:1–46.

53. Hamer, D. H., and Leder, P. (1979): Splicing and the formation of stable RNA. *Cell*, 18:1299–1302.

54. Ivarie, R. D., and O'Farrell, P. H. (1978): The glucocorticoid domain: Steroid-mediated changes in the rate of synthesis of rat hepatoma proteins. *Cell*, 13:41–55.

55. Baxter, J. D., Eberhardt, N. L., Apriletti, J. W., Johnson, L. K., Ivarie, R. D., Schachter, B. S., Morris, J. A., Seeburg, P. H., Goodman, H. M., Latham, K. R., Polansky, J. R., and Martial, J. A. (1979): Thyroid hormone receptors and responses. *Recent Prog. Horm. Res.*, 35:97–153.

56. Seo, H., Vassart, G., Brocas, H., and Refetoff, S. (1977): Triiodothronine stimulates specifically growth hormone mRNA in rat pituitary tumor cells. *Proc. Natl. Acad. Sci. USA*, 74:2053–2058.

57. Chan, L., Means, A. R., and O'Malley, B. W. (1978): Steroid hormone regulation of specific gene expression. *Vitam. Horm.*, 36:259–295.

58. Palmiter, R. D., Moore, P. B., Mulvihill, E. R., and Emtage, S. (1976): A significant lag in the induction of ovalbumin messenger RNA by steroid hormones: A receptor translocation hypothesis. *Cell*, 8:557–572.

59. Dugaiczyk, A., Inglis, A. S., Strike, P. M., Burley, R. W., Beattie, W. G., and Chan, L. (1981): Comparison of the nucleotide sequence of cloned DNA coding for an apoprotein (apo VLDL-II) from avian blood and the amino acid sequence of an egg yolk protein (apovitellenin I). Equivalence of the two sequences gene. *Gene*, 14:175–182.

60. Lin, C. T., and Chan, L. (1981): Estrogen regulation of yolk and non-yolk protein synthesis in the avian liver: An immunocytochemical study. *Differentiation*, 18:105–114.

61. Lin, C. T., and Chan, L. (1980): Effects of estrogen on specific protein synthesis in the cockerel liver: An immunocytochemical study on major apoproteins in very low and high density lipoproteins and albumin. *Endocrinology*, 107:70–75.

62. Chan, L., Jackson, R. L., O'Malley, B. W., and Means, A. R. (1976): Synthesis of very low density lipoproteins in the cockerel. Effects of estrogen. *J. Clin. Invest.*, 58:368–379.

63. Deeley, R. G., Udell, D. S., Burns, A. T. H., Gordon, J. I., and Goldberger, R. F. (1977): Kinetics of avian vitellogenin messenger RNA induction: Comparison between primary and secondary response to estrogen. *J. Biol. Chem.*, 252:7913–7915.

64. Tsai, S. Y., Tsai, M.-J., Lin, C. T., and O'Malley, B. W. (1979): Effect of estrogen on ovalbumin gene expression in differentiated nontarget tissues. *Biochemistry*, 18:5726–5731.

65. Morgan, E. H. (1969): Factors affecting the synthesis of transferrin by rat tissue slices. *J. Biol. Chem.*, 244:4193–4199.

66. Lee, D. C., McKnight, G. S., and Palmiter, R. D. (1978): The action of estrogen and progesterone on the expression of the transferrin gene. A comparison of the response in chick liver and oviduct. *J. Biol. Chem.*, 253:3494–3503.

67. Savouret, J.-J. Loosfelt, H., Atger, M., and Milgrom, E. (1980): Differential hormonal control of a messenger RNA in two tissues: Uteroglobin mRNA in the lung and the endometrium. *J. Biol. Chem.*, 255:4131–4136.

68. Roop, D. R., Nordstrom, J. L., Tsai, S. Y., Tsai, M.-J., and O'Malley, B. W. (1978): Transcription of structural and intervening sequences of the ovalbumin gene and identification of probable precursors to ovalbumin mRNA. *Cell*, 15:671–685.

69. Roop, D. R., Tsai, M.-J., and O'Malley, B. W. (1980): Definition of the 5' and 3' ends of transcripts of the ovalbumin gene. *Cell*, 19:53–68.

70. Tsai, M. J., Ting, A. C., Noodstrom, J. L., Zimmer, W., and O'Malley B. W. (1980): Processing of high molecular weight ovalbumin and ovomucoid precursor RNAs to messenger RNA. *Cell*, 22:219–230.

71. Swaneck, G. E., Nordstrom, J. L., Kreuzeler, F., Tsai, M.-J., and O'Malley, B. W. (1979): Effect of estrogen on gene expression in chicken oviduct: Evidence for transcriptional control of ovalbumin gene. *Proc. Natl. Acad. Sci. USA*, 76:1049–1053.

72. Ernest, M. J., and Feigelson, P. (1978): Increase in hepatic tyrosine aminotransferase mRNA during enzyme induction by N^6,O^2-dibutyryl cyclic AMP. *J. Biol. Chem.*, 253:319–322.

73. Iynedjian, P. B., and Hanson, R. W. (1977): Increase in level of functional messenger RNA coding for phosphoenolpyruvate carboxykinase (GTP) during induction by cyclic adenosine 3':5'-monophosphate. *J. Biol. Chem.*, 252:655–662.

74. Matusik, R. J., and Rosen, J. M. (1978): Prolactin induction of casein mRNA in organ culture: A model system for studying peptide hormone regulation of gene expression. *J. Biol. Chem.*, 253:2343–2347.

74a. Terry, P. M., Banerjee, M. R., and Lui, R. M. (1977): Hormone-inducible casein messenger RNA in a serum-free organ culture of whole mammary gland. *Proc. Natl. Acad. Sci. USA*, 74:2441–2445.

75. Wicks, W. D. (1974): Regulation of protein synthesis by cyclic AMP. *Adv. Cyclic Nucleotide Res.*, 4:335–438.

76. Guyette, W. A., Matusik, R. J., and Rosen, J. M. (1979): Prolactin-mediated transcriptional and posttranscriptional control of casein gene expression. *Cell*, 17:1013–1023.

77. Dugdale, M., and Masi, A. T. (1971): Hormonal contraception and thromboembolic disease: Effects of the oral contraceptives on hemostatic mechanisms: A review of the literature. *J. Chronic Dis.*, 23:775–790.

78. Conrad, J., Samama, M., and Salomon, Y. (1972): Antithrombin III and the oestrogen content of combined oestro-progestagen contraceptives. *Lancet*, 2:1148–1149

79. Wynn, V., Doar, J. W. H., Mills, G. L., and Stokes, T. (1969): Fasting serum triglyceride, cholesterol, and lipoprotein levels during oral contraceptive therapy. *Lancet*, 2:756–760.

80. Laragh, J. H., Baer, L., Brunner, H. R., Buhler, F. R., Sealey,

J. E., and Vaughan, E. D. (1972): Renin, angiotensin and aldosterone system in pathogenesis and management of hypertensive vascular disease. *Am. J. Med.*, 52:633–649.

81. Ingbar, S. H., Braverman, L. E., Darober, N. A., and Lee, G. Y. (1965): A new method for measuring the free thyroid hormone in human serum and an analysis of the factors that influence its concentration. *J. Clin. Invest.*, 44:1679–1689.

82. Bennion, K. J., Ginsberg, R. L., Garnick, M. B., and Bennett, P. H. (1976): Effects of oral contraceptives on the gallbladder bile of normal women. *N. Engl. J. Med.*, 294:189–193.

83. Klatskin, G. (1977): Hepatic tumors: Possible relationship to use of oral contraceptives. *Gastroenterology*, 73:386–394.

84. Hillyard, L. A., Entennan, C., and Chaikoff, I. L. (1956): Concentration and composition of serum lipoproteins of cholesterol-fed and stilbestrol-injected birds. *J. Biol. Chem.*, 223:359–368.

85. Chan, L., Snow, L. D., Jackson, R. L., and Means, A. R. (1979): Hormonal regulation of lipoprotein synthesis in the cockerel. In: *Ontogeny of Receptors and Reproductive Hormone Action*, edited by T. H. Hamilton, J. H. Clark, and W. A. Sadler, pp. 331–351. Raven Press, New York.

86. Chao, Y., Windler, E. E., Chen, G. C., and Havel, R. J. (1979): Hepatic catabolism of rat and human lipoproteins in rats treated with 17-ethinyl estradiol. *J. Biol. Chem.*, 254:11360–11366.

87. Kovanen, P. T., Brown, M. S., and Goldstein, J. L. (1979): Increased binding of low density lipoprotein to liver membranes from rats treated with 17-ethyl estradiol. *J. Biol. Chem.*, 254:11367–11373.

88. Dickson, R. B., and Eisenfeld, A. J. (1979): Estrogen receptor in rat liver: Translocation to the nucleus in isolated parenchymal cells. *Endocrinology*, 105:627–635.

89. Milin, B., and Roy, A. K. (1973): Androgen "receptor" in rat liver: Cytosol "receptor" deficiency in pseudohermaphrodite male rats. *Nature [New Biol.]*, 242:248–250.

90. Greene, G. L., Fitch, F. W., and Jensen, E. V. (1980): Monoclonal antibodies to estrophilin: Probes for the study of estrogen receptors. *Proc. Natl. Acad. Sci. USA*, 77:157–161.

91. Manley, J. L., Fire, A., Cans, A., Sharp, P. A., and Gefter, M. L. (1980): DNA-dependent transcription of adenovirus genes in a soluble whole-cell extract. *Proc. Natl. Acad. Sci. USA*, 77:3855–3859.

92. Weil, P. A., Luse, D. S., Segall, J., and Roeder, R. G. (1979): Selective and accurate initiation of transcription at the Ad2 major late promotor in a soluble system dependent on purified RNA polymerase II and DNA. *Cell*, 18:469–489.

93. Wu, G. J. (1978): Adenovirus DNA directed transcription of 5.5S RNA *in vitro*. *Proc. Natl. Acad. Sci. USA*, 2175–2179.

94. Wasylyk, B., Kedinger, C., Corden, J., Brison, O., and Chambon, P. (1980): Specific *in vitro* initiation of transcription on conalbumin and ovalbumin genes and comparison with adenovirus-2 early and late genes. *Nature*, 285:367–373.

95. Tsai, S. Y., Tsai, M.-J., and O'Malley, B. W. (1981): Specific 5'-flanking sequences are required for faithful initiation of *in vitro* transcription of the ovalbumin gene. *Proc. Natl. Acad. Sci. USA*, 78:879–883.

96. Cheng, S.-Y., Maxfield, F. R., Robbins, J., Willingham, M. C., and Pastan, I. H. (1980): Receptor-mediated uptake of 3,3',5-triodo-L-thyronine by culture fibroblasts. *Proc. Natl. Acad. Sci. USA*, 77:3425–3429.

97. Chan, L., and O'Malley, B. W. (1978): Steroid hormone action: Recent advances. *Ann. Intern. Med.*, 89(1):694–701.

The Liver: Biology and Pathobiology, edited by
I. Arias, H. Popper, D. Schachter, and D. A. Shafritz.
Raven Press, New York © 1982.

Chapter 11

Regulation of Membrane Proteins in Hepatocytes

Darrell Doyle, Janet Cook, and Heinz Baumann

This chapter presents a succinct and critical analysis of current knowledge concerning regulation of membrane protein biogenesis and turnover in mammalian liver. In the study of membrane biogenesis in mammalian tissues, the liver has received considerable attention because the hepatocyte constitutes about 80% of the liver cell mass (1). A recent review by Evans (2) gives a rather comprehensive treatment of the biochemistry of the hepatocyte plasma membrane. Also, we (3) have presented a comprehensive treatment of overall cell plasma membrane biochemistry, including all components of the membrane. We restrict our attention here to those studies that provide insight into the mechanism(s) used by hepatocytes to regulate the concentration of specific proteins and glycoproteins in the different membrane systems of this rather complex cell.

The membrane systems of the cell include the nuclear membrane, the smooth and rough endoplasmic reticulum (ER), the Golgi systems and Gerl structures (4), peroxisomes, lysosomes, mitochondria, a variety of not well-defined intracellular vesicular-like structures (which probably include endocytic and secretory and/or exocytic vesicles and possibly other vesicles serving as yet unknown functions), and the plasma membrane (see Fig. 1). Many of these organelles, most obviously the Golgi (5–7) and the plasma membrane, contain regional specializations of their membranes that differ from each other in both structure and function. For example, the plasma membrane of the hepatocyte consists of at least the following domains: a sinusoidal or perisinusoidal region, where exchanges between the hepatocyte and tissue fluids and the circulation take place. This domain of plasma membrane would be expected to contain receptors that facilitate these exchanges, such as the specific receptors for insulin, glucagon, other hormones, growth factors, and other large and small molecular weight material in the blood. Some of these receptors may be involved in promoting optimal regeneration following hepatocyte necrosis. The lateral or intercellular domain of the plasma membrane might contain different proteins,

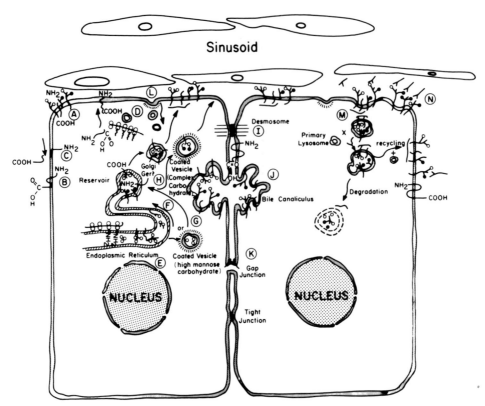

FIG. 1. Idealized hepatocytes. The plasma membrane is segregated into the following regional specializations: sinusoidal/perisinusoidal domain; lateral domain; bile canaliculus (J); tight and gap junctions (K); desmosome (I); and coated pits (L). (A) denotes a unit or domain of perisinusoidal membrane containing a set of proteins and glycoproteins embedded in the lipid bilayer. (B) denotes a transmembrane integral protein with C-terminal outside and N-terminal residue inside the cell. This orientation is in contrast to that of the protein in (A), which has its N-terminal residue outside of the cell. In (C), a serum or surface protease has cleaved the externally oriented protein, one mechanism of plasma membrane protein turnover in hepatocytes. Proteins either individually or in units in the lipid bilayer could also be shed from the cell into the circulation. Most integral transmembrane plasma membrane proteins are usually synthesized on mRNAs on membrane-bound polysomes. If they are glycoproteins, they are core glycosylated via the dolichol pathway while still nascent on the polysome. They then traverse the Golgi/Gerl system, where additional glycosylation occurs (E,F,G,H,). Coated vesicles (G,H) may be involved in the transfer of these proteins from the ER to the Golgi (high mannose intermediate) and from the Golgi to the plasma membrane (complex carbohydrate intermediate). Some more widely distributed integral membrane proteins can also be synthesized on free polysomes (D). The major pathway for membrane protein degradation is via interiorization of units of membrane, which fuse with lysosomes. The contents of the interiorized membrane vesicle are then degraded, but the membrane itself usually escapes degradation and recycles back to the surface, possibly via the Golgi or Gerl structures. An externally oriented plasma membrane glycoprotein can interact with a ligand, such as a hormone, serum macromolecule, growth factor, or antibody and be concentrated in the membrane (sometimes but not always in a coated pit region) before being interiorized (N). The fate of these interiorized units of membrane is discussed in the text.

perhaps proteins or protein channels that facilitate exchange between cells. Similarly, the membrane domains of the bile canalículus (J in Fig. 1), the tight and gap junctional complexes (K in Fig. 1), and coated pit regions (L in Fig. 1) would contain at least some proteins and glycoproteins that differ from each other and from the other domains of the membrane. These specific proteins would endow these structures with their specific functions. Certain drugs, e.g., chlorpromazine and phenothiazine, may interact with components of tight junctions, thus altering their physiology. The mechanism(s) used by the hepatocyte to establish the differentiated state of its membranes and the mechanism(s) used to modulate the composition of these

membranes in response to different cues in the environment is the primary subject of this chapter. We cannot discuss in detail every membrane system of this cell. Discussion of mitochondrial and peroxisomal biogenesis has been excluded almost completely because these topics are covered in other chapters. To date, little is known about either the composition or the route of biogenesis of the nuclear membrane (however, see refs. 8 and 9). More is known regarding the composition and regulation of composition of the plasma membrane and the ER of the hepatocyte. We concentrate our attention primarily on these organelles, particularly the plasma membrane, since the ER is discussed elsewhere in this volume.

PATHWAY OF BIOSYNTHESIS OF PLASMA MEMBRANE PROTEINS

The basic mechanism(s) used by mammalian cells for synthesis of membrane proteins is similar, regardless of the particular membrane in which the protein resides or the particular cell in which the membrane resides. The mechanism is similar to that used by the cell to synthesize proteins destined for secretion (10–13).

Vectorial Transport of Secretory Proteins

Like secretory proteins, most membrane proteins are probably synthesized in the membrane-bound ribosomes of the rough endoplasmic reticulum (RER). In fact, there is probably no difference in composition between those ribosomes that are membrane-bound and those that are free in the cytoplasm. It is the information contained in the sequence of the mRNA for the secretory protein that directs the ribosome to bind to the ER, as postulated by Blobel and Sabatini in 1971 (12) and demonstrated experimentally by Milstein et al. (13), and Blobel and Dobberstein (10,11). The mRNAs for proteins destined for secretion from the cell contain information for hydrophobic amino acid sequences or signals that endow the free ribosomes containing the growing nascent secretory or membrane polypeptide with the ability to become associated with the membrane of the ER.

The signal amino acid sequence for many secretory proteins consists of about 25 residues at the amino terminal end of the protein molecule. These residues are encoded by bases at the 5' end of the specific mRNA molecule. These hydrophobic residues, while nascent on free polysomes, become spontaneously embedded in the bilayer of the ER. The association of the ribosome with its growing nascent secretory protein then becomes stabilized by specific proteins, termed ribophorins, in the membrane of the ER of the hepatocyte (14,15). The net result of these initial events in secretory protein biogenesis is formation of a "pore" in the lipid bilayer, such that the growing polypeptide chain, while the mRNA is still being translated, is unidirectionally transported across the bilayer and into the lumen of the ER. Whether or not energy is required for transport, or the source of such energy, is not yet known. As part of the translocation mechanism, there may be a modification of the secretory protein in that the signal hydrophobic sequences for many but not all secretory proteins are cleaved, most likely by an endopeptidase associated with the membrane of the ER (16). However, cleavage of the signal peptide is not essential for translocation, nor need the signal sequence be located at the N-terminal region of the secretory protein. The signal sequence for chicken ovalbumin is present as an internal domain of the polypeptide; there is no cleavage during translocation of this secretory protein (17).

Biosynthesis of Immunoglobulin μ Heavy Chain

The biosynthesis of an authentic or integral membrane protein (18) that indeed penetrates the lipid bilayer is similar to that described above for secretory proteins. The main difference is that the membrane protein stays associated with the bilayer rather than being transported into the lumen of the ER. In fact, it is possible to compare the early steps in biosynthesis of membrane and secreted forms of the same protein, the immunoglobulin (IgM) μ-heavy chain. This protein is either membrane bound or secreted from B-lymphocytes, depending on the stage of differentiation. Several groups (19–21) have shown that there are two different mRNAs, one of 2.4 Kb and one of 2.7 Kb, that specify two forms of μ heavy chain, one the secreted form (MW 64,000) and the other, the membrane-bound form (MW 67,000).

The two mRNAs encoding the secreted and membrane-bound μ heavy chains are identical throughout the coding region up to the 3' end of the fourth constant domain, the Cμ 4 domain. The larger 2.7 Kb mRNA for the membrane-bound form contains additional bases at the 3' edge of the Cμ 4 domain. From the nucleotide sequence of a cDNA clone of the mRNA for the membrane-bound form of the μ heavy chain, Rogers et al. (20) could predict the amino acid sequence of the carboxy terminal portion of the membrane polypeptide. In contrast to the 20 residue hydrophilic C-terminal segment of the Cμ 4 domain of the secreted form of μ heavy chain, the membrane-bound form was predicted to have a 41 residue C-terminal segment containing a hydrophobic sequence. This additional hydrophobic sequence or signal would then lock the μ heavy chain into the lipid bilayer and stop the transfer of the polypeptide into the lumen of the ER.

Membrane Glycoproteins Synthesized on Membrane-Bound Polysomes

The phenobarbital-inducible cytochrome P450, a major transmembrane glycoprotein in the ER of rat liver hepatocytes, also is synthesized on membrane-bound polysomes of the RER (22–24). This protein also contains an N-terminal sequence of hydrophobic amino acids that may provide the membrane insertion signal, but there is no proteolytic cleavage of the signal during translocation. Interestingly, 3'-methyl-cholanthrene-inducible cytochrome P448, also of rat ER, appears to be synthesized on membrane-bound ribosomes but with a cleavable signal sequence (24). Similarly, the major histocompatability complexes of both mice and humans contain genes specifying the structure of plasma membrane glycoproteins, denoted D and K antigens in the mouse and HLA antigens in humans. The mRNAs for these relatively abundant membrane glycoproteins are also translated on membrane-bound polysomes. In this case, the proteins are probably synthesized as larger molecular weight precursors containing signals that are subsequently cleaved to the final product (25–27). The ultimate orientation and conformation of these membrane proteins in the lipid bilayer, although not completely known, is probably also determined by the presence in the polypeptide of one or more amino acid signal sequences. Depending on the location of these hydrophobic regions in relationship to more hydrophilic residues in the polypeptide, the membrane protein could traverse the bilayer not at all or completely, or attain a complex but thermodynamically favored orientation in the bilayer similar to that attained by some erythrocyte membrane proteins (B in Fig. 1) (28,29).

Are all membrane proteins synthesized on membrane-bound polysomes? For glycoproteins, such as cytochrome P450, HLA or H2 antigens, or immunoglobulins, the answer is probably yes. The pathway of glycoprotein biogenesis practically dictates that this class of proteins must be synthesized by membrane-bound polysomes of the ER. The essential steps of this pathway are as follows:

Glycosylation of glycoproteins through linkage of oligosaccharides to the amide of asparagine residues occurs within the lumen of the ER, while the growing polypeptide chain is still nascent on the membrane-bound polysome (30). Events involved in glycosylation are quite complex and still being analyzed by several groups using a variety of eukaryotic systems (3,31–48). A dolichol pyrophosphate oligosaccharide is involved in the transfer of a large oligosaccharide to an asparagine residue of the growing polypeptide (in correct sequence with other amino acids to act as an acceptor). The dolichol pyrophosphate oligosaccharide is probably synthesized in the membranes of the ER. The structure of this core oligosaccharide for many but not all glycoproteins is (glucose 3; mannose 9; N-acetylglucosamine 2 bound to ASN) in the following configuration:

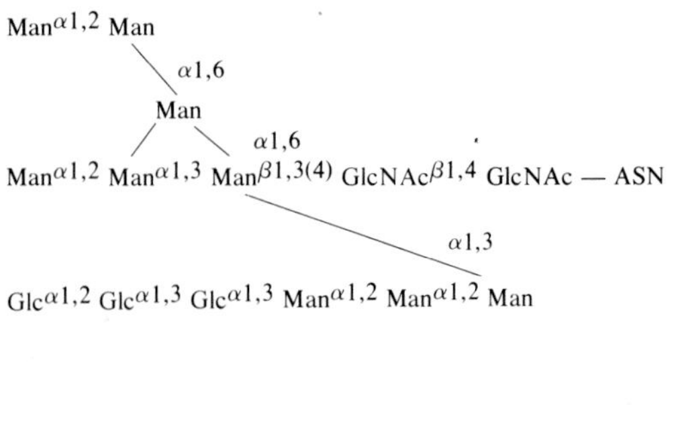

$$\text{Man}^{\alpha1,2}\text{Man}$$
$$\searrow \alpha1,6$$
$$\text{Man}$$
$$\nearrow \qquad \searrow \alpha1,6$$
$$\text{Man}^{\alpha1,2}\text{Man}^{\alpha1,3}\ \text{Man}^{\beta1,3(4)}\text{GlcNAc}^{\beta1,4}\text{GlcNAc}-\text{ASN} \qquad [1]$$
$$\searrow \alpha1,3$$
$$\text{Glc}^{\alpha1,2}\text{Glc}^{\alpha1,3}\text{Glc}^{\alpha1,3}\text{Man}^{\alpha1,2}\text{Man}^{\alpha1,2}\text{Man}$$

Following *en bloc* transfer of the oligosaccharide to the growing polypeptide, there is a series of processing or trimming reactions catalyzed by at least two glucosidases and one or more mannosidases leading to the structure mannose 5; GlcNAc 2; ASN.

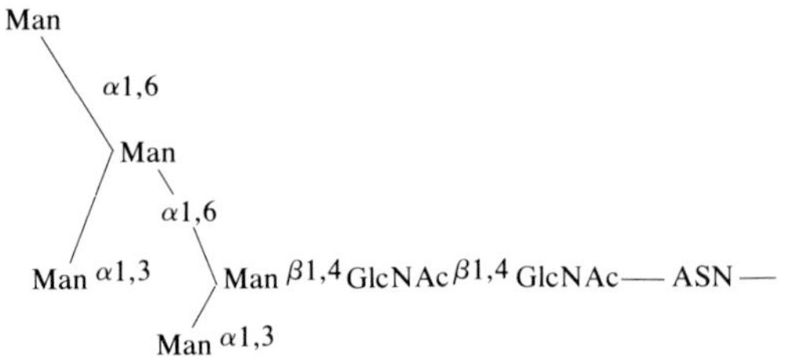

$$\text{Man}$$
$$\searrow \alpha1,6$$
$$\text{Man}$$
$$\searrow \alpha1,6$$
$$\text{Man}^{\alpha1,3}\ \text{Man}^{\beta1,4}\text{GlcNAc}^{\beta1,4}\text{GlcNAc}-\text{ASN}- \qquad [2]$$
$$\text{Man}^{\alpha1,3}$$

These enzymes are localized in microsomal fractions consisting of rough and smooth ER and/or Golgi membranes. Structure [2] is then modified by the addition of an N-acetylglucosamine residue catalyzed by a UDP transferase (in the Golgi membranes?) to yield:

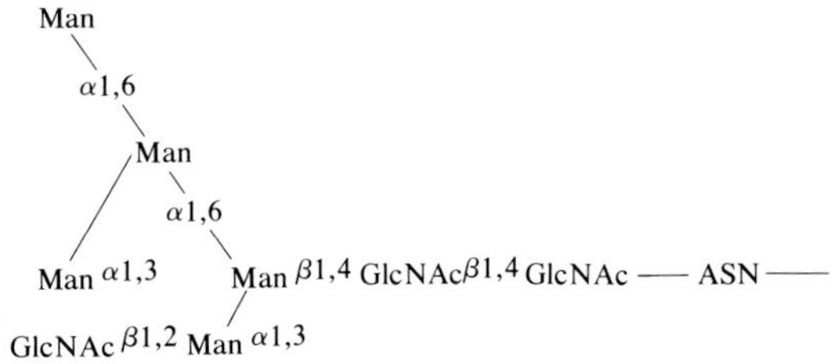

$$\text{Man}$$
$$\searrow \alpha1,6$$
$$\text{Man}$$
$$\nearrow \qquad \searrow \alpha1,6$$
$$\text{Man}^{\alpha1,3}\ \text{Man}^{\beta1,4}\text{GlcNAc}^{\beta1,4}\text{GlcNAc}-\text{ASN}- \qquad [3]$$
$$\text{GlcNAc}^{\beta1,2}\text{Man}^{\alpha1,3}$$

One or more enzymes in the Golgi membranes then remove an additional two mannosyl residues to yield:

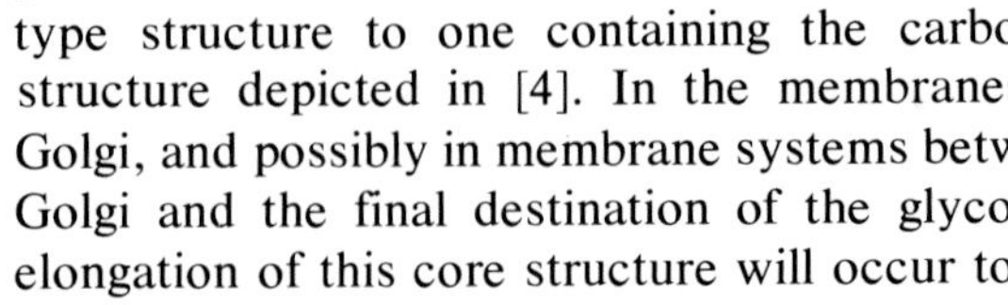

$$\text{Man}$$
$$\searrow \alpha1,6$$
$$\text{Man}^{\beta1,4}\text{GlcNAc}^{\beta1,4}\text{GlcNAc}-\text{ASN}- \qquad [4]$$
$$\text{GlcNAc}^{\beta1,2}\text{Man}^{\alpha1,3}$$

After transfer from the membranes of the rough and smooth ER to the membranes of the Golgi, the glycoprotein has been transformed from a high mannose type structure to one containing the carbohydrate structure depicted in [4]. In the membranes of the Golgi, and possibly in membrane systems between the Golgi and the final destination of the glycoprotein, elongation of this core structure will occur to change the N-linked oligosaccharide to the complex type characteristic of mature membrane and secretory glycoproteins. As part of these elongation reactions, N-acetyl glucosamine, galactose, sialic acid, fucose, and possibly other sugar residues will be added by nucleotide-linked transferase enzymes in these membrane systems.

This sequence of reactions in the glycoprotein synthetic pathway predicts that little if any glycoprotein should be found, other than membrane bound in mammalian cells (49–57; but see also ref. 58 for an example of a reported exception). Furthermore, the oligosaccharide moieties of membrane and secretory glycoproteins should not be on the cytoplasmic side but on the luminal side of rough and smooth ER, Golgi membranes, and other intracellular membranes and vesicles. Enzymatic, lectin, and other topologic probes have suggested that this is the case (30,51,56,57,59). If the sequence of reactions just described is used by the cell for the biosynthesis of a glycoprotein having the complex N-linked oligosaccharide structure, and if this protein is resident in the membrane of the ER, (e.g., as with cytochrome P450), then during synthesis this protein must traverse the ER and the Golgi membrane and return to the ER. Hence a carrier system would be required to transport the completed glycoprotein to its final destination. Membrane vesicles were thought to pinch off from the Golgi to transport membrane and/or secretory proteins to their final destination in the cell (53–55,60–62).

Coated Vesicles in the Transport of Membrane Glycoproteins Through the Cell

Recently, Rothman and Fine (63) have presented evidence implicating clathrin-coated vesicles as the vehicle for transport of the envelope glycoprotein of vesicular stomatitis virus (VSV) to the plasma membrane of Chinese hamster ovary (CHO) cells. The transport occurred in two distinct stages (see sequences denoted G and H in Fig. 1). In the first (earlier) stage, the coated vesicles contained the viral envelope glycoprotein with the high mannose oligosaccharide structure referred to earlier. In the second (later) stage, the viral envelope glycoprotein in the coated vesicles was resistant to digestion with endoglycosidase H and presumably had the mature complex oligosaccharide structure.

Clathrin-coated vesicles of the first stage, carrying the high mannose glycoprotein, presumably represented a stage in the transport of the glycoprotein between the ER and the Golgi apparatus. Clathrin-coated vesicles containing the mature glycoprotein was presumed to represent a stage in the transport of the viral envelope glycoprotein from the Golgi to the plasma membrane. Such vesicles (whether coated or not), having different specificities for different membrane systems of the hepatocyte, could provide part of the mechanism for attaining membrane differentiation. For example, a vesicle carrying the mature cytochrome P450 glycoprotein after processing in the Golgi might be able to recognize and fuse specifically with the ER, while a glycoprotein destined for the lysosome, the plasma membrane, or some other intracellular organelle or for secretion would be transported from the Golgi in a different vesicle with a different recognition marker. In fact, Smilowitz (64) has shown that the routes of intracellular transport of two glyco-

proteins (one a secreted esterase and one the acetylcholine receptor, an integral membrane protein) were different in skeletal muscle. Both glycoproteins are found in the Golgi membrane after synthesis. In the presence of low concentrations of monovalent ionophores, however, the acetylcholine receptor continues to accumulate in the plasma membrane, while secretion of the esterase is markedly inhibited, suggesting differential transport through the intracellular membranes of these two glycoproteins.

Rodrigues-Boulan and Sabatini (65) showed a polarity in the maturation of enveloped virus in monolayer cultures of canine kidney (MDCK) cells. The apical and basolateral plasma membranes of these cells are separated by tight junctional barriers between adjacent cells. VSV virus (and its membrane glycoprotein) is released from the basolateral membrane, while influenza virus and parainfluenza virus are released at the apical surface. Thus the envelope glycoproteins of these viruses might also be carried in vesicles coated or not coated to two different domains of the plasma membrane. Hepatitis viral antigens could also become incorporated into hepatocyte membranes by a similar mechanism leading to a pathologic state.

What are the signals that specifically direct vesicles carrying glycoproteins from the Golgi membrane to different regions in the cell? The answer to this question is not yet known, but various possibilities are discussed in a later section. Glycosylation of viral glycoproteins, which may be involved in signal generation, does not appear to be involved here; inhibition of N-glycosylation with tunicamycin had no affect on polarity of virus maturation (57).

Time Required to Synthesize and Insert Glycoproteins in the Plasma Membrane

The partitioning of steps in glycosylation of membrane glycoproteins into different intracellular membrane systems should allow an estimation of the time required by the cell to synthesize and transport proteins to their respective plasma membrane locations. Similar transit times have been estimated for viral glycoprotein maturation (38,39,44) and for the maturation of the plasma membrane glycoproteins of rat hepatoma tissue culture (HTC) cells and mouse liver. We discuss only the HTC cell system.

Monolayer cultures of HTC cells contain a complex set of externally oriented plasma membrane glycoproteins. This set was identified by two-dimensional acrylamide gel electrophoresis of membranes obtained from cells that had been labeled *in situ* by reduction with tritiated sodium borohydride after the cells were treated with neuraminidase and galactose oxidase (50,51,66,67). This procedure labels specifically galactose and galactosamine residues of glycoproteins and glycolipids. A representative sample of these plasma membrane glycoproteins is also accessible *in situ* to trypsin, and the release of certain glycopeptide fragments from HTC cells by trypsin is reproducible (68). Baumann (50) used the accessibility to trypsin to probe the time required for mannose- or fucose-labeled glycoproteins to become externally oriented on the plasma membrane of these cells. Most of the mannose label should be added to asparagine residues of the growing membrane polypeptide on the ER via the dolichol oligosaccharide pathway. In contrast, labeled fucose should be added to membrane glycoproteins in the Golgi membranes after trimming of the high mannose structures. Most of the plasma membrane glycoproteins in HTC cells exist as charge heterogeneous forms, primarily due to differences in extent of sialylation of the glycoprotein with a common amino acid backbone (51,68–70). Sialylation of membrane glycoproteins also occurs in the membranes of the Golgi; in fact, in HTC cells, sialylation may occur before fucosylation. The HTC cell glycoproteins, therefore, should not show much charge heterogeneity until they pass through the Golgi system during biogenesis.

Baumann (50) was able to show that a period of 40 min to 2 hr was required for the glycoproteins to reach (by coated or other type vesicle) the plasma membrane and be trypsin sensitive from the site where fucosylation occurred (the Golgi). It required from 2.5 to 3 hr for glycoproteins to reach the plasma membrane from the site where mannosylation occurred (the ER). Hence the time required to transfer (by vesicles or by some type of membrane flow mechanism) the glycoprotein from the ER (mannose but not fucose labeled, and reduced charge heterogeneity) to the Golgi (fucose labeled, accumulation of charge heterogeneity via addition of sialic acids) was about 1 hr.

Tunicamycin will inhibit the *en bloc* transfer of the high mannose oligosaccharide to the growing nascent polypeptide. The growing polypeptide does not have the accepting substrate for further glycosylation. Experiments with tunicamycin were done to confirm that about 1 hr was required to transfer an HTC cell glycoprotein from the ER to the Golgi membrane.

This temporal sequence of events for the biogenesis of glycoproteins in HTC cells was obtained without recourse to cell fractionation, which is sometimes difficult to effect with hepatic cells in culture or in the animal.

Nonglycosylated Membrane Proteins Synthesized on Free Polysomes

Thus far we have discussed only the biosynthesis of membrane glycoproteins. The questions arise of whether all membrane proteins are glycosylated and whether all membrane proteins are synthesized on membrane-bound polysomes of the RER. It is clear that not all integral membrane proteins are glycosylated. For example, the large subunit of the ouabain-sensitive NaK-ATPase (71), a set of externally oriented (and accessible to lactoperoxidase-catalyzed iodination) plasma membrane proteins, including a highly purified 55,000 MW protein of HTC cells (72–74), and also the cytochrome b5 (75,76) and NADH cytochrome b5 reductase (77–80) of hepatocytes do not contain carbohydrate residues in detectable amounts. While the synthesis of N-glycosylated membrane glycoproteins on membrane-bound ribosomes of the ER is obligate for the reasons discussed above, nonglycosylated membrane proteins could be made by a different biosynthetic pathway. In fact, cytochrome b5 (75) and NADH cytochrome b5 reductase (77–80) of rat liver hepatocytes are both made on free polysomes; the polypeptide, after release from the free polysomes, is transferred in a nonprocessed form to the membrane system in which it resides (D in Fig. 1). There is, however, no significant pool of these proteins in the soluble fraction of the liver; the proteins, after release from the free polysome, must find their way to the membrane quickly and efficiently. In fact, both proteins are rather ubiquitously distributed among several membrane systems of the hepatocyte.

Factors Controlling Localization of Proteins in Different Membranes of the Cell

Both these proteins are found as integral membrane proteins in the ER, the Golgi apparatus, and the mitochondria. Cytochrome b5 also may be present in the plasma membrane, the peroxisome, and the nuclear envelope. This type of distribution is consistent with a site of synthesis on free polysomes for both hepatocyte proteins. The carboxy terminal end of both of these proteins (76,81,82) is enriched in hydrophobic amino acid residues; it is this region that provides the membrane binding site. Either protein, after being released from the polysome, likely can be inserted into any membrane with a lipid composition with affinity for the accessible hydrophobic carboxy terminal end of the protein. Most of the information for membrane insertion must be contained within the amino acid sequence of the protein. However, the fact that both cytochrome b5 and the NADH cytochrome b5 reductase are not present in the same concentration in each of the membranes in which they reside suggests that some other determinant may be involved in specifying localization. Lipid composition, some other membrane component, or some as yet unknown modification of the protein may be required for insertion into the proper membrane.

Because of their mode of biogenesis, N-glycosylated membrane glycoproteins would be expected to be less ubiquitous in their distribution than the membrane proteins synthesized on free polysomes. As discussed below, however, many glycoproteins of the plasma membrane are not unique to this organelle and are present on intracellular membranes. Furthermore, at least one lysosomal hydrolase, β-glucuronidase, is present in about equal amounts in both lysosomes and ER of liver. Genetic studies have shown rather unequivocably that a single structural gene specifies the protein in both membrane systems of mice (83–85).

β-Glucuronidase, a glycoprotein probably like most lysosomal hydrolases, is made on membrane-bound polysomes of the ER as a precursor with a signal amino acid extension (10–12). During N-glycosylation at the ER, a mannose 6-phosphate residue is formed as part of the oligosaccharide structure (86). As initially proposed by Kaplan et al. (87), many and probably all lysosomal hydrolases contain this phosphorylated sugar, which may act as a recognition marker responsible for the incorporation of these enzymes into lysosomes (88–91). A specific high affinity receptor for mannose 6-phosphate is present on the membranes of fibroblasts. About 80% of the total specific binding of this receptor for β-glucoronidase is present on intracellular membranes (92); a finding that led Sly (90) to propose a role for the receptor in regulating intracellular traffic of acid hydrolases from their initial site of synthesis on membrane-bound polysomes of the RER through the Golgi and/or Gerl systems to the lysosomes. Consistent with this proposed role of the mannose 6-phosphate receptor is the observation that fibroblasts from patients with I cell disease secrete their acid hydrolases rather than incorporating them into lysosomes (93). This genetic defect results in lysosomal hydrolases that lack the mannose 6-phosphate signal, although they do have the receptor. Hence the I cell fibroblast treats the acid hydrolases as secretory glycoproteins rather than delivering them to lysosomes (93).

The same mannose 6-phosphate-specific receptor is also present externally on the plasma membrane of fibroblasts, which has led to the suggestion that the plasma membrane itself may be an intermediate in the biogenesis of the lysosome. This suggestion is actually a variation of the secretion-recapture hypothesis originally proposed by Neufeld and collaborators (93,94). The proposed mechanism for biogenesis is as follows: Lysosomal hydrolases are synthesized and processed with the mannose 6-phosphate recognition signal. The intracellular receptor for this signal then binds the hydrolases, possibly in the Golgi or Gerl region of the cell, and transports membrane-bound hydrolase to the plasma membrane. The unit of plasma membrane containing the hydrolase is then interiorized and fuses with an already existing lysosome. If this mechanism is correct, the time that the lysosomal hydrolase spends on the plasma membrane must be short, be-

cause it has not been possible to compete for the presumably externally accessible hydrolase with mannose 6-phosphate.

Most evidence is consistent with either of the above hypotheses concerning the pathway of lysosomal hydrolase biogenesis and the role of mannose 6-phosphate as a recognition signal in this pathway. However, none of the data provides unequivocal proof that either of the proposed mechanisms is correct. Most, and again possibly all, lysosomal hydrolases undergo a peculiar secondary modification in which an additional processing step involving further cleavage of the enzymes occurs (89,95). The kinetics of this process suggest that the cleavage occurs after the acid hydrolases reach the lysosome (95). Recently, Frisch and Neufeld (96) have shown that processing can be accomplished in a cell-free membrane-derived system of fibroblasts at acid pH, again suggesting that processing *in vivo* occurs in the lysosome. It might be predicted, therefore, that plasma membrane forms of the hydrolases, if in transit to the lysosome, would not yet be processed. Regardless of which mechanism delivers the acid hydrolases to the lysosome, because of the advantageous properties of this system and the progress made to date on the signals targeting these enzymes to lysosomes, resolution of this biogenetic pathway may be expected in the foreseeable future.

The mechanism specifying the localization of glucuronidase in the ER of mammalian cells, including hepatocytes, may be completely different from that specifying lysosomal localization. Paigen and colleagues (84,85,97,98) have shown that two different polypeptides are precipitated from detergent extracts of ER of mouse liver by an F(ab)² fragment of an antibody specific for β-glucuronidase. Only one polypeptide is precipitated by the same antibody from extracts of lysosomes. The immune precipitate from lysosomes contains only the 75,000 MW catalytic subunit of the acid hydrolase. In contrast, the immune precipitate from microsomes contains, in addition to a slightly modified form of the catalytic β-glucuronidase subunit, an accessory polypeptide component of about 50,000 MW. This protein, termed egasyn, is presumably responsible for anchoring β-glucuronidase to the membranes of the ER, since one inbred strain of mice that carries an altered gene, such that there is no microsomal glucuronidase, also lacks egasyn, the anchoring protein.

A question arises from studies of lysosomal hydrolase biogenesis and insertion into the two different membrane systems of the hepatocyte: Does the microsomal form of lysosomal hydrolase carry the mannose 6-phosphate residue that has been proposed as the recognition signal for insertion into lysosomes? Clearly, more information about the structural differences between the β-glucuronidase in lysosomes and ER, and the structure of egasyn, the microsomal binding protein, should provide insight into posttranscriptional modifications that are involved in targeting this enzyme to the different membranes of the hepatocyte.

Some glycoproteins are uniquely distributed to one membrane domain of the hepatocyte. For example, two transmembrane glycoproteins of MW 63,000 and 65,000 are present in the RER and not the SER of rat hepatocytes (14,15). As mentioned previously, these proteins, termed ribophorins, probably are involved in binding of ribosomes to the RER, since they could be preferentially cross linked to ribosomal proteins of the large ribosomal subunit with glutaraldehyde. Most other proteins of the RER are identical to those of the SER, including cytochrome P450. Assuming that the ribophorins are made by a similar mechanism as cytochrome P450, why are they restrained from distributing themselves throughout the ER? It may be, as suggested by Kreibich et al. (14,15), that the ribophorins are associated with each other or with other integral membrane proteins or peripheral cytoskeletal proteins, forming a lattice structure or intramembraneous network that cannot move freely in the plane of the lipid bilayer. Such interactions may occur in erythrocytes (28,29,99,100). For example, erythrocyte band 3, a complex transmembrane glycoprotein, may associate with the peripheral spectrin network on the cytoplasmic side of the plasma membrane. Indirect evidence for similar associations of integral, externally oriented membrane proteins with cytoskeletal elements, such as the proteins of the microfilaments and microtubules, has also been presented for mammalian cells other than erythrocytes (18,100,101).

Mechanisms similar to those responsible for the unique localization of the ribosome-binding proteins in RER may be involved in regulating the specific localization of certain proteins in specialized domains of a membrane. For example, GAP junctions are specialized regions of contact between opposed plasma membranes of adjacent cells (K in Fig. 1). These junctions may be involved in the transfer and regulation of transfer of small molecules and ions between cells. The junctional element is composed of hexagonal units, which are embedded in the opposed membranes in register, forming a channel between the cells (102–105). The major constituent(s) of this junction in rat liver hepatocytes is probably one (or possibly more) protein(s) of 26,000 MW; it is uniquely confined to the GAP junction domain of the hepatocyte plasma membrane (106–109). Whether or not this protein(s) is a glycoprotein and its exact route of biogenesis remain to be elucidated.

Although considerable progress has been made in the last few years to elucidate the signals on membrane proteins that determine the ultimate localization of specific proteins in the different membrane systems of the cell, it is obvious from results to date that more

must be done. The following are some of the parameters that define membrane localization and consequently the differentiated state of the membrane:

1. Is the protein synthesized on free or membrane-bound polysomes?
2. Is the mRNA modified by having additional sequences leading to an additional hydrophobic domain on the protein?
3. The amino acid composition and possibly secondary structure of the protein.
4. Is the protein glycosylated?
5. Are there signal sugars on the glycosylated protein?
6. After insertion into the membrane, does the membrane protein become associated with itself or other integral membrane proteins or peripheral cytoskeletal or exoskeletal type proteins?
7. Do the presumptive vesicles, coated or uncoated, carrying the membrane protein from the Golgi to its final destination, have informational molecules determining the type of membrane to which the vesicle is capable of fusing?

METABOLIC FATE OF PLASMA MEMBRANE PROTEINS AFTER INSERTION INTO THE LIPID BILAYER

Plausible Mechanisms for the Removal of a Protein From the Plasma Membrane

The metabolic fate of membrane proteins and glycoproteins after insertion into their respective domains of the hepatocyte membrane system has received considerable attention in recent years. The results of many of these studies often are difficult to interpret because of the different methodologies employed to measure membrane protein turnover. The results may appear to be conflicting. In an attempt to reconcile the different studies and to develop a framework within which to interpret studies on membrane protein turnover in hepatocytes, we propose three possible mechanisms by which a protein or glycoprotein can be removed from the membrane domain in which it resides. We use as an example (Fig. 1) proteins of the plasma membrane of the hepatocyte: (a) The protein can be shed from the membrane into the external milieu with or without part of the lipid bilayer. (b) The protein can present an accessible site to a protease or some other hydrolase located either outside the hepatocyte or in the membrane of the hepatocyte (C in Fig. 1). (c) The domain of membrane containing the protein can vesiculate and fuse with a lysosome; the protein or glycoprotein then would be made accessible to the acid pH of the lysosomes, allowing digestion of susceptible bonds by acid hydrolases and proteases of the lysosomal milieu (M in Fig. 1).

There must be some restraints on the shedding mechanism (19). It would be difficult in thermodynamic terms because of the hydrophilic nature of the carbohydrate residues for a glycoprotein in the plasma membrane or the ER, for example, to cross the lipid bilayer and enter the cytoplasmic fraction of the cell. Similarly, one or more hydrophobic sequences that strongly lock the protein in the membrane bilayer may prevent shedding without part of the bilayer (protein in region B of Fig. 1). Some sequences that determine orientation of the protein in the membrane, however, may not be so tight; this type of protein might leak from its hydrophobic lipid domain.

Basic Mechanism for Degradation of Plasma Membrane Proteins Via Interiorization of Domains of Membrane Followed by Lysosomal Fusion

The fate of externally oriented plasma membrane proteins in suspension cultures of HTC cells has been examined extensively (53–55,67,68,72–74,110). In this cell, ultimately of rat hepatocyte origin, the plasma membrane is relatively simple and does not show the regional specializations that are characteristic of the hepatocyte in the liver. The turnover of the externally oriented proteins of HTC cells was studied in order to avoid complications arising from the necessity of obtaining a relatively homogeneous preparation of plasma membrane by cell fractionation methods. Lactoperoxidase-catalyzed iodination was used as a general method to label plasma membrane and surface proteins having an externally oriented tyrosine residue accessible for iodination. Indeed, we (73) could show that only externally oriented tyrosine residues were labeled when HTC cells were subjected *in situ* to iodination using a modification (111) of the lactoperoxidase method of cell surface labeling (112,113). Furthermore, neither overall cell metabolism nor turnover of the iodinated proteins was affected significantly by the labeling procedure itself.

It was rather straightforward to show that: (a) the iodinated proteins were lost from the hepatoma cells slowly, with a half-life of 100 hr or more; (b) the iodinated proteins were not shed from the HTC cells but were degraded to acid-soluble material that was released to the medium; and (c) most of the proteins that were accessible to iodination *in situ* were degraded at similar rates, albeit with long half-lives (72). In fact, in HTC cells, quite a few proteins (60 to 100) are present in the plasma membrane or at the surface of the cell in sufficient quantity to be iodinated and easily resolved by one- and two-dimensional electrophoretic methods (55). Uniform turnover of many plasma membrane proteins would be expected if the main mechanism for the removal of these proteins from the surface of the

cell involved interiorization of a domain of membrane containing a random assortment of externally oriented proteins, followed by fusion of the interiorized unit of membrane with a lysosome. In fact, we (67) found that the externally oriented glycolipids of the HTC cell were turned over at the same rate as the iodinated surface proteins, suggesting that after interiorization, the entire unit of membrane was degraded in the phagolysosome. A problem complicating these studies was that the method of labeling, that is, lactoperoxidase-catalyzed iodination, would be expected to label mainly the major externally oriented proteins of the hepatoma cell. Some of these proteins also would be expected to be exoskeletal or peripheral cell proteins, rather than authentic or intrinsic plasma membrane proteins. It is difficult but possible (74) to distinguish between these two types.

Turnover of Externally Oriented Plasma Membrane Glycoproteins

To examine the less abundant glycoproteins that were externally oriented on the HTC cell, Baumann and Doyle (67) treated HTC cells *in situ* first with neuraminadase to expose galactose and galactosamine residues of externally oriented glycoproteins and glycolipids. The cells then were treated with galactose oxidase to oxidize the hydroxyl groups of galactose and galactosamine residues, which were subsequently reduced with tritiated sodium borohydride (114). A complex set of externally oriented glycoproteins was identified by this labeling procedure. These externally oriented glycoproteins were actually a less abundant subset of the proteins identified by lactoperoxidase-catalyzed iodination. When the proteins that were labeled after *in situ* lactoperoxidase-catalyzed iodination of HTC cells were fractionated on columns of concanavalin A, the iodinated proteins that bound to the plant lectin were similar to those glycoproteins that were labeled *in situ* after HTC cells were subjected to the galactose oxidase-sodium borohydride-labeling regimen. These proteins were lost from the cell with biphasic kinetics. Again, loss was by degradation to acid-soluble material that was released to the medium. A slow phase of loss corresponded to the half-life of 100 hr or more seen for the total iodinated proteins or the glycolipids of the membrane; but 50% or more of the externally oriented glycoproteins were degraded at a rate corresponding to a half-life of 1 day or less. Contributing to this rapid phase of turnover was a glycoprotein of 85,000 MW. This was a major externally oriented glycoprotein of the HTC cell. Its mode of turnover (68) was by a mechanism that involved a protease that acted at the surface of the HTC cell to release from the 85,000 MW glycoprotein, a 55,000 MW glycopeptide fragment which accumulated in the medium. The 85,000 MW glycoprotein *in situ* was sensitive to trypsin. Trypsin also released from this glycoprotein a 55,000 MW glycopeptide which was similar in composition to the glycopeptide that accumulated in serum-free medium as a normal consequence of the mode of turnover of the 85,000 MW glycoprotein.

The 85,000 MW plasma membrane glycoprotein was turned over by a different mechanism than the bulk of surface protein that was accessible to iodination. The latter class of proteins probably was turned over via an endocytic mechanism, while the 85,000 MW glycoprotein was removed from the HTC cell by a surface-acting protease. The faster rate of degradation of the 85,000 MW glycoprotein, which accounted for about 10 to 15% of the incorporated label, could not alone account for the biphasic kinetics exhibited for the loss of label incorporated into surface glycoproteins after treatment of HTC cells with galactose oxidase and sodium borohydride.

Many of the other labeled glycoproteins in the more rapidly turning over fraction of surface-labeled glycoproteins were also turning over synchronously. The half-life of 24 hr, however, was in contrast to the 100-hr synchronous half-lives exhibited by the total surface iodinated proteins. Synchronous turnover of the more rapidly turning over fraction of surface glycoproteins again suggests an endocytic mechanism. Similar results were obtained by Hubbard and Cohn (115) and Kaplan et al. (116) for the turnover of externally oriented glycoproteins of mouse peritoneal macrophages and fibroblasts. That is, these proteins were lost from the macrophage or fibroblast in a biphasic fashion. One component demonstrated a rapid rate of turnover with a half-life of 1 day or less; the other fraction showed a slow rate of turnover corresponding to a half-life of about 100 hr. Most of the proteins turning over at the slower rate were in fact turning over synchronously. The rapid phase of protein loss in macrophages was due largely to low molecular weight species (116).

The same externally oriented protein in some cells shows biphasic turnover kinetics whether iodinated in its tyrosine backbone or tritium labeled in its galactose residues. For example, we have shown (A. V. Le and D. Doyle, *unpublished*) that the H2D and H2K antigens, which are externally oriented glycoproteins on the mouse macrophage, turn over with biphasic kinetics corresponding to a rapid half-life of 1 day or less and a slow half-life of 100 hr or more. These results suggest that the same glycoprotein may be turned over by more than one mechanism in some cells. Part of the H2 antigens on macrophages or hepatocytes may be turned over by the endocytic mechanism at a slow rate (half-life 100 hr) and part at a faster rate by a different mechanism, possibly patching on the surface and interiorization in coated pits or shedding.

Redistribution of Membrane Proteins Before Interiorization

The observation that most of the major externally oriented proteins in HTC cells and mouse peritoneal macrophages turn over synchronously suggests that these proteins are distributed randomly in the membrane and that one (or only a few) major domains in terms of turnover exists on the plasma membrane of these two cell types. For a protein to be turned over faster (or slower) than the other proteins of the domain, it would have to be removed from its domain and concentrated in the plane of the membrane, forming a new domain; the new domain would be interiorized and fused with a lysosome at a different rate than that of the previous unit of membrane (see region N of Fig. 1). It is known that certain macromolecules external to the cell can bring about such redistributions of externally oriented plasma membrane proteins (117–121). For example, receptors for the polypeptide hormones insulin and epidermal growth factor, as well as receptors for some serum proteins, are uniformly distributed on the plasma membrane. The ligands for these receptors, however, can bring about a redistribution or clustering of the receptor in the plane of the membrane. The receptor/ligand complex then becomes interiorized, possibly in a coated pit. The interiorized unit can fuse with a lysosome, which may lead to degradation not only of the ligand but also (but not always) of the receptor. This type of mechanism may be involved in the so-called "down regulation" of hormone receptors for such physiologically important ligands as insulin and epidermal growth factor (119,121). It may also be involved in hepatic diseases brought about by the lipopolysaccharide toxin of certain bacterial cell walls. As part of the receptor clustering to form a new domain and interiorization steps, the receptor may become cross linked to either some other protein in the membrane or some peripheral cytoplasmic protein (66). Transglutaminases are intracellular enzymes that can covalently cross link proteins; Davies and colleagues (117) have shown that inhibitors of transglutaminase also inhibit ligand (and receptor?) clustering and internalization.

The preceding studies suggest that the main (but not the only) mode by which plasma membrane proteins are turned over involves interiorization of domains of membrane, followed by fusion of the interiorized unit of membrane with subsequent degradation of the membrane protein. Most studies suggesting this mechanism have been performed with tissue culture cells, including hepatoma cells. Does the same (or similar) mechanism function in hepatocytes?

Studies of Hepatocyte Protein Turnover *In Situ* and *In Vitro*

Studies on the turnover of proteins constituting the plasma membrane and the membranes of the ER of rat liver by Dehlinger and Schimke (122,123) suggested that the proteins of these membranes were turning over rather slowly (half-life 3 to 5 days) and at heterogeneous rates. Higher molecular weight components appeared to be turned over at faster rates than polypeptides of lower molecular weight. Similar results were reported by Gurd and Evans (124) and Tauber and Reutter (125). These studies utilized intact animals and relied on cell fractionation methods to isolate the membrane of interest. In rat liver, the proteins of the soluble fraction show the most pronounced correlation between subunit or polypeptide molecular weight and rate of degradation. Hence any contamination of the membrane fraction with soluble proteins would tend to exaggerate the size-turnover correlation, especially if most of the proteins of the membrane fraction are turning over relatively slowly and with more uniform rates. In the study by Tauber and Reutter (125), most of the membrane proteins, as resolved from the plasma membrane fraction by dodecyl sulfate-polyacrylamide gel electrophoresis, had similar rates of degradation. Only a few proteins appeared to be turning over faster than the bulk of labeled membrane protein. Some of these could have been secretory proteins.

To overcome certain problems inherent in using intact animals and cell fractionation methods to examine the turnover of liver plasma membrane proteins, Warren and Doyle (126) attempted to study the turnover of plasma membrane proteins in isolated rat liver hepatocytes by following the loss of radioactivity incorporated *in situ* into externally oriented surface proteins via lactoperoxidase-catalyzed iodination. The radioactivity incorporated into externally oriented proteins having accessible tyrosine residues was lost with biphasic kinetics. There was a rapid phase of turnover corresponding to a half-life of less than 1 day and a slow phase corresponding to a half-life of about 80 to 100 hr. There was enrichment for smaller molecular weight polypeptides in the rapidly turning over fraction, as there is for macrophages. Many of the polypeptides in the slowly turning over fraction were degraded at synchronous rates. Warren and Doyle (126) also examined the turnover of a major externally oriented glycoprotein that is specifically confined to liver hepatocytes (127,128), the hepatic binding protein. This protein binds, interiorizes, and delivers to

lysosomes serum glycoproteins that have exposed penultimate galactose residues (49,129,130). It turned over with a half-life of about 20 hr, a turnover time faster than that of the bulk iodinated surface proteins of the hepatocyte. These results are similar to results already discussed for the turnover of the plasma membrane proteins of HTC cells and macrophages; that is, the externally oriented proteins of the cells are turned over in a biphasic fashion.

Most of the proteins comprising the slower class in terms of degradation are turned over synchronously, suggesting degradation of membrane units in lysosomes following endocytosis. Some proteins in the slower turnover class may be peripheral exoskeletal proteins. The glycoproteins of HTC cells and hepatocytes are enriched in the more rapidly turning over class of membrane proteins (half-life 1 day or less). Most of the glycoproteins in this class also are turning over synchronously, albeit at a faster rate than the bulk of externally accessible plasma membrane protein. Again, the bulk of plasma membrane glycoproteins probably are removed from the surface in domains and degraded via the endocytic-lysosomal fusion mechanism. The domain in which the protein resides may be a regional specialization of the membrane, such as the gap junction or sinusoidal face of the hepatocyte plasma membrane; or the domain may be formed by clustering in the lipid bilayer brought about by a ligand, such as a polypeptide hormone or a serum component. A possible explanation for the more rapid turnover of glycoproteins relative to the non- (or minimally) glycosylated proteins is given in a later section on membrane recycling.

Finally, some plasma membrane proteins of the hepatocyte are turned over by a different mechanism, one that involves surface-acting proteases to degrade accessible proteins and glycoproteins. Some as yet unidentified hepatocyte proteins may be lost by being shed into the circulation.

Elovson (143) has examined the biogenesis of two externally oriented plasma membrane glycoproteins present in the same region or domain of the rat hepatocyte plasma membrane. He used antibodies to the purified proteins to isolate the labeled enzyme from rat liver extracts. One protein, dipeptidyl peptidase IV, was turned over slowly, with a half-life of about 5 days; the other plasma membrane glycoprotein, nucleotide pyrophosphatase, was turned over rapidly (or in a biphasic manner), with a half-life of only 1 day. The mechanism(s) responsible for the differential turnover of these two proteins is not yet known.

Similarly, half-life values measured for the turnover of a set of ER enzymes indicate heterogeneous turnover, with half-lives varying from 3 to more than 100 hr (see ref. 131 for review). In fact, the turnover of a single enzyme in two different membrane systems can vary. For example, Borgese et al. (79) have shown that NADH-cytochrome b5 reductase has a faster rate of turnover in ER relative to its turnover in its mitochondrial domain.

Clearly, much work remains to be done to clarify the mechanism of membrane protein turnover in hepatocytes. For example, knowledge about the turnover properties of the whole set of membrane proteins comprising each of the various domains of the hepatocyte plasma membrane would help to determine which of the three most plausible mechanisms (endocytosis of a domain, surface-acting proteases, or shedding) is responsible for the turnover of each of the proteins within the domain. In fact, better methods for specific labeling of plasma membrane proteins, as well as better methods for membrane fractionation and for resolving complex mixtures of membrane proteins, are being developed.

RECYCLING OF PLASMA MEMBRANE

If the major mode for the removal of plasma membrane proteins and glycoproteins involves interiorization of a unit or domain of membrane followed by fusion with a lysosome, as we suggest, the question arises of whether every interiorized unit of membrane is degraded; the answer probably is no.

Rates of Interiorization of Plasma Membrane Faster Than Rates of Degradation

Steinman et al. (132) showed that mouse macrophages and L cells in culture, during pinocytosis of horseradish peroxidase, interiorize the equivalent of their entire cell surface every 30 min and 2 hr, respectively. The interiorized membrane vesicles fuse with lysosomes, and the horseradish peroxidase is degraded. As discussed above, however, the surface proteins of these cells are stable and are degraded with relatively long half-lives. Also, the size of the intracellular pinocytotic vesicle and lysosomal compartments of these cells did not increase, nor did the surface area of the cell decrease during the course of the experiment. Based on this stereologic analysis, Steinman et al. (132) proposed that the plasma membrane constituents of the pinocytotic vesicle must recycle back to the surface. More direct evidence for recycling was obtained recently by Mellman et al. (133), who allowed cells in culture to pinocytose lactoperoxidase and glucose oxidase. The cells then were administered ^{125}I and glucose. The authors showed that the labeled iodide became incorporated into proteins of the pinosome. The plasma membrane was not labeled; the pinosome proteins were identical or similar to the proteins comprising the plasma membrane of

the cell. Hence the pinosome probably represents a random and representative assortment of the plasma membrane proteins of the cell, or the plasma membrane acts as a single domain in terms of forming the pinocytotic vesicle. When the cells were placed in culture at 37° C, the label in the pinosomes moved (or recycled) back to the surface, as demonstrated by autoradiography of cell thin sections.

HTC cells also interiorize an area equivalent to the entire surface area every hour (134,135). Yet, as we demonstrated (67,72), the turnover rate for the proteins and glycoproteins of the plasma membrane is slow in this cell type. All cells, including hepatocytes *in vivo,* probably are continually interiorizing domains of their plasma membrane at prodigious rates (136,137). Much of the interiorized membrane will fuse with a lysosome or with some other intracellular membrane and recycle back to the surface. The mechanism by which the proteins and glycoproteins of the plasma membrane escape degradation after fusion with a lysosome is not yet known, but some clues toward understanding this process have been obtained recently and are discussed later.

Differential Turnover of the Sugar and Amino Acid Moieties of Membrane Proteins

The glycoproteins of the plasma membrane may not escape degradation completely while traversing the lysosomal compartment during recycling. Kreisel et al. (138) have shown that the carbohydrate and protein moieties of a 110,000 MW glycoprotein of the plasma membrane of rat liver had different rates of turnover. The amino acid backbone of this protein turned over, with a long half-life of 70 to 80 h, characteristic of hepatocyte plasma membrane proteins (126). Fucose was lost from the protein, however, with a half-life of about 12 hr. N-acetyl neuraminic acid also was lost, with a half-life of 33 hr, as was galactose, with a half-life of 20 hr. It may be, as suggested by Kreisel et al. (138) and by Doyle and Baumann (53,67), that during each recycling event, some carbohydrate is digested off the protein by lysosomal hydrolases. If this is correct, it could provide an explanation for the more rapid turnover of glycoproteins relative to total externally oriented plasma membrane proteins observed by Baumann and Doyle (67) in hepatoma cells. These authors followed the turnover of the glycoprotein using metabolic labeling with fucose or external labeling with the galactose oxidase and the sodium borotritide regimen. The glycoproteins were also labeled metabolically in their amino acid backbone with methionine or externally via lactoperoxidase-catalyzed iodination. In the latter cases, the glycoproteins were isolated using affinity chromatography on columns of concanavalin A. If the carbohydrate residues are removed at a different rate than the degradation of the protein backbone during recycling, then the glycoproteins, as labeled with fucose or as isolated based on carbohydrate (mannose) content on concanavalin A, would appear to turn over faster than the non- or minimally glycosylated proteins of the membrane if the mannose were removed.

Plasma Membrane Proteins on Intracellular Membranes

If continual recycling of the plasma membrane is a normal property of eukaryotic cells, a finite compartment of plasma membrane should also be present inside of the cell. Doyle et al. (55) searched for this intracellular fraction of plasma membrane protein in hepatoma cells using cell fractionation in combination with metabolic labeling with fucose and external labeling via lactoperoxidase-catalyzed iodination to distinguish between a plasma membrane and an intracellular localization. An intracellular membrane system was found, which was identical or nearly identical in glycoprotein composition to the plasma membrane. This result was confirmed by Baumann and Doyle (51) using a method not dependent on cell fractionation. The total membrane glycoproteins of hepatoma cells were labeled to steady state by growing cells for several generations in [^{3}H]fucose. The set of glycoproteins so labeled was identified by two-dimensional polyacrylamide gel electrophoresis. Most of the labeled membrane glycoproteins show charge heterogeneity in this system, due mainly to different extents of sialyation to a common protein backbone.

Baumann and Doyle (51), taking advantage of these properties of the glycoproteins, showed that when intact fucose-labeled cells were treated *in situ* with neuraminidase, the accessible glycoproteins, because of the loss of sialic acid residues, migrated to a new, more basic position after electrophoresis in the two-dimensional system. However, only a portion (30 to 40%) of each glycoprotein species was accessible when intact cells were treated with neuraminidase. In contrast, all the glycoprotein was accessible to neuraminidase when cells were disrupted and the glycoproteins removed from the membrane. That is, 60 to 70% of the glycoprotein was not accessible at the surface because it was inside the cell.

Reservoir of Plasma Membrane Proteins on Intracellular Membranes

Both cell fractionation and the neuraminidase probe analysis showed the presence of an intracellular membrane system that was nearly identical in glycoprotein composition to the plasma membrane. The size of this intracellular membrane reservoir was twice as large as

the plasma membrane and was too large to represent recycling membrane. Furthermore, the intracellular membrane did not readily exchange with the plasma membrane because it could not be labeled readily by external labeling of the plasma membrane followed by incubation of the cells at 37° C. Light and electron microscopic autoradiography of fucose-labeled hepatoma cells showed the intracellular compartment to be either the Golgi or Gerl systems of the cell and membrane-limited vesicles associated with these systems (see Figs. 2 and 3). Although the size of this intracellular reservoir of plasma membrane may be unusually large in hepatoma cells, probably because of the large amount of Golgi/Gerl/vesicular structure relative to plasma membrane in this cell type (132), the presence of an intracellular reservoir of plasma membrane is not unique. In many cells, including normal liver, significant quantities of the following plasma membrane proteins are present as authentic constituents (that is, not in transit to the plasma membrane) in intracellular membranes, most likely Golgi/Gerl and vesicular components (5,92,129,139–142): hepatic receptors for insulin and galactose-terminated glycoproteins, receptors for mannose-6-phosphate containing acid hydrolases, the enzymes 5'-nucleotidase and adenyl cyclase, and glucose transport proteins. Not all plasma membrane proteins have been found in intracellular membranes (143).

What is the metabolic function of this intracellular reservoir of plasma membrane protein? We (53–55) proposed that at certain times in its lifetime, the cell may have to put proteins into its surface membrane in a time interval too short to allow *de novo* synthesis. The reservoir would be used in these cases. Evidence that this is indeed the function of the intracellular reservoir of plasma membrane is discussed below.

Some of the intracellular fraction of plasma membrane protein may be involved in carrying out the function of the externally oriented plasma membrane protein. For example, the hepatic receptor for asialo- or, more correctly, galactose-terminated glycoproteins functions to deliver these glycoproteins to the lysosome to be degraded. Actually, the true function of this hepatocyte plasma membrane receptor may be to clear unknown complexes from the circulation (144).

Ashwell and colleagues (49,129,130) and we (70, 126,145) have examined the mechanism by which this receptor performs its function in both isolated hepatocytes in culture and in intact rats. For example, we have shown that in the isolated hepatocyte, during its lifetime (half-life for turnover, 20 hr), each molecule of receptor can deliver about 1,000 molecules of asialoorosomucoid to the lysosome to be degraded. Available evidence, including electron microscopic autoradiographic studies (127,128), is consistent with but does not prove a mechanism for the action of this receptor involving interiorization of the membrane re-

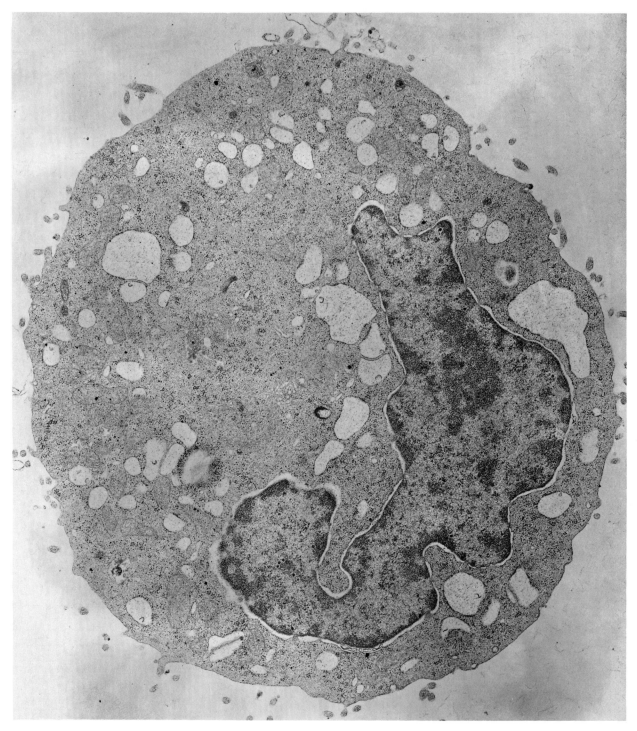

FIG. 2. Electron micrograph of a thin section of HTC cell. Note numerous intracellular vesicles and distended membrane structures that are characteristic of this cell in culture.

ceptor: galactose-terminated glycoprotein complex followed by fusion of the interiorized membrane domain with a lysosome and degradation of the galactose-terminated glycoprotein while the receptor is spared and recycled back to the surface of the cell. The mechanism by which the cell segregates receptor from its ligand in this process is discussed below.

Reconstitution of Membrane Proteins and Transfer to Foreign Cells

The hepatocyte receptor for galactose-terminated glycoproteins is not present exclusively on the plasma membrane. In intact liver, only 10% of the total receptor is externally oriented on the plasma membrane;

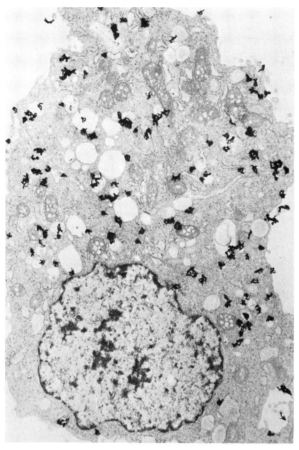

FIG. 3. Autoradiograph of a thin section of an HTC cell labeled for three days in culture with [³H]fucose. Note that a large number of the grains originating from [³H]fucose are over Golgi- or Gerl-derived structures and other vesicles characteristic of the HTC cell.

the rest is present on intracellular membranes, again primarily Golgi/Gerl and associated membrane-limited vesicles. The intracellular fraction of receptor is not necessary for the receptor to carry out its function to deliver galactose-terminated glycoproteins to the lysosome. We (70,145) have isolated from rat liver right-side out membrane vesicles which are enriched in the receptor for galactose-terminated glycoproteins. We also have separated these vesicles into their phospholipid and glycoprotein components and completely reconstituted a right-side out membrane vesicle, into which was inserted purified and iodinated receptor. Using either the right-side out liver membrane vesicle or the completely reconstituted vesicle, we transferred the hepatic receptor to mouse L cells using polyethylene glycol to effect fusion. Before fusion, the mouse L cell was unable to carry out receptor-mediated endocytosis of asialoorosomucoid because the receptor is normally found only on hepatocytes. After transfer of the receptor, however, the L cell was able to bind, interiorize, and deliver to lysosomes asialoorosomucoid, which was subsequently degraded to acid-soluble material. The L cell performed this complex set of reactions at the same rate as hepatocytes.

The receptor after transfer was stable in the L cell turning over with a half-life of 3 to 4 days. This indicated that as in the hepatocyte, each molecule of receptor delivers many hundreds of molecules of ligand to the lysosome, probably because the receptor can recycle. Hence the L cell had been changed into an exact phenocopy of the hepatocyte with respect to the function of this receptor ("cellular engineering"). After transfer to the L cell, however, the receptor did not redistribute itself in the 90:10 intracellular/plasma membrane ratio typical of hepatocytes. Most of the receptor remained localized in the plasma membrane of the L cell. The intracellular fraction of receptor is not required for the receptor to carry out its function of delivering galactose-terminated glycoproteins to the lysosome for degradation. The intracellular reservoir of the hepatocyte plasma membrane proteins, including the receptors for galactose-terminated glycoproteins and for insulin, may serve a regulatory function to be used when the cells need to rapidly increase the concentration of these proteins at the surface. The necessity for rapid replacement of specific proteins in the plasma membrane might occur for example (a) at certain stages of the cell cycle, (b) when a large, acute concentration of an extracellular ligand brings about a significant reduction in the concentration of the plasma membrane receptor for that ligand, (c) when the concentration of a polypeptide hormone, such as insulin or a growth factor, is changed rapidly from a chronic high level, resulting in fewer surface receptors for the hormone (down-regulated state) to a low level, resulting in a requirement for up-regulation, or (d) when the concentration of one or more plasma membrane proteins increases rapidly in response to some change in the environment, i.e., steroid hormone (69,146) or the increase in glucose transport in response to insulin (140,147).

Intracellular Reservoir of Plasma Membrane Proteins Serves a Regulatory Function

Evidence is presented here that indicates a regulatory role for the intracellular reservoir of plasma membrane proteins. We (110) tried to bring about a significant reduction in the concentration of plasma membrane glycoproteins by adding goat immunoglobulin directed against a complex subset of externally oriented glycoproteins to hepatoma cells at 4° C. These cells then were subsequently incubated at 37° C in medium containing rabbit antibody directed against goat IgG. As a result of treatment with the two antibodies, the membrane glycoprotein antigens with the attached fluorescently labeled or iodinated specific antibodies first became patched on the surface. Within a few hours, complete interiorization of antigen and antibodies had occurred. About 40% of the total externally oriented glycoproteins of the hepatoma cell moved from a surface to an intracellular location. We could show that some but not all the plasma membrane glycoprotein was directed to lysosomes in the intracellular compartment. Surprisingly, however, antibody-induced interiorization of the membrane glycoproteins had no effect on their turnover. That is, the glycoproteins were being turned over at the same rate of 1 day or so in either the presence or absence of the antibodies. In fact, the turnover of the iodinated specific antibody was indistinguishable from that of the membrane glycoprotein antigen to which the goat IgG was directed.

These studies shed some light on the mechanism by which the cell could segregate a ligand from its membrane receptor during recycling. The binding of antibody to plasma membrane antigen *in situ* is of a high affinity similar to the binding of asialoorosomucoid to its receptor. After binding, both antibody and asialoorosomucoid are delivered to lysosomes; whereas the asialoorosomucoid is degraded in the lysosome, however, the IgG is not. The difference between the binding characteristics of the two ligands is that while the binding of asialoorosomucoid to its receptor is pH- and calcium ion-dependent, the binding of antibody to antigen is not. When the asialoorosomucoid receptor membrane complex fuses with the lysosome, the drop in pH would promote dissociation, leaving the ligand to be degraded in the lysosome while the receptor recycles (via the Golgi/Gerl?) back to the surface. In contrast, after lysosomal fusion, the antibody would not dissociate from its membrane antigen, and the cell would be unable to distinguish between the membrane antigen and attached antibody. However, the antibody/antigen complex on the interiorized membrane cannot recycle and accumulates in the different constituents of the recycling pathway. In hepatoma cells, these constituents include lysosomes and possibly pinosomes and Golgi/Gerl-like structures. Schneider and colleagues (135,136) used a similar protocol to trap components of the recycling membrane in fibroblasts.

Although 40% of the surface glycoprotein in hepatoma cells was interiorized as a result of antibody treatment, the surface area of the cell did not decrease. *De novo* protein synthesis may not be required to maintain the surface area of these cells, because the glycoproteins are replaced rapidly from the intracellular reservoir.

When Warren and Doyle (126) compared the number of receptors for galactose-terminated glycoproteins that were externally oriented on the plasma membrane of isolated hepatocytes to the total number of receptors in these cells, they found about 60 to 70% of the receptors on the surface. In contrast, Pricer and Ashwell (129) found that 10% of the receptors for galactose-terminated proteins were on the plasma membrane in extracts of rat liver; the rest were in intracellular membranes. The discrepancy between the two studies could be explained by a rapid mobilization and delivery to the plasma membrane of the intracellular receptors when the hepatocytes are isolated from the liver with collagenase and placed in culture. Weigel (148) has shown that the number of binding sites for asialoorosomucoid increases from 7×10^4 to 2×10^5 per cell rapidly after the isolated hepatocytes were cultured at 37° C. The source of this new surface receptor may be the intracellular reservoir.

Finally, a primary effect of insulin on adipose and muscle cell physiology is to rapidly increase the rate of glucose transport. Two groups (140,147) have shown independently that the increased numbers of glucose transport systems on the plasma membrane of the fat cells is attributable to a translocation of glucose transport systems from an as yet unidentified intracellular membrane pool (Golgi/Gerl or vesicles derived therefrom?) to the plasma membrane.

CONCLUSION

The eukaryotic cell can regulate the concentration of specific proteins in its plasma membrane. Many membrane proteins of the hepatoma cell (54,55) and the macrophage (116) are synthesized and delivered to the plasma membrane at synchronous rates to replace those domains of membrane lost in a synchronous manner via the endocytotic mechanism of degradation. The concentration of some proteins is increased by an increase in specific rate of synthesis. For example, the insulin receptor is regulated in 3T3 cells that are differentiating to fat cells by an increase in the rate of synthesis of this relatively short-lived protein or by mobilization and translocation of the membrane protein held in an intracellular reservoir. The latter may be the mechanism of choice if the cell must increase the concentration of a relatively long-lived protein that has been lost from the surface or is needed at the surface in a relatively short time.

Much has been learned in the past few years about the pathway of plasma membrane biogenesis and the dynamic behavior of this complex organelle during normal cell physiology. Still lacking is knowledge about the details of the mechanism by which the hepatocyte can regulate the concentration of individual components of its membrane. Therefore, research must be done to pinpoint what is occurring at the cellular and molecular level in those pathobiologic states in which the liver is the affected organ.

ACKNOWLEDGMENTS

Work from the authors' laboratories has been supported by the National Institutes of Health (GM 24147) and by the National Cancer Institute (CA 26122 and CA 17149).

We thank A. Cairo of the Department of Cell and Tumor Biology, and Dr. Carl Porter of the Department of Experimental Therapeutics, Roswell Park Memorial Institute, for electron microscopy and radioautography of HTC cells. We thank Dr. K. C. Gaines of the Department of Cell and Tumor Biology for teaching us something about liver disease.

REFERENCES

1. Blovin, A., Bolender, R. P., and Weibel, E. (1977): Distribution of organelles and membranes between hepatocytes and nonhepatocytes in the rat liver parenchyma. *J. Cell Biol.*, 72:441–455.
2. Evans, W. H. (1980): A biochemical dissection of the functional polarity of the plasma membrane of the hepatocyte. *Biochim. Biophys. Acta*, 604:27–64.
3. Turco, S. J., and Robbins, P. W. (1979): The initial stages of processing of protein-bound oligosaccharides *in vitro*. *J. Biol. Chem.*, 254:4560–4567.
4. Novikoff, A. B. (1976): The endoplasmic reticulum: A cytochemical review. *Proc. Natl. Acad. Sci. USA*, 73: 2784–2787.
5. Bergeron, J. J. M., Ehrenreich, J. H., Siekevitz, P., and Palade, G. E. (1973): Golgi fractions prepared from rat liver homogenates. II. Biochemical characterization. *J. Cell Biol.*, 59:73–88.
6. Bretz, R., Bretz, H., and Palade, G. (1980): Distribution of terminal glycosyltransferases in hepatic Golgi fractions. *J. Cell Biol.*, 84:87–101.
7. Ehrenreich, J. H., Bergeron, J. J. M., Siekevitz, P., and Palade, G. E. (1973): Golgi fractions prepared from rat liver homogenates. I. Isolation procedure and morphological characterization. *J. Cell Biol.*, 59:45–72.
8. Franke, W. W. (1974): Structure, biochemistry, and functions of the nuclear envelope. *Int. Rev. Cytol. [Suppl.]*, 4:71–236.
9. Gerace, L., and Blobel, G. (1980): The nuclear envelope lamina is reversibly depolymerized during mitosis. *Cell*, 19:277–287.
10. Blobel, G., and Dobberstein, B. (1975): Transfer of proteins across membranes. I. Presence of proteolytically processed and unprocessed nascent immunoglobulin light chains on membrane-bound ribosomes of murine myeloma. *J. Cell Biol.*, 67:835–851.
11. Blobel, G., and Dobberstein, B. (1975): Transfer of proteins across membranes. II. Reconstruction of functional rough microsomes from heterologous components. *J. Cell Biol.*, 67:852–862.
12. Blobel, G., and Sabatini, D. D. (1971): Ribosome-membrane interactions in eukaryotic cells. In: *Biomembranes, Vol. 2*, edited by L. A. Manson, pp. 193–195. Plenum, New York.
13. Milstein, C., Brownlee, G. G., Harrison, T. M., and Mathews, M. B. (1972): A possible precursor of immunoglobulin light chains. *Nature [New Biol.]*, 239:117–120.
14. Kreibich, G., Freienstein, C. M., Pereyra, B. N., Ulrich, B. L., and Sabatini, D. D. (1978): Proteins of rough microsomal membranes related to ribosome binding. II. Cross-linking of bound ribosomes to specific membrane proteins exposed at the binding sites. *J. Cell Biol.*, 77:488–506.
15. Kreibich, G., Ulrich, B. L., and Sabatini, D. D. (1978): Proteins of rough microsomal membranes related to ribosome binding. I. Identification of ribophorins I and II, membrane proteins characteristic of rough microsomes. *J. Cell Biol.*, 77:464–487.
16. Mumford, R. A., Strauss, A. W., Powers, J. C., Pierzchala, P. A., Nishino, N., and Zimmerman, M. (1980): A zinc metalloendopeptidase associated with dog pancreatic membranes. *J. Biol. Cehm.*, 255:2227–2230.
17. Lingappa, V. R., Lingappa, J. R., and Blobel, G. (1979): Chicken ovalbumin contains an internal signal sequence. *Nature*, 281:117.
18. Singer, S. J. (1974): The molecular organization of membranes. *Ann. Rev. Biochem.*, 43:805–833.
19. Alt, F. W., Bothwell, A. L. M., Knapp, M., Siden, E., Mather, E., Koshland, M., and Baltimore, D. (1980): Synthesis of secreted and membrane-bound immunoglobulin Mμ heavy chains is directed by mRNAs that differ at their 3' ends. *Cell*, 20:293–301.
20. Rogers, J., Early, P., Carter, C., Calame, K., Bond, M., Hood, L., and Wall, R. (1980): Two mRNAs with different 3' ends encode membrane-bound and secreted forms of immunoglobulin μ chain. *Cell*, 20:303–312.
21. Singer, P. A., Singer, H. H., and Williamson, A. R. (1980): Different species of mRNA encode receptor and secretory IgM μ chains differing at their carboxy termini. *Nature*, 285: 294–300.
22. Bar-Nun, S., Kreibich, G., Adesnik, M., Alterman, L., Negishi, M., and Sabatini, D. D. (1980): Synthesis and insertion of cytochrome P450 into endoplasmic reticulum membranes. *Proc. Natl. Acad. Sci. USA*, 77:965–969.
23. Fujii-Kuriyama, Y. M., Negishi, R., Mikawa, R., and Tashiro, Y. (1979): Biosynthesis of cytochrome p450 on membrane-bound ribosomes and their subsequent incorporation into

rough and smooth microsomes in rat hepatocytes. *J. Cell Biol.*, 81:510–519.

24. Kumar, A., and Padmanaban, G. (1980): Studies on the synthesis of cytochrome P450 and cytochrome P-448 in rat liver. *J. Biol. Chem.*, 255:522–525.

25. Dobberstein, B. H., Garoff, G., Warren, G., and Robinson, P. J. (1979): Cell-free synthesis and membrane insertion of mouse H2D^d histocompatibility antigen and microglobulin. *Cell*, 17:759–770.

26. Jay, G., Ferrinl, U., Robinson, E. A., Khoury, G., and Appela, E. (1979): Cell free synthesis of mouse H-2 histocompatibility antigens. *Proc. Natl. Acad. Sci. USA*, 76:6562–6566.

27. Ploegh, H. C., Cannon, L. E., and Strominger, J. L. (1979): Cell free translation of the mRNAs for the heavy and light chains of HCA-A and HCA-B antigens. *Proc. Natl. Acad. Sci. USA*, 76:2273–2277.

28. Steck, T. L. (1974): The organization of proteins in the human red blood cell membrane. *J. Cell Biol.*, 62:1–19.

29. Steck, T. L., Koziarz, J. J., Singh, M. K., Reddy, G., and Kohler, H. (1978): Preparation and analysis of seven major topographically defined fragments of band 3, the predominant polypeptide of human erythrocyte membrane. *Biochemistry*, 17:1216–1222.

30. Hanover, J. A., and Lennarz, W. J. (1980): N-linked glycoprotein assembly. Evidence that oligosaccharide attachment occurs within the lumen of the endoplasmic reticulum. *J. Biol. Chem.*, 255:3600–3604.

31. Baynes, J., Hsu, A. F., and Heath, E. C. (1973): The role of mannosylphosphoryl-dehydropolyisoprenol in the synthesis of mammalian glycoproteins. *J. Biol. Chem.*, 248:5693–5704.

32. Chen, W. W., and Lennarz, W. J. (1977): Metabolism of lipid-linked N-acetylglucosamine intermediates. *J. Biol. Chem.*, 252:3473–3479.

33. Chen, W. W., Lennarz, W. J., Tarentino, A. L., and Maley, F. (1975): A lipid-linked oligosaccharide intermediate in glycoprotein synthesis in oviduct. *J. Biol. Chem.*, 250:7006–7013.

34. Elting, J. J., Chen, W. W., and Lennarz, W. J. (1980): Characterization of a glucosidase involved in an initial step in the processing of oligosaccharide chains. *J. Biol. Chem.*, 255:2325–2331.

35. Grinna, L. S., and Robbins, P. W. (1980): Substrate specificities of rat liver microsomal glucosidases which process glycoproteins. *J. Biol. Chem.*, 255:2255–2258.

36. Harpaz, N., and Schachter, H. (1980): Control of glycoprotein synthesis. *J. Biol. Chem.*, 255:4894–4902.

37. Herscovics, H., Golovtchenko, A. M., Warren, C. D., Bugge, B., and Jeanloz, R. W. (1977): Mannosyltransferase activity in calf pancreas microsomes. *J. Biol. Chem.*, 252:224–234.

38. Hubbard, S. C., and Robbins, P. W. (1979): Synthesis and processing of protein-linked oligosaccharides *in vivo*. *J. Biol. Chem.*, 254:4568–4576.

39. Kornfeld, S., Li, E., and Tabas, I. (1978): The synthesis of complex-type oligosaccharides. II. Characterization of the processing intermediates in the synthesis of the complex oligosaccharide units of the vesicular stomatitis virus G protein. *J. Biol. Chem.*, 253:7771–7778.

40. Lin, T., Stetson, B., Turco, S. J., Hubbard, S. C., and Robbins, P. W. (1979): Arrangement of glucose residues in the lipid-linked oligosaccharide precursor of asparaginyl oligosaccharides. *J. Biol. Chem.*, 254:4554–4559.

41. Lucas, J. J., Waechter, C. J., and Lennarz, W. J. (1975): The participation of lipid-linked oligosaccharide in synthesis of membrane glycoproteins. *J. Biol. Chem.*, 250:1992–2002.

42. Parodi, A. J., Behrens, N. H., LeLoir, L. F., and Carmnatti, H. (1972): The role of polyprenol-bound saccharides as intermediates in glycoprotein synthesis in liver. *Proc. Natl. Acad. Sci. USA*, 69:3268–3272.

43. Pless, D. D., and Lennarz, W. J. (1975): A lipid-linked oligosaccharide intermediate in glycoprotein synthesis. *J. Biol. Chem.*, 250:7014–7019.

44. Robbins, P. W., Hubbard, S. C., Turco, S. J., and Wirth, D. F. (1977): Proposal for a common oligosaccharide intermediate in the synthesis of membrane glycoproteins. *Cell*, 12:889–900.

45. Struck, D. K., and Lennarz, W. J. (1977): Evidence for the participation of saccharide-lipids in the synthesis of the oligosaccharide chain of ovalbumin. *J. Biol. Chem.*, 252:1007–1013.

46. Tabas, I., and Kornfeld, S. (1978): The synthesis of complex-type oligosaccharides. III. Identification of an α-D-mannosidase activity involved in a late state of processing of complex-type oligosaccharides. *J. Biol. Chem.*, 253:7779–7786.

47. Turco, S. J., Stetson, B., and Robbins, P. W. (1977): Comparative rates of transfer of lipid-linked oligosaccharides to endogenous glycoprotein acceptors *in vitro*. *Proc. Natl. Acad. Sci. USA*, 74:4411–4414.

48. Waechter, C. J., and Lennarz, W. J. (1976): The role of polyprenol-linked sugars in glycoprotein synthesis. *Ann. Rev. Biochem.*, 45:95–112.

49. Ashwell, G., and Morell, A. G. (1974): The role of surface carbohydrates in the hepatic recognition and transport of circulating glycoproteins. *Adv. Enzymol.*, 41:99–128.

50. Baumann, H. (1980): Biosynthesis of membrane glycoproteins in rat hepatoma tissue culture cells. *J. Supramol. Struct.*, 12:151–164.

51. Baumann, H., and Doyle, D. (1979): Localization of membrane glycoproteins by *in situ* neuraminidase treatment of rat hepatoma tissue culture cells and two-dimensional gel electrophoretic analysis of the modified proteins. *J. Biol. Chem.*, 254:2542–2550.

52. Carey, D. J., and Hirschberg, C. B. (1980): Kinetics of glycosylation and intracellular transport of sialoglycoproteins in mouse liver. *J. Biol. Chem.*, 255:4348–4354.

53. Doyle, D., and Baumann, H. (1979): Turnover of the plasma membrane of mammalian cells. *Life Sci.*, 24:951–966.

54. Doyle, D., Baumann, H., England, B., Friedman, E., Hou, E., and Tweto, J. (1978): Biogenesis of plasma membrane glycoproteins in hepatoma tissue culture cells. *J. Biol. Chem.*, 253:965–973.

55. Doyle, D., Baumann, H., England, B., Friedman, E., Hou, E., and Tweto, J. (1978): Turnover and biogenesis of the plasma membrane proteins of hepatoma tissue culture cells. In: *Protein Turnover and Lysosome Function*, edited by H. Segal and D. Doyle, pp. 689–716. Academic Press, New York.

56. Rodriguez-Boulan, E., Kreibich, G., and Sabatini, D. D. (1978): Spatial orientation of glycoproteins in membranes of rough microsomes. I. Localization of lectin-binding sites in microsomal membranes. *J. Cell Biol.*, 78:874–893.

57. Roth, M. G., Fitzpatrick, J. P., and Compans, R. W. (1979): Polarity of influenza and vesicular stomatitis virus maturation in MDCK cells: Lack of a requirement for glycosylation of viral glycoproteins. *Proc. Natl. Acad. Sci. USA*, 76:6430–6434.

58. Kalish, F., Chovick, N., and Dice, J. F. (1979): Rapid *in vivo* degradation of glycoproteins isolated from cytosol. *J. Biol. Chem.*, 254:4475–4481.

59. Nicolson, G. L., and Singer, S. J. (1974): The distribution and asymmetry of mammalian cell surface saccharides utilizing ferritin-conjugated plant agglutinins as specific saccharide strains. *J. Cell Biol.*, 60:236–248.

60. Farquhar, M. G. (1978): Traffic of products and membranes through the golgi complex. In: *Transport of Macromolecules in Cellular Systems*, edited by S. C. Silverstein, p. 341. Dahlem Konferenzen, Berlin.

61. Jamieson, J. D., and Palade, G. E. (1977): Production of secretory proteins in animal cells. In: *International Cell Biology, 1976–1977*, edited by B. B. Brinkley and K. R. Porter, p. 326. Rockefeller University Press, New York.

62. Palade, G. E. (1975): Intracellular aspects of the process of protein synthesis. *Science*, 189:347–353.

63. Rothman, J. E., and Fine, R. E. (1980): Coated vesicles transport newly synthesized membrane glycoproteins from endoplasmic reticulum to plasma membrane in two successive stages. *Proc. Natl. Acad. Sci. USA*, 77:780–784.

64. Smilowitz, H. (1980): Routes of intracellular transport of acetylcholine receptor and esterase are distinct. *Cell*, 19:237–244.

65. Rodriguez-Boulan, E., and Sabatini, D. D. (1978): Asymmetric budding of viruses in epithelial monolayers: A model system

for study of epithelial polarity. *Proc. Natl. Acad. Sci. USA*, 75:5071–5075.

66. Baumann, H., and Chu, F. F. (1979): Altered composition of membrane glycoconjugates in rat hepatoma tissue culture cells after dexamethasone treatment or *in vivo* growth. *Cancer Res.*, 39:3540–3548.

67. Baumann, H., and Doyle, D. (1978): Turnover of plasma membrane glycoproteins and glycolipids of hepatoma tissue culture cells. *J. Biol. Chem.*, 253:4408–4418.

68. Baumann, H., and Doyle, D. (1979): Effect of trypsin on the cell surface proteins of hepatoma tissue culture cells. *J. Biol. Chem.*, 254:3935–3946.

69. Baumann, H., Gelehrter, T. D., and Doyle, D. (1980): Dexamethasone regulates the program of secretory glycoprotein synthesis in hepatoma tissue culture cells. *J. Cell Biol.*, 85:1–8.

70. Baumann, H., Hou, E., and Doyle, D. (1980): Insertion of biologically active membrane proteins from rat liver into the plasma membrane of mouse fibroblasts. *J. Biol. Chem.*, 255:10001–10012.

71. Kyte, J. (1971): Purification of the sodium- and potassium-dependent adenosine triphosphatase from canine renal medulla. *J. Biol. Chem.*, 246:4157.

72. Tweto, J., and Doyle, D. (1976): Turnover of the plasma membrane proteins of hepatoma tissue culture cells. *J. Biol. Chem.*, 251:872–882.

73. Tweto, J., Friedman, E., and Doyle, D. (1976): Proteins of the hepatoma tissue culture cell plasma membrane. *J. Supramol. Struct.*, 4:141–159.

74. Tweto, J., Hou, E., and Doyle, D. (1979): Purification and characterization of an externally accessible 55,000 molecular weight protein of hepatoma tissue culture cells. *Arch. Biochem. Biophys.*, 193:422–430.

75. Rachubinski, R. A., Verma, P. S., and Bergeron, J. J. M. (1980): Synthesis of rat liver microsomal cytochrome b₅ by free ribosomes. *J. Cell Biol.*, 84:705–716.

76. Strittmatter, P., Rogers, M. J., and Spatz, L. (1972): The binding of cytochrome b₅ to liver microsomes. *J. Biol. Chem.*, 247:7188–7194.

77. Borgese, N., and Gaetani, S. (1980): Site of synthesis of NADH-cytochrome b₅ reductase, an integral membrane protein in rat liver cells. *FEBS Lett.*, 112:216–220.

78. Borgese, N., and Meldolesi, J. (1980): Localization and biosynthesis of NADH-cytochrome b₅ reductase, and integral membrane protein, in rat liver cells. I. Distribution of the enzyme activity in microsomes, mitochondria, and golgi complex. *J. Cell Biol.*, 85:501–515.

79. Borgese, N., Pietrini, G., and Meldolesi, J. (1980): Localization and biosynthesis of NADH-cytochrome b₅ reductase, an integral membrane protein, in rat liver cells. III. Evidence for the independent insertion and turnover of the enzyme in various subcellular compartments. *J. Cell Biol.*, 86:38–45.

80. Meldolesi, J., Corti, G., Pietrini, G., and Borgese, N. (1980): Localization and biosynthesis of NADH-cytochrome b₅ reductase, an integral membrane protein, in rat liver cells. II. Evidence that one single enzyme accounts for the activity in its various subcellular locations. *J. Cell Biol.*, 85:516–526.

81. Fleming, P. J., and Strittmatter, P. (1978): The nonpolar peptide segment of cytochrome b₅: Binding to phospholipid vesicles and identification of the fluorescent tryptophonyl residue. *J. Biol. Chem.*, 253:8198–8202.

82. Mihara, K. S., Sato, R., Sakakibara, R., and Wada, H. (1978): Reduced nicatinamide adenine denucleotide-cytochrome b₅ reductase location of the hydrophobic membrane-binding region of the carboxyl terminal end and the masked amino terminus. *Biochemistry*, 17:2829–2834.

83. Lalley, P. A., and Shows, T. B. (1974): Lysosomal and microsomal glucuronidase: Genetic variant alters electrophoretic mobility of both hydrolases. *Science*, 185:442–444.

84. Paigen, K. (1979): Acid hydrolases as models of genetic control. *Ann. Rev. Genet.*, 13:417–466.

85. Swank, R. T., and Paigen, K. (1973): Biochemical and genetic evidence for a macromolecular β-glucuronidase complex in microsomal membranes. *J. Mol. Biol.*, 77:371–389.

86. Tabas, I., and Kornfeld, S. (1980): Biosynthetic intermediates of β-glucuronidase contain high mannose oligosaccharides with blocked phosphate residues. *J. Biol. Chem.*, 255:6633–6639.

87. Kaplan, P., Achord, D. T., and Sly, W. S. (1977): Phosphohexosyl components of a lysosomal enzyme are recognized by pinocytosis receptors on human fibroblasts. *Proc. Natl. Acad. Sci. USA*, 74:2026–2030.

88. Hasilik, A., and Neufeld, E. F. (1980): Biosynthesis of lysosomal enzymes in fibroblasts. Phosphorylation of mannose residues. *J. Biol. Chem.*, 255:4946–4957.

89. Hasilik, A., and Neufeld, E. F. (1980): Biosynthesis of lysosomal enzymes in fibroblasts. Synthesis as precursors of higher molecular weight. *J. Biol. Chem.*, 255:4937–4945.

90. Sly, W. S. (1980): Saccharide traffic signals in receptor-mediated endocytosis and transport of acid hydrolases. In: *Structure and Function of the Gangliosides,* edited by L. Suennerholm, P. Mandel, H. Dreyfus, and P. F. Urban, pp. 433–451. Plenum, New York.

91. Sly, W. S., and Stahl, P. (1978): Receptor-mediated uptake of lysosomal enzymes. In: *Transport of Macromolecules in Cellular Systems,* edited by S. C. Silverstein, pp. 229–244. Dahlem Konferenzen, Berlin.

92. Fischer, H. D., Gonzalez-Noriega, A., and Sly, W. S. (1980): β-Glucuronidase binding to human fibroblast membrane receptors. *J. Biol. Chem.*, 255:5069–5074.

93. Hickman, S., and Neufeld, E. F. (1972): A hypothesis for I cell disease: Defective hydrolases that do not enter lysosomes. *Biochem. Biophys. Res. Commun.*, 49:992–999.

94. Neufeld, E. F., Lin, T. W., and Shapiro, L. J. (1975): Inherited disorders of lysosomal metabolism. *Ann. Rev. Biochem.*, 44:357–376.

95. Skudlarek, M. D., and Swank, R. T. (1979): Biosynthesis of two lysosomal enzymes in macrophages: Evidence for a precursor of β-galactosidase. *J. Biol. Chem.*, 254:9939–9942.

96. Frisch, A., and Neufeld, E. F. (1980): Limited proteolysis of B hexosaminidase in a cell free system. *Fed. Proc.*, 1866.

97. Lusis, A. J., Tomino, S., and Paigen, K. (1976): Isolation, characterization, and radioimmunoassay of murine egasyn, a protein stabilizing glucuronidase membrane binding. *J. Biol. Chem.*, 251:7753–7760.

98. Tomino, S., and Paigen, K. (1974): Egasyn, a protein complexed with microsomal β-glucuronidase. *J. Biol. Chem.*, 250:1146–1148.

99. Marchesi, V. T., Furthmayr, H., and Tomita, M. (1976): The red cell membrane. *Ann. Rev. Biochem.*, 45:667–698.

100. Tilney, L. G., and Detmers, P. (1975): Actin in erythrocyte ghosts and its association with spectrin. *J. Cell Biol.*, 66:508–520.

101. Edelman, G. M. (1976): Surface modulation in cell recognition and cell growth. *Science,* 192:218–226.

102. Goodenough, D. A. (1974): Bulk isolation of mouse hepatocyte gap junctions. *J. Cell Biol.*, 61:557–563.

103. Makowski, L., Caspor, D. L. D., Phillips, W. C., and Goodenough, D. A. (1977): GAP junction structures. II. Analysis of the X-ray diffraction data. *J. Cell Biol.*, 74:629–645.

104. Robertson, J. D. (1963): The occurrence of a subunit pattern in the unit membranes of club endings in Mauthner cell synapses in goldfish brains. *J. Cell Biol.*, 19:201–221.

105. Unwin, P. N. T., and Zampighi, G. (1980): Structure of the junction between communicating cells. *Nature*, 283:545–549.

106. Finbow, M., Yancey, S. B., Johnson, R., and Revel, J.-P. (1980): Independent lines of evidence suggesting a major gap junctional protein with a molecular weight of 26,000. *Proc. Natl. Acad. Sci. USA*, 77:970–974.

107. Gilula, N. B. (1974): Isolation of rat liver gap junctions and characterization of the polypeptides. *J. Cell Biol.*, 63:111a.

108. Henderson, D., Eibl, H., and Weber, K. (1979): Structure and biochemistry of mouse hepatic gap junctions. *J. Mol. Biol.*, 132:193–218.

109. Hertzberg, E. L., and Gilula, N. B. (1979): Isolation and characterization of gap junction from rat liver. *J. Biol. Chem.*, 254:2138–2147.

110. Baumann, H., and Doyle, D. (1980): Metabolic fate of cell

surface glycoproteins during immunoglobulin-induced internalization. *Cell*, 21:897–907.

111. Hubbard, A. L., and Cohn, Z. A. (1972): The enzymatic iodination of the red cell membrane. *J. Cell Biol.*, 55:390–405.

112. Marchalonis, J. J., Cone, R. E., and Santer, V. (1971): Enzymic iodination, a probe for accessible surface proteins of normal and neoplastic lymphocytes. *Biochem. J.*, 124:921–927.

113. Phillips, D. R., and Morrison, M. (1971): Exposed protein on the intact human erythrocyte. *Biochemistry*, 10:1766–1771.

114. Gahmberg, C. G., and Hakomori, S. (1973): External labeling of cell surface galactose and galactosamine in glycolipid and glycoprotein of human erythrocytes. *J. Biol. Chem.*, 248: 4311–4317.

115. Hubbard, A., and Cohn, Z. A. (1975): Externally disposed plasma membrane proteins. II. Metabolic fate of iodinated polypeptides of mouse L cells. *J. Cell Biol.*, 64:461–479.

116. Kaplan, G., Unkeless, J. C., and Cohn, Z. A. (1979): Insertion and turnover of macrophage plasma membrane proteins. *Proc. Natl. Acad. Sci. USA*, 76:3824–3828.

117. Davies, P. J. A., Davies, D. R., Levitzki, A., Maxfield, F. R., Milhaud, P., Willingham, M. C., and Pastan, I. (1980): Transglutaminase is essential in receptor mediated endocytosis of α_2-macroglobulin and polypeptide hormones. *Nature,* 283: 162–167.

118. Goldstein, L. L., Anderson, R. G. W., and Brown, M. S. (1979): Coated pits, coated vesicles, and receptor mediated endocytosis. *Nature*, 279:679–684.

119. Kosmakos, F. C., and Roth, J. (1978): Regulation of insulin and growth hormone receptors *in vitro* and *in vivo*. In: *Protein Turnover and Lysosome Function*, edited by H. L. Segal and D. Doyle, pp. 763–777. Academic Press, New York.

120. Levitzki, A., Willingham, M., and Pastan, I. (1980): Evidence for participation of transglutaminase in receptor-mediated endocytosis. *Proc. Natl. Acad. Sci. USA*, 77:2706–2710.

121. McKanna, J. A., Haigler, H. T., and Cohen, S. (1979): Hormone receptor topology and dynamics: Morphological analysis using ferritin-labeled epidermal growth factor. *Proc. Natl. Acad. Sci. USA*, 76:5689–5693.

122. Dehlinger, P. J., and Schimke, R. T. (1970): Effect of size on the relative rate of degradation of rat liver soluble proteins. *Biochem. Biophys. Res. Commun.*, 40:1473–1480.

123. Dehlinger, P. J., and Schimke, R. T. (1971): Size distribution of membrane proteins of rat liver and their relative rates of degradation. *J. Biol. Chem.*, 246:2574–2583.

124. Gurd, J. W., and Evans, W. H. (1973): Relative rates of degradation of mouse liver surface membrane proteins. *Eur. J. Biochem.*, 36:273–279.

125. Tauber, R., and Reutter, W. (1978): Protein degradation in the plasma membrane of regenerating liver and Morris hepatomas. *Eur. J. Biochem.*, 83:37–45.

126. Warren, R., and Doyle, D. (1981): Turnover of the surface proteins and the receptor for serum asialoglycoproteins in primary cultures of rat hepatocytes. *J. Biol. Chem.*, 256:1346–1355.

127. Hubbard, A. L., and Stukenbrok, H. (1979): An electron microscope autoradiographic study of the carbohydrate recognition systems in rat liver. II. Intracellular fates of the ^{125}I ligands. *J. Cell Biol.*, 83:65–81.

128. Hubbard, A. L., Wilson, G., Ashwell, G., and Stukenbrok, H. (1979): An electron microscope autoradiographic study of the carbohydrate recognition systems in rat liver. I. Distribution of ^{125}I-ligands among the liver cell types. *J. Cell Biol.*, 83:47–64.

129. Pricer, W. E., and Ashwell, G. (1976): Subcellular distribution of asialoglycoprotein receptor. *J. Biol. Chem.*, 251:7539.

130. Tanabe, T., Pricer, W. E., Jr., and Ashwell, G. (1979): Subcellular membrane topology and turnover of rat hepatic receptor. *J. Biol. Chem.*, 254:1038.

131. Omura, T., and Harano, T. (1977): Biogenesis of endoplasmic reticulum membrane in the liver cell. In: *Structure and Function of Biomembranes*, edited by K. Yagi, pp. 117–125. Japan Scientific Societies Press, Tokyo.

132. Steinman, R. M., Brodie, S. E., and Cohn, Z. A. (1976): Membrane flow during pinocytosis, a stereologic analysis. *J. Cell Biol.*, 68:665–687.

133. Mellman, I., Steinman, R. M., Unkeless, J. C., and Cohn, Z. A. (1981): Selective iodination and polypeptide composition of pinocytotic vesicles. *J. Cell Biol.*, 86:1346–1355.

134. Leroy-Houyet, M.-A., Quintart, J., and Baudhuin, P. (1981): Morphometry and characterization of endocytosis in exponentially growing hepatoma cells in culture. *J. Ultrastruct. Res.*, 69:68–85.

135. Quintart, J., Bartholeyns, J., and Baudhuin, P. (1979): Characterization of subcellular components in synchronized hepatoma cells as a function of the cell cycle. *Biochem. J.*, 184:133–141.

136. Schneider, Y.-J., Tulkens, P., deDuve, C., and Trouet, A. (1979): Fate of plasma membrane during endocytosis. I. Uptake and processing of antiplasma membrane and control immunoglobulins by cultured fibroblasts. *J. Cell Biol.*, 82: 449–465.

137. Silverstein, S. C., Steinman, R. M., and Cohn, Z. A. (1977): Endocytosis. *Ann. Rev. Biochem.*, 46:669–722.

138. Kreisel, W., Volk, B. A., Buchsel, R., and Reutter, W. (1980): Different half-lives of the carbohydrate and protein moieties of a 110,000 dalton glycoprotein isolated from plasma membranes of rat liver. *Proc. Natl. Acad. Sci. USA*, 77:1828–1831.

139. Bergeron, J. J. M., Sikstrom, R., Hand, A. R., and Posner, B. I. (1979): Binding and uptake of ^{125}I-insulin into rat liver hepatocytes and endothelium. *J. Cell Biol.*, 80:427–443.

140. Cushman, S. W., and Wardzala, L. J. (1980): Potential mechanism of insulin action on glucose transport in the isolated rat adipose cell. *J. Biol. Chem.*, 255:4758–4762.

141. Howell, K. E., Ito, A., and Palade, G. E. (1978): Endoplasmic reticulum marker enzymes in golgi fractions—What does this mean? *J. Cell Biol.*, 79:581–589.

142. Ito, A., and Palade, G. E. (1978): Presence of NADPH-cytochrome p-450 reductase in rat liver golgi membranes. *J. Cell Biol.*, 79:590–597.

143. Elovson, J. (1980): Biogenesis of plasma membrane glycoproteins. Tracer kinetic study of two rat liver plasma membrane glycoproteins *in vivo*. *J. Biol. Chem.*, 255:5816–5825.

144. Thornburg, R. W., Day, J. F., Baynes, J. W., and Thorpe, S. R. (1980): Carbohydrate-mediated clearance of immune complexes from the circulation *J. Biol. Chem.*, 255: 6820–6825.

145. Doyle, D., Hou, E., and Warren, R. (1979): Transfer of the hepatocyte receptor for serum asialo-glycoproteins to the plasma membrane of a fibroblast: Acquisition of the hepatocyte receptor functions by mouse L cells. *J. Biol. Chem.*, 254:6853–6856.

146. Rousseau, G. G., Amar-Costesee, A., Verhaegen, M., and Granner, D. K. (1980): Glucocorticoid hormones increase the activity of plasma membrane alkaline phosphodiesterase I in rat hepatoma cells. *Proc. Natl. Acad. Sci. USA*, 77:1005–1009.

147. Suzuki, K., and Kono, T. (1980): Evidence that insulin causes translocation of glucose transport activity to the plasma membrane from an intracellular storage site. *Proc. Natl. Acad. Sci. USA*, 77:2542–2545.

148. Weigel, P. H. (1980): Characterization of the asialoglycoprotein receptor on isolated rat hepatocytes. *J. Biol. Chem.*, 255:6111–6120.

The Liver: Biology and Pathobiology, edited by
I. Arias, H. Popper, D. Schachter, and D. A. Shafritz.
Raven Press, New York © 1982.

Chapter 12

Endocytosis of Glycoproteins

Richard J. Stockert and Anatol G. Morell

All plasma glycoproteins in mammals possess highly branched N-glycoside-linked oligosaccharide units. The intravascular survival of these glycoproteins is critically dependent on the integrity of the outer sequence of their carbohydrate chains. This chapter (a) summarizes the relationship between structure of the oligosaccharide unit of glycoproteins and their metabolic fate, (b) describes the hepatic receptors that recognize specific carbohydrate moieties and initiate removal of glycoproteins from the circulation, and (c) indicates the intracellular pathway which is followed.

METABOLIC FATE OF ASIALOGLYCOPROTEINS

The prototype example in which carbohydrate structure was shown to play a decisive role in regulating the serum survival of glycoproteins was provided by studies of the circulatory fate of the plasma copper-containing glycoprotein, ceruloplasmin. To prepare ceruloplasmin doubly labeled with copper and tritium to study the role of this protein in copper metabolism, sialic acid was removed from the oligosaccharide moiety of the glycoprotein, exposing subterminal galactose-residues. Sequential oxidation of the terminal galactosyl residues and their reduction with tritiated borohydride resulted in formation of sialic acid-free ceruloplasmin, which was selectively labeled in its galactosyl residues (1). The significance of this seemingly minor modification in the oligosac-

charide composition first became apparent in experiments in which desialylated ceruloplasmin was injected into rabbits. Native rabbit ceruloplasmin has a physiologic half-life of 55 hr; when its sialic acid residues were removed, it disappeared from the circulation within minutes (2,3).

Rapidity of circulatory clearance of asialoceruloplasmin was shown to be due to the presence of newly exposed terminal galactosyl residues. Removal by β-galactosidase of the galactose end-groups exposed by neuraminidase, or oxidation of the primary hydroxyl group of these terminal galactose units with galactose oxidase, increased the survival time of asialoceruloplasmin toward that exhibited by the native glycoprotein (2). Further studies established that, although native ceruloplasmin contains approximately 10 sialic acid-galactose sequences per molecule, the exposure of any two galactosyl residues is sufficient to produce immediate clearance of the glycoprotein from the circulation (3,4).

The generality of terminal galactose recognition was demonstrated by the analogously rapid clearance from the circulation of asialo-derivatives of a wide variety of glycoproteins (5–8), a number of which are shown in Fig. 1, and of glycopeptide hormones (1–13). The common feature in all these asialoglycoproteins is the presence of an exposed β-galactosyl residue-terminating sequence in their carbohydrate chains. Of notable exception is transferrin, the iron-transporting glycoprotein of plasma, in which the exposure of galactose residues does not result in an appreciable

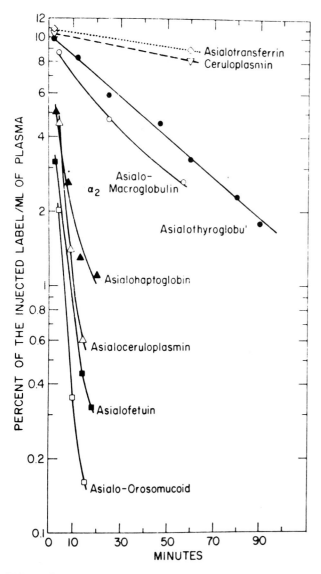

FIG. 1. Survival of intravenously injected native ceruloplasmin and desialylated plasma proteins in the rat.

native glycoprotein, failure to recognize the terminal galactosyl residues of asialotransferrin is attributable to a unique structure of its oligosaccharide moiety.

Hepatic Uptake

Rapid clearance from the circulation of asialoglycoproteins was accompanied by their equally rapid accumulation in liver. Within minutes after doubly labeled asialoceruloplasmin was injected into rabbits, radioactivity was recovered from the liver with less than 1% localized in all other organs. The parallel rates of disappearance from serum and recovery by immunoprecipitation from the liver of the tritiated galactose and copper-64 in the same proportion as that present in the injection provided strong evidence that the intact protein was transferred from plasma into liver (1).

The cell type responsible for this recognition process was established by histoautoradiography of a biopsy specimen of liver following injection of tritiated asialoceruloplasmin (Fig. 2). The labeled protein could be demonstrated exclusively in hepatocytes with no radioactivity in Kupffer cells. This unique cellular localization has been confirmed and extended quantita-

reduction of its circulatory survival. This indicates that, although necessary, the presence of terminal galactose is not a sufficient condition for this recognition phenomenon.

It was demonstrated recently that the composition and structure of the oligosaccharide chains of asialoglycoproteins are indeed the sole determinants of this process (14). Asialoglycopeptides and the protein-free asialooligosaccharides prepared by enzymatic hydrolysis from α_1-antitrypsin were fully potent in prolonging the plasma survival of intact asialo-α_1-antitrypsin. Consistent with the previous observation that asialotransferrin was not rapidly cleared from the circulation, neither the asialoglycopeptides nor the asialooligosaccharides prepared from transferrin inhibited the rapid clearance of asialo-α_1-antitrypsin. Since these derivatives no longer retained the secondary structure of the

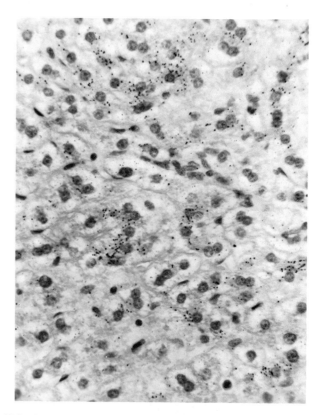

FIG. 2. Autoradiograph of histologic section of liver 3 min following injection of tritium-labeled asialoceruloplasmin into a rabbit. Silver granules overlie the parenchymal cells but are absent in the Kupffer cells.

tively using electron microscopic autoradiography to assess the hepatic distribution of several iodinated asialoglycoproteins (15).

Lysosomal Catabolism

When asialoceruloplasmin doubly labeled with tritium and copper-64 was injected, the almost instantaneous hepatic uptake resulted in pulse labeling of the parenchymal liver cells. This permitted observation of the details of the catabolic sequence which would normally be obscured by the slow, continual production of catabolites (16). Six minutes after intravenous injection of asialoceruloplasmin, immunoprecipitable glycoprotein was recovered from fractions that migrated together with particles, possessing lysosomal enzyme markers. Prior treatment of rats with Triton WR 1339 or dextran, thus varying the specific gravity of the lysosomal fraction, resulted in density shifts of both the immunoprecipitable asialoceruloplasmin and lysosomal enzyme markers. By 30 min, 80% of the copper had been cleaved from the molecule; the ratio of tritium-labeled galactose to copper-64 in the immunochemically recovered protein fell to half the original value. From these results, it was inferred that enzymatic hydrolysis of galactose preceded proteolysis, resulting in the loss of copper. The peptide component of asialoglycoproteins is ultimately hydrolyzed to free amino acids (17).

The role of lysosomes as the major site of degradation was further established by studies of asialofetuin metabolism in both isolated hepatocytes and the perfused liver system (18,19). In both cases, prior treatment with known inhibitors of lysosomal proteinases resulted in a reduction of asialofetuin catabolism and a progressive accumulation of undegraded asialofetuin in a subcellular fraction identified as lysosomal.

HEPATIC RECEPTOR

Membrane Binding

Characteristic of carrier-mediated endocytosis, the hepatic uptake of asialoglycoproteins was shown to be saturable, suggesting the presence of a specific receptor at the hepatocyte cell surface. To permit a more detailed examination of this recognition phenomenon, a sensitive *in vitro* binding assay was developed (20). Specific binding of asialoglycoproteins was shown to be uniquely associated with the particulate fraction of rat liver homogenates. Subsequent fractionation of a low-speed pellet by sucrose-density-gradient centrifugation identified the plasma membrane fractions as the primary locus of binding activity (21). Binding was maximal at a neutral pH and exhibited an absolute requirement for the presence of calcium ions. Although bound asialoglycoproteins could be dissociated readily by lowering the pH below 6 or by addition of a calcium chelating agent, no evidence could be obtained for substantial dissociation of labeled ligand by the addition of a large excess of nonradiolabeled asialoglycoprotein.

Treatment of the membrane preparations with neuraminidase results in the loss of their capacity to bind desialylated glycoproteins. This effect was shown to be reversible by the enzymatic replacement of sialic acid. Effective binding was shown to require not only the absence of sialic acid on the glycoprotein but also its presence in the plasma membrane.

Hepatic Binding Protein

Binding activity was solubilized with Triton X-100 from a lyophilized preparation of a particulate fraction of rabbit liver (22). This crude preparation exhibited specific binding affinity for desialylated glycoprotein comparable to that found in rat liver plasma membranes. A specific binding protein was subsequently isolated and purified by affinity chromatography on columns of Sepharose to which asialoglycoprotein had been covalently coupled (23). The hepatic binding protein with receptor specificity for desialylated glycoproteins proved to be a glycoprotein itself. The minimal molecular weight of the active water-soluble oligomeric protein was about 250,000 daltons, comprised of a mixture of two subunits with estimated molecular weights of 48,000 and 40,000 daltons (24). One-tenth of its weight consisted of sialic acid, galactose, mannose, and N-acetylglucosamine present as two distinctly different oligosaccharides (25). Although the hepatic binding protein is purified as a 250,000 molecular weight complex, *in situ* determination of molecular size by radiation target analysis indicates that only a 105,000 molecular component is essential for ligand binding (26).

Analogous binding proteins have now been isolated and purified from rat and human liver (27,28). Unlike rabbit protein, both rat and human receptors are monomeric, with estimated molecular weights of about 47,000 and 40,000 daltons, respectively. Although binding to both rabbit and rat receptor is essentially irreversible, in the case of the human receptor, reversibility was demonstrated, with a dissociation rate for asialoorosomucoid of 1.7×10^{-3} sec^{-1}. In the other parameters examined, such as the specificity for terminal sugar ligands and the absolute requirement for calcium, the properties of the three mammalian binding proteins were indistinguishable.

As was characteristic of rat plasma membrane preparations, treatment with neuraminidase of the purified protein from either rabbit or rat resulted in the complete loss of their capacity to bind asialoglycoproteins. The effect of neuraminidase was subsequently clarified by the demonstration that the apparent loss of binding activity was due to competition for the binding sites of the protein by its own newly exposed galactosyl residues. When the terminal galactosyl residues of the binding protein are either enzymatically oxidized, hydrolyzed, as shown in Fig. 3, or masked through resialylation, binding activity was restored (29,30).

Lectin Activity

The ability of the purified rabbit protein to agglutinate human and rabbit erythrocytes (as well as desialylated erythrocytes from rat, mouse, and guinea pig) identified the binding protein as a lectin, the first such protein of mammalian origin (31). As was the case for the binding of asialoglycoproteins, the presence of calcium ion was necessary for erythrocyte agglutination. Lower concentrations of rabbit liver lectin were required to agglutinate human type A erythrocytes than type B, with type O being the least agglutinable. Its similarity to plant lectins was extended by the subsequent demonstration that the receptor was a potent mitogen for desialylated human peripheral thymus-derived lymphocytes (32). This recognition by the hepatic lectin of cell surface glycoproteins suggests that, in addition to its possible role in glycoprotein metabolism, it may be a factor in certain cellular interactions as well. The ability of the purified lectin to induce desialylated human peripheral-blood lymphocytes to mediate mitogen-induced cellular cytotoxicity is an example of such possible cell-to-cell interactions (33).

Lectin activity is not limited to preparations of

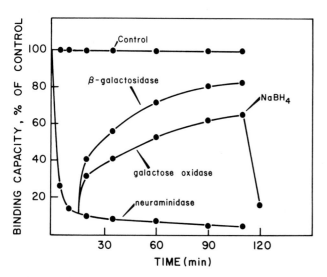

FIG. 3. Effect of enzymes on binding capacity of the purified receptor protein for desialylated orosomucoid.

purified receptor protein. Agglutination was demonstrated with freshly isolated rat hepatocytes incubated with desialylated erythrocytes, spleen lymphocytes, and asialo or normal thymocytes (34). Most hepatocytes were surrounded by a single layer of cells forming rosettes. Almost no rosette formation occurred when hepatocytes were mixed with untreated erythrocytes or spleen lymphocytes. Normal thymocytes, however, adhered to hepatocytes, although rosette formation was less than with asialothymocytes.

In view of the proposed role of glycosyltransferases in the recognition and association of cells (35) the purified binding protein was examined for the presence of glycosyltransferase activity (36). Under optimally determined conditions, however, no transferase activity could be detected for sialic acid, galactose, N-acetylglucosamine, or fucose.

Carbohydrate Specificity

The quantitative differences in agglutinability of the three human blood groups suggested the lectin reacting with blood group antigens. It was inferred that N-acetylgalactosaminyl residues, the antigenic determinants of blood group A, as well as galactosyl residues, determinants of group B, were both recognized by the binding protein. Indeed, agglutination may be reversed by the addition of either of these two monosaccharides or, to a lesser extent, by L-fucose, the determinant of group O red cells. N-acetylgalactosamine proved to be the most potent monosaccharide inhibitor; when present as the terminal sugar of a macromolecule, such as desialylated ovine submaxillary mucin, it is capable of displacing galactose-terminated glycoproteins from the receptor binding site (31). Subsequent studies using agarose-immobilized rabbit binding protein established the order of glycoside inhibitory capacity as α-methyl-N-acetylgalactosamine > β-methyl-N-acetylgalactosamine > β-methylgalactose > α-methylgalactose. Based on the relative inhibitory power of these and other defined carbohydrate structures, the lectin binding site is relatively small, involving a terminal and extending to at least part of the penultimate sugar residue (37).

Although glucose was ineffective in reversing agglutination of erythrocytes by purified rabbit protein or inhibiting rosette formation between isolated hepatocytes and desialylated lymphocytes, when attached to bovine serum albumin, the glucosyl-albumin derivative proved to be as good (or better) an inhibitor than the galactosyl derivative (38). Since there are no known examples of glucose-containing circulatory glycoproteins, the functional significance of glucose recognition by rabbit lectin is unclear.

Intracellular Distribution and Topology

The original identification of the liver plasma membrane as the major locus of the receptor protein was subsequently expanded to include membranes of the Golgi, a smooth microsomal fraction, and the lysosomes (39–41). Binding proteins associated with subcellular fractions enriched with these organelles were isolated and analyzed. Although these preparations were not purified to homogeneity, similar banding patterns were obtained following polyacrylamide gel electrophoresis; antibody prepared against purified binding protein gave rise to a single coincidence line on double immunodiffusion. Based on these results and their common binding characteristics, it was concluded that the binding proteins isolated from the several rat liver subfractions were of common origin.

Detergents, such as Triton X-100, commonly are added to membrane assay mixtures to enhance the activity being measured. It is presumed that the increase results from the exposure of the latent activity associated with membrane proteins localized on the internal surface of the organelles. Binding activity for asialoglycoprotein by the various subcellular fractions differed in their response to the presence or absence of Triton X-100. There was a more than twofold stimulation in binding activity when detergent was added to membrane preparations enriched in either Golgi elements or smooth microsomes but not in the lysosomal fraction (40). Incubation prior to solubilization with detergent of the various fractions with purified antibody to the receptor protein, blocking all external surface binding activity, was used to assign the topographic distribution of the binding protein (27). The antibody titration of binding sites indicated that the receptor binding protein associated with the Golgi and the smooth microsomes is present largely, if not entirely, on the internal or lumenal surface. In contrast, binding sites on intact lysosomes appear to be oriented toward the external or cytosolic surface of these organelles.

INTRACELLULAR PATHWAYS

Ligand Translocation

The rate-limiting step in the catabolism of asialoglycoproteins was shown to be the translocation between the plasma membrane and lysosomes, a process with mean transit time of approximately 7 min (19). In the isolated perfused liver, this intracellular transport was shown to be temperature dependent (42). Uptake and catabolism of asialofetuin continued but were progressively slowed as the temperature decreased from 35° to 20°C. Subcellular fractionation and *in situ*

electron microscopic autoradiography showed that at 20°C, while internalization of asialofetuin continued, fusion with lysosomes of pinocytic vesicles containing radioiodinated glycoprotein did not occur. Such pinocytic vesicles isolated immediately after injection of asialoglycoprotein are apparently devoid of lysosomal enzyme markers (43); with time, however, the asialoglycoprotein is recovered in association with low density particles clearly identifiable as lysosomal. These organelles progressively acquire a higher density during the catabolic process.

Translocation of these vesicles through the cytoplasm appears to involve the hepatic cytoskeleton structures. Direct participation of the hepatocytic microtubular and microfilament elements during transport of asialoglycoproteins was investigated using isolated hepatocytes (44). Treatment of isolated cells with colchicine, an inhibitor of microtubular function, slowed the uptake and degradation of asialofetuin, which could be accounted for by a reduction of plasma membrane binding capacity. In contrast, cytochalasin B, a microfilament inhibitor, selectively reduced asialoprotein degradation with no effect on the uptake process, suggesting an inhibition of intracellular transport to the sites of catabolism.

At the ultrastructural level, the sequential steps involved in this pathway, was described using desialylated glycoproteins covalently coupled to cytochemically demonstrable enzymes, horseradish peroxidase, and tyrosinase (45). The electron microscopic findings document the rapidity of the uptake of the asialoglycoprotein by hepatocytes. At 1 min with coupled proteins still present in the sinusoids, reaction product is observed in endocytic structures at the space of Disse in coated pits and vesicles (Fig. 4) and pleomorphic tubular structures (Fig. 5). Uptake was also observed along the lateral surfaces of hepatocytes, indicating that receptors for asialoglycoproteins are not restricted to the sinusoidal surface of the cell (Fig. 6).

As early as 5 min after injection, marker enzyme was found in pericanalicular residual bodies, which possess morphologic characteristics of secondary lysosomes (Figs. 7 and 8). Smooth membrane extensions were evident on many of the enzyme marker-positive organelles, suggesting that their origin was the smooth endoplasmic reticulum. Regardless of shape or details of origin, the residual bodies correspond to the lysosomes that catabolize asialoglycoproteins, as suggested by earlier cell fractionation studies.

The transition of ligand in the coated pit on the cell surface to intracellular coated vesicles provides the major system for the selective uptake of most macromolecules and peptide hormones that bind to cells (46–49). The asialoglycoprotein receptors appear to be concentrated at these specialized regions of the

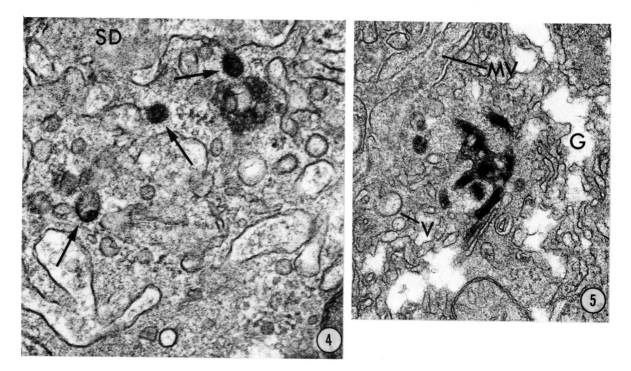

FIG. 4. One minute after injection of ASFT-HRP. DAB reaction product is seen in structures at the sinusoidal border of a hepatocyte, including a coated pit (*uppermost arrow*) showing the hepatocyte plasma membrane most clearly at the right. Probable coated pits, or vesicles sectioned so that their relationships to the plasma membrane are not evident, are indicated by the other two arrows. SD, space of Disse. ×62,000.

FIG. 5. One minute after injection of ASFT-HRP. DAB reaction product fills a pleomorphic tubular structure in the cytoplasm near the sinusoidal border of a periportal hepatocyte. V, vesicle attached to the plasma membrane; MV, microcilli; G, extracted or unstained glycogen. ×41,000.

plasma membrane (50). The coat, composed of polymerized protein, is released from the vesicles by partial or total dissociation as a prelude to fusion with a new intercellular membrane. Such smooth-membraned vesicles continue to migrate and accumulate in the Golgi region of the cells. Ultimately, ligand is found in lysosomes, where degradation takes place. So characteristic is this sequence of cellular events that it suggests that once any ligand is bound to the plasma membrane, internalization and intracellular translocation are mediated by a common biologic process. Coated structures have been suggested to play a decisive role in determining which molecules should be transferred and which retained at any step in communication between different cell compartments (51).

Receptor Reutilization

Subsequent to the demonstration that the hepatic binding protein was associated with internal membranes as well as the plasma membrane of the hepatocyte, it was shown that only a small fraction of total receptor activity was present at the cell surface of intact hepatocytes (18,52). Since amounts of desialylated glycoproteins far in excess of the binding capacity of the surface receptor protein are transported intracel-

lularly under conditions in which neither synthesis nor degradation of the receptor is enhanced (27,53), the cell surface receptor must either be reutilized or replenished from the large pool of intracellular binding protein.

To differentiate between these two alternatives, receptors on the surface of isolated hepatocytes were uniquely marked by neuraminidase treatment (54). This enzyme abolishes binding of galactose-terminated and not desialylated ovine submaxillary mucin. Since only cell surface-associated receptors were modified by neuraminidase treatment, the binding activity of only the cell surface was selectively restricted to desialylated ovine submaxillary mucin, thereby providing the means to distinguish plasma membrane-associated receptors from those associated with intracellular membranes.

Following a period of endocytosis of desialylated ovine submaxillary mucin by neuraminidase-treated hepatocytes, during which time the amount of ligand transported intercellularly exceeded the cell surface binding capacity by at least 20-fold, there was no change in the distribution of receptor protein as determined by differential binding activities. Had native, sialylated, receptor protein from intracellular membranes provided a pool for replenishing the cell surface

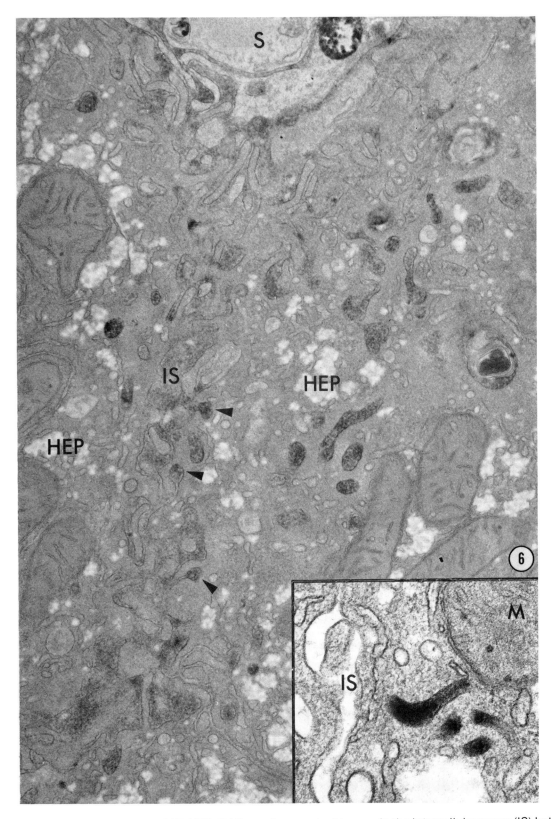

FIG. 6. One minute after injection of ASFT-HRP. DAB reaction product is seen in the intercellular space (IS) between two hepatocytes (HEP) and in vermiform pinocytic channels within the cytoplasm. *Arrowheads,* regions where the continuities are seen between channels and plasma membrane. S, sinusoid, ×41,000. **Inset:** 10 min after injection of ASFT-HRP; reaction product fills tubular pinocytic channels in the lateral cytoplasm of a hepatocyte. M, mitochondrion. ×72,000.

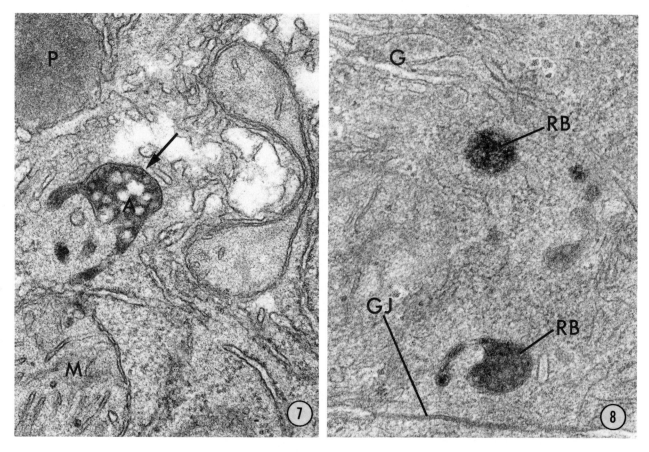

FIGS. 7 and 8. Portions of hepatocytes with residual bodies (RB or arrows) containing reaction product at 5 or 10 min after injection of one of the asialylated conjugates. Note the electron-lucent particles, probably lipoprotein particles, in the residual bodies and the smooth-membraned extensions from the residual bodies. G, Golgi stack; M, mitochondrion; P, peroxisome and the gap junction (GJ). Fig. 7, ×57,000; Fig. 8, ×68,000.

receptor during endocytosis, at least some of the original asialoorosomucoid binding capacity would have been expected to be restored to the cell surface. These results are compatible with the lack of restoration of binding capacity once the initial complement of surface receptors is blocked with specific antibody, as was demonstrated in the isolated perfused liver (55). This is also consistent with the recent demonstration of unaltered endocytosis of asialoorosomucoid when functional hepatic receptors are fused into the plasma membrane of cultured fibroblasts which lack a pre-existing internal receptor pool (56).

It can be inferred from these studies that any reutilization mechanism in the endocytotic process appears to involve only cell surface receptors that remain effectively segregated from intracellular receptors during endocytosis. The plasma membrane receptors may never leave the cell surface as they bind and transfer asialoglycoproteins into the cell, or they may carry their ligand intracellularly and return to the cell surface by a membrane-recycling mechanism (57). In either case, it appears that the large intracellular pool of receptor protein, which may represent more than 90% of

total hepatocytic binding capacity, is not involved in the endocytosis of extracellular glycoproteins.

ALTERATION OF RECEPTOR FUNCTION

Pathologic Liver

Serum for normal persons and patients with a variety of illnesses was tested for its ability to inhibit asialoglycoprotein binding to plasma membranes (13). The small amounts of inhibitory substances in the serum of controls or patients with liver disease, which were presumed to represent a low level of circulating asialoglycoproteins, were significantly increased in sera obtained from patients with clinically confirmed cirrhosis or hepatitis. Serum inhibitors were isolated and identified as asialoglycoproteins (58) by affinity chromatography on the column containing purified receptor covalently linked to agarose.

Increased serum titer from patients with hepatocellular disease could result from either the retention in the circulation of asialoglycoproteins due to reduced receptor activity or from a defect in the terminal stages of glycosylation during biosynthesis of serum glyco-proteins. If the former were true, it would support the concept that the hepatic binding of asialoglycoproteins is an obligatory step in regulating plasma protein metabolism *in vivo*.

Direct evidence for a reduction in receptor protein as a consequence of hepatocellular pathology was obtained in studies using the chemical carcinogen *N*-2-acetylaminofluorene (59). The level of asialoorosomucoid binding capacity of neoplastic nodules induced by this carcinogen was approximately 37% that of normal rat liver homogenates. The binding capacity of primary hepatocellular carcinomas that resulted from this regimen was reduced by 95%. This loss was proportional to the decreased concentration of antigenically detectable receptor present in the altered tissues. These results indicate that a loss of synthesizing capacity of binding protein occurs during exposure to the carcinogen and is almost complete in primary hepatocellular carcinoma.

Cell Proliferation

The effects of cellular replication on expression of receptor function were studied (60), prompted by the observation that rapidly growing liver obtained from human and rabbit embryos was essentially devoid of asialoglycoprotein binding activity (61). While the rat hepatocyte divides approximately once per year, rapid cellular proliferation occurs throughout the liver remnant following a two-thirds hepatectomy. Analyses of influx rate constants for asialoorosomucoid decreased dramatically during the first 48 hr of regeneration, with values falling to approximately 20% of sham-operated controls. Transport function remained depressed for 4 days, with a gradual return to normal by the sixth day. These results suggested that following cellular division, the liver cell undergoes a maturation process resulting in restoration of this specific hepatocytic function.

To determine whether the reduction of asialoglycoprotein binding after hepatectomy is restricted to plasma membrane receptors, surface binding was selectively measured in isolated hepatocytes (62). Two days after hepatoectomy, surface binding of asialoglycoprotein was reduced to 20% of the control level, while homogenized cells exhibited more than 80% of their normal binding capacity. Thus during the peak time of cell division following hepatectomy, binding activity of plasma membranes was disproportionately reduced. With regeneration substantially completed, cell surface binding returned to normal, indicating that the hepatic binding protein, and perhaps other plasma membrane receptors (63), undergo cell cycle-dependent modulation of their expression.

OTHER CARBOHYDRATE-SPECIFIC RECOGNITION SYSTEMS

Although the rapid clearance from the circulation of asialoceruloplasmin could be markedly prolonged by enzymatic hydrolysis of its terminal galactosyl residues, similar prolongation of intravascular survival times was not obtained with the agalacto-derivative of orosomucoid (64). Further enzymatic hydrolysis of the agalacto-orosomucoid to an ahexosamino-derivative, the mannose core glycoprotein, was also without effect on its rapid clearance from the circulation. As was the case with the galactose-terminated asialoorosomucoid, uptake was effected predominately by the liver; however, a substantial portion of the injected mannose-terminated glycoprotein also was localized to the kidneys. Since the rate of plasma clearance of neither the *N*-acetylglucosamine-terminating agalacto-orosomucoid nor the mannose-terminating ahexosamino-orosomucoid was inhibited by the simultaneous infusion of a saturating amount of galactose-terminating asialoorosomucoid, the existence of other hepatic receptor(s) for *N*-acetylglucosamine/mannose was proposed (64).

N-acetylglucosamine-terminated agalactoorosomucoid was shown to be a potent inhibitor of plasma clearance of a number of lysosomal enzymes, including β-glucuronidase (65). Subsequently it was demonstrated that the hepatic uptake of β-glucuronidase was likewise inhibited by mannan, the mannose-terminated glycoprotein of yeast cell wall (66). Recognition of these two sugar residues by a single endocytotic mechanism was confirmed by the cross-inhibition of clearance by mannans and agalactoorosomucoid (67). In contrast to galactose recognition, which is characteristic of hepatocytes, uptake of glycoproteins terminating in either *N*-acetylglycosamine or mannose was localized to the sinusoidal cells of the liver (65,68).

The strong presumptive evidence provided by these *in vivo* and *in vitro* studies was confirmed by the isolation of a membrane protein that recognizes both sugars (69). The protein isolated from rabbit liver homogenates by solubilization with Triton X-100 and affinity chromatography on a mannin-agarose column was assayed by its ability to bind mannin. Inhibitors of binding included both *N*-acetylglycosamine and mannose, but more provocative were far greater inhibitions displayed by native α-mannosidase and β-glucuronidase. These two lysosomal glycosidases, as well as other glycoproteins with terminal *N*-acetylglucosamine or mannose, have been shown to be rapidly cleared from the circulation and taken up by the liver following intravenous injection into rats (70,71). It seems likely that the hepatic uptake of these glycoproteins was mediated by an analogous rat *N*-acetylglucosamine/mannose receptor.

As was the case for the galactose receptors, while the presence of specific terminal residues is necessary, it is not sufficient for recognition. Both IgM and IgE and possibly IgA contain terminal mannose, yet these classes of immunoglobulins continue to survive in the circulation. This apparent paradox was resolved by the demonstration that the long circulatory half-life of IgM is a result of its mannose-terminating oligosaccharide being sterically inaccessible to the receptor (72). Upon antigen binding, soluble IgM immune complexes are rapidly cleared from the circulation. Digestion of the immune complex with a mannosidase abolished both binding by the mannose-specific lectin concanavalin A and rapid clearance from the circulation. From these observations, it was suggested that an antigen-induced conformational change resulted in exposure of the mannose-rich oligosaccharide, which signals the clearance of soluble immune complexes from the circulation.

Evidence of yet another mammalian receptor, this one for fucose, was provided by comparison of the serum survival of two closely related iron-carrying human glycoproteins (73). Transferrin from serum and lactoferrin from milk differ in their oligosaccharide unit by only one fucose residue which is linked α-1-3 to N-acetylglucosamine of the milk protein. This difference is sufficient to effect the rapid clearance of lactoferrin from the plasma. Ten minutes after intravenous injection of iodinated lactoferrin into mice or rats, 85% of the radiolabel was recovered in the liver. The cellular distribution was determined by preparing isolated hepatocytes directly following injection of radiolabeled lactoferrin. Of the total hepatic radioactivity recovered, 98% was localized to the hepatocytes, with less than 2% in the sinusoidal cells (Kupffer and endothelial).

The specificity of fucose recognition was confirmed by *in vivo* uptake inhibition studies. Neither mannan nor derivatives of orosomucoid that are cleared by receptors for galactose, N-acetylglucosamine, or mannose inhibit clearance of lactoferrin, although clearance is inhibited by the fucose-containing glycoprotein fucoiden. Hepatic recognition was shown to be dependent on the α-1-3 linkage since glycoproteins with fucose linked α-1-2 to galactose or α-1-6 to N-acetylglucosamine do not inhibit lactoferrin clearance.

High levels of circulating partially desialylated orosomucoid in the serum of chickens led to the speculation that the galactose-specific receptor was absent in avian species (74). This hypothesis was confirmed by the demonstration that the avian liver was totally deficient in this hepatic binding protein (75). Of even greater significance, however, was the identification by these investigators of an avian hepatic binding activity for N-acetylglucosamine-terminating glycoprotein.

This receptor was subsequently isolated and purified from chicken liver by affinity chromatography procedures analogous to those used for the rabbit liver protein (76). The purified avian receptor protein shares many properties with those of the mammalian protein. Both are glycoproteins forming aggregates in aqueous solution recognizing only the terminal sugar residues of the ligand and requiring calcium for binding. As expected, exposure to neuraminidase was without effect, while subsequent treatment with β-galactosidase resulted in complete loss of binding activity, presumably through autoinhibition of newly exposed N-acetylglucosamine residues. In contrast to the rabbit or rat binding protein and more like the human, binding of ligand was readily reversible. The dissociation rate constant was calculated to be 1.3×10^{-3} sec^{-1}, similar to 1.7×10^{-3} sec^{-1} observed for the human asialoglycoprotein binding receptor.

SUMMARY AND CONCLUSION

The original findings describing a galactose-specific receptor in the liver were extended by numerous investigators to reveal a remarkable collection of cellular receptors for glycoproteins. Four recognition systems have been described for receptor-mediated endocytosis of glycoproteins in the liver alone. In mammals, both the galactose and fucose receptors are localized to the parenchymal cells, while receptors for N-acetylglucosamine or mannose are present in the reticuloendothelial cells. An analogous binding protein, specific for N-acetylglucosamine only, has been isolated from avian liver. Recognition of specific carbohydrate residues is not limited to the cells of the liver; a striking example of this kind of carbohydrate-specified cellular recognition phenomenon has been described in cultured fibroblasts (77). The ability of these cells to internalize lysosomal enzymes has been shown to be a receptor-mediated system dependent on the recognition of mannose-6-phosphate. Several other carbohydrate-binding proteins have been isolated from bovine heart and lung (78), chick embryo muscle (79), and the electric organ of the eel (80). This list will grow further, pointing to the significant role of carbohydrate structure as a means of information storage and retrieval.

Any discussion of the possible physiologic function of membrane-associated lectins must be approached with caution. As pointed out in a recent review by Neufeld and Ashwell (81) of receptor-mediated endocytosis, the tendency is to ascribe a biologic significance to the measurable characteristics that lead to their discovery. Thus binding of asialoglycoproteins to cell surface receptors, as a prelude to their lysosomal catabolism, has implicated the hepatic binding protein in the regulation of glycoprotein homeostasis. The circumstantial evidence for this hypothesis is provided by the presence of galactose-terminated glycoproteins in the circulation of patients with hepatic dysfunction and in avian species lacking the galactose-specific receptor. Several investigators extended the potential posed by carbohydrate-specific receptors to other cellular recognition systems. For example, hepatocytes isolated from rats and chickens exhibit carbohydrate-determined adhesion properties during reaggregation, which reflect the known terminal sugar specificity of their respective hepatocellular receptors (82,83). Furthermore, if it may be assumed that specific carbohydrates provide determinants at the cell surface, the same principle could apply on the subcellular level. The diverse intracellular distribution of the galactose-specific receptor led to the suggestion that it may play a role in membrane or organelle fusion as part of the overall process of intracellular recognition (84).

However attractive these extrapolations may be, in the absence of experimental confirmation, the physiologic function of mammalian lectins remains speculative.

REFERENCES

1. Morell, A. G., Van den Hamer, C. J. A., Scheinberg, I. H., and Ashwell, G. (1966): Physical and chemical studies on ceruloplasmin. Preparation of radioactive sialic acid-free ceruloplasmin labeled with tritium on terminal D-galactose residues. *J. Biol. Chem.*, 241:3745–3749.
2. Morell, A. G., Irvine, R. A., Sternlieb, I., Scheinberg, I. H., and Ashwell, G. (1968): Physical and chemical studies on ceruloplasmin. Metabolic studies on sialic acid-free ceruloplasmin *in vivo*. *J. Biol. Chem.*, 243:155–159.
3. Hickman, J., Ashwell, G., Morell, A. G., Van den Hamer, C. J. A., and Scheinberg, I. H. (1970): Physical and chemical studies on ceruloplasmin. Preparation of N-acetylneuraminic acid-1-^{14}C-labeled ceruloplasmin. *J. Biol. Chem.*, 245:759–766.
4. Van den Hamer, C. J. A., Morell, A. G., Scheinberg, I. H., Hickman, J., and Ashwell, G. (1970): Physical and chemical studies on ceruloplasmin. IX. The role of galactosyl residues in the clearance of ceruloplasmin from the circulation. *J. Biol. Chem.*, 245:4397–4403.
5. Morell, G. A., Gregoriadis, G., Scheinberg, I. H., Hickman, J., and Ashwell, G. (1971): The role of sialic acid in determining the survival of glycoproteins in the circulation. *J. Biol. Chem.*, 246:1461–1467.
6. Conway, T. P., Morgan, W. T., Liem, H. H., and Muller-Eberhard, V. (1975): Catabolism of photo-oxidized and desialylated hemopexin in the rabbit. *J. Biol. Chem.*, 250:3067–3073.
7. Glaser, C. B., Karic, L., Fallat, R. J., and Stockert, R. J. (1977): *Biochim. Biophys. Acta*, 495:87–92.
8. Hildenbrandt, G. R., and Aronson, N. N., Jr. (1980): Uptake of asialoglycophorin liposomes by the perfused rat liver. *Biochim. Biophys. Acta*, 631:499–502.
9. Braunstein, G. D., Reichert, L. E., Van Hall, E. V., et al. (1971): The effects of desialylation on the biologic and immunologic activity of human pituitary lutenizing hormone. *Biochem. Biophys. Res. Commun.*, 42:962–967.
10. Nelsetuen, G. L., and Suttie, J. W. (1971): Properties of asialo and aglycoprothrombin. *Biochem. Biophys. Res. Commun.*, 45:198–203.
11. Lukowsky, W. A., and Painter, R. H. (1972): Studies on the role of sialic acid in the physical and biological properties of erythropoietin. *Can. J. Biochem.*, 50:909–917.
12. Goldwasser, E., Kung, C. K. H., and Eliason, J. (1974): The role of sialic acid in erythropoietin action. *J. Biol. Chem.*, 249:4202–4206.
13. Marshall, J. S., Green, A. M., Pensky, J., Williams, S., Zinn, A., and Carlson, D. M. (1974): Measurement of circulating desialylated glycoproteins and correlation with hepatocellular damage. *J. Clin. Invest.*, 54:555–562.
14. Gan, J. C. (1979): Inhibitory effects of α_1-antitrypsin derived asialooligosaccharide on the liver uptake on the asialyglycoproteins. *Int. J. Biochem.*, 11:481–486.
15. Hubbard, A. L., Wilson, G., Ashwell, G., and Stukenbrok, H. (1979): An electron microscope autoradiographic study of the carbohydrate recognition systems in rat liver. *J. Cell. Biol.*, 83:47–64.
16. Gregoriadis, G., Morell, A. G., Sternlieb, I., and Scheinberg, I. H. (1970): Catabolism of desialylated ceruloplasmin in the liver. *J. Biol. Chem.*, 245:5833–5837.
17. La Badie, J. H., Chapman, K. P., and Aronson, N. N. (1975): Glycoprotein catabolism in rat liver. *Biochem. J.*, 152:271–279.
18. Tolleshaug, H., Berg, T., Nilsson, M., and Norum, K. R. (1977): Uptake and degradation of ^{125}I-labeled asialofetuin by isolated rat hepatocytes. *Biochim. Biophys. Acta*, 499:73–84.
19. Dunn, W. A., La Badie, J. H., and Aronson, N. N. (1979): Inhibition of ^{125}I-asialofetuin catabolism by leupeptin in the perfused rat liver and *in vivo*. *J. Biol. Chem.*, 254:4191–4196.
20. Pricer, W. E., Jr., and Ashwell, G. (1971): The binding of desialylated glycoproteins by plasma membranes of rat liver. *J. Biol. Chem.*, 246:4825–4833.
21. Van Lenten, L., and Ashwell, G. (1972): The binding of desialylated glycoproteins by plasma membranes of rat liver. Development of a quantitative inhibition assay. *J. Biol. Chem.*, 247:4633–4640.
22. Morell, A. G., and Scheinberg, I. H. (1972): Solubilization of hepatic binding sites for asialoglycoproteins. *Biochem. Biophys. Res. Commun.*, 48:808–815.
23. Hudgin, R. L., Pricer, W. E., Jr., Ashwell, G., Stockert, R. J., and Morell, A. G. (1974): The isolation and properties of a rabbit liver binding protein specific for asialoglycoproteins. *J. Biol. Chem.*, 249:5536–5543.
24. Kawasaki, T., and Ashwell, G. (1976): Chemical and physical properties of an hepatic membrane protein that specifically binds asialoglycoproteins. *J. Biol. Chem.*, 251:1296–1302.
25. Kawasaki, T., and Ashwell, G. (1976): Carbohydrate structure of glycopeptides isolated from an hepatic membrane-binding protein specific for asialoglycoproteins. *J. Biol. Chem.*, 251:5292–5299.
26. Steer, C. J., Harmon, J. T., and Kempner, E. S. (1980): Radiation target analysis to determine the minimal structural assembly of the hepatic asialoglycoprotein receptor. *Gastroenterology*, 79A.
27. Tanabe, T., Pricer, W. E., Jr., and Ashwell, G. (1979): Subcellular membrane topology and turnover of a rat hepatic binding protein specific for asialoglycoproteins. *J. Biol. Chem.*, 254:1038–1043.
28. Baenziger, J. U., and Maynard, Y. (1980): Human hepatic lectin. *J. Biol. Chem.*, 255:4607–4613.
29. Stockert, R. J., Morell, A. G., and Scheinberg, I. H. (1977): Hepatic binding protein: The protective role of its sialic acid residues. *Science*, 197:667–668.
30. Paulson, J. C., Hill, R. L., Tanabe, T., and Ashwell, G. (1977): Reactivation of asialo-rabbit liver binding protein by resialylation with β-D-galactoside α 2-6 sialyltransferase. *J. Biol. Chem.*, 252:8624–8628.
31. Stockert, R. J., Morell, A. G., and Scheinberg, I. H. (1974): Mammalian hepatic lectin. *Science*, 186:365–366.
32. Novogrodsky, A., and Ashwell, G. (1977): Lymphocyte mitogenesis induced by a mammalian liver protein that specifically binds desialylated glycoproteins. *Proc. Natl. Acad. Sci. USA*, 74:676–678.
33. Vierling, J. M., Steer, C. J., Hickman, J. W., James, S. P., and Jones, E. A. (1978): Cell-mediated cytotoxicity of desialylated human lymphocytes induced by a mitogenic mammalian liver protein. *Gastroenterology*, 75:456–461.
34. Kolb, H., Kolb-Bachofen, U., and Schlepper-Schafer, J. (1979):

Cell contacts mediated by D-galactose-specific lectins on liver cells. *Biol. Cell.*, 36:301–308.

35. Roseman, S. (1970): The synthesis of complex carbohydrates by multiglycosyltransferase systems and their pontential function in intercellular adhesion. *Chem. Phys. Lipids*, 5:270–274.

36. Hudgin, R. L., and Ashwell, G. (1974): Studies on the role of glycosyl transferases in the hepatic binding of asialoglycoproteins. *J. Biol. Chem.*, 249:7369–7372.

37. Sarkar, M., Liao, J., Kabat, E. A., Tanabe, T., and Ashwell, G. (1979): The binding site of rabbit hepatic lectin. *J. Biol. Chem.*, 254:3170–3174.

38. Stowell, C. P., and Lee, C. Y. (1978): The binding of D-glucosyl-neoglycoproteins to the hepatic asialoglycoprotein receptor. *J. Biol. Chem.*, 258:6107–6110.

39. Riordan, J. R., Mitchell, L., and Slavik, M. (1974): The binding of asialoglycoprotein to isolated golgi apparatus. *Biochem. Biophys. Res. Commun.*, 59:1373–1379.

40. Pricer, W. E., Jr., and Ashwell, G. (1976): Subcellular distribution of a mammalian hepatic binding protein specific for asialoglycoproteins. *J. Biol. Chem.*, 251:7539–7544.

41. Sawamura, T., Nakada, H., Fujii-Kurujama, Y., and Tashiro, Y. (1980): Some properties of a binding protein specific for asialoglycoproteins and its distribution in rat liver microsomes. *Cell. Struct. Function*, 5:133–146.

42. Dunn, W. A., Hubbard, A. L., and Aronson, N. N., Jr. (1980): Low temperature selectively inhibits fusion between pinocytic vesicles and lysosomes during heterophagy of ^{125}I-asialofetuin by the perfused rat liver. *J. Biol. Chem.*, 255:5971–5978.

43. Pertoft, H., Warmegard, B., and Hook, M. (1978): Heterogeneity of lysosomes originating from rat liver parenchymal cells. *Biochem. J.*, 174:309–317.

44. Kolset, S. O., Tolleshaug, H., and Berg, T. (1979): The effect of colchiceine and cytochalasin B on uptake and degradation of asialoglycoproteins in isolated rat hepatocytes. *Exp. Cell Res.*, 122:159–167.

45. Stockert, R. J., Haims, H. B., Morell, A. G., et al. (1980): Endocytosis of asialoglycoprotein-enzyme conjugates by hepatocytes. *Lab. Invest.*, 43:556–563.

46. Golstein, J. L., Anderson, R. G. W., and Brown, M. S. (1979): Coated pits, coated vesicles, and receptor mediated endocytosis. *Nature*, 279:679–685.

47. Maxfield, F. R., Schlessinger, J., Schechter, Y., Pastan, I. H., and Willingham, M. C. (1978): Collection of insulin, EGF and α_2-macroglobin in the same patches on the surface of cultured fibroblasts and common internalization. *Cell*, 14:805–810.

48. Willingham, M. C., and Pastan, I. H. (1980): The receptosome: An intermediate organelle of receptor-mediated endocytosis in cultured fibroblasts. *Cell*, 21:67–77.

49. Gorden, P., Carpentier, J., Cohen, S., and Orci, L. (1978): Epidermal growth factor: Morphological demonstration of binding internalization and lysosomal association in human fibroblasts. *Proc. Natl. Acad. Sci. USA*, 57:5025–5029.

50. Wall, D. A., and Hubbard, A. L. (1980): Distribution of asialoglycoprotein binding sites on rat hepatocyte cell surfaces. *J. Cell. Biol.*, 84:91a.

51. Pearse, B. (1980): Coated pits. *TIBS*, 5:131–134.

52. Steer, C., and Clarenburg, R. (1979): Unique distribution of glycoprotein receptors on parenchymal and sinusoidal cells of rat liver. *J. Biol. Chem.*, 254:4457–4461.

53. Steer, C. J., and Ashwell, G. (1980): Studies on a mammalian binding protein specific for asialoglycoproteins. *J. Biol. Chem.*, 255:3008–3013.

54. Stockert, R. J., Howard, D. J., Morell, A. G., and Scheinberg, I. H. (1980): Functional segregation of hepatic receptors for asialoglycoproteins during endocytosis. *J. Biol. Chem.*, 255:9028–9029.

55. Stockert, R. J., Gartner, U., Morell, A. G., and Wolkoff, A. W. (1980): Effect of receptor-specific antibody on the uptake of desialylated glycoproteins in the isolated perfused rat liver. *J. Biol. Chem.*, 255:3830–3831.

56. Doyle, D., Hou, E., and Warren, R. (1979): Transfer of the hepatocyte receptor for serum asialoglycoproteins to the plasma membrane of a fibroblast. *J. Biol. Chem.*, 254:6853–6856.

57. TulRens, P., Schneider, E. J., and Trouet, A. (1977): The fate of the plasma membrane during endocytosis. *Biochem. Soc. Trans.*, 5:1809–1814.

58. Lunney, J. (1976): Studies on the regulation of serum glycoprotein homeostasis. Doctoral dissertation, Johns Hopkins University, Baltimore.

59. Stockert, R. J., and Becker, F. F. (1980): Diminished hepatic binding protein for desialylated glycoproteins during chemical hepatocarcinogenesis. *Cancer Res.*, 40:3632–3634.

60. Gartner, U., Stockert, R. J., Morell, A. G., and Wolkoff, Q. W. (1981): Modulation of the transport of bilirubin and asialo-orosomucoid during liver regeneration. *Hepatology*, 1:99–106.

61. Hickman, J., and Ashwell, G. (1974): Studies on the hepatic binding of asialoglycoproteins by hepatoma tissue and by isolated hepatocytes. In: *Enzyme Therapy in Lysosomal Storage Diseases*, edited by J. M. Tager, G. J. M. Hooghwinkel, and W. Th., Daems, North-Holland, Amsterdam.

62. Howard, D. J., Stockert, R. J., and Morell, A. G. (1980): Altered expression of a plasma membrane receptor during hepatic regeneration. *Gastroenterology*, 79A: 1026.

63. Leffert, H., Alexander, N. M., Faloona, G., Rubalcava, B., and Unger, R. (1975): Specific endocrine and hormonal receptor chances associated with liver regeneration in adult rats. *Proc. Natl. Acad. Sci. USA*, 72:4033–4036.

64. Stockert, R. J., Morell, A. G., and Scheinberg, I. H. (1976): The existence of a second route for the transfer of certain glycoproteins from the circulation into the liver. *Biochem. Biophys. Res. Commun.*, 68:988–993.

65. Stahl, P., Schlesinger, P. H., Rodman, J. S., and Doebber, T. (1976): Evidence for specific recognition sites mediating clearance of lysosomal enzymes *in vivo*. *Proc. Natl. Acad. Sci. USA*, 73:4045–4051.

66. Achord, D. T., Brot, F. E., Gonzalez-Noriega, A., Sly, W. W., and Stahl, P. (1977): Human β-glucuronidase. II. Fate of infused human placental β-glucuronidase in the rat. *Pediatr. Res.*, 11:816–822.

67. Achord, D. T., Brot, F. E., and Sly, W. S. (1977): Inhibition of the rat clearance system for agalactoorosomucoid by yeast mannans and mannose. *Biochem. Biophys. Res. Commun.*, 77:409–415.

68. Achord, D. T., Brot, F. E., Bell, C. E., and Sly, W. W. (1978): Human β-glucuronidase: *In vivo* clearance and *in vitro* uptake by a glycoprotein recognition system on reticulo endothelial cells. *Cell*, 15:269–278.

69. Kawasaki, T., Etoh, R., and Yamashina, I. (1978): Isolation and characterization of a mannan-binding protein from rabbit liver. *Biochem. Biophys. Res. Commun.*, 81:1018–1024.

70. Windelhake, J. I., and Nicolson, G. L. (1976): Aglycosyl antibody. *J. Biol. Chem.*, 251:1074–1080.

71. Baynes, J. W., and Wold, F. (1976): Effect of glycosylation on the *in vivo* circulating half-life of rebonuclease. *J. Biol. Chem.*, 251:6016–6024.

72. Day, J. F., Thornburg, R. W., Thorpe, S. R., and Baynes, J. W. (1980): Carbohydrate-mediated clearance of antibody-antigen complexes from the circulation. *J. Biol. Chem.*, 255:2360–2365.

73. Prieel, J. P., Pizzo, S. V., Glagow, L. R., Paulson, J., and Hill, R. L. (1978): Hepatic receptor that specifically binds oligosaccharides containing fucosyl × 1-3 N-acetylglucosamine linkages. *Proc. Natl. Acad. Sci. USA*, 75:2215–2219.

74. Regoeczi, E., Hatton, M. W. C., and Charlwood, P. A. (1975): Carbohydrate-mediated elimination of avian plasma glycoproteins in mammals. *Nature*, 254:699–701.

75. Lunney, J., and Ashwell, G. (1975): A hepatic receptor of avian origin capable of binding specifically modified glycoproteins. *Proc. Natl. Acad. Sci. USA*, 73:341–343.

76. Kawasaki, T., and Ashwell, G. (1977): Isolation and characterization of an avain hepatic binding protein specific for N-acetyl glucosamine-terminated glycoproteins. *J. Biol. Chem.*, 252:6536–6543.

77. Neufeld, E. F., Lim, T. W., and Shapiro, L. J. (1975): Inherited

disorders of lysosomal metabolism. *Annu. Rev. Biochem.,* 44:357.

78. DeWaard, A., Hickman, S., and Dornfeld, S. (1976): Isolation and properties of β-galactoside binding lectins of calf heart and lung. *J. Biol. Chem.,* 251:7581–7586.

79. Den, H., and Malinzak, D. A. (1977): The isolation and properties of a β-D-galactoside specific lectin from chick embryo thigh muscle. *J. Biol. Chem.,* 252:5444–5450.

80. Teichberg, V. I., Silman, I., Beitsch, D. D., and Resheff, C. (1975): A β-D-galactoside binding protein from electric organ tissue of *Electrophorus electricus. Proc. Natl. Acad. Sci. USA,* 72:1383–1390.

81. Neufeld, E. F., and Ashwell, G. (1980): Carbohydrate recognition systems for receptor mediated pinocytosis. In: *The Biochemistry of Glycoproteins and Proteoglycans,* edited by W. J. Lemarz, pp. 241–266.

82. Obrink, B., Kuhlenschmidt, M. S., and Roseman, S. (1977): Adhesive specificity of juvenile rat and chicken liver cells and membranes. *Proc. Natl. Acad. Sci. USA,* 74:1077–1081.

83. Weigel, P. H., Schmell, E., Lee, Y. C., and Roseman, H. (1978): Specific adhesion of rat hepatocytes to β-galactosides linked to polyacrylamide gels. *J. Biol. Chem.,* 25:330–335.

84. Ashwell, G. (1977): A functional role for lectins. *Trends Biol. Sci.,* 2:N-186.

The Liver: Biology and Pathobiology, edited by
I. Arias, H. Popper, D. Schachter, and D. A. Shafritz.
Raven Press, New York © 1982.

Chapter 13

Energy Metabolism

Sam Seifter and Sasha Englard

The liver serves as an intermediary between the dietary sources of energy and the extrahepatic tissues that are the main users of energy. In that capacity the liver receives, by way of the portal circulation, the various small molecules arising from digestion, sorts them for metabolism and storage, and distributes some to the peripheral circulation for use by other tissues. To carry out those functions and to maintain a structural apparatus for their performance, the liver extracts a significant portion of the nutrients to provide energy for its own macromolecular syntheses, transport of materials in and out of liver cells, and metabolic conversions within the cells.

The liver also receives metabolites transported by the blood from other tissues. Thus in relation to provision of energy, the liver obtains fatty acids and glycerol from adipose tissues, lactate and pyruvate from skeletal muscle and blood cells, alanine and certain other amino acids from muscle, and branched chain α-keto acids from skeletal muscle where they arise by transamination of leucine, isoleucine, and valine (1). In turn, the liver exports two principal substrates that can be oxidized in peripheral tissues to provide energy. The first is glucose; this arises by glycogenolysis of stored glycogen and by gluconeogenesis from lactate, pyruvate, glycerol, propionate, and alanine. Many other amino acids whose carbon chains can give rise to pyruvate, oxaloacetate, fumarate, malate, succinate, or α-ketoglutarate can contribute to production of glucose by gluconeogenesis. The second substrate made by the liver for transport

to other tissues is acetoacetate (or its reduced derivative, 3-hydroxybutyrate). Acetoacetate arises from acetyl-CoA coming from the oxidation of fatty acids transported to the liver from adipose tissue. The liver also synthesizes storage lipids in the form of triacylglycerols and phospholipids; these are packaged with lipoproteins and delivered to the blood for use in peripheral tissues. The scheduling of synthesis and transport of these substrates is exquisitely regulated by hormones and coordinated with the amounts and nature of fuels from the diet, with the length of time after feeding, and with the quantity of glucose available in relation to the requirements of tissues that have an obligate need for glucose. Those tissues are the blood cells, especially erythrocytes, and renal medulla. Thus the liver is sensitive to the kinds of fuels needed by specific tissues under different physiological conditions and, in cooperation with other tissues, is programmed to provide those fuels.

In addition to manufacturing and exporting fuels that can be oxidized directly for energy in other tissues, the liver provides critical compounds to be used by those tissues in enabling and permissive capacities relative to the release and storage of energy arising from substrate oxidation. Thus the liver carries out the final steps in the synthesis of carnitine and creatine, respectively, both of which are sent to the peripheral circulation to be concentratively absorbed by target organs that utilize them in their energy machinery. Carnitine, 4-N-trimethyl-3-hydroxy-aminobutyric acid, is synthesized as follows (2):

L-Lysine→protein peptidyl lysine $\xrightarrow[\text{L-methionine}]{\text{S-adenosyl-}}$ protein

peptidyl 6-N-trimethyl-L-lysine→free 6-N-trimethyl-L-

lysine→3-hydroxy-6-N-trimethyl-L-lysine $\xrightarrow{\text{glycine}}$ 4-N-

trimethylaminobutyraldehyde→4-N-trimethylaminobutyric

acid→L-carnitine

The final hydroxylation step in humans is performed in the liver and kidneys (3,4). Some of the resulting carnitine is used both in mitochondria and peroxisomes of hepatocytes for the transport of fatty acids across membranes, but most is exported for use in other tissues that metabolize fatty acids for energy, i.e., skeletal and cardiac muscle. Deficiency of carnitine can result in poor performance of muscle, since it effectively deprives the tissue of capacity to oxidize fatty acids (5,6).

The liver is also the site of the final synthesis of creatine which occurs by methylation of guanidinoacetate by S-adenosylmethionine (7). Although the liver has little creatine kinase (8), and therefore hardly uses creatine for its own energy balance, it exports creatine to tissues such as skeletal muscle, heart, and brain. These tissues have mechanisms for concentrative absorption of creatine from extracellular fluid and use creatine as an acceptor of the terminal high energy phosphate group of ATP as governed by the action of creatine kinase. If the liver were not to make creatine, the entire energy balance of those tissues would be upset, not only because a reserve of high energy phosphate would be diminished, but the nature of the adenine nucleotide pool would be affected. The presence of creatine helps regulate the ATP:ADP ratio, which in turn affects the oxidative capacity of a tissue.

The liver makes other compounds for export that, in one way or another, affect energy release and utilization in other tissues; these are not considered in detail here. This chapter is primarily concerned with the nature of substrates that the liver uses to provide energy for its many transport and biosynthetic functions, the metabolic pathways open to these substrates, the interrelationships among the pathways, and finally, the regulation of those pathways to allow the liver a choice among them in relation to the physiological state of the whole organism. We also examine the several ways in which the liver provides specific fuels for different extrahepatic tissues according to their requirements; this includes consideration of the signals to the liver which make it sensitive to the needs of other tissues.

NATURE OF FUELS PROVIDED TO THE LIVER BY THE INTESTINE

We first discuss some general considerations about the nature of diets that provide the fuels. Human diets vary depending on economic factors, climate, geographical location, development of agriculture and other technologies, and the cultural habits and energy requirements of different peoples. Our examples are chosen largely from the diets eaten in the United States, Canada, and many parts of Europe, where the level of protein is higher than in the diets of peoples in tropical areas and the level of cereal carbohydrates (mainly starches) is lower. Also, the peoples of those areas ingest a large percentage of their carbohydrate in the form of highly refined sugars such as sucrose; in fact, the annual per capita consumption of refined sugars and syrups in the United States and Great Britain averages about 115 pounds, as compared to about 146 pounds of cereal carbohydrate (9). The following discussion deals largely with diets of that kind.

If one assumes a diet that provides 3,000 kilocalories[1] per day, the average adult working person in the United States partitions the provision of energy as approximately 13 to 15% from proteins, 40% from carbohydrates, and 40% from fats. About 7% of calories is derived from ethanol (10), a consideration of importance for the biochemistry of the liver (11). (In a significant number of people, the percentage of calories due to ethanol is much higher.) Translated in terms of amount of nutrients provided, the average person daily ingests about 100 g protein, 130 g fat, 300 g carbohydrate, and 30 g ethanol. Taking into account the further partitioning of dietary carbohydrate, that individual consumes about 120 g sucrose, of which 60 g appears as fructose. Thus the liver of the average person must metabolize two special compounds, fructose and ethanol, from which a significant amount of energy is derived. Foodstuffs are ingested intermittently; consequently, the metabolism of the liver has evolved in relation to that circumstance and is characterized by poorly understood circadian rhythms and diurnal cycles.

After digestion and absorption of foodstuffs, the liver, through the portal circulation, is presented with a mixture of amino acids, monosaccharides, short-chain fatty acids, and occasionally, ethanol. The liver is able to process most of the amino acids through a combination of transamination and oxidative deamination but poorly transaminates the branched chain amino acids leucine, isoleucine, and valine (12). The latter primarily are sent into the peripheral circulation, from which they are extracted especially by skeletal muscle where they can be used in protein synthesis or, under condition of short supply of glucose, transaminated with pyruvate to form the corresponding branched chain α-keto acids and alanine (12). These keto acids and alanine, again under conditions of glucose lack, may be sent to the liver to be processed into

---

[1] One kilocalorie (kcal) is equivalent to 4.184 kilojoules (kJ).

energy sources for the liver itself and for other tissues; the processes involved are considered subsequently.

In addition to long-chain fatty acids, dietary lipids contain a variety of short-chain fatty acids. When released by lipolytic digestion, these are relatively easily absorbed into the intestinal cells, having the advantage of smaller molecular weight and greater water solubility as compared with long-chain fatty acids. Resynthesis of triacylglycerols from monoacylglycerols occurs in the intestinal cells with preference given to the incorporation of long-chain fatty acids. Accordingly, the short-chain acids remain free, are easily transferred to the portal circulation, and are carried to the liver (13). Immediately after digestion of a meal containing fats, the liver is presented primarily with short-chain fatty acids and utilizes them for its energy metabolism through oxidation in the mitochondrial fatty acid oxidation system. Nevertheless, the liver ultimately receives some of the long-chain fatty acids released by digestion, but the process is circuitous. The triacylglycerols reconstituted in the intestinal absorbing cells are incorporated into chylomicrons together with cholesterol esters and phospholipids and sent into the lymph (14). The lymph empties into the circulation at the thoracic duct, and the chylomicrons are then circulated throughout the organism. Chylomicrons presented to the adipose tissue are acted on by an endothelial lipoprotein lipase (not to be confused with the hormone-sensitive lipase in adipocytes), releasing long-chain fatty acids (which originated in the dietary lipids) and diacylglycerols (14). The latter may be taken into adipocytes where they can be resynthesized into triacylglycerols, but the fatty acids are transferred to plasma albumin and carried in the blood to the various tissues. Some of the fatty acid is extracted by the liver, so that the organ eventually does derive some fraction of long-chain fatty acids from the dietary lipids. Furthermore, the remnants of chylomicrons, which still contain some triacylglycerols, are also carried by the blood to the liver where hepatic triacylglycerol lipase may provide an additional fraction of the dietary long-chain fatty acids. However, most long-chain fatty acids are brought to the liver after lipolysis of triacylglycerols stored in adipocytes.

USE OF OXYGEN BY THE LIVER FOR ENERGY FUNCTIONS

The hepato-portal system is highly aerobic. Constituting only about 4% of the total body weight, it receives about 28% of the total blood flow in 1 min and consumes about 20% of the total oxygen used by the human organism (15).

In the basal state, a 70-kg man uses about 400 liters of oxygen per day (16), of which about 80 liters are consumed by the liver. This occurs in relation to the 340–360 kcal of energy expended by the liver under basal conditions (20% of a total of 1,800 kcal used by the whole organism) (17).

The oxygen is used primarily for the oxidation of fuels, most of which results in the preservation of free energy as the high energy pyrophosphate bonds of ATP; the standard free energy of ATP is 7.3 kcal/mole, or 30.5 kJ/mole. Perhaps about 90% of the oxygen consumed by the liver is used in reactions that can be poisoned by cyanide, constituting the so-called cyanide-sensitive respiration, most of which is related to the mitochondrial electron transport system or respiratory chain in which cytochrome oxidase is the iron hemoprotein sensitive to cyanide.

Cyanide-insensitive respiration is principally associated with enzymes present in peroxisomes or microbodies; these enzymes utilize flavin nucleotides as coenzymes, the oxidation-reduction potentials of which are modified so that they can couple directly with molecular oxygen (18); hydrogen peroxide is formed instead of water, as produced in the mitochondrial respiratory chain. Examples of such flavin nucleotide-containing enzymes are xanthine oxidase, uricase, D-amino acid oxidase, and fatty acyl-CoA oxidase. Hydrogen peroxide produced in peroxisomes is rapidly metabolized by the action of catalase which, in the absence of a suitable oxidizable substrate, catalyzes the release of molecular oxygen; in the presence of such a substrate (e.g., ethanol or methanol), catalase causes reduction of hydrogen peroxide (19).

Under most conditions, the liver obtains the largest fraction of its ATP through the oxidation of fatty acids; considerably less is derived from the oxidation of pyruvate formed in glycolysis or from lactate brought from skeletal muscle and blood cells. If the liver were oxidizing only fatty acids, its theoretical respiratory quotient (R.Q.), defined as the ratio of volumes of carbon dioxide produced to volumes of oxygen consumed, would be approximately 0.71. In reality, that figure would be modified upward if the liver were simultaneously synthesizing fatty acids from glucose and glucose by gluconeogenesis. In fact, energy derived from oxidation of fatty acids is used for driving gluconeogenesis.

Glycogen stored in the liver is used primarily to provide glucose to the blood for distribution to tissues that require it for energy metabolism. However, some glucose 1-phosphate derived from glycogen by glycogenolysis is directed into the glycolytic pathway and completely oxidized in the tricarboxylic acid cycle, ultimately yielding some ATP for use by the liver. Some of the triose phosphate produced in glycolysis, however, is diverted for synthesis of L-α-glycerol phosphate used in the production of triacylglycerols.

The liver, like other fatty acid-synthesizing tissues, including adipose tissue and mammary gland, has the enzymes of the pentose phosphate cycle (hexose monophosphate pathway), the oxidative branch of which provides NADPH for reductive synthesis of fatty acids. Although much experimental difficulty is encountered in evaluating the amount of glucose that goes through the oxidative arm of the pentose phosphate cycle as opposed to the glycolytic pathway (and indeed much effort has been expended for that purpose), such an estimation for the liver may have little physiological significance. Normally, the liver does not have a significant rate of glycolysis from glucose resulting in production of pyruvate or lactate; also, the oxidative branch of the pentose phosphate cycle is virtually suppressed. However, under conditions of lipogenesis which cause NADPH to be drawn off for fatty acid synthesis, the pentose phosphate cycle would become active. Artificially, an increased flux of glucose 6-phosphate through the oxidative pentose phosphate pathway can be made to occur by addition of phenazine methosulfate which can oxidize NADPH directly (20). In any case, glucose oxidation by the pentose phosphate cycle does not result in formation of ATP.

One can obtain some measure of the dependence of the liver on oxygen by examining two energy-requiring biosynthetic functions carried out by hepatocytes: production of albumin and creatine. In humans, albumin is manufactured exclusively by hepatocytes in an amount of approximately 12 g or 0.18 mmoles/day (17). Since a molecule of albumin contains 585 amino acid residues, about that many peptide bonds are formed. The synthesis of each peptide bond requires the input of about five high energy pyrophosphate bonds; accordingly, the total daily synthesis of albumin requires about 0.526 moles ATP. The complete oxidation of a molecule of glucose to carbon dioxide and water can produce up to 38 molecules of ATP; the complete oxidation of a molecule of palmitic acid yields 129 molecules of ATP. To make 0.18 mmoles albumin, the liver must oxidize 13.8 mmoles glucose (2.48 g) or 4.0 mmoles palmitic acid (1.02 g). The oxidation of that amount of glucose entails the consumption of about 82 mmoles or 1.9 liters oxygen; the corresponding figure for palmitic acid is 85 mmoles or 2.0 liters oxygen. These values are simply for polypeptide synthesis and do not include the additional energy needed for processing and transport of albumin.

The second example deals with creatine, the daily synthesis of which can be estimated from the daily excretion of creatinine in the urine. For an average man, the amount is approximately 25 mg creatinine per kilogram body weight; the figure for an average woman is about 5 mg less. One can estimate the daily synthesis of creatine by a 70-kg man to be approximately 1.75 g or 13.3 mmoles. The liver performs the last step in the synthesis of creatine, namely, the N-methylation of guanidinoacetate. The reaction requires the donation of a methyl group from S-adenosylmethionine. S-adenosylmethionine is made in the liver by a reaction in which a molecule of ATP is split with formation of one molecule each of inorganic phosphate and inorganic pyrophosphate. The resynthesis of ATP from adenosine would require the input of three high energy pyrophosphate bonds; essentially, methylation of guanidinoacetate requires the equivalent of three molecules of ATP, which means that the daily synthesis of creatine requires about 50 mmoles ATP just for the methylation step. That, in turn, requires the oxidation of 1.32 mmoles glucose (238 mg) using 7.9 mmoles (177 ml) oxygen. Alternatively, it requires oxidation of about 0.38 mmoles (97 mg) palmitic acid using about 8 mmoles (180 ml) oxygen.

HIGH ENERGY COMPOUNDS USED BY THE LIVER

Ultimately, all the energy used by animal organisms arises from oxidation of substrates. The principal form in which energy is preserved is the pyrophosphate bond of ATP; a minor fraction of the energy is conserved in GTP formed in a substrate level phosphorylation in the tricarboxylic acid cycle when α-ketoglutarate is oxidatively decarboxylated to succinate. A second generation of high energy bonds can be formed by the transfer of the terminal phosphate group of ATP to a suitable acceptor molecule such as a nucleoside diphosphate; in that case, little free energy is lost and new nucleoside triphosphates are formed that can be used in specific syntheses. In that category of reactions, for example, UDP is converted to UTP by reaction with ATP; the UTP so formed can be used in synthesis of nucleic acids or uridine diphosphateglucose (UDP glucose). Similarly, CDP can be phosphorylated by ATP to form CTP; and the latter can be used in synthesis of nucleic acids or cytidine diphosphatecholine (CDP choline).

A third generation of high energy phosphoanhydride bonds is formed when a nucleoside triphosphate transfers its nucleotidyl moiety to the acyl group of an organic acid to form an acylphosphoanhydride with little change of free energy; another product of the reaction is inorganic pyrophosphate. The nucleoside triphosphate used most frequently is ATP, although reactions are known also with CTP, UTP, and GTP. The general reaction with ATP is:

$$ATP + R \cdot COOH \rightleftharpoons R \cdot \overset{\overset{\displaystyle O}{\|}}{C} - AMP + PP_i$$

This reaction can be driven to the right by hydrolysis of the high energy inorganic pyrophosphate producing inorganic phosphate; an inorganic pyrophosphatase catalyzes this cleavage.

The formation of acylphosphoanhydrides occurs in the activation of amino acids to form aminoacyl adenylates used in protein biosynthesis, and in formation of fatty acyl adenylates in prelude to oxidation of fatty acids. The activated acyl group can then be transferred to a specific intermediate in the process. Thus, in protein biosynthesis, the activated aminoacyl group is transferred to the terminal adenylate residue of a specific tRNA molecule; in fatty acid oxidation, the fatty acyl moiety is transferred to the sulfur atom of CoASH. Both kinds of reactions occur with little change in free energy, thus keeping the newly formed acyl derivatives in an activated state:

Aminoacyl adenylate + tRNA $\rightleftharpoons$ aminoacyl-tRNA + adenylate

and

fatty acyl adenylate + CoASH $\rightleftharpoons$ fatty acyl-CoA + adenylate.

Except for one substrate level phosphorylation step and one internal oxidation-reduction step in glycolysis, and one substrate level phosphorylation reaction in the tricarboxylic acid cycle that results in formation of GTP, the reactions leading to synthesis of high energy pyrophosphate bonds (ATP) occur in conjunction with the mitochondrial respiratory chain. That requires oxidation of a substrate to occur with reduction of either NAD^+ or FAD to form NADH and $FADH_2$, respectively, and reoxidation of the coenzyme through the electron transport chain in the presence of molecular oxygen, ADP, and inorganic phosphate. NADPH, which is formed in a reaction utilizing $NADP^+$, cannot be reoxidized directly by the mitochondrial respiratory chain and, therefore, cannot be coupled with production of ATP. Table 1 shows the steps in glycolysis, the tricarboxylic acid cycle including oxidation of pyruvate, and fatty acid oxidation that lead to production of ATP and GTP.

In the liver, the generation of ATP resulting from the reoxidation of NADH formed in the glutamate dehydrogenase reaction may, under certain circumstances, be of quantitative significance. For instance, when the amount of protein in the diet is in excess of that needed to provide amino acids for protein and nucleic acid synthesis, many of the amino acids can be transaminated with α-ketoglutarate to form glutamate and their corresponding α-keto acids; the glutamate can be oxidatively deaminated to ammonia and α-ketoglutarate, while NAD^+ is simultaneously reduced to NADH. NADH can be reoxidized in the presence of molecular oxygen, ADP, and inorganic phosphate with production of three molecules of ATP by oxidative phosphorylation. This amount of ATP is almost equivalent to the energy required for synthesis of urea from ammonia formed in the deamination reaction. However, should the glutamate dehydrogenase operate with $NADP^+$ instead of with NAD^+, as can occur (21,22), no ATP would be generated with reoxidation of the coenzyme. Instead, the energy made available by oxidation of substrate is preserved as described below.

When a substrate is oxidized by a dehydrogenase that uses $NADP^+$, the NADPH formed cannot be directly reoxidized through the electron transport chain. The energy remains resident in the C-H bond formed when the pyridinium ring of the coenzyme is reduced. In certain highly specific reactions, constituting direct or indirect transhydrogenation systems, the following overall reaction occurs:

$$NADPH + H^+ + NAD^+ \rightleftharpoons NADP^+ + NADH + H^+$$

NADH then can be sent through the respiratory chain to produce three molecules of ATP. Thus the C-H bond in NADPH has energy equivalent to three ATP pyrophosphate bonds that can be made available biologically. In fact, most of the NADPH produced in the liver does not undergo transhydrogenation with NAD^+ but is employed directly for certain reductive syntheses that bypass the use of ATP. Two such reductive steps requiring the input of energy and of H atoms occur in synthesis of fatty acids from acetyl-CoA, a major activity of the liver. These reactions are concerned with, respectively, reduction of a keto to an alcohol group and reduction of a carbon-carbon double bond to a carbon-carbon single bond (see Fig. 5). The NADPH used for these syntheses arises primarily from three oxidative reactions, as shown below:

$$\text{Glucose 6-phosphate} + NADP^+ \xrightarrow{\text{glucose 6-phosphate dehydrogenase}} \text{6-phosphogluconolactone} + NADPH + H^+$$

$$\text{6-Phosphogluconate} + NADP^+ \xrightarrow{\text{phosphogluconate dehydrogenase}} \text{D-ribulose 5-phosphate} + CO_2 + NADPH + H^+$$

$$\text{L-Malate} + NADP^+ \xrightarrow[\substack{\text{(decarboxylating) } (NADP^+) \\ \text{E.C. 1.1.1.40}}]{\substack{\text{"Malic" enzyme,} \\ \text{malate dehydrogenase}}} \text{pyruvate} + CO_2 + NADPH + H^+$$

GENERAL USES OF ENERGY IN THE LIVER

Approximately one-half the energy available to the liver is utilized in various kinds of transport (especially Na^+) and secretory functions (17,23); ions and substrates are carried into and out of cells, end products are removed, bile is formulated and secreted, and osmotic equilibrium is maintained by movement of water between extracellular and intracellular compartments. Some substances move across barriers by passive or facilitated diffusion without expenditure of energy, as is probably the case for fatty acids, glucose, and urea. For purposes of export, however, triacylglycerols, phospholipids, and cholesterol esters are incorporated into specific lipoproteins whose synthesis requires investment of energy.

Another utilization of energy is in the storage of fuels. Formation of glycogen, triacylglycerols, and phospholipids requires energy, as does the intrahe-

TABLE 1. *Total ATP yield for the oxidation of glucose and of various fatty acids*

Function	Reactions	ATP yield
Glycolysis	1. Glucose→glucose 6-phosphate	−1
	2. Fructose-6-phosphate→fructose 1,6-bisphosphate	−1
	3.[a] [2]Glyceraldehyde-3-phosphate + [2]P_i + [2]NAD^+→[2]3-phosphoglyceroylphosphate + [2]NADH + [2] H^+:	
	a. [2]3-phosphoglyceroylphosphate→ [2]3-phosphoglycerate	+2
	b. [2]NADH + [2]H^+ + O_2→[2]NAD^+ + 2[H_2O]	+6[c]
	4.[b] [2]Phosphoenolpyruvate→[2]pyruvate	+2
	Total for glucose→ [2]pyruvate	+8
Pyruvate dehydrogenase and tricarboxylic acid cycle	1. NADH-generating reactions with subsequent reoxidation of reduced coenzyme by electron transport system	
	a. Pyruvate→acetyl-CoA + CO_2	+3
	b. Isocitrate→α-ketoglutarate + CO_2	+3
	c. α-Ketoglutarate→succinyl-CoA + CO_2	+3
	d. Malate→oxaloacetate	+3
	2. $FADH_2$-generating reaction with subsequent reoxidation of reduced coenzyme by electron transport system	
	a. Succinate→fumarate	+2
	3. Substrate level phosphorylation reaction generating GTP followed by transphosphorylation to ADP	
	a. Succinyl-CoA→succinate	+1
	Total for pyruvate→$3CO_2$	+15
	Total for glucose→$6CO_2$	+38

patic synthesis of glucose by gluconeogenesis. The synthesis of proteins and nucleic acids, urea, and a multitude of other substances are all highly energy-requiring reactions. Indeed, the biosynthetic activity of the liver reads like a litany of biochemistry. Biotransformation reactions of metabolites and drugs, such as the formation of bilirubin glucuronides, are energy consuming.

The following discussion mainly concerns reactions that occur in the parenchymal cells of the liver. Kupffer, endothelial, and other cells in the liver are more specialized in function than is the hepatocyte and generate much of their energy (as ATP and NADPH) by the metabolism of glucose. An ongoing discussion concerning hepatocytes is whether they constitute a metabolically homogeneous population (24). Do hepatocytes partition their functions in relation to their proximity to a blood supply of oxygen? Do some hepatocytes engage chiefly in gluconeogenesis, while others devote their energies to lipogenesis? See Gumucio and Miller, *this volume.*

UTILIZATION OF SUGARS BY THE LIVER

The carbohydrates presented to the liver after digestion are principally glucose, fructose, and, especially in infancy and childhood, galactose. In preparation for its metabolism, each is phosphorylated by a kinase in hepatocytes (Fig. 1). The principal phosphorylating enzyme for glucose in hepatocytes of rats, and probably of humans (although this is not yet fully settled), is glucokinase (25–29). Glucokinase differs from hexokinases, which are present in many other kinds of cells including Kupffer cells, in that it is more specific for glucose, operates with a much higher K_m for glucose (10^{-2} M compared to 10^{-5} M), and is not inhibited by one of the products of its reaction, glucose 6-phosphate. Glucokinase operates in the presence of high concentrations of glucose and probably evolved in relation to the synthesis of glycogen. Thus, large amounts of glucose coming to the liver are deposited as glycogen; relatively little immediately enters the glycolytic pathway. Large concentrations of glucose

TABLE 1.—*Continued*

Function		Reactions	ATP yield
Fatty acid oxidation[d]	1.	Hexanoate + ATP + CoA→hexanoyl-CoA + AMP + PP	−2
	2.	Hexanoyl-CoA→*trans*-Δ^2-hexanoyl-CoA (followed by reoxidation of $FADH_2$-protein by electron transport system)	+2
	3.	L-3-Hydroxyhexanoyl-CoA→3-ketohexanoyl-CoA (followed by reoxidation of NADH by electron transport system)	+3
	4.	3-Ketohexanoyl-CoA→butyryl-CoA + acetyl-CoA	0
	5.	Butyryl-CoA→crotonyl-CoA (followed by reoxidation of $FADH_2$-protein by electron transport system)	+2
	6.	L-3-Hydroxybutyryl-CoA→acetoacetyl-CoA (followed by reoxidation of NADH by electron transport system)	+3
	7.	Acetoacetyl-CoA→[2]acetyl-CoA	0
	8.	[3]Acetyl-CoA oxidized via tricarboxylic acid cycle	+36
		Total for hexanoate→$6CO_2$	+44

[a] Considered to be the substrate level phosphorylation reaction with the esterification of inorganic phosphate that ultimately leads to the generation of ATP in reaction 3a.

[b] The phosphate groups of phosphoenolpyruvate that are transphosphorylated to ADP originate from the ATP used in the phosphorylation of glucose and fructose 6-phosphate.

[c] Assuming that this cytosolic NADH transfers its reducing equivalents to oxaloacetate and that the malate thus produced is transported into and oxidized in the mitochondria. The alternative dihydroxyacetone phosphate-L-α-glycerolphosphate shuttle mechanism for the O_2-coupled reoxidation of cytosolic NADH yields only 2ATPs/NADH, with a consequent lowering of that ATP yield for the complete oxidation of glucose to 36.

[d] For a fatty acid containing n carbon atoms and x double bonds, McGilvery (162), from the sequence of reactions as formulated in the table, derives the equation $8.5n - 2x - 7$ for the net yield of ATP on complete oxidation. Thus for hexanoic acid (C_6), this would be $(8.5 \times 6) - 0 - 7$, or 44, as shown in the table; for palmitate (C_{16}), one obtains a value of $(8.5 \times 16) - 0 - 7$ or 129 ATPs. For palmitoleate (*cis*-Δ^9-hexadecanoate), oleate (*cis*-Δ^9-octadecenoate), linoleate (*cis*-*cis*-$\Delta^{9,12}$-octadecadienoate), linolenate (*all cis*-$\Delta^{9,12,15}$-octadecatrienoate), and arachidonate (*all cis*-$\Delta^{5,8,11,14}$-eicosatetraenoate), the ATP yields calculated from the equation would be 127, 144, 142, 140, and 155, respectively.

depress the active form of phosphorylase and stimulate glycogen synthase (30); the net effect is in favor of glycogen deposition. Glucokinase is under control of glucose and insulin; apparently, its synthesis is increased by diets high in glucose and by the consequent secretion of insulin (25).

Fructose is phosphorylated in hepatocytes by a fructokinase or ketohexokinase, with participation of ATP (31–36). The product is fructose 1-phosphate. Fructokinase is highly active in liver. Although fructose can ultimately form glycogen by conversion to glucose 6-phosphate by the pathway shown in Fig. 2, fructose 1-phosphate can traverse the glycolytic pathway more readily than can glucose. Glycolysis results in the production of pyruvate that can then be oxidized to acetyl-CoA, a precursor of fatty acid synthesis; and a side reaction of glycolysis results in formation of L-α-glycerol phosphate required in the synthesis of triacylglycerols. Thus fructose, because of its greater flux through glycolysis than glucose, is a better substrate for lipogenesis in the liver.

METABOLISM OF GALACTOSE IN THE LIVER

Galactose occurs in the diet primarily in the form of the disaccharide lactose. Human milk contains about 7% of lactose and bovine milk about 5%. Galactose consumed in excess of the need of the organism for biosynthesis of glycoproteins and galactolipids is metabolized chiefly in the liver. It can ultimately be incorporated as glucosyl units in glycogen or be converted to glucose 6-phosphate and enter the glycolytic pathway for oxidation and provision of energy.

Pyruvate formed from galactose in that manner obviously can be oxidized further to produce acetyl-CoA, with the options open to acetyl-CoA for additional production of energy through oxidation in the tricarboxylic acid cycle or for biosynthesis of fatty acids. Some features of galactose metabolism are shown in Fig. 1.

The first reaction of galactose in the liver is with ATP to form galactose 1-phosphate; the governing enzyme is a specific galactokinase. The metabolism of

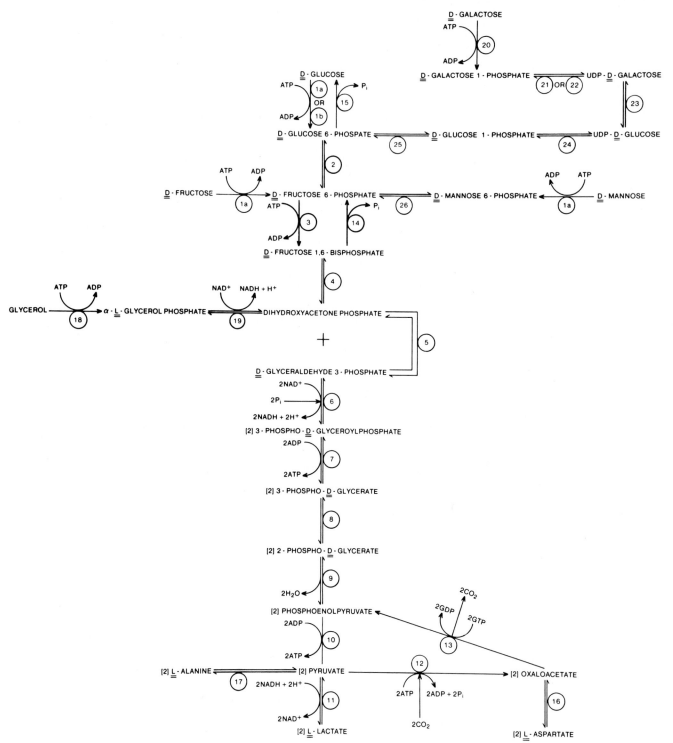

FIG. 1. Pathways of glycolysis and gluconeogenesis, including points of entry of D-fructose, D-mannose, and D-galactose. *1a:* Hexokinase (E.C.2.7.1.1); *1b:* glucokinase (E.C.2.7.1.2); *2:* glucosephosphate isomerase (E.C.5.3.1.9); *3:* 6-phosphofructokinase (E.C.2.7.1.11); *4:* fructose-bisphosphate aldolase (E.C.4.1.2.13); *5:* triosephosphate isomerase (E.C.5.3.1.1); *6:* glyceraldehyde-phosphate dehydrogenase (E.C.1.2.1.12); *7:* phosphoglycerate kinase (E.C.2.7.2.3); *8:* phosphoglyceromutase (E.C.2.7.5.3); *9:* enolase (E.C.4.2.1.11); *10:* pyruvate kinase (E.C.2.7.1.40); *11:* lactate dehydrogenase (E.C.1.1.1.27); *12:* pyruvate carboxylase (E.C.6.4.1.1); *13:* phosphoenolpyruvate carboxykinase (E.C.4.1.1.32); *14:* fructose-bisphosphatase (E.C.3.1.3.11); *15:* glucose-6-phosphatase (E.C.3.1.3.9); *16:* alanine aminotransferase catalyzing the reaction L-alanine + α-ketoglutarate = pyruvate + L-glutamate (E.C.2.6.1.2); *17:* asparate aminotransferase catalyzing the reaction L-asparate + α-ketoglutarate = oxaloacetate + L-glutamate (E.C.2.6.1.1); *18:* glycerol kinase (E.C.2.7.1.30); *19:* glycerol-3-phosphate dehydrogenase (E.C.1.1.1.8); *20:* galactokinase (E.C.2.7.1.6); *21:* galactose-1-phosphate uridylyltransferase (E.C.2.7.7.10) catalyzing the reaction UTP + α-D-galactose 1-phosphate = pyrophosphate + UDPgalactose; *22:* UDP glucose-hexose 1-phosphate uridylyltransferase (E.C.2.7.7.12) catalyzing the reaction UDP glucose + α-D-galactose 1-phosphate = α-D-glucose 1-phosphate + UDP galactose; *23:* UDP glucose 4-epimerase (E.C.5.1.3.2); *24:* glucose-1-phosphate uridylyltransferase (E.C.2.7.7.9) catalyzing the reaction UTP + α-D-glucose 1-phosphate = pyrophosphate + UDP glucose; *25:* phosphoglucomutase (E.C.2.7.5.1); *26:* mannosephosphate isomerase (E.C.5.3.1.8).

galactose in human liver follows the Leloir pathway (37,38):

(a)

$$\text{Galactose} + \text{ATP} \xrightarrow{\text{galactokinase}} \text{galactose 1-phosphate} + \text{ADP}$$

(b)

$$\begin{array}{c}\text{Galactose 1-phosphate} \\ + \text{ UDPglucose}\end{array} \xrightarrow[\text{uridylyltransferase}]{\text{UDPglucose-hexose 1-phosphate}} \begin{array}{c}\text{UDPgalactose} \\ + \text{ glucose 1-phosphate}\end{array}$$

(c)

$$\text{UDPgalactose} \xrightarrow{\text{UDPglucose 4-epimerase}} \text{UDPglucose}$$

Depending on the metabolic state of the liver, glucose 1-phosphate formed in the transferase reaction can be converted to glucose 6-phosphate and enter the glycolytic pathway for production of energy. Also, UDP-glucose arising in the epimerase reaction may be directed toward glycogenesis.

With respect to the epimerase, its action requires NAD^+ as a coenzyme. NAD^+ removes a hydrogen atom from C-4 of the UDP hexose as well as one from the -OH on C-4; an intermediate UDP ketohexose forms. The NADH also produced in the reaction remains bound to the enzyme, which then transfers the hydrogen atom to a molecule of UDP ketohexose in such a way as to produce a UDP hexose with the -OH at C-4 in an opposite configuration. In the human, if ethanol has been consumed with galactose, its oxidation by alcohol dehydrogenase in the liver significantly increases the amount of coenzyme in the form of NADH and consequently increases the ratio of NADH to NAD^+. Such increase can inhibit the epimerase and decrease conversion of UDP galactose to UDP glucose. The overall effect is diminished clearance of galactose by the liver and from blood (39). In this situation, decreased tolerance to galactose has a metabolic basis without overt pathology.

METABOLISM OF FRUCTOSE (AND GLYCERALDEHYDE)

Unlike the phosphorylation of fructose in extrahepatic tissues, which occurs through the agency of a general hexokinase and results in formation of fructose 6-phosphate, phosphorylation in the liver (Fig. 2) occurs with a specific fructokinase, called ketohexokinase; the product is fructose 1-phosphate (31–36). Accordingly, fructose in the liver cannot directly enter glycolysis to any significant degree. Instead, the liver is equipped with a special aldolase, called fructose 1-phosphate aldolase or aldolase B to distinguish it from the aldolase A that acts on fructose 1,6-bisphosphate in the glycolytic pathway (35,41–44). Although

aldolase B can also effectively catalyze the reversible reaction between fructose 1,6-bisphosphate and the two triose phosphates (3-phosphoglyceraldehyde phosphate and dihydroxyacetone phosphate), aldolase A acts only weakly on the reversible conversion of fructose 1-phosphate to dihydroxyacetone phosphate and glyceraldehyde.

Glyceraldehyde formed by aldolase B can be phosphorylated by a specific triokinase (glyceraldehyde kinase) to produce glyceraldehyde 3-phosphate (35,41, 45). As shown in Fig. 2, the aldolases form fructose 1,6-bisphosphate and eliminate the need for participation of 6-phosphofructokinase in the metabolism of fructose in the liver. The importance of that circumstance is that the early steps of fructose utilization in the liver are free from many controls. One may recall that the flux of glucose through glycolysis is regulated largely at the level of 6-phosphofructokinase; the activity of that enzyme is modulated by many allosteric effectors (ATP, ADP, AMP, P_i, citrate) and by glucagon and epinephrine (46–48). Recently, the most potent effector has been found to be fructose 2,6-bisphosphate (49–55), whose synthesis is diminished by the action of glucagon (56). Since fructose 2,6-bisphosphate stimulates the 6-phosphofructokinase reaction and, therefore, the flux of glucose through glycolysis, the action of glucagon is to diminish that flux. The great significance of this for the metabolism of fructose is that the bypass of 6-phosphofructokinase allows fructose to go through glycolysis with fewer restraints than those imposed on glucose. The result is more ready formation of pyruvate and, accordingly, of acetyl-CoA for synthesis of fatty acids. It also allows more ready formation of a byproduct of glycolysis, namely, the L-α-glycerol phosphate that is used in esterification of fatty acids to form triacylglycerols. Thus, it is clear why lipogenesis in the liver is greater from fructose than from glucose.

If the only action of glucagon were at the level of the phosphofructokinase reaction, the therapeutic use of fructose would seem to have justification in diabetic persons with a glucagon/insulin imbalance. However, glucagon also indirectly decreases the flux of pyruvate through the pyruvate dehydrogenase system, where insulin is important as a countervailing hormone. In any case, the use of intravenous alimentation with fructose has important side effects that make its use questionable and perhaps dangerous. The side effects can be observed in normal animals and humans taking a large fructose meal but are exaggerated in patients with hereditary fructose intolerance in whom liver aldolase B is lacking. Accumulation of fructose 1-phosphate occurs in both cases (35,36,57,58). The phenomenon can be duplicated and studied in isolated livers of rats perfused with solutions containing fructose; in this case, accumulation of fructose 1-phos-

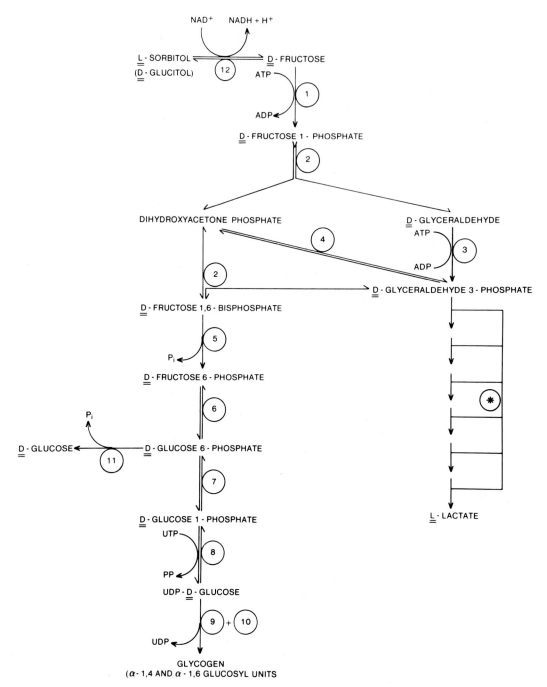

FIG. 2. Pathway of *D*-fructose metabolism in the liver. *1:* Ketohexokinase (E.C.2.7.1.3); *2:* fructose-bisphosphate aldolase (E.C.4.1.2.13); *3:* triokinase (E.C.2.7.1.28); *4:* triosephosphate isomerase (E.C.5.3.1.1); *5:* fructose-bisphosphatase (E.C.3.1.3.11); *6:* glucosephosphate isomerase (E.C.5.3.1.9); *7:* phosphoglucomutase (E.C.2.7.5.1); *8:* glucose-1-phosphate uridylyltransferase (E.C.2.7.7.9); *9:* glycogen synthase (E.C.2.4.1.11); *10:* 1,4-α-glucan branching enzyme (E.C.2.4.1.18); *11:* glucose-6-phosphatase (E.C.3.1.3.9); *12:* L-iditol dehydrogenase (E.C.1.1.1.14). (✱) : Reactions of glycolysis catalyzed by enzymes 6–11 as shown in Fig. 1.

phate occurs coordinately with depletion of ATP and P_i (42,58,59). Of course, in normal humans (or rats) the effect is not due to lack of aldolase B, as in hereditary fructose intolerance, nor to an imbalance between ketohexokinase activity and aldolase B activity, since these are normally about the same order of magnitude. The initial depletion of ATP is caused by rapid phosphorylation of fructose with ATP catalyzed

by ketohexokinase. Ultimately, that leads to sequestration of P_i into fructose 1-phosphate. The initial depletion of ATP and P_i constitutes removal of two important restraints on the catabolism of adenine nucleotides, since both inhibit 5'-nucleotidase and adenosine deaminase (42,59). Accordingly, degradation of adenine nucleotides is enhanced, resulting in diminution of the total pool of adenine nucleotides. For instance, the perfused rat livers referred to above show a decrease in that pool to a level of one-third to one-quarter of normal. The metabolic consequences of that kind of decrease coupled with diminution of the concentration of P_i can be very severe. Thus under such conditions of diminished adenine nucleotides, the liver behaves almost as though it were severely hypoxic, and in fact becomes a lactate-producing organ (60). In the human, it could cause lactic acidosis. The mechanisms for those effects are not fully understood, but the dangers are sufficient to discourage the use of parenteral fructose solutions for nutritional purposes (36,60–62).

GLYCOLYSIS

The glycolytic pathway, also known as the Embden-Meyerhof-Parnas pathway (Fig. 1), is the only mechanism by which glucose (or sugars interconvertible with it) can be oxidized anaerobically with production of ATP. Thus when tissue such as liver, which normally operates under highly aerobic conditions, is rendered hypoxic, production of ATP by oxidative phosphorylation is greatly diminished and glycolysis greatly increased. Glycolysis can operate as a cycle under hypoxic or anaerobic conditions when pyruvate is transformed to lactate by lactate dehydrogenase; NADH is thereby reoxidized to NAD^+ to allow the critical step of oxidation of 3-phosphoglyceralde to continue (see Fig. 1). The total capacity for glycolysis can be estimated by measurement of lactate production in the absence of oxygen when suspensions of cells, slices of tissues, or whole perfused organs are permitted to metabolize glucose (63–68). The potential for glycolysis of the liver of a fed adult rat is about 150 μmoles/g as determined from lactate production of isolated perfused livers under anaerobic conditions (69). The glycolytic potential of human liver would not be so high because the metabolic rates of larger animals are less than those of smaller animals. However, no uncomplicated estimate of glycolytic potential of human liver has been made. The value is probably in the range of production of 100 to 200 g lactate per day (60).

Under normal aerobic conditions, the liver primarily uses fatty acids as substrates for oxidation, and the glycolytic rate is low. Glycolysis occurs mainly from stored glycogen; little proceeds directly from glucose per se. Higher rates of glycolysis are associated with lipogenesis from carbohydrate. The carbon atoms of the sugar provide both acetyl-CoA for synthesis of fatty acids and L-α-glycerol phosphate for their esterification. Glycolysis starting with fructose or sorbitol is more efficient than glucose for lipogenesis.

Flux of glucosyl units through the glycolytic pathway initially depends on controls imposed on glycogen

metabolism. For example, high concentrations of glucose entering hepatocytes activate glycogen synthase and diminish the activity of phosphorylase, thus favoring glycogenesis over glycogenolysis (30) and resulting in less substrate available for glycolysis. Normal levels of glucose are compatible with glycogenolysis, but much of the resulting glucose 6-phosphate is hydrolyzed to free glucose by glucose 6-phosphatase and becomes available as blood glucose. However, control at the level of glycogen metabolism is coordinated with controls on the irreversible reactions in the glycolytic pathway.

As shown in Fig. 1, starting with free glucose, the pathway has three irreversible reactions catalyzed by, respectively, glucokinase (hexokinase), 6-phosphofructokinase, and pyruvate kinase. Hexokinase, but not glucokinase, is inhibited by glucose 6-phosphate. 6-Phosphofructokinase is inhibited by ATP and, when citrate is present with ATP, more strongly than by ATP alone. Inhibition of 6-phosphofructokinase by ATP is relieved by P_i, AMP, ADP, fructose 6-phosphate, or fructose 1,6-bisphosphate (46–48). The most significant activation of 6-phosphofructokinase, however, occurs in the presence of a newly discovered metabolite, fructose 2,6-bisphosphate (49–54). On a micromolar basis, this compound is 1,000 times more active than fructose 1,6-bisphosphate (55); it acts by increasing the affinity of fructose 6-phosphate for 6-phosphofructokinase, thereby relieving inhibition by ATP.

Fructose 2,6-bisphosphate is synthesized in the liver by a specific kinase using ATP as the phosphorylating substrate (70,71). The activity of the kinase is governed by glucagon; the hormone appears to stimulate a protein kinase to phosphorylate the kinase that catalyzes the synthesis of fructose 2,6-bisphosphate (56,71,72). Phosphorylation causes inactivation of the enzyme and a decrease in concentration of fructose 2,6-bisphosphate, which decreases the flux of fructose 6-phosphate through glycolysis. In turn, the decrease in 6-phosphofructokinase activity causes less production of fructose 1,6-bisphosphate, which is a feedforward activator of pyruvate kinase toward the end of the glycolytic pathway. The overall result is that glucagon diminishes glycolysis and favors gluconeogenesis (the latter effect is considered subsequently).

The third irreversible reaction in glycolysis is catalyzed by pyruvate kinase; that enzyme is activated by fructose 1,6-bisphosphate and inhibited by ATP and some amino acids, notably alanine, which is an important precursor in gluconeogenesis (73). The enzyme can also be phosphorylated by a protein kinase, which results in its inactivation; dephosphorylation by a phosphatase results in reactivation (74).

In the liver, glycolysis is closely related to glycogen deposition (synthesis and glycogenolysis), lipogenesis, and gluconeogenesis. Normally, both glycolysis and gluconeogenesis occur simultaneously. Each of the irreversible steps in glycolysis is matched by an irreversible step in gluconeogenesis (see Fig. 1). Thus interconversion of pyruvate and phosphoenolpyruvate occurs because the action of pyruvate kinase in glycolysis is countered by the combined actions of pyruvate carboxylase and phosphoenolpyruvate carboxykinase in gluconeogenesis; interconversion of fructose 6-phosphate and fructose 1,6-bisphosphate is a result of the action of 6-phosphofructokinase in glycolysis countered by the action of fructose 1,6-bisphosphatase in gluconeogenesis; interconversion of glucose and glucose 6-phosphate occurs because the action of glucokinase is opposed by the action of glucose 6-phosphatase in gluconeogenesis. At each of those levels, "futile cycling" of a substrate could occur, the net balance of which would be the hydrolysis of ATP with production of ADP and P_i (30,75). The direction in which a substrate will go at each of these levels is determined by its concentration, and controls exerted on the enzymes by allosteric effectors. The relatively small amount of energy expended in the cycling of a substrate is not a great price to pay for the control of metabolism at that point. In the case of phosphoenolpyruvate, normal cycling can be pushed in the direction of gluconeogenesis by the action of glucagon which, acting through a cyclic AMP-dependent protein kinase, causes inactivation of pyruvate kinase; that results in an increase in the amount of phosphoenolpyruvate and stimulation of the gluconeogenic pathway.

No significant substrate cycling has been found in livers of mice or rats at the level of interconversion of fructose 6-phosphate and fructose 1,6-bisphosphate. However, such cycling does occur in hepatocytes isolated from rat livers. Glucagon has a profound effect on this cycle, strongly favoring the gluconeogenic pathway (76). Since glucagon interferes with the synthesis of the powerful effector, fructose 2,6-bisphosphate, the flux of fructose 6-phosphate through the 6-phosphofructokinase reaction is slowed considerably by glucagon. Moreover, fructose 2,6-bisphosphate inhibits fructose 1,6-bisphosphatase, so that the action of glucagon removes a restraint on the enzyme and increases the concentration of fructose 6-phosphate (77), which also favors gluconeogenesis.

Recycling between glucose and glucose 6-phosphate in the liver is catalyzed by glucokinase and glucose 6-phosphatase; since the former is a "soluble cytosolic" enzyme and the latter is associated with the endoplasmic reticulum (ER), cycling in this case must include the movement of glucose 6-phosphate into the ER and movement of glucose out. Both enzymes are characterized by relatively high K_m values for their substrates; in the short term, both are controlled principally by the concentration of substrate. This system offers an excellent example of the effect of substrate level per se on flux through the glycolytic pathway. Thus, it has been determined that no net flux of the two metabolites occurs when the blood level of glucose is about 100 mg/100 ml (5.7 mmoles/liter) because the activity of glucokinase becomes equal to the activity of glucose 6-phosphatase (30). An increase of the concentration of either substrate has no influence on the net flux, since the product of the first reaction is returned by the reverse reaction. In the hepatocyte, the presence of systems for metabolism of glycogen, which can be controlled by factors other than substrate concentrations, produces a coordinate control on the level of glucose 6-phosphate. Thus an increased concentration of glucose gives a transient increase in the level of glucose 6-phosphate, but since glucose also depresses phosphorylase and stimulates glycogen synthase, glucose 6-phosphate is drawn off for formation of glycogen, and its level undergoes a secondary decrease. With the decrease of glucose 6-phosphate, the activity of glucose 6-phosphatase is decreased. A large difference occurs in the activity of glucokinase as opposed to the phosphatase. This permits active uptake of glucose for glycogen synthesis. When glycogenolysis is active, as caused by glucagon, glucose 6-phosphate concentration increases considerably and causes increased activity of glucose 6-phosphatase. The glucose that forms diffuses rapidly out of the hepatocytes into the circulation for distribution to other tissues. The change in concentration of glucose is small. What then is the advantage of recycling of these substrates? Hers (30) states that it allows large changes in glucose uptake and output to be regulated only by substrate concentration; however, it requires cooperation of the phosphorylase-glycogen synthase system.

GLUCONEOGENESIS

The pathway for gluconeogenesis in the liver is shown together with that for glycolysis in Fig. 1. The major similarities and differences between the two pathways, and the interactions of the two, are considered in the discussion of glycolysis.

Gluconeogenesis, the production of glucose principally from amino acids and lactate, is carried out solely in liver and kidney cortex; in liver, it apparently is limited to hepatocytes. Although the rates of gluconeogenesis are similar in the two tissues, because of their relative sizes, total production by the liver is probably about nine times as great. However, because gluconeogenesis in the kidney serves special functions relative to maintenance of ammonia production and acid-base balance, and because conditions occur in which gluconeogenesis increases in that organ, the significance of the renal process cannot be discounted. The discussion here, however, is limited to the liver.

Major extrahepatic tissues utilize glucose obligatorily (blood cells and renal medulla); others use it preferentially (brain); however, only liver and kidney make glucose. In the postabsorptive period or during periods of fast, the extrahepatic tissues send precursors to the liver via the blood to be converted to glucose, which is distributed to the tissues to be used as fuel. Two interorgan cycles of that kind have been described, namely, the lactic acid or Cori cycle (78) and the glucose-alanine cycle (79,80). By the process of gluconeogenesis, liver can produce at least 240 g glucose per day (60), which is about twice the amount consumed by nervous tissue and erythrocytes in one day of fasting (81). In most cases, it is not the gluconeogenic capacity of the liver that is limiting, but the supply of precursors. A major fraction of amino acid precursors for gluconeogenesis during fasting or starvation arises by degradation of functional muscle protein and protein in visceral organs, including the liver itself. The process of gluconeogenesis, if not regulated at the precursor level, becomes tissue wasting and can have dire consequences. The degradation of muscle protein in an extended fast declines to a relatively constant level and primarily is spared not by provision of a different pool of precursors for glucose synthesis but by replacing the use of glucose in nervous tissue and in skeletal muscle by another fuel, acetoacetate (82–85). As discussed later, the production of acetoacetate, a fuel that spares conversion of protein to glucose, also occurs in the liver.

Both the obligate users of glucose, erythrocytes and renal medulla, have high rates of glycolysis and produce considerable lactate. Thus the liver has available, from blood cells, a relatively constant and limiting amount of substrate for gluconeogenesis. To this is added a more variable supply of precursors, including gluconeogenic amino acids, glycerol from lipolysis in the adipose tissue, and propionyl-CoA from oxidation in hepatocytes of fatty acids with an odd number of carbon atoms. A fatty acid with an odd number of carbon atoms is oxidized by β-oxidation in which, starting from the carboxyl terminus, two carbon atoms at a time are removed sequentially as acetyl-CoA. At the other end of the chain, β-oxidation ceases with production of a three carbon product, propionyl-CoA. Propionyl-CoA can be converted to methylmalonyl-CoA, which, by enzymatic rearrangement to succinyl-CoA, is able to enter the tricarboxylic acid cycle.

Almost all amino acids, with the exception of leucine, can contribute some carbon atoms to the net synthesis of glucose in the liver; some also contribute carbon atoms to the synthesis of acetoacetate. The points at which the amino acids enter the several pathways are shown in Figs. 1 and 9.

Although alanine coming from muscle is a major precursor of glucose, serine and other amino acids also are important in that regard. Amino acids are a principal source of glucose after liver glycogen has been depleted by glycogenolysis.

Gluconeogenesis, as can be seen in Fig. 1, is both an energy-consuming and a reductive process. For two molecules of pyruvate to traverse the pathway for formation of a molecule of glucose requires investment of the energy of six pyrophosphate bonds of ATP. Also the H atoms of two molecules of NADH and two protons are required at the level of formation of 3-phosphoglyceraldehyde from 3-phospho-D-glyceroyl-phosphate. One may estimate that a 70-kg man uses about 17 kcal/day (about 5% of the approximate total of 340 kcal energy used by the liver in its functions) for gluconeogenic conversion of lactate plus glycerol (17,23). The liver also uses about 48 kcal energy per day (14% of its total) for the degradation of amino acids; this includes the energy expended in synthesis of urea from the ammonia produced by oxidative deamination and the synthesis of both glucose and ketone bodies (17,23). Although all that energy utilization cannot be ascribed directly to the requirement of gluconeogenesis, it may reasonably be considered a necessary concomitant. Much of the energy required for gluconeogenesis is provided by oxidation of fatty acids in hepatocytes.

The control of gluconeogenesis is considered in some detail in the preceding section on glycolysis. Pyruvate carboxylase, at low concentrations of pyruvate, has an almost complete dependence on the presence of acetyl-CoA for activity (73,86). Also, phosphoenolpyruvate carboxykinase, which can be activated by its substrate, oxaloacetate, is controlled most effectively by changes at the transcriptional level in its rate of synthesis. Glucagon and glucocorticoids promote induction of the enzyme, whereas insulin represses its synthesis (87–90).

Overall, gluconeogenesis is stimulated by glucagon and epinephrine and inhibited by insulin, as observed most dramatically in insulin-dependent diabetes mellitus, in which uninhibited gluconeogenesis contributes significantly to the hyperglycemia. Gluconeogenesis also can be affected indirectly by the level of activity of the pyruvate dehydrogenase reaction, which determines the flux of pyruvate away from glucose synthesis and toward oxidative decarboxylation to form acetyl-CoA. Insulin favors oxidative decarboxylation of pyruvate and, therefore, indirectly tends to diminish gluconeogenesis.

Any disease in which carbohydrate metabolism in the liver is disturbed may have an effect on the capacity for gluconeogenesis and its regulation. Conditions in which oxygenation of the liver is diminished, as in congestive heart failure, affect almost all hepatocytes and cause them to turn to glycolysis for production of energy. Consequently, the liver becomes a lactate-producing organ instead of one that directs lactate into gluconeogenesis. Lactic acidosis may ensue, but is not likely to happen in cirrhosis, in which sufficient numbers of hepatocytes may still function normally (60).

In humans, at least two inherited enzyme deficiencies have a major effect on the gluconeogenic pathway. These are type I glycogenosis (von Gierke's disease), in which there is a deficiency of glucose 6-phosphatase, and hexose bisphosphatase deficiency. Both are characterized by severe hypoglycemia and lactic acidosis. Patients with type I glycogenosis do not accumulate hepatic glucose 6-phosphate; Hers (30) has suggested that an unknown feedback mechanism inhibits gluconeogenesis. Patients with diabetes mellitus may have gluconeogenesis in the face of hyperglycemia, indicating that a feedback control on the output of glucose from the liver is affected. Finally, in many experimental hepatomas, dedifferentiated liver cells have a graded loss of gluconeogenic capacity (91).

THE PENTOSE PHOSPHATE CYCLE

This cycle, also called the hexose monophosphate pathway or shunt, consists of two branches that serve different functions in metabolism. Those branches are shown in Fig. 3, where they are designated A and B. The A arm, often called the oxidative pathway, catalyzes two successive dehydrogenations of glucose 6-phosphate, in which some of the energy of oxidation and one of the hydrogen atoms are retained in NADPH. Indeed the primary function of the oxidative branch is production of NADPH for use in reductive syntheses, such as those involved in synthesis of fatty acids from acetyl-CoA. The final step in the oxidative branch also produces ribulose 5-phosphate, which becomes the starting substrate for the B branch. The latter, constituting an almost labyrinthal series of interconversions and rearrangements, has as its main function the production of ribose 5-phosphate for use in synthesis of nucleotides and nucleic acids. It also allows for production of glucose 6-phosphate that can be recycled into the A branch. Thus, the pentose phosphate cycle is not an "alternate" pathway for the oxidation of glucose. It cannot replace the functions of glycolysis, chief of which is the preservation of energy of oxidation in the form of pyrophosphate bonds of ATP; nor can glycolysis replace the functions of the pentose phosphate cycle as outlined.

Not all tissues contain the enzymatic equipment necessary for the pentose phosphate cycle; thus the enzymes of that cycle notably are absent or deficient in the skeletal muscle. The liver, however, has all the enzymes in sufficient amount so that under certain physiological conditions, significant metabolism of glucose can occur through the pentose phosphate cycle (20). Hepatocytes are the main locus of the cycle, but other hepatic cells contain some or all of the necessary elements.

Since the liver has the capacity to produce more ribose 5-phosphate than required for its own metabolic needs, the liver may export derived ribose or ribose nucleosides to other tissues (92). Such nonphosphorylated forms can cross liver cell membranes, appear in the blood, and then be extracted by various cells of the organism. Thus adenosine, the nucleoside of adenine arising from degradation of nucleotides or from S-adenosyl-homocysteine, can be treated in that manner.

The pentose phosphate cycle is under both coarse (slow) and fine (rapid) control. Thus carbohydrates coming to the liver in excess of the amount that can be deposited as glycogen or utilized in glycolysis can cause adaptive changes in the liver resulting in an increased flux of glucose 6-phosphate through the pentose phosphate cycle. Those changes are mediated by as much as 10-fold increase in synthesis of two enzymes of the oxidative branch of the cycle, glucose 6-phosphate dehydrogenase and phosphogluconate dehydrogenase; the increase occurs maximally at about 3 days of high carbohydrate feeding (94).

Fine control is exerted at the level of the reaction catalyzed by glucose 6-phosphate dehydrogenase; this reaction is irreversible in the presence of the lactonase and rate-limiting for the entire sequence. Thus NADPH, ATP, and long-chain acyl-CoA thioesters inhibit that enzyme (93,95). Complete inhibition of the dehydrogenase is considered to occur when NADPH is present in a concentration only one-third of that occurring in normal liver; accordingly, the enzyme would be in a state of complete inactivity under usual metabolic conditions. The question then becomes: how is that inhibition relieved? Withdrawal of NADPH to lower its concentration could achieve deinhibition; this could occur with its utilization in synthesis of fatty acids. Krebs and Eggleston (94), however, proposed a second mechanism for relief of inhibition, which involves a reaction of the dehydrogenase with oxidized glutathione (GSSG) in cooperation with another, as yet unidentified, dialyzable factor.

Glucose 6-phosphate, the substrate of the dehydrogenase reaction, is at the crossroads of three other pathways of carbohydrate metabolism in the liver: glycogen synthesis, glycolysis, and gluconeogenesis. The physiological significance of the rapid control mechanisms applied to the activity of glucose 6-phosphate dehydrogenase perhaps may be that inhibition shuts off access of glucose 6-phosphate to one of the pathways (the pentose phosphate cycle) and dein-

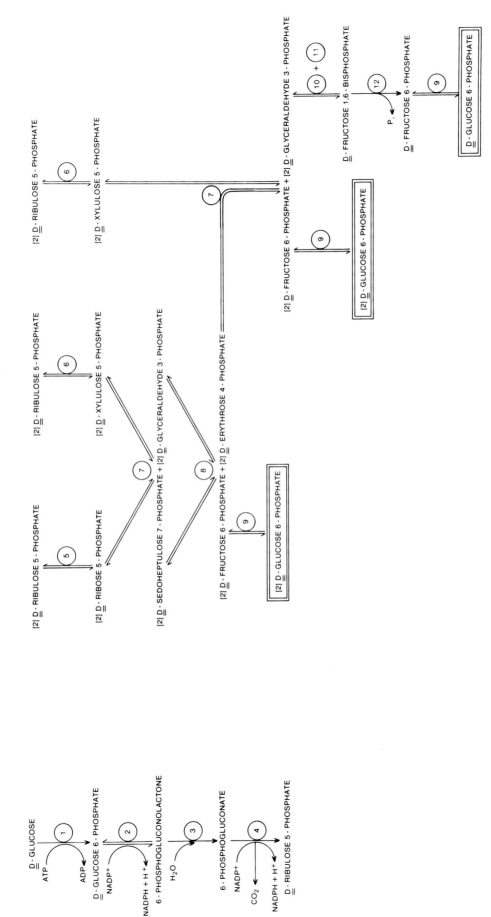

FIG. 3. Pentose phosphate cycle. **A.** Oxidative branch. *1*: Hexokinase (E.C.2.7.1.2) or glucokinase (E.C.2.7.1.1); *2*: glucose-6-phosphate dehydrogenase (E.C.1.1.1.49); *3*: 6-phosphogluconolactonase (E.C.3.1.1.31); *4*: phosphogluconate dehydrogenase, decarboxylating (E.C.1.1.1.44). **B.** Nonoxidative branch. *5*: Ribosephosphate isomerase (E.C.5.3.1.6); *6*: ribulosephosphate 3-epimerase (E.C.5.1.3.1); *7*: transketolase (E.C.2.2.1.1); *8*: transaldolase (E.C.2.2.1.2); *9*: glucosephosphate isomerase (E.C.5.3.1.9); *10*: triosephosphate isomerase (E.C.5.3.1.1); *11*: fructose-bisphosphate aldolase (E.C.4.1.2.13); *12*: fructose-bisphosphatase (E.C.3.1.3.11).

hibition opens it up (94). It is one way of specific channeling for the substrate; others are considered in the sections of this chapter on glycolysis and gluconeogenesis.

In the discussion of gluconeogenesis, a point was made of the remarkable fact that no accumulation of glucose 6-phosphate occurs in the livers of persons with type I glycogenosis due to glucose 6-phosphatase deficiency. A notable feature of that disease, however, is hyperuricemia frequently resulting in gout (96,97). Although a contributing factor to the elevated blood level of uric acid is diminished secretion in the kidney, perhaps due to competition by lactate, a major cause is considered to be increased *de novo* synthesis of purine nucleotides in the liver. Biosynthesis of purines is initiated with phosphoribosylpyrophosphate (PRPP), which serves as a scaffold for stepwise assembly of inosinic acid. In glucose 6-phosphatase deficiency, apparently glucose 6-phosphate is pushed through the pentose phosphate pathway concurrently with inhibition of gluconeogenesis, thus stimulating increased *de novo* synthesis of purine nucleotides. Because the latter synthesis occurs with obligate and coordinate utilization of ribose 5-phosphate to form PRPP, its regulation depends in the first instance on the activity of the pentose phosphate cycle.

GLYCOGEN METABOLISM IN THE LIVER

The pathways for metabolism of glycogen in the liver are shown in Fig. 4. The immediate precursor that donates a glucosyl group to a growing chain of glycogen is uridinediphosphate glucose (UDP glucose). UDP glucose is formed from glucose 1-phosphate, which in turn arises from glucose 6-phosphate in a reaction catalyzed by phosphoglucomutase. Glucose 6-phosphate, in hepatocytes, forms directly from glucose in a reaction with ATP catalyzed by glucokinase. Also, other hexoses, including fructose and galactose, ultimately can be isomerized to glucose in the form of glucose 6-phosphate, so that they too are capable of contributing to the synthesis of glycogen. Finally, all the gluconeogenic substances, including most amino acids, can contribute carbon atoms to the synthesis of glucose 6-phosphate and, therefore, are potentially glycogenic. Formation of glycogen is in general favored by insulin and glucocorticoids. Since the latter are known to promote the secretion of insulin, their effects on glycogen metabolism to a major degree are probably mediated through the pancreatic hormone (98,99). In addition, glucose promotes deposition of glycogen both by inhibition of phosphorylase and stimulation of glycogen synthase.

After a meal containing carbohydrate, the liver can deposit as much as 7% of its weight as glycogen. That, of course, does not represent the full potential of hepatocytes for storage of glycogen, since the feeding of protein-free, glucose-rich diets can cause that figure to reach about 10% (100); and in glycogen storage diseases, as, for example, type I glycogenosis, the figure can reach about 17% (101). In the normal case, however, soon after cessation of feeding, in the so-called postabsorptive period, glycogenolysis increases so that a major part of the glycogen store is depleted in about 4 hr; after 24 hr, less than 1% of liver weight is glycogen (102).

The cost in energy for the storage of glucosyl units into glycogen is modest relative to the functions served. As indicated, having a supply of glycogen in the liver allows the organism, in the postabsorptive state, to provide glucose for other tissues that are either obligate or facultative users of that fuel. Casting of glucose into its polymeric form allows a relatively large amount of the fuel to be stored in hepatocytes without loss by diffusion and without the osmotic consequences that would attend the presence of high concentrations of the monosaccharide. Beginning with glucose and proceeding to formation of UDPglucose, the activated intermediate that can transfer a glucosyl unit to a growing chain of glycogen with little loss of free energy, the equivalent of only one high energy bond of ATP is used for glycogen synthesis; two such bonds should be counted if one considers the enzymatic hydrolysis of inorganic pyrophosphate formed in the reaction between UTP and glucose 1-phosphate. In the repayment of that energy, glycogenolysis utilizes inorganic phosphate to make glucose 1-phosphate that is converted to glucose 6-phosphate, thus making the pivotal phosphorylated intermediate of carbohydrate metabolism without the direct investment of energy from ATP. If glucose 6-phosphate is then hydrolyzed by glucose 6-phosphatase, and the glucose exits the hepatocyte into the peripheral circulation, no additional input of energy will have been required beyond the initial investment considered above. For cells such as the erythrocytes that receive the glucose, the liver will have supplied the energy that allows them to get a maximum net production of ATP from glycolysis.

The erythrocyte, in fact, is a special case in its dependence on the liver. The red blood cells store no significant amount of glycogen, use only glucose for energy, and obtain that energy only by glycolysis, since they have neither a tricarboxylic acid cycle nor an electron transport system. Thus the two net molecules of ATP coming from glycolysis represent the major energy supply of the erythrocyte. If it stored glycogen, the erythrocyte could lose the equivalent of one of those molecules of ATP as noted previously. Instead, the liver has paid the energy of storage. Furthermore, the lactate formed in glycolysis in the red blood cells is carried to the liver where, by gluconeogenesis involving the utilization of two molecules of

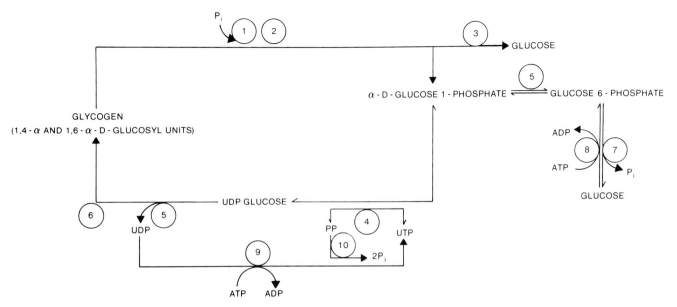

FIG. 4. Schematic representation of reactions in glycogen synthesis and degradation. *1:* Phosphorylase (E.C.2.4.1.1); *2:* 4-α-D-glucanotransferase (E.C.2.4.1.25) catalyzes the transfer of a segment (three residues from the stubs of glycogen α-1,6 branches) to a new 4-position in an acceptor, such as a 1,4-α-D-glucan; *3:* amylo-1,6-glucosidase (E.C.3.2.1.33) catalyzes the endohydrolysis of 1,6-α-D-glucoside linkages at points of branching in chains of 1,4-linked α-D-glucose residues. *2* and *3* are otherwise known as the debranching enzymes. *4:* Glucose-1-phosphate uridylyltransferase (E.C.2.7.7.9); *5:* glycogen synthase (E.C.2.4.1.11) catalyzes formation of 1,4-α-D-glucosyl linkages; *6:* 1,4-α-glucan branching enzyme (E.C.2.4.1.18) catalyzes the transfer of a 7-residue segment of a 1,4-α-D-glucan chain to a primary hydroxyl in a similar glucan chain forming an α-1,6 branch; *7:* glucose-6-phosphatase (E.C.3.1.3.9); *8:* hexokinase (E.C.2.7.1.1) or glucokinase (E.C.2.7.1.2); *9:* nucleoside diphosphate kinase (E.C.2.7.4.6); *10:* inorganic pyrophosphatase (E.C.3.6.1.1).

ATP, it is converted to glucose that once again goes to the erythrocyte. That example demonstrates how, in matters of energy, other tissues may depend on the liver.

On the other hand, when glucose 6-phosphate arising from glycogenolysis is used in the liver itself, not only is the energy of glycolysis obtained as ATP, but considerably more ATP may result if the acetyl-CoA formed by oxidation of pyruvate is sent through the tricarboxylic acid cycle and the respiratory chain. Under some metabolic circumstances, however, the acetyl-CoA may be used preferentially for synthesis of fatty acids.

The hormonal control of glycogen metabolism, mediated through cyclic nucleotide systems or calcium ion fluxes, or both, has been reviewed extensively with particular emphasis on phosphorylation-dephosphorylation modifications of the enzymes concerned (103–115). Although most of the experimental work reviewed deals with metabolism of glycogen in muscle, several of these excellent articles are concerned specifically with events in the liver (106,108,114,115). The following discussion highlights some of those events.

Glycogen synthase is the enzyme governing the transfer of glucosyl units of UDP glucose to a growing chain of glycogen, forming new α-1,4-glucosidic linkages. The enzyme occurs in a nonphosphorylated active form, designated *a*, which can be converted to a phosphorylated inactive form, designated *b*. The conversion may be catalyzed by a cAMP-dependent protein kinase utilizing ATP. A phosphatase may hydrolytically cleave the phosphate group of *b*, thus restoring the enzyme to the *a* species.

In contrast, phosphorylase, the enzyme that catalyzes glycogenolysis, occurs in an active phosphorylated form, called *a*, which can be cleaved hydrolytically by a phosphatase to an inactive, nonphosphorylated form, called *b*. The enzyme catalyzing the phosphorylation of glycogen phosphorylase is phosphorylase kinase, which exists as an inactive unphosphorylated *b* form and is converted into fully active *a* form by a cAMP-dependent protein kinase that utilizes ATP; phosphorylase kinase also phosphorylates glycogen synthase *a* to render it inactive. Thus, any hormone or effector, such as glucagon, that causes the production of cAMP and thereby the activation of the cAMP-dependent protein kinase, will stimulate glycogenolysis and reciprocally inhibit glycogen synthesis.

The control of glycogen synthesis and glycogenolysis has been most clearly delineated for skeletal muscle; although the enzymes involved have been studied extensively in the liver, they have not been isolated with the same degree of purity as those from muscle.

Nevertheless, the processes of glycogen metabolism appear to be similar in the two tissues, with some notable differences occurring with respect to hormonal control.

A variety of hormones and peptides, in concentrations of 10^{-7} to 10^{-11} M, can promote glycogenolysis. They act by binding to specific receptors on the surface of the hepatocyte, an event which in some cases initiates the cAMP cascade involving the protein kinases or in others causes a movement of calcium ions to provide a sufficient local concentration to turn on or off one of the enzymes involved. Experiments with muscle have shown that the local change in calcium ion concentration that occurs intracellularly when a muscle is made to contract, initiates and sustains glycogenolysis without the participation of cAMP and its dependent protein kinase. Such movements of calcium ions in hepatocytes could also promote glycogenolysis. Of the various hormones that promote glycogenolysis in the liver, glucagon is known with certainty to act through the cAMP cascade. Possibly secretin and vasoactive intestinal polypeptide (VIP) act in a similar manner.

Epinephrine, which promotes glycogenolysis in muscle by binding to β-receptors and thereby triggers the cAMP cascade, may not act in that way in hepatocytes of all species. Indeed, it appears to act through β-receptors in the liver of the dog; in the liver of the rat, however, catecholamines probably act through binding to α-receptors. In the latter case, the effect on glycogenolysis probably is mediated through changes in concentration of calcium ions and not through the cAMP system.

Other polypeptides that stimulate glycogenolysis in the liver are vasopressin, angiotensin II, and oxytocin. Their effects do not occur by initiation of a cyclic nucleotide system; nor is there sufficient evidence that they act by causing movements of calcium ions.

Regardless of which mechanism transduces the glycogenolytic effect of a hormone or peptide, the final result is an activation of phosphorylase. Under most conditions, sufficient active form of phosphorylase is present in the liver to catalyze a significant degree of glycogenolysis, but its action is exalted or damped by various noncovalent modifiers. Thus AMP (adenylate) activates phosphorylase b; however, it also inhibits the phosphatase that inactivates phosphorylase a. Its overall effect, then, is to sustain glycogenolysis. Under anaerobic (anoxic) conditions, AMP accumulates in the liver at the expense of ATP and ADP, and glycogenolysis accordingly is promoted. In contrast, the presence of a large concentration of glucose can inhibit both forms of phosphorylase and stimulate phosphorylase a phosphatase; the net result is inhibition of glycogenolysis, which occurs in the liver shortly after ingestion of a meal containing relatively large amounts of glucose.

Although glucagon may promote glycogenolysis by the mechanisms just discussed, the actual output of glucose from the liver may be partially suppressed by the presence of insulin. Thus the ratio of glucagon to insulin may determine whether glycogenolysis results in hyperglycemia.

In addition to the release of glucose from glycogen through the agency of phosphorylase, phosphoglucomutase, and glucose 6-phosphatase, additional formation may occur through the action of hydrolytic enzymes classified as amylases. Two principal amylases are the amylo-1,6-glucosidase and the lysosomal acid α-1,4-glucosidase.

FATTY ACID METABOLISM AND KETOGENESIS

The pathways in the liver for biosynthesis of fatty acids in the cytosol and of fatty acid oxidation and ketogenesis in the mitochondria are shown in Figs. 5 and 6, respectively. Control of these processes, and indeed of parallel and reciprocal relationships among them, is discussed in several excellent reviews (116–121). The biosynthesis of unsaturated fatty acids in liver, and its control, also has been reviewed (122).

Normally, the liver obtains most of its energy by metabolism of fatty acids. When an animal ingests carbohydrate in large excess, the liver responds with increased lipogenesis; both fatty acid and glycerol moieties can be derived from absorbed hexoses. The newly formed triacylglycerols are incorporated into lipoproteins and sent into the peripheral blood; if the rate of lipogenesis exceeds that of lipoprotein synthesis, excess triacylglycerols are stored within liver cells in membrane-enclosed cytoplasmic vesicles (123). During a subsequent restriction of carbohydrate, the triacylglycerols in the vesicles undergo lipolysis, perhaps with the participation of lysosomal enzymes (123). Accordingly, fatty acids are released to be taken up by the mitochondria, where they are oxidized with formation of acetyl-CoA and ketone bodies. One should note that hepatocytes can form triacylglycerols utilizing either exogenous fatty acids or those synthesized *de novo* in the liver.

In periods of short supply of carbohydrate, as in fasting, starvation, and diabetes mellitus, lipogenesis is repressed, glycolysis inhibited, and oxidation of fatty acids greatly stimulated. A prodigious formation of acetoacetate and its reduced derivative, D-3-hydroxybutyrate, ensues. In the first instance, the ketogenesis is made possible by the availability of fatty acid substrates; these arise from lipolysis in adipose tissue and are brought to the liver in the form of complexes with albumin. In the physiological and pathological states of carbohydrate deprivation mentioned above, however, changes occur in the concentrations

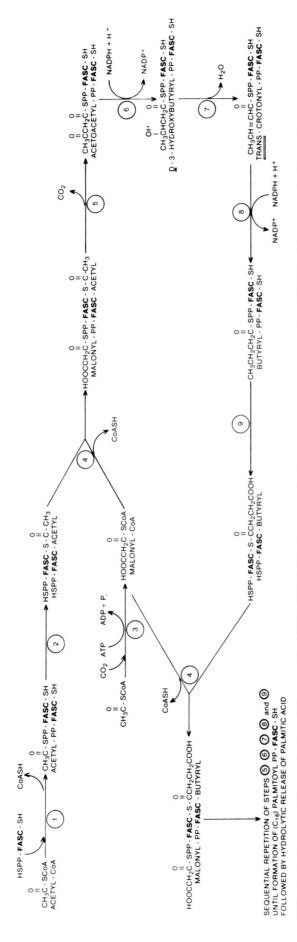

FIG. 5. Pathway of biosynthesis of fatty acid. HSPP-FASC-SH denotes the fatty acid synthase complex (FASC) with one critical cysteine sulfhydryl residue (SH) and a phosphopantetheine (HSPP) moiety covalently linked to a serine residue of the polypeptide chain. *1:* Enzyme with activity like that of [acyl-carrier-protein] acetyltransferase (E.C.2.3.1.38); *2:* transacetylation of the acetyl group from the phosphopantetheinyl to the cysteinyl residue; *3:* acetyl-CoA carboxylase (E.C.6.4.1.2); *4:* enzyme with activity like that of [acyl-carrier-protein] malonyltransferase (E.C.2.3.1.39); *5:* enzyme with activity like that of 3-ketoacyl-[acyl-carrier-protein] synthase (decarboxylating) (E.C.2.3.1.41); *6:* enzyme with activity like that of 3-ketoacyl-[acyl-carrier-protein] reductase (E.C.1.1.1.100); *7:* enzyme with activity like that of crotonoyl-[acyl-carrier-protein] hydratase (E.C.4.2.1.58), (cf. E.C.4.2.1.59, E.C.4.2.1.60, and E.C.4.2.1.61 for 3-hydroxyoctanoyl-, 3-hydroxydecanoyl-, and 3-hydroxypalmitoyl-[acyl-carrier-protein] dehydratases, respectively); *8:* enzyme with activity like that of enoyl-[acyl-carrier-protein] reductase (E.C.1.3.1.10); *9:* transacylation of the butyryl group from the phosphopantetheinyl to the cysteinyl residue.

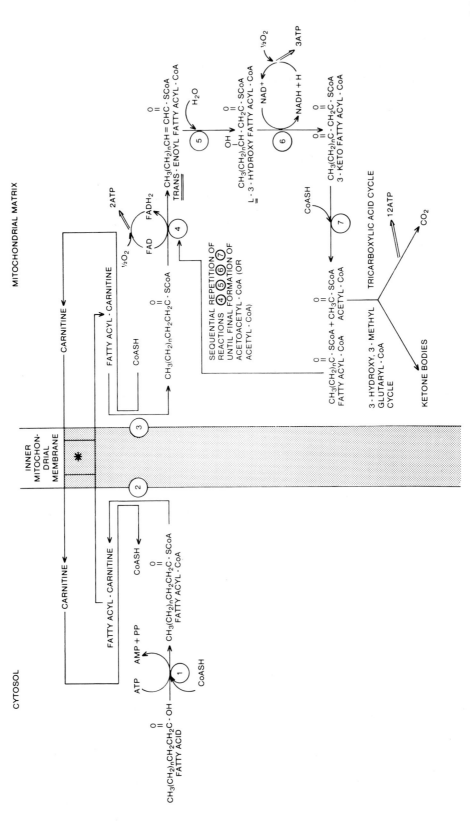

FIG. 6. Mitochondrial pathways of fatty acid oxidation and ketogenesis. *1:* Acyl-CoA synthetase (E.C.6.2.1.3); *2:* carnitine palmitoyltransferase (E.C.2.3.1.21) on the outer surface of the inner mitochondrial membrane; *3:* carnitine palmitoyltransferase (E.C.2.3.1.2.1) on the inner surface of the inner mitochondrial membrane; carnitine-*O*-acylcarnitine antiport; *4:* acyl-CoA dehydrogenase (E.C.1.3.99.3); *5:* enoyl-CoA hydratase (E.C.4.2.1.17); *6:* 3-hydroxyacyl-CoA dehydrogenase (E.C.1.1.1.35); *7:* acetyl-CoA acyltransferase (3-ketoacyl-CoA thiolase) (E.C.2.3.1.16).

of glucagon and insulin in the blood and, accordingly, in their ratio. That appears to be a main mechanism by which the liver becomes a ketogenic organ, since glucagon in an imbalance with insulin represses glycolysis and causes decreased production of malonyl-CoA, oxaloacetate, and citrate. How diminished concentrations of those metabolites channel acetyl-CoA into the ketogenic pathway is considered below. Since most of those effects can be reproduced experimentally with dibutyryl cAMP (121,124,125), glucagon is considered to act by increasing the synthesis of cAMP in hepatocytes.

The remarkable capacity of the liver to oxidize fatty acids and produce acetoacetate is emphasized in an estimate made by McGarry and Foster (119) that the liver, in 1 day, can synthesize half its weight of ketone bodies (approximately 900 g/day). That seemingly exorbitant potential probably is tapped only in a few conditions, such as severe diabetes. One may compare that amount with the quantity of glucose that the liver can produce in a day of fasting after a meal that had resulted in storage of glycogen at a level of about 7%; first about 150 g glucose would result from glycogenolysis, followed by perhaps an equal quantity from gluconeogenesis from lactate.

Acetoacetate should not be considered a product of incomplete oxidation of fatty acids nor a waste product of fat metabolism. It is formed from 3-hydroxy-3-methylglutaryl-CoA, which in turn is formed from the reaction of acetoacetyl-CoA and acetyl-CoA; as seen in Fig. 6, acetyl-CoA can form at all stages of β-oxidation of fatty acids. Acetoacetate is generated in response to signals from extrahepatic tissues mediated by glucagon and insulin informing the liver that glucose must be conserved for its obligate users and that other tissues are prepared to use the ketone bodies for energy. Subsequently, the ketone bodies, acting in a feed-back mechanism, may modulate the release of fatty acids from adipose tissue and the turnover of protein in muscle (120,126,127).

The regulation of fatty acid oxidation and ketogenesis in liver has been studied extensively. Some attempts have been made to understand that regulation in terms of the redox state of hepatocytes as reflected in the ratio of $NAD^+/NADH$; the increased oxidation of fatty acids would result in a decrease of this ratio, theoretically causing a shift of the reaction catalyzed by malate dehydrogenase in favor of malate production at the expense of oxaloacetate (128,129). Another way in which the concentration of oxaloacetate in hepatocytes could be decreased is by diversion of that metabolite into the pathway of gluconeogenesis (130). In both cases, diminished concentration of oxaloacetate was postulated to result in diminished synthesis of citrate, the precursor of fatty acid synthesis, as seen in the following scheme.

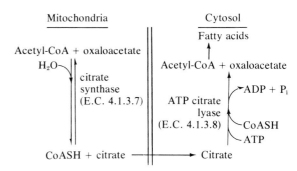

Some investigators, however, have obtained evidence that neither of those explanations can rationalize all the ketogenic situations encountered experimentally and clinically (119,121).

Accordingly, two additional but not mutually exclusive hypotheses have been proposed for control of fatty acid oxidation and ketogenesis when carbohydrate is in short supply. One proposal (121) accepts the concept that oxaloacetate becomes the limiting substrate but pinpoints the cause more remotely in the glycolytic pathway at the level of the 6-phosphofructokinase reaction. Deactivation of that enzyme would diminish the flux of substrate through glycolysis, decrease the amount of pyruvate formed, and hence reduce the amount of oxaloacetate that can form from pyruvate. The second proposal (119) places the control of fatty acid oxidation and ketogenesis at the level of transport of fatty acids into the mitochondria, more specifically in the activity of carnitine acyltransferase I. Both the proposed mechanisms are considered to be regulated strongly by glucagon.

With respect to the first proposal, Lane and Mooney (121) focus on the branch point of reactions of acetyl-CoA in the mitochondria. This is shown in the scheme below:

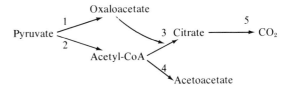

1, 2, 3, 4, and 5 refer to pyruvate carboxylase, pyruvate dehydrogenase, citrate synthase, the 3-hydroxy-3-methylglutaryl-CoA cycle, and the tricarboxylic acid cycle, respectively.

Acetyl-CoA in the mitochondria has the option of condensing with oxaloacetate to form citrate; the citrate then can exit to the cytosol where, at the site of fatty acid synthesis, it can be cleaved to yield acetyl-CoA once again. Alternatively, acetyl-CoA in the mitochondria can form 3-hydroxy-3-methylglutaryl-CoA that can be cleaved to form acetoacetate. Thus at the fork indicated above, the pathway taken by acetyl-CoA could be determined by the concentration of oxaloacetate.

Lane and Mooney (121) found that either dibutyryl cAMP or glucagon caused chick liver cells to suffer precipitous diminution of cytosolic citrate and of mitochondrial oxaloacetate; this was coincident with decreased synthesis of fatty acids and increased ketogenesis. Decrease of citrate concentration in the cytosol would be expected to inactivate the enzyme that catalyzes the committed and rate-limiting step in fatty acid synthesis, namely, acetyl-CoA carboxylase; the reaction involved is the carboxylation of acetyl-CoA to form malonyl-CoA. The carboxylase is active only when it is in a polymeric, filamentous form, as favored by citrate; it is inactive when it is depolymerized, as in the absence of citrate. Thus citrate is both the precursor for acetyl-CoA and the allosteric activator for conversion of acetyl-CoA to fatty acids.

In the experiments described above, the fall in citrate level could be overcome by addition of pyruvate or lactate; concomitantly, the inhibitory effects on fatty acid synthesis and the activating effects on ketogenesis were reversed. The effects of cAMP or glucagon noted previously must then have been mediated in glycolysis at some point before formation of pyruvate. The actual locus was determined to be at the level of the reaction catalyzed by 6-phosphofructokinase. Whether fructose 2,6-bisphosphate (the principal activator of 6-phosphofructokinase, whose synthesis is inhibited by glucagon) can stimulate fatty acid synthesis and inhibit ketogenesis remains to be determined.

The proposal of Lane and Mooney (121) can be summarized as follows: Carbohydrate feeding promotes glycolysis with formation of pyruvate, the major anaplerotic (replenishing) precursor of oxaloacetate in the liver. Oxaloacetate produced in the mitochondria reacts with acetyl-CoA to form citrate; citrate is sent into the cytosol, where, acting as both substrate and allosteric regulator, it favors fatty acid synthesis. Diversion of acetyl-CoA into that pathway, which depends on an adequate supply of oxaloacetate, tunes down the entry of acetyl-CoA into the ketogenic pathway. Glucagon, operating through cAMP, reverses those processes by limiting the formation of pyruvate in glycolysis.

McGarry and Foster (119,125), in whose laboratories the alternative proposal of regulation was developed, place the control by carbohydrate of fatty acid synthesis and ketogenesis at the point of entry of fatty acids into the mitochondria where they can be oxidized. Under conditions of carbohydrate feeding, increased glycolysis occurs, more acetyl-CoA forms from pyruvate, and more malonyl-CoA forms from that acetyl-CoA. Malonyl-CoA has a direct inhibitory effect on the carnitine acyltransferase I reaction, thus preventing the transport of long-chain fatty acids into the mitochondria and, therefore, their oxidation to

acetyl-CoA and subsequent formation of ketone bodies. Glucagon, or dibutyryl cAMP, activates the translocation of long-chain fatty acids across the inner mitochondrial membrane. This is thought to occur by an inhibition of acetyl-CoA carboxylase, the enzyme that catalyzes formation of malonyl-CoA. The sequence of events is then as follows: Carbohydrate feeding causes increased production of pyruvate and, therefore, of malonyl-CoA. Malonyl-CoA inhibits the translocation of long-chain fatty acids into the mitochondria by inactivating the carnitine acyltransferase. Thus fatty acid oxidation and ketogenesis in the mitochondria are inhibited, while fatty acid synthesis can proceed in the cytosol. Should a glucagon/insulin imbalance occur, as when carbohydrate feeding or utilization is curtailed, glucagon causes deactivation of acetyl-CoA carboxylase, production of malonyl-CoA is diminished, inhibition of translocation of long-chain fatty acids is relieved, and fatty acids enter the mitochondria and are oxidized with formation of acetyl-CoA and, subsequently, ketone bodies.

Although the liver is the major organ for production of ketone bodies, it has little 3-ketoacid-CoA transferase, one of the two enzymes that allows a tissue to utilize acetoacetate for energy; thus the liver does not itself oxidize nonthiolated acetoacetate. In many peripheral tissues, including brain, heart and skeletal muscle, kidney, and intestine, acetoacetate may be prepared for oxidation by the following set of reactions, although the activity of 3-ketoacid-CoA transferase is generally more than 10-fold greater than that of acetoacetyl-CoA synthetase:

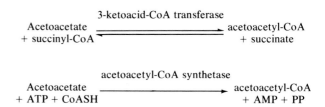

Acetoacetyl-CoA is acted on by acetoacetyl-CoA thiolase to give acetyl-CoA for entrance into the tricarboxylic acid cycle. That enzyme is present in liver but, because of the absence of 3-oxoacid-CoA transferase, is used mainly in the reverse reaction, as required in the process of ketogenesis:

$$\text{2 Acetyl-CoA} \xrightleftharpoons{\text{acetoacetyl-CoA thiolase}} \text{acetoacetyl-CoA} + \text{CoASH}$$

The ketone bodies have been considered to be more than substrates for oxidation in certain peripheral tissues. Emphasis is being placed on acetoacetate and 3-hydroxybutyrate as signals of carbohydrate lack and, therefore, as agents for integration of different fuels for use in the entire body. The subject is discussed by Stanley (127) and reviewed more extensively by Robinson and Williamson (120).

PEROXISOMAL OXIDATION OF FATTY ACIDS

The nature and functional capacities of peroxisomes are described elsewhere in this volume, with particular emphasis on morphology and cytochemistry. The present discussion provides some perspective of the β-oxidation of fatty acids in peroxisomes *vis à vis* their major path of oxidation in the mitochondria. In this regard, the recent review by Tolbert (131) is most helpful.

In 1969, Cooper and Beevers (132,133), studying the endosperm of germinating castor bean, described a nonmitochondrial system of β-oxidation of fatty acids occurring in the class of microbodies known as glyoxysomes. They proposed a pathway involving a fatty acyl-CoA oxidase different from the fatty acyl-CoA dehydrogenase present in mitochondria of many tissues, although both enzymes are FAD-linked. The authors noted a chief difference in the way the reduced FAD is reoxidized. In the mitochondria, the enzyme couples with the electron transport chain, eventually passing the hydrogen atoms and electrons of FADH$_2$ to oxygen to form water; in the peroxisomes, the oxidase couples directly with molecular oxygen, passing hydrogen atoms and electrons through to form hydrogen peroxide. The authors considered that the hydrogen peroxide is then removed by the action of catalase.

Subsequently, similar systems of fatty acid oxidation were described in protozoal ciliates (134–136). Pioneer work by Lazarow and de Duve (137) and Lazarow (138) established that such systems were operative in liver peroxisomes, and the pathway was formulated in considerable detail. Others (139–141) studied the system in livers of several species, including the human (142). Especially important was the finding that administration of clofibrate or other hypolipidemic drugs to animals caused their livers to respond with induction of enzymes of the peroxisomal system of fatty acid oxidation (138,143–147). The scheme for β-oxidation of fatty acids in peroxisomes is shown in Fig. 7 and may be compared with the mitochondrial pathway shown in Fig. 6.

Both pathways are initiated with an investment of high energy from ATP to activate the carboxyl group of a fatty acid, in the following reaction:

Fatty acid + ATP + CoA→fatty acyl-CoA + AMP + PP$_i$

The reaction is catalyzed by an enzyme called fatty acyl-CoA synthetase. One species of the enzyme is linked with the mitochondrial system of fatty acid oxidation, and the locus of its action in the cytosol makes necessary a means of translocation of the activated fatty acid into the mitochondria. This is accomplished by the formation of a fatty acyl-carnitine derivative catalyzed by a carnitine fatty acyl-CoA transferase located in the inner membrane of the mitochondria:

Fatty acyl-CoA + carnitine ⇌ fatty acyl-carnitine + CoA

In the matrix of the mitochondria, then, the fatty acyl group is again transferred to CoA to make fatty acyl-CoA that can be oxidized. In contrast, the translocation of the fatty acid into peroxisomes is independent of carnitine, because the fatty acyl-CoA synthetase to which it is linked is located in the peroxisomes per se. Thus the activated fatty acyl-CoA is generated within the organelle in which its oxidation is to occur. Apparently, however, the translocation of the free fatty acid from the cytosol into the peroxisome requires the participation of a fatty acid binding protein; some have suggested that the so-called Z protein is indeed the binding protein (148).

From the standpoint of energy metabolism, the differences in the first oxidative step between mitochondrial and peroxisomal pathways are critical. The mitochondrial enzyme is an FAD-linked fatty acyl-CoA dehydrogenase that couples with the electron transport chain, so that the energy released in the subsequent reoxidation of the reduced FAD is preserved in pyrophosphate bonds of ATP; in the course of that reoxidation, hydrogen atoms and electrons of FADH$_2$ are transferred to oxygen to form water. In peroxisomes, the enzyme catalyzing the oxidation of fatty acyl-CoA is an FAD-linked oxidase; reoxidation of the reduced flavin occurs directly with molecular oxygen without participation of a respiratory chain. Thus no ATP is produced, and the hydrogen atoms of FADH$_2$ are passed on to oxygen to produce hydrogen peroxide. The latter substance may be decomposed by the action of catalase also present in the peroxisomes, although alternatively, the catalase-hydrogen peroxide complex could oxidize a second substrate, such as ethanol or methanol, if indeed such were present. Because of the two different ways by which the FADH$_2$ coenzyme is reoxidized, the mitochondrial dehydrogenase is cyanide-sensitive, while the peroxisomal oxidase is cyanide-insensitive.

Proceeding down the pathway, the next enzymes show significant differences as between the two organelles. In the mitochondrial pathway, the enoylhydratase and L-3-hydroxy fatty acyl-CoA dehydrogenase activities are exhibited by separate enzymes. In the peroxisomal pathway, the two activities are associated with a single bifunctional enzyme. In the mitochondria, NADH produced by the dehydrogenase can enter the respiratory chain and yield three molecules of ATP by oxidative phosphorylation. NADH produced in the dehydrogenation reaction in peroxisomes must be

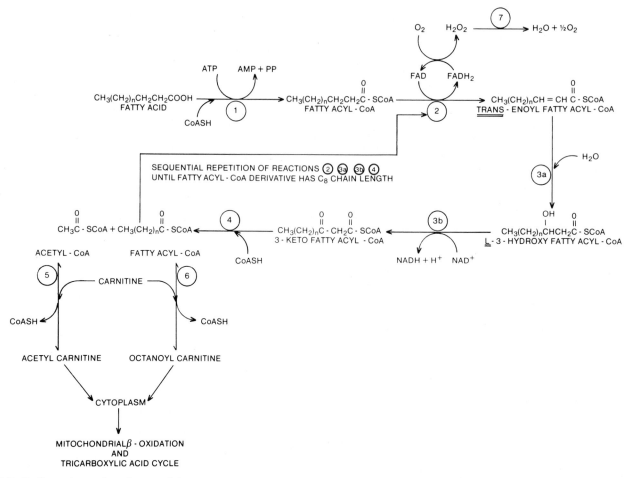

FIG. 7. Peroxisomal pathway of fatty acid oxidation. *1:* Acyl-CoA synthetase (E.C.6.2.1.3); *2:* fatty acyl-CoA oxidase; *3:* bifunctional protein with (a) enoylhydratase (E.C.4.2.1.17) and (b) L-3-hydroxy fatty acyl-CoA dehydrogenase (E.C.1.1.1.35) activities; *4:* acetyl-CoA acyltransferase (3-ketoacyl-CoA thiolase) E.C.2.3.1.16); *5:* carnitine acetyltransferase (E.C.2.3.1.7); *6:* carnitine octanoyltransferase; *7:* catalase (E.C.1.11.1.6). (Adapted from refs. 131 and 137.)

shuttled out. Perhaps eventually its reducing equivalents would be transferred to the mitochondria; depending on the shuttling mechanism employed, either two or three molecules of ATP could be produced.

Another difference between the two systems is exhibited by the corresponding enzymes catalyzing the thiolytic cleavage of 3-keto fatty acyl-CoA to yield acetyl-CoA. The mitochondrial and peroxisomal thiolases differ in specificity and other properties.

Hepatic peroxisomal β-oxidation is specific for long-chain fatty acyl-CoA derivatives, whereas the mitochondrial system utilizes both long- and short-chain fatty acyl-CoA substrates. However, the peroxisomal system appears to be most active with fatty acids containing 10 to 22 carbon atoms and is particularly active with monounsaturated fatty acids, such as erucic acid (C22:1) (131,149).

Peroxisomal oxidation of long-chain fatty acids stops at the level of octanoyl-CoA, whereas mitochondrial oxidation continues to formation of acetoacetyl-CoA. The further oxidation of octanoyl-CoA could

then proceed by one of two mechanisms. First, the substrate could be hydrolyzed by a hydrolase to form octanoic acid and CoA; the octanoic acid could diffuse out to the cytosol and again be activated for oxidation in the mitochondria. Although some studies have indicated that indeed peroxisomal hydrolases exist (150), a more recent publication (151) reports that hydrolases separating with preparations of peroxisomes are probably contaminants arising from lysosomes. Accordingly, the hydrolytic mechanism is not viable. The second mechanism for the transfer of medium- and short-chain acyl groups out of peroxisomes could perhaps involve peroxisomal carnitine fatty acyl-CoA transferases. Indeed, these have been found to exist for the formation of acetyl-carnitine and octanoyl-carnitine. The carnitine derivatives could diffuse out to the cytosol and eventually transfer their fatty acyl groups to mitochondria for oxidation or be used in synthetic reactions. Thus, although the oxidation of long-chain fatty acids in peroxisomes does not begin with a transfer reaction requiring carnitine, exit of the medium-chain fatty acyl groups formed in oxidation may require the participation of carnitine.

In the mitochondria, control is exerted on fatty acid oxidation at the level of the carnitine fatty acyl-CoA transferase reaction that aids in translocation of the fatty acyl group; thus malonyl-CoA formed as a result of carbohydrate metabolism inhibits the transferase reaction (119) and, therefore, diminishes the oxidation of fatty acids. The peroxisomal system is free of such control and apparently is regulated only by the concentration of fatty acid substrate.

The energetics of oxidation are different in the two systems. In the peroxisomes, oxidation of palmitic acid (C16) would occur in four repetitive stages, with formation of octanoyl-CoA, four acetyl-CoA, and four NADH. Those products would leave the peroxisomes by the mechanisms described previously and ultimately could be oxidized in the mitochondria to yield about 121 molecules of ATP. If palmitic acid were to be oxidized directly by the mitochondrial system, about 129 molecules of ATP would result. Carried to completion with subsequent help from the mitochondrial system, oxidation of palmitic acid in the peroxisomes produces only eight fewer ATP molecules. These eight are lost at the four steps in which the fatty acyl-CoA oxidase operates. As explained by Tolbert (131), that relatively small amount of energy would not be a great price to pay if use of the peroxisomal pathway confers some important advantages to the organism. Although the advantages are not known for the existence of the parallel peroxisomal pathway, partition of total oxidation between the two pathways has been studied. Thus about 22% of the total oxidation of palmitate (in terms of acetyl-CoA formed) was found to occur in the peroxisomes of hepatocytes (152). It may be conjectured that the peroxisomal pathway provides a mechanism for the production of acetyl-CoA outside the mitochondria without the participation of citrate formed in the mitochondria. Furthermore, from knowledge obtained concerning induction of most of the enzymes of the peroxisomal pathway by hypolipidemic drugs (138,143−147) and by excessive fat intake (153), even the marginal loss of energy occurring when that pathway is used instead of the mitochondrial system could, under certain circumstances, contribute to removal of lipid and loss of body weight. Finally, oxidation of fatty acyl-CoA derivatives by the oxidase allows generation of hydrogen peroxide that may be used by catalase for oxidation of substrates such as ethanol.

OXIDATION OF PYRUVATE AND ACETYL-CoA

Lactate is produced in liver cells when glycolysis occurs anaerobically. That process results in net for-

mation of two molecules of ATP for each molecule of glucose oxidized. The change in free energy ($\Delta G°'$) occurring when glucose is converted to two molecules of lactate is −47 kcal mol^{-1}; that occurring when glucose is oxidized completely to carbon dioxide and water is −686 kcal mol^{-1}. Thus glycolysis unlocks only about 6% of the total free energy available from glucose metabolized by the glycolytic, pyruvate dehydrogenase, and tricarboxylic acid systems. The total oxidation of glucose results in formation of about 36 to 38 molecules of ATP. One may then calculate the efficiency of energy preservation to be about 31% for anaerobic glycolysis and about 38 to 40% for the complete oxidation of glucose by the combined actions of glycolysis and the tricarboxylic acid cycle. Thus, although the oxidation of pyruvate yields many more times the amount of ATP than produced in glycolysis, the efficiencies of the two pathways are not too disparate.

The oxidation of pyruvate is an aerobic process. Pyruvate formed in glycolysis enters the mitochondria, where it is oxidatively decarboxylated by the pyruvate dehydrogenase system (Fig. 8). The acetyl-CoA that forms can then enter the Krebs tricarboxylic acid cycle (Fig. 9), where its carbon atoms are oxidized to carbon dioxide. The energy of oxidation of pyruvate is preserved in the pyrophosphate bonds of ATP, as shown in Table 1. A single substrate level phosphorylation in the tricarboxylic acid cycle results in formation of GTP.

Acetyl-CoA arising from fatty acid oxidation in the mitochondria can also enter the tricarboxylic acid cycle and be treated identically with acetyl-CoA coming from pyruvate. That is true also for acetyl-CoA deriving from the oxidation of the carbon chain of leucine.

The tricarboxylic acid cycle is regulated by events in the pyruvate dehydrogenase system, which controls the conversion of pyruvate to acetyl-CoA. The subject of that regulation has been dealt with in several reviews (73,154−157) and primary publications (158, 159). However, control of the cycle also depends on factors that determine how much acetyl-CoA will be produced from fatty acids and which of the metabolic options open to acetyl-CoA will be taken.

The pyruvate dehydrogenase system, shown in Fig. 8, consists of several different components that participate in three integrated reactions summed up in the following equation:

$$\text{Pyruvate} + \text{CoA} + \text{NAD}^+ \rightarrow \text{acetyl-CoA} + \text{CO}_2 + \text{NADH} + \text{H}^+$$

The reoxidation of NADH by the respiratory chain can give rise to three molecules of ATP. The continual functioning of the system, which requires reoxidation of NADH, thus depends on the presence of molecular

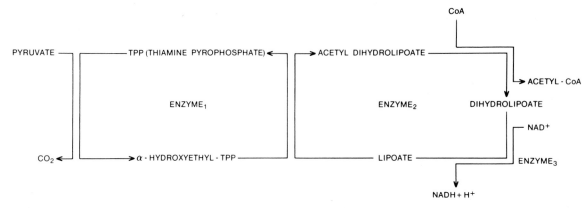

FIG. 8. Schematic representation of the pyruvate dehydrogenase system. Enzyme$_1$ of pyruvate dehydrogenase complex: pyruvate:lipoamide oxidoreductase (decarboxylating and acceptor-acetylating), E.C.1.2.4.1; enzyme$_2$ of pyruvate dehydrogenase complex: dihydrolipoamide acetyltransferase, E.C.2.3.1.12; enzyme$_3$ of pyruvate dehydrogenase complex: dihydrolipoamide reductase, E.C.1.6.4.3.

oxygen. Failing that, pyruvate would be reconverted to lactate, and the full energy benefit of oxidation of carbohydrate would not be attained. The fine control of pyruvate oxidation, however, is achieved in several different ways, most of which relate to enzyme$_1$ of the complex. As the reaction proceeds, the ratios of acetyl-CoA/CoA and NADH/NAD$^+$ increase coordinately; and the activity of enzyme$_1$ decreases by a kind of end-product inhibition of the sequence of reactions. However, enzyme$_1$ is regulated mainly by alternate phosphorylation and dephosphorylation reactions catalyzed, respectively, by a protein kinase and a phosphatase. The kinase, whcih is independent of cAMP, is not activated by glucagon. It is bound to the pyruvate dehydrogenase complex and uses ATP.Mg as the phosphorylating substrate. Phosphorylation of enzyme$_1$ causes inactivation, and dephosphorylation results in reactivation. Pyruvate itself inhibits the kinase and favors the active form of enzyme$_1$; accordingly, it promotes flux of substrate through the pyruvate dehydrogenase system and the tricarboxylic acid cycle. In conditions such as starvation and diabetes, where oxidative carbohydrate metabolism would be diminished, some accumulation of lactate would occur, and fatty acid oxidation and ketogenesis would be favored.

CONCLUSION

Any review of the biochemistry and physiology of the liver that attempts a coherent synthesis of available facts is hindered because the relevant information has been obtained from studies performed with several different animal species and use of different kinds of preparations. Most investigations have been performed in rodents, especially the rat, although chicks, dogs, and humans also have been used. The prepara-

tions employed have been isolated perfused livers, liver homogenates, liver slices, and suspensions of hepatocytes. Obviously, the use of any of those preparations removes the tissue from highly important interactions with other organs and, in many instances, provides only a description of existing pathways of metabolism and an evaluation of the potential capacities of these pathways. By using livers from animals in various physiological states, e.g., after feeding of particular kinds of meals or after fasting, inferences can be made about the effects of different nutrients on the direction of specific metabolic pathways. Study of livers from animals with endocrine deficiencies similarly may provide information about the hormonal control of metabolism. Since the metabolism of the liver greatly depends on minute-by-minute changes in the activity and metabolism of the whole organism, however, the limitations imposed by use of isolated organs, tissues, or cells are severe. Furthermore, findings in one species may not apply to others.

The difficulties and limitations noted above have recently been illustrated in a study of hepatocytes obtained from an avian source, the Japanese quail (160). Although the animals had been fed, the hepatocytes obtained after perfusion of the liver were low in glycogen and were almost depleted of alanine and glutamine. Incubation of the cells with a medium containing alanine caused remarkable increases in glucose uptake, glucose oxidation, and conversion of glucose carbon to fatty acids. Thus alanine was able to reverse the so-called ''glucose paradox'' (160) that appears to be so prominent in rat liver. The paradox is considered to be that rat hepatocytes, under conditions of lipogenesis after a carbohydrate meal, apparently incorporate little of glucose carbon into fatty acids; that is, they show limited utilization of glucose. The difficulty of extrapolating these observations to the whole animal is apparent; they show a potential but do not

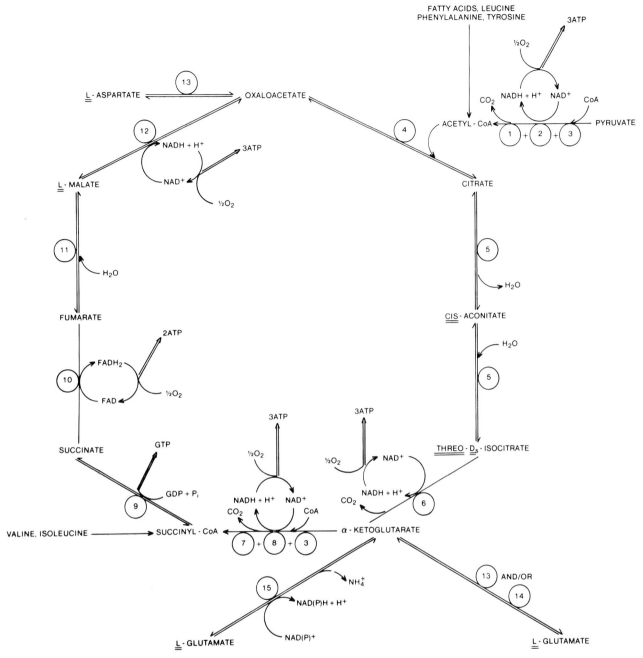

FIG. 9. Krebs tricarboxylic acid cycle. *1:* Pyruvate:lipoamide oxidoreductase (decarboxylating and acceptor-acetylating) (E.C.1.2.4.1); *2:* dihydrolipoamide acetyltransferase (E.C.2.3.1.12); *3:* dihydrolipoamide reductase (E.C.1.6.4.3). *1, 2,* and *3* are components of the pyruvate dehydrogenase complex. *4:* Citrate synthase (E.C.4.1.3.7); *5:* aconitate hydratase (E.C.4.2.1.3); *6:* isocitrate dehydrogenase (E.C.1.1.1.41); *7:* α-ketoglutarate:lipoamide oxidoreductase (decarboxylating and acceptor succinylating) (E.C.1.2.4.2); *8:* dihydrolipoamide succinyltransferase (E.C.2.3.1.61). *7, 8,* and *3* are components of the α-ketoglutarate dehydrogenase complex. *9:* Succinyl-CoA synthetase (E.C.6.2.1.4); *10:* succinate dehydrogenase (E.C.1.3.99.1); *11:* fumarate hydratase (E.C.4.2.1.2), *12:* malate dehydrogenase (E.C.1.1.1.37); *13:* aspartate aminotransferase (E.C.2.6.1.1); *14:* alanine aminotransferase (E.C.2.6.1.2); *15:* glutamate dehydrogenase (E.C.1.4.1.3).

reveal how it would be modified by whole body hormonal and substrate influences.

This chapter has attempted to show how the liver obtains energy to conduct a large number of functions related to transport, biosynthesis of macromolecules and special small molecules, and biotransformation of metabolites and drugs. Many syntheses are performed in service to other organs or tissues, for example, the manufacture of plasma proteins, carnitine, and creatine. On the other hand, the liver collects and transforms substrates to meet the specific fuel requirements of other tissues in response to metabolic signals coming from the whole organism. Remarkably, the liver is probably the only organ that produces acetoacetate for use by muscle, brain, and kidney cortex, yet it does not use that substrate for its own energy metabolism. Also, the liver is the major organ for production of glucose by gluconeogenesis and yet uses little glucose for its own metabolic requirements. The liver expends energy in the storage of glycogen, which subsequently is degraded to yield glucose for other tissues, such as the brain and erythrocytes, while it again uses little of that glucose for its own requirements. The liver makes fatty acids for export as triacylglycerols and phospholipids but uses fatty acids originating from the diet and the adipose tissue for its own energy needs.

The liver does not have much capacity for transamination of leucine, isoleucine, and valine but can actively oxidize the corresponding branched chain α-keto acids arising from transamination in the muscle. It has special capacity for conducting gluconeogenesis from alanine arising in muscle, where the amino groups of the branched chain amino acids are transferred to pyruvate by transamination. All these energy-related functions of the liver are accomplished in ways that are highly regulated by hormones and other agonists, especially by glucagon and insulin. The substrates coming from the liver, such as glucose and acetoacetate, in turn may be primary signals to other tissues to activate or inhibit pathways in the utilization of one or another fuel. Thus acetoacetate produced in the liver may signal the adipose tissue to reduce the extent of lipolysis that provides fatty acids to the liver for production of ketone bodies; and it may signal the muscle to limit proteolysis and activate the pathways for use of ketone bodies for energy. The liver can be said to sense the fuel needs of all of the other tissues in the body and respond by adjusting its metabolism accordingly.

The contribution of the energy metabolism of the liver to the maintenance of acid-base balance in the liver has been explored only tentatively. The production of glucose, a neutral molecule, from lactate and pyruvate is an energy-consuming process that also removes protons. The kidney, also a glucose-producing organ, probably uses the gluconeogenic pathway not only for facilitating ammonia production but for taking up protons. The possible function of the urea cycle in acid-base balance is the subject of a forthcoming review (161).

One cannot doubt that current descriptive knowledge of the metabolic functions of the liver is profound, and something is known of the integration of pathways. However, understanding the dynamic, rapid responses of the liver to changes in the physiologic condition of the total organism in a continuum of time is only beginning to be obtained.

REFERENCES

1. Walser, M., and Williamson, J. R. (editors) (1981): *Metabolism and Clinical Implications of Branched Chain Amino and Ketoacids*. Elsevier, New York.
2. Frenkel, R. A., and McGarry, J. D. (editors) (1980): *Carnitine Biosynthesis, Metabolism and Functions*. Academic Press, New York.
3. Englard, S. (1979): Hydroxylation of γ-butyrobetaine to carnitine in human and monkey tissues. *FEBS Lett.*, 102:297.
4. Rebouche, C. J., and Engel, A. G. (1980): Tissue distribution of carnitine biosynthetic enzymes in man. *Biochim. Biophys. Acta*, 630:22.
5. Engel, A. G. (1980): Possible causes and effects of carnitine deficiency in man. In: *Carnitine Biosynthesis, Metabolism and Functions*, edited by R. A. Frenkel and J. D. McGarry, p. 271. Academic Press, New York.
6. Chapoy, P. R., Angelini, C., Brown, W. J., Stiff, J. E., Shug, A. L., and Cederbaum, S. D. (1980): Systemic carnitine deficiency—A treatable inherited lipid-storage disease presenting as Reye's syndrome. *N. Engl. J. Med.*, 303:1389.
7. Walker, J. B. (1979): Creatine: Biosynthesis, regulation, and function. *Adv. Enzymol.*, 50:177.
8. Dawson, D. M., and Fine, I. H. (1967): Creatine kinase in human tissues. *Arch. Neurol.*, 16:175.
9. Davidson, S., Passmore, R., Brock, J. F. B., and Truswell, A. S. (1979): Carbohydrates. In: *Human Nutrition and Dietetics*. pp. 26–32. Churchill Livingstone, Edinburgh.
10. Davidson, S., Passmore, R., Brock, J. F. B., and Truswell, A. S. (1979): Alcohol. In: *Human Nutrition and Dietetics*, pp. 59–62. Churchill Livingstone, Edinburgh.
11. Li, T.-K. (1977): Enzymology of human alcohol metabolism. *Adv. Enzymol.* 45:427.
12. Harper, A. E., and Zapalowski, C. (1981): Interorgan relationships in the metabolism of the branched-chain amino and α-ketoacids. In: *Metabolism and Clinical Implications of Branched Chain Amino and Ketoacids*, edited by M. Walser, and J. R. Williamson, p. 195. Elsevier, New York.
13. Alfin-Slater, R. B., and Kritchevsky, D. (editors) (1980): *Human Nutrition, A Comprehensive Treatise, Vol. 3A, Nutrition and the Adult: Macronutrients*. Plenum, New York.
14. Nilsson-Ehle, P., Garfinkel, A. S., and Schotz, M. C. (1980): Lipolytic enzymes and plasma lipoprotein metabolism. *Ann. Rev. Biochem.*, 49:667.
15. Cohen, J. J., and Kamm, D. E. (1976): Renal metabolism: Relation to renal function. In: *The Kidney, Vol. 1*, edited by B. M. Brenner and F. C. Rector, Jr., p. 126. Saunders, Philadelphia.
16. Consolazio, C. F., Johnson, R. E., and Pecora, L. J. (editors) (1963): *Physiological Measurements of Metabolic Functions in Man*. McGraw-Hill, New York.
17. Baldwin, R. L., and Smith, N. E. (1974): Molecular control of energy metabolism. In: *The Control of Metabolism*, edited by J. D. Sink, p. 17. The Pennsylvania State University Press, University Park.
18. Tolbert, N. E. (1981): Metabolic pathways in peroxisomes and glyoxysomes. *Ann. Rev. Biochem.*, 50:133.
19. Oshino, N., Jamieson, D., Sugano, T., and Chance, B. (1975): Optical measurement of the catalase-hydrogen peroxide intermediate (compound I) in the liver of anaesthetized rats and its implication to hydrogen peroxide production *in situ*. *Biochem. J.*, 146:67.
20. Cohen, S. M., Rognstad, R., Shulman, R. G., and Katz, J. (1981): A comparison of ^{13}C nuclear magnetic resonance and ^{14}C tracer studies of hepatic metabolism. *J. Biol. Chem.*, 256:3428.
21. Rife, J. E., and Cleland, W. W. (1980): Kinetic mechanism of glutamate dehydrogenase. *Biochemistry*, 19:2321.
22. Cook, P. F. (1982): Kinetic studies to determine the mechanism of regulation of bovine liver glutamate dehydrogenase by nucleotide effectors. *Biochemistry*, 21:113.
23. Crist, K. A., Baldwin, R. L., and Stern, J. S. (1980): Energetics and the demands for maintenance. In: *Human Nutrition, A*

Comprehensive Treatise, Vol. 3A, Nutrition and the Adult: Macronutrients, edited by R. B. Alfin-Slater and D. Kritchevsky, p. 159. Plenum, New York.

24. Katz, J., and Rognstad, R. (1978): Compartmentation of glucose metabolism in liver. In: *Microenvironments and Metabolic Compartmentation,* edited by P. A. Srere and R. W. Estabrook, p. 227. Academic Press, New York.

25. Weinhouse, S. (1976): Regulation of glucokinase in liver. *Curr. Top. Cell. Regul.,* 11:1.

26. Lauris, V., and Cahill, G. F., Jr. (1966): Hepatic glucose phosphotransferases. Variations among species. *Diabetes,* 15:475.

27. Borrebaek, B., Hultman, E., Nilsson, L. H., Jr., Roch-Norlund, A. E., and Spydevold, O. (1970): Adaptable glucokinase activity of human liver. *Biochem. Med.* 4:469.

28. Willms, B., Ben-Ami, P., and Söling, H. D. (1970): Hepatic enzyme activities of glycolysis and gluconeogenesis in diabetes of man and laboratory animals. *Horm. Metab. Res.,* 2:135.

29. Pilkis, S. J. (1968): Identification of human hepatic glucokinase and some properties of the enzyme. *Proc. Soc. Exp. Biol. Med.,* 129:681.

30. Hers, H. G. (1980): Carbohydrate metabolism and its regulation. In: *Inherited Disorders of Carbohydrate Metabolism,* edited by D. Burman, J. B. Holton, and C. A. Pennock, p. 3. University Park Press, Baltimore.

31. Leuthardt, F., and Testa, E. (1951): Die phosphorylierung der fructose in der leber. *Helv. Chim. Acta,* 34:931.

32. Hers, H. G. (1952): La fructokinase du foie. *Biochem. Biophys. Acta,* 8:416.

33. Parks, R. E., Ben-Gershom, E., and Lardy, H. A. (1957): Liver fructokinase. *J. Biol. Chem.,* 227:231.

34. Adelman, R. C., Ballard, F. J., and Weinhouse, S. (1967): Purification and properties of rat liver fructokinase. *J. Biol. Chem.,* 242:3360.

35. Heinz, F., Lamprecht, W., and Kirsch, J. (1968): Enzymes of fructose metabolism in human liver. *J. Clin. Invest.,* 47:1826.

36. Woods, H. F. (1980): Pathogenic mechanisms of disorders in fructose metabolism. In: *Inherited Disorders of Carbohydrate Metabolism,* edited by D. Burman, J. B. Holton, and C. A. Pennock, p. 191. University Park Press, Baltimore.

37. Leloir, L. F. (1951): The enzymatic transformation of uridine diphosphate glucose into a galactose derivative. *Arch. Biochem. Biophys.,* 33:186.

38. Gitzelmann, R., and Hansen, R. G. (1980): Galactose metabolism, hereditary defects and their clinical significance. In: *Inherited Disorders of Carbohydrate Metabolism,* edited by D. Burman, J. B. Holton, and C. A. Pennock, p. 61. University Park Press, Baltimore.

39. Isselbacher, K. J., and Krane, S. M. (1961): Studies on the mechanism of the inhibition of galactose oxidation by ethanol. *J. Biol. Chem.,* 236:2394.

40. Leuthardt, F., Testa, E., and Wolf, H. P. (1953): Der enzymatische Abbau des fructose-1-phosphate in der leber. *Helv. Chim. Acta,* 36:227.

41. Sillero, M. A. G., Sillero, A., and Sols, A. (1969): Enzymes involved in fructose metabolism in liver and the glyceraldehyde metabolic crossroads. *Eur. J. Biochem.,* 10:345.

42. Woods, H. F., Eggleston, L. V., and Krebs, H. A. (1970): The cause of hepatic accumulation of fructose-1-phosphate on fructose loading. *Biochem. J.,* 119:501.

43. Horecker, B. L., Tsolas, O., and Lai, C. Y. (1972): Aldolases. In: *The Enzymes, Vol. 7,* 3rd edition, edited by P. D. Boyer, p. 213. Academic Press, New York.

44. Horecker, B. L., MacGregor, J. S., Singh, V. N., Melloni, E. and Pontremoli, S. (1981): Aldolase and fructose bisphosphatase: Key enzymes in the control of gluconeogenesis and glycolysis. *Curr. Top. Cell. Regul.,* 18:181.

45. Hue, L., and Hers, H. G. (1972): The conversion of (4-^{3}H) fructose and of (4-^{3}H) glucose to liver glycogen in the mouse. An investigation of the glyceraldehyde crossroads. *Eur. J. Biochem.,* 29:268.

46. Goldhammer, A. R., and Paradies, H. H. (1979): Phospho-

fructokinase: Structure and function. *Curr. Top. Cell. Regul.,* 15:109.

47. Uyeda, K. (1979): Phosphofructokinase. In: *Advances in Enzymology, Vol. 48,* edited by A. Meister, p. 193. Wiley, New York.

48. Hers, H. G., Hue, L., and Van Schaftingen, E. (1981): The fructose 6-phosphate/fructose 1,6-bisphosphate cycle. *Curr. Top. Cell. Regul.* 18:199.

49. Van Schaftingen, E., Hue, L., and Hers, H. G. (1980): Fructose 2,6-bisphosphate, the probable structure of the glucose- and glucagon-sensitive stimulator of phosphofructokinase. *Biochem. J.,* 192:897.

50. Claus, T. H., Schlumpf, J., Pilkis, J., Johnson, R. A., and Pilkis, S. J. (1981): Evidence for a new activator of rat liver phosphofructokinase. *Biochem. Biophys. Res. Commun.,* 98:359.

51. Furuya, E., and Uyeda, K. (1980): An activation factor of liver phosphofructokinase. *Proc. Natl. Acad. Sci. USA,* 77:5861.

52. Van Schaftingen, E., and Hers, H. G. (1981): Formation of fructose 2,6-bisphosphate from fructose 1,6-bisphosphate by intramolecular cyclisation followed by alkaline hydrolysis. *Eur. J. Biochem.,* 117:319.

53. Hesbain-Frisque, A.-M., Van Schaftingen, E., and Hers, H. G. (1981): Structure and configuration of fructose 2,6-bisphosphate by ^{31}P and ^{13}C nuclear magnetic resonance. *Eur. J. Biochem.,* 117:325.

54. Pilkis, S. J., El-Maghrabi, M. R., Pilkis, J., Claus, T. H., and Cumming, D. A. (1981): Fructose 2,6-bisphosphate: A new activator of phosphofructokinase. *J. Biol. Chem.,* 256:3171.

55. Van Schaftingen, E., Jett, M. F., Hue, L., and Hers, H. G. (1981): Control of liver 6-phosphofructokinase by fructose 2,6-bisphosphate and other effectors. *Proc. Natl. Acad. Sci. USA,* 78:3483.

56. Van Schaftingen, E., Hue, L., and Hers, H. G. (1980): Control of the fructose 6-phosphate/fructose 1,6-bisphosphate cycle in isolated hepatocytes by glucose and glucagon. *Biochem. J.,* 192:887.

57. Kjerulf-Jensen, K. (1942): The phosphate esters formed in the liver tissue of rats and rabbits during assimilation of hexoses and glycerol. *Acta Physiol. Scand.,* 4:249.

58. Burch, H. B., Max, P., Chyu, K., and Lowry, O. H. (1969): Metabolic intermediates in liver of rats given large amounts of fructose or dihydroxyacetone. *Biochem. Biophys. Res. Commun.,* 34:619.

59. Maenpaa, P. H., Raivio, K. O., and Kekomaki, M. P. (1968): Liver adenine nucleotides; fructose-induced depletion and its effect on protein synthesis. *Science,* 161:1253.

60. Krebs, H. A. Woods, H. F., and Alberti, K. G. M. M. (1975): Hyperlactataemia and lactic acidosis. *Essays Med. Biochem.,* 1:81.

61. Hers, H. G. (1970): Misuses for fructose. *Nature,* 227:421.

62. Woods, H. F., and Alberti, K. G. M. M. (1972): Dangers of intravenous fructose. *Lancet,* 2:1354.

63. Wu, R. (1965): Rate-limiting factors in glycolysis and inorganic orthophosphate transport in rat liver and kidney slices. *J. Biol. Chem.,* 240:2373.

64. Gaja, G., Ragnotti, G., Cajone, F., and Bernelli-Zazzera, A. (1968): Changes in the concentrations of some phosphorylated intermediates and stimulation of glycolysis in liver slices. *Biochem. J.,* 109:867.

65. Woods, H. F., and Krebs, H. A. (1971): Lactate production in the perfused rat liver. *Biochem. J.,* 125:129.

66. Brunengraber, H., Boutry, M., and Lowenstein, J. M. (1973): Fatty acid and 3-β-hydroxysterol synthesis in the perfused rat liver. *J. Biol. Chem.,* 248:2656.

67. Zehner, J., Loy, E., Mullhofer, G., and Bucher, Th. (1973): The problem of cell heterogeneity of liver tissue in the study of fructose metabolism. *Eur. J. Biochem.,* 34:248.

68. Seglen, P. O. (1974): Autoregulation of glycolysis, respiration, gluconeogenesis and glycogen synthesis in isolated parenchymal rat liver cells under aerobic and anaerobic conditions. *Biochim. Biophys. Acta,* 338:317.

69. Walli, R. A. (1978): Interrelation of aerobic glycolysis and

lipogenesis in isolated perfused liver of well-fed rats. *Biochim. Biophys. Acta,* 539:62.

70. El-Maghrabi, M. R., Claus, T. H., Pilkis, J., and Pilkis, S. J. (1981): Partial purification of a rat liver enzyme that catalyzes the formation of fructose 2,6-bisphosphate. *Biochem. Biophys. Res. Commun.,* 101:1071.

71. Van Schaftingen, E., and Hers, H. G. (1981): Phosphofructokinase 2: The enzyme that forms fructose 2,6-bisphosphate from fructose 6-phosphate and ATP. *Biochem. Biophys. Res. Commun.,* 101:1078.

72. Hue, L., Blackmore, P. F., and Exton, J. H. (1981): Fructose 2,6-bisphosphate. *J. Biol. Chem.,* 256:8900.

73. Denton, R. M., and Halestrap, A. P. (1978): Regulation of pyruvate metabolism in mammalian tissues. *Essays Biochem.,* 15:37.

74. Engström, L. (1980): Regulation of liver pyruvate kinase by phosphorylation-dephosphorylation. In: *Molecular Aspects of Cellular Regulation, Vol. 1, Recently Discovered Systems of Enzyme Regulation by Reversible Phosphorylation,* edited by P. Cohen, p. 11. Elsevier, Amsterdam.

75. Hue, L. (1981): The role of futile cycles in the regulation of carbohydrate metabolism in the liver. *Adv. Enzymol.,* 52:247.

76. Clark, M. G., Kneer, N. M., Bosch, A. L., and Lardy, H. A. (1974): The fructose 1,6-diphosphatase-phosphofructokinase substrate cycle. *J. Biol. Chem.,* 249:5695.

77. Van Schaftingen, E., and Hers, H. G. (1981): Inhibition of fructose-1,6-bisphosphatase by fructose 2,6-bisphosphate. *Proc. Natl. Acad. Sci. USA,* 78:2861.

78. Cori, C. F. (1981): The glucose-lactic acid cycle and gluconeogenesis. *Curr. Top. Cell. Regul.* 18:377.

79. Felig, P. (1973): Progress in endocrinology and metabolism. The glucose-alanine cycle. *Metabolism,* 22:179.

80. Garber, A. J., Karl, I. E., and Kipnis, D. M. (1976): Alanine and glutamine synthesis and release from skeletal muscle. I. Glycolysis and amino acid release. II. The precursor role of amino acids in alanine and glutamine synthesis. *J. Biol. Chem.,* 251:826.

81. Coleman, J. E., and Rosenberg, L. E. (1980): *Molecular Mechanisms of Disease,* 3rd edition. Yale University Press, New Haven.

82. Cahill, G. F., Jr., and Owen, O. E. (1968): Some observations on carbohydrate metabolism in man. In: *Carbohydrate Metabolism and its Disorders, Vol. 1,* edited by F. Dickens, W. J. Whelan, and P. J. Randle, p. 497. Academic Press, London.

83. Felig, P., Marliss, E., Pozefsky, T., and Cahill, G. F., Jr. (1970): Amino acid metabolism in the regulation of gluconeogenesis in man. *Am. J. Clin. Nutr.,* 23:986.

84. Ruderman, N. B., Aoki, T. T., and Cahill, G. F., Jr. (1976): Gluconeogenesis and its disorders in man. In: *Gluconeogenesis: Its Regulation in Mammalian Species,* edited by R. W. Hanson and M. A. Mehlman, p. 515. Wiley, New York.

85. Owen, O. E., Patel, M. S., Block, B. S. B., Kreulen, T. H., Reichle, F. A., and Mazzoli, M. A. (1976): Gluconeogenesis in normal, cirrhotic, and diabetic humans. In: *Gluconeogenesis: Its Regulation in Mammalian Species,* edited by R. W. Hanson and M. A. Mehlman, p. 533. Wiley, New York.

86. Barritt, G. J., Zander, G. L., and Utter, M. F. (1976): The regulation of pyruvate carboxylase activity in gluconeogenic tissues. In: *Gluconeogenesis: Its Regulation in Mammalian Species,* edited by R. W. Hanson and M. A. Mehlman, p. 3. Wiley, New York.

87. Tilghman, S. M., Hanson, R. W., and Ballard, F. J. (1976): Hormonal regulation of phosphoenolpyruvate carboxykinase (GTP) in mammalian tissues. In: *Gluconeogenesis: Its Regulation in Mammalian Species,* edited by R. W. Hanson and M. A. Mehlman, p. 47. Wiley, New York.

88. Iynedjian, P. B., Kioussis, D., Garcia Ruiz, J. P., and Hanson, R. W. (1978): Hormonal regulation of phosphoenolpyruvate carboxykinase (GTP) synthesis. In: *11th Meeting (Copenhagen, 1977) of Fed. European Bioch. Soc. Vol. 42 (Symposium Al), Regulatory Mechanisms of Carbohydrate Metabolism,* edited by V. Esmann, p. 83. Pergamon Press, Oxford.

89. Lardy, H. A., MacDonald, M. J., Huang, M-T., and Bentle, L. A. (1978): Regulation of phosphopyruvate synthesis in normal and pathological states. In: *11th Meeting (Copenhagen, 1977) of Fed. European Bioch. Soc. Vol. 42 (Symposium Al), Regulatory Mechanisms of Carbohydrate Metabolism,* edited by V. Esmann, p. 93. Pergamon Press, Oxford.

90. Nelson, K., Cimbala, M. A., and Hanson, R. W. (1980): Regulation of phosphoenolpyruvate carboxykinase (GTP) mRNA turnover in rat liver. *J. Biol. Chem.,* 255:8509.

91. Weber, G., Kizaki, H., Shiotani, T., Tzeng, D., and Williams, J. C. (1978): The molecular correlation concept of neoplasia: Recent advances and new challenges. *Adv. Exp. Med. Biol.,* 92:89.

92. Lerner, M. H., and Lowy, B. A. (1974): The formation of adenosine in rabbit liver and its possible role as a direct precursor of erythrocyte adenine nucleotides. *J. Biol. Chem.,* 249:959.

93. Bonsignore, A., and DeFlora, A. (1972): Regulatory properties of glucose-6-phosphate dehydrogenase. *Curr. Top. Cell. Regul.,* 6:21.

94. Krebs, H. A., and Eggleston, L. V. (1974): The regulation of the pentose phosphate cycle in rat liver. *Adv. Enzyme Regul.,* 12:421.

95. Levy, H. R. (1979): Glucose-6-phosphate dehydrogenases. In: *Advances in Enzymology, Vol. 48,* edited by A. Meister, p. 97. Wiley, New York.

96. Wyngaarden, J. B., and Kelley, W. N. (1978): Gout. In: *The Metabolic Basis of Inherited Disease,* fourth edition, edited by J. B. Stanbury, J. B. Wyngaarden, and D. S. Fredrickson, p. 916. McGraw-Hill, New York.

97. Howell, R. R. (1978): The glycogen storage diseases. In: *The Metabolic Basis of Inherited Disease,* fourth edition, edited by J. B. Stanbury, J. B. Wyngaarden, and D. S. Frederickson, p. 137. McGraw-Hill, New York.

98. Van Lan, V., Yamaguchi, N., Garcia, M. J., Ramey, E. R., and Penhos, J. C. (1974): Effect of hypophysectomy and adrenalectomy on glucagon and insulin concentration. *Endocrinology,* 94:671.

99. Whitton, P. D., and Hems, D. A. (1976): Glycogen synthesis in the perfused liver of adrenalectomized rats. *Biochem. J.,* 156:585.

100. Seifter, S., Harkness, D. M., Rubin, L., and Muntwyler, E. (1948): The nicotinic acid, riboflavin, D-amino acid oxidase, and arginase levels of the livers of rats on a protein-free diet. *J. Biol. Chem.,* 176:1371.

101. Stetten, DeW., Jr., and Stetten, M. R. (1960): Glycogen metabolism. *Physiol. Rev.,* 40:505.

102. Ruderman, N. B., Aoki, T. T., and Cahill, G. F., Jr. (1976): Gluconeogenesis and its disorders in man. In: *Gluconeogenesis: Its Regulation in Mammalian Species,* edited by R. W. Hanson and M. A. Mehlman, p. 515. Wiley, New York.

103. Fischer, E. H., Heilmeyer, L. M. G., Jr., and Haschke, R. H. (1971): Phosphorylase and the control of glycogen degradation. *Curr. Top. Cell. Regul.,* 4:211.

104. Larner, J., and Villar-Palasi, C. (1971): Glycogen synthase and its control. *Curr. Top. Cell. Regul.,* 3:195.

105. Stalmans, W., and Hers, H. G. (1973): Glycogen synthesis from UDPG. In: *The Enzymes, Vol. IX,* third edition, edited by P. D. Boyer, p. 309. Academic Press, New York.

106. Hers, H. G. (1976): The control of glycogen metabolism in the liver. *Ann. Rev. Biochem.,* 45:167.

107. Nimmo, H., and Cohen, P. (1977): Hormonal control of protein phosphorylation. *Adv. Cyclic Nucleotide Res.,* 8:145.

108. Larner, J., Lawrence, J. C., Walkenbach, R. J., Roach, P. J., Hazen, R. J., and Huang, L. C. (1978): Insulin control of glycogen synthesis. *Adv. Cyclic Nucleotide Res.,* 9:425.

109. Cohen, P. (1978): The role of cyclic-AMP-dependent protein kinase in the regulation of glycogen metabolism in mammalian skeletal muscle. *Curr. Top. Cell. Regul.,* 14:117.

110. Cohen, P. (1979): The hormonal control of glycogen metabolism in mammalian muscle by multivalent phosphorylation. *Biochem. Soc. Trans.,* 7:16.

111. Cohen, P. (1980): Well established systems of enzyme regulation by reversible phosphorylation. In: *Molecular Aspects of Cellular Regulation, Vol. 1, Recently Discovered Systems of Enzyme Regulation by Reversible Phosphorylation,* edited by P. Cohen, p. 1. Elsevier, Amsterdam.

112. Cohen, P. (1980): The role of calmodulin and troponin in the regulation of phosphorylase kinase from mammalian skeletal muscle. In: *Calcium and Cell Function, Vol. 1, Calmodulin,* edited by W. Y. Cheung, p. 183. Academic Press, New York.

113. Cohen, P. (1980): Protein phosphorylation and the coordinated control of intermediary metabolism. In: *Molecular Aspects of Cellular Regulation, Vol. 1, Recently Discovered*

Systems of Enzyme Regulation by Reversible Phosphorylation, edited by P. Cohen, p. 255. Elsevier, Amsterdam.

114. Hems, D. A., and Whitton, P. D. (1980): Control of hepatic glycogenolysis. *Physiol. Rev.,* 60:1.

115. Roach, P. J. (1981): Glycogen synthase and glycogen synthase kinases. *Curr. Top. Cell. Regul.,* 20:45.

116. Unger, R. H. (1974): Alpha- and beta-cell interrelationships in health and disease. *Metabolism,* 23:581.

117. Van Golde, L. M. G., and Van Den Bergh, S. G. (1977): Liver. In: *Lipid Metabolism in Mammals-1,* edited by F. Snyder, p. 35. Plenum, New York.

118. McGarry, J. D., and Foster, D. W. (1977): Hormonal control of ketogenesis. Biochemical considerations. *Arch. Intern. Med.,* 137:495.

119. McGarry, J. D., and Foster, D. W. (1980): Regulation of hepatic fatty acid oxidation and ketone body production. *Ann. Rev. Biochem.,* 49:395.

120. Robinson, A. M., and Williamson, D. H. (1980): Physiological roles of ketone bodies as substrates and signals in mammalian tissues. *Physiol. Rev.,* 60:143.

121. Lane, M. D., and Mooney, R. A. (1981): Tricarboxylic acid cycle intermediates and the control of fatty acid synthesis and ketogenesis. *Curr. Top. Cell. Regul.,* 18:221.

122. Jeffcoat, R. (1979): The biosynthesis of unsaturated fatty acids and its control in mammalian liver. In: *Essays in Biochemistry, Vol. 15,* edited by P. N. Campbell and R. D. Marshall, p. 1. Academic Press, New York.

123. Mooney, R. A., and Lane, M. D. (1981): Formation and turnover of triglyceride-rich vesicles in the chick liver cell. *J. Biol. Chem.,* 256:11724.

124. McGarry, J. D., Takabayashi, Y., and Foster, D. W. (1978): The role of malonyl-CoA in the coordination of fatty acid synthesis and oxidation in isolated rat hepatocytes. *J. Biol. Chem.,* 253:8294.

125. McGarry, J. D., and Foster, D. W. (1979): In support of the roles of malonyl-CoA and carnitine acyltransferase I in the regulation of hepatic fatty acid oxidation and ketogenesis. *J. Biol. Chem.,* 254:8163.

126. Green, A., and Newsholme, E. A. (1979): Sensitivity of glucose uptake and lipolysis of white adipocytes of the rat to insulin and effects of some metabolites. *Biochem. J.,* 180:365.

127. Stanley, J. C. (1981): The glucose-fatty acid-ketone body cycle. *Br. J. Anaesth.,* 53:131.

128. Wieland, O., Weiss, L., and Eger-Neufeldt, I. (1964): Enzymatic regulation of liver acetyl-CoA metabolism in relation to ketogenesis. *Adv. Enzyme Regul.,* 2:85.

129. Williamson, J. R., Kreisberg, R. A., and Felts, P. W. (1966): Mechanism for the stimulation of gluconeogenesis by fatty acids in perfused rat liver. *Proc. Natl. Acad. Sci. USA,* 56:247.

130. Krebs, H. A. (1966): The regulation of the release of ketone bodies by the liver. *Adv. Enzyme Regul.,* 4:339.

131. Tolbert, N. E. (1981): Metabolic pathways in peroxisomes and glyoxysomes. *Ann. Rev. Biochem.,* 50:133.

132. Cooper, T. G., and Beevers, H. (1969): Mitochondria and glyoxysomes from castor bean endosperm. Enzyme constituents and catalytic capacity. *J. Biol. Chem.,* 244:3507.

133. Cooper, T. G., and Beevers, H. (1969): β-Oxidation in glyoxysomes from castor bean endosperm. *J. Biol. Chem.,* 244:3514.

134. Graves, L. B., and Becker, W. M. (1974): Beta-oxidation in glyoxysomes from *Euglena. J. Protozool.,* 21:771.

135. Blum, J. J. (1973): Localization of some enzymes of β-oxidation of fatty acids in the peroxisomes of *Tetrahymena. J. Protozool.,* 20:688.

136. Hyrb, D. J., and Hogg, J. F. (1976): A peroxisomal fatty acyl-coenzyme A oxidase in *Tetrahymena pyriformis. Fed. Proc.,* 35:1501.

137. Lazarow, P., and de Duve, C. (1976): A fatty acyl-CoA oxidizing system in rat liver peroxisomes; enhancement by clofibrate, a hypolipidemic drug. *Proc. Natl. Acad. Sci. USA,* 73:2043.

138. Lazarow, P. B. (1978): Rat liver peroxisomes catalyze the beta oxidation of fatty acids. *J. Biol. Chem.,* 253:1522.

139. Osumi, T., and Hashimoto, T. (1978): Acyl-CoA oxidase of rat liver: A new enzyme for fatty acid oxidation. *Biochem. Biophys. Res. Commun.,* 83:479.

140. Osumi, T., and Hashimoto, T. (1978): Enhancement of fatty acyl-CoA oxidizing activity in rat liver peroxisomes by di-(2-ethylhexyl) phthalate. *J. Biochem.,* 83:1361.

141. Murphy, P. A., Krahling, J. B., Gee, R., Kirk, J. R., and Tolbert, N. E. (1979): Enzyme activities of isolated hepatic peroxisomes from genetically lean and obese male mice. *Arch. Biochem. Biophys.,* 193:179.

142. Bronfman, M., Inestrosa, N. C., and Leighton, F. (1979): Fatty acid oxidation by human liver peroxisomes. *Biochem. Biophys. Res. Commun.,* 88:1030.

143. Moody, D. E., and Reddy, J. K. (1974): Increase in hepatic carnitine acyltransferase activity associated with peroxisomal (microbody) proliferation induced by the hypolipidemic drugs clofibrate, nafenopin, and methyl clofenapate. *Res. Commun. Chem. Pathol. Pharmacol.,* 9:501.

144. Markwell, M. A. K., McGroarty, E. J., Bieber, L. L., and Tolbert, N. E. (1973): The subcellular distribution of carnitine acyltransferases in mammalian liver and kidney. A new peroxisomal enzyme. *J. Biol. Chem.,* 248:3426.

145. Markwell, M. A. K., Bieber, L. L., and Tolbert, N. E. (1977): Differential increase of hepatic peroxisomal, mitochondrial and microsomal carnitine acyltransferases in clofibrate-fed rats. *Biochem. Pharmacol.,* 26:1697.

146. Osumi, T., and Hashimoto, T. (1979): Subcellular distribution of the enzymes of the fatty acyl-CoA beta-oxidation system and their induction by di(2-ethylhexyl) phthalate in rat liver. *J. Biochem.,* 85:131.

147. Osmundsen, H., Neat, C. E., and Norum, K. R. (1979): Peroxisomal oxidation of long chain fatty acids. *FEBS Lett.,* 99:292.

148. Appelkvist, E. L., and Dallner, G. (1980): Possible involvement of fatty acid binding protein in peroxisomal β-oxidation of fatty acids. *Biochim. Biophys. Acta,* 617:156.

149. Osmundsen, H., and Neat, C. E. (1979): Regulation of peroxisomal fatty acid oxidation. *FEBS Lett.,* 107:81.

150. Osmundsen, H., Neat, C. E. and Borrebaek, B. (1980): Fatty acid products of peroxisomal β-oxidation. *Int. J. Biochem.,* 12:625.

151. Bieber, L. L., Krahling, J. B., Clarke, P. R. H., Valkner, K. J., and Tolbert, N. E. (1981): Carnitine acyltransferases in rat liver peroxisomes. *Arch. Biochem. Biophys.,* 211:599.

152. Kondrup, J., and Lazarow, P. B. (1981): Flux of palmitoyl-CoA through peroxisomal and mitochondrial β-oxidation in isolated hepatocytes. International Conference on Peroxisomes and Glyoxysomes, Sept. 9–11. *NY Acad. Sci. (Abstr.).*

153. Neat, C. E., Thomassen, M. S., and Osmundsen, H. (1980): Induction of peroxisomal β-oxidation in rat liver by high-fat diets. *Biochem. J.,* 186:369.

154. Reed, L. J. (1969): Pyruvate dehydrogenase complex. *Curr. Top. Cell. Regul.* 1:233.

155. Wieland, O. H., Siess, E. A., Weiss, L., Löffler, G., Patzelt, C., Portenhauser, R., Hartman, V., and Schirmann, A. (1973): Regulation of the mammalian pyruvate dehydrogenase complex by covalent modification. *Symp. Soc. Exp. Biol.,* 27:371.

156. Numa, S. and Yamashita, S. (1974): Regulation of lipogenesis in animal tissues. *Curr. Top. Cell. Regul.,* 8:197.

157. Reed, L. J. (1981): Regulation of mammalian pyruvate dehydrogenase complex by a phosphorylation-dephosphorylation cycle. *Curr. Top. Cell. Regul.,* 18:95.

158. Pratt, M. L., and Roche, T. E. (1979): Mechanism of pyruvate inhibition of kidney pyruvate dehydrogenase kinase and synergistic inhibition by pyruvate and ADP. *J. Biol. Chem.,* 254:7191.

159. Saltiel, A., Jacobs, S., Siegel, M., and Cuatrecasas, P. (1981): Insulin stimulates the release from liver plasma membranes of a chemical modulator of pyruvate dehydrogenase. *Biochem. Biophys. Res. Commun.,* 102:1041.

160. Riesenfeld, G., Wals, P. A., Golden, S., and Katz, J. (1981): Glucose, amino acids, and lipogenesis in hepatocytes of Japanese quail. *J. Biol. Chem.,* 256:9973.

161. Atkinson, D. E., and Camien, M. E. (1982): The role of urea synthesis in the removal of metabolic bicarbonate and the regulation of blood pH. *Curr. Top. Cell. Regul.,* 21:261.

162. McGilvery, R. W. (1970): *Biochemistry, a Functional Approach,* first edition. Saunders, Philadelphia.

The Liver: Biology and Pathobiology, edited by
I. Arias, H. Popper, D. Schachter, and D. A. Shafritz.
Raven Press, New York © 1982.

Chapter 14

Urea Synthesis and Ammonia Metabolism

Sue G. Powers and Alton Meister

Ammonia plays a central role in nitrogen metabolism. It is both a product of protein and nucleic acid catabolism and a precursor of nonessential amino acids, nucleic acids, and certain other nitrogenous compounds. The liver is a major site of ammonia metabolism. The steady-state level of ammonia in liver is about 0.7 mM; that in blood plasma is about 10-fold lower. These values represent the total of NH_3 (the form that can freely diffuse across cell membranes) and NH_4^+. About 1% of ammonia is uncharged at physiological pH ($pK_a = 9.25$).

A general scheme for the metabolism of ammonia in the liver is given in Fig. 1. The major features include: (a) release of nitrogen from amino acids, nucleic acid bases, and amines in the form of ammonia or glutamate; (b) deamination of glutamate through the action of glutamate dehydrogenase; (c) conversion of ammonia to urea; (d) conversion of urea to ammonia in the gastrointestinal tract by the action of bacterial urease, and (e) synthesis of glutamine (glutamine serves as a storage and transport form of ammonia).

SOURCES OF AMMONIA IN THE LIVER

Ammonia Derived from the Degradation of Amino Acids, Amines, and Nucleic Acids

Substantial amounts of hepatic ammonia arise from the oxidative deamination of glutamate catalyzed by glutamate dehydrogenase (1), which catalyzes reaction [1]. Glutamate dehydrogenase is localized primarily in the mitochondrial matrix, and under these conditions, the system seems to be close to equilibrium. Although the position of the equilibrium is unfavorable for deamination, the reaction is pulled toward ammonia formation by removal of the products. As discussed below, glutamate dehydrogenase, by the reverse of reaction [1], may also function to remove

$$^-OOC-CH_2-CH_2-\overset{\overset{\displaystyle NH_3^+}{|}}{C}H-COO^- + NAD(P)^+ \rightleftharpoons {}^-OOC-CH_2-CH_2-\overset{\overset{\displaystyle O}{\|}}{C}-COO^- + NH_4^+ + NAD(P)H + H^+ \qquad [1]$$

glutamate α-ketoglutarate

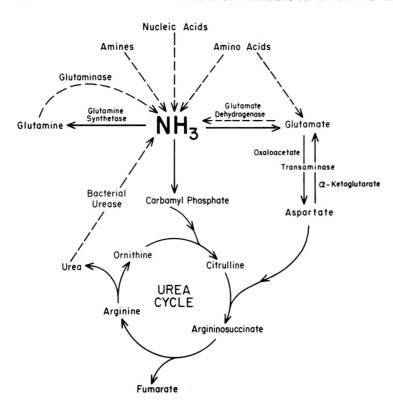

FIG. 1. General scheme of ammonia metabolism in the liver. *Broken arrows*, pathways of ammonia formation; *solid arrows*, pathways of ammonia utilization.

hepatic ammonia. Definition of the exact metabolic role of this enzyme is complicated by a number of factors that regulate its activity (2). NAD and NADP function about equally well as coenzymes. Guanosine nucleotides and ATP strongly inhibit activity, whereas AMP and ADP activate. These purine nucleotide effects vary depending on whether NAD or NADP is the coenzyme and whether other purine nucleotides are present. The enzyme undergoes reversible polymerization, which influences the activity of the enzyme and is affected by the presence of pyrimidine and purine nucleotides.

Other enzymatic reactions that take place in liver and lead to release of significant amounts of ammonia are listed in Table 1. Deamidation reactions comprise one class of ammonia-producing reactions (3). Ammonia may be cleaved from the amide group of glutamine (no. 1, Table 1), asparagine (no. 2, Table 1), or the α-keto analogs of glutamine and asparagine (no. 3, Table 1). Glutamine and asparagine residues within proteins are also subject to deamidation, but the mechanisms of such reactions are not yet known. The utilization of free glutamine constitutes another major source of hepatic ammonia.

The pyridoxal-phosphate-dependent deamination reactions form a second category of ammonia-producing reactions (3); thus ammonia is eliminated from serine, threonine, cysteine, cystathionine, and homoserine (nos. 4–6, Table 1). Ammonia is also released from histidine in a nonoxidative deamination reaction (no. 7, Table 1), but histidine ammonia lyase

acts by an active site dehydroalanine residue and does not use pyridoxal phosphate.

A flavin-dependent enzyme catalyzing oxidative deamination reactions, D-amino acid oxidase (no. 8, Table 1), acts on a number of D-amino acids and on the nonchiral amino acid, glycine (3); presumably, this oxidase serves to degrade D-amino acids derived from exogenous sources, such as the diet and bacterial cell walls. An L-amino acid oxidase activity is also present in liver, but its low activity suggests that it is probably not quantitatively significant in producing ammonia. Amino oxidase(s) (no. 9, Table 1) deaminate a number of mono- and diamines including epinephrine, norepinephrine, and serotonin.

Another category of ammonia-releasing reactions is hydrolytic deamination of nucleic acid bases and their derivatives (nos. 10–13, Table 1). Of these reactions, AMP-deaminase is quantitatively most significant (1,4).

Ammonia Derived from Glutamate via Glutamate Dehydrogenase

Initially the catabolism of protein leads to much more glutamate than ammonia. As discussed above, ammonia may be derived directly from such glutamate by the action of glutamate dehydrogenase. Glutamate is formed by transamination reactions between α-ketoglutarate and amino acids released by hydrolysis of proteins (reaction [2]). Although the number, specificity, and subcellular localization of amino acid trans-

TABLE 1. *Ammonia-producing hepatic enzymatic reactions*

1. Glutaminase

$$\underset{\text{Glutamine}}{H_2N-\overset{\overset{\displaystyle O}{\|}}{C}-CH_2-CH_2-\overset{\overset{\displaystyle NH_3^+}{|}}{CH}-COO^-} \rightarrow \underset{\text{Glutamate}}{^-OOC-CH_2-CH_2-\overset{\overset{\displaystyle NH_3^+}{|}}{CH}-COO^-} + NH_4^+$$

2. Asparaginase

$$\underset{\text{Asparagine}}{H_2N-\overset{\overset{\displaystyle O}{\|}}{C}-CH_2-\overset{\overset{\displaystyle NH_3^+}{|}}{CH}-COO^-} \rightarrow \underset{\text{Aspartate}}{^-OOC-CH_2-\overset{\overset{\displaystyle NH_3^+}{|}}{CH}-COO^-} + NH_4^+$$

3. ω-Amidase

$$\underset{\alpha\text{-Ketoglutaramate}}{H_2N-\overset{\overset{\displaystyle O}{\|}}{C}-CH_2-CH_2-\overset{\overset{\displaystyle O}{\|}}{C}-COO^-} + H_2O \rightarrow \underset{\alpha\text{-Ketoglutarate}}{^-OOC-CH_2-CH_2-\overset{\overset{\displaystyle O}{\|}}{C}-COO^-} + NH_4^+$$

$$\underset{\alpha\text{-Ketosuccinamate}}{H_2N-\overset{\overset{\displaystyle O}{\|}}{C}-CH_2-\overset{\overset{\displaystyle O}{\|}}{C}-COO^-} + H_2O \rightarrow \underset{\text{Oxaloacetate}}{^-OOC-CH_2-\overset{\overset{\displaystyle O}{\|}}{C}-COO^-} + NH_4^+$$

4. Serine, threonine dehydrases

$$\underset{\text{Serine}}{^-OOC-\overset{\overset{\displaystyle NH_3^+}{|}}{CH}-CH_2OH} \rightarrow \underset{\text{Pyruvate}}{^-OOC-\overset{\overset{\displaystyle O}{\|}}{C}-CH_3} + NH_4^+$$

$$\underset{\text{Threonine}}{^-OOC-\overset{\overset{\displaystyle NH_3^+}{|}}{CH}-\underset{\underset{\displaystyle OH}{|}}{CH}-CH_3} \rightarrow \underset{\alpha\text{-Ketobutyrate}}{^-OOC-\overset{\overset{\displaystyle O}{\|}}{C}-CH_2-CH_3} + NH_4^+$$

5. Cysteine desulfhydrase

$$\underset{\text{Cysteine}}{HS-CH_2-\overset{\overset{\displaystyle NH_3^+}{|}}{CH}-COO^-} + H_2O \rightarrow \underset{\text{Pyruvate}}{CH_3-\overset{\overset{\displaystyle O}{\|}}{C}-COO^-} + NH_4^+ + H_2S$$

6. Cystathionine γ-lyase

$$\underset{\text{Cystathionine}}{^-OOC-\overset{\overset{\displaystyle NH_3^+}{|}}{CH}-CH_2-CH_2-S-CH_2-\overset{\overset{\displaystyle NH_3^+}{|}}{CH}-COO^-} + H_2O \rightarrow \underset{\alpha\text{-Ketobutyrate}}{^-OOC-\overset{\overset{\displaystyle O}{\|}}{C}-CH_2-CH_3} + \underset{\underset{\displaystyle \underset{NH_3^+}{|}}{\text{Cysteine}}}{HS-CH_2-CH-COO^-} + NH_4^+$$

$$\underset{\text{Homoserine}}{^-OOC-\overset{\overset{\displaystyle NH_3^+}{|}}{CH}-CH_2-CH_2-OH} \rightarrow \underset{\alpha\text{-Ketobutyrate}}{^-OOC-\overset{\overset{\displaystyle O}{\|}}{C}-CH_2-CH_3} + NH_4^+$$

Table 1—continued

TABLE 1—*Continued*

7. Histidine ammonia-lyase

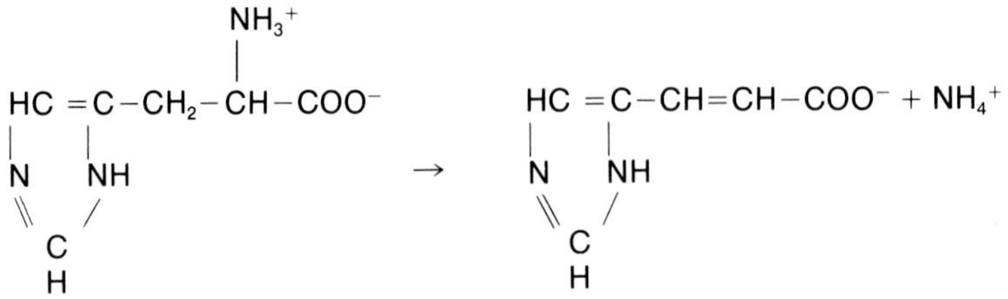

$$HC=C-CH_2-\overset{\overset{\displaystyle NH_3^+}{|}}{CH}-COO^- \quad \rightarrow \quad HC=C-CH=CH-COO^- + NH_4^+$$

Histidine   Urocanate

8. D-Amino acid oxidase (acts on many D-amino acids and on glycine)

$$H_3^+N-CH_2-COO^- + 1/2\,O_2 \rightarrow H-\overset{\overset{\displaystyle O}{\|}}{C}-COO^- + NH_4^+$$

Glycine   Glyoxalate

9. Amine oxidase

$$RCH_2NH_3^+ + O_2 + H_2O \rightarrow RCHO + NH_4^+ + H_2O_2$$

10. AMP deaminase

$$AMP + H_2O \rightarrow IMP + NH_4^+$$

11. Adenosine deaminase

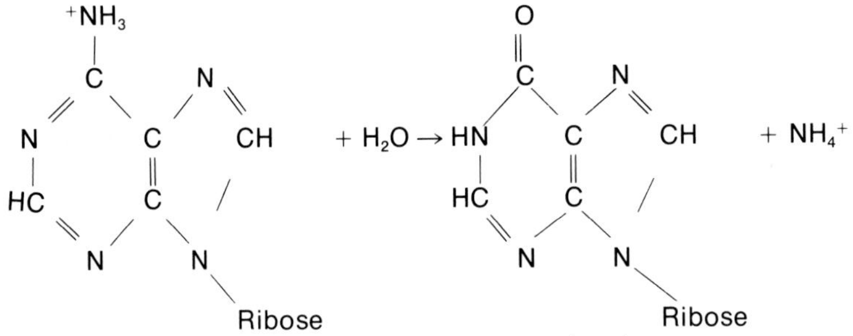

Adenosine $+ H_2O \rightarrow$ Inosine $+ NH_4^+$

12. Guanine deaminase

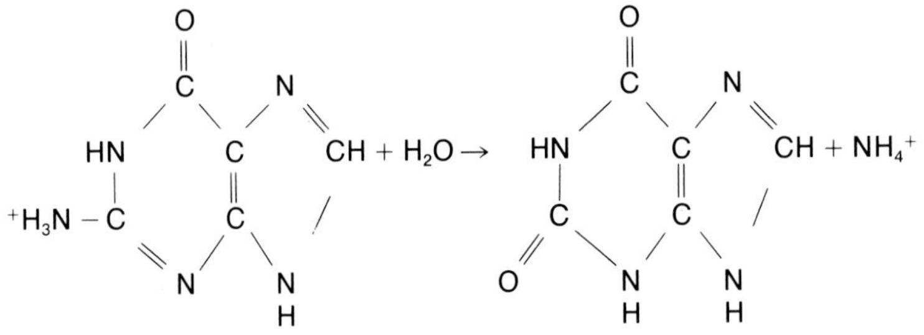

Guanine $+ H_2O \rightarrow$ Xanthine $+ NH_4^+$

13. Cytosine deaminase

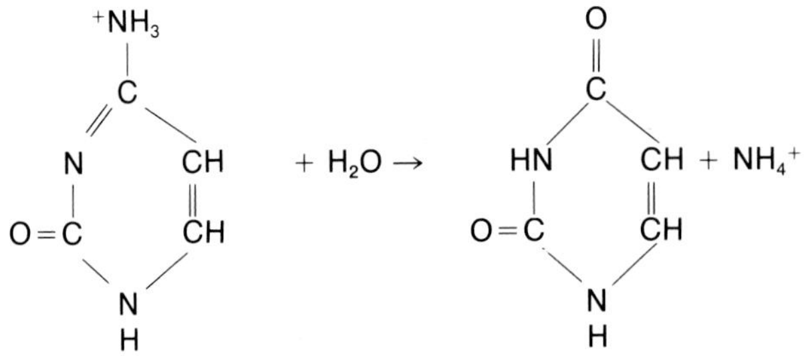

Cystosine $+ H_2O \rightarrow$ Uracil $+ NH_4^+$

$$\overset{O}{\overset{\|}{^-OOC-C-CH_2-CH_2-COO^-}} + \overset{NH_3{}^+}{\overset{|}{^-OOC-CH-R}} \rightleftharpoons \overset{NH_3{}^+}{\overset{|}{^-OOC-CH-CH_2-CH_2-COO^-}} + \overset{O}{\overset{\|}{^-OOC-C-R}} \qquad [2]$$

α-ketoglutarate　　　　　　amino acid　　　　　　　　　glutamate　　　　keto acid

aminases are still not fully defined, it has been clear since Schoenheimer's pioneering work with heavy isotopes (5) that all of the amino acids except lysine and threonine undergo reversible transamination. The deamination of amino acids occurs largely through transfer of the amino group to α-ketoglutarate to form glutamate. Glutamate is also derived directly from the hydrolysis of protein and in the degradation of proline, histidine, and glutamine.

Ammonia Derived from Bacterial Degradation of Urea in the Gastrointestinal Tract

The hydrolysis of urea by organisms of the intestinal flora is a quantitatively significant source of hepatic ammonia; at least 25% of the urea produced is degraded by bacterial urease. It appears that urea diffuses from the liver into the circulating blood, is hy-

drolyzed by bacteria at a mucosal or juxtamucosal location in the colon and elsewhere in the gastrointestinal tract, and the ammonia thus generated diffuses into the portal blood and is transported to the liver, where it is reconverted to urea (6).

OVERVIEW OF UREA SYNTHESIS

The urea cycle operates in a tightly controlled manner to dispose of approximately 90% of the surplus nitrogen in ureotelic organisms. As shown in Fig. 2, urea is formed from ammonia and CO_2 in a cyclical process in which ornithine, citrulline, argininosuccinate, and arginine are carrier compounds. The five steps of the urea cycle are catalyzed by the following enzymes: (a) carbamylphosphate synthetase, (b) ornithine transcarbamylase, (c) argininosuccinate synthetase, (d) argininosuccinase, and (e) arginase. *N*-

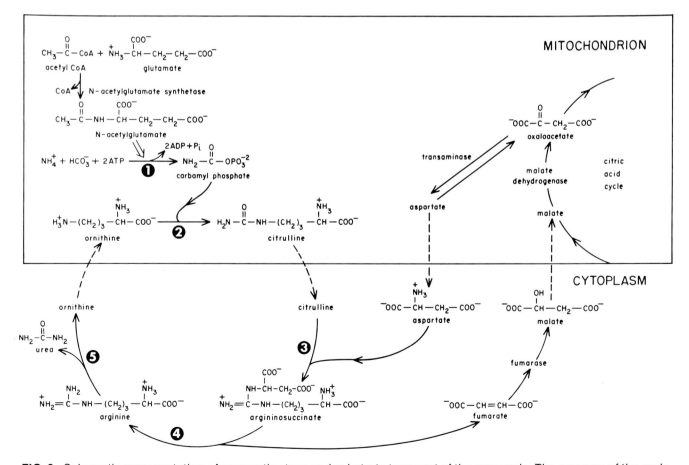

FIG. 2. Schematic representation of enzymatic steps and substrate transport of the urea cycle. The enzymes of the cycle are **(1)** carbamylphosphate synthetase I, **(2)** ornithine transcarbamylase, **(3)** argininosuccinate synthetase, **(4)** argininosuccinase, and **(5)** arginase. *Broken arrows,* transport across the mitochondrial membrane; *double arrow,* essential activation of reaction [1] by *N*-acetylglutamate.

Acetylglutamate synthetase catalyzes an essential auxiliary step of the cycle; the product of this reaction, N-acetylglutamate, is a required cofactor (see below) for carbamylphosphate synthetase. Half of the urea nitrogen is derived from free NH_3 (step 1) and half from aspartate (step 3). The aspartate is replenished by way of the citric acid cycle (Fig. 2); the fumarate released at step 4 of the urea cycle yields oxaloacetate via the citric acid cycle. The oxaloacetate is then transaminated to aspartate (by glutamate-aspartate transaminase, reaction 2). A total of four high-energy phosphate equivalents is thus required per urea molecule synthesized. Two molecules of ATP are cleaved to two molecules of ADP and inorganic phosphate in step 1, and one molecule of ATP is cleaved to AMP and pyrophosphate in step 3. Pyrophosphate is cleaved by pyrophosphatase to yield orthophosphate. The synthesis of urea may seem inefficient from the energetic standpoint. In the course of evolution, however, the single enzymatic step catalyzed by arginase may have been added to a preexisting multienzyme biosynthetic pathway for arginine.

The liver is the only organ quantitatively important in urea synthesis, although arginine biosynthesis, by steps 3–4 of the urea cycle (Fig. 2) occurs in many extrahepatic tissues. Subcellular localization also plays an important role in the functioning of the urea cycle in that the first two steps of the urea cycle, as well as that catalyzed by N-acetylglutamate synthetase, occur in the mitochondrial matrix, whereas the remaining enzymes are cytosolic. This split localization requires that, during operation of the urea cycle, ornithine enters and citrulline leaves the mitochondrion. It seems that ornithine can be transported across the mitochondrial membrane by two unidirectional processes, an ornithine/citrulline exchange system and an ornithine/H^+ exchange system, whereas citrulline is transported across the membrane in either direction, via a carrier specific for certain neutral amino acids (7). It is also necessary for fumarate to be converted to malate (Fig. 2), which can be transported into the mitochondrial matrix by several anion carriers (which have been denoted as dicarboxylate, tricarboxylate, or α-ketoglutarate carriers), which promote exchange between anions (7). In the matrix, malate is converted to aspartate, which must then return to the cytoplasm, apparently via either a glutamate/H^+ carrier or an aspartate/glutamate exchange system (7). Moreover, the enzymes, carbamylphosphate synthetase and ornithine transcarbamylase, are synthesized on cytosolic ribosomes in the form of precursors approximately 4,000 to 5,5000 daltons larger than the mitochondrial

forms of the enzymes and are transported, by an as yet undefined process, into the mitochondrial matrix.

In addition to the principal functions of nitrogen disposal and ammonia detoxication, the urea cycle probably plays a role in maintaining pH homostasis, since one proton is released per turn of the urea cycle (reaction [3]).

PROPERTIES OF THE UREA CYCLE ENZYMES

Each of the urea cycle enzymes has been purified to homogeneity from rat and/or bovine liver and has been studied fairly extensively (8). With the exception of argininosuccinase, the enzymes have also been purified from human liver. Preliminary data on their properties agree well with those on the other mammalian enzymes. The catalytic and physical properties of the urea cycle enzymes are outlined in Table 2.

Carbamylphosphate Synthetase

Formation of carbamylphosphate constitutes the first step of two biosynthetic pathways, one leading to urea (and arginine), and the other to pyrimidines, as shown in Fig. 3. Bacteria possess a single carbamylphosphate synthetase that provides carbamylphosphate for both pathways. This enzyme can utilize both ammonia and glutamine as nitrogen donors but has a much higher K_m value for ($NH_3 + NH_4^+$) than for glutamine. Eukaryotes have two carbamylphosphate synthetases, each being pathway specific. The enzyme that provides carbamylphosphate for pyrimidine biosynthesis (carbamylphosphate synthetase II) is localized in the cytoplasm and is present in all of the wide variety of organisms and tissues that have been examined. Carbamylphosphate synthetase II has the same nitrogen donor specificity as the bacterial enzyme. The synthetase involved in the urea cycle (carbamylphosphate synthetase I) is found only in the liver mitochondria of ureotelic vertebrates and in the earthworm. Carbamylphosphate synthetase I (8,9) only utilizes ammonia as the nitrogen donor and requires N-acetyl-glutamate as an allosteric cofactor (reaction [4]).

Early preparations of mammalian carbamylphosphate synthetase I were unstable. Currently used purification procedures start with cell fractionation techniques that yield a clean separation of mitochondria; the previously observed instability was apparently due largely to the presence of proteolytic enzymes derived from lysosomes and other organelles.

$$3\,ATP^{-4} + 2\,NH_4^+ + HCO_3^- \rightarrow NH_2 - \overset{\overset{\textstyle O}{\|}}{C} - NH_2 + 2\,H_2O + H^+ + 2\,ADP^{-2} + AMP^{-1} + 4P_i^{-2} \qquad [3]$$

TABLE 2. *Catalytic and physical properties of the purified urea cycle enzymes*

Enzyme	Source	Cellular localization	Monomeric unit	Oligomeric unit	Specific activity (μmoles/min/ mg, 37°C)	Substrate, K_m (mM)
Carbamylphosphate synthetase I	Rat, bovine, and human liver	Mitochondrial matrix	160,000– 165,000	?	1.87–5	MgATP, 1; NH_4^+, 0.4–2; HCO_3^-, 5
Ornithine trans-carbamylase	Rat, bovine, and human liver	Mitochondrial matrix	36,000– 40,000	Trimer, 108,000– 120,000	233–920	Carbamylphosphate, 0.03; ornithine, 0.4
Argininosuccinate synthetase	Rat, bovine, and human liver	Cytoplasm	45,000	Tetramer, 180,000	2.1–4.2	Citrulline, 0.044; aspartate, 0.02–0.04; MgATP, 0.15–0.32
Argininosuccinase	Bovine liver	Cytoplasm	50,000	Tetramer, 200,000	22.5	Argininosuccinate, 0.01
Arginase	Rat, bovine, and human liver	Cytoplasm	30,000	Tetramer, 120,000	47,000	Arginine, 10

Carbamylphosphate synthetase I not only has the highest molecular weight chain in the mitochondrion, it is also quantitatively the major mitochondrial protein, making up 15 to 20% of the total protein in the mitochondrial matrix and having an estimated *in vivo* concentration of 70 mg/ml (10). As noted earlier, an approximately 170,000 dalton carbamylphosphate synthetase I precursor is synthesized in the cytosol (11).

The reaction catalyzed by carbamylphosphate synthetase is exceptional in that two molecules of MgATP

(12,13) are required to form one molecule of the product carbamylphosphate, and in that biotin is not required for bicarbonate activation (13a). The two molecules of MgATP are used in separate steps. One MgATP is used for activation of bicarbonate to form enzyme-bound carboxyphosphate (14–16). The carboxyphosphate and ammonia then react on the enzyme surface to form carbamate, with release of P_i. The second molecule of MgATP is used for phosphorylation of enzyme-bound carbamate to form carbamylphosphate

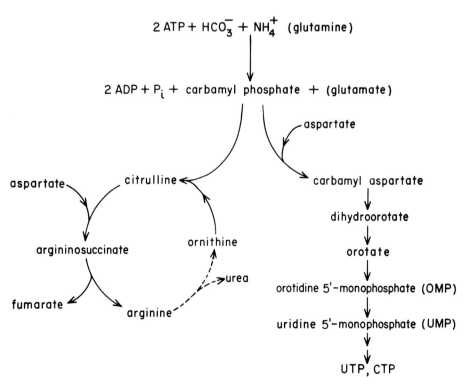

FIG. 3. Generalized biosynthetic pathways for arginine and/or urea and for pyrimidine nucleotides. Arginase, which catalyzes the reaction indicated by the dotted line, occurs in the liver where a complete urea cycle exists.

$$NH_4^+ + HCO_3^- + 2\ MgATP^{-2} \xrightarrow[\text{K}^+,\ \text{Mg}^{2+}]{\text{N-acetylglutamate}} NH_2-\overset{\overset{\displaystyle O}{\|}}{C}-O-\overset{\overset{\displaystyle O}{\|}}{\underset{\underset{\displaystyle O^-}{|}}{P}}-O^- + 2\ MgADP^{-1} + P_i^{-2} + 2\ H^+ \qquad [4]$$

and MgADP. The fact that two molecules of ATP are cleaved makes the reaction essentially irreversible.

K$^+$ and free Mg^{2+} are required for the activity of carbamylphosphate synthetase I and appear to act as allosteric effectors, which increase the affinity of the enzyme for MgATP. An N-acylglutamate compound is absolutely required for carbamylphosphate synthetase I activity; N-acetylglutamate seems to be the natural cofactor since it is the most effective compound tested and shares a mitochondrial localization with carbamylphosphate synthetase I (17). *N*-Acetylglutamate apparently does not function chemically in the carbamylphosphate synthetase I reaction but induces a required conformational change in the enzyme. It has been established that the unprotonated form of ammonia is the true substrate of carbamylphosphate synthetase I (18).

Ornithine Transcarbamylase

The reaction catalyzed by ornithine transcarbamylase (8,19) is given in reaction [5]. The equilibrium of this reaction strongly favors citrulline formation, with a K$_{Eq}$ of 100,000 (37°C, pH 6.7).

Like carbamylphosphate synthetase I, ornithine transcarbamylase is a major protein component of the mitochondrial matrix, constituting 3 to 4% of the matrix protein and having an approximate *in vivo* con-

centration of 15 mg/ml (20). It is synthesized in the cytoplasm as a 4,000 dalton precursor which is transported into the mitochondrion (21). The inhibitors, norvaline and δ-*N*-(phosphonacetyl)-L-ornithine, have served as useful tools in the study of ornithine transcarbamylase. The trimeric structure of ornithine transcarbamylase is noteworthy, since protein trimers have been found to occur only rarely.

Argininosuccinate Synthetase

The reaction catalyzed by argininosuccinate synthetase (8) is given in reaction [6]. In contrast to the first two steps of the urea cycle, this reaction is freely reversible. However, cleavage of the product pyrophosphate by pyrophosphatase pulls the reaction strongly toward argininosuccinate formation. High concentrations of a number of amino acids inhibit the activity of this enzyme (22).

Argininosuccinase

Argininosuccinase (8) catalyzes the freely reversible reaction shown in reaction [7]. Argininosuccinase and argininosuccinate synthetase are found in a variety of tissues rather than being localized in the liver, as are the first two urea cycle enzymes. The conversion of

$$
\begin{array}{c}
\overset{\displaystyle NH_3^+}{|} \\
\overset{\displaystyle (CH_2)_3}{|} \\
\overset{\displaystyle HC-NH_3^+}{|} \\
COO^- \\
\text{Ornithine}
\end{array}
\quad + \;
\begin{array}{c}
\overset{\overset{\displaystyle O}{\|}}{NH_2-C-OPO_3^{-2}} \\
\text{Carbamylphosphate}
\end{array}
\; \rightleftharpoons \;
\begin{array}{c}
\overset{\overset{\displaystyle O}{\|}}{NH-C-NH_2} \\
\overset{\displaystyle |}{(CH_2)_3} \\
\overset{\displaystyle |}{HC-NH_3^+} \\
\overset{\displaystyle |}{COO^-} \\
\text{Citrulline}
\end{array}
\; + \; P_i + H^+ \qquad [5]
$$

$$
\begin{array}{c}
\overset{\displaystyle NH_2}{|} \\
\overset{\displaystyle C=O}{|} \\
\overset{\displaystyle NH}{|} \\
\overset{\displaystyle (CH_2)_3}{|} \\
H_3N^+CHCOO^- \\
\text{Citrulline}
\end{array}
\; + \;
\begin{array}{c}
\overset{\displaystyle COO^-}{|} \\
\overset{\displaystyle H_3\overset{+}{N}CH}{|} \\
\overset{\displaystyle CH_2}{|} \\
COO^- \\
\text{Aspartate}
\end{array}
\; + \; 2\ MgATP^{-2} \; \rightleftharpoons \;
\begin{array}{c}
\overset{\displaystyle ^+NH_2}{\|} \\
\overset{\displaystyle C-NH-}{|} \\
\overset{\displaystyle NH}{|} \\
\overset{\displaystyle (CH_2)_3}{|} \\
H_3^+N-CHCOO^-
\end{array}
\begin{array}{c}
\overset{\displaystyle COO^-}{|} \\
\overset{\displaystyle CH}{|} \\
\overset{\displaystyle CH_2}{|} \\
COO^- \\
\end{array}
\; + \; MgAMP^{-1} + MgPP_i^{-2} + 2\ H^+ \qquad [6] \\
\text{Argininosuccinate}
$$

$$
\begin{array}{ccc}
\overset{+}{\text{N}}\text{H}_2 \quad \text{COO}^- & & \overset{+}{\text{N}}\text{H}_2 \quad \text{COO}^- \\
\| \quad\quad | & & \| \quad\quad | \\
\text{C}-\text{NH}-\text{CH} & & \text{C}-\text{NH}_2 \quad \text{CH} \\
| \quad\quad\quad | & \rightleftharpoons & | \quad\quad\quad \| \quad\quad [7]\\
\text{NH} \quad\quad \text{CH}_2 & & \text{NH} \quad\quad + \quad \text{HC} \\
| \quad\quad\quad | & & | \quad\quad\quad | \\
(\text{CH}_2)_3 \quad \text{COO}^- & & (\text{CH}_2)_3 \quad\quad \text{COO}^- \\
| & & | \\
\text{H}_3^+\text{N}-\text{CHCOO}^- & & \text{H}_3^+\text{N}-\text{CHCOO}^-
\end{array}
$$

Argininosuccinate   Arginine   Fumarate

citrulline to arginine via argininosuccinate is required for the biosynthesis of arginine. Arginine is used as a building block of proteins and as an intermediate in the formation of creatine phosphate and related compounds. Citrulline is presumably transported by the blood from the liver to other tissues.

Arginase

Arginase (8), which catalyzes the reaction given in reaction [8], is most abundant in livers of ureotelic vertebrates although it is present in most other tissues and is found in many organisms. It is a metalloenzyme that contains 1 mole Mn^{2+} per 30,000 dalton subunit. Mn^{2+} is required for its activity.

REGULATION OF THE UREA CYCLE

The urea cycle is subject to strict regulation. Ammonia, toxic when in excess, is an essential precursor of a number of nitrogenous compounds. Thus, although there is a large flux through the urea cycle, the concentration of hepatic ammonia is maintained at a nearly constant level of about 0.7 mM. As discussed below, several types of regulation are exerted on the urea cycle in addition to the expected controls imposed by the required transport of substrates into and out of the mitochondrial matrix and by the near irreversibility of some of the enzymatic reactions.

Long-Term Adaptation: Regulation of the Amounts of Urea Cycle Enzymes

Coordinate changes in the amounts of the urea cycle enzymes carbamylphosphate synthetase I, ornithine transcarbamylase, argininosuccinate synthetase, argininosuccinase, and arginase constitute a slow response to metabolic perturbation (23,24). When the dietary protein intake of rats or primates is varied, the total hepatic content of the five urea cycle enzymes is proportional to both the protein intake and to the rate of urea excretion. Increases of two- to threefold in enzyme levels and in urea excretion rate occur with

high protein intake or starvation (leading to increased protein catabolism), and two- to fivefold decreases in both parameters occur with protein-free diets. It is noteworthy that glutamate dehydrogenase, glutamate-aspartate transaminase, and glutamate-alanine transaminase, auxiliary enzymes required for assimilation of ammonia into urea, also increase in activity during fasting, whereas many other enzymes decrease in activity. When protein intake is increased, both transaminase activities increase, but glutamate dehydrogenase activity is unchanged.

The changes in the amounts of urea cycle enzymes could be due to alterations in either the rate of protein synthesis or of that of protein breakdown, or perhaps a combination of both. The rate of enzyme synthesis is known to be the primary regulatory factor for both argininosuccinate synthetase and arginase; the same form of regulation presumably applies to the other urea cycle enzymes, since the levels are under coordinate control. Increased levels of all five enzymes also result from administration of the hormones glucagon, which is known to increase in starvation, and glucocorticosteroids, which produce tissue breakdown and an increased protein load. Under all of these conditions, 3 to 7 days are required to achieve new steady-state levels of the enzymes. A major reason for the slow response in decreasing the amounts of enzymes is that the urea cycle enzymes have relatively long half-lives, i.e., 5 to 8 days.

The levels of the five urea cycle enzymes also change coordinately during fetal and neonatal development (25). In the rat, the enzymes appear only a few days before birth; activity then increases rapidly for several weeks after birth. In human fetal liver, the enzymes are present much earlier, at about the 50th day of gestation, and the levels gradually increase throughout gestation and for a few weeks after birth.

Under conditions of either excess or limiting arginine, the level of arginase changes in a pattern different from that for the other four urea cycle enzymes. With excess arginine, there is a decrease in the activity of the first four enzymes and an increase in the activity of arginase; with limiting arginine, the changes are in the opposite direction. These findings suggest that arginine biosynthesis, which occurs when only the

$$\begin{array}{c}
\overset{+}{N}H_2 \\
\| \\
C-NH_2 \\
| \\
NH \\
| \\
(CH_2)_3 \\
| \\
H_3^+N-CHCOO^-
\end{array}
\quad + H_2O \rightarrow
\begin{array}{c}
\overset{+}{N}H_3 \\
| \\
(CH_2)_3 \\
| \\
H_3^+N-CHCOO^-
\end{array}
\quad +
\begin{array}{c}
O \\
\| \\
H_2N-C-NH_2
\end{array}
\qquad [8]$$

Arginine   Ornithine   Urea

first four enzymes of the cycle are active, may be increased at the expense of urea synthesis.

Rate-Limiting Reactions of the Urea Cycle

When the enzymes of the urea cycle are assayed in liver homogenates (26) (Table 3), it appears that argininosuccinate synthetase catalyzes the rate-limiting step of the cycle and that carbamylphosphate synthetase I and argininosuccinase activities are also close to being rate limiting, whereas the ornithine transcarbamylase and arginase activities are much higher. The specific activities of the isolated homogeneous enzymes (Table 2) follow the same general pattern.

When urea synthesis is studied *in vivo* in mice (27), the urea cycle intermediates citrulline, argininosuccinate, and arginine are found to be present in constant but very low amounts. Thus, the rate-limiting step must be the first step of the pathway, formation of carbamylphosphate by carbamylphosphate synthetase I. However, to explain the low levels of intermediates found, it appears that the activities of the other four urea cycle enzymes must also be regulated.

Regulation by Alterations of the Intracellular Substrate Levels

The major factor that accounts for the differences between the rate-limiting steps in the whole mouse studies and tissue homogenate experiments appears to be the *in vivo* substrate concentrations. The substrates which are potentially limiting compounds are given in Table 4. Carbamylphosphate synthetase I is apparently the primary site of regulation by variation of substrate concentrations. The hepatic concentrations of ammonia (0.7 mM) and of the essential effector, *N*-acetylglutamate (0.1 mM), are about equal to the K_m values, so that the enzyme can be only half saturated, at most, with each compound. The *in vivo* affinities may differ from the reported ones, however, since the latter are measured with dilute enzyme solutions, and the intracellular concentration of carbamylphosphate synthetase I is 0.4 mM. When a significant proportion of the substrate molecules can be bound to the enzyme, standard Michaelis-Menten kinetic analysis is

invalid (28). The concentrations of MgATP and free Mg^{2+} could also be suboptimal for the functioning of carbamylphosphate synthetase I.

A moderately rapid adaptation of urea cycle activity to amino acid metabolism, requiring 10 to 30 min, is mediated by *N*-acetylglutamate (27). This regulatory scheme involves the enzymes carbamylphosphate synthetase I and *N*-acetylglutamate synthetase and their respective allosteric effectors, *N*-acetylglutamate and arginine. Both *N*-acetylglutamate synthetase and its product *N*-acetylglutamate are localized in the mitochondria, along with carbamylphosphate synthetase I. *N*-Acetylglutamate synthetase interacts with arginine and glutamate, two components of the amino acid pool; glutamate is a substrate for *N*-acetylglutamate synthetase, and arginine is an allosteric effector that can increase the maximal velocity up to sixfold. *In vivo* experiments have confirmed that the synthesis of *N*-acetylglutamate is proportional both to the arginine and glutamate content of the liver and to the flux through the urea cycle. The *N*-acetylglutamate level has been shown to adapt to dietary protein intake in a manner parallel to that of the five urea cycle enzymes but within the much briefer time period of minutes rather than days. A relatively rapid response to a decrease in dietary protein is possible since the half-life of *N*-acetylglutamate in the liver is about 20 min.

TABLE 3. *Relative activity of the urea cycle enzymes in liver homogenates*

Enzyme	Activity relative to argininosuccinate synthetase activity[a]	
	Rat liver	Human liver
Carbamylphosphate synthetase I	2.65	3.1
Ornithine transcarbamylase	53	73
Argininosuccinate synthetase	1	1
Argininosuccinase	1.2	2.4
Arginase	529	956

[a] Each enzyme activity was determined under optimal assay conditions and expressed as units of activity per g liver (26).

TABLE 4. *Potentially limiting substrates of the urea cycle*

Substrate	K_m for purified enzyme (mM)	Concentration *in vivo* (mM)
NH_4^+	0.4–2.0, carbamylphosphate synthetase I	0.7
N-acetylglutamate	0.1, carbamylphosphate synthetase I	0.1
MgATP	1.0, carbamylphosphate synthetase I	8.0
Mg^{2+} (free)	0.2, carbamylphosphate synthetase I	0.3–1.0
Ornithine	1.4, ornithine transcarbamylase	0.3
Arginine	10, arginase	0.05

Ornithine transcarbamylase and arginase are also subject to regulation via substrate concentration since the normal hepatic concentrations of ornithine and arginine are lower than the K_m values for the respective enzymes (Table 4). In addition, ornithine transcarbamylase is present at a sufficiently high concentration that, as is the case with carbamylphosphate synthetase I, the *in vivo* affinities are probably different from the ones measured under *in vitro* conditions.

Immediate Adaptation: Allosteric Regulation of the Enzyme Activities

In allosteric regulation of enzyme activity, the catalytic activity is modified by a change in the conformation of the protein that is induced by the noncovalent binding of a specific metabolite at a site on the protein distinct from the catalytic site. In almost all cases, allosteric enzymes are oligomers; the substrate serves as one allosteric effector by inducing changes in the other monomeric units of the oligomer when it binds to one of the monomers. Allosteric effectors are classified as either positive, which have a stimulatory effect on catalytic activity, or negative, which inhibit the enzymatic activity. The three enzymes of the urea cycle with the lowest intrinsic activity—carbamylphosphate synthetase I, argininosuccinate synthetase, and argininosuccinase—are allosteric enzymes.

In the case of carbamylphosphate synthetase I, *in vitro* studies have shown that MgATP is a positive effector, and that pyrimidine nucleotides are negative effectors (29). These findings are consistent with *in vivo* studies that indicate that, although carbamylphosphate synthetase I functions predominantly in the urea cycle, it also plays a role in the *de novo* synthesis of pyrimidines (Fig. 3) and that the activity of carbamylphosphate synthetase I is regulated by components of the pyrimidine pathway. Carbamylphosphate synthetase I is subject to another type of immediate regulation in that the addition of ammonium salts or ornithine causes an almost instantaneous increase in the production of carbamylphosphate, and thus also of urea, *in vivo* and in liver slices, isolated hepatocytes, and perfused liver (27). Ammonia can function as a substrate to increase carbamylphosphate production,

as previously discussed. However, the mechanism of ornithine activation is not known.

Each of the three substrates of argininosuccinate synthetase—citrulline, aspartate, and MgATP—serves as a negative allosteric effector (8). The affinity of the enzyme for citrulline and aspartate increases 10- to 20-fold in going from high to low substrate concentrations; the affinity for MgATP increases threefold with decreasing MgATP concentrations. Negative allosteric regulation of enzyme activity thus greatly extends the minimum substrate concentration necessary for appreciable catalytic activity. In addition to allosteric regulation, argininosuccinate synthetase is subject to strong product inhibition by all three products—AMP, argininosuccinate, and inorganic pyrophosphate.

Argininosuccinase is also regulated by negative allosterism; thus, the affinity for argininosuccinate increases as the substrate concentration decreases (8). The number of substrate binding sites shows similar negative allosteric changes. There are two tight binding sites at low argininosuccinate concentration and four lower affinity binding sites at higher substrate concentration.

OTHER END PRODUCTS OF HEPATIC AMMONIA METABOLISM

Glutamine

Glutamine (3) is quantitatively the second major product of hepatic ammonia metabolism and serves the additional important function of storing and transporting ammonia. Glutamine synthetase catalyzes the formation of glutamine by coupling the exergonic cleavage of ATP to ADP and inorganic phosphate to the endergonic coupling of glutamate and ammonia (30), as shown in reaction [9]. The equilibrium of this reaction strongly favors glutamine synthesis. Utilization of ammonia is made even more efficient by the fact that glutamine synthetase has a low K_m (approximately 0.18 mM) for ammonia. Glutamine is transported out of the liver into the peripheral blood, where it represents approximately 20% of the total amino acid pool, and is delivered to other organs where

$$^-OOC-CH_2-CH_2-\overset{\overset{\displaystyle +NH_3}{|}}{CH}-COO^- + MgATP^{-2} + NH_4^+ \rightarrow H_2N-\overset{\overset{\displaystyle O}{\|}}{C}-CH_2-CH_2-\overset{\overset{\displaystyle +NH_3}{|}}{CH}-COO^- + MgADP^{-1} + P_i^{-2} + H^+$$

Glutamate   Glutamine   [9]

glutaminases (no. 1, Table 1) can release ammonia as needed.

Glutamate

As discussed above, glutamate dehydrogenase may utilize ammonia to form glutamate (reversal of reaction [1]). That the K_m value of this enzyme for ammonia is about 20 times that of glutamine synthetase, as well as about fivefold higher than the *in vivo* concentration of ammonia, suggests that glutamate dehydrogenase is not a quantitatively significant ammonia-utilizing enzyme.

Pyrimidine Nucleotide Biosynthesis

In vivo studies (31) have indicated that, although the main role of carbamylphosphate synthetase I is in the urea cycle, it may also be involved in the biosynthesis of pyrimidine nucleotides (Fig. 3). Increased formation and excretion of orotate and other intermediates in the pyrimidine pathway have been found in experimentally induced hyperammonemia, arginine deficiency, and congenital deficiencies of ornithine transcarbamylase and argininosuccinate synthetase. It has also been demonstrated that carbamylphosphate can cross the mitochondrial membrane. Administration of ammonium salts was found to induce an increased rate of pyrimidine biosynthesis; tissues lacking carbamylphosphate synthetase I do not exhibit such a response to ammonia. Studies with rat liver slices indicate that pyrimidine nucleosides or their metabolites are effective inhibitors of carbamylphosphate synthetase I activity, unless high levels of ammonia are also present. These observations are consistent with the shunting of excess carbamylphosphate from the mitochondria into the cytoplasm where it functions in pyrimidine biosynthesis. The extent of carbamylphosphate synthetase I participation in pyrimidine biosynthesis under normal physiological conditions is still controversial; some workers find only negligible participation, whereas others believe that carbamylphosphate synthetase I can provide about 80% of the carbamylphosphate that is utilized for pyrimidine biosynthesis.

REFERENCES

1. Krebs, H. A., Hems, R., Lund, P., Halliday, D., and Read, W. W. C. (1978): Sources of ammonia for mammalian urea synthesis. *Biochem. J.*, 176:733–737.

2. Frieden, C. (1976): The regulation of glutamate dehydrogenase. In: *The Urea Cycle*, edited by S. Grisolia, R. Baguena, and R. Mayor, pp. 59–71. John Wiley, New York.

3. Meister, A. (1965): *Biochemistry of the Amino Acids*, 2nd edition. Academic Press, New York.

4. McGivan, J. D., and Chappell, J. B. (1975): On the metabolic function of glutamate dehydrogenase in rat liver. *FEBS Lett.* 52:1–7.

5. Schoenheimer, R. (1942): *The Dynamic State of Body Constituents.* Harvard University Press, Cambridge.

6. Wolpert, E., Phillips, S. J., and Summerskill, W. H. J. (1971): Transport of urea and ammonia production in the human colon. *Lancet*, II:1387–1390.

7. LaNoue, K. F., and Schoolwerth, A. C. (1979): Metabolite transport in Mitochondria. *Ann. Rev. Biochem.*, 48:871–922.

8. Ratner, S. (1973): Enzymes of arginine and urea synthesis. *Adv. Enzymol.*, 39:1–90.

9. Meijer, A. J. (1979): Regulation of carbamyl-phosphate synthase (ammonia) in liver in relation to urea cycle activity. *Trends Biochem. Sci.*, 4:83–86.

10. Clarke, S. (1976): A major polypeptide component of rat liver mitochondria: Carbamyl phosphate synthetase. *J. Biol. Chem.*, 251:950–961.

11. Shore, G. C., Carignan, P., and Raymond, Y. (1979): *In vitro* synthesis of a putative precursor to the mitochondrial enzyme, carbamyl phosphate synthetase. *J. Biol. Chem.*, 254:3141–3144.

12. Jones, M. E. (1965): Amino acid metabolism. *Ann. Rev. Biochem.*, 34:381–418.

13. Meister, A., and Powers, S. G., (1978): Glutamine-dependent carbamyl phosphate synthetase: Catalysis and regulation. *Curr. Top. Cell. Regul.*, 16:289–315.

13a. Andersen, P. M., Wellner, V. P., Rosenthal, G. A., and Meister, A. (1970): Carbamyl phosphate synthetase. In: *Methods in Enzymology*, edited by H. A. Tabor and C. W. Tabor, Vol. 17A, pp. 235–243.

14. Powers, S. G., and Meister, A. (1976): Identification of enzyme-bound activated CO_2 as carbonic-phosphoric anhydride: Isolation of the corresponding trimethyl derivative from the active site of glutamine-dependent carbamyl phosphate synthetase. *Proc. Natl. Acad. Sci. USA*, 73:3020–3024.

15. Powers, S. G., and Meister, A. (1978): Carbonic-phosphoric anhydride (carboxy phosphate): Significance in catalysis and regulation of glutamine-dependent carbamyl phosphate synthetase. *J. Biol. Chem.*, 253:1258–1265.

16. Wimmer, M. J., Rose, I. A., Powers, S. G., and Meister, A. (1979): Evidence that carboxy phosphate is a kinetically competent intermediate in the carbamyl phosphate synthetase reaction. *J. Biol. Chem.*, 254:1854–1859.

17. Cohen, P. P. (1962): Carbamyl group synthesis. In: *The Enzymes*, Vol. 6, 2nd edition, edited by P. D. Boyer, H. Lardy, and K. Myrback, pp. 477–494. Academic Press, New York.

18. Rubio, V., and Grisolia, S. (1977): Mechanism of mitochondrial carbamyl phosphate synthetase. Synthesis and properties of active CO_2, precursor of carbamyl phosphate. *Biochemistry*, 16:321–329.

19. Marshall, M. (1976): Ornithine transcarbamylase from bovine liver. In: *The Urea Cycle*, edited by S. Grisolia, R. Baguena, and R. Mayor, pp. 169–179. John Wiley, New York.

20. Clarke, S. (1976): The polypeptides of rat liver mitochondria: Identification of a 36,000 dalton polypeptide as the subunit of ornithine transcarbamylase. *Biochem. Biophys. Res. Commun.*, 71:1118–1124.

21. Conboy, J. G., Kalousek, F., and Rosenberg, L. E. (1979): *In vitro* synthesis of a putative precursor of mitochondrial ornithine transcarbamylase. *Proc. Natl. Acad. Sci. USA*, 76:5724–5727.

22. Takada, S., Saheki, T., Igarashi, Y., and Katsunuma, T. (1979): Studies on rat liver argininosuccinate synthetase. Inhibition by various amino acids. *J. Biochem.*, 85:1309–1314.

23. Schimke, R. T., (1962): Differential effects of fasting and protein-free diets on levels of urea cycle enzymes in rat liver. *J. Biol. Chem.*, 237:1921–1924.

24. Aebi, H. (1976): Coordinated changes in enzymes of the ornithine cycle and response to dietary conditions. In: *The Urea Cycle*, edited by S. Grisolia, R. Baguena, and R. Mayor, pp. 275–296. John Wiley, New York.

25. Raiha, N. C. R. (1976): Developmental changes of urea-cycle enzymes in mammalian liver. In: *The Urea Cycle*, edited by S. Grisolia, R. Baguena, and R. Mayor, pp. 261–274. John Wiley, New York.

26. Nuzum, C. T., and Snodgrass, P. J. (1976): Multiple assays of the five urea-cycle enzymes in human liver homogenates, In: *The Urea Cycle*, edited by S. Grisolia, R. Baguena, and R. Mayor, pp. 325–349. John Wiley, New York.

27. Tatibana, M., and Shigesada, K. (1976): Regulation of urea biosynthesis by the acetylglutamate-arginine system. In: *The Urea Cycle*, edited by S. Grisolia, R. Baguena, and R. Mayor, pp. 301–317. John Wiley, New York.

28. Henderson, P. J. F. (1973): Steady-state enzyme kinetics with high-affinity substrates or inhibitors. *Biochem. J.*, 135:101–107.

29. Kerson, L. A. and Appel, S. H. (1968): Kinetic studies on rat liver carbamylphosphate synthetase. *J. Biol. Chem.*, 243:4279–4285.

30. Meister, A. (1974): Glutamine synthetase of mammals. *The Enzymes*, Vol. 10, 3rd edition, edited by P. D. Boyer, pp. 699–754. Academic Press, New York.

31. Pausch, J. G., Keppler, D. O. R., and Gerok, W. (1977): Increased *de novo* pyrimidine nucleotide synthesis in liver induced by ammonium ions in amounts surpassing the urea cycle capacity. *Eur. J. Biochem.*, 76:157–163.

The Liver: Biology and Pathobiology, edited by
I. Arias, H. Popper, D. Schachter, and D. A. Shafritz.
Raven Press, New York © 1982.

Chapter 15

Oxidative Biotransformation of Drugs

Alvito P. Alvares

In order to exert its biological effect, a drug or foreign compound must interact with receptors in suitable concentrations. The intensity and duration of action of a pharmacologically active substance is dependent on absorption, binding, metabolism, and excretion. Numerous foreign compounds, including drugs, are so hydrophobic that they would remain in the body indefinitely were it not for phase I and phase II enzymes of biotransformation. During phase I metabolism, one or more polar groups (e.g., hydroxyl, carboxyl, or amino) are introduced into the parent molecule, thereby presenting the phase II conjugating enzymes (e.g., glucuronyltransferases) with a substrate. The conjugated products are sufficiently hydrophilic to be readily excreted through the kidney or bile. The biotransformation of drugs can occur in several tissues, including the portals of entry and excretion, namely, lung, intestine, skin, and kidney. The liver, however, is the major site of biotransformation of drugs and other foreign chemicals.

This biotransformation in the liver is accomplished by enzymes that can metabolize a wide variety of structurally unrelated drugs, toxic agents, and environmental pollutants which the body may be exposed to. The enzymes of biotransformation are primarily localized in the membranes of the endoplasmic reticulum (ER) of liver cells, a network of interconnected channels present in the cytoplasm. Unlike some other cellular organelles, the ER cannot be separated from cells as an intact structure. When liver cells are homogenized and then centrifuged, the tubular reticulum breaks up, and bits of the membranes are

"pinched off" to form tiny vesicles called microsomes. These microsomal fractions, which contain the rough and smooth ER, are a convenient natural source of enzymes for laboratory studies of xenobiotic biotransformation.

Oxidative reactions account for most of the liver phase I transformations, largely because there are so many different ways in which a compound can be oxidized. These reactions are carried out primarily by enzymes localized in the ER. The liver also contains enzymes that catalyze the reduction of nitro and azo compounds. The relative importance of these enzymes is not clear. Although some differences have been noted between the nitro and azo reductase enzymes, both involve anaerobic reactions, requiring NADPH. Prontosil, an azo dye originally used for the treatment of streptococcal and pneumococcal infections, is reduced to an active metabolite, sulfanilamide. The antibacterial agent chloramphenicol is also reduced in part by the nitro reductase system to an amine. Because of the requirements of anaerobic conditions, it has been postulated that the nitro and azo reduction observed *in vivo* is probably caused by bacterial flora in the anaerobic environment of the gut. In addition to reductive enzyme pathways, a heterogeneous group of enzymes catalyzes the hydrolysis of esters and amide. Although many of these phase I hydrolytic enzymes are localized in blood plasma, some are localized in the ER of the liver. For example, liver microsomes catalyze the conversion of meperidine to meperidinic acid and ethanol. Most hydrolytic reactions, however, are nonmicrosomal. Procaine, a local anesthetic, is cleaved readily to *p*-aminobenzoic acid and diethylaminoethanol by plasma esterases. The hydrolytic cleavage of amides, such as procainamide, results in the liberation of carboxylic and amine groups. Such carboxyl, alcohol, and amine groups may then undergo a variety of conjugation (phase II) reactions.

The oxidative biotransformations catalyzed by liver microsomal enzyme systems are the most important enzymic reactions involved in phase I metabolism of drugs. Examples are summarized in Table 1. Certain drug oxidations are mediated by soluble, cystolic enzymes rather than the microsomal oxidative enzymes. The best known examples of these oxidations include the metabolism of aliphatic alcohols, such as ethanol and methanol. Alcohol and aldehyde dehydrogenases present in the cytosolic fraction of the liver metabolize ethanol to acetaldehyde and acetate, and methanol to formaldehyde and formic acid. Other studies (1) indicate that microsomal enzyme systems can also oxidize ethanol and methanol to their corresponding aldehydes, although evidence still indicates that cytosolic alcohol dehydrogenase is the major enzyme involved in the conversion of ethanol to acetaldehyde.

Although many drugs are metabolized to substances of little or no pharmacologic activity by enzymes localized in the ER, these enzymes are capable of converting drugs to metabolites that do possess measurable activity. They also possess the ability to convert biologically inactive compounds to compounds of considerable pharmacologic or toxicological activity. Some examples are depicted in Table 2. The principal metabolite of pentobarbital is a pharmacologically inactive derivative. Both imipramine and its principal N-demethylated metabolite, desmethylimipramine are tricyclic antidepressants. Similarly, phenylbutazone, a drug with antiinflammatory and uricosuric properties, is metabolized to two major metabolites, one possessing the antiinflammatory properties and the other the uricosuric effects of the parent compound. Cyclophosphamide is a prodrug that is oxidized *in vivo* to the pharmacologically active aldophosphamide. An example of the oxidative metabolism of a biologically inactive compound to a toxic metabolite is the conversion of the insecticide parathion to paraoxon. Certain polycyclic aromatic hydrocarbon carcinogens require oxidative metabolism *in vivo* to produce proximate carcinogens. The oxidative enzyme systems that metabolize drugs also metabolize endogenous substrates. Both endogenous and synthetic steroids and other endogenous compounds, such as fatty acids, biogenic amines, cholesterol, thyroxin, and prostaglandins, have been shown to be substrates of the liver and other nonhepatic microsomal enzyme systems (see refs. 2–4). It should be emphasized that a particular drug or endogenous substrate may not necessarily be metabolized to only one metabolite. A given compound usually undergoes several reactions and thus is converted to several different metabolites. Toxic effects of some

TABLE 1. *General types of oxidative reactions catalyzed by hepatic microsomal enzymes*

Reaction	Example
1. Side-chain oxidation	$R-CH_2-CH_2-CH_3 \longrightarrow R-CH_2-CHOH-CH_3$
2. Aromatic hydroxylation	$R-\bigcirc \longrightarrow R-\bigcirc-OH$
3. N, O, or S-dealkylation	$R-NH-CH_3 \longrightarrow R-NH_2 + HCHO$
4. Deamination	$R-\underset{CH_3}{CH}-NH_2 \longrightarrow R-\underset{CH_3}{CHO} + NH_3$
5. Epoxidation	$R-\bigcirc \longrightarrow R-\bigcirc^O$
6. Sulfoxidation	$R-S-R' \longrightarrow R-\overset{O}{\underset{\parallel}{S}}-R'$
7. Desulfuration	$R-\underset{\underset{S}{\parallel}}{P}\langle^{R_1}_{R_2} \longrightarrow R-\underset{\underset{O}{\parallel}}{P}\langle^{R_1}_{R_2} + S$
8. N-hydroxylation	$R-NH-\overset{O}{\underset{\parallel}{C}}-CH_3 \longrightarrow R-NOH-\overset{O}{\underset{\parallel}{C}}-CH_3$

TABLE 2. *Ability of oxidative enzymes to inactivate or activate foreign chemicals*

Pharmacological action	Example
1. Active compound → inactive metabolite	Pentobarbital → Hydroxypentobarbital
2. Active compound → active metabolite	Imipramine → Desmethylimipramine
3. Inactive compound → active metabolite	Parathion → Paraoxon

drugs and other foreign compounds may be due entirely or in part to metabolic products.

MICROSOMAL DRUG-METABOLIZING ENZYME SYSTEM

The microsomal oxidative drug-metabolizing enzymes are membrane bound and function as a multicomponent electron transport system. This enzyme system has an absolute requirement for NADPH and molecular oxygen and is also known as microsomal hydroxylases, monooxygenases, or mixed-function oxidases. In early studies with liver microsomal suspensions, it was shown that this enzyme consists of at least two protein components: a hemeprotein called cytochrome P-450 and a flavoprotein called NADPH-cytochrome P-450 reductase. The latter enzyme has also been termed NADPH-cytochrome c reductase. Cytochrome P-450 is the substrate- and oxygen-binding site of the enzyme system, while the reductase serves as an electron carrier, shuttling electrons from NADPH to the cytochrome P-450-substrate complex. In 1968, this liver microsomal enzyme system was solubilized with detergent and resolved chromatographically into three components (5), which were identified as cytochrome P-450, NADPH-cytochrome P-450 reductase, and phospholipid. Another hemeprotein, cytochrome b_5, is present in liver microsomes and may participate in drug and endogenous substrate

oxidations. Its precise function is not clear, however, nor is it known just how the various components of the monooxygenase or mixed-function oxidase complex are arrayed in the tubular membranes of the ER.

Cytochrome P-450 gets its designation from the fact that in the reduced form it binds with carbon monoxide, yielding a complex with an absorbance maximum at 450 nm. Cytochrome P-450-dependent oxidations have been termed mixed-function oxidases because in its reduced form the hemeprotein catalyzes the consumption of a molecule of oxygen, with one atom of oxygen appearing in the oxidized form of the substrate and the other atom being reduced to form water. A general scheme for the cytochrome P-450 reduction-oxidation cycle is shown in Fig. 1. The substrate combines with the oxidized form of cytochrome P-450 to form a ferric hemeprotein-substrate complex. The complex then undergoes a one-electron reduction via the NADPH-dependent transport chain forming the ferrous-substrate complex. The latter reacts with molecular oxygen to form an oxygenated intermediate. This oxygenated-P-450 intermediate then undergoes a second electron reduction and through an internal rearrangement, one atom of oxygen is reduced to water, while the other atom of oxygen is introduced into the substrate molecule.

The presence of more than one liver microsomal monooxygenase system was first postulated about 25 years ago by Axelrod (6), who showed species differ-

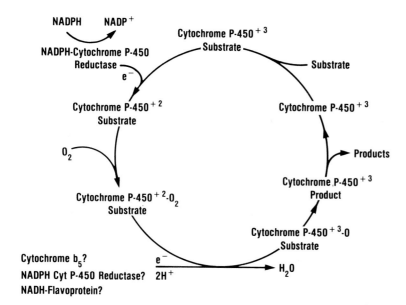

FIG. 1. Mechanism of cytochrome P-450 enzyme system.

ences in the N-demethylation of methadone and meperidine. The rabbit metabolized these compounds faster than the rat. Studies by Conney et al. (7) and by Takemori and Mannering (8) suggested not only that drug-metabolizing enzymes in various species differ, but that the liver of a single species may contain more than one monooxygenase enzyme system.

The use of microsomal enzyme inducers, such as phenobarbital and 3-methylcholanthrene, administered to rats demonstrated in the late 1960s the presence of at least two forms of microsomal cytochromes P-450, which differed in their spectral and catalytic properties (9,10). The form induced by 3-methylcholanthrene was termed cytochrome P-448 (9) or cytochrome P_1-450 (10). The data accumulated to date using these and other enzyme inducers have demonstrated the presence of several cytochrome P-450 isozymes differing in spectral, catalytic, and immunologic properties, as well as in electrophoretic patterns on sodium dodecyl sulfate gels, and in partial amino acid sequencing (see review, ref. 11). More than 20 cytochrome P-450 isozymes have been isolated from different species and tissues of experimental animals, with molecular weights ranging from 48,000 to 56,000. Some forms, such as cytochrome P-450b in rats (12) and cytochrome $P-450_{LM2}$ in rabbits (13), are primarily induced by phenobarbital, a potent inducer of drug-metabolizing enzymes in experimental animals, as well as in humans. Due to a lack of uniform nomenclature and structural information, it is possible that these two forms of cytochrome P-450 are similar if not identical.

More recently, human liver microsomal cytochrome P-450 has been purified to homogeneity by Wang et al. (14). However, the cytochromes P-450 isolated from different individuals had significantly different molecular weights. These differences may have been due to

genetic and environmental influences in the individuals studied. Other catalytic studies with human liver microsomes (15) also suggest that human liver contains multiple forms of cytochrome P-450 and that the relative proportion of each form varies among individuals. The relative amounts of various forms of the hemeprotein, which may be involved in the metabolic activation or detoxification of drugs and other foreign chemicals, will play a significant role in determining drug and carcinogen metabolism and their related toxicities. It should be noted that the substrate specificities of various forms of cytochrome P-450 are broad and overlapping, although the rate of metabolism by the different forms is different.

FACTORS INFLUENCING DRUG METABOLISM

Age

The newborn infant is more sensitive than the adult to many drugs. Obstetricians and pediatricians, therefore, exert great care in administering drugs to pregnant mothers and infants. Barbiturates, alcohol, narcotics, and other drugs that cross the placenta occasionally produce neonatal toxicity and even death. An explanation for the sensitivity of infants to drugs came from the observation that newborn animals lack liver microsomal enzyme systems for the metabolism of many drugs. Impaired drug metabolism can be demonstrated *in vitro* by comparison of the liver homogenate from neonatal and adult animals. In experimental animals, the development of drug-metabolizing enzymes with age parallels drug metabolism *in vivo* and results in decreased duration of drug action.

Although in laboratory animals cytochrome P-450-dependent monooxygenase activities are low and practically absent during the fetal development, human fetal liver contains significant levels of monooxygenase activities (between 35 and 40% of adult liver activities) (16). This disparity between laboratory animals and human fetal hydroxylases may be due to differences in dietary factors, as well as exposures to environmental chemicals that may cross the placental barrier. Unlike the human, experimental animals are bred and housed in rather carefully controlled environmental conditions.

Systematic studies on the age dependence of hepatic drug-metabolizing enzymes in humans are lacking. Scattered reports indicate that children may metabolize drugs faster than adults. Previous studies have shown that children metabolize certain drugs, such as diazoxide (17), phenobarbital (18), antipyrine, and phenylbutazone (19), at a faster rate than adults. In children (19) ranging in age from 1 to 8 years, the mean antipyrine half-life (6.6 hr) was significantly lower than the mean half-life obtained in adults (13.6 hr). The mean phenylbutazone half-lives in children and adults, 1.7 and 3.2 days, respectively, also differed significantly (Fig. 2). Both test drugs are metabolized primarily through oxidative pathways. Studies with theophylline administered to asthmatic children showed that children eliminated the bronchodilator at a considerably faster rate than adults (20), thus requiring higher dosages to achieve therapeutic concentrations.

It has long been recognized that aging is associated with alterations in pharmacological variables, and an age-related decline in the metabolism of a number of xenobiotics is observed in old rats (21). The plasma half-lives and pharmacological effects of drugs in the elderly differ from those in healthy young adults. Although part of the changes may be due to changes in renal function, plasma protein binding, volume of distribution, and regional blood flow, O'Malley et al. (22) and Vestal et al. (23) have indirectly provided evidence for reduced metabolic activity in the elderly. The mean plasma half-life values with antipyrine and phenylbutazone were found to be 45 and 29% greater, respectively, in geriatric patients than in young controls (Fig. 3). This decreased ability to metabolize drugs may contribute to the known high incidence of adverse drug reactions in the elderly.

Nutrition

In addition to age, under certain conditions, diet can markedly affect the hepatic microsomal drug-metabolizing enzyme activities and hence the pharmacological action of drugs. Alterations in dietary intake can produce pathological states, or vice versa. Recent studies, however, have shown that acute fasting in patients with classic, confirmed anorexia nervosa resulted in antipyrine pharmacokinetic parameters that were similar to healthy female controls (24). When allowance was made for body weight, neither half-life nor clearance was changed in obese patients administered antipyrine and tolbutamide (25) or sulfisoxazole, isoniazid, and procaine (26).

The protein/carbohydrate ratio of calorically adequate diets has shown consistent effects on drug metabolism in experimental animals. Dietary protein levels that are not adequate for maintaining maximal growth rates are also inadequate for synthesis of the drug-metabolizing enzymes. In contrast, a high-protein diet fed to rats increased the metabolism of pentobarbital, strychnine, and aminopyrine by liver microsomes (27). On the other hand, a high carbohydrate diet decreases liver monooxygenase activities (28). Such dietary manipulations have been shown to alter the rate of metabolism of antipyrine and theophylline in man (29,30), both drugs being extensively oxidized by the hepatic monooxygenase systems.

Significant changes in drug oxidation rates are observed in control subjects administered an isocaloric diet who are initially fed a high protein-low carbohydrate diet followed by a high carbohydrate-low protein diet. The rate of antipyrine and theophylline metabolism was prolonged twofold as the percentage of total calories represented by carbohydrate doubled from 35 to 70% and the percentage of protein decreased from 44 to 10% (30). The fat content in the diets was maintained constant. Pharmacokinetic parameters showed that dietary changes in the protein/carbohydrate ratio affected only theophylline and antipyrine half-lives and clearances without altering the volume of dis-

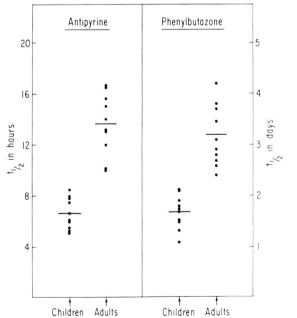

FIG. 2. Differences in antipyrine and phenylbutazone half-lives in children and adults. (Data taken from ref. 19.)

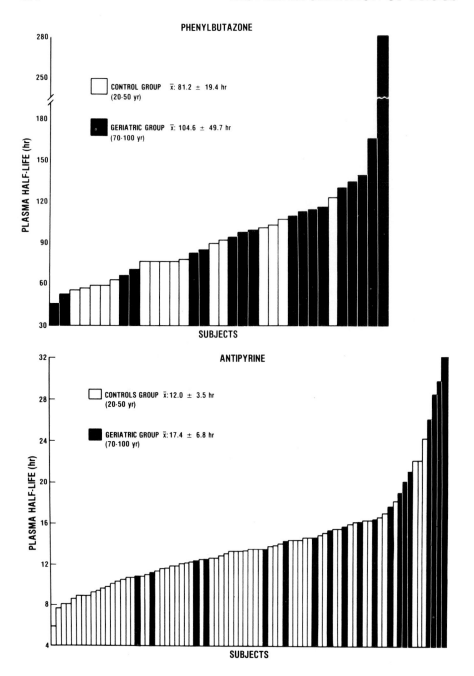

FIG. 3. Individual plasma antipyrine and phenylbutazone half-lives in control and geriatric patients. (Data taken from ref. 22.)

tribution of the drugs. Plasma elimination rates of theophylline following the dietary manipulations in the same subjects are shown in Fig. 4. These findings have been confirmed by Feldman et al. (29), who investigated the effect of similar dietary manipulations on theophylline biotransformation in children with bronchial asthma during long-term theophylline administration.

Other macronutrients in the diet may also influence rates of drug metabolism. In rats, a diet containing certain cruciferous vegetables, such as brussels sprouts, cabbage, cauliflower, or spinach, has been shown to enhance the intestinal metabolism of the hexobarbital, phenacetin, 7-ethoxycoumarin, and of the

polycylic aromatic carcinogen benzo(a)pyrene (31). Following the feeding of cabbage and brussels sprouts to humans, small but statistically significant changes in antipyrine metabolism were observed. In the same study, mean plasma concentrations of phenacetin were decreased by 34 to 67% (32).

Populations in different parts of the world and individuals within these populations differ widely in their diets. The nutritional-pharmacological interactions described may explain in part the interindividual differences in rates of drug metabolism. In addition, these interactions may occur in those individuals who undertake weight-reducing regimens, in vegetarians, in malnourished subjects, in postoperative patients who

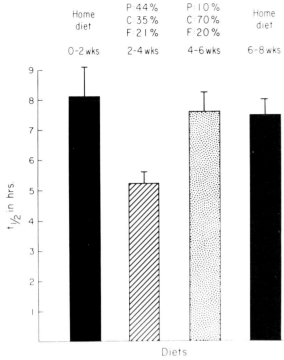

| Home diet | P 44% C 35% F 21% | P 10% C 70% F 20% | Home diet |
| 0-2 wks | 2-4 wks | 4-6 wks | 6-8 wks |

FIG. 4. Theophylline half-lives in six normal subjects maintained on their usual home diets, on a high protein (P)-low carbohydrate (C) diet, and on a low protein-high carbohydrate diet. Fat (F) content during the two test diets was maintained constant. (Data taken from ref. 30.)

receive glucose intravenously as a sole form of nourishment, and in large numbers of patients whose disease processes (e.g., diabetes, atherosclerosis) require significant nutritional restrictions. The experimental findings described here raise the possibility that these various groups might show substantial deviations from normal in the rates at which they metabolize or respond therapeutically to drugs.

Inter- and Intraindividual Variation in Drug Oxidations

Marked interindividual differences exists in the rates of drug metabolism. Although most drugs are metabolized in the liver, the clinically used laboratory procedures for liver function have no general predictive value for an individual's ability to metabolize drugs. Studies by Sjoqvist and von Bahr (33) showed 10- to 30-fold interindividual differences in the steady-state plasma concentrations of the antidepressant drugs, desmethylimipramine and nortryptyline. In 1968, Vesell and associates showed five- to 10-fold interindividual variations in such frequently used drugs as phenylbutazone and bishydroxycoumarin (34); these variations, shown to be under genetic control, vanished within monozygotic twins, where no genetic differences exist, but were preserved within dizygotic twins. Interindividual variations of four- to sixfold in plasma

half-lives of diazepam and oxazepam have also been reported (33).

Recent studies have shown that both genetic and environmental factors control the rates and pathways of drug biotransformation in humans. An approach for assessing the role of environment in regulating the metabolism of a drug is to study the metabolism of the drug on several occasions in normal volunteers who are allowed to pursue a normal lifestyle and to eat an unrestricted diet (35). The amount of intraindividual variability depends on the drug studied. A study of the plasma elimination rates of drugs that undergo oxidative metabolism showed greater day-to-day variations for the metabolism of phenacetin than for the metabolism of phenylbutazone (35). A small amount of variability occurred in the metabolism of phenylbutazone administered on five different occasions to the same subject. The difference between the lowest and highest plasma half-life for each subject ranged from 12% in one subject to 55% in another. When phenacetin was administered to the seven subjects on five occasions, the percent difference between the minimum and maximum values in the plasma half-lives of the drug varied from 30% in one subject to 100% in two subjects studied (35). The mean intraindividual variation observed with antipyrine was intermediate between phenylbutazone and phenacetin. These intraindividual differences in rates of drug metabolism are to be ascribed to the subject's external environment and/or physiologic factors (internal environment).

Effect of Enzyme Inducers on Oxidative Metabolism of Drugs

It is now established that a wide variety of environmental agents can induce the oxidative drug-metabolizing enzymes in the liver and in several extrahepatic tissues. The enhanced rate of drug biotransformation was often associated with a faster termination of drug action. More recently, however, extensive data have showed that in some instances, induction of microsomal monooxygenase activities can also result in the formation of electrophilic metabolites of drugs and chemical carcinogens, which are biologically more active and are often responsible for the acute or chronic toxicity associated with certain foreign compounds. It should be noted that induction does not affect oxidative (phase I) reactions only; phase II reactions also can be affected. For example, certain inducers of cytochrome P-450 and associated enzymic activities will also induce glucuronyl transferases.

The stimulating effect of foreign compounds on liver microsomal enzyme activity was first observed by the Millers at Wisconsin. They and their associates (36,37) showed the stimulatory effects of polycyclic aromatic hydrocarbons on liver microsomal enzymic activities. Evidence was also presented in these early studies that polycyclic hydrocarbons increase enzyme activity by inducing the synthesis of more enzyme protein (36,37). The stimulating effect of barbiturates and other drugs was then discovered by Remmer (38) and by Conney and Burns (39). Further studies on induction by phenobarbital revealed that the enhanced rate of metabolism of drugs was associated with proliferation of smooth ER in the hepatocytes (40) and increased concentrations of the components of the monooxygenase enzyme system, cytochrome P-450, and NADPH-cytochrome P-450 reductase activity (41). Since these pioneering studies, more than 200 steroid hormones, drugs, insecticides, chemical carcinogens, and other environmentally derived chemicals are known to stimulate drug metabolism in experimental animals; many have been shown to do the same thing in man.

Inducers of hepatic monooxygenases have been categorized into two main groups (see review in ref. 2). One group, of which phenobarbital and the insecticide DDT are prototypes, enhances the metabolism of a large variety of substrates by these liver enzymes. In rats, this group of enzyme inducers has been shown to markedly increase liver cytochrome P-450 content and associated enzyme activities, such as ethylmorphine N-demethylase activity (Fig. 5). In control subjects administered sedative dosages of phenobarbital, the barbiturate causes an enhanced rate of plasma elimination of the test drug antipyrine (Fig. 5).

Polycyclic aromatic hydrocarbons, such as benzo(a)pyrene and 3-methylcholanthrene, comprise a second major group of enzyme inducers. This group induces the synthesis of cytochrome P-448, a hemeprotein that differs in spectral and catalytic properties from cytochrome P-450 present in untreated rats or in rats pretreated with phenobarbital (9,10,42). The two classes of inducing substances can be distinguished by differences in catalytic activities. Phenobarbital is a potent inducer of ethylmorphine and benzphetamine N-demethylase and testosterone 16α-hydroxylase activities in liver microsomes, whereas aryl hydrocarbon (benzo(a)pyrene) hydroxylase activity is preferentially induced by polycyclic aromatic hydrocarbons in experimental animals as well as in human tissues, such as the skin (Fig. 6). It should be noted that certain other environmentally derived chemicals can induce other forms of cytochrome P-450. Purified forms of cytochromes P-450 and P-448 from rat liver microsomes have been termed cytochromes P-450b and P-450c, respectively. Differences in substrate specificities of these two purified hemeproteins, and a third form of cytochrome P-450 termed cytochrome P-450a, are shown in Table 3. Other environmentally derived chemicals, such as 2,3,7,8-tetrachlorodibenzo-p-dioxin (TCDD) and polychlorinated biphenyls (PCBs), can induce other distinct forms of these hemeproteins.

The mechanisms of induction of drug-metabolizing enzymes by phenobarbital and 3-methylcholanthrene involve stimulation of mRNA synthesis followed by *de*

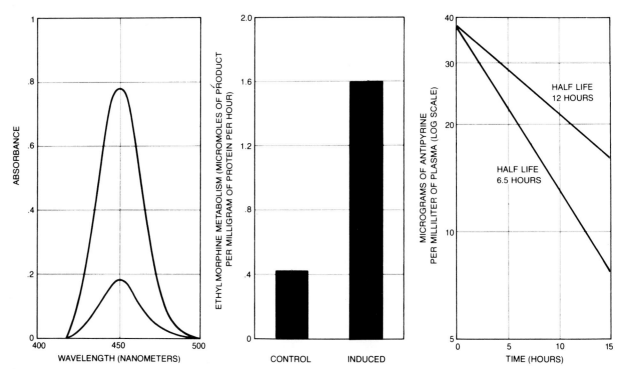

FIG. 5. Effect of pretreatment of rats with phenobarbital on hepatic cytochrome P-450 (*left panel*); ethylmorphine metabolism (*center panel*); and on mean plasma half-lives of antipyrine (*right panel*) before (*top line*) and after (*lower line*) administration of phenobarbital, 2 mg/kg/day for 21 days, to five normal human subjects. (Data taken from ref. 65.)

TABLE 3. *Catalytic activity of various purified forms of rat liver cytochrome P-450[a]*

Substrate[b]	Phenobarbital		3-Methyl-cholanthrene	
	P-450a	P-450b	P-450a	P-450c
Benzphetamine	2.2	216.6	2.6	5.0
Benzo(a)pyrene	0.04	0.2	0.3	24.5
7-Ethoxycoumarin	0.2	13.9	1.1	67.5
Zoxazolamine	0.48	2.2	2.0	29.7
Testosterone				
7 α-OH	4.1	0.06	5.4	0.08
16 α-OH	0.08	1.3	0.04	0.02
6 β-OH	0.11	0.04	0.08	0.36

[a] Data from Ryan et al. (12).

[b] Activity expressed as nanomoles product formed per minute per mole cytochrome P-450.

novo synthesis of new enzyme protein. Induction by phenobarbital also appears to produce stabilization of enzyme protein and decreases the rate of degradation of mRNA and of microsomal protein, including NADPH-cytochrome P-450 reductase (43). A cytosolic receptor protein is involved in induction by 3-methylcholanthrene; however, no such receptor protein has yet been detected for phenobarbital.

Drug-drug interactions involving microsomal oxidative enzyme induction can have important clinical applications. Patients often are given several drugs at the same time without proper consideration of the possibility that one drug may interact with another. Adding or subtracting a drug can have serious consequences for the metabolism and action of other drugs being given to the patient. Anticoagulant therapy in man is attended by risks of this kind. Daily administration of 2 mg/kg phenobarbital antagonized the anticoagulant response to warfarin (44). When a patient treated chronically with 75 mg/day bishydroxycoumarin was administered 65 mg/day phenobarbital for 4 weeks in addition to the bishydroxycoumarin, there was a substantial decrease in plasma level of bishydroxycoumarin and a shortening of prothrombin time (45).

An important interaction first reported in 1971 involved the interaction of drugs with contraceptive steroids. Rifampicin, a drug used in the treatment of tuberculosis, stimulates hepatic microsomal enzymes. Several pregnancies have been reported in women taking rifampicin in conjunction with contraceptive steroids. There is now good evidence that rifampicin increases the rate of metabolism of both estrogenic and progestogenic components of oral contraceptives (46). Chronic ethanol consumption also produces enhanced microsomal enzyme activities, resulting in increased metabolism of ethanol and drugs, such as meprobamate, pentobarbital, aminopyrine, antipyrine, and tolbutamide (1).

Humans may also be exposed to enzyme-inducing chemicals in the environment or through occupational exposure. Studies by Poland et al. (47) have shown that intensive occupational exposure to DDT re-

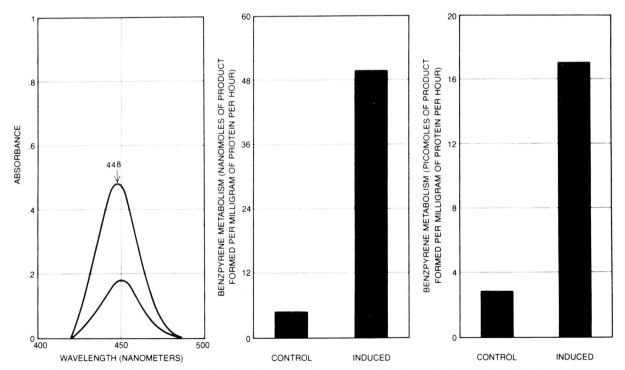

FIG. 6. Effect of pretreatment of rats with 3-methylcholanthrene on hepatic cytochrome P-450 (*left panel*); benzo(a)pyrene hydroxylase activity (*center panel*); and on hydroxylase activity (*right panel*) in human skin grown in tissue culture in presence and absence of benzanthracene. (Data taken from ref. 65.)

sulted in significantly lower serum half-life of phenyl-butazone and a marked increase in urinary excretion of 6β-hydroxycortisol in workers occupationally exposed to the insecticide. The urinary excretion of 6β-hydroxycortisol has been used as a test for the induction of hepatic drug-metabolizing enzymes in man (2). PCBs, another class of chlorinated hydrocarbons, are widely used industrial chemicals. Their uses include application as dielectric fluids in capacitors and transformers, as hydraulic fluids, and as heat transfer fluids. Workers exposed to PCBs showed a significantly lower mean antipyrine half-life (10.8 hr) when compared with the mean half-life of 15.6 hr in subjects not exposed. Metabolic clearance rates for the drug were 52.4 and 34.4 ml/min in PCB-exposed and normal subjects, respectively (48). Such occupational exposure can also lead to exposure of other family members through contaminated clothing of the workers involved. Similarly, communities surrounding industrial plants that pollute the surrounding environment through waste disposal may have unusually high exposure risks to chemicals, which may alter the activities of liver monooxygenases of exposed individuals.

Cigarette smoke contains a wide variety of polycyclic hydrocarbons, including benzo(a)pyrene, 1,2-benzanthracene, 1,2,5,6-dibenzanthracene, chrysene, anthracene, and phenanthrene. In addition, it contains carbon monoxide, cadmium, nicotine, acrolein, and some pesticides. Previous studies have shown that cigarette smoking results in lowered plasma levels of phenacetin, theophylline, imipramine, antipyrine, and pentazocine. The interaction of theophylline and cigarette smoking is potentially one of the most clinically important effects of smoking because theophylline, widely used as a bronchodilator, has a low therapeutic index and large interindividual variability in elimination rates in man (49). In studies carried out by Hunt et al. (50), the mean plasma half-life of theophylline was 4.3 hr in smokers, compared with 7.0 hr in nonsmokers (Fig. 7). Theophylline is metabolized largely in the liver, with a minor fraction excreted unchanged. The decrease in plasma half-life was accompanied by a significant increase in total body clearance of the drug in smokers. Chronic marijuana smoking seems to have a similar magnitude of inducing effect on theophylline clearance as tobacco smoking (51). It should be emphasized that the inductive effects of cigarette or marijuana smoking on drug metabolism may be selective. As pointed out earlier, the polycyclic hydrocarbon class of inducing substances induces the metabolism of fewer substrates than the barbiturate class of inducers.

Nonnutrient components of the diet are a major source of exposure of man to foreign chemicals. In addition to being present in cigarette smoke and polluted city air, polycyclic hydrocarbons are present in smoked foods, such as charcoal-broiled meats (52). In a recent study (53), normal volunteers were placed on

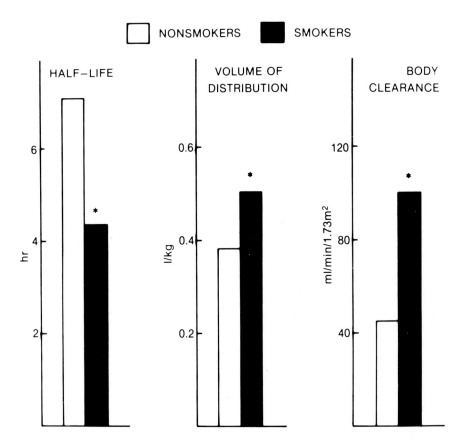

FIG. 7. The pharmacokinetics of theophylline disposition in smokers and nonsmokers. *Bar,* mean for eight subjects; *asterisk,* value significantly different from respective control value. (Data taken from ref. 50.)

a control diet for 7 to 10 days, then on a charcoal-broiled meat diet for 4 days; the same subjects then were placed back on the control diet for 7 days. During the control diets, the meat was cooked over burning charcoal with aluminum foil placed between the meat and burning charcoal. During the charcoal-broiled beef diet period, the meat was cooked directly over the burning charcoal in the absence of aluminum foil. At the end of each diet period, 900 mg phenacetin was administered orally to each subject, and the plasma concentrations of phenacetin were determined at various times. As shown in Table 4, feeding the charcoal-broiled meat for 4 days markedly lowered the plasma concentrations of phenacetin. Such nonnutrient contamination of food may play a role in regulating drug metabolism. Feeding of charcoal-broiled beef has also been shown to enhance the metabolism of antipyrine and theophylline (54).

The clinical consequences of enzyme induction will be determined by the therapeutic index of the drug. For example, marked changes in plasma clearance of antipyrine, phenacetin, or phenylbutazone will probably have little or no clinical consequence, whereas small changes in clearance rates of theophylline and the oral anticoagulants may prove critical. Furthermore, the fact that an interaction occurs does not preclude the use of two drugs simultaneously. For example, appropriate manipulation of the dose of an anticoagulant, based on prothrombin times and on administration or discontinuation of an enzyme-inducing drug, is acceptable and safe. Occupational and other environmental factors, such as smoking and dietary habits, may necessitate the individualization of certain drug therapies.

Inhibition of Oxidative Metabolism of Drugs

Inhibition of drug metabolism may result in exaggerated and prolonged response with an increased risk of toxicity. Many interactions of this type involve liver monooxygenases; mechanisms include substrate competition and functional impairment of enzyme activity. *In vitro* studies using liver microsomal enzyme preparations have shown that competitive inhibition kinetics

are observed with many drugs that are metabolized by the oxidative enzymes. Acute ethanol ingestion has been shown to significantly retard the disappearance of pentobarbital and meprobamate from the blood of normal human subjects (55). *In vitro* studies showed that this interaction involved competitive or partial inhibition by ethanol of the metabolism of several substrates. In contrast to the acute effects, chronic administration of ethanol enhances the activity of hepatic monooxygenases (1). The acute ethanol interaction explains in part the increased sensitivity of inebriated persons to the effects of certain drugs.

Chronic administration of allopurinol and nortriptyline (56) and of disulfiram (57) to humans has been shown to cause impairment of drug metabolism. Recent reports have shown that cimetidine, a drug widely used in the treatment of peptic ulcer disease, may potentiate the effects of oral anticoagulants (58) and impair the elimination of benzodiazepines, such as diazepam (59), or theophylline and antipyrine (60) in man. The interaction of cimetidine with theophylline and oral anticoagulants has considerable clinical importance since the latter drugs have a low therapeutic index. In a recent study (63) in seven healthy volunteers taking daily subtherapeutic doses of warfarin, the addition of cimetidine, 200 mg three times a day and 400 mg at night for 3 weeks, resulted in a marked increase in prothrombin time; plasma warfarin concentration increased from 0.96 to 1.76 μg/ml (Fig. 8). The prothrombin time at the end of the study was not significantly different from that before the addition of cimetidine. Animal studies have shown that cimetidine inhibits N-demethylase and benzo(a)-pyrene hydroxylase activities in liver microsomes of untreated, phenobarbital-treated, and 3-methylcholanthrene-treated rats (64).

Effects of Liver Disease

The hepatic drug elimination of many drugs may be impaired in patients with liver disease. Alterations observed depend on the drug studied, the stage of the disease, the presence of collateral circulation, and concurrent drug intake. For example, the changes are

TABLE 4. *Effect of charcoal-broiled beef diet on the plasma concentration of phenacetin in man* [a]

| Diet | Phenacetin in plasma (ng/ml) at intervals after administration (hr) [b] | | | | | |
	1	2	3	4	5	7
Control	1,328 ± 481	925 ± 166	313 ± 60	149 ± 27	66 ± 14	17 ± 4
Charcoal-broiled beef	319 ± 90	163 ± 32	74 ± 17	34 ± 9	15 ± 4	7 ± 2
Control	1,827 ± 661	623 ± 128	271 ± 76	99 ± 24	40 ± 11	14 ± 4

[a] Data from Conney et al. (53).
[b] Phenacetin, 900 mg, was administered to nine subjects after each dietary regimen. Each value represents the mean ± SE for nine subjects.

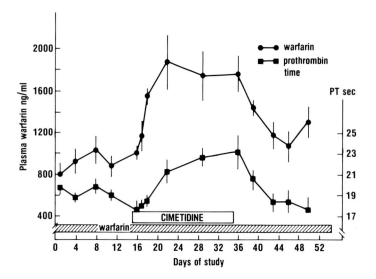

FIG. 8. Effect of cimetidine on steady-state warfarin concentration and prothrombin time in seven normal subjects. (Data taken from ref. 63.)

somewhat less dramatic in acute viral hepatitis than in cirrhosis. Many of the reported changes can be rationalized in terms of the pathophysiology of the disease. Defects in drug metabolism correlate poorly with routine liver-function tests, except perhaps with reduced serum albumin, which may reflect poor protein synthesis, including the drug-metabolizing enzymes. Values for several indices of the drug-metabolizing enzyme system in the liver vary greatly, but the mean values in groups of patients with mild hepatitis or inactive cirrhosis do not differ significantly from those of controls. In contrast, hepatic cytochrome P-450 and associated enzymic activities are significantly lower in patients with severe hepatitis, active cirrhosis, and other severe liver disease.

METABOLIC ACTIVATION OF DRUGS TO TOXIC SUBSTANCES

An important result of drug metabolism studies in recent years has been the realization that many foreign compounds are metabolized by the liver and other tissues to potent alkylating or arylating agents. Such studies have demonstrated how chemically stable compounds can produce serious tissue lesions in man, including neoplasia, hepatic and renal necrosis, bone marrow aplasia, and other adverse reactions. This is because potent intermediates that are formed during biotransformation can bind covalently to tissue macromolecules. A number of hepatotoxic drugs, such as acetaminophen, acetanilide, phenacetin, and furosemide have been shown to cause hepatic necrosis. These drugs, when ingested in large doses, may be activated by cytochrome P-450-dependent oxidations, resulting in the formation of metabolites that bind to tissue macromolecules, such as DNA and RNA. Autoradiograms show that covalent binding occurs preferentially in the necrotic areas of the liver. Further-

more, pretreatment of animals with inducers or inhibitors of cytochrome P-450-dependent metabolism similarly altered the metabolism of the hepatotoxins, the severity of the hepatic necrosis, and the extent of hepatic binding of radiolabeled metabolites. Many of these concepts of metabolic activation were developed during studies of chemical carcinogenesis.

Although many adverse drug reactions involving the liver are of minor clinical concern, some can cause hepatic failure and death. The mechanism of toxicity attributable to overdoses of acetaminophen has been studied extensively. This commonly used analgesic and antipyretic drug is safe at therapeutic doses. In large doses, however, it is hepatotoxic in both man and experimental animals, producing primarily centrilobular necrosis (see reviews, refs. 61 and 62). Acetaminophen is primarily excreted as a sulfate or glucuronide conjugate. It is also metabolized by the hepatic monooxygenase system to a reactive metabolite. Glutathione plays an important role in the detoxification of this metabolite (Fig. 9). The chemical nature of the reactive metabolite has been an area of investigation by several laboratories. Recent studies suggest that N-hydroxylation is an important metabolic step, which is catalyzed by the cytochrome P-450 system. N-Hydroxyacetaminophen then undergoes a spontaneous dehydration to form the reactive metabolite, N-acetylimidoquinone. This metabolite then conjugates with glutathione; the resulting conjugate is subsequently excreted as a mercapturic acid derivative in the urine. It is not until a significant amount (about 70%) of glutathione in the liver is depleted that covalent binding and subsequent liver necrosis is seen (61). Several investigators have postulated that the reactive metabolite of acetaminophen may be an arene oxide in the 3,4-position.

The involvement of cytochrome P-450 in the formation of the reactive metabolite is based on the following experimental evidence. The formation of the me-

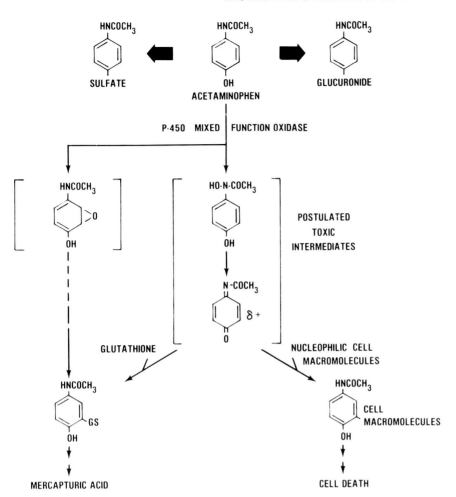

FIG. 9. Metabolic pathways of acetaminophen.

tabolite can be demonstrated *in vitro* by measuring the covalent binding of the metabolite in a microsomal incubation mixture containing hepatic microsomes with NADPH. Anaerobic conditions, deletion of NADPH, or an atmosphere containing CO decreased covalent binding. Inducers of microsomal enzymes, such as phenobarbital, or inhibitors, such as piperonyl butoxide, markedly increased or decreased, respectively, the severity of liver necrosis and covalent binding of acetaminophen administered to mice. The finding that glutathione serves as a protective mechanism for the reactive metabolite(s) has led to the use of N-acetylcysteine as an antidote in acetaminophen poisoning. Although the sulfhydryl compound is effective in the early stages of poisoning, its exact mechanism of action is not well understood.

The concept of drug metabolism causing toxicity applies not only to drugs taken in large doses but also to certain drugs taken in therapeutic doses. Genetic slow acetylators of procainamide, isoniazid, and hydralazine are likely to develop drug-induced systemic lupus erythematosus. In addition, the incidence of polyneuropathy for patients receiving isoniazid is higher in slow than in rapid acetylators. In fast acetylators, isoniazid may cause hepatic injury. Iso-

niazid is acetylated to acetylisoniazid. Administration of acetylisoniazid to rats or mice caused no significant hepatic necrosis; however, marked necrosis is seen in rats pretreated with phenobarbital. This necrosis is prevented by simultaneous inhibitors of hepatic monooxygenases, such as piperonyl butoxide or cobaltous chloride (61). It has been shown in other experiments that acetylisoniazid is hydrolyzed to acetylhydrazine and that acetylhydrazine is metabolically activated to cause covalent binding to macromolecules and a striking midzonal and centrilobular necrosis. The nature of the metabolic toxic intermediate has not been identified. The involvement of hepatic monooxygenases is strengthened by the clinical observation of increased incidence of isoniazid injury in patients with tuberculosis also receiving the microsomal enzyme inducer rifampicin (62).

The above examples demonstrate the role of hepatic monooxygenases in drug-induced toxicity. A major gap in our knowledge of this process is the site of binding of the toxic intermediates and the sequence of events between binding and the clinical manifestation of the toxicity. In addition to genetic factors, environmental factors or concomitant ingestion of other drugs may influence the qualitative and quantitative composition of microsomal hemeproteins, which activate foreign compounds, including drugs. These factors may determine why some people show a toxic reaction to a drug whereas others do not.

SUMMARY

Most drugs and other foreign compounds, including carcinogens, that the body is exposed to are detoxified by the oxidative enzymes, as well as by the conjugating enzymes localized in liver cells. In recent years, attention has focused on the metabolites or pathways of drug metabolism that result in pharmacologically or toxicologically active intermediates. Several of the methodologic approaches utilized, such as the determination of covalent binding to tissue macromolecules and its correlation with tissue damage, originated in the studies of chemical carcinogenesis. Many questions remain to be resolved in explaining drug toxicity; for example, why are some individuals more susceptible and why are some more resistant to drug toxicity?

The duration and action of drugs metabolized by the liver monooxygenases, as well as their toxicity, may be determined by genetic as well as environmental factors. Unfortunately, no single animal species metabolizes drugs exactly as do humans. There are interspecies differences in both the rates and pathways of drug metabolism. Furthermore, the experimental animal is not exposed to a variety of environmental factors facing humans. These factors, such as differences in dietary and/or alcohol intake, smoking habits, and occupational exposure to enzyme inducers and inhibitors, definitely play a role in the marked individual variations in the rates of drug metabolism. Some of these differences are undoubtedly of genetic origin. For example, a small proportion of the human population has an abnormal pseudocholinesterase enzyme that does not metabolize succinylcholine as rapidly as does the normal enzyme. A large number of cytochrome P-450 isozymes have been isolated and purified. Genetic or environmental factors may cause some individuals to possess one or more aberrant hemeproteins which can cause toxicity or which may make one smoker more susceptible to chemical carcinogenesis than the other.

The causes of most individual differences in drug metabolism are not well defined. Nevertheless, it is well known that even in relatively small groups of patients, the plasma levels of drugs given to patients in the same dose may vary. In addition to such interindividual differences, an important finding is that even within the same individual, the rates of metabolism of some drugs, such as theophylline or phenacetin, may vary markedly in a temporal manner, when the same drug is administered on different occasions. This observation strongly suggests that in humans there may not be a "basal" level of drug-metabolizing activity. Such basal levels are more prevalent in experimental animals, such as the rat or mouse, within a laboratory or between different laboratories assaying the same cytochrome P-450-dependent enzymic activity.

Exposure to various environmental chemicals, including drugs, may explain some of the adverse reactions or tolerance observed when drugs are administered to humans. Such chemical exposures should be considered as one of the primary sources of drug interactions observed in man. It should be emphasized that such chemical exposure may have physiologic consequences other than those affecting the rates of metabolism of drugs or other foreign substances. They may alter the metabolism of endogenous substrates, such as steroid hormones or prostaglandins. Although most of the research with monooxygenases has been carried out with liver enzymic systems, these chemical exposures can induce or inhibit monooxygenases in other tissues. The balance between the products of detoxification and bioactivation may determine organ-specific toxicity to certain chemicals; for example, why is the liver particularly susceptible to acetaminophen toxicity and not the red cell?

Finally, the therapeutic implications of drug-induced enzyme induction or inhibition will be most obvious clinically for those drugs with a low therapeutic index, such as theophylline, oral anticoagulants, and antiarrhythmic drugs. The action of these drugs must be carefully monitored whenever other drugs are coadministered. It would be useful to have a reliable marker drug or an endogenous excretory product that would predict whether the functional capacity of a subject's cytochrome P-450 system(s) is impaired. This would greatly facilitate the individualization of human drug therapy.

REFERENCES

1. Lieber, C. S., Teschke, R., Hasumura, Y., and DeCarli, L. M. (1975): Differences in hepatic and metabolic changes after acute and chronic alcohol consumption. *Fed. Proc.*, 34:2060–2074.
2. Conney, A. H. (1967): Pharmacological implications of microsomal enzyme induction. *Pharmacol. Rev.*, 19:317–366.
3. Gillette, J. R. (1966): Biochemistry of drug oxidation and reduction by enzymes in hepatic endoplasmic reticulum. In: *Advances in Pharmacology, Vol. 4*, edited by S. Garattini and P. A. Shore, pp. 219–266. Academic Press, New York.
4. Kupfer, D. (1980): Endogenous substrates of monooxygenases: Fatty acids and prostaglandins. *Pharmacol. Ther.*, 11:469–496.
5. Lu, A. Y. H., and Coon, M. J. (1968): Role of hemoprotein P-450 in fatty acid ω-hydroxylation in a soluble enzyme system from liver microsomes. *J. Biol. Chem.*, 243:1331–1332.
6. Axelrod, J. (1956): The enzymatic N-demethylation of narcotic drugs. *J. Pharmacol. Exp. Ther.*, 117:322–330.
7. Conney, A. H., Gillette, J. R., Inscoe, J. K., Trams, E. G., and Posner, H. S. (1959): 3,4-Benzpyrene-induced synthesis of liver microsomal enzymes which metabolize foreign compounds. *Science*, 130:1478–1479.
8. Takemori, A. E., and Mannering, G. J. (1958): Metabolic N- and O-demethylation of morphine- and morphinan-type analgesics. *J. Pharmacol. Exp. Ther.*, 123:171–179.

9. Alvares A. P., Schilling, G., Levin, W., and Kuntzman, R. (1967): Studies on the induction of CO-binding pigments in liver microsomes by phenobarbital and 3-methylcholanthrene. *Biochem. Biophys. Res. Commun.*, 29:521–526.

10. Sladek, N. E., and Mannering, G. J. (1966): Evidence for a new P-450 hemoprotein in hepatic microsomes from methylcholanthrene-treated rats. *Biochem. Biophys. Res. Commun.*, 24:668–674.

11. Lu, A. Y. H., and West, S. B. (1980): Multiplicity of mammalian microsomal cytochromes P-450. *Pharmacol. Rev.*, 31:277–295.

12. Ryan, D. E., Thomas, P. E., Korzeniowski, D., and Levin, W. (1979): Separation and characterization of highly purified forms of liver microsomal cytochrome P-450 from rats treated with polychlorinated biphenyls, phenobarbital and 3-methylcholanthrene. *J. Biol. Chem.*, 254:1365–1374.

13. Haugen, D. A., and Coon, M. J. (1976): Properties of electrophoretically homogeneous phenobarbital-inducible and β-naphthoflavone-inducible forms of liver microsomal cytochrome P-450. *J. Biol. Chem.*, 251:7929–7939.

14. Wang, P., Mason, P. S., and Guengerich, F. P. (1980): Purification of human liver cytochrome P-450 and comparison to the enzyme isolated from rat liver. *Arch. Biochem. Biophys.*, 199:206–219.

15. Kapitulnik, J., Poppers, P. J., and Conney, A. H. (1977): Comparative metabolism of benzo(a)pyrene and drugs in human liver. *Clin. Pharmacol. Ther.*, 21:166–176.

16. Rane, A., and Ackerman, E. (1971): Metabolism of ethylmorphine and aniline in human fetal liver. *Clin. Pharmacol. Ther.*, 13:663–670.

17. Pruitt, A. W., Dayton, P. G., and Patterson, J. H. (1973): Disposition of diazoxide in children. *Clin. Pharmacol. Ther.*, 14:73–82.

18. Garrettson, L. K., and Dayton, P. G. (1970): Disappearance of phenobarbital and diphenylhydantoin from serum of children. *Clin. Pharmacol. Ther.*, 11:674–679.

19. Alvares, A. P., Kapelner, S., Sassa, S., and Kappas, A. (1975): Drug metabolism in normal, lead-poisoned children and normal adults. *Clin. Pharmacol. Ther.*, 17:179–183.

20. Ellis, E. F., Koysooko, R., and Levy, G. (1976): Pharmacokinetics of theophylline in children with asthma. *Pediatrics*, 58:542–547.

21. Kato, R., and Takanaka, A. (1968): Metabolism of drugs in old rats: Activities of NADPH-linked electron transport and drug-metabolizing enzyme systems in liver microsomes of old rats. *Jpn. J. Pharmacol.*, 18:381–388.

22. O'Malley, K., Crooks, J., Duke, E., and Stevenson, I. H. (1971): Effect of age and sex on human drug metabolism. *Br. Med. J.*, 3:607–609.

23. Vestal, R. E., Norris, A. H., Tobin, J. D., Cohen, B. H., Shock, N. W., and Andres, R. (1975): Antipyrine metabolism in man: Influence of age, alcohol, caffeine, and smoking. *Clin. Pharmacol. Ther.*, 18:425–432.

24. Bakke, O. M., Aanderud, S., Syversen, G., Bassoe H. H., and Myking, O. (1978): Antipyrine metabolism in anorexia nervosa. *Br. J. Clin. Pharmacol.*, 5:341–343.

25. Reidenberg, M. M., and Vesell, E. S. (1975): Unaltered metabolism of antipyrine and tolbutamide in fasting man. *Clin. Pharmacol. Ther.*, 17:650–656.

26. Reidenberg, M. M. (1977): Obesity and fasting: Effects on drug metabolism and drug action in man. *Clin. Pharmacol. Ther.*, 22:729–734.

27. Kato, R., Oshima, T., and Tomizawa, S. (1968): Toxicity and metabolism of drugs in relation to dietary protein. *Jpn. J. Pharmacol.*, 18:356–366.

28. Strother, A., Throckmorton, J. K., and Herzer, C. (1971): The influence of high sugar consumption on the duration of action of barbiturates and in vitro metabolism of barbiturates, aniline and p-nitroanisole. *J. Pharmacol. Exp. Ther.*, 179:490–498.

29. Feldman, C. H., Hutchinson, V. E., Pippenger, C. E., Blumenfeld, T. A., Feldman, D. R., and Davis, W. J. (1980): Effect of dietary protein and carbohydrate on theophylline metabolism in children. *Pediatrics*, 66:956–962.

30. Kappas, A., Anderson, K. E., Conney, A. H., and Alvares, A. P. (1976): Influence of dietary protein and carbohydrate on antipyrine and theophylline metabolism in man. *Clin. Pharmacol. Ther.*, 20:643–653.

31. Pantuck, E. J., Hsiao, K.-C., Loub, W. D., Wattenberg, L. W., Kuntzman, R., and Conney, A. H. (1976): Stimulatory effect of vegetables on intestinal drug metabolism in the rat. *J. Pharmacol. Exp. Ther.*, 198:278–283.

32. Pantuck, E. J., Pantuck, C. B., Garland, W. A., Min, B. H., Wattenberg, L. W., Anderson, K. E., Kappas, A., and Conney A. H. 1979): Stimulatory effect of brussels sprouts and cabbage on human drug metabolism. *Clin. Pharmacol. Ther.*, 25:88–95.

33. Sjoqvist, F., and von Bahr, C. (1973): Interindividual differences in drug oxidation: Clinical importance. *Drug. Metab. Dispos.*, 1:469–482.

34. Vesell, E. S. (1979): Intraspecies differences in frequency of genes directly affecting drug disposition: The individual factor in drug response. *Pharmacol. Rev.*, 30:555–563.

35. Alvares, A. P., Kappas, A., Eiseman, J. L., Anderson, K. E., Pantuck, C. B., Pantuck, E. J., Hsiao, K.-C., Garland, W. A., and Conney, A. H. (1979): Intraindividual variation in drug disposition. *Clin. Pharmacol. Ther.*, 26:407–419.

36. Conney, A. H., Miller, E. C., and Miller, J. A. (1956): The metabolism of methylated aminoazo dyes. V. Evidence for induction of enzyme synthesis in the rat by 3-methylcholanthrene. *Cancer Res.*, 16:450–459.

37. Conney, A. H., Miller, E. C., and Miller, J. A. (1957): Substrate-induced synthesis and other properties of benzo(a)-pyrene hydroxylase in rat liver. *J. Biol. Chem.*, 228:753–766.

38. Remmer, H. (1959): Der beschleunigte Abbau von Pharmaka in den Lebermikrosomen unter dem Einfluss von Luminal. *Naunyn Schmiedebergs Arch. Exp. Pathol. Pharmakol.*, 235:279–290.

39. Conney, A. H., and Burns, J. J. (1959): Stimulatory effect of foreign compounds on ascorbic acid biosynthesis and on drug-metabolizing enzymnes. *Nature*, 184:363–366.

40. Fouts, J. R., and Rogers, L. A. (1965): Morphological changes in the liver accompanying stimulation of microsomal drug metabolizing enzyme activity by phenobarbital, chlordane, benzpyrene or methylcholanthrene in rats. *J. Pharmacol. Exp. Ther.*, 147:112–119.

41. Orrenius, S., and Ernster, L. (1964): Phenobarbital-induced synthesis of the oxidative demethylating enzymes of rat liver microsomes. *Biochem. Biophys. Res. Commun.*, 16:60–65.

42. Ryan, D., Lu, A. Y. H., Kawalek, J., West, S. B., and Levin, W. (1975): Highly purified cytochromes P-448 and P-450 from rat liver microsomes. *Biochem. Biophys. Res. Commun.*, 64:1134–1141.

43. Rees, D. E. (1979): The mechanism of induction of the microsomal drug hydroxylation system in rat liver by phenobarbital. *Gen. Pharmacol.*, 10:341–350.

44. Robinson, D. S., and MacDonald, M. G. (1966): The effect of phenobarbital administration in the control of coagulation achieved during warfarin therapy in man. *J. Pharmacol. Exp. Ther.*, 153:250–253.

45. Cucinell, S. A., Conney, A. H., Sansur, M., and Burns, J. J. (1965): Drug interactions in man: 1. Lowering effect of phenobarbital on plasma levels of bishydroxycoumarin (Dicoumarol) and diphenylhydantoin (Dilantin) *Clin. Pharmacol. Ther.*, 6:420–429.

46. Breckenridge, A. M., Back, D. J., Cross, K., Crawford, F., MacIver, M., Orme, M. L. E., Rowe, P. H., and Smith, E. (1980): Influence of environmental chemicals on drug therapy in humans: Studies with contraceptive steroids. In: *Environmental Chemicals, Enzyme Function and Human Disease*, Ciba Foundation Symposium 76, pp. 289–302. Excerpta Medica, New York.

47. Poland, A., Smith, D., Kuntzman, R., Jacobson, M., and Conney, A. H. (1970): Effect of intensive occupational exposure to DDT on phenylbutazone and cortisol metabolism in human subjects. *Clin. Pharmacol. Ther.*, 11:724–732.

48. Alvares, A. P., Fischbein, A., Anderson, K. E., and Kappas, A. (1977): Alterations in drug metabolism in workers exposed to polychlorinated biphenyls. *Clin. Pharmacol. Ther.*, 22:140–146.

49. Ogilvie, R. I. (1978): Clinical pharmacokinetics of theophylline. *Clin. Pharmacokinet.*, 3:267–293.

50. Hunt, S. N., Jusko, W. J., and Yurchak, A. M. (1976): Effect of

smoking on theophylline disposition. *Clin. Pharmacol. Ther.,* 19:546–551.

51. Jusko, W. J., Schentag, J. J., Clark, J. H., Gardner, M., and Yurchak, A. M. (1978): Enhanced biotransformation of theophylline in marihuana and tobacco smokers. *Clin. Pharmacol. Ther.,* 24:406–410.

52. Lijinsky, W., and Shubik, P. (1964): Benzo(a)pyrene and other polynuclear hydrocarbons in charcoal-broiled meat. *Science,* 145:53–55.

53. Conney, A. H., Pantuck, E. J., Hsiao, K.-C., Garland, W. A., Anderson, K. E., Alvares, A. P., and Kappas, A. (1976): Enhanced phenacetin metabolism in humans fed charcoal-broiled beef. *Clin. Pharmacol. Ther.,* 201:663–642.

54. Kappas, A., Alvares, A. P., Anderson, K. E., Pantuck, E. J., Pantuck, C. B., Chang, R., and Conney, A. H. (1978): Effect of charcoal-broiled beef on antipyrine and theophylline metabolism. *Clin. Pharmacol. Ther.,* 23:445–450.

55. Rubin, E., Gang, H., Misra, P. S., and Lieber, C. S. (1970): Inhibition of drug metabolism by acute ethanol intoxication. *Am. J. Med.,* 49:801–806.

56. Vesell, E. S., Passananti G. T., and Greene, F. E. (1970): Impairment of drug metabolism in man by allopurinol and nortryptyline. *N. Engl. J. Med.,* 283:1484–1488.

57. Vesell, E. S., Passananti, G. T., and Lee, C. H. (1971): Impairment of drug metabolism by disulfiram in man. *Clin. Pharmacol. Ther.,* 12:785–792.

58. Silver, B. A., and Bell, W. R. (1979): Cimetidine potentiation of the hypothrombinamic effect of warfarin. *Ann. Intern. Med.,* 90:348–349.

59. Klotz, U., and Reimann, I. (1980): Delayed clearance of diazepam due to cimetidine. *N. Engl. J. Med.,* 301:1012–1014.

60. Roberts, R. K., Grice, J., Wood, L., Petroff, V., and McGuffie, C. (1981): Cimetidine impairs the elimination of theophylline and antipyrine. *Gastroenterology,* 81:19–21.

61. Mitchell, J. R., and Jollow, D. J. (1975): Metabolic activation of drugs to toxic substances. *Gastroenterology,* 68:392–410.

62. Hinson, J. A., Pohl, L. R., Monks, T. J., and Gilette, J. R. (1981): Acetaminophen-induced hepatotoxicity. *Life Sci.,* 29:107–116.

63. Serlin, M. J., Sibeon, R. G., Mossman, S., Breckenridge, A. M., Williams, J. R. B., Atwood, J. L., and Willoughby, J. M. T. (1979): Cimetidine: Interactions with oral anticoagulants in man. *Lancet,* II:317–319.

64. Puurunen, J., and Pelkonen, O. (1979): Cimetidine inhibits microsomal drug metabolism in the rat. *Eur. J. Pharmacol.,* 55:335–336.

65. Kappas, A., and Alvares, A. P. (1975): How the liver metabolizes foreign substances. *Sci. Am.,* 232:21–31.

The Liver: Biology and Pathobiology, edited by
I. Arias, H. Popper, D. Schachter, and D. A. Shafritz.
Raven Press, New York © 1982.

Chapter 16

Conjugation Reactions in the Metabolism of Xenobiotics

John Caldwell

The enormous range of metabolic transformations that foreign compounds may undergo in the body can be conveniently classified into two distinct types: (a) phase I reactions of oxidation, reduction, and hydrolysis, and (b) phase II reactions (1). The latter are syntheses in which a drug or metabolite is combined with an endogenous molecule to form a conjugate (1,2). The conjugation reactions were the first reactions of drug metabolism to be discovered because, in many cases, they produce the final elimination products of drugs. Since the development of drug metabolism as a subdiscipline in the 1950s, phase I reactions, particularly microsomal oxidations, however, have attracted the most attention. Most research on conjugation reactions has been in biochemistry rather than biochemical pharmacology, because they are frequently reactions of importance in intermediary metabolism and biosynthesis.

The above historic sequence probably is responsible for the assumption that conjugation processes are inherently less interesting than are phase I reactions. Thus phase I reactions may (a) produce pharmacologically active metabolites, (b) generate harmful reactive metabolites, and (c) liberate drugs from prodrugs. In contrast, conjugation reactions are considered to terminate the biologic activity of a compound and frequently cause a pronounced increase in drug polarity and acidity, thereby aiding in its excretion. Although much energy and effort is expended on rigorous identification and characterization of the products of phase

I metabolism, the same is not true for conjugation reactions which have been fully characterized in only a few cases.

Many accounts of conjugation reactions deal mainly with biochemistry; pharmacologic and toxicologic implications have been largely overlooked. The importance of these reactions, however, is now beginning to be appreciated. This chapter concerns the biochemistry of various conjugation reactions and their significance in biochemical pharmacology and toxicology.

The conjugation reactions are a group of synthetic metabolic reactions in which a compound foreign to the energy-yielding metabolism of the body, or a metabolite thereof, is combined with an endogenous molecule or grouping to give a product known as a conjugate. The major conjugation reactions are catalysed by a transferase enzyme which is specific for the particular endogenous conjugating agent. The compound undergoing conjugation must have within its structure a suitable functional group for combination with the conjugation agent. This may be a chemically stable group, such as hydroxyl (phenolic, alcoholic, or carboxylic), amino, heterocyclic ring nitrogen, or thiol, or a chemically reactive group, such as epoxide, arene oxide, or carbonium ion.

The products of the principal conjugation reactions are generally biologically inactive or possess markedly reduced activity. They are commonly more water-soluble than are their precursors, and thus these reactions favor elimination of the compound from the body through urine and/or bile. The main function of some conjugations is to protect against chemically reactive intermediates which are produced during oxidative metabolism.

CLASSIFICATION OF THE CONJUGATION REACTIONS

Eight major classes of conjugation reactions are listed in Table 1, where they are divided into two types according to their reaction sequences. Being synthetic reactions, the conjugation reactions involve high-energy activated intermediates. Thus the sequences involve either combination of the xenobiotic with an activated conjugating agent, commonly a nucleotide, or, alternatively, preliminary activation of the xenobiotic to a high-energy intermediate which can interact with the conjugating agent. The former is more common.

Reactions Involving Activated Conjugating Agents

Glucuronic Acid Conjugation

Glucuronic acid conjugation is the most versatile reaction in terms of the wide range of xenobiotic substrates it may accept and its wide distribution through species and tissues. The glucuronic acid found in the conjugate derives from the nucleotide, uridine diphosphate glucuronic acid (UDPGA), in which glucuronic

acid is in the α-form (protons on C-1 and C-2 cis to each other). This is transferred to the acceptor substrate by UDP glucuronyltransferase (UDPGT) with inversion of the configuration of the glucuronic acid, so that, in the conjugate, the sugar acid is present in the β-form (protons on C1 and C-2 trans to each other). A wide range of functional groups may combine with glucuronic acid (Table 2).

The enzyme UDPGT is principally found in the liver and is membrane bound in the endoplasmic reticulum (ER). UDPGT activity is recovered in the microsomal fraction of tissue homogenates and is, at least in part, latent, being activated by a variety of agents that disrupt membrane structure (3). UDP-N-acetyl glucosamine appears to control its latency in vivo (3). Being membrane bound, heterogeneity of the enzyme has been hard to establish, but evidence accumulated over many years, based on studies of species and strain differences, tissue distribution, induction, and inhibition, suggests that more than one form of the enzyme is present (4).

TABLE 1. Classification of the major conjugation reactions

Reaction	Conjugating agent	Functional groups involved
Reactions involving activated conjugating agents		
Glucuronidation	UDP glucuronic acid	−OH, −COOH, −NH₂, −NR₂, −SH, ≳C-H
Glucose conjugation	UDP glucose	−OH, −COOH, −SH
Sulfation	PAPS	−OH, −NH₂, −SH
Methylation	S-Adenosyl-methionine	−OH, −NH₂
Acetylation	Acetyl CoA	−OH, −NH₂
Cyanide detoxication	Sulfane sulfur	CN⁻
Reactions involving activated foreign compounds		
Glutathione conjugation	Glutathione	Arene oxide, epoxide, alkyl- and arylhalide
Amino acid conjugation	Glycine, Glutamine, Ornithine, Taurine	−COOH

TABLE 2. Types of compounds forming glucuronic acid conjugates[a]

Functional group	Example
Hydroxyl	
Primary alcohol	Trichloroethanol
Secondary alcohol	Propranolol
Tertiary alcohol	Tert-butanol
Alicyclic secondary alcohol	Cyclohexanol
Phenol	Phenol
Enol	4-Hydroxycoumarin
Aromatic hydroxylamine	2-Naphthylhydroxylamine
Aliphatic hydroxylamine	N-Hydroxychlorphentermine
Hydroxamic acid	N-Hydroxy-2-acetamido-fluorene
Carboxyl	
Alkyl	2-Ethylhexanoic acid
Aromatic	Benzoic acid
Heterocyclic	Nicotinic acid
Arylalkyl	Indole-3-acetic acid
Aryloxyacetic	Clofibric acid
Amine	
Aromatic	Aniline
Azaheterocycle	Sulfisoxazole
Carbamate	Meprobamate
Sulfonamide	Sulfadimethoxine
Hydroxylamine N-	N-Hydroxy-2-acetamido-fluorene
Tertiary aliphatic	Cyproheptadine
Sulfur	
Thiol	2-Mercaptobenzothiazole
Carbodithioic acid	N,N-Diethyldithiocarbamic acid
Carbon	
Heterocyclic ring	Phenylbutazone

[a] Taken from refs. 2, 9, and 11.

At present, it is clear that there are two UDPGTs, one responsible for conjugation of small planar compounds and the other for nonplanar compounds. The two enzymes are differentially inducible (5), have separate ontogenesis (6), and were separated by column chromatography (7). Other evidence from studies of the inducibility of UDPGT activity suggest the existence of at least two more forms (5).

Glucuronic acid conjugation occurs in mammals, birds, amphibians, reptiles, and fish, but not in insects (8). Cats are relatively defective among mammals in their ability to form many glucuronides which are readily produced by other species. Although originally thought to be completely unable to perform this reaction, the cat has been shown to form glucuronides of large molecules but not smaller ones. This is illustrated in Table 3 with respect to ester and ether glucuronides. This defect in glucuronidation is a biochemical characteristic of cat-like carnivores, the *Feloidea,* and extends to the lion, lynx, civet, cat, and forest genet (8). A comprehensive review of glucuronic acid conjugation has been provided by Dutton and his colleagues (4,9,10).

Sugar Conjugations

At least three sugars may be involved in conjugation reactions of xenobiotics: glucose, ribose, and xylose. These reactions are, in many ways, analogous with the glucuronic acid conjugation, since the sugars are derived from high-energy UDP sugars and transferred to the xenobiotic by a specific transferase located principally in the ER of the liver (12). The functional groups of xenobiotics involved in such conjugations are the same as those for glucuronidation, but the range of xenobiotics involved and species occurrence of other sugar conjugations is restricted in comparison with glucuronidation.

TABLE 3. *Structural dependence of defective glucuronide formation in the cat*[a]

Group	Percent of dose excreted as glucuronide in:	
	Cat	Rat
Phenols		
Phenol	1	44
1-Naphthol	1	47
Paracetamol	3	24
Phenolphthalein	60	98
Carboxylic acids		
1-Naphthylacetic acid	0	79
Clofibric acid	2	82
Diphenylacetic acid	76	95

[a] Adapted from ref. 8.

Glucose Conjugation

In glucose conjugation, the functional group of the xenobiotic is linked to C-1 of glucose derived from UDP glucose to form a β-glucoside. It appears that this mechanism replaces glucuronidation in insects and other invertebrates; many phenols, carboxylic acids, and aromatic thiols may undergo this reaction in these species (2). The occurrence of glucose conjugation in mammals is a more recent observation and is more restricted in terms of acceptor substrate (11). Only four compounds have been reported to form glucosides in mammals: bilirubin (12) and oxinepac (an arylacetic acid) form ester glucosides at the carboxyl group, and two heterocyclic compounds give rise to N-glucosides, 3-(4-pyridyl)-5-(4-pyrimidinyl)-1,2,4-triazole (a xanthine oxidase inhibitor), and amobarbital (11). The tissue and subcellular location and cofactor requirements of these reactions have not been well studied; they appear mainly in microsomal preparations of liver and require UDP glucose (11).

Ribose Conjugation

Ribose conjugation of certain nitrogen-containing heterocycles to give N-ribosides occurs in mammals (11). Little is known of the enzymology of such conjugations, but N-riboside formation is important in the metabolism of 2-hydroxynicotinic acid, purine and pyrimidine base analogs, and imidazole acetic acid, a metabolite of histamine.

Xylose Conjugation

Thus far, no xenobiotic has been shown to undergo conjugation with xylose. Detailed studies have shown that bilirubin gives rise to an ester xyloside (12), in addition to its well-known ester glucuronide and glucoside. The reaction uses UDP xylose as the sugar source and is catalyzed by a transferase which is present in the hepatic ER. Bilirubin xyloside is present in the bile of man, rat, rabbit, dog, cat, chicken, and mouse.

Sulfate Conjugation

Sulfate conjugation is a reaction of hydroxyl (and occasionally amino or thiol) groups in which they are linked to sulfate anion to form a highly polar, highly ionized sulfate ester (13,14). To participate in this reaction, inorganic sulfate must be activated to the high-energy sulfate donor 3'-phosphoadenosine-5'-phosphosulfate (PAPS), from which sulfate is transferred to the xenobiotic by a sulfotransferase (14).

The sulfate-activating enzymes are closely associated with the sulfotransferase. Sulfate conjugation has the following three-step reaction sequence:

1. $ATP + SO_4^{2-} \xrightarrow{\text{ATP-sulfurylase}}$

Adenosine-5'-phosphosulfate (APS)

2. $ATP + APS \xrightarrow{\text{ATP-phosphokinase}}$

PAPS

3. $PAPS + R\text{-}OH \xrightarrow{\text{Sulfotransferase}}$

$R\text{-}OSO_3 H$ + 3'-phosphoadenosine-
5'-phosphate (PAP)

These enzymes are all located in the cell cytoplasm of liver and other organs (14).

The xenobiotic substrates undergoing sulfation are mainly hydroxyl compounds of a variety of types, including alcohols, phenols, catechols, and hydroxylamines; some examples are given in Table 4. Sulfation may, in certain cases, also be a metabolite route of thiols (thiophenol may be converted to its S-sulfate) and aromatic amines (aniline and 1- and 2-naphthylamine gives rise to small amounts of corresponding sulfamic acids) (14).

The sulfotransferases, which are responsible for conjugation of phenolic xenobiotics, are different from those which conjugate sulfate steroids. The two types of enzyme can be separated by ammonium sulfate precipitation (15). Recent work has shown that there are four distinct enzymes in the phenol sulfotransferase fraction; two are active toward true phenols, one is active toward N-hydroxy-2-acetamidofluorene, and one is active toward estrone (16).

The importance of sulfate conjugation in xenobiotic metabolism depends on the dose of the compound administered. Sulfate conjugation is readily saturated and, therefore, is more important at low doses (11,13). It has always been assumed that saturation of this reaction is caused by the small amount of PAPS and inorganic sulfate available within the body. Although administration of inorganic sulfate or cysteine (which can also function as a PAPS precursor) reverses the reduction in sulfation caused by coadministration of another compound metabolized by that reaction, administration of PAPS precursors has little effect on normal conjugation with sulfate. It has been suggested that the kinetic properties of the sulfotransferases give rise to the saturation and not sulfate depletion. When challenged by a compound conjugated with sulfate, the extracellular inorganic sulfate pool is readily supplemented from other body pools (13).

For many compounds, notably phenols, sulfation is a metabolic alternative to glucuronidation, and the relative extent of the two pathways are determined by chemical structure which determines the affinity for enzymes involved in conjugation (11,13). Sulfation is a

TABLE 4. *Types of compounds forming sulfates* [a]

Functional group (Hydroxyl)	Example
Primary alcohol	Ethanol
Secondary alcohol	Butan-2-ol
Phenol	Phenol
Catechol	α-Methyl-DOPA
Alicyclic	Dehydroepiandrosterone
Heterocyclic	3-Hydroxycoumarin
Hydroxyamide	N-hydroxy-2-acetamidofluorene
Aromatic hydroxylamine	2-Naphthylhydroxylamine

[a] Taken from refs. 2, 11, 13, and 14.

feature of the metabolism of small, chemically simple molecules of low lipid solubility which have a subcellular distribution in favor of the cytosol, where the sulfotransferases are located. Additionally, sulfation is relatively more important at low dose levels. Reviews of the various aspects of sulfation are given by Dodgson and Rose (14) and Mulder (17).

Methylation

A variety of compounds containing -OH, $-NR_2$, and -SH groups can be methylated in the body. Although of great importance in the metabolism of endogenous compounds (18), methylation is only rarely of quantitative importance in the fate of xenobiotics (11). A list of the types of compounds undergoing methylation is shown in Table 5.

Xenobiotic phenols, which undergo methylation, are generally either catechols or phenols with bulky substituents *ortho* to the -OH. A variety of nitrogen centers may be methylated; in the case of the tertiary amines and aromatic azaheterocycles, the product is a quaternary ammonium compound. Only in the case of those compounds converted to quaternary ammonium compounds is the water solubility and polarity of the xenobiotic increased by methylation. Methylation of phenols, thiols, and primary and secondary amines reduces polarity and water solubility (11). Thus the function of methylation must be sought elsewhere than

TABLE 5. *Types of compounds undergoing methylation* [a]

Functional group	Example
Primary amine	Amphetamine
Secondary amine	Desmethylimipramine
Tertiary amine	Dimethylaminoethanol
Azaheterocycle	Pyridine
Phenol	4-Hydroxy-3,5-diiodobenzoic acid
Catechol	α-Methyl-DOPA
Thiol	Thiouracil

[a] Taken from refs. 11 and 18.

simple facilitation of excretion. In the case of the catecholamines, which are methylated at the 3-hydroxy group, the products have markedly reduced activity at adrenergic receptors (11).

The methyl group used in methylation is derived from the body pool of activated C-1 intermediates (11,18). In most cases, the source is the nucleotide S-adenosylmethionine, but methylation of primary and secondary amines in the brain involves 5-methyltetrahydrofolic acid. The source of the methyl group in formation of quaternary ammonium compounds is unknown. The enzymology of various methylation reactions has been reviewed recently by Borchardt (19).

The zoologic distribution of various methylation reactions has been poorly studied (8). O-methylation of catechols and N-methylation of histamine and norepinephrine occur throughout the Mammalia, but O-methylation of 4-hydroxy-3,5-diiodobenzoic acid is quantitatively more important in primates, including man, than in nonprimate species (8). Considerable interspecies variations occur in N-methylation of pyridine to the more toxic N-methylpyridinium; the reaction is extensive (>25% of dose methylated) in rabbit, guinea pig, and cat but low (2 to 10% of dose) in rat, mouse, and man (20).

Acetylation

Acetylation is an important route of metabolism for many compounds containing a primary amine function, including amines, amino acids, sulfonamides, hydrazines, and hydrazides. Examples are listed in Table 6. Endogenous compounds containing the hydroxyl (e.g., choline) and thiol (e.g., coenzyme A) groups may also be acetylated; with respect to xenobiotics, however, the reaction is restricted to -NH$_2$ functions (11).

Acetylation involves formation of an amide bond between an -NH$_2$ function in the xenobiotic and the acetyl moiety; the latter is derived from the high-energy compound acetyl CoA. Acetyl CoA is derived from intermediary metabolism within the cell, and the reaction is catalyzed by the enzyme N-acetyltransferase (21). This transferase exists in two distinct forms under separate regulatory control, as revealed by a genetic polymorphism controlling the rate of drug acetylation (22). This polymorphism can be easily demonstrated in man and in outbred animal populations of rabbits and squirrel monkeys (21). The rate of acetylation is a trait showing autosomal mendelian genetics, with two alleles acting at a single locus. The two alleles are for fast (H^F) or slow (H^S) acetylation; thus three phenotypes may be discerned in the population: homozygous fast (H^F H^F), homozygous slow (H^S H^S), and heterozygotes (H^F H^S) of intermediate acetylation capacity. In most studies, heterozygotes are hard to distinguish from homozygous fast acetylators (21). The incidence of these alleles, and thus phenotypes, varies in different populations, from 50% fast/50% slow in the United States to 90% fast/10% slow in Orientals (22).

A number of compounds undergoing acetylation, however, do not exhibit genetic polymorphism; comparatively little interindividual variation is seen in their acetylation, which shows unimodal (monomorphic) distribution in the population. Examples include para-aminobenzoic acid and sulfanilamide. Genetic control over acetylation permits classification of substrates into monomorphic and polymorphic substrates, which are in general bulkier than are the monomorphic ones.

Polymorphic acetylation of many substrates occurs in man and in several laboratory animals species, including mice, rabbits, and squirrel monkeys (21). In addition, two marked species defects in N-acetylation reactions have been described (8). Thus the dog and related carnivores, such as the fox and hyena, are unable to acetylate most of the various classes of substrate for this reaction with the exception of S-substituted cysteines and the sulfonamide (N^1) nitrogen of sulfonamides. The guinea pig is unable to catalyze the final step of mercapturic acid synthesis, the N-acetylation of S-substituted cysteines.

The enzymology of N-acetylation and the molecular basis of the acetylation polymorphism is poorly understood (21). The reaction appears to proceed via a "ping-pong" Bi-Bi mechanism, in which acetyl CoA acetylates the N-acetyltransferase, followed by acetylation of the amine with enzyme regeneration. Many unsuccessful attempts have been made to demonstrate variant forms of N-acetyltransferase in human tissue (23). A single enzyme appears to acetylate monomorphic and polymorphic substrates; the difference between the phenotypes lies in flexibility of the active site (23). It has been suggested that there is an induced fit of substrate to the active site so that, in the case of the slow acetylators, acetyl CoA may be brought close to the NH$_2$ group of compounds, such as para-aminobenzoic acid, but not to that of bulkier molecules, such as sulfamethazine. The more flexible

TABLE 6. Types of compounds undergoing acetylation[a]

Functional group	Example
Aromatic amine	para-Aminobenzoic acid
Sulfonamide	Sulfanilamide
Hydrazine	Hydrazine
Hydrazide	Isoniazid
S-substituted cysteine	Cysteine conjugate of ethacrynic acid

[a] Taken from refs. 8, 11, and 23.

active site of the enzyme from fast acetylators can catalyze the acetylation of both types of substrates.

Cyanide Detoxication

The highly toxic pseudohalogen cation cyanide (CN⁻) is detoxified by conjugation with a sulfane sulfur atom to yield thiocyanate (SCN⁻), which is much less toxic. Thiocyanate, however, is not devoid of biologic properties and is thyrotoxic because of its ability to compete with iodide for uptake into the thyroid. Although the toxicity of cyanide is well recognized and exposure to it in the Western World is carefully controlled, native foodstuffs of many African peoples are rich in cyanogenetic glycosides. Cassava, which is a main caloric source for millions of people, is rich in these glycosides; chronic cyanide poisoning is a feature of such populations (24).

It has been known for many years that rhodanese (thiosulfate-cyanide sulfur-transferase), an enzyme able to convert cyanide to thiocyanate, is able to catalyze the following reaction:

$$S{=}SO_3^{2-} + CN^- \rightarrow SO_3^{2-} + SCN^-$$

The outer sulfur atom of thiosulfate is a so-called sulfane, a divalent sulfur atom which is readily removed enzymically, as above, or chemically by dilute acid. Rhodanese is found in the mitochondrial matrix of most tissues; it is present in greatest quantity in liver and is widely distributed in living organisms.

It has become clear that the total cyanide detoxication capacity of an organism is not attributable to rhodanese, and that other mechanism(s) must be involved. It appears that sulfane sulfur from 3-mercaptopyruvate can also be used in formation of thiocyanate, catalyzed by 3-mercaptopyruvate sulfur transferase, thus

$$HS-CH_2 - \overset{\overset{\displaystyle O}{\|}}{C} -COO^- + CN^-$$

$$\rightarrow H_3C- \overset{\overset{\displaystyle O}{\|}}{C} -COO^- + SCN^-$$

The kinetics of this reaction are extremely complicated, and there is less overall thiocyanate formed than pyruvate. This enzyme is phylogenetically of wide distribution and occurs in a range of tissues in addition to liver and kidney. A full discussion of the fate of cyanide, its interactions with the sulfane pool of the body, and toxicologic sequelae are provided by Westley (25).

Although detoxication of cyanide does not involve high-energy nucleotide intermediates, it must be considered as involving an activated conjugating agent, since the sulfane sulfur used to form thiocyanate is chemically labile.

Reactions Involving Activated Foreign Compounds

Glutathione Conjugation

Conjugation with the nucleophilic tripeptide glutathione (γ-glutamyl cysteinylglycine) (see Fig. 4) is a reaction of a variety of xenobiotics with considerable toxicologic significance. The products of glutathione conjugation, which are S-substituted glutathiones, undergo extensive metabolism to yield mercapturic (or premercapturic) acids (S-substituted N-acetyl cysteines) as the final urinary elimination products.

Xenobiotic substrates for glutathione conjugation are electrophiles. Two types may be distinguished: (a) those sufficiently electrophilic to be conjugated per se, and (b) those requiring metabolic conversion to an electrophile. The first group of reactions involves halo- and nitroalkanes, sulfonic acid esters, and halo- and nitrobenzenes. In each case, displacement of the electron-withdrawing group by the sulfur of glutathione occurs. Michael addition of glutathione across a double bond with strongly electronegative substituents also occurs. Typical mechanisms are seen in Fig. 1. The second group of substrates includes reactive oxidation products, such as arene oxides, aliphatic and alicyclic epoxides, and reactive N-oxidation products. Glutathione opens the strained oxirane ring (Fig. 2) or attacks an electron-deprived center in the molecule.

As well as reactions giving rise to conjugates as final products, glutathione and its associated conjugating enzymes may be involved in the metabolism of nitrite

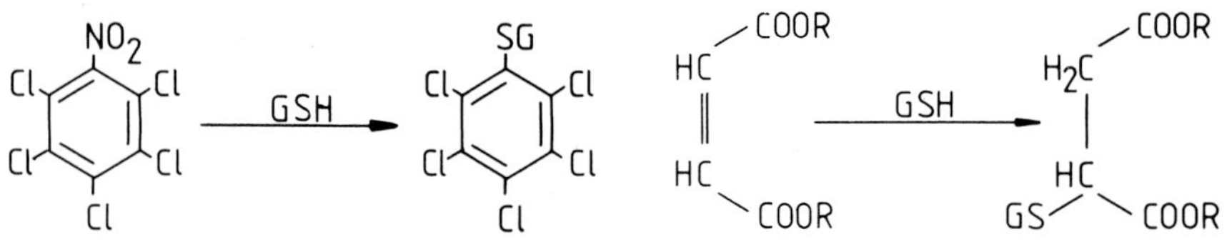

FIG. 1. Glutathione conjugation involving (**left**) displacement of an electrophilic substituent by glutathione (GSH) or (**right**) Michael addition of GSH across a carbon-carbon double bond.

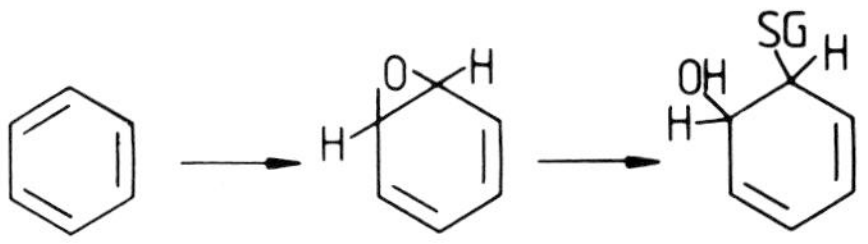

FIG. 2. Oxidation of an aromatic system to give an epoxide, followed by opening of the oxirane ring by glutathione.

esters and alkyl thiocyanates. In such cases, however, the only conjugate formed is the homoconjugate, oxidized glutathione. Two molecules of glutathione are consumed successively (Fig. 3). Similar reactions occur in the detoxication of peroxides, leading to formation of oxidized glutathione.

These various types of glutathione conjugations are catalyzed by a series of enzymes, the glutathione S-transferases, which are located in the cytosol of many tissues and were early recognized to exist in multiple forms. More recently, up to six forms, depending on the tissue source, have been separated. The enzymes have two subunits; one is constant and possesses the glutathione binding site, and the other is variable, having the drug substrate binding site. The reaction mechanism involves the existence of the thiolate ion glutathione S^- as the reactive species at the active site of the enzyme.

Glutathione conjugates are rarely excreted in urine because their polarity and molecular weight favor biliary excretion. They are extensively metabolized (Fig. 4), resulting in formation of S-substituted N-acetylcysteines or mercapturic acids. This transformation of the peptide moiety occurs in liver, intestinal wall, and kidney. In the case in which a glutathione conjugate arises from opening of an arene oxide ring, the final products are nonaromatic, premercapturic acids, which may be converted to aromatic mercapturic acids by proton-catalyzed dehydration (Fig. 5).

The zoologic distribution of glutathione conjugation, which occurs in most mammals, has not been well studied. Guinea pigs do not excrete mercapturic acids as metabolites of compounds conjugated with glutathione, but this is not attributable to their inability to form glutathione conjugates. Rather, the defect arises from the absence in this species, of the final step of mercapturic acid synthesis, N-acetylation of the S-substituted cysteines. A more detailed discussion of the biologic role of glutathione is given elsewhere in this volume. Other comprehensive reviews on glutathione conjugations have been provided by Chasseaud (26) and Jerina and Bend (27).

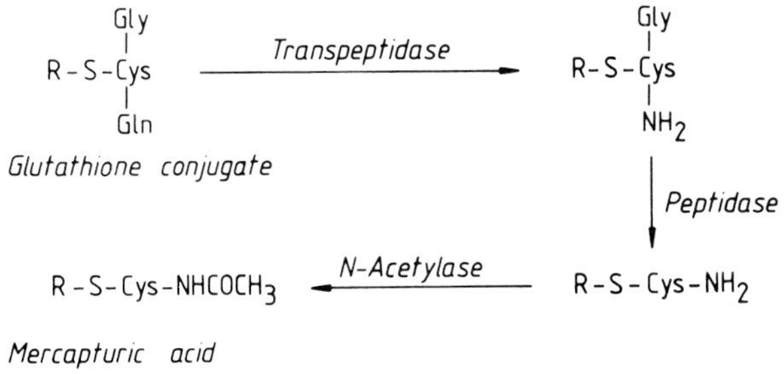

FIG. 4. Conversion of a glutathione conjugate to a mercapturic acid.

Epoxide Hydration

Epoxides are common initial products of microsomal oxidation. Although they generally undergo spontaneous chemical rearrangement, they are reactive species which can be toxic. Many can undergo conjugation with glutathione, a reaction of great importance for their detoxication. The other means of inactivating epoxides by metabolism is by hydration to a dihydrodiol. This reaction,

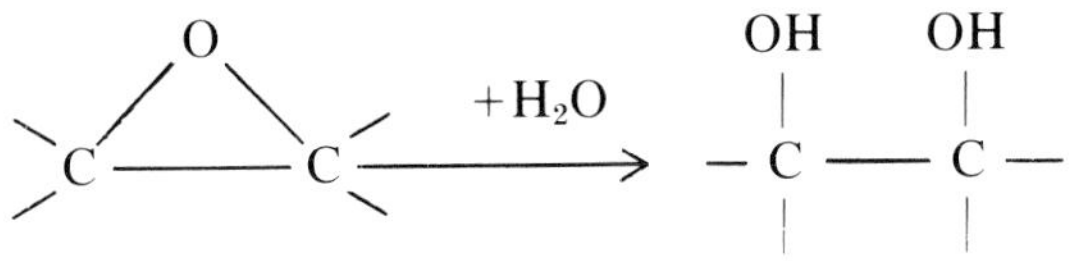

is performed by epoxide hydrolase, an enzyme in the microsomal fraction of liver and other organs. Epoxide hydrolase activity toward some substrates also occurs in cytosol.

A wide range of epoxide substrates may undergo hydration, ranging from simple molecules, such as octene 1,2-oxide and styrene 7,8-oxide, to large structures, such as benzo(a)pyrene 4,5-oxide and carbamazepine 10,11-oxide. Despite this range of substrates, there appears to be a single form of epoxide hydrolase which has been purified to apparent homogeneity. Evidence from induction, inhibition, ontogenesis, and other studies supports the existence of one form of this enzyme. The enzyme has an essential histidine residue in its active site which functions as a base catalyst by removing a proton from the attacking

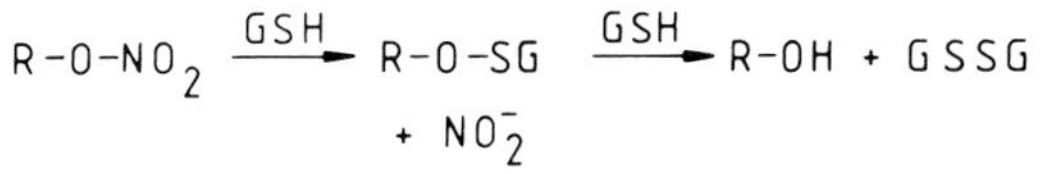

FIG. 3. Glutathione (GSH)-catalyzed denitration of a nitrite ester.

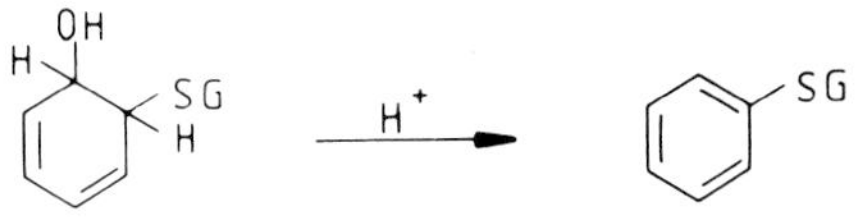

FIG. 5. Proton-catalyzed dehydration of a premercapturic acid to a mercapturic acid.

water molecule without actually producing free OH^- (28).

Cytosolic epoxide hydrolase was first discovered by Hammock et al. (29) and has a different range of substrate specificities than does that found in the ER. It appears to be more concerned with metabolism of endogenous epoxides of fatty acids, terpenes, and steroids. A fuller account of epoxide hydrolase and its reactions is given by Oesch (30).

Amino Acid Conjugations

Many xenobiotic carboxylic acids may undergo conjugation with one of a variety of amino acids, which are usually small, aliphatic, and nonessential. The products of these reactions are conjugates in which an amide (peptide) bond links the carboxyl group of the acid with the α-amino function of the amino acid. These reactions apparently involve activation of the acid to its CoA thioester via an adenylate intermediate, followed by transfer of the activated acyl moiety to the amino acid. The three steps of the conjugation are:

1. $R.COOH + ATP$
   $\rightarrow R.CO{\sim}AMP + PPi$
2. $R.CO{\sim}AMP + CoA.SH$
   $\rightarrow R.CO{\sim}S.Co.A + AMP$
3. $R.CO{\sim}S.CoA + H_2N.R^1COOH$
   $\rightarrow R.CONH. R^1COOH + CoA.SH$

The range of structures undergoing amino acid conjugation is small; these reactions are restricted to aromatic, heteroaromatic, cinnamic, and arylacetic acids. Even within this limited range of substrates, the extent of amino acid conjugation depends on steric hindrance around the carboxyl group by the aryl grouping and side chain substituents.

Major amino acid conjugations occur with glycine, glutamine, taurine, and ornithine. In addition, isolated cases of conjugation with glutamic acid, serine, histidine, alanine, and aspartic acid have been reported. The particular amino acid used for conjugation of a given acid depends on the structure of the acid and the

animal species. Examples of utilization of these various amino acids in the conjugation of xenobiotic acids in various species are given in Tables 8 (glycine), 9 (glutamine), 10 (taurine), 11 (ornithine), and 12 (others).

Although structure of the acid is the major determinant of overall amino acid conjugation, the nature of the amino acid used depends on species. For aromatic (benzoic), heterocyclic, and cinnamic acids, most species use glycine; ornithine is found in the anseriform and galliform birds (chicken, duck). With arylacetic acid and aryloxyacetic acids, glycine conjugation occurs in subprimate mammals and is replaced by glutamine in primates. Taurine conjugation also occurs with these acids, and is frequent in carnivorous mammals.

The enzymology of these conjugations remains largely unknown. The reaction sequence for glycine, glutamine, and ornithine conjugation follows that seen above; little is known about the other amino acid conjugations. Indeed, it has been impossible to achieve taurine conjugation of arylacetic acids in broken cell preparations from liver and kidney. The enzymes of amino acid conjugation are in mitochondria; although the exact location of the acyl-CoA-forming enzymes is uncertain, the amino acid N-acyl-transferases are soluble in the mitochondrial matrix.

Virtually all amino acid conjugations involve single amino acids; rarely are dipeptide conjugates found. Examples include the glycylglycine and glycyltaurine conjugates of quinaldic and kynurenic acids formed by cats and the glycylvaline conjugate of 3-phenoxybenzoic acid in ducks. Nothing is known of the enzymology of these dipeptide conjugations, nor of the mode of addition of the amino acid residues.

Carboxylic acids may be metabolized by amino acid conjugation or by glucuronidation. The relative extent of these two reactions is a function of the structure of

TABLE 7. *"Monomorphic" and "polymorphic" substrates for N-acetylation in man*[a]

Monomorphic (variation within population is normally distributed)	Polymorphic (variation within population exhibits two or more modes)
para-Aminobenzoic acid	Sulfamethazine
Sulfanilamide	Isoniazid
	Dapsone
	Hydrallazine
	Procainamide

[a] Taken from ref. 23.

TABLE 8. *Species and structure dependence of the conjugation of xenobiotic acids with glycine*[a]

Type of acid	Example	Species
Aliphatic	Propionic	Man
Aromatic	Benzoic, naphthoic, and nuclear-substituted derivatives	Mammals
Heterocyclic	Isonicotinic	Mammals
Arylacetic	Phenylacetic and nuclear-substituted derivatives	Subprimate mammals
β-Arylpropionic	Phenylpropionic	Mammals
Aryloxyacetic	2,4-Dichlorophenoxy-acetic	Mammals
Acrylic	Cinnamic	Mammals
Bile (steroid) acids	Cholic	Mammals

[a] Drawn from ref. 31.

TABLE 9. *Species and structure dependence of the conjugation of carboxylic acids with glutamine*[a]

Type of acid	Example	Species
Arylacetic	Phenylacetic and nuclear-substituted derivatives, naphthyl	Primates
	Phenylacetic	Ferret
	2-Naphthylacetic	Several non-primates
Aryloxyacetic	Diphenylmethoxy-acetic	Rhesus monkey

[a] Drawn from ref. 31.

TABLE 10. *Species and structure dependence of the conjugation of carboxylic acids with taurine*[a]

Type of acid	Example	Species
Aromatic	3-Phenoxybenzoic	Mouse
Arylacetic	Phenylacetic and nuclear-substituted derivatives, naphthylacetic	Many mammals, notably carnivores
Aryloxyacetic	2,4-Dichloro- and 2,4,5-trichloro-phenoxyacetic	Rat, mouse (minor)
	Clofibric	Dog, cat, ferret

[a] Drawn from ref. 31.

TABLE 11. *Species and structure dependence of the conjugation of carboxylic acids with ornithine*[a]

Type of acid	Example	Species
Aromatic	Benzoic and nuclear-substituted derivatives	Anseriform (ducks, geese) and galliform (hens, turkeys) birds, reptiles
Heterocyclic	Nicotinic	Hen
Arylacetic	Phenylacetic and nuclear-substituted derivatives	Hen

[a] Drawn from ref. 31.

TABLE 12. *Some unusual amino acid conjugations of carboxylic acids*[a]

Amino acid	Acid	Species
Arginine		Arthropoda
Glutamic acid	Benzoic	Indian fruit bat
Histidine		*Peripatus*
Aspartic acid	o,p'-DDA	Rat
Alanine		Mouse, hamster
Serine	Xanthurenic	Mammals
Glycylglycine		
Glycyltaurine	Quinaldic	Cat
Glycylvaline	3-Phenoxybenzoic	Mallard duck

[a] Drawn from ref. 31.

the acid in question; acids whose structures preclude amino acid conjugation are conjugated with glucuronic acid. This is due to structure-related differences in affinity of the acids for mitochondria and the amino acid-conjugating enzymes on the one hand, and the ER and glucuronyltransferase on the other. Recent comprehensive reviews of various amino acid conjugations in the metabolism of carboxylic acids are found elsewhere (31,32). Enzymologic aspects of these reactions are described by Killenberg and Webster (33).

Unusual Conjugation Reactions

As analytic techniques improve and the catalog of compounds studied from a metabolic viewpoint grows, new types of conjugation reactions are discovered. Some represent novel reactions of well-known conjugating agents, e.g., the C- and quaternary-N-glucuronides; others involve previously unknown conjugating agents. In some cases, available evidence shows that the novel reaction does not involve any well-known conjugating agent, but the exact nature of the conjugating agent remains to be elucidated. This section briefly mentions some novel conjugating agents that occur in xenobiotic conjugates.

Acylation and Acyl Group Transfer

Acetylation is a well-recognized reaction; recently, however, three other acylation reactions have been reported. The N-deethylated metabolite of an anorectic drug, para-chloro-2-ethylaminopropiophenone, is conjugated at its nitrogen center with succinate, whereas 11-hydroxy-Δ9-tetrahydrocannabinol forms O-stearoyl and O-palmitoyl conjugates. Other acylations involve many of the acyl-CoAs found in the body. Acidic compounds converted to acyl-CoAs may participate in synthetic reactions analogous to those of lipid biosynthesis. Thus 3-phenoxybenzoic acid is incorporated into a mixed triglyceride, dipalmitoyl-3-phenoxy-benzoylglycerol (34). Benzoic acid undergoes addition of an acetyl group to its carboxyl group in the same way as does acetyl-CoA; and benzoylacetic acid (3-phenyl-3-oxopropionic acid) and the corresponding β-hydroxy acid are found as minor metabolites (35).

Phosphate Conjugates

In view of the importance of activated phosphate, it is surprising that phosphate conjugation is encountered rarely. The best examples are formation of monophenylphosphate from phenol in the cat and di-(2-amino-1-naphthyl)-phosphate from 2-naphthylamine in the dog.

Methylthio (R-S-CH₃) Conjugates

A wide range of compounds can give rise to methylthio conjugates, including naphthalene, bromazepam, caffeine, propranolol, and carbamazepine. These probably arise from methylation of thiols, produced by thiol transfer or cleavage of a glutathione conjugate by cysteine conjugate β-lyase (36).

Other examples of unusual conjugations are given by Caldwell (11), Israili et al. (37), and Jenner and Testa (38). At present, these unusual reactions appear to be restricted to particular combinations of substrate and species; little is known of their mechanisms. Some may prove to be general routes of foreign compound metabolism.

BIOLOGIC SIGNIFICANCE OF THE CONJUGATION REACTIONS

The various conjugation reactions are fruitful fields for biochemical investigation, but the same is not true of pharmacologic and toxicologic studies. In the eyes of many workers concerned with implications of the various pathways of drug metabolism, conjugates are of lesser interest than phase I reactions, notably oxidation. Oxidation may result in formation of pharmacologically active metabolites or chemically reactive metabolites of toxicologic significance. The conjugations, in contrast, are seen as detoxication reactions, which effectively terminate xenobiotic activity and which, by increasing the water solubility and acidity of drugs, facilitate their elimination. The biologic significance of these reactions is as follows: (a) although they result in detoxication, they may be saturable or defective and thereby fail in this task; (b) they may produce biologically active metabolites, which contribute to toxicology of the drug in question; and (c) they have important pharmacokinetic consequences for many compounds.

Detoxication Function of Conjugation

The considerable physicochemical changes produced by conjugation lead to a loss of ligand interaction with receptors for the parent compound and to its facile elimination from the body. Since there are many active and reactive oxidized metabolites of numerous compounds, the conjugation reactions may be the true detoxication mechanisms. This can be seen for phenolic compounds, which generally undergo glucuronidation, and aromatic amines, which are commonly N-acetylated. The presence of a glucuronidation defect in the cat and of a N-acetylation defect in the dog has been alluded to (8); comparison of the toxicities of appropriate substrates in deficient and normal spe-

cies gives an indication of the toxicologic significance of these reactions.

Table 13 shows that the cat is more susceptible to lethal effects of several phenols than is the rabbit; Table 14 shows that the LD_{50}s of several amino compounds are lower in dogs than in other species. Only in rare cases is it possible to subject xenobiotic conjugates to toxicity testing; the few instances of such tests illustrate that glucuronidation, sulfation, and amino acid conjugations result in marked reductions in toxicity as compared with the parent compounds (11). In addition, the role of glutathione conjugation in the detoxication of chemically reactive intermediates capable of causing tissue injury by covalent binding must be stressed (26).

Conjugation has an important role in detoxication mechanisms; any change in the ability of an organism to effect conjugation will be harmful. This occurs when the conjugation reaction becomes saturated, in genetically determined inter- or intraspecies differences in conjugation, and when drug interactions reduce the capacity of a conjugation reaction. Conjugations may be saturated as a consequence of the limited availability of the endogenous conjugating agent or by the quantity of enzyme becoming rate-limiting. Several conjugations exhibit limited capacity (Table 15); Table 16 lists some examples where failure of detoxication arises from saturation of conjugation for the compound in question (11). The examples shown include cases where the parent compound is toxic (benzoic acid, phenol), where failure to conjugate allows formation of toxic metabolites by alternative, generally minor, pathways (chloramphenicol), and failure of conjugation of reactive intermediates (acetaminophen, bromobenzene).

There are several so-called species defects of drug conjugation in which particular animal species are unable to perform a conjugation of otherwise widespread zoologic distribution (8); some are listed in Table 17. The toxicologic significance of the defects in cat and dog has been discussed; in each case, however, the defect must be considered when extrapolating data from species to species. This is especially true of reac-

TABLE 13. *Importance of glucuronidation in the detoxication of phenolic compounds*[a]

Compound	LD₅₀ (mg/kg)	
	Cat	Rabbit
Phenol	80	250
Acetaminophen	250	1,200
1-Naphthol	100	9,000
2-Naphthol	100	3,000

[a] Adapted from ref. 11.

TABLE 14. *Importance of N-acetylation in the detoxication of amines, hydrazines, and hydrazides* [a]

	LD$_{50}$ (mg/kg)	
Compound	Dog	Rat
para-Aminobenzoic acid	1,000	2,000
Sulfanilamide	2,000	3,900
1,1-Dimethylhydrazine	60	250
Isoniazid	250	1,500

[a] Adapted from ref. 11.

tions which are defective in nonprimate mammals and which occur only in man and other primate species (8).

The best example of the significance of intraspecies differences in conjugation occurs with N-acetylation. This reaction is subject to genetic control by two alleles acting at a single locus, and the population exhibits a bimodal distribution into fast and slow acetylators (22). It is not surprising that the incidence of adverse reactions to drugs undergoing acetylation varies between the two phenotypes. In general, the compounds are both more effective (lower dose requirement) and more toxic in slow acetylators (39). Acetylation polymorphism also occurs in mice, rabbits, and squirrel monkeys (21).

Certain inborn errors of metabolism are associated with reduced capacity for drug conjugation. Thus patients with the Crigler-Najjar syndrome or Gilbert's disease, both of which are characterized by low glucuronidation of bilirubin, exhibit reduced glucuronidation of many drugs *in vivo* and *in vitro* in liver biopsies (40). A reduced capacity for glycine conjugation of salicylate occurs in mongolism (Down's syndrome). (11).

Compounds can exert a toxic action indirectly by depleting the body of appropriate endogenous conjugation agents which have important functions in intermediary metabolism (11). Examples are naphthalene, certain halobenzenes, and nicotinamide. The former compounds undergo glutathione conjugation and can deplete the lens of the eye of this tripeptide, causing opacity. Nicotinamide is N-methylated; high doses cause growth failure due to depletion of methyl group donors of the one-carbon pool.

TABLE 15. *Relative capacities of some conjugation reactions*

Capacity	Reaction
High	Glucuronidation
Medium	Acetylation of monomorphic substrates, amino acid conjugation
Low	Sulfation, glutathione conjugation
Variable	Acetylation of polymorphic substrates

TABLE 16. *Failure of detoxication arising from the saturation of conjugation reactions* [a]

Compound	Saturable reaction	Toxic reaction
Benzoic acid Phenol	Glycine conjugation	Death in cats as no glucuronidation to compensate
Chloramphenicol	Glucuronidation	"gray syndrome" in human neonate
Acetaminophen Bromobenzene	Glutathione conjugation	Hepatocellular necrosis

[a] Adapted from ref. 11.

CONJUGATION RESULTING IN METABOLIC ACTIVATION

In most but not all cases, conjugation results in detoxication of xenobiotics. Several examples demonstrate that conjugates contribute to the biologic activity of foreign compounds; these fall into three types: (a) chemically stable conjugates with biologic activity arising from reversible interaction with tissues, (b) chemically reactive conjugates, which may bind irreversibly to tissues, and (c) conjugates which become active subsequent to further metabolism, generally following cleavage of the bond linking xenobiotic and conjugating agent (Table 18).

The first type of active conjugate, which is stable and has intrinsic activity *per se*, is not discussed further, except to note that this possibility must always be considered, particularly with molecules able to be N-acetylated. The second type, the chemically reactive conjugates, are especially noteworthy in view of the essential contribution of conjugation to formation of a reactive electrophilic species responsible for a variety of toxic sequelae, including tumor initiation.

Arylamines, arylacetamides, and ally benzenes require a two-step metabolic activation to their ultimate carcinogens. This involves initial hydroxylation at nitrogen or at C-1 of the allyl side chain and subsequent conjugation of the products with sulfate or glucuronic

TABLE 17. *Species defects of conjugation reactions*

Reaction	Species
Glucuronidation	Cat and other *Feloidea*
Sulfation	Pig
Hippuric acid formation	Indian fruit bat
N-acetylation of aromatic amines and hydrazines	Dog
N-acetylation of S-substituted cysteines	Guinea pig
N^1-glucuronidation of sulfonamides	Nonprimate mammals
Glutamine conjugation	Nonprimate mammals

TABLE 18. *Conjugation reactions leading to metabolic activation*

Conjugation reaction	Compound	Activity of product and comments
Conjugation producing stable active metabolites		
Glucuronidation	Morphine (at 6-position)	Potent analgesic
N-acetylation	Sulfanilamide	Antibacterial (metabolite also used as a drug)
	Procainamide	Potent antiarrhythmic (metabolite also used as a drug)
	Acebutolol	β-Blocker
O-methylation	Isoproterenol (at 3-position)	β-Blocker (opposes action of parent drug)
Conjugation contributing to formation of reactive metabolites		
Glucuronidation	N-hydroxyoryl-amines and amides (e.g., N-hydroxy-2-acetamidofluorene) 1′-Hydroxyallylbenzenes (e.g., safrole, estragole)	Conjugation favors formation of reactive electrophilic ultimate carcinogens
Glutathione Conjugation	Dihaloalkanes	Products can act as sulfur mustards, causing mutagenesis and perhaps carcinogenesis
Conjugates active after further metabolism		
Glucuronidation	N-hydroxy-2-acetamidofluorene (N-glucuronide)	Transport form of proximate carcinogen to bladder, giving cancer at that site
N-acetylation	Isoniazid	Cleavage to N-acetylhydrazine in the first step in conversion to an hepatotoxic metabolite

acid. The O-sulfate and O-glucuronide moieties are excellent leaving groups, better than hydroxyl; thus formation of the electrophilic arylnitrenium or carbonium ions is facilitated by conjugation. These matters are discussed elsewhere (41).

The activation of vicinal dihaloalkanes by conjugation follows a different sequence. These compounds are readily conjugated with glutathione; one halogen is displaced by the S of glutathione, giving an S-monohaloalkylglutathione. Formation of the thioether activates the second halogen; the product is a sulfur mustard, which readily dissociates, giving the halide ion and a reactive carbonium ion on the terminal carbon of the alkane chain, as depicted in Fig. 6. This reaction sequence can occur with a range of dihaloalkanes. The greatest activation is seen in compounds where the halogens are *cis* (42). This phenomenon is responsible for the mutagenic potential of these compounds *in vitro* and may contribute to their toxicity in the whole animal.

Conjugation reactions also contribute to the overall effects of foreign compounds after further metabolism; in some cases, this may result from their acting as transport forms resulting in a toxic reaction, particularly with conjugates which are cleaved by one of the various hydrolytic enzymes. Thus the N-glucuronides of certain N-hydroxyarylamines, which have a free N-OH group and are not reactive metabolites, are stable in the liver and are excreted in the urine. They are broken down in the urinary bladder by β-glucuronidases and may initiate tumor formation at a site different from that at which the metabolite was formed (43). The consequences of hydrolysis and further metabolism of conjugates excreted in bile are presented below.

An excellent example of toxicity of a conjugate arising from its further metabolism occurs with isoniazid (44). N-Acetylation of this antitubercular drug is under genetic control; hepatotoxicity, which closely resembles acute viral hepatitis, is due to a reactive metabolite produced by further biotransformation of N-acetylisoniazid, which is first hydrolyzed to give isonicotinic acid and N-acetylhydrazine; the latter compound is N-hydroxylated and is dehydrated to acetyldiazene, which binds covalently to liver macromolecules and causes necrosis. The extent of binding of material derived from N-acetylisoniazid and the severity of liver necrosis show a strong positive correlation. It has been suggested that isoniazid is more hepatotoxic to fast acetylators, but this is doubtful, and there may not be a relationship between acetylator status and liver injury.

PHARMACOKINETIC IMPLICATIONS OF CONJUGATION

The various conjugation reactions that xenobiotics can undergo have important implications for their disposition and excretion and may also be involved in the etiology of drug interactions. These matters may be termed pharmacokinetic implications.

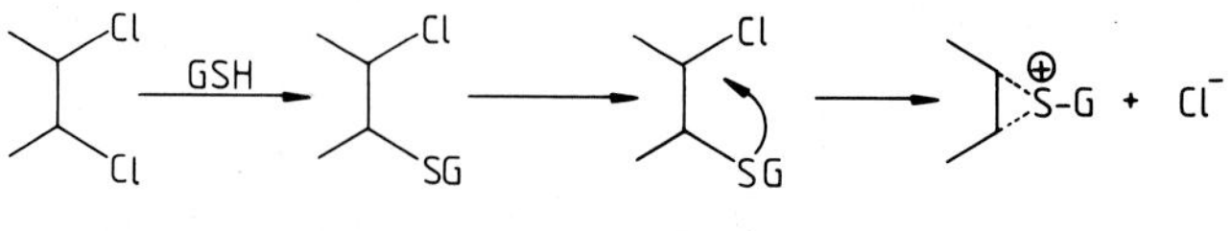

FIG. 6. Formation of a sulfur mustard from a dihaloalkane by glutathione (GSH) conjugation.

Total Body Clearance

The products of the major conjugation reactions are polar and are eliminated in the urine and/or bile. It is a matter of common experience that the ultimate excretion products of the majority of xenobiotics are conjugates. These reactions are responsible for the major fraction of total body clearance of xenobiotics. Many glucuronides, sulfates, and amino acid conjugates are actively secreted by the kidney tubule (11). Detailed pharmacokinetic studies on drugs, such as aspirin, show that their various conjugates are eliminated faster than are the unchanged compound or their phase I metabolites (11).

Saturation of Conjugation

Most simple pharmacokinetic equations consider only situations in which compounds exhibit first-order kinetics. When any of the processes under consideration is capacity-limited, however, expressions involving Michaelis-Menten terms must be derived. This results in variation in pharmacokinetics with dose (nonlinear kinetics), which has important consequences (45): (a) nonexponential elimination kinetics, (b) increasing elimination half-life with dose, (c) area under the plasma-concentration-time curve (AUC) after oral dose not proportional to the fraction of the dose absorbed, (d) pattern of metabolites varies with dose (i.e., the fraction of excreted material metabolized by the saturable pathway falls with dose), and (e) competitive interaction with other drugs handled by the saturable route may occur.

Although phase I metabolism of a few drugs exhibits dose-dependent kinetics (e.g., the 4-hydroxylation of diphenylhydantoin), the ease with which conjugation reactions may be saturated has been mentioned. There are many examples of extensively conjugated drugs exhibiting dose-dependent metabolism and kinetics within the human therapeutic range (11), including acetaminophen and salicylamide (both conjugated with glucuronic acid and sulfate), salicylate (conjugated with glycine and glucuronic acid), and isoniazid (which is N-acetylated).

Biliary Elimination

To undergo biliary excretion, anionic molecules must be amphipathic and of sufficient molecular weight; the latter exhibits species variation (rat 325 ± 50, rabbit 475, man 500) (46). Since most drugs are relatively small and lipid-soluble, conjugation is critical in their acquisition of characteristics for biliary excretion (46). This is most notable for the glucuronic acid and glutathione mechanisms. In addition to a role

in the fecal elimination of xenobiotics, biliary excretion has other consequences. It exposes compounds and/ or metabolites to the gastrointestinal microflora, which have a wide range of metabolic activities (46). Metabolism by the gut flora can involve routes of metabolism not normally occurring within tissues, such as reductive dealkylation and heterocyclic ring fission. Compounds excreted in the bile may cause localized toxicity within the gut, such as occurs with indomethacin. This drug is excreted in the bile as its ester glucuronide, and the conjugate is cleared by bacterial enzymes. The indomethacin so liberated is ulcerogenic to the small intestine (11).

Many compounds excreted in the bile are subsequently reabsorbed from the gut and undergo enterohepatic circulation (46). This can result in secondary peaks in plasma level time curves of drugs, sustained body levels due to recirculation, and slowing of elimination. Secondary plasma level peaks may be associated with rebound effects of drugs (46).

Conjugations as a Cause of Route of Administration-Related Variation in Metabolism

Although the liver is generally the major site of drug metabolism, other organs have considerable capacity to effect many of these reactions. The intestinal mucosa is such an organ; while its contribution to the metabolism of parenterally administered compounds is minimal, it may be more important than the liver in the metabolism of compounds absorbed from the gut (47). This is especially notable for compounds undergoing conjugation and is well illustrated by the bronchodilator isoproterenol. When given intravenously, it is excreted in the urine largely unchanged, with the 3-O-methyl conjugate also present. When given orally, however, the major metabolite is the 3-O-sulfate, which is formed in the gut wall. Other reactions occurring in the gut mucosa include glucuronidation, N-acetylation, and glycine conjugation (48). Compounds handled by these routes in the gut show variations in metabolism with route of administration, as occurs with isoproterenol.

Drug Interactions Due to Competition for Conjugation

The relatively low substrate specificity and capacity of conjugation enzymes lead to the expectation that drug interactions occur due to competition for the enzymes. This is particularly true when either or both compounds is at a concentration close to the K_m. Examples (11) include salicylate/salicylamide and acetaminophen/salicylamide (competition for glucuronidation), ascorbic acid/salicylate (competition for sulfation), and acetaminophen/salicylamide (competition for glucuronidation and sulfation).

The foregoing suggests that conjugation interactions which reduce the capacity of the organism to effect conjugation carry the potential for hazard. This may be seen in the interaction between acetaminophen and salicylamide. Acetaminophen is hepatotoxic at high doses but innocuous at normal therapeutic doses. The major routes of its metabolism are conjugation with glucuronic acid and sulfate, and a small amount is converted to a hepatotoxic reactive metabolite, which is normally detoxified by glutathione conjugation. When salicylamide is coadministered, glucuronidation and sulfation of acetaminophen are reduced by competition, and there is an increase in the proportion undergoing metabolic activation. The dose required to elicit hepatotoxicity is reduced by this interaction (49).

CONCLUSION

The significance of conjugation reactions for the biochemical pharmacology and toxicology of xenobiotics is highlighted. These reactions are critical in detoxication and excretion of foreign compounds but may on occasion be involved in their activation. Alteration in the ability of an organism to effect these reactions will have important consequences for biologic activity, pharmacokinetics, and elimination of compounds which are substrates for conjugation.

Drug metabolism as a subdiscipline has shown comparatively little interest in the conjugation reactions. It is often thought that conjugation is inevitable, leading only to excretion. Indeed, one may hear statements to the effect that a drug "is not metabolized, only conjugated." That conjugation is not inevitable is illustrated by examples of species defects, genetic defects, and ready saturability of certain reactions.

The descriptions given of the biochemistry of the various conjugation reactions show that our knowledge of them is unevenly distributed. Thus glucuronidation attracts considerable interest, but reactions such as amino acid conjugations and methylation remain largely unknown. Our knowledge of the plethora of genetic, physiologic, and environmental factors potentially influencing the conjugation reactions is poor.

Conjugation reactions are virtually unexplored from the viewpoint of their impact on intermediary metabolism, despite their essential role in the inactivation of endogenous compounds (e.g., bilirubin) and in biosynthesis (e.g., heparin). What are the implications of depletion of active sulfate caused by a phenolic substrate for synthesis of connective tissue macromolecules involving sulfation? Conjugation makes use of several essential compounds, including high-energy nucleotides; alterations in intermediary metabolism along the lines alluded to above may be expected to occur.

Individual susceptibility to disease may arise from variations in the capacity of conjugation reactions. Several examples of drug toxicity originating in such a way may be relevant to idiopathic disease. Many diseases originate in unrecognized exposure to environmental toxins or in faulty metabolism of endogenous toxins. As well as being more at risk from drug-induced systemic lupus erythematosus (SLE), slow acetylators are also predisposed to spontaneous SLE (39). Although the basis of this is unknown, the finding has implications for this and other conjugation pathways.

Division of the various reactions of xenobiotic metabolism into two distinct phases is useful but should not be regarded as a "law of drug metabolism." Without a proper appreciation of the significance of conjugation reactions in their various ways, it is impossible to discern relationships between the metabolism of foreign compounds and the effects they elicit. A fresh look at conjugation reactions and their interrelationships with intermediary metabolism could provide advances in biochemistry and pathology.

ACKNOWLEDGMENTS

I am grateful to my colleagues Mary Varwell Marsh, Keith Sinclair, John O'Gorman, and Andrew Hutt for many discussions and literature references, and to Nicholas Oates for help with the illustrations. I wish to thank Jill Rogers and Jill Spencer for typing the manuscript. The encouragement of Professor Robert Smith is gratefully acknowledged.

REFERENCES

1. Williams, R. T. (1959): *Detoxication Mechanisms*, second edition. Chapman and Hall, London.
2. Williams, R. T. (1967): The biogenesis of conjugation and detoxication products. In: *Biogenesis of Natural Compounds*, second edition, edited by P. Bernfeld, pp. 590–639. Pergamon, Oxford.
3. Kasper, C. B., and Henton, D. (1980): Glucuronidation. In: *Enzymatic Basis of Detoxication, Vol. 2*, edited by W. B. Jakoby, pp. 4–36. Academic Press, New York.
4. Dutton, G. J., and Burchell, B. (1977): Newer aspects of glucuronidation. *Prog. Drug. Metab.*, 2:1–70.
5. Bock, K. W., Clausbruck, U. C. V., Kaufmann, R., Libienblum, W., Oesch, F., Pfeil, H., and Platt, K. L. (1980): Functional heterogeneity of UDP-glucuronyl transferase in rat tissue. *Biochem. Pharmacol.*, 29:495–500.
6. Wishart, G. J., Campbell, M. T., and Dutton, G. J. (1978): Functional heterogeneity of UDP-glucuronyltransferase. In: *Conjugation reactions in drug biotransformation*, edited by A. Aitio, pp. 179–187. Elsevier, Amsterdam.
7. Bock, K. W., Josting, D., Lilenblum, W., and Pfeil, H. (1979): Purification of rat liver glucuronyltransferase—Separation of two enzyme forms inducible by 3-methylcholanthrene or phenobarbital. *Eur. J. Biochem.*, 98:19–26.
8. Caldwell, J. (1980): Comparative aspects of detoxication in mammals. In: *Enzymatic Basis of Detoxication, Vol. 1*, edited by W. B. Jakoby, pp. 85–114. Academic Press, New York.

9. Dutton, G. J., Wishart, G. J., Leakey, J. E. A., and Goheer, M. A. (1977): Conjugation with glucuronic acid and other sugars. In: *Drug Metabolism from Microbe to Man*, edited by D. V. Parke and R. L. Smith, pp. 71–90. Taylor and Francis, London.

10. Dutton, G. J. (1981): *Glucuronidation of Drugs and Related Compounds*. C.R.C. Press, Boca Raton, Florida.

11. Caldwell, J. (1980): Conjugation reactions. In: *Concepts in Drug Metabolism*, edited by P. Jenner and B. Testa, pp. 211–250. Marcel Dekker, New York.

12. Heirwegh, K. P. M. (1978): Formation, metabolism and significance of bilirubin-IX glucosides. In: *Conjugation Reactions in Drug Biotransformation*, edited by A. Aitio, pp. 67–76. Elsevier, Amsterdam.

13. Mulder, G. J. (1981): Conjugation of phenols. In: *Metabolic Basis of Detoxication*, edited by W. B. Jakoby, J. R. Bend, and J. Caldwell, Academic Press, New York (*in press*).

14. Dodgson, K. S., and Rose, F. A. (1970): Sulfoconjugation and sulfohydrolysis. In: *Metabolic Conjugation and Metabolic Hydrolysis, Vol. 1*, edited by W. H. Fishman, pp. 239–325. Academic Press, New York.

15. Nose, Y., and Lipmann, F. (1958): Separation of steroid sulfokinases. *J. Biol. Chem.*, 233:1348–1351.

16. Jakoby, W. B., Sekura, R. D., Lyon, E. S., Marcus, C. J., and Wang, C. J. (1980): Sulfotransferases. In: *Enzymatic Basis of Detoxication, Vol. 2*, edited by W. B. Jakoby pp. 199–228. Academic Press, New York.

17. Mulder, G. J. (editor) (1981): *Sulfation of Drugs and Related Compounds*. C.R.C. Press, Boca Raton, Florida.

18. Usdin, E., Borchardt, R. T., and Creveling, C. R. (1979): *Transmethylations*. American Elsevier, New York.

19. Borchardt, R. T. (1980): N- and O-methylation. In: *Enzymatic Basis of Detoxication, Vol. 2*, edited by W. B. Jakoby, pp. 43–62. Academic Press, New York.

20. D'Souza, J., Caldwell, J., and Smith R. L. (1980): Species variations in the N-methylation and quarternization of [^{14}C]pyridine. *Xenobiotica*, 10:151–157.

21. Weber, W. W., and Glowinski, I. B. (1980): Acetylation. In: *Enzymatic Basis of Detoxication, Vol. 2*, edited by W. B. Jakoby, pp. 169–186. Academic Press, New York.

22. Weber, W. W. (1973): Acetylation of drugs. In: *Metabolic Conjugation and Metabolic Hydrolysis, Vol. 3*, edited by W. H. Fishman, pp. 249–296. Academic Press, New York.

23. Weber, W. W., Hein, D. W., Hirata, M., and Patterson, E. (1978): Genetics of drug acetylation: Molecular nature of the INH acetylation polymorphism. In: *Conjugation Reactions in Drug Biotransformation*, edited by A. Aitio, pp. 145–153. Elsevier, Amsterdam.

24. Osuntokun, B. O. (1980): A degenerative neuropathy with blindness and chronic cyanide intoxication of dietary origin: The evidence in the Nigerians. In: *Toxicology in the Tropics*, edited by R. L. Smith and E. A. Bababunmi, pp. 16–52. Taylor and Francis, London.

25. Westley, J. (1980): Rhodanese and the sulfane pool. In: *Enzymatic Basis of Detoxication, Vol. 2*, edited by W. B. Jakoby, pp. 245–262. Academic Press, New York.

26. Chasseaud, L. F. (1979): The role of glutathione and glutathione S-transferases in the metabolism of chemical carcinogens and other electrophilic agents. *Adv. Cancer Res.*, 29:175–274.

27. Jerina, D. M., and Bend, J. R. (1977): Glutathione S-transferases. In: *Biological Reactive Intermediates*, edited by D. J. Jollow, J. J. Kocsis, R. Snyder, and H. Vainio, pp. 207–236. Plenum, New York.

28. Levin, W., Jerina, D. M., Thomas, P. E., and Lu, A. Y. H. (1978): Physical and catalytic properties of purified rat liver epoxide hydrase. In: *Conjugation Reactions in Drug Biotransformation*, edited by A. Aitio, pp. 337–346. Elsevier, Amsterdam.

29. Hammock, B. D., Gill, S. S., Stamoudis, V., and Gilbert, L. I. (1976): Soluble mammalian epoxide hydrolase: Action on juvenile hormone and other terpenoid epoxides. *Comp. Biochem. Physiol.*, 53:263–265.

30. Oesch, F. (1980): Epoxide hydrolase. In: *Enzymatic Basis of Detoxication, Vol. 2*, edited by W. B. Jakoby, pp. 277–290. Academic Press, New York.

31. Caldwell, J., Idle, J. R., and Smith, R. L. (1980): The amino acid conjugations. In: *Extrahepatic Metabolism of Drugs and Other Foreign Compounds*, edited by T. E. Gram, pp. 435–492. SP Medical and Scientific Books, Jamaica, N.Y.

32. Caldwell, J. (1982): The conjugation of xenobiotic carboxylic acids in mammals. In: *Metabolic Basis of Detoxication*, edited by W. B. Jakoby, J. R. Bend, and J. Caldwell. Academic Press, New York (*in press*).

33. Killenberg, P. G., and Webster, L. T., Jr. (1980): Conjugation by peptide bond formation. In: *Enzymatic Basis of Detoxication, Vol. 2*, edited by W. B. Jakoby, pp. 141–167. Academic Press, New York.

34. Crayford, J. V., and Hutson, D. H. (1980); Xenobiotic triglyceride formation. *Xenobiotica*, 10:349–354.

35. Marsh, M. V., Hutt, A. J., Caldwell, J., Smith, R. L., Horner, M. W., Houghton, E., and Moss M. S. (1981): Evidence for the formation of a novel pathway of benzoic acid metabolism involving the addition of a two-carbon fragment. *Biochem. Pharmacol.* (*in press*).

36. Weisiger, R. A., and Jakoby, W. B. (1980): S-Methylation: Thio S-Methyltransferase. In: *Enzymatic Basis of Detoxication, Vol. 2*, edited by W. B. Jakoby, pp. 131–140. Academic Press, New York.

37. Israili, Z. H., Dayton, P. G., and Kiechel, J. R. (1977): Novel routes of drug metabolism. *Drug Metab. Dispos.*, 5:411–415.

38. Jenner, P., and Testa, B. (1978): Novel pathways in drug metabolism. *Xenobiotica*, 8:1–25.

39. Reidenberg, M. M., and Drayer, D. E. (1977): Clinical consequences of polymorphic acetylation of basic drugs. *Clin. Pharmacol. Ther.*, 22:251–258.

40. Schmid, R., and McDonagh, A. F. (1978): Hyperbilirubinaemia. In: *Metabolic Basis of Inherited Disease*, edited by J. B. Stanbury, J. B. Wyngaarden, and D. S. Fredrickson, pp. 1221–1257. McGraw-Hill, New York.

41. Miller, J. A., and Miller, L. C. (1977): The concept of reactive electrophilic metabolites in chemical carcinogenesis. In: *Biological Reactive Intermediates*, edited by D. J. Jollow, J. J. Kocsis, R. Snyder, and H. Vainio, pp. 6–24. Plenum, New York.

42. Van Bladeren, P. J., van der Gen, A., Breimer, D. D., and Mohn, G. R. (1979): Stereoselective activation of vicinal dihalogen compounds to mutagens by glutathione conjugation. *Biochem. Pharmacol.*, 28:2521–2524.

43. Kadlubar, F. F., Miller, J. A., and Miller, E. C. (1977): Hepatic microsomal N-glucuronidation and nucleic acid binding of N-hydroxyarylamines in relation to urinary bladder carcinogenesis. *Cancer Res.*, 37:805–814.

44. Mitchell, J. R., Zimmerman, H. J., Ishak, K. G., Thorgeirsson, S. S., Timbrell, J. A., Snodgrass, W. R., and Nelson, S. D. (1976): Isoniazid liver injury: Clinical spectrum, pathology and probable pathogenesis. *Ann. Intern. Med.*, 84:181–192.

45. Wagner, J. G. (1974): A modern view of pharmacokinetics. In: *Pharmacology and Pharmacokinetics*, edited by T. Teorell, R. L. Dedrick, and R. G. Condliffe, pp. 27–67. Plenum, New York.

46. Smith, R. L. (1973): *The Excretory Function of Bile*. Chapman and Hall, London.

47. Connolly, M. E., Davies, D. S., Dollery, C. T., Morgan, C. D., Paterson, J. W., and Sandler, M. (1972): Metabolism of isoprenaline in dog and man. *Br. J. Pharmacol.*, 46:458–472.

48. Caldwell, J., and Smith, R. L. (1977): Metabolism of drugs and the routes of administration. In: *Formulation and Preparation of Dosage Forms*, edited by J. Polderman, pp. 169–181. Elsevier, Amsterdam.

49. Jollow, D. J., and Smith, C. (1977): Biochemical aspects of toxic metabolites: Formation, detoxication and covalent binding. In: *Biological Reactive Intermediates*, edited by D. J. Jollow, J. J. Kocsis, R. Snyder, and H. Vainio, pp. 43–59. Plenum, New York.

The Liver: Biology and Pathobiology, edited by
I. Arias, H. Popper, D. Schachter, and D. A. Shafritz.
Raven Press, New York © 1982.

Chapter 17

Glutathione

Alton Meister

Glutathione [L-γ-glutamyl-L-cysteinylglycine (GSH)] is found in virtually all mammalian cells in concentrations that range from about 0.1 to 10 mM. It is the major intracellular thiol, often the most abundant low molecular weight peptide, and, except perhaps for glutamine, the most abundant γ-glutamyl compound found in cells. It occurs predominantly within cells where its concentration is substantially higher than that of glutathione disulfide (GSSG). GSH is also found in extracellular fluids, such as blood plasma, in relatively low concentrations; in rat blood plasma, the concentration of GSH + GSSG is about 25 to 35 μM GSH equivalents; in man, this value is about 1 to 3 μM. The GSH molecule has two characteristic structural features: a γ-glutamyl linkage and a sulfhydryl group, moieties that promote the intracellular stability of GSH and which are intimately involved in the several functions of this tripeptide. Thus the sulfhydryl group of GSH participates in several types of reactions, and transfer of the γ-glutamyl group of GSH is a significant step in its utilization.

GSH performs a variety of physiological and metabolic functions. These include thiol transfer reactions which seem to protect cell membranes and proteins, to promote thiol-disulfide reactions involved in protein assembly, protein degradation, and catalysis, to provide reducing capacity for other reactions (e.g., the formation of deoxyribonucleotides from ribonucleotides), and to detoxify hydrogen peroxide, organic peroxides, free radicals, and foreign compounds. GSH also participates by several chemical mechanisms in the metabolism of various endogenous compounds; it serves catalytically in some instances and as a reactant in others. It also functions in the transport of amino acids (and perhaps also of certain amines and peptides): GSH itself is transported across cell membranes. The intracellular concentration of GSH + GSSG is greater than those of cysteine and cystine: therefore, it serves as a storage form of these sulfur-containing amino acids. Some tissues, e.g., the liver, are very active in GSH biosynthesis and translocate GSH to the blood plasma; other tissues, especially the kidney, are active in removing GSH from blood plasma. Thus GSH appears to be a major interorgan transport form of cysteine.

Although the reactions of glutathione metabolism occur in many tissues, including the liver, there are significant quantitative differences in the various reactions in different tissues, some of which are noted below. The literature on GSH is extensive, and it is not possible to cite here all the findings that have been recorded. The wide distribution of GSH and of many of the enzymes involved in its metabolism and function attest to its significance in many aspects of cellular function. Although many important roles have long been ascribed to this ubiquitous tripeptide, insights into the detailed chemical mechanisms involved in its metabolic and physiological functions have only recently been achieved. In this chapter, emphasis is given to phenomena that have been well characterized biochemically. The reader is referred to the published proceedings of recent conferences and reviews (1–6).

BIOSYNTHESIS OF GSH

GSH is synthesized in most if not all mammalian cells (5,7). The liver is particularly active and has relatively high (4 to 10 mM) levels of GSH. The synthesis of GSH is catalyzed by the successive actions of γ-glutamylcysteine synthetase and GSH synthetase, which catalyze reactions [1] and [2], respectively.

L-Glutamate + L-cysteine + ATP
$$\underset{Mg^+}{\rightleftharpoons} \text{L-}\gamma\text{-glutamyl-L-cysteine} + \text{ADP} + \text{P}_i \quad [1]$$

L-γ-Glutamyl-L-cysteine + ATP + glycine
$$\underset{Mg^+}{\rightleftharpoons} \text{GSH} + \text{ADP} + \text{P}_i \quad [2]$$

Both reactions take place by mechanisms involving the intermediate formation of enzyme-bound acyl phosphates. Thus γ-glutamylphosphate is formed on γ-glutamylcysteine synthetase, and γ-glutamylcysteinylphosphate is formed in analogous fashion on GSH synthetase. Both enzymes have been highly purified from several sources, and the properties of the purified enzymes have been studied extensively (7). γ-Glutamylcysteine does not usually occur in high concentrations in liver or other tissues, probably because it is effectively utilized. This dipeptide not only is a substrate of GSH synthetase but can be utilized by γ-glutamyltranspeptidase and γ-glutamylcyclotransferase (see below). It has been suggested that the two synthetases are coupled or linked to facilitate the utilization of γ-glutamylcysteine by GSH synthetase. Under normal conditions, the activity of γ-glutamylcysteine synthetase is less than maximal, since this enzyme is feedback-inhibited by GSH (8). In the inborn error 5-oxoprolinuria (9), in which there is a block of GSH synthetase activity, there is overproduction of γ-glutamylcysteine, and this dipeptide is extensively converted to 5-oxoproline and cysteine, a reaction catalyzed by γ-glutamylcyclotransferase. Although the tissue level of GSH undoubtedly plays a significant role in the regulation of GSH biosynthesis, the tissue levels of cysteine also influence GSH synthesis. It is well known that the level of GSH in the liver decreases in experimental animals (e.g., rat, mouse) from about 8 mM to almost half this value on fasting, and the level rises appreciably when feeding is resumed.

INTERCONVERSION BETWEEN GSH AND GSSG

That the intracellular concentrations of GSH are substantially higher (about 20-fold or more) than those of GSSG is consistent with the presence of effective enzyme activity that catalyzes the reduction of GSSG. The enzyme GSH reductase is highly active in liver, kidney, and virtually all other mammalian tissues. The physiological function of this enzyme is to regenerate GSH, which has been converted to GSSG by oxidation and by thiol transfer reactions. GSH reductase has been obtained in highly purified form from several

sources and has been extensively studied (10–15). The enzyme is a flavoprotein containing one mole of flavin adenine dinucleotide (FAD) per enzyme subunit; the prosthetic group is linked noncovalently to the enzyme. GSH reductase catalyzes reaction [3], which is essentially irreversible.

$$\text{GSSG} + \text{NADPH} + \text{H}^+ \rightarrow 2\,\text{GSH} + \text{NADP}^+ \quad [3]$$

The specificity of GSH reductase has not yet been fully defined. GSSG, the mixed disulfide between GSH and γ-glutamylcysteine and the mixed disulfide between GSH and coenzyme A are substrates. The mixed disulfide between GSH and cysteine is not a substrate. Other disulfides, including mixed disulfides between GSH and various proteins, have been reported to be substrates of GSH reductase. Such findings, however, may be ascribed to the occurrence of nonenzymatic transhydrogenation between GSH and mixed disulfides to form GSSG, which is the actual substrate of the enzyme.

Several hematological disorders are associated with reduced levels of GSH reductase in erythrocytes (1). In some instances, there may be an abnormal GSH reductase whose affinity for FAD is reduced. In others, the situation is apparently more complex and not yet well understood. Reduced levels of GSH reductase have been observed occasionally in apparently normal individuals; addition of FAD to erythrocyte extracts increases the reductase activity, which may also increase after oral administration of riboflavin (16–18).

GSH may be converted to GSSG by reactions involving oxidation or transhydrogenation. The enzyme GSH peroxidase was first found in erythrocytes (19–21), where it was considered to function in the protection of hemoglobin against oxidation by hydrogen peroxide. The enzyme catalyzes the decomposition of hydrogen peroxide according to reaction [4].

$$2\,\text{GSH} + \text{H}_2\text{O}_2 \rightarrow \text{GSSG} + 2\,\text{H}_2\text{O} \quad [4]$$

The reduction of hydrogen peroxide in erythrocytes is coupled to the oxidation of glucose-6-phosphate and 6-phosphogluconate, according to the scheme given in Fig. 1. GSH peroxidase subsequently was found in many mammalian tissues, including liver and kidney, where it probably functions in a manner similar to that shown in Fig. 1. In certain cells, NADPH can be formed by the action of other dehydrogenases. Both GSH peroxidase and catalase function to destroy hydrogen peroxide; GSH peroxidase acts on relatively low levels of hydrogen peroxide, whereas catalase acts to remove high concentrations or bursts of hydrogen peroxide formation. The two enzymes thus appear to complement each other in protecting against oxidative reactions caused by hydrogen peroxide.

GSH peroxidase also interacts with other hydro-

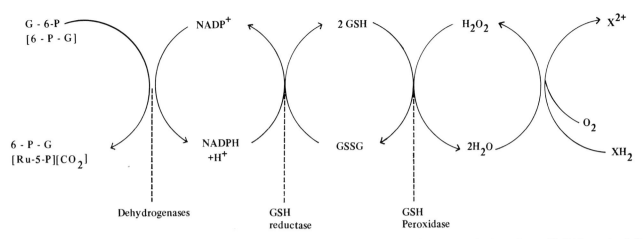

FIG. 1. Scheme for coupling of the reduction of H_2O_2 to the oxidation of glucose-6-phosphate (G-6-P) and of 6-phosphogluconate (6-P-G).

peroxides and reduces them to the corresponding alcohols (reaction [5]).

$$2\ GSH + ROOH \rightarrow ROH + H_2O + GSSG \quad [5]$$

The enzyme is active with a wide variety of acceptor hydroperoxides, including such compounds as ethyl hydroperoxide, cumene hydroperoxide, linoleic acid hydroperoxide, and others (1–3,22). It has been suggested that the marked lack of specificity of GSH peroxidase enables it to initiate a repair mechanism to overcome peroxidation of complex molecules, such as lipids or nucleic acids. In support of this view, it has been found that GSH peroxidase prevents lipid peroxidation and functional impairment of isolated mitochondria. There is also evidence that GSH deficiency can lead to lipid peroxidation, and that this reaction can cause hepatocellular lysis (23–26).

It has long been known that selenium is an essential trace element for animals, and it has been believed that selenium is involved in a protection mechanism. GSH peroxidase contains about 4 g atoms selenium per mole enzyme (27), and there is evidence that the enzyme selenium functions in the catalytic mechanism. The observation that selenium-deficient rats have decreased GSH peroxidase activity is in accord with the view that selenium is an essential component of the enzyme (28,29).

Some GSH probably is oxidized to GSSG intracellularly, for example, in erythrocytes. There is also evidence that GSH is oxidized to GSSG extracellularly, and that this reaction is largely nonenzymatic (30). The finding that purified preparations of γ-glutamyltranspeptidase can catalyze apparent oxidation of GSH led to the finding that such oxidation is mediated by cysteinylglycine (a product of the transpeptidation reaction), which reacts rapidly and nonenzymatically with oxygen to form cystinyl-bis-glycine. Nonenzymatic transhydrogenation between cystinyl-bis-glycine and GSH yields GSSG. These and similar reactions prob-

ably contribute to the extracellular formation of GSSG as well as to formation of disulfide forms of cysteine and γ-glutamylcysteine.

Many thiol-disulfide exchange reactions undoubtedly occur, but the detailed enzymology of these events is not yet clear. Close coupling between the reactions catalyzed by GSH reductase (reaction [3]) and various thiol-exchange reactions may be envisioned as indicated in reactions [6] to [9].

$$GSH + RSSR' \rightleftharpoons RSSG + R'SH \quad [6]$$
$$GSH + RSSR' \rightleftharpoons R'SSG + RSH \quad [7]$$
$$R'SSG + GSH \rightleftharpoons GSSG + R'SH \quad [8]$$
$$RSSG + GSH \rightleftharpoons GSSG + RSH \quad [9]$$

Some such reactions are known to occur rapidly in the absence of an enzyme, but there is evidence for the existence of several enzymes that catalyze the reduction of particular disulfides by GSH. The first GSH transhydrogenase to be described (31), obtained from beef liver, catalyzes the reduction of homocystine, according to reaction [10].

$$2\ GSH + \text{homocystine} \rightleftharpoons GSSG + 2\ \text{homocysteine} \quad [10]$$

Subsequent studies suggest that cystine, the mixed disulfide between GSH and coenzyme A (32), and several other mixed disulfides may be reduced in this manner. It has been reported that the liver contains a GSH-insulin transhydrogenase that promotes the reductive cleavage of the disulfide bonds of insulin by GSH and closely related thiols (33–35). Reactions of this type probably are involved in the biosynthesis, aggregation, and folding of proteins, i.e., by forming specific disulfide linkages. They may also be involved in the degradation of proteins. Such reactions probably are also important to form and maintain specific protein thiol groups, or disulfide linkages, that are critical for protein structure and catalysis. They may also be involved in regulatory phenomena. Reactions of this type are probably also mediated by thioredoxin and glutaredoxin, low molecular weight acidic proteins that contain an "active" disulfide linkage capable of being reduced by certain low molecular weight thiols (36). These proteins, which do not exhibit catalytic activity themselves, probably function together with GSH and various dehydrogenases in a variety of processes involving interconversions between protein sulfhydryl and disulfide groups (37). At least several enzymes catalyze such thiol-disulfide exchange reactions; more studies are needed on the purification and characterization of these catalysts.

Dehydroascorbate is known to react with GSH to form ascorbate, according to reaction [11].

$$\text{Dehydroascorbate} + 2\ \text{GSH} \rightleftharpoons \text{ascorbate} + \text{GSSG} \qquad [11]$$

An enzyme that catalyzes this reaction has been obtained from plants and bacteria (38–41), but it is not clear whether such activity exists in mammalian tissues, where the reaction may be at least partly non-enzymatic (42,43).

FUNCTION OF GSH AS A COENZYME

GSH functions as a coenzyme in several enzyme-catalyzed reactions. The first of these to be discovered was the glyoxalase reaction, which is catalyzed by two widely distributed enzymes (4,44–51). In this reaction, methylglyoxal is converted to D-lactate, as indicated in reactions [12] to [14] [R = methyl]:

$$\text{G–SH} + \underset{\underset{\text{O}\ \ \text{O}}{\|\ \ \|}}{\text{H–C–C–R}} \xrightarrow{\text{nonenzymatic}}$$

$$\underset{\underset{\text{OH}\ \ \text{O}}{|\ \ \ \|}}{\text{G–S–CH–C–R}} \qquad [12]$$

$$\underset{\underset{\text{OH}\ \ \text{O}}{|\ \ \ \|}}{\text{G–S–CH–C–R}} \xrightarrow{\text{glyoxalase I}} \underset{\underset{\text{O}\ \ \text{H}}{\|\ \ \ |}}{\overset{\overset{\text{OH}}{|}}{\text{G–S–C–C–R}}} \qquad [13]$$

$$\underset{\underset{\text{O}\ \ \text{H}}{\|\ \ \ |}}{\overset{\overset{\text{OH}}{|}}{\text{G–S–C–C–R}}} \xrightarrow{\text{glyoxalase II}} \text{G–SH} + \qquad [14]$$

$$\underset{\underset{\text{H}}{|}}{\overset{\overset{\text{OH}}{|}}{\text{HOOC–C–R}}}$$

The hemimercaptal formed nonenzymatically by interaction of methylglyoxal with GSH (reaction [12])

serves as the substrate in reaction [13], which is catalyzed by glyoxalase I. S-lactyl-GSH, formed in reaction [13], is converted by glyoxalase II into GSH and D-lactate (reaction [14]). Several analogs of methylglyoxal also are active in this system. The biologic significance of the glyoxalase reactions has long been a mystery. The provocative suggestion has been made that keto-aldehydes play a significant role in the regulation of cell division; according to this idea, methylglyoxal retards cell growth, and glyoxalase promotes growth by destruction of methylglyoxal (52–54). Although some evidence is consistent with this hypothesis, additional studies are needed. The glyoxalase system occurs in liver and a number of other mammalian tissues.

GSH also functions as a coenzyme for formaldehyde dehydrogenase, a pyridine nucleotide-dependent enzyme, present in liver and also in other tissues, that converts formaldehyde to formic acid (55,56). The actual substrate is thought to be the hemimercaptal formed between formaldehyde and GSH. The hemimercaptal is converted to formate, and GSH is regenerated.

The oxidation of homogentisate in liver leads initially to the formation of maleylacetoacetate. The conversion of this compound to its geometric isomer fumarylacetoacetate is catalyzed by an isomerase, which is markedly activated by GSH (44,57). GSH catalyzes the isomerization at a slow rate in the absence of enzyme. A similar cis-trans-isomerization occurs in the degradation of gentisic acid in bacteria; GSH is a coenzyme in this pathway for the isomerization of maleylpyruvate to fumarylpyruvate (58).

There is evidence that GSH also functions catalytically in certain other reactions, e.g., in the isomerization of prostaglandin H and of Δ^5-3-ketosteroids (see below). GSH also may function as a cofactor in the conversion of thyroxine to 3,3',5'-triiodothyronine (59–60).

UTILIZATION OF GSH BY THE MERCAPTURIC ACID PATHWAY AND BY SIMILAR PATHWAYS OF ENDOGENOUS METABOLISM

Mercapturic acids are S-substituted derivatives of N-acetyl L-cysteine, which are formed by a series of reactions initiated by the interaction of GSH with electrophilic compounds. The conjugation of such compounds with GSH may take place nonenzymatically or may be catalyzed by GSH S-transferases. The γ-glutamyl moiety of the GSH conjugate is removed by the action of γ-glutamyl transpeptidase, and the C-terminal glycine moiety is cleaved by the action of peptidase. This is followed by N-acetylation of the cysteine conjugate (Fig. 2).

A wide variety of foreign compounds, including

$$X + \gamma\text{-GLU} - \text{CySH} - \text{GLY} \xrightarrow{\quad 1 \quad} \gamma\text{-GLU} - \text{CyS} - \text{GLY}$$
$$\begin{array}{c} | \\ X \end{array}$$

$$\xrightarrow[\text{-glu}]{\quad 2 \quad} \underset{\underset{X}{|}}{\text{CyS} - \text{GLY}} \xrightarrow[\text{-gly}]{\quad 3 \quad} \text{CyS} - X$$

$$\xrightarrow{\quad 4 \quad} \text{N-Acetyl-Cys} - X \text{ (a mercapturic acid)}$$

FIG. 2. Formation of mercapturic acids. X, Compounds with an electrophilic center. Enzymes: (1) GSH S-transferases; (2) γ-Glutamyltranspeptidase; (3) Dipeptidase; (4) N-acetylase (acetyl-coenzyme A).

many drugs, can be detoxified by the mercapturic acid pathway (2,61,62). Compounds with an electrophilic center can readily conjugate with GSH; in some instances, an electrophilic center may be introduced into a molecule by another reaction; for example, naphthalene is converted by the action of microsomal oxygenase to an epoxide, which reacts with GSH.

The liver, as well as other tissues, contains high levels of GSH S-transferase activity. Administration of compounds that readily form mercapturic acids typically leads to a decrease in the level of GSH in the liver, and also to biliary excretion of the corresponding GSH conjugate as well as the related cysteinylglycine, cysteine, and N-acetyl cysteine derivatives. Such compounds may be converted to other products within the intestinal lumen, or they may be excreted in the feces. Mercapturic acids have been found most often in the urine. The pathway of metabolism and mode of excretion depends on a number of factors, including the nature of the foreign compound and the species. The formation of mercapturic acid after administration of various compounds to animals has been investigated by many workers since this phenomenon was first observed in 1879 (63,64); a voluminous literature is available on this subject (1,61,62). Some examples taken from the long list of compounds (61) that interact with GSH in this manner are halogenonitrobenzenes, 2-chloro-s-triazines, aryl nitrocompounds, phenoltetrabromphthaleins (including bromsulfophthalein), aralkyl halides, alkyl halides, certain allyl compounds, alkyl methanesulfonates, certain organophosphorus compounds, arene oxides, and isothiocyanates. Two major types of reactions have been observed: (a) replacement (for example, the conjugation of GSH with benzyl chloride) (reaction [15]), and (b) conjugation of GSH with epoxides (reaction [16]).

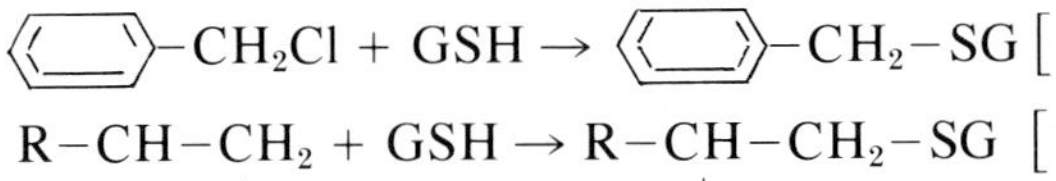

$$\langle\!\!\!\langle \underline{\phantom{\text{O}}} \rangle\!\!\!\rangle\text{-CH}_2\text{Cl} + \text{GSH} \rightarrow \langle\!\!\!\langle \underline{\phantom{\text{O}}} \rangle\!\!\!\rangle\text{-CH}_2\text{-SG} \quad [15]$$

$$\underset{\underset{O}{\diagdown\diagup}}{R-\text{CH}-\text{CH}_2} + \text{GSH} \rightarrow \underset{\underset{OH}{|}}{R-\text{CH}-\text{CH}_2\text{-SG}} \quad [16]$$

The GSH S-transferases of rat liver, human liver, and a number of other tissues have been purified and their substrate specificities examined (62). The GSH S-transferases of rat liver account for about 10% of the soluble protein of this tissue. Six different proteins that exhibit GSH S-transferase activity were obtained in essentially homogeneous form from rat liver. All these are composed of two apparently identical subunits of molecular weight 24,000, but they differ with respect to isoelectric point, antigenic properties, and substrate specificity. In addition to catalyzing the formation of GSH conjugates, purified GSH S-transferase proteins have been found to bind a number of ligands that are not substrates. The GSH S-transferases apparently are identical with proteins known as ligandins, first recognized as proteins that bind a variety of anionic compounds (2,65,66). Ligandins may function in the process by which these compounds are transferred from plasma into the liver cell (66). Ligandins can bind bilirubin, certain carcinogens and steroids, and azo dyes. It has been proposed that the "ligandin-GSH S-transferase" family of proteins has three detoxification functions: (a) catalysis, (b) binding of ligands that are not substrates, and (c) covalent bond formation with very reactive compounds leading to inactivation and destruction of the protein (2,62,67–69).

More must be learned about the details of metabolism of various GSH conjugates. Removal of the γ-glutamyl group undoubtedly is catalyzed by γ-glutamyltranspeptidase, an enzyme that appears to be localized on the external surface of certain cell membranes (see below). This suggests that this step in the mercapturic acid pathway, as well as the cleavage of the C-terminal glycine moiety (which is probably cleaved by the activity of membrane-bound dipeptidase), may take place predominantly extracellularly. The N-acetylation reaction, which utilizes acetyl-coenzyme A, takes place intracellularly, indicating that there is transport of the cysteine conjugate into the cell. Removal of the γ-glutamyl group by γ-glutamyltranspeptidase probably is accelerated by amino acids and thus coupled with the formation of γ-glutamyl amino acids, as discussed below.

It is generally believed that the GSH S-transferases function in a protective capacity against compounds that might otherwise be toxic or carcinogenic; indeed, conjugation with GSH usually results in the formation of less toxic products. Foreign compounds may be transformed, often by oxidation, to carcinogenic species, which may conjugate readily with GSH. The evidence that GSH and GSH S-transferases protect against carcinogenesis is as yet incomplete, although the idea is attractive. It is of interest that liver GSH S-transferases (ligandins) are induced by phenobarbital, polycyclic hydrocarbons, and certain other compounds (61,70). A number of studies indicate a connection between GSH metabolism and carcinogenesis (71). Thus the concentration of GSH in male rat liver was found to increase after administration of 3'-methyl-4-dimethylaminoazobenzene (72), and good correlation was found between the relative carcinogenic activities of azo dyes and the ability of these compounds to increase the concentration of liver GSH (73).

γ-Glutamyltranspeptidase activity of liver increases after administration of 3'-methyl-4-dimethylaminoazobenzene, 2-acetylaminofluorene, thioacetamide, ethionine, and dimethylnitrosamine (74,75). Certain rat hepatomas (76), as well as several other types of tumors (77,78), have high levels of γ-glutamyltranspeptidase activity; in contrast, normal liver has relatively little transpeptidase activity. Administration of certain carcinogens leads to increased γ-glutamyltranspeptidase activity (79–81). Isolated normal hepatocytes have relatively low γ-glutamyltranspeptidase activity; in contrast, hepatoma tissue culture cells have much higher activity. Enzymatic and histochemical procedures carried out on different cell populations during induction of liver cancer by carcinogens have shown a marked increase in γ-glutamyltranspeptidase activity in tumor nodules as compared to controls. Transpeptidase activity increases in foci of early putative preneoplastic hepatocytes induced by a single dose of carcinogen. These and other studies (82) have led to the conclusion that increased γ-glutamyltranspeptidase activity is a marker for early, as well as late, putative liver preneoplastic and neoplastic cells. At this stage of our knowledge, it appears that GSH, GSH S-transferases (ligandins), and perhaps other enzymes involved in GSH metabolism, including γ-glutamyltranspeptidase, are closely associated with the process of carcinogenesis. The detailed nature of these relationships must be elucidated.

Although many studies have emphasized conjugation (and thus detoxication) of a large number of foreign compounds, including drugs, with GSH, there is increasing evidence that certain compounds formed endogenously follow similar metabolic pathways. Thus there is evidence for conjugation of estradiol-17-β with GSH in rat liver preparations and in vivo (83–88). Administration of the GSH conjugate of 2-hydroxy-estradiol-17-β to rats led to biliary excretion of the corresponding cysteinylglycine, cysteine, and N-acetylcysteine derivatives. There is also evidence for the formation of GSH conjugates of prostaglandins (89,90). GSH peroxidase may function in prostaglandin metabolism, for example, in the conversion of a 15-hydroperoxy group to a hydroxy group (91). GSH seems also to function in other aspects of prostaglandin metabolism (92–94).

Conjugation with GSH also plays a significant role in the metabolism of the leukotrienes. Leukotriene A, an epoxide derived from arachidonic acid, forms the GSH adduct leukotriene C; removal of the γ-glutamyl moiety of leukotriene C by γ-glutamyltranspeptidase yields leukotriene D, a slow-reacting substance of anaphylaxis (95,96). Details of these metabolic pathway must be worked out. Some of the GSH, cysteinylglycine, and cysteine derivatives of these compounds may be physiologically important. Given the wide variety of foreign compounds and drugs known to react with GSH (either nonenzymatically or enzymatically), one may expect that many compounds formed in endogenous metabolism will form GSH adducts and possibly to metabolized by the mercapturic pathway. In this connection, there is evidence that 5-S-GSH-DOPA formed in melanocytes is an intermediate in the incorporation of cysteine sulfur into melanin pigments (97); 5-S-cysteinyl-DOPA often is excreted in large amounts in the urine of patients with melanoma metastases (98).

The enzymatic conversion of Δ^5-3-ketosteroids to the corresponding α,β-unsaturated Δ^4-3-ketosteroids is catalyzed by proteins of human and rat liver which appear to be identical with GSH S-transferases (99). Δ^5-3-Ketosteroid isomerase activity of human liver was found to be distributed among the five different GSH S-transferases that have been found in this tissue. These findings suggest that the GSH S-transferases may have additional catalytic functions.

γ-Glutamyltranspeptidase activity is found normally in human serum, but the activity is extremely low compared to that found in certain tissues, e.g., kidney. Clinical studies have shown that serum γ-glutamyltranspeptidase activity is elevated in many alcoholic subjects. Determinations of serum γ-glutamyltranspeptidase may serve as a sensitive test of impaired liver function. γ-Glutamyltranspeptidase activity of serum is elevated in many types of liver disease; its association with hepatic disease is of interest because the liver, compared to other tissues (e.g., kidney) has relatively little γ-glutamyltranspeptidase activity. The transpeptidase activity of adult liver is localized in the bile ductules and the fine biliary tracts. It has been postulated that the enzyme may be solubilized from its membraneous location by increased hepatic bile salt concentration (100). This interpretation is consistent with the finding in experimental systems of increased serum bile salt concentrations together with increased serum γ-glutamyltranspeptidase activity soon after experimental bile duct obstruction.

In the human disease hereditary tyrosinemia, there is an apparent block in tyrosine metabolism at the step catalyzed by fumarylacetoacetase (101). It has been postulated that the accumulation of maleylacetoacetate, which presumably occurs in this condition, leads to toxicity by reacting with GSH and thus making the liver more vulnerable to other toxic compounds. Patients with the chronic form of hereditary tyrosinemia commonly develop hepatocellular tumors. Consistent with this interpretation is the finding that such patients have low levels of liver GSH.

There has been some success in the development of histochemical procedures for the localization of GSH (102,103). In one study, it was found that the hepatocytes relatively close to the central vein contain much less GSH than do those in other regions of the rat liver lobule (103). This might explain why these cells are evidently more susceptible to attack by electrophilic compounds.

The ability of GSH to complex with various metals and metal-containing molecules has been noted by various investigators (see, for example ref. 104); one of the protective functions of GSH may lie in its affinity for certain heavy metals. The possibility that GSH functions in normal metabolism by chelating metals must be considered.

FUNCTION AND METABOLISM OF GSH BY THE γ-GLUTAMYL CYCLE

The synthesis of GSH and its degradation to its constituent amino acids take place by the reactions of the γ-glutamyl cycle (Fig. 3) (5,105). There is good evidence that the cycle functions *in vivo*, and that it is one of the systems that mediates the transport of amino acids. The cycle involves synthesis of GSH; therefore, its operation is closely connected with other functions and reactions of this tripeptide. GSH is synthesized intracellularly by reactions [1] and [2]. The initial step in the utilization of GSH is catalyzed by γ-glutamyltranspeptidase, a membrane-bound enzyme that catalyzes the transfer of the γ-glutamyl moiety of GSH to amino acids to yield γ-glutamyl amino acids and cysteinylglycine. γ-Glutamyl amino acids, formed in close association with the cell membrane, are translocated into the cell. Such transport of a dipeptide apparently is analogous to the transport of certain

other dipeptides (106). There is evidence that kidney and probably other cells have a transport mechanism for γ-glutamyl amino acids which is separate from systems that transport free amino acids (107). Cysteinylglycine is cleaved to cysteine and glycine by the action of dipeptidase; such activity is present on the cell membrane and also is found intracellularly. γ-Glutamyl amino acids are converted to the corresponding free amino acids and 5-oxoproline by the action of the intracellular enzyme γ-glutamylcyclotransferase (reaction [17]).

$$\text{L-}\gamma\text{-Glutamyl-L-amino acid} \rightarrow \text{5-oxo-L-proline} \\ + \text{L-amino acid} \qquad [17]$$

$$\text{5-Oxo-L-proline} + \text{ATP} + 2\ H_2O \rightarrow \text{L-glutamate} \\ + \text{ADP} + \text{Pi} \qquad [18]$$

5-Oxoproline is decyclized to yield glutamate in a reaction coupled to the cleavage of ATP to ADP and inorganic phosphate (reaction [18]).

γ-Glutamyltranspeptidase is widely distributed in mammalian tissues (108). The enzyme is especially concentrated in certain epithelial structures involved in transport processes, e.g., the epithelia of the proximal renal tubule, jejunal villi, choroid plexus, bile ductules, seminal vesicles, and the ciliary body. It is present in many other locations in lesser amounts, including certain central nervous system neurons. Histochemical studies show that the transpeptidase is localized in the brush border of the proximal renal tubule, and that it is bound to the external (luminal) surface of the cell membrane. In the liver, γ-glutamyltranspeptidase is localized in the bile duct epithelium and in the canalicular regions of hepatocytes. It is notable that fetal liver exhibits much higher γ-glutamyltranspeptidase activity than does adult liver. On the other hand, the kidneys of fetal and newborn rats exhibit low transpeptidase activity; the activity increases during development, ultimately leading to the high activity levels typical of adult kidney.

Although γ-glutamyltranspeptidase can catalyze hydrolysis of GSH and other γ-glutamyl compounds *in vitro*, there is substantial evidence that transpeptidation is a major function of the enzyme *in vivo* (109). A variety of neutral amino acids and dipeptides are active as acceptors of the γ-glutamyl group; the most active amino acid acceptors include cystine (110), glutamine, and methionine. Transpeptidase may be inhibited *in vivo* by injecting animals with inhibitors of this enzyme, leading to extensive glutathionuria (111). Such findings and other studies indicate that intracellular renal GSH is transported to the membrane-bound transpeptidase. Similar transport of GSH undoubtedly occurs at the other anatomic sites at which this enzyme is localized. It thus appears that transport of GSH is a discrete step in the γ-glutamyl cycle. Trans-

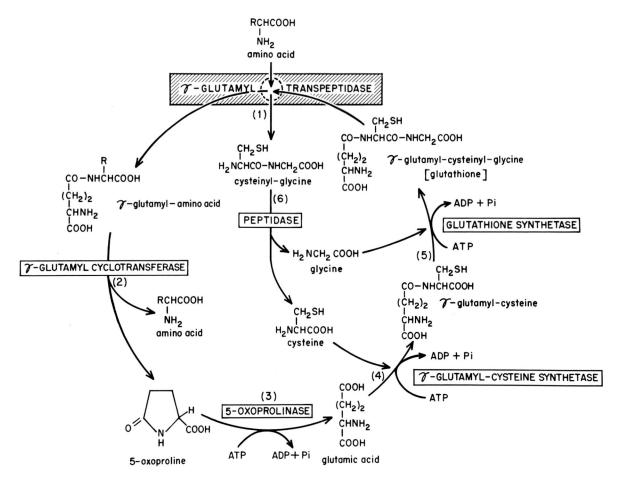

FIG. 3. The γ-glutamyl cycle (105).

port out of the liver has also been observed (112); thus there is evidence that the concentration of GSH in the hepatic vein is substantially higher than that found in other major blood vessels of the rat (113). GSH is also found in the bile. Tissues that have relatively low transpeptidase activity, such as liver and muscle, transport GSH to the blood plasma, whereas in the kidney and at other sites at which transpeptidase is highly concentrated, GSH is transported to the membrane-bound enzyme, and the products of enzyme action are taken up by the cell (114).

Adminstration of an inhibitor of GSH synthesis to mice results in a prompt decrease in tissue levels, and thus a marked decrease in plasma levels, of GSH (115). When an inhibitor of transpeptidase is given, however, the plasma GSH level increases. The kidney uses GSH that is transported from renal cells (intraorgan cycle) as well as GSH present in plasma (which originates from liver and other tissues). Translocation of GSH from the liver appears to be a significant pathway for the transport of amino acid sulfur from liver to kidney (interorgan cycle).

Blocks of the γ-glutamyl cycle have been found in certain inborn errors of metabolism and have been

achieved by the administration of inhibitors to experimental animals. Administration of a competitive inhibitor of 5-oxoprolinase to mice decreases the metabolism of 5-oxoproline; therefore, this compound accumulates in the tissues (116). The accumulation of 5-oxoproline is greater after giving both the inhibitor and amino acids, especially amino acids that are good acceptor substrates of γ-glutamyltranspeptidase. Administration of a competitive inhibitor of γ-glutamylcyclotransferase leads to a marked decrease in the level of 5-oxoproline in the kidney, an effect attributable to *in vivo* inhibition of γ-glutamylcyclotransferase (116).

Blockage of the γ-glutamyl cycle at the step of γ-glutamylcysteine synthetase has been observed in patients deficient in this enzyme activity (118,119). These patients have GSH deficiency, a tendency to hemolysis, various central nervous system disturbances, and aminoaciduria. In patients with 5-oxoprolinuria, an inborn error associated with mental deficiency, hemolysis, acidosis, and GSH synthetase deficiency, there is massive urinary excretion of 5-oxoproline and increased blood levels of this compound leading to acidosis (9,120). Since GSH normally regulates its own biosynthesis by feedback inhibition of γ-glutamylcys-teine synthetase (8), the low levels of GSH in this disease lead to overproduction of γ-glutamylcyste-ine and to increased conversion of this dipeptide to 5-oxoproline and cysteine, a reaction catalyzed by γ-glutamylcyclotransferase. The formation of 5-oxo-proline exceeds the capacity of 5-oxoprolinase, lead-ing to excretion of 5-oxoproline in the urine. There is thus a futile cycle of γ-glutamylcysteine synthesis followed by its conversion to 5-oxoproline and cysteine.

Animals treated with inhibitors of γ-glutamyltrans-peptidase and patients with γ-glutamyltranspeptidase deficiency excrete, in addition to GSH and GSSG, large amounts of γ-glutamylcysteine and cysteine moieties (determined after reduction and derivatiza-tion) in their urine (121). This observation indicates that the function of γ-glutamyltranspeptidase is closely associated with the metabolism or transport, or both, of cyst(e)ine and γ-glutamylcyst(e)ine. It has been shown that the γ-glutamylcyst(e)ine found in the urine of animals treated with transpeptidase inhibitors is formed by the action of the residual transpeptidase rather than by cleavage of the C-terminal glycine moiety of GSH (122). The findings suggest that γ-glutamylcystine, formed by the action of γ-glutamyl-transpeptidase and cystine, is poorly transported into cells in γ-glutamyltranspeptidase deficiency (or inhibi-tion), and therefore is excreted. Transport of γ-gluta-mylcystine into cells appears to be inhibited by the high levels of GSH that accompany reduced transpep-tidase activity. The finding of urinary γ-glutamylcyst-eine and cysteine moieties in transpeptidase deficiency or inhibition reflects accumulation of γ-glutamylcyst-ine and is in accord with the fact that cystine is an excellent acceptor substrate of γ-glutamyltrans-peptidase (110). After transport into the cell γ-gluta-mylcystine may be reduced to γ-glutamylcysteine and cysteine, both of which are substrates for GSH syn-thesis (reactions [1] and [2]).

Of the several blocks of the γ-glutamyl cycle that have been studied, defects in amino acid transport have been observed in two instances: (a) γ-gluta-mylcysteine synthetase deficiency, and (b) γ-gluta-myltranspeptidase deficiency. Dramatic amino acid transport defects have not been observed in the blocks of 5-oxoprolinase, GSH synthetase, and γ-glutamyl-cyclotransferase that have been examined; however, most of the inhibitions thus far achieved or observed are far from complete. Since there are multiple amino acid transport systems that overlap in specificity, it may be expected that blockage of one system may not invariably produce an easily detectable transport defect. The accumulated data support the view that one of the functions of GSH, through its metabolism, is connected with a pathway of amino acid transport.

REFERENCES

1. *Symposium on Glutathione,* edited by L. Flohé, H. Ch. Ben-ohr, H. Sies, H. D. Waller, and A. Wendel. (Tubingen, 1973), Thieme, Stuttgart.
2. Arias, I. M., and Jakoby, W. B. (editors) (1976): *Glutathione, Metabolism and Function.* Raven Press, New York.
3. Sies, H., and Wendel, A. (editors) (1978): *Glutathione, Func-tions in Liver and Kidney.* Springer-Verlag, Berlin.
4. Meister, A. (1975): Biochemistry of glutathione. In: *Metabo-lism of Sulfur Compounds, Metabolic Pathways,* 3rd edition, edited by D. M. Greenberg, vol. 7, pp. 101–188. Academic Press, New York.
5. Meister, A., and Tate, S. S. (1976): Glutathione and related γ-glutamyl compounds; biosynthesis and utilization. *Ann. Rev. Biochem.,* 45:559–604.
6. Meister, A. (1981): On the cycles of glutathione metabolism and transport. In: *Symposium on Biological Cycles (Honoring Sir Hans A. Krebs), Current Topics in Cellular Regulation, Volume 18,* edited by B. Horecker and E. Stadtman, pp. 21–57.
7. Meister, A. (1974): Glutathione synthesis. *The Enzymes,* (3rd edition, vol. 10, pp. 671–697, edited by Paul D. Boyer. Academic Press, New York.
8. Richman, P., and Meister, A. (1975): Regulation of γ-glutamyl-cysteine synthetase by nonallosteric feedback inhi-bition by glutathione. *J. Biol. Chem.,* 250:1422–1426.
9. Meister, A. (1977): 5-Oxoprolinuria (pyroglutamic aciduria) and other disorders of glutathione biosynthesis. In: *The Meta-bolic Basis of Inherited Diseases,* 4th edition, edited by J. B. Stanbury, J. B. Wyngaarden, and D. S. Frederickson, pp. 328–336. Mc-Graw Hill, New York.
10. Mapson, L. W., and Goddard, D. R. (1951): The reduction of glutathione by plant tissues. *Biochem. J.,* 49:592–601.
11. Conn, E. E., and Vennesland, B. (1951): Glutathione reduc-tase of wheat germ. *J. Biol. Chem.,* 192:17–28.
12. Rall, T. W., and Lehninger, A. L. (1952): Glutathione reduc-tase of animal tissues. *J. Biol. Chem.,* 194:119–130.
13. Racker, E. (1955): Glutathione reductase from bakers' yeast and beef liver. *J. Biol. Chem.,* 217:855–865.
14. Colman, R. F., and Black, S. (1965): On the role of flavin adenine dinucleotide and thiol groups in the catalytic mecha-nism of yeast glutathione reductase. *J. Biol. Chem.,* 240:1796–1803.
15. Staal, G. E. J., Visser, J., and Veeger, C. (1969): Purification and properties of glutathione reductase of human erythro-cytes. *Biochim. Biophys. Acta,* 185:39–48.
16. Beutler, E. (1969): Glutathoine reductase: Stimulation in nor-mal subjects by riboflavin supplementation. *Science,* 165:613–615.
17. Beutler, E. (1969): Effect of flavin compounds on glutathione reductase activity: In vivo and in vitro studies. *J. Clin. Invest.,* 48:1957–1966.
18. Paniker, N. V., Srivastava, S. K., and Beutler, E. (1970): Glutathione metabolism of the red cells effect of glutathione reductase deficiency on the stimulation of hexose monophos-phate shunt under oxidative stress. *Biochim. Biophys. Acta,* 215:456–460.
19. Mills, G. C. (1957): Hemoglobin catabolism I. Glutathione peroxidase, an erythrocyte enzyme which protects hemoglo-bin from oxidative breakdown. *J. Biol. Chem.,* 229:189–197.
20. Mills, G. C. (1960): Glutathione peroxidase and the destruction of hydrogen peroxide in animal tissues. *Arch. Biochem. Biophys.,* 86:1–5.
21. Mills, G. C. (1959): The purification and properties of glutathione peroxidase of erythrocytes. *J. Biol. Chem.,* 234:502–506.
22. Sies, H., Wahlländer, A., Waydhas, C., Soboll, S., and Häberle, D. (1980): Functions of intracellular glutathione in hepatic hydroperoxide and drug metabolism and the role of extracellular glutathione. *Adv. Enzyme Regul.,* 18:303–320.
23. Anundi, I., Högberg, J., and Stead, A. H. (1979): Glutathione depletion in isolated hepatocytes: Its relation to lipid peroxi-dation and cell damage. *Acta Pharmacol. Toxicol.* 45:45–51.

24. Little, C., and O'Brien, P. J. (1968): An intracellular GSH-peroxidase with a lipid peroxide substrate. *Biochem. Biophys. Res. Commun.*, 31:145–150.

25. Christophersen, B. O. (1968): Formation of monohydroxy-polyenic fatty acids from lipid peroxides by a glutathione peroxidase. *Biochim. Biophys. Acta*, 164:35–46.

26. Christophersen, B. O. (1969): Reduction of linolenic acid hydroperoxide by a glutathione peroxidase. *Biochim. Biophys. Acta*, 176:463–470.

27. Flohé, L., Gunzler, W. A., and Shock, H. H. (1973): Glutathione peroxidase: A selenoenzyme. *FEBS Lett.*, 32:132–134.

28. Rotruck, J. T., Pope, A. L., Ganther, H. E., Swanson, A. B., Hafeman, D. G., and Hoekstra, W. G. (1973): Selenium: Biochemical role as a component of glutathione peroxidase. *Science*, 179:588–590.

29. Smith, P. J., Tappel, A. L., and Chow, C. K. (1974): Glutathione peroxidase activity as a function of dietary selenomethionine. *Nature*, 247:392–393.

30. Griffith, O. W., and Tate, S. S. (1980): The apparent glutathione oxidase activity of γ-glutamyl transpeptidase. *J. Biol. Chem.*, 255:5011–5014.

31. Racker, E. (1955): Glutathione-homocystine transhydrogenase. *J. Biol. Chem.*, 217:867–874.

32. Chang, S. H., and Wilken, D. R. (1966): Participation of the unsymmetrical disulfide of coenzyme A and glutathione in an enzymatic sulfhydryl-disulfide interchange. *J. Biol. Chem.*, 241:4251–4260.

33. Katzen, H. M., Tietze, F., and Stetten, D. W., Jr. (1963): Further studies on the properties of hepatic glutathione-insulin transhydrogenase. *J. Biol. Chem.*, 238:1006–1011.

34. Tomizawa, H. H. (1962): Properties of glutathione insulin transhydrogenase from beef liver. *J. Biol. Chem.*, 237:3393–3396.

35. Varandani, P. T. (1973): Insulin degradation. VII. Sequential degradation of insulin by rat liver homogenates at physiologic concentrations of insulin and in the absence of exogenous glutathione. *Biochim. Biophys. Acta*, 320:249–257.

36. Holmgren, A. (1981): Thiredoxin: Structure and functions. *Trends Biochem. Sci.*, 6(1):26–29.

37. Freedman, R. B. (1979): How many distinct enzymes are responsible for the several cellular processes involving thiol: protein-disulphide interchange? *FEBS Lett.*, 97:201–210.

38. Crook, E. M., and Morgan, E. J. (1944): The reduction of dehydroascorbic acid in plant extracts. *Biochem. J.*, 38:10–15.

39. Esselen, W. B. Jr., and Fuller, J. E. (1939): The oxidation of ascorbic acid as influenced by intestinal bacteria. *J. Bacteriol.*, 37:501–521.

40. Gero, E. (1964): Le role de l'acide ascorbique dans l'oxydation enzymatique du diphosphopyridine nucleotide reduit. *Biochim. Biophys. Acta*, 92:160–163.

41. Mapson, L. W. (1959): Enzyme systems associated with the oxidation and reduction of glutathione in plant tissues. In: *Glutathione*, edited by E. M. Crook, pp. 28–42. Cambridge University, Press, London.

42. Hughes, R. E. (1964): Reduction of dehydroascorbic acid by animal tissues. *Nature*, 203:1068–1069.

43. Grimble, R. F., and Hughes, R. E. (1967): A dehydroascorbic acid "reductase" factor in guinea-pig tissues. *Experientia*, 23:362.

44. Knox, W. E. (1960): Glutathione. In: *The Enzymes, Vol. 2*, edited by P. D. Boyer, H. Lardy, and K. Myrback, pp. 253–294. Academic Press, New York.

45. Neuberg, C. (1913): Uber die Zerstorung von Milchsaurealdehyd und Methylglyoxal durch tierische Organe. *Biochem. Z.*, 39:501–506.

46. Dakin, H. D., and Dudley, H. W. (1913): An enzyme concerned with the formation of hydroxy acids from ketonic aldehydes. *J. Biol. Chem.*, 14:155–157.

47. Dakin, H. D., and Dudley, H. W. (1913): On glyoxalase. *J. Biol. Chem.*, 14:423–431.

48. Lohmann, K. (1932): Beitrag zur enzymatischen Umwandlung von synthetischem Methylglyoxal in Milchsaure. *Biochem. Z.*, 254:332–354.

49. Behrens, O. K. (1941): Coenzymes for glyoxalase. *J. Biol. Chem.*, 141:503–508.

50. Racker, E. (1951): The mechanism of action of glyoxalase. *J. Biol. Chem.*, 190:685–696.

51. Vander Jagt, D. L., Han. L.-P. B., and Lehman, C. H. (1972): Kinetic evaluation of substrate specificity in the glyoxalase-I-catalyzed disproportionation of α-ketoaldehydes. *Biochemistry*, 11:3735–3740.

52. Szent-Gyorgyi, A. (1965): Cell division and cancer. *Science*, 149:34–37.

53. Egyud, L. G. (1965): Studies on autobiotics: Chemical nature of retine. *Proc. Natl. Acad. Sci. USA*, 54:200–202.

54. Egyud, L. G., and Szent-Gyorgyi, A. (1966): On the regulation of cell division. *Proc. Natl. Acad. Sci. USA*, 56:203–207.

55. Strittmatter, P., and Ball, E. G. (1955): Formaldehyde dehydrogenase, a glutathione-dependent enzyme system. *J. Biol. Chem.*, 213:445–461.

56. Kinoshita, J. H., and Masurat, T. (1958): The effect of glutathione on the formaldehyde oxidation in the retina. *Am. J. Ophthalmol.* 46:42–46.

57. Knox, W. E., and Edwards, S. W. (1955): The properties of maleylacetoacetate, the initial product of homogentisate oxidation in liver. *J. Biol. Chem.*, 216:489–498.

58. Lack, L. (1961): Enzymic cis-trans isomerization of maleylpyruvic acid. *J Biol. Chem.*, 236:2835–2840.

59. Balsam, A., and Ingbar, S. H. (1979): Observations on the factors that control the generation of triiodothyronine from thyroxine in rat liver and the nature of the defect induced by fasting. *J. Clin. Invest.*, 63:1145–1156.

60. Visser, T. J. (1980): Deiodination of thyroid hormone and the role of glutathione. *Trends Biochem. Sci.*, 5:222–224.

61. Chasseaud, L. F. (1979): The role of glutathione and glutathione S-transferases in the metabolism of chemical carcinogens and other electrophilic agents. *Adv. Cancer Res.*, 29:175–274.

62. Jakoby, W. B. (editor) (1980): *Enzymatic Basis of Detoxication*. Academic Press, New York.

63. Baumann, E., and Preusse, C. (1879): Ueber Bromphenylmercaptursaure. *Ber. Dtsch. Ges.*, 12:806–810.

64. Jaffe, M. (1879): Ueber die nach Einfubrung von Brombenzol und Chlorbenzol im Organismus entstehenden schwefelhaltigen Sauren. *Ber. Dtsch. Chem. Ges.*, 12:1092–1098.

65. Levi, A. J., Gatmaitan, Z., and Arias, I. M. (1969): Two hepatic cytoplasmic protein fractions, Y and Z, and their possible role in the hepatic uptake of bilirubin, sulfobromophthalein, and other anions. *J. Clin. Invest.*, 48:2156–2167.

66. Reyes, H., Levi, A. J., Gatmaitan, Z., and Arias, I. M. (1971): Studies of Y and Z, two hepatic cytoplasmic organic anion-binding proteins: Effect of drugs, chemicals, hormones and cholestasis. *J. Clin. Invest.*, 50:2242–2252.

67. Habig, W. H., Pabst, M. J., and Jakoby, W. B. (1974): Glutathione S-transferases. The first enzymatic step in mercapturic acid formation. *J. Biol. Chem.*, 249:7130–7139.

68. Habig, W. H., Pabst, M. J., Fleischner, G., Gatmaitan, Z., Arias, I. W., and Jakoby, W. B. (1974): The identity of glutathione S-transferase B with ligandin, a major binding protein of liver. *Proc. Natl. Acad. Sci. USA*, 71:3879–3882.

69. Ketley, J. N., Habig, W. H., and Jakoby, W. B. (1975): Binding of nonsubstrate ligands to the glutathione S-transferases. *J. Biol. Chem.*, 250:8670–8673.

70. Benson, A. M., Cha, Y.-N., Bueding, E., Heine, H. S., and Talalay, P. (1979): Elevation of extrahepatic glutathione S-transferase and epoxide hydratase activities by 2(3)-tert-butyl-4-hydroxyanisole. *Cancer Res.*, 39:2971–2977.

71. Meister, A., and Griffith, O. W. (1979): Effects of methionine sulfoximine analogs on the synthesis of glutamine and glutathione: Possible chemotherapeutic implications. *Cancer Treat. Rep.*, 63:1115–1121.

72. Neish, W. J. P., and Rylett, A. (1963): Azo dyes and rat liver glutathione. *Biochem. Pharmacol.*, 12:893–903.

73. Neish, W. J. P., Davies, H. M., and Reeve, P. M. (1964): Carcinogenic azo dyes, dye-binding and liver glutathione. *Biochem. Pharmacol.*, 13:1291–1303.

74. Fiala, S., and Fiala, E. S. (1973): Activation by chemical car-

cinogens of γ-glutamyl transpeptidase in rat and mouse liver. *J. Natl. Cancer Inst.*, 51:151–158.

75. Fiala, S., and Fiala, E. S. (1971): Activation of γ-glutamyl transpeptidase in rat liver by toxic doses of dimethylnitrosamine. *Naturwissenschaften*, 4:330–331.

76. Fiala, S., Fiala, A. E., and Dixon, B. (1972): γ-Glutamyl transpeptidase in transplantable, chemically induced rat hepatomas and "spontaneous" mouse hepatomas. *J. Natl. Cancer Inst.*, 48:1393–1401.

77. Engin, A. (1976): Glutathione content of human skin carcinomas. *Arch. Dermatol. Res.*, 257:53–55.

78. Fiala, S., Fiala, A. E., Keller, R. W., and Fiala, E. S. (1977): γ-Glutamyl transpeptidase in colon cancer induced by 1,2-dimethylhydrazine. *Arch. Geschwulstforsch.*, 47:117–122.

79. Cheng, S., Nassar, K., and Levy, D. (1978): γ-Glutamyltranspeptidase activity in normal regenerating and malignant hepatocytes. *FEBS Lett.*, 85:310–312.

80. Cameron, R., Kellen, J., Kolin, A., Malkin, A., and Farber, E. (1978): "γ-Glutamyltransferase in putative premalignant liver cell populations during hepatocarcinogenesis. *Cancer Res.*, 38:823–829.

81. Fiala, S., Mohndru, A., Kettering, W. G., Fiala, A. E., and Morris, H. P. (1976): Glutathione and γ-glutamyl transpeptidase in rat liver during chemical carcinogenesis. *J. Natl. Cancer Inst.*, 57:591–598.

82. Wirth, P. J., and Thorgeirsson, S. S. (1978): Glutathione synthesis and degradation in fetal and adult rat liver and Novikoff hepatoma. *Cancer Res.*, 38:2681–2685.

83. Kuss, E. (1967): Kurzmitteilung. Wasserlosliche Metabolite des 17β-Ostradiols. *Hoppe Seylers Z. Physiol. Chem.*, 348:1707–1708.

84. Kuss, E. (1968): Kurzmitteilung. Wasserlosliche Metabolite des Ostradiols-17β, II. *Hoppe Seylers Z. Physiol. Chem.*, 349:1234–1236.

85. Kuss, E. (1969): Kurzmitteilung. Wasserlosliche Metabolite des Ostradiols-17β, III. Trennung und Identifizierung der 1- and 4-Glutathionthioather von 2,3-Dihydroxy-ostratrienen. *Hoppe Seylers Z. Physiol. Chem.*, 350:95–97.

86. Kuss, E. (1971): Mikrosomale Oxidation des Ostradiols-17β. 2-Hydroxylierung und 1-bzw. 4-Thioatherbildung mit und ohne 17-Hydroxyl-Dehydrogenierung. *Hoppe Seylers Z. Physiol. Chem.*, 352:817–836.

87. Jellinck, P. H., Lewis, J., and Boston, F. (1967): Further evidence for the formation of an estrogen-peptide conjugate by rat liver in vitro. *Steroids*, 10:329–346.

88. Elce, J. S., and Harris, J. (1971): Conjugation of 2-hydroxy-estradiol-17β (1,3,5(10)-estratriene-2,3,17β-triol) with glutathione in the rat. *Steroids*, 18:583–591.

89. Cagen, L. M., Fales, H. M., and Pisano, J. J. (1976): Formation of glutathione conjugates of prostaglandin A₁ in human red blood cells. *J. Biol. Chem.*, 251:6550–6554.

90. Cagen, L. M., and Pisano, J. J. (1979): The glutathione conjugate of prostaglandin A₁ is a better substrate than prostaglandin E for partially purified avian prostaglandin E 9-ketoreductase. *Biochim. Biophys. Acta*, 573:547–551.

91. Chaudhari, A., Anderson, M. W., and Eling, T. E. (1978): Conjugation of 15-keto-prostaglandins by glutathione S-transferases. *Biochim. Biophys. Acta*, 531:56–64.

92. Nugteren, D. H., and Hazelhof, E. (1973): Isolation and properties of intermediates in prostaglandin biosynthesis. *Biochim. Biophys. Acta*, 326:448–461.

93. Ogino, N., Miyamoto, T., Yamamoto, S., and Hayaishi, O. (1977): Prostaglandin endoperoxide E isomerase from bovine vesicular gland microsomes, a glutathione-requiring enzyme. *J. Biol. Chem.*, 252:890–895.

94. Raz, A., Kenig-Wakshal, R., and Schwartzman, M. (1977): Effect of organic sulfur compounds on the chemical and enzymatic transformations of prostaglandin endoperoxide H₂. *Biochim. Biophys. Acta*, 488:322–329.

95. Orning, L., Hammarstrom, S., and Samuelsoon, B. (1980): Leukotriene D: A slow reacting substance from rat basophilic leukemia cells. *Proc. Natl. Acad. Sci. USA*, 77:2014–2017.

96. Hammarstrom, S., Samuelsson, B., Clark, D. A., Goto, G., Marfat, A., Mioskowski, C., and Corey, E. J. (1980):

97. Prota, G. (1979): Cysteine and glutathione in mammalian pigmentation. In: *Natural Sulfur Compounds*, edited by D. Cavallini, G. E. Gaull, and V. Zappia, pp. 391–398. Plenum, New York.

98. Agrup, G., Agrup, P., Andersson, T., Falck, B., Hansson, J.-A., Jacobsson, S., Rorsman, H., Rosengren, A.-M., and Rosengren, E. (1975): *Acta Derma. Venereol. (Stockh.)*, 55:337–341.

99. Benson, A. M., Talalay, P., Keen, J. H., and Jakoby, W. B. (1977): Relationship between the soluble glutathione-dependent Δ⁵-3-ketosteroid isomerase and the glutathione S-transferases of the liver. *Proc. Natl. Acad. Sci. USA*, 74:158–162.

100. Huseby, N.-E., and Vik, T. (1978): The activity of γ-glutamyltransferase after bile duct ligation in guinea pig. *Clin. Chim. Acta*, 88:385–392.

101. Lindblad, B., Lindstedt, S., and Steen, G. (1977): On the enzymic defects in hereditary tyrosinemia. *Proc. Natl. Acad. Sci. USA*, 74:4641–4645.

102. Asghar, K., Reddy, B. G., and Krishna, G. (1975): Histochemical localization of glutathione in tissues. *J. Histochem. Cytochem.*, 23:774–779.

103. Smith, M. T., Loveridge, N., Wills, E. D., and Chayen, J. (1979): The distribution of glutathione in the rat liver lobule. *Biochem. J.*, 182:103–108.

104. Omata, S., Sakimura, K., Ishi, T., and Sugano, H. (1978): Chemical nature of a methylmercury complex with a low molecular weight in the liver cytosol of rats exposed to methylmercury chloride. *Biochem. Pharmacol.*, 27:1700–1702.

105. Meister, A. (1973): On the enzymology of amino acid transport. *Science*, 180:33–39.

106. *Peptide Transport and Hydrolysis* (1977): CIBA Foundation Symposium Vol. 50, (New Series). edited by K. Elliott and M. O'Connor. Elsevier, Amsterdam.

107. Griffith, O. W., Bridges, R. J., and Meister, A. (1979): Transport of γ-glutamyl amino acids; role of glutathione and γ-glutamyl transpeptidase. *Proc. Natl. Acad. Sci. USA*, 76:6319–6322.

108. Meister, A., Tate, S. S., and Ross, L. L. (1976): Membrane-bound γ-glutamyl transpeptidase. In: *The Enzymes of Biological Membranes*, edited by A. Martinosi, vol. 3, pp. 315–347. Plenum Press, New York.

109. Allison, D., and Meister, A. (1981): Evidence that transpeptidation is a significant function of γ-glutamyl transpeptidase. *J. Biol. Chem.*, 256:2988–2992.

110. Thompson, G. A., and Meister, A. (1975): Utilization of L-cystine by the γ-glutamyl transpeptidase-γ-glutamyl cyclotransferase pathway. *Proc. Natl. Acad. Sci. USA*, 72:1985–1988.

111. Griffith, O. W., and Meister, A. (1979): Translocation of intracellular glutathione to membrane-bound γ-glutamyl transpeptidase as a discrete step in the γ-glutamyl cycle; glutathionuria after inhibition of transpeptidase. *Proc. Natl. Acad. Sci. USA* 76:268–272.

112. Bartoli, G. M., and Sies, H. (1978): Reduced and oxidized glutathione efflux from liver. *FEBS Lett.*, 86:89–91.

113. Anderson, M. E., Bridges, R. J., and Meister, A. (1980): Direct evidence for inter-organ transport of glutathione and that the non-filtration renal mechanism for glutathione utilization involves γ-glutamyl transpeptidase. *Biochem. Biophys. Res. Commun.*, 96:848–853.

114. Griffith, O. W., and Meister, A. (1979): Glutathione: Interorgan translocation, turnover and metabolism. *Proc. Natl. Acad. Sci. USA*, 76:5606–5610.

115. Griffith, O. W., Bridges, R. J., and Meister, A. (1978): Evidence that the γ-glutamyl cycle functions in vivo using intracellular glutathione; effects of amino acids and selective inhibition of enzymes. *Proc. Natl. Acad. Sci. USA*, 75:5405–5408.

116. Van Der Werf, P., Stephani, R. A., and Meister, A. (1974): Accumulation of 5-oxoproline in mouse tissues after inhibition of 5-oxoprolinase and administration of amino acids; evidence

for function of the γ-glutamyl cycle. *Proc. Natl. Acad. Sci. USA,* 71:1026–1029.

117. Bridges, R. J., Griffith, O. W., and Meister, A. (1980): L-γ-(threo-β-methyl) glutamyl-L-α-aminobutyrate, a selective substrate of γ-glutamyl cyclotransferase; inhibition of enzymic activity by β-aminoglutaryl-L-γ-aminobutyrate. *J. Biol. Chem.,* 255: 10,787-10,792.

118. Konrad, P. N., Richards, F., II, Valentine, W. N., and Paglia, D. E. (1972): γ-Glutamyl-cysteine synthetase deficiency. A cause of hereditary hemolytic anemia. *N. Engl. J. Med.,* 286:557–561.

119. Richards, F., II, Cooper, M. R., Pearce, L. A., Cowan, R. J., and Spurr, C. L. (1974): Familial spinocerebellar degenera-tion, hemolytic anemia, and glutathione deficiency. *Arch. Intern. Med.,* 134:534–537.

120. Wellner, V. P., Sekura, R., Meister, A., and Larsson, A. (1974): Glutathione synthetase deficiency, an inborn error of metabolism of involving the γ-glutamyl cycle in patients with 5-oxoprolinuria (pyroglutamic aciduria). *Proc. Natl. Acad. Sci. USA,* 71:2505–2509.

121. Griffith, O. W., and Meister, A. (1980): Excretion of cysteine and γ-glutamylcysteine moieties in human and experimental animal γ-glutamyl transpeptidase deficiency. *Proc. Natl. Acad. Sci. USA,* 77:3384–3387.

122. Griffith, O. W., Bridges, R. J., and Meister, A. (1981): Formation of γ-glutamylcyst(e)ine *in vivo* is catalyzed by γ-glutamyl transpeptidase. *Proc. Natl. Acad. Sci. USA,* 78:2777–2781.

The Liver: Biology and Pathobiology, edited by
I. Arias, H. Popper, D. Schachter, and D. A. Shafritz.
Raven Press, New York © 1982.

Chapter 18

Heme and Bile Pigment Metabolism

Jayanta Roy Chowdhury, Allan W. Wolkoff, and Irwin M. Arias

SOURCES OF BILIRUBIN

Approximately 75% of bilirubin, a breakdown product of heme, is derived from senescent erythrocytes (1). This has been established by studies of the incorporation of radiolabeled glycine or delta-aminolevulinic acid into bilirubin in man and rat. Following injection of these compounds, two peaks of circulating radioactive bilirubin are found. The first or early labeled peak is seen within 3 days; the second appears between 40 and 80 days. Further investigation has revealed that the early labeled peak has two components. The initial component, comprising two-thirds of early labeled bilirubin is hepatic in origin; cytochrome P-450 and catalase may be important sources of this initial bilirubin. The terminal component is enhanced in conditions associated with ineffective erythropoiesis. Unlike glycine, delta-aminolevulinic acid is preferentially incorporated into hepatic hemoproteins. When radiolabeled delta-aminolevulinic acid is injected, there is no incorporation of radioactivity into the second component of early labeled bilirubin (2).

Conversion of Heme to Bilirubin

Heme is a complex of iron with protoporphyrin IX. Formation of bilirubin from heme involves selective cleavage of the porphyrin ring at the α-methene bridge (Fig. 1). This reaction is catalyzed by the microsomal enzyme heme oxygenase in a reaction requiring Fe^{2+} and a reducing agent, such as NADPH. This enzyme appears to be rate limiting in formation of bilirubin, and the highest activity is found in such organs as the spleen, in which sequestration of senescent erythrocytes occurs (3). Heme oxygenase has been purified from pig spleen (4) and rat liver (5). An alternative mechanism for conversion of heme to bilirubin has been proposed. This involves a quasienzymatic reaction in which heme combines with a microsomal apoenzyme to produce an enzyme, such as cytochrome P-450. Oxygen bound to this heme-apoprotein complex may undergo reductive activation in the presence of NADPH, and may react with the α-methene carbon of heme (6). Nonenzymatic oxidation of the α-oxyheme formed by heme oxygenase results in lib-

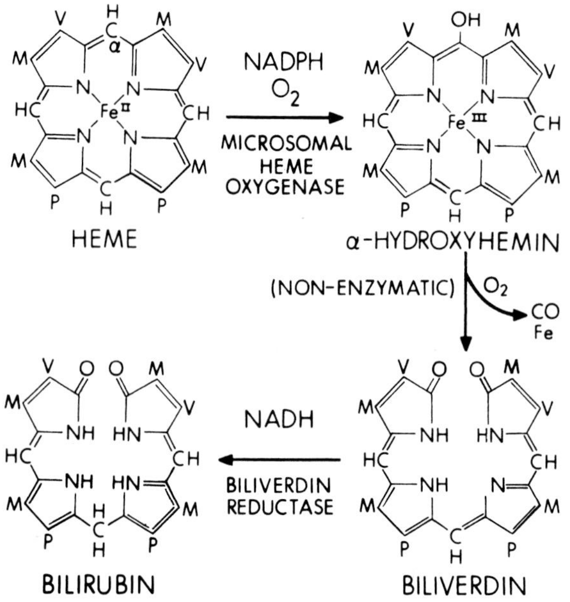

FIG. 1. Mechanism of heme ring opening and subsequent reduction of biliverdin to bilirubin.

eration of carbon monoxide and iron and opening of the porphyrin ring with subsequent formation of the green pigment, biliverdin. In mammals and fish, which excrete bilirubin, biliverdin is converted to bilirubin by biliverdin reductase, a soluble enzyme requiring NADH or NADPH for activity (7).

These chemical reactions result in formation of bilirubin IX_α, which is the most abundant naturally occurring isomer (8). Small amounts of non-α isomers of bilirubin have been detected (9); the mechanism of formation of these bilirubins is unknown.

PHYSICAL CHARACTERISTICS OF BILIRUBIN

X-ray diffraction data have confirmed that bonds between the pyrrolenone rings A and B, and C and D are in the Z or *trans*-configuration, and that the oxygen attached to the outer ring is in lactam rather than lactim configuration (10). The bilirubin molecule has four acidic groups. The two carboxyl groups have pKs of 4.4, and the two lactam groups have pKs of 13.0. Despite these acidic groups, the bilirubin molecule is poorly soluble in aqueous solutions and tends to form colloids or surface films (11). Recent X-ray diffraction studies have provided an explanation for the solubility characteristics of this molecule. The bilirubin IX_α molecule has internal hydrogen bonding between each propionic acid side chain and the pyrrolic and lactam sites in the opposite half of the molecule. The resulting molecule has the form of a "ridge tile"; because both carboxylic groups, all NH groups, and the two lactam oxygens are engaged by hydrogen bonding, the mole-

cule is insoluble in water (10). Internal hydrogen bonding may be disrupted by esterification of the propionic acid side chains; the resulting molecule (conjugated bilirubin) is water-soluble. Because of the differences in configuration, bilirubin IX_β, IX_γ, and IX_δ isomers, as well as biliverdin, are unable to form internal hydrogen bonds and are more soluble in aqueous solutions than is bilirubin IX_α.

Bilirubin is light sensitive and undergoes photooxidation and degradation to colorless fragments (12). It may also undergo geometric isomerization on exposure to light. The two dipyrroles, which are normally in a *trans* or Z configuration, may convert to a *cis* or E configuration, forming bilirubin ZE, EZ, or EE photoisomers. These photoisomers are relatively stable at room temperature in the absence of light, and slowly revert to bilirubin IX_α ZZ (13). Photoisomerization of bilirubin interferes with internal hydrogen bonding, resulting in a more water-soluble molecule. When injected into rats, bilirubin photoisomers are readily excreted into bile, where they revert to bilirubin IX_αZZ. Photoisomerization of bilirubin may be responsible for excretion of unconjugated bilirubin into bile during phototherapy of neonates with unconjugated hyperbilirubinemia (14). A third effect of light on the bilirubin molecule is dipyrrolic scrambling, in which the bilirubin IX_α molecule is converted to nonphysiologic symmetrical III_α and XIII_α isomers (12).

Ultraviolet/Visible Absorption Spectra

The position of the main absorption band (λ_{max}) of bilirubin depends on the bile pigment and on the solvent. Bilirubin isomers (III_α, IX_α, and XIII_α) form strong internal hydrogen bonds and have absorption maxima which lie within a narrow range in most organic solvents. In contrast, the spectrum of bilirubin IX_α dimethylester, in which the hydrogen bond-forming propionic acid carboxyl groups are blocked, is sensitive to change in solvents (15).

Unconjugated bilirubin IX_α has a λ_{max} of 450 to 474 nm in most organic solvents (Fig. 2) and an extinction coefficient (OD_{1cm}^{max} or E_{max}) of 48.0 to 63.4/mM. In alkaline aqueous solutions, there is a 10 to 30 nm shift of the λ_{max} toward shorter wavelengths (hypsochromic shift) and a weaker absorption band at 280 to 300 nm. A shoulder appears at 520 nm with increasing bilirubin concentration due to dimerization of bilirubin. At neutral pH, an increase in the concentration of bilirubin above its solubility results in a slow decrease in absorption and gradual appearance of a shoulder at 490 nm, which is followed by an abrupt increase in light scattering due to self aggregation of bilirubin. Persistence of a negative charge at the surface of aggregated bilirubin molecules may explain the temporary stability of the colloid solution. Lee and Gartner propose

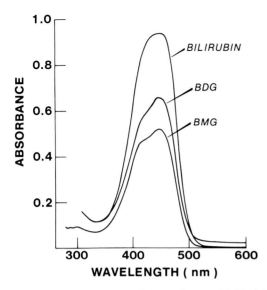

FIG. 2. Absorption spectra of unconjugated bilirubin IX$_\alpha$, bilirubin IX$_\alpha$ monoglucuronide (BMG), and bilirubin IX$_\alpha$ diglucuronide (BDG) in methanol.

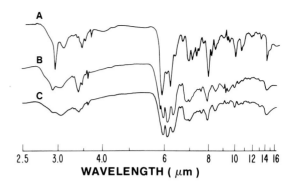

FIG. 3. The infrared spectra of bilirubin IX$_\alpha$ (A), a bilirubin "pigment stone" from a patient with sickle cell disease (B), and synthesized calcium bilirubinate (C) in potassium bromide. The ordinate shows percent transmittance in a logarithmic scale. (Courtesy of Bruce W. Trotman.)

that bilirubin toxicity may result from interaction of the colloidal sol of bilirubin with the surface of cells (15a).

Infrared Spectra

The characteristic infrared (IR) spectra of bilirubins are due to N–H (lactam or pyrrole), C=O (lactam or carboxyl), and C=C stretching vibrations. The IR spectra for bilirubin IX$_\alpha$ contains bands at 3,412 and 3,265 cm^{-1} corresponding to the lactam and pyrrole N–H stretching frequency (Fig. 3). These bands are reduced to a single 3,330 cm^{-1} band in bilirubin dimethyl ester (15). The band at 1,686 cm^{-1} represents the carboxylic C=O, and shifts to 1,735 in the dimethylester. The bands at 1,645 and 1,611 cm^{-1} are due to lactam C=O and C=C stretching vibrations, respectively.

The characteristic carboxylic C=O stretching vibrations are recognizable in calcium bilirubinate and even in crude specimens such as pigment gallstones, and have been used to quantitate the proportion of bilirubin in these stones (16).

Circular Dichroism Spectra

Bilirubin in solution in achiral solvents, such as chloroform and water, is not optically active. In the presence of certain proteins, such as albumin, ligandin, Z-protein, and myelin basic protein (15), bilirubin displays large Cotton effects in the region of the bilirubin absorption band. Optical activity is also observed in sodium deoxycholate (22) and poly (L-lysine) (23). Optically active bilirubin complexes usually show two

CD maxima: one at 400 to 440 nm and the other at 446 to 488 nm. Most optically active bilirubin complexes can be assigned as either type I, where the 400 to 440 nm band is negative and 446 to 448 m band is positive, or type II, where the opposite is true. CD offers a sensitive method of studying bilirubin binding to albumin and ligandin (17).

Proton Magnetic Resonance Spectra

Proton magnetic resonance spectra (^{1}H-nmr) of bilirubin IX$_\alpha$ (Fig. 4) shows broad singlets at 9.3 to 11.2 ppm due to lactam and pyrrole protons and at 11.9 ppm due to COOH protons. Both signals disappear on exchange with D$_2$O, but the N–H signals are not affected by small amounts of water. This supports a lactam configuration of bilirubin, since N–H protons exchange more slowly than do OH protons. The central bridge proton (C-10) and the protons of the other two bridges (C-5 and C-15) give rise to signals at 3.9 and 5.9 to 6.6 ppm, respectively. The vinyl and methyl substituents give rise to signals in the regions of 5 to 7 and 1.6 to 2.2 ppm, respectively. A change of solvent from DMSO-d$_6$ to CHCl$_3$ does not affect the position of the exomethyl (C-2) signal of bilirubin IX$_\alpha$ but causes a −0.2 ppm shift in the case of bilirubin dimethyl ester (15). This is consistent with a preferred configuration of the internally hydrogen bonded bilirubin IX$_\alpha$ in both solvents and conformational mobility of the dimethyl ester, which cannot form internal hydrogen bonds since the propionic acid groups are blocked.

Mass Spectra

Electron impact mass spectrometry has been used most frequently. A major peak at M584 represents the intact molecule, and peaks at M286 and M299 represent the dipyrrolic fragments. Since bilirubin is rela-

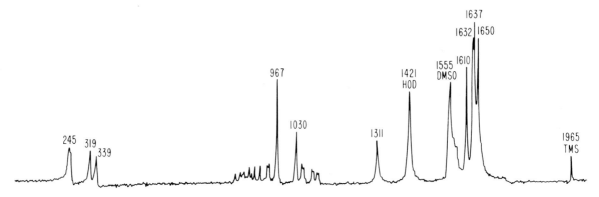

FIG. 4. The ¹H nuclear magnetic resonance spectrum of bilirubin IX$_\alpha$ in deuteriated dimethylsulfoxide (100 MHz). (Courtesy of George Wu.)

tively involatile, high source temperatures required for this technique may cause misleading artifacts. Field desorption techniques are more gentle and give rise to a predominant peak representing the intact molecule (15).

TOXICITY OF BILIRUBIN

The potential toxicity of bilirubin is well known. In mutant Gunn rats and patients with Crigler-Najjar syndrome type I, serum bilirubin levels are greatly elevated, resulting in premature death. Bilirubin inhibits RNA synthesis, protein synthesis (18), and carbohydrate metabolism in brain (19), and protein synthesis in liver (20). Bilirubin may also uncouple oxidative phosphorylation and inhibit ATPase activity of brain mitochondria (21). Studies *in vitro* reveal that bilirubin inhibits hydrolytic enzymes (22), dehydrogenases (23), and enzymes involved in electron transport (24).

QUANTITATION OF BILIRUBIN PRODUCTION

Normally, bilirubin is excreted almost entirely in bile; bilirubin production, therefore, can theoretically be quantitated from biliary excretion. This is not feasible in man, and other methods are employed. Bacteria in the lower gastrointestinal tract convert bilirubin to urobilinogen; fecal urobilinogen excretion approximates bilirubin production. A more reliable estimate of bilirubin production is from studies of the turnover of intravenously injected radiolabeled bilirubin (25). Following injection, blood samples are collected at frequent intervals, and radioactivity in plasma is determined. Plasma bilirubin clearance (the fraction of plasma from which bilirubin is irreversibly extracted) is inversely proportional to the area under the radiobilirubin disappearance curve. Bilirubin removal is quantitated as the product of plasma bilirubin concentration and clearance of radiolabeled bilirubin. In the steady state, removal of bilirubin must equal the amount of newly synthesized bilirubin entering the plasma pool. This method slightly underestimates bilirubin production, because it does not quantitate that small portion of bilirubin which is produced in the liver and excreted directly into bile without appearing in the circulation. More accurate quantitation of bilirubin production can be obtained from studies of carbon monoxide production. It should be borne in mind that a small portion of carbon monoxide in expired air may be produced from nonheme sources, such as halogenated methane and polyphenolic compounds, including catecholamines. In addition, some carbon monoxide may be produced by intestinal bacteria (26).

BINDING OF BILIRUBIN TO ALBUMIN

Bilirubin circulates bound to albumin (27), which protects cells against the potential toxicity of bilirubin. Albumin protects against an otherwise lethal dose of bilirubin following intravenous injection in puppies (28). Because most of the toxic effects of bilirubin are caused by the free ligand, albumin binding plays a protective role. Toxicity of bilirubin on isolated brain mitochondria is abolished by an equimolar amount of albumin (29). Sulfonamide administration to newborns enhances bilirubin encephalopathy, probably because of dissociation of bilirubin from binding to albumin (30). Infusion of albumin into hyperbilirubinemic individuals increases plasma bilirubin concentration due to transfer of bilirubin from tissues to plasma (31).

Under physiologic conditions, bilirubin is present almost exclusively bound as the dianion to a primary binding site on albumin, with smaller amounts on one or two secondary sites (11,32,33). The reaction is fast and reversible; the binding affinity is high, and equilibrium is independent of pH. Below pH 7.4, albumin molecules aggregate with nonionized bilirubin acid (11). These aggregates occur in hyperbilirubinemic states that are accompanied by acidosis (11).

Interaction of bilirubin with albumin has been studied by ultrafiltration, ultacentrifugation, gel chromatography, affinity chromatography on albumin agarose polymers, dialysis, and electrophoresis (11). Following addition of H_2O_2 and horseradish peroxidase to a bilirubin-albumin solution, unbound bilirubin is rapidly destroyed as compared with bound bilirubin. Binding of bilirubin to albumin results in bilirubin fluorescence, circular dichroism, quenching of protein fluorescence, and shift in absorbance spectra (11). Using these techniques, the equilibrium binding of bilirubin to albumin has been determined. The K_a for the primary binding site is approximately 10^8 M^{-1}, whereas that for the secondary site is 10 times less (11).

Binding of bilirubin to peptides derived by enzymatic hydrolysis or cyanogen bromide cleavage of albumin has also been studied. Bilirubin binds only to fragments containing amino acid residues 186 to 248 (34), 1 to 386, 49 to 307 (35), and 182 to 585 (36). Affinity labeling studies indicate that bilirubin is primarily bound to a fragment containing residues 124 to 297 and, to a lesser extent, to residues 446 to 547 (37). Studies of covalent binding of bilirubin to albumin reveal binding to lysine 240 in human albumin and to lysine 238 in bovine serum albumin (38).

Binding of other ligands to albumin may influence its binding capacity for bilirubin. Binding may competitively displace bilirubin or produce conformational changes which enhance (cooperative binding) or decrease (anticooperative) bilirubin binding (39). Sulfonamides, antiinflammatory drugs, and cholangiographic contrast media displace bilirubin competitively from albumin and increase the risk of kernicterus in jaundiced newborn babies (40). Some benzodiazepine drugs and long chain fatty acids in low concentrations bind to human albumin without affecting bilirubin binding (41). Albumin binding of medium chain fatty acids, such as laureate and myristate, increases the binding constant for bilirubin (39). Short chain fatty acids bind to albumin anticooperatively with bilirubin (42). When large amounts of fatty acid bind to albumin, major conformational changes occur, which generally decrease the binding of other ligands, including bilirubin.

Because of the influence of many metabolites and drugs on albumin binding of bilirubin and its transfer from plasma to the central nervous system, measurement of total rather than free plasma bilirubin concentration does not accurately estimate the risk of brain damage from unconjugated bilirubin (27). Efforts have been made to quantitate unbound bilirubin in serum by gel chromatography (43), peroxidase treatment (44), electrophoresis on cellulose acetate (45), and fluorimetry of serum with or without detergent treatment (46); none of these methods is reliable (11). An alternative approach is to determine the amount of unoc-

cupied bilirubin binding sites on albumin. Titration of serum with bilirubin or a dye that binds to albumin has been used. Binding to secondary binding sites occurs before primary sites are saturated, however, and some dyes bind at sites other than the bilirubin binding site. Binding of bilirubin to erythrocytes depends on the albumin/bilirubin ratio in serum and indirectly reflects reserve bilirubin binding sites on albumin (47). Competitive binding by a ^{14}C-labeled ligand (monoacetyl-4,4'-diaminodiphenyl sulfone) (48) or a spin-labeled ligand ([1-N-2,6,6-tetramethyl-1-oxyl-4-piperidinyl) 5-N(1-aspartate)-2,4-dinitrobenzene]) (49) has been used to determine reserve binding capacity. A recently developed fluorimetric method for determination of bound albumin and reserve bilirubin binding capacity (46) in small quantities of whole blood is simple and promising. Despite inaccuracies, several empirical tests for determination of reserve bilirubin binding capacity of serum albumin clinically correlate with brain damage (50) and may be useful in clinically assessing the risk of bilirubin toxicity. Although the newer methods are more accurate and theoretically sounder, clinical experience is needed for their evaluation.

UPTAKE OF BILIRUBIN BY THE LIVER

Despite high-affinity binding to albumin, bilirubin is rapidly transferred from plasma into the liver. Because the ability of the liver to transfer bilirubin from the circulation does not reflect hepatic blood flow, uptake appears to be a specific hepatic function which requires recognition of bilirubin by a plasma membrane receptor (51). Kinetic studies in isolated perfused dog (52) and rat liver (53) and in rats *in vitro* (51) reveal that bilirubin uptake is saturable. The process has other features of a carrier-mediated transport system: preloading, countertransport, and competition. Following an intravenous loading dose of bilirubin, the plasma disappearance of a subsequent tracer dose of ^{3}H-bilirubin is enhanced (51). Efflux of radiolabeled ligand from liver after subsequent infusion with unlabeled ligand has been claimed (51); however, the data may represent ligand efflux from intracellular binding sites. Competition for hepatic uptake *in vivo* occurs among bilirubin, indocyanine green (ICG) (51), sulfobromophthalein (BSP) (51), and conjugated bilirubin (54) but not with bile acids (51,53,54).

Albumin does not accompany bilirubin into the hepatocyte; bilirubin is completely extracted from albumin before hepatocellular uptake occurs. Five minutes after injection of ^{3}H-bilirubin and ^{131}I-albumin in rats, approximately 60% of injected bilirubin is intrahepatic, whereas only 10% of injected albumin is in liver, probably in the vascular space (55). Simultaneous injection of ^{125}I-albumin and ^{3}H-bilirubin in isolated perfused liver reveals rapid uptake of bilirubin with no removal of albumin from the perfusate (52,53,56). Similar results were observed after analysis of plasma disappearance of labeled bilirubin and albumin in man (57).

Whether free or albumin-bound bilirubin interacts with the hepatocyte prior to hepatic uptake is controversial. Based on kinetic studies, Weisiger et al. (58,59) proposed that the albumin-bilirubin complex interacts with an albumin receptor on the hepatocyte; additional studies to quantitate free and bound bilirubin are necessary. When rat liver was perfused with protein-free fluorocarbon, bilirubin uptake was unaffected by infusion of bilirubin as a complex with albumin or ligandin, or with fluorocarbon alone (60). These results suggest that albumin binding does not facilitate hepatic bilirubin uptake. Previously Barnhart and Clarenburg (61) observed that organic anion uptake rates in isolated perfused liver vary inversely with the perfusate albumin concentration. In hypoalbuminemic patients, the plasma albumin concentration and hepatic BSP removal related inversely (62). These studies suggest that albumin binding may prevent bilirubin from nonspecific diffusion into tissues but does not directly contribute to the hepatic uptake mechanism.

Based on these studies, hepatic uptake of bilirubin is believed to represent a carrier-mediated process. The nature of the presumed "carrier" and its mechanism are unknown. Uptake does not appear to require energy or to be Na^+ dependent (53). ICG, BSP, probenecid (63), rifampicin (64), and cholecystographic agents (66) compete with bilirubin for hepatic uptake. Uptake of some of these compounds may be independent from that of bilirubin (67).

The hypothesis that ligandin, an abundant intrahepatocellular organic anion binding protein, mediates hepatic bilirubin uptake was tested in isolated perfused rat liver (56); bilirubin influx and efflux rates were quantitated using a multiple indicator dilution technique in normal and thyroidectomized rats before and after treatment with phenobarbital. Because ligandin is induced after phenobarbital administration and stabilized in the absence of thyroid hormone, these treatments increase liver ligandin levels two- to threefold (56,68). There was no positive correlation between hepatic ligandin concentration and the influx rate of bilirubin; however, the efflux rate of bilirubin from liver back to plasma varied inversely with hepatic ligandin concentration (56,69). This study suggests that intracellular protein binding of bilirubin plays no role in the extraction of bilirubin from serum albumin and subsequent transport into the hepatocyte; however, binding to ligandin influences the net uptake of bilirubin by regulating the efflux of bilirubin from the liver into plasma.

Several studies have quantitated the binding of bilirubin and other organic anions to rat liver cell plasma membrane preparations (LPM). Cornelius et al. (70) demonstrated saturable binding of 200 nmoles BSP bound/mg rat liver LPM protein; bilirubin had no effect on BSP binding. Reichen et al. (71) determined the K_a of BSP binding to LPM as 5.5×10^7 M^{-1} with saturation at 0.035 nmoles/mg protein. Tiribelli et al. (72) studied BSP binding to rat LPM and described high affinity binding with a K_d of 4.88 μM and saturation at 40.4 nmoles BSP/mg protein. Bilirubin (0.5 mM) competitively inhibited BSP binding, resulting in an apparent K_d of 10.5 μM, indicating approximately 100-fold lower affinity of membrane for bilirubin.

Subsequently, a protein was isolated by gel chromatography from an acetone powder of LPM (73). This 170,000 dalton protein binds over 100 nmoles BSP/mg, implying at least 17 binding sites for BSP. Whether these 17 binding sites represent only high affinity binding sites is not clear. Wolkoff and Chung (74) studied the interaction of BSP with rat LPM and described high affinity (K_a, 0.27 μM^{-1}) saturable (6.3 nmoles/mg protein) binding of ^{35}S-BSP, which was eliminated after preincubation of membrane with trypsin. To identify specific membrane binding proteins, a photoaffinity probe was devised, in which ^{35}S-BSP was covalently bound to LPM after exposure to ultraviolet light. SDS-polyacrylamide gel electrophoresis and fluorography revealed radioactivity predominantly associated with a single 55,000 dalton protein. A protein with identical electrophoretic mobility was purified from deoxycholate-solubilized LPM after affinity chromatography on glutathione (GSH)-BSP-agarose gel. This protein is immunologically distinct from rat serum albumin and ligandin and binds bilirubin (K_d, 20 μM). The relationship of this protein to that isolated by Tiribelli and colleagues (73) is unknown. A protein of similar molecular weight was purified by Reichen and Berk (75) following affinity chromatography of Triton X-100-solubilized liver cell plasma membrane on bilirubin agarose gel. Although these proteins avidly bind organic anions, their role as LPM receptors for organic anions and their relationship to transmembrane transport of these compounds await further study.

Evidence in support of carrier-mediated hepatic uptake of bilirubin comes from study of uptake in regenerating rat liver. The normal rat hepatocyte divides approximately once per year (76). Following two-thirds hepatectomy, rapid cellular replication occurs throughout the liver remnant and is associated with expression of oncofetal antigens (77). These findings suggest that hepatic regeneration is accompanied by transient "retrodifferentiation" of hepatocytes. Using a multiple indicator dilution technique, single-pass transport of ^3H-bilirubin was determined in isolated perfused rat liver from 6 hr to 6 days after two-thirds hepatectomy or sham surgery. In this procedure, influx of bilirubin is independent of liver mass. Within 6 hr of two-thirds hepatectomy, influx of bilirubin decreased by 50% as compared to that in sham-operated controls and returned to normal 4 days later. The fact that influx of bilirubin and asialoorosomucoid reached a nadir at the time of greatest cellular proliferation and subsequently returned to normal suggests "maturation" of liver cell function for restoration of specific hepatocyte function.

INTRAHEPATOCELLULAR STORAGE OF BILIRUBIN

Fifteen minutes after the intravenous injection of ^{3}H-bilirubin into rats, plasma ^{3}H-bilirubin declines by more than 90%, and 25 to 30% of the injected dose remains in liver (78). Radioactivity does not appear in bile until 3 to 4 min after injection and subsequently appears at approximately 3%/min of the injected dose (78). Thus from the time bilirubin is cleared from plasma and subsequently excreted into bile, it is accumulated or stored within the hepatocyte.

At all times after intravenous injection, a large proportion of ^{3}H-bilirubin is associated with the 100,000 × g cytosol of liver homogenates (78). Bilirubin is only slightly soluble in aqueous solution at physiologic pH, suggesting that it is bound in the cytosol. Gel filtration of cytosol containing ^{3}H-bilirubin or ^{35}S-BSP reveals that radioactivity is associated with two protein peaks, termed Y and Z (79). These proteins differ from albumin and each other with respect to biochemical and immunologic characteristics (80). When a tracer quantity of radiolabeled anion is added to liver homogenate, binding is almost exclusively to the Y protein, whereas with larger amounts, binding to the Z protein becomes more apparent (79). This result suggests that, under physiologic conditions, Y protein is the principal cytoplasmic protein to which organic anions bind.

Y protein has been purified to homogeneity (80) and avidly binds many compounds, including various drugs, hormones, and organic anions (79,81−84). Similar proteins were identified by other investigators: Morey and Litwack (85) identified a protein by its ability to bind a cortisol metabolite, and Ketterer et al. (86) identified a protein that bound an azo-dye carcinogen. These three proteins proved to be identical by structural and immunologic techniques, and the protein was termed "ligandin" (87). Ligandin accounts for approximately 5% of liver cytosol protein (88) and also has GSH transferase (89), ketosteroid isomerase (90), and GSH peroxidase activities (91). In the rat, ligandin is identical to GSH transferase B, the major member of a class of six distinct basic GSH transferases which were purified from rat liver cytosol (92). Five GSH transferases have been isolated from human liver, but unlike the comparable rat proteins, the human proteins have identical amino acid composition and cross react immunologically (92). Each of the rat and human GSH transferases avidly binds bilirubin and other organic anions as nonsubstrate ligands (92,93).

The high affinity of these proteins for organic anions suggested that they may play a role in transport by the liver (94). Circumstantial evidence for this hypothesis was provided by studies of ontogeny and phylogeny. Addition of BSP to liver cytosol followed by Sephadex G-75 chromatography revealed that in elasmobranchs, teleosts, and the gill-breathing amphibia, there was no detectable Y peak; the Z peak was either undetectable or present in trace amounts. Prominent Y and Z peaks were found in lung-breathing amphibians, reptiles, birds, and mammals (95).

A developmental study of the soluble organic anion binding proteins in three species of frog during metamorphosis revealed undetectable Y and Z peaks in the youngest forms. During development, a prominent Z peak was seen, and both Y and Z peaks were present in adults (95). Similar results were obtained in guinea pigs (96) and monkeys (97); "maturation" of ligandin coincided with normalization of hepatic organic anion transport. Additional studies of organic anion transport in elasmobranchs revealed that the relationship of ligandin and other GSH transferases to hepatic organic anion transport may be complex (98). These animals have low but detectable levels of GSH transferase activity in liver (99); 24 hr after injection, however, 75 to 85% of ^{35}S-BSP was recovered in bile and liver.

The ability to bind to ligandin does not imply that a given ligand will be removed from the circulation by the liver. For example, Evans blue is slowly excreted by the liver *in vivo*. After intravenous injection of Evans blue into a rat, no binding to the Y and Z fractions of rat liver cytosol occurs; addition of the dye to liver cytosol *in vitro* reveals abundant binding to the Y peak (79).

Although bilirubin and other organic anions are stored in the liver primarily bound to ligandin, the selectivity of organic anion uptake by the liver cell is probably a function of the plasma membrane. Serum albumin has a greater affinity for bilirubin than does purified ligandin (100); the affinity of ligandin for bilirubin may decrease during purification (101). That this view is incorrect was demonstrated in a circular dichroism study of bilirubin-ligandin interaction in rat liver cytosol and fractions obtained during purification of ligandin (102). Ligandin but not albumin retained the capacity to bind bilirubin in liver supernatant components. In their respective physiological milieus, albumin and ligandin are structurally adapted to bind ligands, albumin in serum and ligandin in the cytosol of the liver cell. With respect to organic anion transport, ligandin may function within the hepatocyte much as albumin does in the circulation, binding bilirubin and preventing efflux from the hepatocyte back into the circulation (56) and nonspecific diffusion of bilirubin into compartments of the hepatocyte. This hypothesis is supported by the finding that bilirubin inhibits mitochondrial respiration *in vitro;* this effect is completely prevented by ligandin (103). The relationship of ligandin binding of bilirubin and its conjugates to intracellular transport and conjugation and biliary excretion is not known.

CONJUGATION OF BILIRUBIN

Before bilirubin is excreted in bile, its propionic acid carboxyl groups are esterified, forming mono- or diconjugates. Studies of human T-tube bile (104) and bile from dogs (105), alligators, cats, chickens, horses, opossums, rabbits, and snakes (106) show xylosyl and glucosyl conjugates. More complex conjugating sugar groups, including glucuronosyl-glucosyl, glucuronosyl-glucuronosyl, and glucosyl-glucosyl-glucuronosyl, were characterized in human T-tube bile (107). Glucuronic acid is the major conjugating group in normal mammalian bile (104).

Although the existence of bilirubin monoglucuronide as a chemical entity was questioned (108), bilirubin glucuronides are now known to be present as mono- and diconjugates (Fig. 5) (109). Because bilirubin IX_α is an asymmetrical molecule, bilirubin IX_α monoglucuronide exists as two isomers, depending on where the glucuronyl group is attached. The two isomers have been separated by thin-layer or high performance liquid chromatography after substitution of the conjugating group by NH_2 (109) or CH_3 groups (110).

QUANTITATION OF BILIRUBIN AND ITS CONJUGATES

Since bilirubin conjugates are structurally unstable and undergo oxidation, their quantitation and characterization have been primarily performed using two dipyrrolic derivatives formed by reaction of bilirubin with a diazo reagent. The reaction begins with electrophilic attack by a diazonium ion at the 9 and 11 positions of bilirubin (111) and converts the tetrapyrrole to diazotized azopyrroles and formaldehyde. Unconjugated bilirubin is converted to two unconjugated dipyrroles; bilirubin diconjugates form two conjugated azodipyrroles, and bilirubin monoconjugates form one conjugated and one unconjugated azodipyrrole.

In 1916, van den Bergh and Muller (112) discovered that serum contains two species of bilirubin. One reacts with sulfanilic acid diazo reagent within minutes; the other reacts rapidly only when accelerator substances, such as methanol or caffeine, are present (112). The first type of reaction is called direct; the second is the indirect diazo reaction. Later, it was realized that indirect-reacting bilirubin represents unconjugated bilirubin, and that direct-reacting bilirubin largely represents conjugated bilirubin (113). The direct diazo reaction overestimates the levels of conjugated bilirubin. For example, solutions of crystalline bilirubin may show as much as 10% of total pigment as direct reacting. In most clinical laboratories, a direct-reacting bilirubin concentration of less than 15% of total is normal. Various modifications of the van den Bergh reaction are commonly used for clinical determination of bilirubin conjugates.

More recently, ethyl anthranilate and *p*-iodoaniline diazo reagents were used in place of sulfanilic acid diazo reagent. These methods are more sensitive, accurate, and selective, and the azodipyrroles formed can be extracted and analyzed by thin-layer (105) and high pressure liquid chromatography. The conjugated azopyrrole formed by reaction of bilirubin conjugates with ethylanthranilate diazonium reagent has been characterized as the 1-0-acylglucopyranuric acid glycoside (114). When bile flow is impeded, bilirubin IX_α-1-0-acyl glucuronides rearrange with formation of 2-, 3-, and 4-acyl glucuronides (114). This sequential migration of the bilirubin 0-acyl group from position 1 to positions 2, 3, and 4 of glucuronic acid is nonenzymatic, base catalyzed and occurs on incubation of bile or isolated bilirubin IX_α glucuronides at 37°C (115).

The azo method cannot be applied to quantitate accurately the parent tetrapyrroles in a complex mixture of mono- and diconjugates. Methods for separation and quantitation of intact bilirubin tetrapyrroles have been developed. In 1954, Cole et al. (116) separated serum bile pigment into unconjugated bilirubin and two direct-reacting components, pigments I and II, by column chromatography. Pigment II was characterized as bilirubin diglucuronide. The exact nature of pigment I, which yielded equimolar amounts of conjugated and unconjugated azodipyrroles on diazo reaction, remained controversial. Subsequently, Heirwegh and associates (105) developed highly resolving thin-layer chromatographic systems for separation of bilirubin and its conjugates. Analysis of tetrapyrrole azoderivatives revealed predominantly bilirubin IX_α conjugates in the bile of various species. In addition, a small amount of bilirubin IX_β, IX_γ, and IX_δ occur in dog bile (116). Small amounts of sulfate, phosphate, and taurine conjugates of bilirubin have also been described in bile (15). Although separation of intact bilirubin tetrapyrroles by thin-layer chromatography has led to better understanding of bilirubin conjugates, the methods are tedious, and quantitative pigment recovery is not possible.

High performance liquid chromatography (HPLC) offers high resolution and quantitative recovery of bile pigments. Methyl esters formed by alkaline methanolysis of bilirubin mono- and diconjugates have been separated and quantitated by HPLC (117). In this method, the conjugating moieties are replaced by methyl groups, and the pigments cannot be separated on the basis of their conjugating moieties. Methods for separation and quantitation of intact bilirubin tetrapyrrole conjugates by HPLC have been developed (118–121) and offer accurate and sensitive means to identify and quantitate bilirubin conjugates in body fluids and *in vitro* (Fig. 5).

Bilirubin diglucuronide is the major pigment in human, dog, and rat bile (122). Conjugation of bilirubin with glucuronic acid is catalyzed by the microsomal enzyme uridine diphosphoglucuronate glucuronosyltransferase (UDP-glucuronyl transferase, EC 2.4.1.17), which catalyzes transfer of the glucuronyl moiety of UDP-glucuronide (123). UDP-glucuronyl transferases have an important role in glucuronidation and disposition of many other endogenous substances, such as thyroxine, tetrahydrocortisol, and steroid hormones, and various exogenous compounds (124). The enzyme activity is present in mammalian liver (124) and in the liver of many salt- and fresh-water fish (125). Highest specific enzyme activity is in the microsomal fraction of liver homogenates (124); the enzyme is also present in renal cortex, gastrointestinal mucosa, epidermis, and adrenal tissue. Activities in these tissues are lower than in liver (124).

UDP-glucuronyltransferase is an integral part of the microsomal membrane, and function depends on its lipid environment. Treatment of microsomes with phospholipase A inactivates the enzyme; activity is restored on addition of phospholipid micelles (126). Delipidation of deoxycholate-solubilized enzyme inactivates the enzyme. Virtually complete reactivation was obtained following dialysis of the delipidated enzyme preparation with lecithin (127).

The activity of UDP-glucuronyltransferase *in vitro* is influenced by membrane-perturbing agents. Detergents, such as Triton X-100, Lubrol, digitonin, tween, and low concentrations of deoxycholate, enhance enzyme activity (128). An increase in enzyme activity occurs after sonication of microsomal preparations (129), storage at 0° C in potassium chloride solution (130), and brief incubation with phospholipase A (131). Two models have been proposed to explain this activation. In the compartmental model, the catalytic site of the enzyme is partially separated from its substrates by the lipid membranes. Membrane perturbation enhances enzyme activity *in vitro* by increasing accessi-

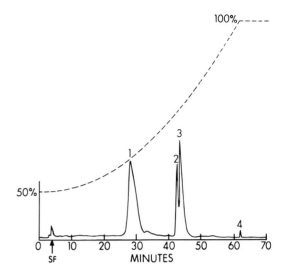

FIG. 5. Separation of bilirubin diglucuronide (*1*), bilirubin monoglucuronide C_{12} (*2*) and C_8 (*3*), and unconjugated bilirubin (*4*) on HPLC of Wistar rat bile. Bile (0.025 ml) was chromatographed on a reverse phase (μ-Bondapak C-18, Waters') column. Pigments were eluted with a concave gradient (*interrupted line*) of methanol (50 to 100% in 60 min) in sodium acetate (0.1 M, pH 4.0) containing 5 mM 1-heptane sulfonic acid at 1 ml/min. SF, solvent front.

bility of substrates to the catalytic site (132). In the allosteric model, enzyme activity is constrained by the membrane. Activating agents release the enzyme from constraint and increase enzyme activity (133).

UDP-glucuronyltransferase appears to consist of a group of related enzymes. Following treatment of rats with methylcholanthrene, hepatic UDP-glucuronyltransferase activity is influenced differently toward different aglycone substrates (134). Attempts to solubilize enzyme activity from rat liver microsomes with detergents yield different results with bilirubin and *p*-nitrophenol as substrates (135). UDP-glucuronyltransferase activity toward *p*-aminophenol and other xenobiotics develops in late fetal rat liver, whereas bilirubin and steroid hormone glucuronidating activity develops postnatally (136).

Treatment of pregnant rats with glucocorticoids results in precocious development of fetal UDP-glucuronyltransferase activity with phenolic substrates but not with bilirubin (136). Homozygous Gunn rats cannot form bilirubin glucuronides but form acyl- and N-glucuronides and glucuronides of several phenolic substrates, such as thyroxine and tetrahydrocortisol (137, 138). Glucuronidating activity toward *o*-aminophenol is deficient *in vitro* but is restored to normal by pretreatment of microsomes with diethylnitrosamine (138). The effect of diethylnitrosamine does not depend on microsomal membranes, since the effect persists in UDP-glucuronyltransferase purified from Gunn rat liver. These studies suggest functional heterogeneity of UDP-glucuronyltransferase.

At least two functionally different UDP-glucuronyl transferases have been purified to apparent homogeneity from rat liver microsomes (139–141). l-Naphthol, p-nitrophenol, and 3-hydroxybenzo(a)pyrene are substrates for a class of UDP-glucuronyltransferase which is inducible by methylcholanthrene in rats (142). Bilirubin and several steroid hormones are substrates for a second class of UDP-glucuronyltransferase which is inducible by phenobarbital (142). There may be other functional classes and subclasses. Classification on the basis of inducibility may be species specific. For example, methylcholanthrene induces UDP-glucuronyltransferase activity toward bilirubin in mice (143) but not in rats (142). Although much evidence suggests heterogeneity of UDP-glucuronyltransferase, there are similarities among the different classes of the enzyme. Gunn rats have not only a deficiency in UDP-glucuronyltransferase activity toward bilirubin but also have defective glucuronidation of p-nitrophenol, o-aminophenol, l-naphthol, and methylumbelliferone (144). Antibody prepared against pure rat p-nitrophenol UDP-glucuronyltransferase precipitates p-nitrophenol and bilirubin glucuronidating activity from solubilized rat liver microsomes. This result suggests structural similarity of at least a portion of the enzyme molecule. Although Gunn rat liver microsomes cannot convert bilirubin to bilirubin glucuronides, incubation of bilirubin dimethylester with Gunn rat liver microsomes and UDP-glucuronic acid results in sequential formation of bilirubin and bilirubin glucuronides (145).

Formation of Bilirubin Diglucuronide

Since the discovery of UDP-glucuronyltransferase, formation of bilirubin diglucuronide, the major pigment in man, rat, and dog bile, has been presumed to be catalyzed by this enzyme. The major product formed on incubation of bilirubin, UDP-glucuronic acid, and rat liver microsomes is bilirubin monoglucuronide rather than diglucuronide (146). UDP-glucuronyltransferase accepts many aglycones as substrates; theoretically, bilirubin monoglucuronide could be a substrate. In studies of the separate conversion of bilirubin to monoglucuronide and monoglucuronide to bilirubin diglucuronide by cat liver microsomes, the two reactions differed in pH optima and inhibition by competitive substrates (147). UDP-glucuronic acid-dependent conversion of bilirubin monoglucuronide to diglucuronide has been shown in rat and human liver microsomal systems (121,148). A second enzyme-catalyzing conversion of bilirubin monoglucuronide to diglucuronide was purified from plasma membrane-

enriched fractions of rat liver homogenate (149). The enzyme catalyzes dismutation of 2 moles bilirubin monoglucuronide to 1 mole bilirubin diglucuronide and 1 mole unconjugated bilirubin (150). The mechanism may involve either transesterification or enzyme-catalyzed rearrangement of dipyrroles. Neither mechanism has been established. The product of the reaction retains the IX_α configuration, which is the configuration of bilirubin conjugates in bile (150). The highest specific activity of the enzyme is in the canalicular-enriched subfraction of rat liver plasma membrane preparations.

Enzyme activity is normal in Gunn rat liver and in patients with the Crigler-Najjar syndrome who lack UDP-glucuronyltransferase activity toward bilirubin (151). The function of the enzyme has been tested *in vivo*. The major bilirubin conjugate in the liver cell is almost exclusively bilirubin monoglucuronide, even in rats that excrete predominantly bilirubin diglucuronide in bile (78). When unconjugated bilirubin is infused intravenously in rats at rates exceeding the maximum excretory capacity, conjugated bilirubin accumulates in blood. Bilirubin conjugates in serum are mostly bilirubin monoglucuronide, whereas bilirubin diglucuronide is the predominant pigment in bile (150). Bilirubin monoglucuronide infused in Gunn rats was excreted in bile partly as bilirubin diglucuronide (149, 151). When bilirubin monoglucuronide with ^3H label on bilirubin and ^{14}C label on glucuronic acid was infused in Gunn rats, bilirubin diglucuronide excreted in bile had twice the $^{14}C:^3H$ ratio compared to the injected pigment. When double-labeled bilirubin monoglucuronide was infused in normal rats, the $^{14}C:^3H$ ratio in the bilirubin diglucuronide excreted in bile was greater than (but not double) the ratio in injected bilirubin monoglucuronide. This may be due to partial conversion of ^3H-bilirubin produced in the dismutation reaction to bilirubin diglucuronide. When an excess of unconjugated bilirubin is injected with the double-labeled bilirubin monoglucuronide, the $^{14}C:^3H$ ratio in bilirubin diglucuronide in bile is the same as the ratio in the injected pigment. This suggests that dismutation of bilirubin monoglucuronide is inhibited by high intrahepatic unconjugated bilirubin concentration (152). Other authors infused double-labeled bilirubin in monoglucuronide with an excess of unconjugated bilirubin and found no difference in the $^{14}C:^3H$ ratio in bilirubin diglucuronide excreted in bile and in the injected bilirubin monoglucuronide.

Conversion of bilirubin monoglucuronide to bilirubin diglucuronide has also been observed in isolated perfused Gunn rat liver in which the intrahepatic bilirubin concentration was depleted by perfusion with an albumin-containing solution. Conversion to diglucuronide was reduced when the intrahepatic bilirubin was repleted by perfusion with a bilirubin-containing solution. These results suggest that bilirubin monoglucuronide is converted to bilirubin diglucuronide by both UDP-glucuronyltransferase and enzymatic dismutation. When the intrahepatic concentration of unconjugated bilirubin is high, dismutation is inhibited, UDP-glucuronyltransferase mechanism persists, and bilirubin diglucuronide formation proceeds at a slower rate than normal. The problem is complex because spontaneous dismutation involving formation of non-physiologic III_α and XII_α isomers can occur in the absence of protein (153).

BILIARY EXCRETION OF BILIRUBIN

Canalicular excretion of bilirubin is thought to be an energy-dependent process that transports the pigment against a concentration gradient. In fish, unconjugated bilirubin is excreted in bile; in mammals, conjugation is essential for bilirubin excretion. For example, Gunn rats and patients with the Crigler-Najjar syndrome, type I, lack UDP-glucuronyltransferase activity and manifest lifelong unconjugated hyperbilirubinemia. Accumulation of conjugated bilirubin in serum following intravenous infusion of unconjugated bilirubin at a rate exceeding the maximal excretory capacity of bilirubin suggests that canalicular transport rather than conjugation is rate limiting in bilirubin excretion (150, 154). When UDP-glucuronyltransferase activity is partially or totally deficient, however, conjugation may be rate limiting in bilirubin excretion (155).

Patients with the Dubin-Johnson syndrome and mutant Corriedale sheep with an analogous functional defect have reduced capacity to transport conjugated bilirubin, BSP, ICG, iopanoic acid, phylloerythrin, and metanephrine glucuronide into the bile. Affected patients and sheep have normal transport maximum for infused taurocholate (156). A dissociation between bilirubin and bile salt excretory capacity also occurs in the primate fetus (157). These observations suggest that there are at least two mechanisms for organic anion excretion by the liver: one for bile salts, another for other organic anions.

Maximal bilirubin excretory capacity (T_{max}) depends on bile flow, which is increased by infusion of bile salts (158), or phenobarbital treatment, which enhances bile flow rate by a nonbile salt-dependent mechanism (159). T_{max} of bilirubin is enhanced in both cases. Several other bile salt-dependent choleretics increase bile flow but not T_{max} for organic anions.

It has been proposed that incorporation of bilirubin conjugates in bile salt mixed micelles in bile reduces the concentration of bilirubin in bile and results in canalicular excretion of bilirubin along a downhill gradient into a "micellar sink" (160). Infusion of non-micelle-forming bile salts also enhances bilirubin ex-

cretory capacity (161). The relationship of bile salt excretion, bile flow, and bilirubin excretion has been studied in patients with gallstones (162). Approximately one-third of bilirubin excretion has been calculated to be bile salt independent, which suggests that bile salt micelles are not essential for canalicular transport of conjugated bilirubin in man. Excretion of unconjugated bilirubin, which comprises about 3% of bilirubin excreted in man, may depend on interaction with mixed micelles. Kinetic studies of taurocholate and BSP excretion suggest that there may be an interaction of bile salt receptors and receptors for other organic anions at the level of canalicular excretion (163). Self aggregation and incorporation of bilirubin in mixed micelles (160) may occur in bile and decrease the bilirubin concentration in the aqueous phase.

Bilirubin, BSP, and ICG apparently compete for biliary excretion. Since these anions compete for hepatic uptake and share intracellular binding proteins, it cannot be assumed that they share a common receptor in the bile canaliculus. Combined bilirubin and BSP infusion studies in rats indicate that BSP may be excreted by two canalicular pathways. Bilirubin competes for only one of these (164).

The enzyme-catalyzing dismutation of bilirubin monoglucuronide is concentrated in the canalicular subfraction of rat liver plasma membrane preparations (151). Since little bilirubin diglucuronide is found within the hepatocyte despite a high affinity for ligandin (124), a possible linkage may exist between bilirubin monoglucuronide dismutase and biliary secretion of diglucuronide (165).

Fate of Bilirubin in the Gastrointestinal Tract

Bilirubin reaches the intestinal tract mainly conjugated and is not substantially absorbed (166). In some circumstances, there may be enhanced excretion of unconjugated bilirubin into the intestine. Absorption of unconjugated bilirubin from the intestine may contribute to neonatal hyperbilirubinemia (167). Absorption of bilirubin from the gallbladder occurs in animals (168).

Bilirubin is degraded into a series of urobilinogen and related products by intestinal bacteria (169). Urobilinogens are present in deconjugated states. It is not known whether deconjugation precedes or follows bilirubin degradation, but bacterial β-glucuronidase plays a role in the deconjugation (167). Most of the urobilinogen reabsorbed from the intestine is reexcreted in the bile; a small fraction is excreted by the kidney. Enhanced tubular absorption and instability of the pigment in acid urine makes urobilinogen excretion in urine an unreliable indicator of the status of bilirubin metabolism. In a jaundiced patient, absence of urobilinogen in stool and urine suggests complete obstruction of the bile duct. In liver disease and increased bilirubin production, urinary urobilinogen excretion is increased. Urobilinogen is colorless. Oxidation leads to formation of urobilin, which contributes to the color of normal urine and stool.

Alternate Pathways of Bilirubin Elimination

After injection of labeled unconjugated bilirubin in man, only 3% is excreted by the kidney. Even in the presence of marked hyperbilirubinemia, bile remains the main route of bilirubin excretion (165).

In patients with the Crigler-Najjar syndrome and in Gunn rats, a small amount of unconjugated bilirubin is secreted in bile. Additional unconjugated bilirubin may reach the intestinal lumen by passage across the intestinal wall or by desquamation of intestinal epithelial cells (170). Ambient light or phototherapy forms geometric isomers of bilirubin (EE, EZ, or ZE forms), which are excreted in unconjugated form and converted to bilirubin $IX_{\alpha}ZZ$ in the bile (13). Considerable bilirubin is degraded to polar diazo-negative compounds, which are excreted in both bile and urine (170). A fraction of pigment is converted to tetrapyrrole-dihydroxyl derivatives and dipyrroles (171). Bilirubin catabolism in the liver is enhanced by induction of mixed function oxidases (172).

In intrahepatic or extrahepatic cholestasis, the plasma conjugated bilirubin concentration increases. After injection of radiolabeled bilirubin in animals with experimentally ligated bile ducts (173) and in children with biliary atresia (174), 50 to 90% of injected radioactivity is excreted in urine. In total biliary obstruction, urinary excretion becomes the major pathway of bilirubin excretion (175). Renal excretion of conjugated bilirubin depends on glomerular filtration of a small, nonprotein-bound fraction of conjugated bilirubin (175). There is evidence for tubular reabsorption but not for tubular secretion of bilirubin (176).

DISORDERS OF BILIRUBIN METABOLISM

As described above, the hepatic transport of bilirubin involves four distinct but probably interrelated stages (Fig. 6): (a) uptake from the circulation, (b) intracellular binding or storage, (c) conjugation, largely with glucuronic acid, and (d) biliary excretion. Abnormalities in any of these processes may result in hyperbilirubinemia. Complex clinical disorders, such as hepatitis or cirrhosis, affect multiple processes. In several inheritable disorders, the transfer of bilirubin from blood to bile is disrupted at a specific step. Study of these disorders has permitted better understanding

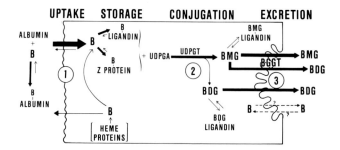

FIG. 6. Schematic summary of hepatic transport and metabolism of bilirubin (B). In the circulation, bilirubin is bound avidly to albumin. This complex dissociates, and bilirubin alone enters the liver cell by a process with characteristics of facilitated diffusion (1). A fraction of bilirubin within the liver cell is derived from breakdown of hepatic heme proteins. Bilirubin inside the hepatocyte binds to cytosolic proteins (ligandin and Z protein), which prevents its efflux from the cell. Bilirubin is conjugated with glucuronic acid (2) in the presence of bilirubin UDP-glucuronyl transferase (UDPGT) and UDP-glucuronic acid (UDPGA) to form bilirubin monoglucuronide (BMG) and bilirubin diglucuronide (BDG), both of which may bind to ligandin in the cytosol. Normally, conjugation is virtually obligatory for biliary excretion of bilirubin (3), although small amounts of unconjugated bilirubin are found in bile in some circumstances. The hepatocyte plasma membranes are enriched in an enzyme, bilirubin glucuronoside glucuronsyltransferase (BGGT), which dismutates BMG to BDG and unconjugated bilirubin. The relationship of BGGT to biliary excretion is unknown. Canalicular excretion is thought to be an energy-requiring process that normally is rate-limiting in bilirubin throughput and may be shared by other organic anions, except bile salts.

of bilirubin metabolism in health and disease. Each disorder is characterized by varied degrees of hyperbilirubinemia of the unconjugated or conjugated type.

DISORDERS OF BILIRUBIN METABOLISM RESULTING IN PREDOMINANTLY UNCONJUGATED HYPERBILIRUBINEMIA

Neonatal Hyperbilirubinemia

By adult standards, every newborn baby has hyperbilirubinemia, and about 50% of neonates are clinically jaundiced during the first 5 days of life. Serum bilirubin is predominantly unconjugated. Exaggeration of this "physiologic jaundice" can result in marked hyperbilirubinemia with risk of kernicterus. In 4,000 consecutive infants, 16% had maximal serum bilirubin concentrations of 10 mg/dl or above; in 5%, bilirubin concentrations exceeded 15 mg/dl (177). In normal, full-term human neonates, serum bilirubin concentrations increase rapidly from 1−2 to 5−6 mg/dl in approximately 72 hr and subsequently decrease to normal within 7 to 10 days (178). Physiologic jaundice of the newborn appears to result from a combination of increased bilirubin production and delayed maturation in the capability of the liver to dispose of bilirubin. Severe neonatal unconjugated hyperbilirubinemia results from exaggeration in one or more of the regularly occurring developmental restrictions characteristic of the newborn period and/or superimposition of additional mechanisms.

Increased Bilirubin Load

Increased bilirubin production due to premature breakdown of erythrocytes or to ineffective erythropoiesis causes hyperbilirubinemia in the presence of normal liver function. Hemolytic disorders, such as sickle cell disease and hereditary spherocytosis, and toxic or idiosyncratic drug reactions are common causes of hemolytic jaundice. Ineffective erythropoiesis occurs in thalassemia, vitamin B_{12} deficiency, and congenital dyserythropoietic anemias. Serum bilirubin is mostly unconjugated and rarely exceeds 4 mg/dl, except when there is an associated hepatobiliary disorder (165). Rarely, the rate of bilirubin production exceeds the bile canalicular excretory capacity, and conjugated bilirubin accumulates in serum (179).

Syndromes Associated with UDP-Glucuronyltransferase Deficiency

Crigler-Najjar Syndrome, Type I

The rare disorder described by Crigler and Najjar in 1952 (180) is characterized by severe unconjugated hyperbilirubinemia due to the absence of bilirubin UDP-glucuronyltransferase activity (Table 1). The syndrome occurs in all races and is inherited as an autosomal recessive trait; there may be a family history of consanguinity and an increased incidence of other disorders inherited as autosomal recessive traits. Most infants die with kernicterus during the neonatal period (181); some have survived to early adulthood only to succumb to kernicterus later in life (181,182).

Serum bilirubin is virtually all unconjugated; the concentration is 20 to 25 mg/dl but may be as high as 50 mg/dl (183). Serum bilirubin tends to be lower in summer due to exposure to sunlight and higher during intercurrent illness (184). Bile may be pale (183), fecal urobilinogen excretion is reduced, and the urine is yellow due to uncharacterized pigments (185), although no bilirubin is present in urine. Bilirubin production is normal (184), as are liver function tests, including oral cholecystography and BSP and ICG clearance (182). Liver biopsy reveals normal histology by light and electron (181) microscopy. In some patients, canalicular and bile ductular cholestasis occur (181), possibly because of enhanced excretion of unconjugated bilirubin in bile during phototherapy (181).

Mutant Wistar rats with nonhemolytic unconjugated hyperbilirubinemia were described by Gunn in 1938 (186), and a colony of the mutant animals was maintained by W. E. Castle for over 15 years. Homozygous Gunn rats lack bilirubin UDP-glucuronyltransferase activity and are prototypes of Crigler-Najjar syndrome, type I. Study of these animals has resulted in major advances in the understanding of bilirubin transport, metabolism, and encephalopathy. Homozygous Gunn rats have 3 to 20 mg bilirubin/dl serum, all of which is unconjugated. Heterozygous Gunn rats are anicteric. As in Crigler-Najjar syndrome, type I, there is no bilirubinuria, and the bile contains only small amounts of unconjugated bilirubin, with traces of bilirubin conjugates (187). Homozygous Gunn rats cannot concentrate urine due to high renal medullary bilirubin concentration, which interferes with sodium transport (188). Similar concentration defects have not been described in the kidneys of patients with Crigler-Najjar syndrome, type I, although bilirubin is deposited in the kidneys (189).

Homozygous Gunn rats develop cytoplasmic neuronal changes on the third day of life; many mitochondria contain glycogen by the eighth day; and degeneration of Purkinje and other neuronal cells is evident by 2 weeks. The brain of a healthy Gunn rat does not have yellow staining. Administration of sulfadimethoxine, a drug that competes for albumin binding, to 14-day-old animals results in yellow staining of selective areas of the brain, with neurologic deterioration (190). The basis of the selectivity of bilirubin staining for certain neurons is unknown. In addition to lack of bilirubin glucuronidation, Gunn rats have partial deficiency for conjugation of several xenobiotics, although enzyme activity is normal for other substrates.

Treatment of patients with this disorder is aimed at reduction of plasma unconjugated bilirubin concentration for prevention or reversal of bilirubin encephalopathy. Unfortunately, currently available methods are ineffective or impractical on a long-term basis. Plasmapheresis effectively reduces plasma bilirubin concentration by removing albumin-bound bilirubin (181,182). Phototherapy, which is the major treatment for severe neonatal unconjugated hyperbilirubinemia, becomes less effective when children reach the age of 3 to 4 years because of thickening of the skin, pigmentation, and decreased surface area comparative to body mass (181). Chronic phlebotomy in one patient decreased bilirubin production by reducing the average age of the erythrocytes, but the effect was offset by an unexpected reduction in plasma bilirubin clearance (191).

Crigler-Najjar syndrome, type I, is a single enzyme deficiency disease, and UDP-glucuronyltransferase replacement is a possible future treatment. Transplantation of a normal Wistar rat kidney, which con-

TABLE 1. *Principal differential characteristics of chronic unconjugated hyperbilirubinemias*

Characteristic	Crigler-Najjar syndrome		Gilbert syndrome
	Type I	Type II	
Histology of liver	Normal	Normal	Normal
Serum bilirubin concentration	20–50 mg%	<20 mg%	Usually <3 mg%
Routine liver function tests	Normal	Normal	Normal
45-Min plasma BSP retention	Normal	Normal	Usually normal, may be elevated in some patients
Bile	Usually pale; contains trace of unconjugated bilirubin and mono-conjugates	Increased proportion of bilirubin monoglucuronide	Increased proportion of bilirubin monoglucuronide
Hepatic bilirubin UDP-glucuronyl transferase activity	Absent	Reduced	Reduced
Effect of phenobarbital on serum bilirubin concentration	None	Reduction	Reduction
Mode of inheritance	Autosomal recessive	Autosomal recessive?	Autosomal dominant?
Prevalence	Rare	Uncommon	Common (≤5% of the population)
Prognosis	Kernicterus	Usually benign	Benign
Animal model	Homozygous Gunn rat	Heterozygous Gunn rat?	Mutant Southdown sheep?

tains bilirubin UDP-glucuronyltransferase activity, in homozygous Gunn rats results in excretion of bilirubin glucuronides in bile and rapid decrease in serum bilirubin concentration (151). Since enzyme activity is undetectable in human kidney, however, renal transplantation cannot be recommended for the treatment of Crigler-Najjar syndrome, type I. Subcutaneous transplantation of rat hepatoma cells (192) and portal venous infusion of hepatocytes (193) isolated from heterozygous Gunn rats resulted in biliary excretion of bilirubin glucuronides in homozygous Gunn rats and reduction of plasma bilirubin concentration. Transplantation of small pieces of normal rat liver into homozygous Gunn rats was also reported to reduce serum bilirubin concentration (194); attempts at confirmation of these results, however, were unsuccessful (195).

Crigler-Najjar Syndrome, Type II

This syndrome, which was described by Arias in 1962 (196), is characterized by marked unconjugated hyperbilirubinemia (8 to 20 mg/dl plasma) and markedly reduced hepatic UDP-glucuronyltransferase activity (Table 1). In contrast to Crigler-Najjar syndrome, type I, the clinical course is almost always benign (196).

Occasionally, neurologic changes resembling kernicterus and brain histology characteristic of bilirubin encephalopathy may be observed (197). In one case, the serum bilirubin concentration increased from 15 to 40 mg/dl after surgery for acute appendicitis, and diplopia, generalized seizures, confusion, and abnormalities on electroencephalogram developed. The patient was treated for hyperbilirubinemia and, following reduction of serum bilirubin concentration to 15 mg/dl, neurologic abnormalities resolved (198).

As in Crigler-Najjar syndrome, type I, abnormalities in laboratory tests are limited to an increased serum bilirubin concentration, which is usually less than 20 mg/dl but may reach 40 mg/dl during fasting or intercurrent illness (199). Serum bilirubin is unconjugated, and there is no bilirubinuria. Bilirubin production is normal; about 50% of estimated bilirubin production is excreted in bile (183). Although more than 90% of conjugated bilirubin in normal bile is bilirubin diglucuronide, bilirubin monoglucuronide is the major pigment in the bile of patients with the Crigler-Najjar syndrome, type II (198, 200). The reason for this interesting biochemical abnormality is not known. Hepatic bilirubin UDP-glucuronyltransferase activity is virtually undetectable by conventional assays (196).

Crigler-Najjar syndrome, type II is differentiated

TABLE 2. *Principal differential characteristics of chronic conjugated hyperbilirubinemias*

Characteristic	Dubin-Johnson syndrome	Rotor syndrome
Appearance of liver	Grossly black	Normal
Histology of liver	Dark pigment; predominantly in centrilobular areas; otherwise normal	Normal; no increase in pigmentation
Serum bilirubin	Elevated, usually between 2 and 5 mg%, occasionally as high as 20 mg%; predominantly direct-reacting	Elevated, usually between 2 and 5 mg%, occasionally as high as 20 mg%; predominantly direct-reacting
Routine liver function tests	Normal except for bilirubin	Normal except for bilirubin
45-min plasma BSP retention	Normal or elevated; secondary rise at 90 min	Elevated; no secondary rise at 90 min
Oral cholecystogram	Usually does not visualize the gall bladder	Usually visualizes the gall bladder
Urinary coproporphyrin	Normal total >80% as coproporphyrin I	Elevated total; elevated proportion of coproporphyrin I but <80%
Mode of inheritance	Autosomal recessive	Autosomal recessive
Prevalence	Uncommon (1:1,300 in Persian Jews)	Rare
Prognosis	Benign	Benign
Animal model	Mutant Corriedale sheep	None

from the Crigler-Najjar syndrome, type I by reduction of serum bilirubin concentration on treatment with phenobarbital (183,201) or other agents which induce hepatic microsomal enzymes (202). However, an increase in hepatic bilirubin UDP-glucuronyltransferase activity has been only rarely demonstrated by the relatively insensitive conventional assay methods (199,202).

Crigler-Najjar syndrome type II commonly occurs in families (183,196). There is neither sex predilection nor evidence of consanguinity. The mode of inheritance is uncertain; both autosomal dominant with incomplete penetrance (183) and autosomal recessive (202) inheritance have been suggested. There is an increased incidence of mild unconjugated hyperbilirubinemia suggestive of Gilbert's syndrome (see below) in family members. Whether Crigler-Najjar syndrome, type II is the homozygous or a more severe form of Gilbert's syndrome or represents a different disease entity is conjectural.

Gilbert Syndrome (Constitutional Hepatic Dysfunction, Familial Nonhemolytic Jaundice)

Gilbert syndrome, described by Gilbert and Lereboullet in 1901 (203), is characterized by mild (usually less than 3 mg/dl) fluctuating hyperbilirubinemia (Table 2). Serum bilirubin concentrations increase during fasting, stress, intercurrent illness, hyperthyroidism, and menstrual periods (204). The only positive physical finding is jaundice. Occasionally, patients have vague constitutional complaints, which are probably manifestations of anxiety. Aside from hyperbilirubinemia, liver function tests are normal. Liver biopsy is usually not necessary for diagnosis. Liver histology is normal, except for a nonspecific accumulation of lipofuscin pigments (205). Bile collected by duodenal intubation shows an increased proportion (20 to 60%) of bilirubin monoglucuronide (200). Although hemolysis is not part of the syndrome, increased bilirubin production in hemolysis often unmasks Gilbert syndrome.

The incidence of Gilbert syndrome is not known, although it is a common disorder. The higher incidence reported in males probably reflects a higher normal serum bilirubin concentration as compared to that in females. An autosomal dominant inheritance has been suggested. Since the serum bilirubin concentration in the normal population follows a skewed (206) or bimodal (207) distribution rather than a Gaussian distribution, diagnosis is often uncertain, and determination of inheritance may be tenuous. Family studies using an increased proportion of bilirubin monoglucuronide in bile as a marker may provide more conclusive evidence for inheritance of this condition. Whether Gilbert syndrome and Crigler-Najjar syndrome, type II, represent distinct pathophysiologic conditions is not clear.

Two apparently unrelated biochemical defects have been reported in Gilbert syndrome. Hepatic bilirubin UDP-glucuronyltransferase activity has been consistently reduced (208,209). Multicompartmental analysis of plasma bilirubin disappearance after intravenous injection of radiolabeled bilirubin suggests a hepatic uptake defect of bilirubin in addition to reduced hepatic bilirubin-conjugating capacity (210,211). In these studies, initial bilirubin concentration was determined by extrapolating the bilirubin disappearance curve to zero time. Other authors who determined the initial space of distribution of bilirubin from the space of distribution of radiolabeled albumin found no abnormality in the initial hepatic uptake of bilirubin (212). Although hepatic bilirubin-UDP-glucuronyltransferase activity is reduced in Gilbert syndrome, the remaining activity exceeds the estimated enzyme activity required to conjugate normal daily bilirubin production. Therefore, the relationship between hyperbilirubinemia and reduced UDP-glucuronyltransferase activity remains unclear. Enzyme activity, however, which is measured in optimized conditions in vitro, may not reflect the enzyme activity in vivo.

Plasma disappearance of organic anions other than bilirubin usually is normal in Gilbert syndrome. In some cases, BSP and ICG uptake are reduced (213). In other cases, the initial uptake of BSP was normal; compartmental analysis showed an excretion defect at a later stage. Thus Gilbert syndrome may represent a heterogeneous group of disorders.

Prolonged, mild, unconjugated hyperbilirubinemia in the absence of other abnormalities of liver function or hemolysis suggests Gilbert syndrome. A 48-hr fast exaggerates hyperbilirubinemia in Gilbert syndrome (214). The hyperbilirubinemia results from decreased hepatic clearance of bilirubin rather than increased production. Although hepatic UDP-glucuronyltransferase activity in vitro is not altered in rats by fasting, enzyme activity may be reduced in vivo due to reduction in hepatic UDP-glucuronic acid content resulting from reduced UDP-glucose dehydrogenase activity (215). Fasting may cause hyperbilirubinemia by mechanisms other than its effect on hepatic UDP-glucuronyltransferase, since it increases plasma bilirubin concentration in homozygous Gunn rats (216). The serum bilirubin concentration in normal individuals and in patients with other hepatobiliary diseases also increases during fasting. Therefore, the fasting test is of limited use in the differential diagnosis.

Intravenous administration of nicotinic acid provokes hyperbilirubinemia in Gilbert syndrome (217). This effect is probably attributable to increased splenic bilirubin production and is abolished by splenectomy (218). As with fasting, the nicotinic acid test does not clearly differentiate patients with Gilbert syndrome from normal individuals and from patients with other hepatobiliary disorders (219). Liver biopsy usually is not needed for the diagnosis; when it is performed, however, reduced bilirubin UDP-glucuronyltransferase activity is found. An increased proportion of bilirubin monoglucuronide in duodenal bile helps to make the diagnosis even in the presence of hemolysis.

The last two tests distinguish Gilbert syndrome from hemolytic jaundice and other hepatobiliary disorders (219), but some overlap exists between Gilbert syndrome and Crigler-Najjar syndrome, type II. No treatment, other than reassurance, is needed for patients with Gilbert syndrome.

Animal Model

Unconjugated hyperbilirubinemia and photodermatitis due to retention of phylloerythrin, the end product of chlorophyll metabolism, was described in mutant Southdown sheep in 1942 (220) in New Zealand. Similar mutant sheep were later found in California (221). Plasma disappearance rates of BSP, ICG, and rose-bengal (221) and transport maximum and relative storage capacity of BSP are reduced (221). Hepatic influx of intravenously administered ^{14}C-bilirubin is decreased. In contrast to Gilbert syndrome, however, efflux of bilirubin from liver to plasma is increased, and hepatic sequestration of bilirubin and UDP-glucuronyltransferase activity are normal (222). Increased bilirubin production from hepatic heme has been suggested (223). Mutant Southdown sheep demonstrate chronic interstitial nephritis (224); its relationship to hyperbilirubinemia is unknown.

Disorders of Bilirubin Metabolism Characterized by Predominantly Conjugated Hyperbilirubinemia

Dubin-Johnson Syndrome

The Dubin-Johnson syndrome, described in 1954 by Dubin and Johnson (225) and Sprinz and Nelson (226), is characterized by mild, predominantly conjugated hyperbilirubinemia and grossly black liver (Table 2). The syndrome frequently occurs in Persian Jews (1:1,300), in whom it is also associated with coagulation factor VII deficiency (227). It has been reported in both sexes and all races (228). Serum bilirubin concentration is usually between 2 and 5 mg/dl but may be as high as 25 mg/dl. More than 50% of serum bilirubin is direct reacting with sulfanilic acid diazo reagent (229,230). The degree of icterus increases during intercurrent illness, intake of oral contraceptives, and pregnancy. The disorder usually is discovered after puberty and often is unmasked by contraceptives or pregnancy. In contrast to findings in many other hepatobiliary disorders, the major serum conjugated bile pigment in Dubin-Johnson syndrome was reported to be bilirubin diglucuronide (231). As in normal individuals, bilirubin diglucuronide is the predominant pigment in bile (231).

Other liver function tests, such as serum albumin, transaminases, cholesterol, alkaline phosphatase, and prothrombin time, and complete blood count are normal. Oral cholecystography usually does not visualize the gallbladder (232). Liver biopsy usually is not needed for a diagnosis; it reveals a grossly black liver due to accumulation of a melanin-like pigment that appears to be in the lysosomes on electron microscopy (233). Several investigators have suggested that these pigments are poorly defined lipofuscins (234). Chemically and by incorporation of ^{3}H-epinephrine, the pigment resembles melanin (235). Electron spin-resonance (ESR) spectroscopy suggests that the pigments differ from authentic melanin, but these studies are compatible with the pigment being composed of melanin-like polymers (236). The pigment disappears after acute viral hepatitis, only to reappear slowly after recovery (237).

Hepatic transport of conjugated bilirubin, BSP, ICG, metanephrine glucuronide, and cholecystographic contrast medium (iopanoic acid) is decreased (238). The initial plasma disappearance of bilirubin, BSP, ICG, and ^{125}I-rose bengal is normal (239), as is hepatic BSP storage (240). Following intravenous injection of BSP, plasma BSP concentration is normal or slightly increased at 45 min, but there is a secondary rise in plasma BSP from liver into the circulation (239). A similar secondary rise is found with bilirubin but not with organic anions which are not conjugated in the liver (238,239). The biphasic BSP disappearance curve is not diagnostic of Dubin-Johnson syndrome and may occur in other hepatobiliary disorders (241). The T_m of BSP in Dubin-Johnson syndrome is reduced to 10% of normal during constant BSP infusion, but relative hepatic storage capacity is normal (240). No augmentation of biliary BSP excretion was found during dehydrocholate-induced choleresis in a patient with Dubin-Johnson syndrome with biliary fistula (242). The organic anion excretion defect is inherited as an autosomal recessive characteristic; carriers cannot be detected, even by constant BSP infusion studies (229).

Coproporphyrins in body fluids exist as either isomer III or isomer I. Isomer III is the normal precursor of heme; isomer I is a byproduct. Approximately 25% of urinary coproporphyrins and 75% of biliary coproporphyrins normally are isomer I (243). In Dubin-Johnson syndrome, total urinary coproporphyrin excretion is normal, but more than 80% is coproporphyrin I (244). In many hepatobiliary disorders, including cholestasis, total urinary coproporphyrin excretion is increased; coproporphyrin I accounts for less than 65% of total. The combination of normal total urinary coproporphyrin excretion with more than 80% as isomer I is diagnostic of Dubin-Johnson syndrome. In obligate heterozygotes (unaffected parents and children of patients with Dubin-Johnson syndrome), total urinary coproporphyrin excretion is reduced by approximately 40%; the ratio of isomer I to isomer III is intermediate between results in control and Dubin-Johnson

syndrome (243). This aspect of Dubin-Johnson syndrome is inherited as an autosomal recessive characteristic.

The mechanism of abnormal urinary coproporphyrin excretion is not known; a defect in hepatic porphyrin biosynthesis has been postulated (243,244). Coproporphyrin content of bile and urine changed little on intravenous delta-aminolevulinic acid infusion in patients with Dubin-Johnson syndrome (245). Reduced hepatic coproporphyrin III cosynthetase activity could result in decreased synthesis of this isomer and concomitant increase in isomer I in urine. However, this enzyme activity was normal in the liver and blood cells of four patients with Dubin-Johnson syndrome (246).

Mutant Corriedale Sheep

In 1965, Cornelius et al. (247) described a mutant strain of Corriedale sheep with hepatic pigmentation and an organic anion excretion defect similar to that seen in Dubin-Johnson syndrome. Taurocholate excretion is normal, and biliary BSP excretion does not increase during taurocholate-induced choleresis (156). The mutants are photosensitive due to accumulation of phylloerythrin (248), a chlorophyll-derived porphyrin which is normally excreted quantitatively and unchanged in the bile of ruminants. Incorporation of radioactivity in hepatic pigments after intravenous infusion of [^{3}H]-epinephrine suggests that these pigments are related to melanin (249).

Rotor Syndrome

Rotor syndrome, a rare and benign disorder, is characterized by chronic, predominantly conjugated hyperbilirubinemia, normal liver histology, and greatly delayed plasma BSP disappearance; it was described in 1948 by Rotor, Manahan, and Florentin (250) (Table 2). In contrast to Dubin-Johnson syndrome, the liver is not pigmented; there is abnormal BSP retention (25% after 45 min of intravenous injection of 5 mg/kg) and no secondary rise of plasma BSP concentration (251). Studies using constant BSP infusion showed a 75 to 90% reduction in relative hepatic storage capacity and a 50% reduction in the T_m of BSP (251). The T_m and storage capacity of BSP in phenotypically normal obligate heterozygotes of Rotor syndrome were intermediate between normal and Rotor syndrome (251). Rotor syndrome and the hepatic storage disease (252) may represent a single pathophysiologic entity.

Total urinary coproporphyrin excretion is 2.5 to five times greater than in normal controls; the proportion of coproporphyrin I is approximately 65%. The pattern of urinary coproporphyrin excretion in Rotor syndrome is similar to that found in other hepatobiliary disorders and differentiates it from the Dubin-Johnson syndrome (253). Similar to the organic anion excretion defect, abnormal urinary coproporphyrin excretion in Rotor syndrome is inherited as a recessive characteristic (253) and is probably attributable to reduced biliary excretion of coproporphyrins with concomitant increase in renal excretion.

Benign, Recurrent Intrahepatic Cholestasis

Benign recurrent intrahepatic cholestasis is a rare disorder characterized by recurrent attacks of cholestasis (254) associated with enlargement and tenderness of the liver and increased serum levels of bile acids, conjugated bilirubin, and alkaline phosphatase. The attacks occur at intervals of several months to years, last a few weeks to several months, and are preceded by a preicteric phase of 2 to 4 weeks in which patients experience malaise, anorexia, and pruritus (255). During cholestasis, plasma disappearance of unconjugated bilirubin is normal, but serum-conjugated bilirubin concentration increases due to reflux out of the liver (256). During attacks, there may be malabsorption of fat and fat-soluble vitamins and prolongation of prothrombin time (256). Light microscopy of the liver shows cholestasis. Electron microscopy reveals distortion and reduction of microvilli in bile canaliculi and in the number of acid phosphatase-rich lysosomes (257). The abnormalities are not specific and occur in other forms of cholestasis. Between attacks, liver function tests and histology are normal (257). The disorder occurs in families. Its mode of inheritance, pathogenesis, and specific means of treatment or prevention are unknown.

REFERENCES

1. Berk, P. D., Howe, R. B. Bloomer, J. R., and Berlin, N. I. (1969): Studies of bilirubin kinetics in normal adults. *J. Clin. Invest.*, 48:2176.
2. Robinson, S. H. (1977): Origins of the early-labeled peak. In: *The Chemistry and Physiology of Bile Pigments*, edited by P. D. Berk and N. I. Berlin, p. 175. U.S. Government Printing Office, Washington, D.C.
3. Tenhunen, R., Marver, H. S., and Schmid, R. (1970): The enzymatic catabolism of hemoglobin: Stimulation of microsomal heme oxygenase by hemin. *J. Lab. Clin. Med.*, 75:410.
4. Yoshida, T., and Kikichi, G. (1977): Heme oxygenase purified to apparent homogeneity from pig spleen microsomes. *J. Biochem.*, 81:265.
5. Maines, M. D., Ibrahim, N. G., and Kappas, A. (1977): Solubilization and partial purification of heme oxygenase from rat liver. *J. Biol. Chem.*, 252:5900.
6. O'Carra, P., and Colleran, E. (1977): Nonenzymic and quasienzymatic models for catabolic heme cleavage. In: *The Chemistry and Physiology of Bile Pigments*, edited by P. D. Berk and N. I. Berlin, p. 26. U.S. Government Printing Office, Washington, D.C.
7. Colleran, E., and O'Carra, P. (1977): Enzymology and comparative physiology of biliverdin reduction. In: *The Chemistry and Physiology of Bile Pigments*, edited by P. D. Berk and

N. I. Berlin, p. 69. U.S. Government Printing Office, Washington, D.C.
8. Blanckaert, N., Fevery, J., and Compernolle, F. (1976): Synthesis and separation by thin-layer chromatography of bilirubin-IX isomers. Their identification as tetrapyrroles and dipyrrol anthranilate azo derivates. *Biochem. J.*, 155:405.
9. Heirwegh, K. P. M., Blanckaert, N., Compernolle, F., Fevery, J., and Zaman, Z. (1977): Detection and properties of the non-α-isomers of bilirubin-IX. *Biochim. Soc. Trans.*, 5:316.
10. Bonnet, R. J., Davis, E., and Hursthouse, M. B. (1976): Structure of bilirubin. *Nature*, 262:326.
11. Broderson, R. (1980): Binding of bilirubin to albumin. CRC critical reviews in Clinical Laboratory. *Sciences*, p. 305.
12. McDonagh, A. F. (1975): Thermal and photochemical reactions of bilirubin IX. *Ann. N.Y. Acad. Sci.*, 244:553.
13. Lightner, D. A., Wooldrige, T. A., and McDonagh, A. F. (1979): Photobilirubin. An early bilirubin photoproduct detected by absorbance difference spectroscopy. *Proc. Natl. Acad. Sci. USA*, 76:29.
14. McDonagh (1976): Phototherapy of neonatal jaundice. *Soc. Trans.*, 4:219.
15. McDonagh, A. F. (1979): Bilatrienes and 5,15-biladienes. In: *The Porphyrins, Vol. VI. Bile Pigments*, edited by D. Dolphin, p. 293. Academic Press, New York.
15a. Lee, K. S. and Gartner, L. M. (1976): Spectrophotometric characteristics of bilirubin. *Pediatr. Res.* 10:782.
16. Trotman, B. W., Bernstein, S. E., Bove, K. E., and Wirt, G. D. (1980): Studies on the pathogenesis of pigment gallstones in hemolytic anemia: Description and characterization of a mouse model. *J. Clin. Invest.*, 65:1301.
17. Kamisaka, K., Listowsky, I., and Arias, I. M.: (1973): Circular dichroism studies of Y protein (lingandin) a major organic anion binding protein in liver, kidney and small intestine. *Ann. N.Y. Acad. Sci.*, 226:148.
18. Nandi Majumdar, A. P. (1974): Bilirubin encephalopathy. Effect on RNA polymerase activity and chromatin template activity in the brain of the Gunn rat. *Neurobiology*, 4:425.
19. Katoh, R., Kashiwamata, S., and Niwa, F. (1975): Studies on cellular toxicity of bilirubin. Effect on the carbohydrate metabolism in the young rat brain. *Brain Res.*, 83:81.
20. Nandi Majumdar, A. P., and Greenfield, S. (1974): Evidence of defective protein synthesis in liver in rats with congenital hyperbilirubinemia. *Biochim. Biophys. Acta*, 335:260.
21. Mustafa, M. G., Cowger, M. L., and King, T. E. (1969): Effects of bilirubin on mitochondrial reactions. *J. Biol. Chem.*, 244:6403.
22. Strumia, E. (1959): Effect of bilirubin on some hydrolases. *Boll. Soc. Ital. Biol. Sper.*, 35:2160.
23. Flitman, R., and Worth, N. H. (1966): Inhibition of hepatic alcohol dehydrogenase by bilirubin. *J. Biol. Chem.*, 241:669.
24. Noir, B. A., Boveris, A., Garazo, Pereipa, A. M., and Stoppani, A. O. M. (1972): Bilirubin: A multi-site inhibitor of mitochondrial respiration. *FEBS Lett.*, 27:270.
25. Bloomer, J. R., Berk, P. D., Howe, R. B., Waggoner, J. G., and Berlin, N. I. (1970): Comparison of fecal urobilinogen excretion with bilirubin production in normal volunteers and patients with increased bilirubin production. *Clin. Chem. Acta*, 29:463.
26. Engel, R. R. (1977): Alternative sources of carbon monoxide. In: *Chemistry and Physiology of Bile Pigments*, edited by P. D. Berk and N. I. Berlin, p. 148. U.S. Department of Health, Education and Welfare, Bethesda, Maryland.
27. Odell, G. B. (1959): The dissociation of bilirubin from albumin and its clinical implications. *J. Pediatr.*, 55:268.
28. Bowen, W. R., Porter, E., and Waters, W. F. (1959): The protective action of albumin in bilirubin toxicity in newborn puppies. *Am. J. Dis. Child.*, 98:568.
29. Mustafa, M. G., Cowger, M. L., and King, T. E. (1969): Effects of bilirubin on mitochondrial reactions. *J. Biol. Chem.*, 244:6403.
30. Odell, G. B. (1973): Influence of binding on the toxicity of bilirubin. *Ann. N.Y. Acad. Sci.*, 226:225.
31. Odell, G. B., Cohen, S. N., and Gordes, E. H. (1962): Admin-

istration of albumin in the management of hyperbilirubinemia by exchange transfusion. *Pediatrics,* 30:613.

32. Brodersen, R. (1979): Bilirubin solubility and interaction with albumin and phospholipid. *J. Biol. Chem.,* 254:2364.

33. Berde, C. B., Hudson, B. S., Simoni, R. D., and Sklar, L. A. (1979): Human serum albumin: Spectroscopic studies of binding and proximity relationships for fatty acid and bilirubin. *J. Biol. Chem.,* 254:391.

34. Reed, R. G., Feldhoff, R. C., Clute, O. L., and Peters, T. (1975): Fragments of bovine serum albumin produced by limited proteolysis. Conformation and ligand binding. *Biochemistry,* 14:4578.

35. Geisow, M. J., and Beaven, G. H. (1977): Large fragments of human serum albumin. *Biochem. J.,* 161:619.

36. Sjodin, T., Hansson, R., and Sjoholm, I. (1977): Isolation and identification of a trypsin-resistant fragment of human serum albumin with bilirubin- and drug-binding properties. *Biochem. Biophys. Acta,* 494:61.

37. Gitzelmann-Cumarasamy, N., Kuenzle, C. C., and Wilson, K. J. (1976): Mapping of the primary bilirubin binding site of human serum albumin. *Experientia,* 32:768.

38. Jacobsen, C. (1978): Lysine residue 240 of human serum albumin is involved in high-affinity binding of bilirubin. *Biochem. J.,* 171:453.

39. Brodersen, R. (1978): Binding of bilirubin and other ligands to human serum albumin. In: *Albumin, Structure, Biosynthesis, Function,* edited by T. Peters, and I. Sjoholm, p. 61. Pergamon, Oxford.

40. Brodersen, R. (1978): Free bilirubin in blood plasma of the newborn. Effects of albumin, fatty acids, pH, displacing drugs and phototherapy. Appendix: A provisional survey of the bilirubin-displacing effect of 150 drugs. In: *Intensive Care in the Newborn, Vol. 2,* edited by L. Stern, p. 331. Masson, New York.

41. Brodersen, R., Sjodin, T., and Sjoholm, I. (1977): Independent binding of benzodiazepines and bilirubin to human serum albumin. *J. Biol. Chem.,* 252:5067.

42. Rudman, D., Bixler, T. J., and Del Rio, A. E. (1971): Effect of free fatty acid on binding of drugs by bovine serum albumin, by human serum albumin and by rabbit serum. *J. Pharmacol. Exp. Ther.,* 176:261.

43. Kapitulnik, J., Valaes, T., Kaufmann, N. A., and Blondheim, S. H. (1974): Clinical evaluation of Sephadex gel filtration in estimation of bilirubin binding in serum in neonatal jaundice. *Arch. Dis. Child.,* 49:886.

44. Brodersen, R., Cashore, W., Wennberg, R. P., Ahlfors, C. E., Rasmussen, L. F., and Shusterman, D. (1979): Kinetics of bilirubin oxidation with peroxidase, as applied to studies of bilirubin-albumin binding. *Scand. J. Clin. Lab. Invest.,* 39:143.

45. Athanassiadis, S., Chopra, D. R., Fisher, M., and McKenna, J. (1974): An electrophoretic method for detection of unbound bilirubin and reserve bilirubin binding capacity in serum of newborns. *J. Lab. Clin. Med.,* 83:968.

46. Lamolla, A. A., Eisinger, J., Blumberg, W. E., Palet, S. C., and Flores, J. (1979): Fluorometric study of the partition of bilirubin among blood components: Basis for rapid microassays of bilirubin and bilirubin binding capacity in whole blood. *Anal. Biochem.,* 15:25.

47. Bratlid, D. (1973): Reserve albumin binding capacity, salicylate saturation index, and red cell binding of bilirubin in neonatal jaundice. *Arch. Dis. Child.,* 48:393.

48. Brodersen, R. (1978): Determination of the vacant amount of high affinity bilirubin binding site on serum albumin. *Acta Pharmacol. Toxicol.,* 42:153.

49. Hsia, J. C., Kwan, N. H., Er, S. S., Wood, D. J., and Chance, G. W. (1978): Development of a spin assay for reserve bilirubin loading capacity of human serum. *Proc. Natl. Acad. Sci. USA,* 75:1542.

50. Porter, E. G., and Waters, W. J. (1966): A rapid micromethod for measuring the reserve albumin binding capacity in serum for newborn infants with hyperbilirubinemia. *J. Lab Clin. Med.,* 67:660.

51. Scharschmidt, B. F., Waggoner, J. G., and Berk, P. D. (1975):

52. Goresky, C. A. (1975): The hepatic uptake process: its implications for bilirubin transport. In: *Jaundice,* edited by C. A. Goresky and M. M. Fisher, p. 159. Plenum, New York.

53. Paumgartner, G., and Reichenn, J. (1976): Kinetics of hepatic uptake of unconjugated bilirubin. *Clin. Sci. Mol. Med.,* 51:169.

54. Shupeck, M., Wolkoff, A. W., Scharschmidt, B. F., Waggoner, J. G., and Berk, P. D. (1978): Studies of the kinetics of purified conjugated bilirubin-^{3}H in the rat. *Am. J. Gastroenterol.,* 70:259.

55. Brown, W. R., Grodsky, G. M., and Carbone, J. V. (1964): Intracellular distribution of tritiated bilirubin during hepatic uptake and excretion. *Am. J. Physiol.,* 207:1237.

56. Wolkoff, A. W., Goresky, C. A., Sellin, J., Gatmaitan, Z., and Arias, I. M. (1979): Role of ligandin in transfer of bilirubin from plasma into liver. *Am. J. Physiol.,* 236:E638.

57. Bloomer, J. R., Berk, P. D., Vergalla, J., and Berlin, N. I. (1973): Influence of albumin on the extravascular distribution of unconjugated bilirubin. *Clin. Sci. Mol. Med.,* 45:517.

58. Weisiger, R., Gollan, J., and Ockner, R. (1981): Receptor for albumin on the liver cell surface may mediate uptake of fatty acids and other albumin-bound substances. *Science,* 211:1048.

59. Weisiger, R., Gollan, J., and Ockner, R. (1980): An albumin receptor on the liver cell may mediate hepatic uptake of sulfobromophthalein and bilirubin: Bound ligand, not free, is the major uptake determinant. *Gastroenterology,* 79:1065 (Abstr.).

60. Wolkoff, A. W., Ohmi, N., and Gartner, U. (1980): Uptake of bilirubin by the liver does not require an albumin receptor. *Gastroenterology,* 79:1068 (Abstr.).

61. Barnhart, J. L., and Clarenburg, R. (1973): Factors determining clearance of bilirubin in perfused rat liver. *Am. J. Physiol.,* 225:497.

62. Grausz, H., and Schmid, R. (1971): Reciprocal relation between plasma albumin level and hepatic sulfobromophthalein removal. *N. Engl. J. Med.,* 284:1403.

63. Vogin, E. E., Scott, W., Boyd, J., Bear, W. T., and Mattis, P. A. (1966): Effect of probenecid on indocyanine green clearance. *J. Pharmacol. Exp. Ther.,* 152:509.

64. Acocella, G., Nicolis, F. B., and Tenconi, L. T. (1965): The effect of an intravenous infusion of rifamycin SV on the excretion of bilirubin, bromsulphalein, and indocyanine green in man. *Gastroenterology,* 49:521.

65. Nosslin, B., and Morgan, E. H. (1965): The effect of phloroglucinol derivatives from male fern on dye excretion by the liver in the rabbit and rat. *J. Lab. Clin. Med.,* 65:891.

66. Bolt, R. J., Dillon, R. S., and Pollard, H. M. (1961): Interference with bilirubin excretion by a gall bladder dye (bunamiodyl). *N. Engl. J. Med.,* 265:1043.

67. Clarenburg, R., and Kao, C. C. (1973): Shared and separate pathways for biliary excretion of bilirubin and BSP in rats. *Am. J. Physiol.,* 225:192.

68. Reyes, H., Levi, A. J., Gatmaitan, Z., and Arias, I. M. (1971): Studies of Y and Z, two hepatic cytoplasmic anion-binding proteins: effect of drugs, chemicals, hormones and cholestasis. *J. Clin. Invest.,* 50:2242.

69. Wolkoff, A. W. (1980): The glutathione S-transferases: their role in the transport of organic anions from blood to bile. In: *Liver and Biliary Tract Physiology I,* edited by N. B. Javitt, p. 151. University Park Press, Baltimore.

70. Cornelius, C. E., Ben-Ezzer, J., and Arias, I. M. (1967): Binding of sulfobromophthalein sodium (BSP) and other organic anions by isolated hepatic cell plasma membranes *in vitro. Proc. Soc. Exp. Biol. Med.,* 124:665.

71. Reichen, J., Blitzer, B. L., and Berk, P. D. (1981): Binding of unconjugated and conjugated sulfobromophthalein to rat liver plasma membrane fractions *in vitro. Biochim. Biophys. Acta,* 640:298.

72. Tiribelli, C., Panfili, E., Sandri, G., Frezza, M., and Sottocasa, G. L. (1976): Liver bromsulphophthalein transport as a carrier mediated process. In: *Diseases of the Liver and Biliary Tract,* edited by C. M. Leevy, p. 55 Karger, Basel.

Hepatic organic anion uptake in the rat. *J. Clin. Invest.,* 56:1280.

73. Tiribelli, C., Lunazzi, G., Luciani, G. L., Panfili, E., Gassin, B., Liut, G., Sandri, G., and Sottocasa, G. (1978): Isolation of a sulfobromophthalein-binding protein from hepatocyte plasma membrane. *Biochim. Biophys. Acta,* 532:105.

74. Wolkoff, A. W., and Chung, C. T. (1980): Identification, purification, and partial characterization of an organic anion binding protein from rat liver cell plasma membrane. *J. Clin. Invest.,* 65:1152.

75. Reichen, J., and Berk, P. D. (1979): Isolation of an organic anion binding protein from rat liver plasma membrane fractions by affinity chromatography. *Biochem. Biophys. Res. Commun.,* 91:484.

76. Steiner, J. W., Perz, Z. M., and Taichman, L. B. (1966): Cell population dynamics in the liver. A review of quantitative morphological techniques applied to the study of physiological growth. *Exp. Mol. Pathol.,* 5:146.

77. Bucher, N. L., and Malt, R. A. (1971): *Regeneration of Liver and Kidney,* Little, Brown, Boston.

78. Wolkoff, A. W., Ketley, J. N., Waggoner, J. G., Berk, P. D., and Jakoby, W. B. (1978): Hepatic accumulation and intracellular binding of conjugated bilirubin. *J. Clin. Invest.,* 61:142.

79. Levi, A. J., Gatmaitan, Z., and Arias, I. M. (1969): Two hepatic cytoplasmic protein fractions, Y and Z, and their possible role in the hepatic uptake of bilirubin, sulfobromophthalein, and other anions. *J. Clin. Invest.,* 48:2156.

80. Fleischner, G., Robbins, J., and Arias, I. M. (1972): Immunological studies of Y protein: a major cytoplasmic organic anion binding protein in rat liver. *J. Clin. Invest.,* 51:677.

81. Lichter, M., Fleischner, G., Kirsch, R., Levi, A. J., Kamisaka, K., and Arias, I. M. (1976): Ligandin and Z protein in binding of thyroid hormones by the liver. *Am. J. Physiol.,* 230:1113.

82. Kamisaka, K., Listowsky, I., Gatmaitan, Z., and Arias, I. M. (1975): Interactions of bilirubin and other ligands with ligandin. *Biochemistry,* 14:2175.

83. Kirsch, R., Kamisaka, K., Fleischner, G., and Arias, I. M. (1975): Structural and functional studies of ligandin, a major renal organic anion binding protein. *J. Clin. Invest.,* 55:1009.

84. Goldstein, E. J., and Arias, I. M. (1976): Interaction of ligandin with radiographic contrast media. *Invest. Radiol.,* 11:594.

85. Morey, K. S., and Litwack, G. (1969): Isolation and properties of cortisol metabolite binding proteins of rat liver cytosol. *Biochemistry,* 8:4813.

86. Ketterer, B., Ross-Mansell, P., and Whitehead, J. K. (1967): The isolation of carcinogen-binding protein from livers of rats given 4-dimethylaminoazobenzene. *Biochem. J.,* 103:316.

87. Litwack, G., Ketterer, B., and Arias, I. M. (1971): An abundant liver protein which binds steroids, bilirubin, carcinogens and a number of exogenous anions. *Nature,* 234:466.

88. Fleischner, G. M., Robbins, J. B., and Arias, I. M. (1977): Cellular localization of ligandin in rat, hamster, and man. *Biochem. Biophys. Res. Commun.,* 74:992.

89. Habig, W. H., Pabst, M. J., Fleischner, G., Gatmaitan, Z., Arias, I. M., and Jakoby, W. B. (1974): The identity of glutathione S-transferase B with ligandin, a major binding protein of liver. *Proc. Natl. Acad. Sci. USA,* 10:3879.

90. Benson, A. M., Talalay, P., and Jakoby, W. B. (1977): Relationship between the soluble glutathione-dependent ^{5}-3-ketosteroid isomerase and the glutathione S-transferases of the liver. *Proc. Natl. Acad. Sci. USA,* 74:158.

91. Prohaska, J. R., and Ganther, H. E. (1977): Glutathione peroxidase activity of glutathione S-transferase purified from rat liver. *Biochem. Biophys. Res. Commun.,* 76:437.

92. Kamisaka, K., Habig, W. H., Ketley, J. N., Arias, M., and Jakoby, W. B. (1975): Multiple forms of human glutathione S-transferase and their affinity for bilirubin. *Eur. J. Biochem.,* 60:153.

93. Bhargava, M. M., Ohmi, N., Listowsky, I., and Arias, I. M. (1980): Structural catalytic, binding, and immunological properties associated with each of the two subunits of rat liver ligandin. *J. Biol. Chem.,* 255:718.

94. Arias, I. M. (1979): Ligandin: a review and update of a multifunctional protein. *Med. Biol.,* 57:328.

95. Levine, R. I., Reyes, H., Levi, A. J., Gatmaitan, Z., and Arias, I. M. (1971): Phylogenetic study of organic anion transfer from plasma into the liver. *Nature [New Biol.],* 231:277.

96. Levi, A. J., Gatmaitan, Z., and Arias, I. M. (1969): Deficiency of hepatic organic anion-binding protein as a possible cause of nonhaemolytic unconjugated hyperbilirubinemia in the newborn. *Lancet,* 2:139.

97. Levi, A. J., Gatmaitan, Z., and Arias, I. M. (1970): Deficiency of hepatic organic anion-binding protein, impaired organic anion uptake by liver and "physiologic" jaundice in newborn monkeys. *N. Engl. J. Med.,* 283:1136.

98. Boyer, J. L., Schwarz, J., and Smith, N. (1976): Biliary secretion in elasmobranchs. II. Hepatic uptake and biliary excretion of organic anions. *Am. J. Physiol.,* 230:974.

99. Bend, J. R., and Fouts, J. R. (1973): Glutathione S-transferase: Distribution in several marine species and partial characterization in hepatic soluble fractions from little skate, *Raja erinaces,* liver. *Bull. Mt. Desert Island Biol. Lab.,* 13:4.

100. Kamisaka, K., Listowsky, I., Fleischner, G., Gatmaitan, Z., and Arias, I. M. (1976): The binding of bilirubin and other organic anions to serum albumin and ligandin (Y protein). In: *Bilirubin Metabolism in the Newborn (II),* p. 156. Excerpta Medica, Amsterdam.

101. Ketterer, B., Tipping, E., Beale, D., and Meuwissen, J. A. T. P. (1976): Ligandin, glutathione transferase, and carcinogen binding. In: *Glutathione: Metabolism and Function,* edited by I. M. Arias and W. B. Jakoby, p. 243. Raven Press, New York.

102. Listowsky, I., Gatmaitan, Z., and Arias, I. M. (1978): Ligandin retains and albumin loses bilirubin binding capacity in liver cytosol. *Proc. Natl. Acad. Sci. USA,* 75:1213.

103. Kamisaka, K., Gatmaitan, Z., Moore, C. L., and Arias, I. M. (1975): Ligandin reverses bilirubin inhibition of liver mitochondrial respiration *in vitro. Pediatr. Res.,* 9:903.

104. Fevery, J., Van Damme, B., Michiels, R., De Groote, J., and Heirwegh, K. P. M. (1972): Bilirubin conjugates in bile of man and rat in the normal state and in liver disease. *J. Clin. Invest.,* 51:2482.

105. Fevery, J., Van Hees, G. P., Leroy, P., Compernolle, F., and Heirwegh, K. P. M. (1971): Excretion in dog bile of glucose and xylose conjugates of bilirubin. *Biochem. J.,* 125:803.

106. Cornelius, C. E., Kelly, K. C., and Himes, J. A. (1975): Heterogeneity of bilirubin conjugates in several animal species. *Cornell Vet.,* 65(1):90.

107. Kuenzle, C. C. (1970). Bilirubin conjugates of human bile. *Biochem. J.,* 119:411.

108. Weber, A., Schalm, L., and Witmans, J. (1963): Bilirubin monoglucuronide (pigment I): A complex. *Acta Med. Scand.,* 173:19.

109. Jansen, F. H., and Billing, B. H. (1971): The identification of monoconjugates of bilirubin in bile as amide derivatives. *Biochem. J.,* 125:917.

110. Blanckaert, N. (1980): Analysis of bilirubin and bilirubin mono and diconjugates. Determination of their relative amounts in biological fluids. *Biochem. J.,* 185:115.

111. Hutchinson, D. W., Johnson, B., and Knell, A. J. (1972): The reaction between bilirubin and aromatic diazo compounds. *Biochem. J.,* 127:907.

112. Van den Bergh, A. A. H., and Muller, P. (1916): Ueber eine direkte und eine indirekte Diazoreaktion auf Bilirubin. *Biochem. Z.,* 77:90.

113. Talafant, E. (1956): Properties and composition of bile pigment giving direct diazo reaction. *Nature [Lond.],* 178:312.

114. Compernolle, F., Van Hees, G. P., Blanckaert, N., and Heirwegh, K. P. M. (1978): Glucuronic acid conjugates of bilirubin IX$_\alpha$ in normal bile compared with post-obstructive bile. *Biochem. J.,* 171:185.

115. Blanckaert, N., Campernolle, F., Leroy, P., Van Hourtte, R., Fevery, J., and Heirwegh, K. P. M. (1978): The fate of bilirubin IX$_\alpha$ glucuronide in cholestasis and during storage *in vitro. Biochem. J.,* 171:203.

116. Cole, P. G., Lathe, G. H., and Billing, B. H. (1954): Separation of the bile pigments of serum, bile and urine. *Biochem. J.,* 57:514.

117. Blanckaert, N., Kabra, P. M., Farina, F. A., Stafford, B. E., Marton, L. M., and Schmidt, R. (1980): Measurement of bilirubin and its mono- and diconjugates in human serum by alkaline methanolysis and high performance liquid chromatography. *J. Lab. Clin. Med.*, 96:198.

118. Onishi, S., Itoh, S., Kawade, N., Isobe, K., and Sugiyama, S. (1980): An accurate and sensitive analysis by high pressure liquid chromatography of conjugated and unconjugated bilirubin IX$_\alpha$ and in various biological fluids. *Biochem. J.*, 185:281.

119. Jansen, P. L. M. (1981): β-Glucuronidase resistant bilirubin glucuronide isomers in cholestatic liver disease—determination of bilirubin metabolites in serum by means of high-pressure liquid chromotography. *Clin. Chim. Acta*, 110:309.

120. Jansen, P. L. M., and Tangerman, A. (1980): Separation and characterization of bilirubin conjugates by high performance liquid chromatography. *J. Chromatogr.*, 182:100.

121. Roy Chowdhury, J., Roy Chowdhury, N., Wu, G., Shouval, R., and Arias, I. M. (1981): Bilirubin mono- and diglucuronide formation by human liver *in vitro*: Assay by high pressure liquid chromatography. *Hepatology*, 1:622.

122. Fevery, J. B., Van Damme, R., Michiels, R., De Groote, J., and Heirwegh, K. P. M. (1972): Bilirubin conjugates in bile of man and rat in the normal state and in liver disease. *J. Clin. Invest.*, 51:2482.

123. Dutton, G. J., and Burchell, B. (1977): New aspects of glucuronidation. *Prog. Drug Metab.*, 2:1.

124. Dutton, G. J. (1966): The biosynthesis of glucuronides. In: *Glucuronic Acid Free and Combined*, edited by G. J. Dutton, p. 185. Academic Press, New York.

125. Roy Chowdhury, J., Roy Chowdhury, N., and Arias, I. M. (1979): Bilirubin conjugation in the spiny dog fish, squalus acanthias, the small skate, *Raja erinaeca*, and the winter flounder, *Pseudopleuronectes americanas*. *Comp. Biochem. Physiol.*, 66B:523.

126. Graham, A. B., Pechey, D. T., Toogood, K. C., Thomas, S. B., and Wood, G. C. (1977): The phospholipid dependence of uridine diphosphate glucuronyl transferase. *Biochem. J.*, 163:117.

127. Jansen, P. L. M., and Arias, I. M. (1975): Delipidation and reactivation of UDP glucuronosyl transferase from rat liver. *Biochim. Biophys. Acta*, 391:28.

128. Jansen, P. L. M. (1972): Studies on UDP glucuronyl transferase. Doctoral dissertation, University of Nijmegen, The Netherlands.

129. Henderson, P. (1970): Activation *in vitro* of rat hepatic UDP glucuronyl transferase by ultra sound. *Life Sci.* 9(II):511.

130. Graham, A. B., and Wood, G. C. (1973): Factors affecting the response of microsomal UDP-glucuronyltransferase to membrane perturbants. *Biochem. Biophys. Acta*, 311:45.

131. Vassey, D. A., and Zakim, D. (1971): Regulations of microsomal enzymes by phospholipids. *J. Biol. Chem.*, 246:4649.

132. Heirwegh, K. P. M., Campbell, M., and Meuwissen, J. A. T. P. (1978): Compartmentation of membrane bound enzymes. Some basic concepts and consequences for kinetic studies. In: *Conjugation Reactions in Drug Biotransformation*, edited by A. Aitio, p. 191. Elsevier, Amsterdam.

133. Hallinan, T. (1978): Comparison of compartmented and of conformational phospholipid-constraint models for the intramembranous arrangement of UDP-glucuronyl transferase. In: *Conjugation Reactions in Drug Biotransformation*, edited by A. Aitio, p. 257. Elsevier, Amsterdam.

134. Bock, K. W., Frohling, W., Remmer, H., and Rexer, B. (1973): Effects of phenobarbital and 3 methyl cholanthrene on substrate specificity of rat liver microsomal UDP glucuronyl transferase. *Biochim. Biophys. Acta*, 327:46.

135. Halac, E., and Reff, A. (1967): Studies on bilirubin UDP glucuronyl transferase. *Biochem. Biophys. Acta*, 139:328.

136. Wishart, G. J. (1978): Functional heterogeneity of UDP glucuronosyl transferase as indicated by its differential development and inducibility by glucocorticoids. *Biochem. J.*, 174:485.

137. Drucker, W. D. (1968): Glucuronic acid conjugation of tetrahydrocortisone p-nitrophenol in the homozygous Gunn rats. *Proc. Soc. Exp. Biol. Med.*, 129:308.

138. Mowat, A. P., and Arias, I. M. (1970): Observations of the effect of diethyl nitrosamine on glucuronide formation. *Biochem. Biophys. Acta*, 212:175.

139. Gorski, J. P., and Kasper, C. B. (1977): Purification and properties of microsomal UDP glucuronyl transferase from rat liver. *J. Biol. Chem.*, 252:1336.

140. Burchell, B. (1977): Purification of UDP glucuronyl transferase from untreated rat liver. *FEBS Lett.*, 78:101.

141. Bock, K. W., Josling, D., Lilenblum, W. M., and Pfeil, H. (1979): Purification of rat liver glucuronyl transferase—separation of two enzyme forms inducible by 3-methylcholanthrene or phenobarbital. *Eur. J. Biochem.*, 98:19.

142. Bock, K. W., Kittel, J., and Josting, D. (1978): Purification of rat liver UDP glucuronyl transferase: Separation of two enzyme forms with different substrate specificity and differential inducibility. In: *Conjugation Reactions in Drug Biotransformation*, edited by A. Aitio, p. 357. Elsevier, Amsterdam.

143. Malik, N., and Owens, I. S. (1978): Induction of bilirubin UDP glucuronosyl transferase (T'ase) activity in mice by 3-methylcholanthrene (MC) and 2,3,7,8-tetrachlorodibenzo-p-dioxin (TCDD). *Pharmacologist*, 20:200 (Abstr.).

144. Nakata, D., Zakim, D., and Vassey, D. A. (1976): Defective function of a microsomal UDP glucuronyl transferase in Gunn rats. *Proc. Natl. Acad. Sci. USA*, 73:289.

145. Odell, G. B., Cukier, J. O., and Gourley, G. R. (1981): The presence of a microsomal UDP-glucuronyl transferase for bilirubin in homozygous jaundiced Gunn rats and in the Crigler-Najjar syndrome. *Hepatology*, 1:307–315.

146. Heirwegh, K. P. M., Van De Vijver, M., and Fevery, J. (1972): Assay and properties of digitonin-activated bilirubin uridine diphosphate glucuronyl transferase from rat liver. *Biochem. J.*, 129:605.

147. Jansen, P. L. M. (1972): Mono and diglucuronidation of bilirubin. *Folia Med. Neurol.*, 15:205.

148. Blanckaert, N., Gollan, J., and Schmid, R. (1979): Bilirubin diglucuronide synthesis by a UDP glucuronide acid dependent enzyme system in rat liver microsomes. *Proc. Natl. Acad. Sci. USA*, 76:2037.

149. Roy Chowdhury, J., Roy Chowdhury, N., Bhargava, M., and Arias, I. M. (1979): Purification and partial characterization of rat liver bilirubin glucuronoside glucuronosyl transferase. *J. Biol. Chem.*, 254:8336.

150. Jansen, P. L. M., Roy Chowdhury, J., Fischberg, E. B., and Arias, I. M. (1977): Enzymatic conversion of bilirubin monoglucuronide to diglucuronide by rat liver plasma membranes. *J. Biol. Chem.*, 252:2710.

151. Roy Chowdhury, J., Fischberg, E. B., Daniller, A., Jansen, P. L. M., and Arias, I. M. (1978): Hepatic conversion of bilirubin monoglucuronide to bilirubin diglucuronide in uridine diphosphate glucuronyl transferase deficient man and rat by bilirubin glucuronoside glucuronosyl transferase. *J. Clin. Invest.*, 21:191.

152. Roy Chowdhury, J., Roy Chowdhury, N., Gartner, U., Wolkoff, A. W., and Arias, I. M. (1980): How is bilirubin diglucuronide formed from bilirubin monoglucuronide? Resolution of a controversy. *Gastroenterology*, 79:1050.

153. Sieg, A., and Heirwegh, K. P. M. (1981): Evidence against enzymatic conversion *in vitro* of bilirubin mono- to bilirubin diglucuronide in preparations from Gunn rat liver. *Gastroenterology*, 80:1349 (Abstr.).

154. Arias, I. M., Johnson, L., and Wolfson, S. (1961): Biliary excretion of injected conjugated and unconjugated bilirubin by normal and Gunn rats. *Am. J. Physiol.*, 200:1091.

155. Robinson, S. H., Yannoni, C., and Nagasawa, S. (1971): Bilirubin excretion in rats with normal and impaired bilirubin conjugation. Effect of phenobarbital. *J. Clin. Invest.*, 50:2606.

156. Alpert, S., Mosher, M., Shanske, A., and Arias, I. M. (1969): Multiplicity of hepatic excretory mechanism for organic anions. *J. Gen. Physiol.*, 53:238.

157. Bernstein, R. B., Novy, M. J., Piasecki, G. J., Lester, R., and Jackson, B. T. (1969): Bilirubin metabolism in the fetus. *J. Clin. Invest.*, 48:1678.

158. Upson, D. W., Gronwall, R. R., and Cornelius, C. E. (1970):

Maximal hepatic excretion of bilirubin in sheep. *Proc. Soc. Exp. Biol. Med.*, 134:9.

159. Barnhart, J., Ritt, S., Ware, A., and Coombes, B. (1973): A comparison of the effects of taurocholate and theophylline on BSP excretion in dogs. In: *The Liver: Quantitative Aspects of Structure and Function*, edited by G. Paumgartner and R. Preisig, p. 315. Karger, Basel.

160. Scharschmidt, B. F., and Schmid, R. (1977): The ''micellar sink.'' *Gastroenterology*, 72:1182 (Abstr.).

161. Binet, S., Delage, Y., and Erlinger, S. (1979): Influence of taurocholate, taurochenodeoxycholate and taurodehydrocholate on sulfobromophthalein transport into bile. *Am. J. Physiol.*, 236:E10.

162. Shull, S. D., Wagner, C. I., Trotman, B. W., and Soloway, R. D. (1977): Factors affecting bilirubin excretion in patients with cholesterol or pigment gallstones. *Gastroenterology*, 72:625.

163. Forker, E. L. (1977): Canalicular anion transport. Effect of bile acid-independent choleretics. In: *Bile Pigments, Chemistry and Physiology*, edited by P. D. Berk and N. I. Berlin, p. 383. U.S. Department of Health, Education and Welfare, Bethesda, Maryland.

164. Clarenburg, R., and Kao, C. C. (1973): Shared and separate pathways for biliary excretion of bilirubin and BSP in rats. *Am. J. Physiol.*, 225:192.

165. Berk, P. D., Jones, E. A., Howe, R. B., and Berlin, N. I. (1980): Disorders of bilirubin metabolism. In: *Metabolic Control and Disease*, 8th edition, edited by P. K. Bondy and L. E. Rosenberg, p. 1009. Saunders, Philadelphia.

166. Lester, R., and Schmid, R. (1963): Intestinal absorption of bile pigments. II. Bilirubin absorption in man. *N. Engl. J. Med.*, 269:178.

167. Brodersen, R., and Herman, L. S. (1963): Intestinal reabsorption of unconjugated bilirubin: a possible contributing factor in neonatal jaundice. *Lancet*, 1:1242.

168. Ostrow, J. D. (1967): Absorption of bile pigments by the gall bladder. *J. Clin. Invest.*, 46:2035.

169. Stoll, M. S., Lim, C. K., and Gray, C. H. (1977): Chemical variants of the uroblins. In: *Chemistry and Physiology, Bile Pigments* edited by P. D. Berk and N. I. Berlin, p. 483. U.S. Government Printing Office, Washington, D.C.

170. Schmid, R., and Hammaker, L. (1963): Metabolism and disposition of C^{14}-bilirubin in congenital nonhemolytic jaundice. *J. Clin. Invest.*, 42:1720.

171. Berry, C. S., Zarembo, J. E., and Ostrow, J. D. (1972): Evidence for conversion of bilirubin to dihydroxyl derivatives in the Gunn rat. *Biochem. Biophys. Res. Commun.*, 49:1366.

172. Kapitulnik, J., and Ostrow, J. D. (1978): Stimulation of bilirubin catabolism in jaundiced Gunn rats by an inducer of microsomal mixed function mono-oxygenases. *Proc. Natl. Acad. Sci. USA*, 75:682.

173. Cameron, J. L., Pulaski, E. J., Abel, T., and Iber, F. L. (1966): Metabolism and excretion of bilirubin C^{14} in experimental obstructive jaundice. *Ann. Surg.*, 163:330.

174. Cameron, J. L., Filler, R. M., Iber, E. L., Abel, T., and Randolph, J. G. (1966): Metabolism and excretion of C^{14} labeled bilirubin in children with biliary atresia. *N. Engl. J. Med.*, 274:231.

175. Fulop, M., Sanson, J., and Brazeau, P. (1965): Dialyzability, protein binding, and renal excretion of plasma conjugated bilirubin. *J. Clin. Invest.*, 44:666.

176. Gollan, J. L., Dallinger, K. J. C., and Billing, B. H. (1978): Excretion of conjugated bilirubin in the isolated perfused rat kidney. *Clin. Sci. Mol. Med.*, 54:381.

177. Hardy, J. B., and Peeples, M. O. (1971): Serum bilirubin levels in newborn infants. Distributions and associations with neurological abnormalities during the first year of life. *Johns Hopkins Med. J.*, 128:265.

178. Gartner, L. M., Lee, K., Vaisman, S., Lane, D., and Zarafu, I. (1977): Development of bilirubin transport and metabolism in the newborn Rhesus monkey. *J. Pediatr.*, 90:513.

179. Snyder, A. L., Satterlee, W., Robinson, S. H., and Schmid, R. (1967): Conjugated plasma bilirubin in jaundice caused by pigment overload. *Nature [Lond.]*, 213:93.

180. Crigler, J. F., and Najjar, V. A. (1952): Congenital familial nonhemolytic jaundice with kernicterus. *Pediatrics*, 10:169.

181. Wolkoff, A. W., Roy Chowdhury, J., Gartner, L. A., Rose, A. L., Biempica, L., Giblin, D. R., Fink, D., and Arias, I. M. (1979): Crigler-Najjar syndrome (type I) in an adult male. *Gastroenterology*, 76:3380.

182. Blaschke, T. F., Berk, P. D., Scharschmidt, B. F., Guyther, J. R., Vergalla, J., and Waggoner, J. G. (1974): Crigler-Najjar syndrome: an unusual course with development of neurologic damage at age eighteen. *Pediatr. Res.*, 8:573.

183. Arias, I. M., Gartner, L. M., Cohen, M., Ben-Ezzer, J., and Levi, A. J. (1969): Chronic nonhemolytic unconjugated hyperbilirubinemia with glucuronyl transferase deficiency: clinical, biochemical, pharmacologic, and genetic evidence foe heterogeneity. *Am. J. Med.*, 47:395.

184. Bloomer, J. R., Berk, P. D., Howe, R. B., and Berlin, N. I. (1971): Bilirubin metabolism in congenital nonhemolytic jaundice. *Pediatr. Res.*, 5:256.

185. Kapitulnik, J., Kaufmann, N. A., Goitein, K., Cividalli, G., and Blondheim, S. H. (1974): A pigment found in the Crigler-Najjar syndrome and its similarity to an ultrafilterable photoderivative of bilirubin. *Clin. Chim. Acta*, 57:231.

186. Gunn, C. H. (1938): Hereditary acholuric jaundice in a new mutant strain of rats. *J. Hered.*, 29:137.

187. Blankaert, N., Fevery, J., Heirwegh, K. P. M., and Compernolle, F. (1977): Characterization of the major diazopositive pigments in bile of homozygous Gunn rats. *Biochem. J.*, 164:237.

188. Call, N. B., and Tisher, C. C. (1975): The urinary concentrating defect in the Gunn strain of rat. Role of bilirubin. *J. Clin. Invest.*, 55:319.

189. Gardner, W. A., and Konigsmark, B. (1969): Familial nonhemolytic jaundice: Bilirubinosis and encephalopathy. *Pediatrics*, 43:365.

190. Schutta, H. S., and Johnson, L. (1969): Clinical signs and morphologic abnormalities in Gunn rats treated with sulfadiethoxine. *J. Pediatr.*, 75:1070.

191. Berk, P. D., Scharschmidt, B. F., Waggoner, J. G., and White, S. C. (1976): The effect of repeated phlebotomy on bilirubin turnover, bilirubin clearance and unconjugated hyperbilirubinaemia in the Crigler-Najjar syndrome and the jaundiced Gunn rat: Application of computers to experimental design. *Clin. Sci. Mol. Med.*, 50:333.

192. Rugstad, H. E., Robinson, S. M., Yannoni, C., and Tasjia, A. H. (1970): Transfer of bilirubin uridine diphosphate glucuronyl transferase to enzyme deficient rats. *Science*, 170:553.

193. Sebrow, O., Gatmaitan, Z., Orlandi, F., Chowdhury, J. R., and Arias, I. M. (1980): Replacement of hepatic UDP glucuronyl transferase activity in homozygous Gunn rats. *Gastroenterology*, 78:1332 (Abstr.).

194. Mukherjee, A. B., and Krasner, J. (1973): Induction of an enzyme in genetically deficient rats after grafting of normal liver. *Science*, 183:68.

195. Van Houwelingen, C. A. J., and Arias, I. M. (1976): Attempts to induce hepatic uridine diphosphate glucuronyl transferase in genetically deficient Gunn rats by grafting of normal liver tissue. *Pediatr. Res.*, 10:830.

196. Arias, I. M. (1962): Chronic unconjugated hyperbilirubinemia without overt signs of hemolysis in adolescents and adults. *J. Clin. Invest.*, 41:2233.

197. Berk, P. D., Wolkoff, A. W., and Berlin, N. I. (1975): Inborn errors of bilirubin metabolism. *Med. Clin. North Am.*, 59:803.

198. Gordon, E. R., Shaffer, E. A., and Sass-Kortsaka, A. (1976): Bilirubin secretion and conjugation in the Crigler-Najjar syndrome type II. *Gastroenterology*, 70:761.

199. Gollan, J. L., Huang, S. M., Billing, B., and Sherlock, S. (1975): Prolonged survival in three brothers with severe type II Crigler-Najjar syndrome. Ultrastructural and metabolic studies. *Gastroenterology*, 68:1543.

200. Fevery, J., Blanckaert, N., Heirwegh, K. P. M., Preaux, A-M., and Berthelot, P. (1977): Unconjugated bilirubin and an increased proportion of bilirubin monoconjugates in the bile of patients with Gilbert's syndrome and Crigler-Najjar syndrome. *J. Clin. Invest.*, 60:970.

201. Arias, I. M., Gartner, L., Furman, M., and Wolfson, S. (1963): Studies of the effect of several drugs on hepatic glucuronide formation in newborn rats and humans. *Ann. N.Y. Acad. Sci.*, 111:274.

202. Black, M., Fevery, J., Parker, D., Jacobson, J., Billing, B. H., and Carson, E. R. (1974): Effect of phenobarbitone on plasma ^{14}C bilirubin clearance in patients with unconjugated hyperbilirubinaemia. *Clin. Sci. Mol. Med.*, 46:1.

203. Gilbert, A., and Lereboullet, P. (1901): La Cholemie simple familiale. *Sem. Med.*, 21:241.

204. Foulk, W. T., Butt, H. R., Owen, C. A., and Whitcomb, F. F. (1959): Constitutional hepatic dysfunction (Gilbert's disease): its natural history and related syndrome. *Medicine*, 38:25.

205. Sagild, U., Dalgaard, O. Z., and Tygstrup, N. (1962): Constitutional hyperbilirubinemia with unconjugated bilirubin in the serum and lipochrome-like pigment granules in the liver. *Ann. Intern. Med.*, 56:308.

206. Bailey, A., Robinson, D., and Dawson, A. M. (1977): Does Gilbert's disease exist? *Lancet*, 1:931.

207. Owens, D., and Evans, J. (1975): Population studies on Gilbert's syndrome. *J. Med. Genet.*, 12:152.

208. Black, M., and Billing, B. H. (1969): Hepatic bilirubin UDP glucuronyltransferase activity in liver disease and Gilbert's syndrome. *N. Engl. J. Med.*, 280:1266.

209. Felsher, B. F., Craig, J. R., and Carpio, N. (1973): Hepatic bilirubin glucuronidation in Gilbert's syndrome. *J. Lab. Clin. Med.*, 81:829.

210. Berk, P. D., Bloomer, J. R., Howe, R. B., and Berlin, N. I. (1970): Constitutional hepatic dysfunction (Gilbert's syndrome): a new definition based on kinetic studies with unconjugated radiobilirubin. *Am. J. Med.*, 49:296.

211. Okolicsanyi, L., Ghidini, O., Orlando, R., Cortellazzo, S., Benedetti, G., Naccarato, R., and Manitto, P. (1978): An evaluation of bilirubin kinetics with respect to the diagnosis of Gilbert's syndrome. *Clin. Sci. Mol. Med.*, 54:535.

212. Goresky, C. A., Gordon, E. R., Shaffer, E. A., Parie, P., Carassavas, D., and Aronoff, A. (1978): Definition of a conjugation dysfunction in Gilbert's syndrome: Studies of the handling of bilirubin loads and of the pattern of bilirubin conjugates secreted in bile. *Clin. Sci. Mol. Med.*, 1:63.

213. Cobelli, C., Ruggeri, A., Toffolo, G., Okolicsanyi, L., Venuti, M., and Orlando, R. (1981): BSP vs bilirubin kinetics in Gilbert's syndrome. In: *Familial Hyperbilirubinemia*, edited by L. Okolicsanyi, p. 121. Wiley, New York.

214. Okolicsanyi, L., Orlando, R., Venuti, M., Dalbrun, G., Cobelli, C., Ruggeri, A., and Salvan, A. (1981): A modeling study of the effect of fasting on bilirubin kinetics in Gilbert's syndrome. *Am. J. Physiol.*, 240:266.

215. Felsher, B. F., Carpio, N. M., and Van Couvering, K. (1979): Effect of fasting and phenobarbital on hepatic UDP-glucuronic acid formation in the rat. *J. Lab. Clin. Med.*, 93:414.

216. Gollan, J. L., Hatt, K. J., and Billing, B. H. (1975): The influence of diet on unconjugated hyperbilirubinemia in the Gunn rat. *Clin. Sci. Mol. Med.*, 49:229.

217. Ohkubo, H., Musha, H., and Okuda, K. (1979): Studies on nicotinic acid interaction with bilirubin metabolism. *Dig. Dis. Sci.*, 24:700.

218. Fromke, V. L., and Miller, D. (1972): Constitutional hepatic dysfunction (CHD: Gilbert's disease): A review with special reference to a characteristic increase and prolongation of the hyperbilirubinemic response to nicotinic acid. *Medicine*, 51:451.

219. Fevery, J., Verwilghen, R., Tan, T. G., and De Groote, J. (1980): Glucuronidation of bilirubin and the occurrence of pigment gallstones in patients with chronic haemolytic diseases. *Eur. J. Clin. Invest.*, 10:219.

220. Cunningham, I. J., Hopkirk, C. S. M., and Filmer, J. F. (1942): Photosensitivity diseases in New Zealand. I. Facial eczema: its clinical pathological and biochemical characteristics. *NZ J. Sci. Tech.*, 24A:185.

221. Cornelius, C. E., and Gronwall, R. R. (1968): Congenital photosensitivity and hyperbilirubinemia in Southdown sheep in the United States. *Am. J. Vet. Res.*, 29:291.

222. Mia, A. S., Gronwall, R. R., and Cornelius, C. E. (1970): Bilirubin ^{14}C turnover in normal and mutant Southdown sheep

with congenital hyperbilirubinemia. *Proc. Soc. Exp. Biol. Med.*, 133:955.

223. Mia, A. S., Cornelius, C. E., and Gronwall, R. R. (1970): Increased bilirubin production from sources other than circulating erythrocytes in mutant Southdown sheep. *Proc. Soc. Exp. Biol. Med.*, 136:227.

224. McGavin, M. D., Gronwall, R. R., Cornelius, C. E., and Mia, A. S. (1972): Renal radial fibrosis in mutant Southdown sheep with congenital hyperbilirubinemia. *Am. J. Pathol.*, 67:601.

225. Dubin, I. N., and Johnson, F. B. (1954): Chronic idiopathic jaundice with unidentified pigment in liver cells: A new clinicopathologic entity with a report of 12 cases. *Medicine (Baltimore)*, 33:155.

226. Sprinz, H., and Nelson, R. S. (1954): Persistent nonhemolytic hyperbilirubinemia associated with lipochrome-like pigment in liver cells: Report of four cases. *Ann. Intern. Med.*, 41:952.

227. Seligsohn, U., Shani, M., Ramot, B., Adam, A., and Sheba, C. (1970): Dubin-Johnson Syndrome in Israel. II. Association with factor-VII deficiency. *Q. J. Med.*, 39:569.

228. Schmid, R. (1972): Hyperbilirubinemia. In: *The Metabolic Basis of Inherited Disease*, third edition, edited by J. B. Stanbury, J. B. Wyngaarden, and D. S. Fredrickson, pp. 1141-1178. McGraw-Hill, New York.

229. Cohen, L., Lewis, C., and Arias, I. M. (1972): Pregnancy, oral contraceptives, and chronic familial jaundice with predominantly conjugated hyperbilirubinemia (Dubin-Johnson syndrome). *Gastroenterology*, 62:1182.

230. Kondo, T., Kuchiba, K., Ohtsuka, Y., Yanagisawa, W., Shiomura, T., and Taminato, T. (1974): Clinical and genetic studies on Dubin-Johnson syndrome in a cluster area in Japan. *Jpn. J. Human Genet.*, 18:378.

231. Rosenthal, P., Kabra, P., Blanckaert, N., Kondo, T., and Schmidt, R. (1981): Homozygous Dubin-Johnson syndrome exhibits a characteristic serum bilirubin pattern. *Hepatology, Abstr.*, 1:540.

232. Morita, M., and Kihava, T. (1971): Intravenous cholecystography and metabolism of meglumin iodipamide (biligrafin) in Dubin-Johnson syndrome. *Radiology*, 99:57.

233. Muscatello, U., Mussini, I., and Agnolucci, M. T. (1967): The Dubin-Johnson syndrome: An electron microscopic study of the liver cell. *Acta Hepatosplenol. (Stuttg.)*, 14:162.

234. Kermarec, J., Duplay, H., and Daniel, R. (1972): Etude histochimique et ultrastrucurale comparative des pigments de la melanose colique et du syndrome de Dubin-Johnson. *Ann. Biol. Clin.*, 30:567.

235. Ehrlich, J. C., Novikoff, A. B., Platt, R., and Essner, E. (1960): Hepatocellular lipofuscin and the pigment of chronic idiopathic jaundice. *Bull. N.Y. Acad. Med.*, 36:488.

236. Swartz, H. M., Sarna, T., and Varma, R. R. (1979): On the nature and excretion of the hepatic pigment in the Dubin-Johnson syndrome. *Gastroenterology*, 76:958.

237. Ware, A., Eigenbrodt, E., Naftalis, J., and Combes, B. (1974): Dubin-Johnson syndrome and viral hepatitis. *Gastroenterology*, 67:560.

238. Schoenfield, L. J., McGill, D. B., Hunton, D. B., Foulk, M. T., and Butt, H. R. (1963): Studies of chronic idiopathic jaundice (Dubin-Johnson syndrome). I. Demonstration of hepatic excretory defect. *Gastroenterology*, 44:101.

239. Erlinger, S., Dhumeaux, D., Desjeux, J. F., and Benhamon, J. P. (1973): Hepatic handling of unconjugated dyes in the Dubin-Johnson syndrome. *Gastroenterology*, 64:106.

240. Wheeler, H. O., Meltzer, J. I., and Bradley, S. E. (1960): Biliary transport and hepatic storage of sulfobromophthalein sodium in the unanesthetized dog, in normal man, and in patients with hepatic disease. *J. Clin. Invest.*, 39:1131.

241. Rodes, J., Zubizarreta, A., and Bruguera, M. (1972): Metabolism of the bromsulphalein in Dubin-Johnson syndrome. Diagnostic value of the paradoxical in plasma levels at BSP. *Dig. Dis.*, 17:545.

242. Gutstein, S., Alpert, S., and Arias, I. M. (1968): Studies of hepatic excretory function. IV. Biliary excretion of sulfobromophthalein in a patient with Dubin-Johnson syndrome and a biliary fistula. *Isr. J. Med. Sci.*, 4:46.

243. Kaplowitz, N., Javitt, N., and Kappas, A. (1972): Corropor-

phyrin I and III excretion in bile and urine. *J. Clin. Invest.*, 51:2895.

244. Wolkoff, A. W., Cohen, L. E., and Arias, I. M. (1973): Inheritance of the Dubin-Johnson syndrome. *N. Engl. J. Med.*, 288:113.

245. Kondo, T., Kuchiba, K., and Shimizu, Y. (1979): Metabolic fate of exogenous delta-aminoleuvulinic acid in Dubin-Johnson syndrome. *J. Lab. Clin. Med.*, 94:421.

246. Shimizu, Y., Kondo, T., Kuchiba, K., and Urata, G. (1977): Uroporphyrin III cosynthetase in liver and blood in the Dubin-Johnson syndrome. *J. Lab. Clin. Med.*, 89:517.

247. Cornelius, C. E., Arias, I. M., and Osburn, B. I. (1965): Hepatic pigmentation with photosensitivity: A syndrome in Corriedale sheep resembling Dubin-Johnson syndrome in man. *J. Am. Vet. Med. Assoc.*, 146:709.

248. Cornelius, C. E., Osburn, B. I., Gronwall, R. R., and Cardinet, G. H. (1968): Dubin-Johnson syndrome in immature sheep. *Am. J. Dig. Dis.*, 13:1072.

249. Arias, I. M., Bernstein, L., Toffler, R., and Ben Ezzer, J. (1965): Black liver disease in Corriedale sheep: Metabolism of tritiated epinephrine and incorporation of isotope into the hepatic pigment *in vivo*. *J. Clin. Invest.*, 44:1026.

250. Rotor, A. B., Manahan, L., and Florentin, A. (1948): Familial nonhemolytic jaundice with direct van den Bergh reaction. *Acta Med. Phil.*, 5:37.

251. Wolpert, E., Pascasio, F. M., Wolkoff, A. W., and Arias, I. M. (1977): Abnormal sulfobromophthalein metabolism in Rotor's syndrome and obligate heterozygotes. *N. Engl. J. Med.*, 296:1091.

252. Dhumeaux, D., and Berthelot, P. (1975): Chronic hyperbilirubinemia associated with hepatic uptake and storage impairment: a new syndrome resembling that of the mutant Southdown sheep. *Gastroenterology*, 69:988.

253. Wolkoff, A. W., Wolpert, E., Pascasio, F. N., and Arias, I. M. (1976): Rotor's syndrome, a distinct inheritable pathophysiologic entity. *Am. J. Med.*, 60:173.

254. Summerskill, W. H. J., and Walshe, J. M. (1959): Benign recurrent intrahepatic obstructive jaundice. *Lancet*, 2:686.

255. De Pagter, A. G. F., Van Berge Henegouwen, G. P., Bokkel-Huinnuk, J. A., and Brandt, K-H. (1976): Familial benign recurrent intrahepatic cholestasis. *Gastroenterology*, 71:202.

256. Summerfield, J. A., Scott, J., Berman, M., Ghent, C., Bloomer, J. R., Berk, P. D., and Sherlock, S. (1980): Benign recurrent intrahepatic cholestasis: Studies of bilirubin kinetics, bile acids, and cholangiography. *Gut*, 21:154.

257. Biempica, L., Gutstein, S., and Arias, I. M. (1967): Morphological and biochemical studies of benign recurrent cholestasis. *Gastroenterology*, 52:521.

The Liver: Biology and Pathobiology, edited by
I. Arias, H. Popper, D. Schachter, and D. A. Shafritz.
Raven Press, New York © 1982.

Chapter 19

Porphyrin Metabolism

Joseph R. Bloomer

The word porphyrin is derived from the Greek word *porphuros* (red-purple) (1). This is an appropriate derivation, because porphyrins impart a spectacular port-wine appearance to the urine when present in high concentrations. They also exhibit red fluorescence when irradiated with ultraviolet light (wavelength, 400 nm). Both properties are due to the conjugated double bond system of the tetrapyrrole ring (Fig. 1), which has the same structure for all porphyrins. The different porphyrins vary in the composition of side chains, which are attached to the tetrapyrrole ring.

The porphyrins and their reduced forms (porphyrinogens) are intermediates of the heme biosynthetic pathway (Fig. 2). The porphyrinogens are colorless and nonfluorescent because the methene bridges of the tetrapyrrole ring are replaced by methane groups. When exposed to air, however, they rapidly and spontaneously oxidize to their porphyrin counterparts.

The liver has two roles in porphyrin metabolism. First, it is a major site of heme biosynthesis because heme is required as a prosthetic group for important hepatic compounds, such as the mitochondrial cytochromes and cytochrome P-450. As a result, the liver may be the principal source of porphyrins and porphyrin precursors which are excreted excessively in genetic disorders of heme biosynthesis. This provides the basis for the classification of several of these disorders, collectively called the porphyrias, as hepatic (2). Second, the liver is a route of excretion for porphyrins. This is an important factor in the pathogenesis of some

of the clinical manifestations of the porphyrias. In addition, hepatobiliary disease may cause an increase in urinary porphyrin excretion, a condition known as secondary porphyrinuria.

In this chapter, features of abnormal hepatic porphyrin metabolism are considered in view of these roles of the liver.

HEPATIC HEME BIOSYNTHESIS AND ITS REGULATION

The rate at which hepatic heme is produced in normal man has not been quantitated directly, but indirect estimates have been made in two ways. From measurement of the incorporation of labeled δ-aminolevulinic acid (ALA) into bilirubin, it is apparent that 10 to 20% of the total bilirubin formed in adults comes from the degradation of hepatic heme (3). In the steady-state situation where the synthesis of heme is equal to its rate of degradation, this places the normal rate of hepatic heme production at 0.7 to 1.4 μmoles/kg body weight/day. Since the heme prosthetic group of some hepatic hemoproteins may be degraded along pathways that do not form bilirubin, this is probably a low estimate. Based on the measurement of hepatic ALA synthase activity in normal adult liver, the rate of hepatic heme production is estimated to be 1.6 μmoles/ kg body weight/day (4).

The pathway by which the liver synthesizes heme is the same as that in the bone marrow and other heme-forming tissues of the body (Fig. 2). Although the

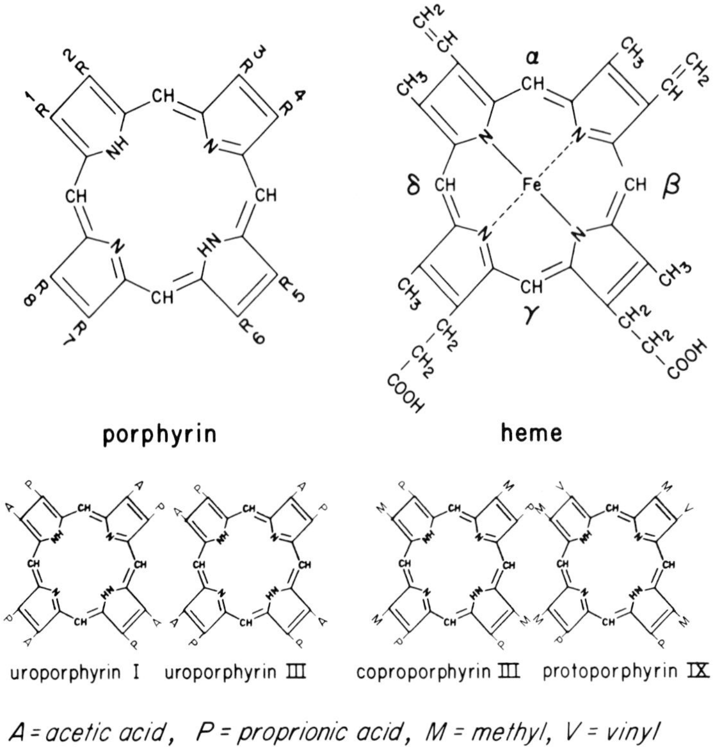

porphyrin

heme

FIG. 1. Structures of porphyrins and heme. All porphyrins have the same basic ring structure. They differ in the composition of the side chains which are attached to the tetrapyrrole ring. Porphyrinogens are the reduced forms of the porphyrins in which the methene bridges linking the pyrroles are replaced by methane groups.

uroporphyrin I   uroporphyrin III   coproporphyrin III   protoporphyrin IX

A = acetic acid,   P = proprionic acid,   M = methyl,   V = vinyl

intermediates of the pathway are identical, it has not been determined that the enzymes that catalyze the steps are structurally the same in the various tissues. If isoenzymes exist, the properties of the hepatic enzymes may differ from those in other heme-forming tissues.

The enzymes of heme biosynthesis are compartmentalized within the cell, such that the first and last steps of the pathway occur in the mitochondria, whereas the intermediate steps take place in the soluble portion of the cell. In the first step of heme

biosynthesis, ALA synthase catalyzes the formation of ALA from glycine and succinyl-CoA in the presence of pyridoxal phosphate. This is the only step in the pathway in which a cofactor participates. Two molecules of ALA condense to form porphobilinogen (PBG), and four molecules of PBG polymerize to form uroporphyrinogen. The coordinate action of uroporphyrinogen I synthase and uroporphyrinogen III cosynthase is required to form the type III isomer of uroporphyrinogen. In the absence of the cosynthase, the type I isomer is formed. Only porphyrinogens of

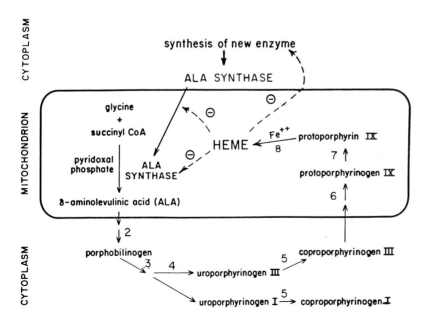

FIG. 2. Heme biosynthetic pathway. Heme may regulate hepatic ALA synthase, which catalyzes the first and rate-limiting step of the pathway, by three mechanisms: (a) repression of the synthesis of enzyme, (b) interference with the translocation of newly synthesized enzyme from cytoplasm to mitochondria, (c) direct inhibition of enzyme activity. Other enzymes of the pathway are numbered as follows: 2—ALA dehydrase, 3—uroporphyrinogen I synthase, 4—uroporphyrinogen III cosynthase, 5—uroporphyrinogen decarboxylase, 6—coproporphyrinogen oxidase, 7—protoporphyrinogen oxidase; 8—heme synthase (ferrochelatase).

type III isomer are intermediates in the biosynthesis of heme; compounds containing heme derived from a type I isomer have not been identified.

The side chains of the porphyrinogen are decarboxylated in the next series of reactions. Uroporphyrinogen III, which has eight carboxylic side chains, is converted to the dicarboxylic acid compound protoporphyrinogen IX. Following the enzymatic oxidation of protoporphyrinogen to protoporphyrin, heme is formed by chelation of ferrous iron to protoporphyrin.

The principal means by which hepatic heme biosynthesis is controlled is through regulation of ALA synthase. This is in keeping with the biochemical principle that the first enzyme in an unbranched biosynthetic pathway controls the flux of substrates down the pathway. Beyond ALA synthase, the kinetics of the enzymes are such that accumulation of intermediates of the heme biosynthetic pathway is minimal under normal conditions.

Hepatic ALA synthase is synthesized in the cytoplasm, where it is associated with other proteins in a large molecular weight aggregate (5). Newly made enzyme is translocated from cytosol to mitochondria and processed in an unknown manner before it becomes functional in heme biosynthesis. The activity of ALA synthase can be induced by drugs and naturally occurring steroids (6,7). Induction is blocked by carbohydrate intake (8), a phenomenon observed for other enzymes in mammalian liver and called the glucose effect.

Heme regulates the level of hepatic ALA synthase activity through negative feedback (Fig. 2) by three different mechanisms: (a) repression of the synthesis of enzyme, (b) interference with the transfer of newly synthesized enzyme from cytosol to mitochondria, and (c) direct inhibition of enzyme activity. These processes have been studied primarily in experimental animals and cultured chick embryo hepatocytes. Sufficient observations have been made to indicate that they probably operate in man as well.

Repression of enzyme synthesis is an important mechanism by which heme regulates hepatic ALA synthase. Proportional increases in enzyme activity and the amount of enzyme protein occur when ALA synthase is chemically induced in cultured chick embryo liver cells (9). Heme blocks the increase in enzyme activity and the amount of new enzyme protein without changing general protein synthesis. A heme concentration of 10^{-7} M in the culture medium of chick embryo liver cells represses the induction of ALA synthase by 50% (10). It is unclear whether this effect is exerted at the level of transcription or at a later step in synthesis of the protein.

Heme also affects hepatic ALA synthase by interfering with the translocation of newly synthesized enzyme from cytosol to the mitochondria. The administration of heme to rats that have had hepatic ALA

synthase activity induced by certain drugs causes the enzyme to accumulate in the extramitochondrial fraction (11). This has not been demonstrated for all types of chemical induction in rats. Moreover, heme does not cause accumulation of soluble ALA synthase in cultured chick embryo liver cells (12).

Direct inhibition of ALA synthase activity by heme has been demonstrated using solubilized, partially purified enzyme (13). Other metalloporphyrins, porphyrins, and bilirubin also inhibit activity. Heme causes 50% inhibition of ALA synthase activity at a concentration of 2×10^{-5} M (13). This is 200 times the concentration required to repress synthesis of the enzyme in tissue culture, indicating that inhibition is a less sensitive mechanism for regulation of ALA synthase. Nevertheless, since both ALA synthase and heme synthase, the enzyme that catalyzes the chelation of ferrous iron to protoporphyrin to form heme, are intramitochondrial enzymes, it is possible that the generation of heme within mitochondria provides a local concentration sufficient to inhibit ALA synthase. When ALA synthase and heme synthase activities are examined simultaneously in isolated rat liver mitochondria, ALA synthase activity is not altered at rates of heme formation estimated to be at least 75 times that occurring *in vivo* (14).

These studies indicate that heme probably does not regulate hepatic ALA synthase physiologically by preventing transfer of newly formed enzyme from cytosol to mitochondria or by directly inhibiting activity of the enzyme. These mechanisms may be important when heme is used to treat patients with acute porphyric attacks. The level of hepatic ALA synthase appears to be modulated by the rate of synthesis of the enzyme. This is possible because ALA synthase and its messenger RNA have a short biological half-life in liver (approximately 70 min in the rat) (15). A portion of hepatic heme presumably enters a regulatory pool, combining with an as-yet unidentified aporepressor to adjust the synthesis of ALA synthase. Depletion of the regulatory pool allows ALA synthase to be synthesized at a greater rate. As the regulatory pool is repleted, synthesis of the enzyme slows. The size of the regulatory heme pool may be affected by the requirement for hemoproteins in the liver. For example, phenobarbital may increase hepatic ALA synthase because the level of drug metabolizing hemoproteins increases, thereby shunting heme from the regulatory pool to serve as a prosthetic group for these compounds. Other factors that may influence the size of the regulatory heme pool are the rate of catabolism of heme in the liver cell, the rate at which heme leaks from the hepatocyte into bile or plasma, and defects in the heme biosynthetic pathway.

This formulation explains in part why compounds of diverse structure, including insecticides, carcinogens, and steroids, induce hepatic ALA synthase. They may have the common property of altering the heme pool in the liver which regulates synthesis of the enzyme. Other compounds may stimulate synthesis of the enzyme directly. However, the manner in which some factors influence the level of the enzyme is not so clearly explained. The mechanism by which glucose represses the induction of hepatic ALA synthase is one such example.

There are other sites in the heme biosynthetic pathway where control may be exerted. Iron affects the pathway at multiple sites (16), and defects in enzymes distal to ALA synthase may cause the steps catalyzed by these enzymes to become rate-limiting in certain circumstances.

EXCRETION OF PORPHYRINS AND PORPHYRIN PRECURSORS

The porphyrin precursors ALA and PBG are excreted in urine (Table 1). When hepatic formation of these compounds increases in patients during acute porphyric attacks, urinary levels are markedly elevated. The amount of biliary excretion under this circumstance is unknown.

Since uroporphyrinogen and coproporphyrinogen are the true intermediates of heme biosynthesis, they should be excreted by the liver and kidney, rather than uroporphyrin and coproporphyrin, unless they are oxidized *in vivo* to porphyrins before excretion. Studies in experimental animals indicate that *in vivo* oxidation occurs under some circumstances (17); the extent to which it occurs in man, however, has not been determined. Nevertheless, it is unnecessary and impractical to measure the excretion rate of porphyrinogens per se for clinical purposes, particularly since these compounds rapidly and spontaneously oxidize when exposed to air. Consequently, urine and fecal extracts are treated with dilute iodine solution to ensure oxidation of the porphyrinogens to their porphyrin counterparts. The porphyrin content of urine increases after oxidation with dilute iodine, indicating that porphyrinogens are present.

The relative amount of an individual porphyrin pres-

ent in urine and feces correlates with the number of carboxyl groups in the compound and hence with its water solubility. Uroporphyrin, which has eight carboxyl groups and is water soluble, is found predominantly in the urine (Table 1). Coproporphyrin has four carboxyl groups and is found in both urine and feces. Protoporphyrin, which is poorly water soluble because it has only two carboxyl groups, is not excreted in urine. The protoporphyrin level in feces is the highest of any porphyrin. The total porphyrin content of feces is variable in type and amount for normal individuals because some porphyrins may be derived from food or may be formed by intestinal bacteria.

Hepatic uptake and excretion of porphyrins has been examined directly in rats using incident ultraviolet illumination and fluorescence microscopy (18). After injection of coproporphyrin into the jugular vein, fluorescence is observed in the hepatic sinusoids in 5 to 15 sec and in the liver cells in 1 to 2 min. The bile canaliculi show brilliant fluorescence a few minutes later. Following injection of protoporphyrin, 25 to 30 min elapse before fluorescence appears in the canaliculi. Uroporphyrin is not taken up by the liver cells but is eliminated rapidly and completely by the kidney.

Studies have been performed with the isolated perfused rat liver to examine the mechanism of protoporphyrin excretion (19). In this system, secretion into bile is the rate-limiting step in excretion, even though protoporphyrin is concentrated in bile. Bile acids facilitate the biliary excretion of protoporphyrin in a manner similar to their effect on biliary lipid excretion. Protoporphyrin also undergoes an enterohepatic circulation (20) probably because of the lipid solubility of the compound, which allows it to cross cellular membranes readily.

In addition to the water solubility of the porphyrin, the nature of its isomeric form influences the route of excretion. The type I isomer of coproporphyrin predominates over the type III isomer in bile, whereas the opposite occurs in urine (21,22). When types I and III isomers of coproporphyrin are infused into bile fistula rats in equimolar amounts, the concentration ratio of the type I to type III isomer in the bile is 2:1. This finding suggests that there is a carrier transport system in the liver that requires a stereospecific

TABLE 1. *Level of porphyrins and porphyrin precursors in normal adults*

Porphyrin	Red cells	Serum	Urine	Feces
ALA	?	ND−10 μg/dl	<4 mg/day	?
PBG	?	ND−4.4 μg/dl	<4 mg/day	?
Uroporphyrin	ND	ND	10−50 μg/day	<4 μg/g dry wt
Coproporphyrin	ND−2 μg/dl	ND	50−280 μg/day	<33 μg/g dry wt
Protoporphyrin	15−60 μg/dl	ND or trace	ND	<107 μg/g dry wt

ND, none detected using currently available technique.
These values are from the Watson Laboratory, Abbott-Northwestern Hospital, Minneapolis, Minnesota. The level shown for a porphyrin includes its porphyrinogen counterpart.

configuration of the porphyrin which favors the symmetrical type I isomer (22).

THE HEPATIC PORPHYRIAS

The porphyrias are a group of disorders in which inborn errors of heme biosynthesis cause excessive accumulation and excretion of porphyrins and porphyrin precursors. Four of the seven types of porphyria are classified as hepatic, because the liver is the major if not sole site of expression of the biochemical abnormality (Table 2). In a fifth disorder, protoporphyria, both the liver and bone marrow may contribute to the biochemical abnormality (23). The two porphyrias that do not have hepatic expression of the disease, congenital erythropoietic porphyria and erythropoietic coproporphyria, are uncommon compared to hepatic porphyrias.

All the hepatic porphyrias (Table 2) are inherited in an autosomal dominant pattern. A rare case of recessive inheritance has been reported (24). Porphyria cutanea tarda is unique in that there is both a familial and a sporadic occurrence. The occasional occurrence of the disorder in more than one family member has long suggested a hereditary form; recent examinations of the enzyme abnormality in the disease substantiate this (25,26). Sporadic cases associated with the use of alcohol or birth control pills, however, are more common. Whether or not there is a genetic predisposition in the sporadic cases of porphyria cutanea tarda remains unclear. The multiple cases that developed after the accidental ingestion of hexachlorobenzine in Turkey in the late 1950s indicate that this disorder can be acquired (27).

The clinical manifestations of the porphyrias encompass many areas of medicine, including neurology, dermatology, and multiple subspecialties of internal medicine. Three major features are considered: (a) neuropsychiatric symptoms, (b) cutaneous symptoms, and (c) structural hepatic disease. The diagnosis of a specific porphyria is frequently suggested by the combination of clinical features (Table 2).

Even though the hepatic porphyrias are inherited, clinical manifestations rarely occur before puberty, except in protoporphyria, where photosensitivity begins in infancy. Clinical symptoms of acute intermittent porphyria and variegate porphyria most frequently have their onset in the third decade. Manifestations of porphyria cutanea tarda usually occur after age 30.

Pathogenesis of the Biochemical Abnormalities in the Porphyrias

The diagnosis of a porphyria is made by demonstrating increased amounts of porphyrins and/or porphyrin precursors in the urine, feces, or blood (Table 2). Screening tests can be used in the initial evaluation of patients suspected to have porphyria (28). The Watson-Schwartz test has been used extensively to detect increased amounts of PBG in the urine. The principle of this test is that PBG reacts with Ehrlich's aldehyde reagent to form a red pigment which remains in the aqueous phase after extraction with chloroform and butanol. The test is useful since urine PBG is increased during acute attacks in those forms of porphyria that manifest neuropsychiatric symptoms. The result must be interpreted cautiously, however, because several compounds interfere with the determination. Urobilinogen in particular will produce a false positive test unless extractions are carefully performed. Quantitative determination of urinary PBG should be done in patients with a positive test. Similarly, quantitative studies should be done when screening tests detect increased amounts of porphyrins in red cells, feces, or urine.

Recent studies have shown that partial enzyme defects in the heme biosynthetic pathway underlie the biochemical abnormalities that characterize the porphyrias. Porphyrins and/or porphyrin precursors accumulate because of these enzyme defects and are excreted in increased amounts, resulting in the array of biochemical abnormalities unique to each porphyria. Acute intermittent porphyria has been most extensively investigated. The livers of patients with this disorder have deficient activity of uroporphyrinogen I synthase, which catalyzes the conversion of PBG to uroporphyrinogen (29). As a result, ALA and PBG are excreted in increased amounts in urine. The enzyme defect is not found in the livers of patients with variegate porphyria and porphyria cutanea tarda (29), in which the patterns of abnormal porphyrin excretion differ from those in acute intermittent porphyria.

The defect in uroporphyrinogen I synthase has also been demonstrated in cultured skin fibroblasts and red cell hemolysates from patients with acute intermittent porphyria (30–34); this reflects the genetic nature of the disease. However, it raises the question of why the disease is not expressed in tissues other than liver. One possibility is that only in liver may the enzyme defect reduce the activity of uroporphyrinogen synthase to a critical level such that ALA and PBG accumulate.

Enzyme defects have been defined in the other porphyrias as well. Deficient activity of heme synthase (ferrochelatase), which catalyzes the chelation of ferrous iron to protoporphyrin to form heme, is found in liver (35), bone marrow cells (36,37), peripheral blood cells (38,39), and cultured skin fibroblasts (11,12) from patients with protoporphyria. Fecal and erythrocyte protoporphyrin levels are elevated in protoporphyria, reflecting this enzyme abnormality. In hereditary co-

TABLE 2. *Porphyrias in which the liver expresses the biochemical abnormality*

Feature	Acute intermittent porphyria		Variegate porphyria		Hereditary coproporphyria		Protoporphyria	Porphyria cutanea tarda
	Remission	Relapse	Remission	Relapse	Remission	Relapse	Symptomatic	Symptomatic
Biochemical abnormalities								
Red cell protoporphyrin	N	N	N	N	N	N	+++	N
Feces								
Coproporphyrin	N	N	++	++	++	+++	N to +	N
Protoporphyrin	N	N	+++	+++	N	+	N to +++	N
Urine								
ALA	+	+	N	++	N	++	N	N
PBG	++	+	N	++	N	++	N	N
Uroporphyrin	N or +	+++	N	+++	N	++	N	+++
Coproporphyrin	N or +	++	N or +	+++	N or +	+++	N	+
Enzyme defect	Uroporphyrinogen I synthase		Heme synthase? Protoporphyrinogen oxidase?		Coproporphyrinogen oxidase		Heme synthase	Uroporphyrinogen decarboxylase
Clinical features								
Inheritance	Autosomal dominant		Autosomal dominant		Autosomal dominant		Autosomal dominant	Familial- autosomal dominant sporadic?
Neuropsychiatric symptoms	Yes		Yes		Yes		No	No
Skin lesions	No		Yes		Yes		Yes	Yes
Structural liver disease	No		No		No		Yes	Yes

N, normal level; +, mild increase; ++, moderate increase; +++, marked increase.

proporphyria, a defect in coproporphyrinogen oxidase is present (24,40,41) and a defect in uroporphyrinogen decarboxylase in porphyria cutanea tarda (25,26,42,43). The defect in uroporphyrinogen decarboxylase is found in red cells and liver tissue of patients with the familial type of porphyria cutanea tarda (26). In sporadic cases, hepatic enzyme activity is deficient (42), but it is uncertain whether the enzyme abnormality is also present in other tissues (42,43). Until the controversy is resolved, it appears that hepatic levels of uroporphyrinogen decarboxylase are deficient in all patients with porphyria cutanea tarda; a generalized tissue defect may be present only in patients with the familial form of the disease.

In variegate porphyria, studies disagree as to whether there is a defect in heme synthase activity or in protoporphyrinogen oxidase activity (36,44). An abnormality at either site could explain why fecal protoporphyrin is constantly elevated in patients with variegate porphyria. Since heme synthase activity is clearly defective in protoporphyria, which has very different features from variegate porphyria, an abnormality in protoporphyrinogen oxidase is the more attractive possibility. Further studies are required to settle the issue.

Recently, a deficiency of ALA dehydrase activity has been found in red cells in some individuals (46,47). Although the majority have been asymptomatic, two patients had increased urinary excretion of ALA and experienced neurological abnormalities (47), suggesting another type of porphyria previously unrecognized.

With the exception of protoporphyria, the residual enzyme activity in tissues of patients with the porphyrias is approximately 50% of normal, indicating that these disorders are probably due to structural gene defects in which one of the alleles codes for synthesis of a protein that has minimal activity. Residual heme synthase activity in protoporphyria tissue is only 10 to 25% of normal. This is still compatible with an autosomal dominant trait, but the enzyme abnormality is probably not merely a reduction in the amount of normal enzyme.

Provided that accessible tissue is suitable for assay, demonstration of an enzyme defect can be used to establish the diagnosis of a specific form of porphyria in a patient whose biochemical studies are equivocal. Since the clinical and biochemical manifestations of several of the porphyrias seldom occur before puberty, children may be screened for the disease at an early age and advised concerning the use of drugs that may bring out the disease. Similarly, genetic counseling of families in which a member has porphyria can be done more effectively. These applications are presently being applied extensively in acute intermittent porphyria.

Since enzyme activity is defective in tissues of some individuals who show neither biochemical nor clinical manifestations of porphyria, it is apparent that the enzyme abnormality alone is not sufficient to cause expression of the disease. Moreover, biochemical manifestations in patients may vary considerably from one period to another. Thus other factors must combine with the enzyme defect to produce biochemical manifestations of the disease. One such factor is the requirement for hepatic heme synthesis. In patients with porphyria, a demand for more heme synthesis may necessitate a large increase of ALA synthase to compensate for the enzyme defect. This will increase the synthesis of intermediates of heme synthesis that precede the enzymatic block and enhance the biochemical abnormalities that characterize the disease. Hepatic ALA synthase activity is increased markedly in patients with acute intermittent porphyria, hereditary coproporphyria, and variegate porphyria during acute attacks (29,48–51). When the patients are in remission, hepatic ALA synthase activity is lower and the excretion of porphyrins and porphyrin precursors is less (29,49).

Other factors may directly modify the enzyme defects. For example, ferrous iron inhibits uroporphyrinogen decarboxylase activity in crude liver extracts (52). That the livers in patients with porphyria cutanea tarda characteristically show hemoiderosis may be an important factor in bringing out the disease in patients who have reduced enzyme activity. Further identification of factors that modify the enzyme defects will contribute to our understanding of the fluctuations that occur in the biochemical manifestations of the porphyrias.

Neuropsychiatric Symptoms in the Porphyrias

Neuropsychiatric abnormalities cause the clinical manifestations that occur in acute attacks of porphyria. Abdominal pain, the most frequent symptom (53,54), is caused by an autonomic neuropathy that causes disturbed gastrointestinal motility. The pain is generally severe, colicky, and localized to the lower quadrants of the abdomen, but it can mimic any intraabdominal process. The presence of dilated bowel loops on abdominal X-rays often suggests the presence of mechanical intestinal obstruction. Other features of the attack attributable to the autonomic neuropathy include tachycardia, labile hypertension with postural hypotension, urinary retention, and excessive diaphoresis (53,54). Overactivity of the sympathetic nervous system has been documented biochemically in a few patients by demonstrating increased urinary excretion of epinephrine and norepinephrine.

Peripheral neuropathy, including cranial nerve involvement, frequently accompanies the autonomic neuropathy (53,54). Total flaccid paralysis may occur, and complications due to respiratory paralysis are a leading cause of death. Although the neuropathy is generally reversible, residual paresis sometimes continues for several years following an acute attack (55).

In some patients, hypothalamic lesions were found at postmortem examinations (54). Inappropriate secretion of antidiuretic hormone, which may result from hypothalamic involvement, has been proposed as a cause of the hyponatremia that is frequently observed during an acute attack of porphyria (56). Gastrointestinal sodium loss and impaired renal sodium transport also contribute to electrolyte abnormalities (57). The demonstration that patients with acute intermittent porphyria frequently have diminished blood volumes suggests that the secretion of antidiuretic hormone may be inappropriate in these situations (58).

Psychiatric manifestations are also common in the porphyrias (53,54). An organic brain syndrome with restlessness, disorientation, and hallucinations occurs frequently during attacks. Other manifestations include schizophrenia, depression, and neuroses. Several patients reside in mental institutions.

Since neuropsychiatric abnormalities occur in porphyrias in which there is increased excretion of ALA and PBG (Table 2), efforts have been made to show that these compounds are neurotoxic. ALA is particularly suspect because other disorders in which there is increased urinary excretion of this compound, such as lead poisoning and hereditary tyrosinemia, also have neurological abnormalities. If ALA is injected into the brain ventricles of the experimental animal, neurotoxicity is produced (59). ALA inhibits human brain ATPase *in vitro* and is a potent agonist of γ-aminobutyric acid receptors (60,61), indicating mechanisms by which the toxicity could be caused.

Despite these experimental studies, the major difficulty in ascribing the nervous system manifestations to the toxic effects of ALA and/or PBG is that the degree of involvement correlates poorly with urinary and serum levels of these compounds; some patients have no symptoms despite excreting large amounts. Moreover, ALA is not consistently found in the spinal fluid of patients with attacks of porphyria. Alternate mechanisms to explain the neuropsychiatric manifestations of the porphyrias have been proposed. Intermittent ischemia, an abnormality in myelin metabolism or heavy metal metabolism, and impaired synthesis of acetylcholine have been postulated but unproved. A kryptopyrrolic compound which bears a structural resemblance to PBG has been measured in the urine of patients with acute intermittent porphyria (62). Since this compound was found in the urine of patients with psychoses of other types, it may be important in the pathogenesis of the psychiatric disturbances. In view of the fact that the biochemical abnormalities in the porphyrias are caused by defects in heme biosyn-

thesis, the neuropsychiatric abnormalities may arise from a deficiency of heme in the nervous system.

Cutaneous Symptoms in the Porphyrias

Cutaneous symptoms occur in those porphyrias in which there is increased excretion of porphyrins (Table 2). Patients with protoporphyria have itching, burning, or stinging when their skin is exposed to sunlight (63). This is followed by erythema and edema of the exposed areas which may persist for several weeks. Window glass does not prevent the reaction. Chronic skin changes consist of thickening and scarring.

Bullous skin lesions are found in the other porphyrias (63). Although the lesions occur principally in sun-exposed areas, they are caused by increased skin fragility rather than a reaction to sunlight per se. Acute photosensitivity reactions, such as those in protoporphyria, are rare. Chronic skin changes are milia, hirsutism (particularly prominent on the upper part of the cheeks and the periorbital areas), areas of hyperpigmentation and depigmentation, and occasionally sclerodermoid changes. In long-standing untreated cases, scarring and alopecia may be prominent.

The photosensitizing effects of the porphyrin compounds have been recognized for many years. Oral ingestion of ALA also causes photosensitivity, probably because it is converted to porphyrins. The wavelength of light that causes skin reactions is approximately 400 nm (64), the point at which the porphyrin compounds absorb maximally (called the Soret band). Porphyrins deposited in skin or circulating in the dermal blood vessels presumably absorb light which is dissipated locally as energy. Damage to the skin may occur because of free radicle formation or singlet oxygen formation (65,66).

Hepatic Disease in the Porphyrias

Although the liver is the major site of the biochemical abnormality in several of the porphyrias, structural liver damage occurs only in protoporphyria and porphyria cutanea tarda. Hepatic dysfunction is not a feature of the acute attack in acute intermittent porphyria and variegate porphyria (53,54). Patients with acute intermittent porphyria have abnormal bromosulfthalein (BSP) excretion, particularly when symptomatic, but the defect does not include other organic anions that are excreted into bile and therefore appears specifically related to BSP metabolism (67). Mild elevations of serum transaminase occur in 10 to 20% of symptomatic patients (54), but this probably reflects nonspecific hepatic reaction to the illness or is of nonhepatic origin.

Liver disease is common in patients with porphyria cutanea tarda, and a variety of histological abnormalities are found in liver biopsy specimens (45,68–71). Hepatic siderosis and fatty infiltration have been observed in all reports. One report indicated that needlelike inclusions are also frequently present in the cytoplasm of hepatocytes (45). The degree of liver necrosis and fibrosis varies in its severity. In the United States, less than 10% of patients have cirrhosis; a much higher incidence has been reported from other countries (71). Hepatoma appears to develop with increased frequency in patients with long-standing porphyria cutanea tarda (69).

Patients with the sporadic form of porphyria cutanea tarda frequently have a history of heavy alcohol consumption. Some of the features in the biopsy specimens, such as fatty infiltration, are compatible with alcohol-induced changes, but the entire constellation of changes is not that of alcoholic liver damage. Moreover, liver damage of similar nature occurs in patients in whom the sporadic form of porphyria cutanea tarda is associated with the use of birth control pills (68). Although hepatic siderosis is common, the degree of hepatic iron deposition is only two to three times normal (70), much less than that observed in patients with hemochromatosis; iron is unlikely to have a direct toxic effect. An unexplored possibility is that uroporphyrin or uroporphyrinogen is somehow toxic to the liver.

Hepatobiliary disease is a potentially serious feature of protoporphyria, as 15 cases have been reported in which death occurred from hepatic failure (72). The patients are generally over the age of 30, but children have also died from liver disease (72); the liver disease is not associated with alcoholism, viral hepatitis, drug use, or exposure to toxins.

Liver biopsy specimens from fatal cases show cirrhosis with massive deposits of dark brown pigment. When examined by polarizing microscopy, the pigment deposits have a distinctive birefringence; on electron microscopy, they are crystalline in nature (72). Although the chemical composition of the pigment deposits has not been defined, they are thought to be composed principally of protoporphyrin, since the protoporphyrin content of the liver is high. Current speculation is that the deposition of protoporphyrin crystals in hepatobiliary structures is an important factor in the pathogenesis of the liver damage. Either extrahepatic or intrahepatic biliary deposition may cause portal inflammation and fibrosis by biliary obstruction or by a toxic effect of the crystalline material on the bile duct epithelium. Crystalline deposits of protoporphyrin may also form within hepatocytes and cause cell death directly. Recent studies with isolated perfused rat liver indicate that protoporphyrin impairs bile formation even when it is in solution (19), possibly because the lipid-soluble compound damages the bile canalicular membrane.

Although only a small fraction of patients with protoporphyria develop fatal hepatic disease, the incidence of hepatobiliary problems in this disorder may be fairly common (72–74). Variable degrees of hepatocellular necrosis and fibrosis, associated with birefringent pigment deposits, have been found in liver biopsy specimens of patients who have minimal biochemical evidence of liver disease (72,73). Prospective evaluation of a large group of patients with protoporphyria is required to determine the incidence of hepatobiliary abnormalities and the prognosis of these changes.

Therapy in the Porphyrias

Prophylaxis is a cornerstone of management in patients with disorders of porphyrin metabolism. Exogenous factors which initiate or exacerbate symptoms must be avoided, particularly in acute intermittent porphyria, variegate porphyria, and hereditary coproporphyria, in which acute attacks are manifested by neuropsychiatric abnormalities. A variety of drugs, infection, fasting, use of alcohol, and hormonal factors have all been implicated as precipitants of acute attacks (75). The use of enzyme assays to identify asymptomatic individuals who carry the gene defect will increase the importance of preventive counseling.

The administration of hematin has been the most exciting advance in treatment of patients with acute neurological symptoms (76–78). Prior to this, high carbohydrate intake offered the only basic approach to therapy (8). The solution of hematin is prepared by dissolving heme (crystallized from human red cells) in 0.25% sodium carbonate and adjusting the pH of the solution to 8.0. Under these conditions, heme is converted to hematin, as iron is in the ferric state, and hydroxyl radicles are ligands to ferric iron. The usual schedule of administration is 3 to 4 mg/kg i.v. every 12 hr for 3 days, repeating the cycle as necessary.

The rationale for this therapy is that hepatic ALA synthase is regulated by heme through negative feedback control (Fig. 2), as previously discussed. Thus administration of heme in the form of hematin is expected to lower hepatic ALA synthase activity and turn off the excessive production of ALA and PBG. If these compounds are neurotoxic, symptoms should abate as the biochemical abnormality is reversed. Alternatively, if the neurological symptoms are caused by a deficiency of heme in the nervous system, heme may be replenished in this tissue, provided that it can be taken up from plasma.

Irrespective of the mechanism by which neurological abnormalities arise in the porphyrias, administration of hematin may be effective in reversing the attack (77,78). Serum and urinary levels of ALA and PBG decrease markedly during the period in which hematin is administered, and clinical manifestations abate. If paresis has been established due to a prolonged attack, however, hematin administration may not be effective, indicating that therapy should be started early. Adverse effects of hematin administration have been rare.

The cutaneous manifestations of the porphyrias may also be managed effectively. Phlebotomy lowers uroporphyrin excretion and causes skin lesions to heal in patients with porphyria cutanea tarda (79). Abnormalities in liver function reverse, even when alcohol intake is continued (79). Chloroquine can be used to mobilize uroporphyrin from the liver, although some patients have a febrile, hepatotoxic reaction. In protoporphyria, photosensitivity can be ameliorated by the oral intake of beta-carotene (80). The mechanism by which cutaneous symptoms reverse is not precisely known in either case. In porphyria cutanea tarda, phlebotomy appears to lower the production of porphyrins, whereas in protoporphyria, beta-carotene may quench free radicals or trap singlet oxygen in skin.

Since fatal hepatic disease in protoporphyria has been recognized only in the past decade, there is little information concerning appropriate therapy. Preliminary reports indicate that cholestyramine administration may reverse the hepatic disease, theoretically because it binds protoporphyrin in the intestine and interrupts its enterohepatic circulation (72). Conceivably, efforts to modify the rate of protoporphyrin production, such as the administration of hematin, will also prove useful. Early recognition of hepatic disease is probably critical if therapy is to be successful to prevent hepatic protoporphyrin deposition from reaching an irreversible stage.

PORPHYRIN METABOLISM IN HEPATOBILIARY DISORDERS

Since the bile is an important route by which porphyrins are excreted, it is not surprising that urinary porphyrin levels increase in various hepatobiliary diseases. This condition is called secondary porphyrinuria to distinguish it from the abnormal porphyrin metabolism that occurs in the inherited porphyrias. Secondary porphyrinuria is not accompanied by the clinical manifestations observed in the porphyrias.

Urinary excretion of coproporphyrin increases prominently in hepatobiliary diseases (81,82). Uroporphyrin may also increase, but ALA and PBG do not. Because of its poor water solubility, protoporphyrin is not excreted in the urine, even in the face of severe cholestasis.

In extrahepatic biliary obstruction, the increase in urinary coproporphyrin excretion is attended by a higher proportion of the type I isomer than normally occurs (Table 3). This reflects the fact that the type I isomer, which is normally excreted preferentially in bile (21,22), is shunted to the urine. In parenchymal liver disease, two patterns are observed (81). Cirrhosis due to alcoholism is usually associated with a proportion of coproporphyrin I in urine that is similar to that in normal individuals, unless there is extensive hemolysis occurring, whereas the pattern in other types of parenchymal disease is similar to that in biliary obstruction (Table 3). Acute ingestion of alcohol can cause a significant increase in the urinary excretion of coproporphyrin in cirrhotic patients, usually beginning 2 to 4 days after intoxication (83).

Disorders of hepatic organic anion excretion also have abnormal urinary coproporphyrin excretion. In the Dubin-Johnson syndrome, the proportion of isomer I in urine is markedly increased, whereas the total excretion of coproporphyrin remains normal or only mildly increased (84–86). This is in sharp contrast to the Rotor syndrome, in which the pattern is like that in biliary obstruction (87). The reason for the distinct pattern observed in the Dubin-Johnson syndrome is unclear. It does not appear to reflect an associated abnormality in the activity of a heme pathway enzyme (88), although this has not been assessed by direct assay in liver biopsy specimens.

Using the urinary coproporphyrin pattern as a marker of the disease, it has been shown that the

TABLE 3. *Secondary porphyrinuria in hepatobiliary disorders* [a]

Disorder	Total urinary coproporphyrin	Percent as isomer I
Normal	50–280 µg/day	10–50
Parenchymal liver disease		
Alcoholic cirrhosis	↑	Usually <40
Postnecrotic cirrhosis	↑	40–60
Hepatitis	↑	40–60
Biliary obstruction	↑↑	40–60
Rotor syndrome	↑↑	40–80
Dubin-Johnson syndrome	Normal or slight ↑	80–100

[a] Data from refs. 21, 81, 84, 85, 87, and 89.

Dubin-Johnson syndrome is inherited as an autosomal recessive disorder (86). Heterozygotes have a percentage of isomer I that is intermediate between normal individuals and those who express the syndrome.

The activities of the various heme pathway enzymes have not been examined to any extent in patients with hepatobiliary diseases. Hepatic ALA synthase activity is modestly increased in homogenates from cirrhotic livers (89), but the effect of this on hepatic heme metabolism in the patients is uncertain. Both the extent and type of liver damage will undoubtedly influence the activities of the enzymes. Thus some manifestations of hepatobiliary diseases may be due to altered hepatic heme biosynthesis.

ACKNOWLEDGMENT

This work was supported by research grant AM 26466 from the National Institutes of Health.

REFERENCES

1. Watson, C. J. (1947): Some aspects of the porphyrin problem in relation to clinical medicine. The Gordon Wilson Lecture for 1947. *Trans. Am. Clin. Climatol. Assoc.*, 59:163–172.
2. Schmid, R., Schwartz, S., and Watson, C. J. (1954): Porphyrin content of bone marrow and liver in the various forms of porphyria. *AMA Arch. Int. Med.*, 93:167–190.
3. Jones, E. A., Bloomer, J. R., and Berlin, N. I. (1971): The measurement of the synthetic rate of bilirubin from hepatic hemes in patients with acute intermittent porphyria. *J. Clin. Invest.*, 50:2259–2265.
4. Kaufman, L., and Marver, H. S. (1970): Biochemical defects in two types of human hepatic porphyria. *N. Engl. J. Med.*, 283:954–958.
5. Ohashi, A., and Kikuchi, G. (1978): Purification and some properties of two forms of δ-aminolevulinate synthase from rat liver cytosol. *J. Biochem.*, 85:239–247.
6. Granick, S. (1966): The induction in vitro of the synthesis of δ-aminolevulinic acid synthetase in chemical porphyria: A response to certain drugs, sex hormones, and foreign chemicals. *J. Biol. Chem.*, 241:1359–1375.
7. Kappas, A., Song, C. S., Levere, R. D., Sachson, R. A., and Granick, S. (1968): The induction of δ-aminolevulinic acid synthetase in vivo in chick embryo liver by natural steroids. *Proc. Natl. Acad. Sci. USA*, 61:509–513.
8. Tschudy, D. P., Welland, P. H., Collins, A., and Hunter, G. W., Jr. (1964): The effect of carbohydrate feeding on the induction of δ-aminolevulinic acid synthetase. *Metabolism*, 13:396–406.
9. Whiting, M. J., and Granick, S. (1976): δ-Aminolevulinic acid synthase from chick embryo liver mitochondria II. Immunochemical correlation between synthesis and activity in induction and repression. *J. Biol. Chem.*, 251:1347–1353.
10. Granick, S., Sinclair, P., Sassa, S., and Grieninger, G. (1975): Effects by heme, insulin, and serum albumin on heme and protein synthesis in chick embryo liver cells cultured in a chemically defined medium, and a spectrofluorometric assay for porphyrin composition. *J. Biol. Chem.*, 250:9215–9225.
11. Yamauchi, K., Hayashi, N., and Kikuchi, G. (1980): Translocation of δ-aminolevulinate synthase from the cytosol to the mitochondria and its regulation by heme in the rat liver. *J. Biol. Chem.*, 255:1746–1751.
12. Whiting, M. J. (1976): Synthesis of δ-aminolaevulinate synthase by isolated liver polyribosomes. *Biochem. J.*, 158:391–400.
13. Scholnick, P. L., Hammaker, L. E., and Marver, H. S. (1969): Soluble hepatic ALA synthetase: End-product inhibition of the partially purified enzyme. *Proc. Natl. Acad. Sci. USA*, 63:65–70.
14. Wolfson, S. J., Bartczak, A., and Bloomer, J. R. (1979): Effect of endogenous heme generation on δ-aminolevulinic acid synthase activity in rat liver mitochondria. *J. Biol. Chem.*, 254:3543–3546.
15. Tschudy, D. P., Marver, H. S., and Collins, A. (1965): A model for calculating messenger RNA half-life: Short-lived messenger RNA in the induction of mammalian δ-aminolevulinic acid synthetase. *Biochem. Biophys. Res. Commun.*, 21:480–487.
16. Bonkowsky, H. L., Sinclair, P. R., and Sinclair, J. F. (1979): Hepatic heme metabolism and its control. *Yale J. Biol. Med.*, 52:13–37.
17. Sano, S., and Rimington, C. (1963): Excretion of various porphyrins and their corresponding porphyrinogens by rabbits after intravenous injection. *Biochem. J.*, 86:203–212.
18. Rimington, C. (1965): Biliary secretion of porphyrins and hepatogenous photosensitization. In: *The Biliary System*, edited by W. Taylor, pp. 325–333. F. A. Davis, Philadelphia.
19. Avner, D. L., and Berenson, M. M. (1979): Protoporphyrin-induced cholestasis. *Gastroenterology*, 77:A2.
20. Ibrahim, G. W., and Watson, C. J. (1968): Enterohepatic circulation and conversion of protoporphyrin to bile pigment in man. *Proc. Soc. Exp. Biol. Med.*, 127:890–895.
21. Aziz, M. A., and Watson, C. J. (1969): An analysis of the porphyrins of normal and cirrhotic human liver and normal bile. *Clin. Chim. Acta*, 26:525–531.
22. Kaplowitz, N., Javitt, N., and Kappas, A. (1972): Coproporphyrin I and III excretion in bile and urine. *J. Clin. Invest.*, 51:2895–2899.
23. Scholnick, P., Marver, H. S., and Schmid, R. (1971): Erythropoietic protoporphyria: Evidence for multiple sites of excess protoporphyrin formation. *J. Clin. Invest.*, 50:203–207.
24. Grandchamp, B., Phung, N., and Nordmann, Y. (1977): Homozygous case of hereditary coproporphyria. *Lancet*, 2:1348–1349.
25. Benedetto, A. V., Kushner, J. P., and Taylor, J. S. (1978): Porphyria cutanea tarda in three generations of a single family. *N. Engl. J. Med.*, 298:358–362.
26. Kushner, J. P., Barbuto, A. J., and Lee, G. R. (1976): An inherited enzymatic defect in porphyria cutanea tarda: Decreased uroporphyrinogen decarboxylase activity. *J. Clin. Invest.*, 58:1089–1098.
27. Schmid, R. (1960): Cutaneous porphyria in Turkey. *N. Engl. J. Med.*, 263:397–398.
28. Cripps, D. J., and Peters, H. A. (1967): Fluorescing erythrocytes and porphyrin screening tests on urine, stool, and blood. *Arch. Dermatol.*, 96:712–720.
29. Strand, L. J., Felsher, B. F., Redeker, A. G., and Marver, H. S. (1970): Heme biosynthesis in intermittent acute porphyria: Decreased hepatic conversion of porphobilinogen to porphyrins and increased delta-aminolevulinic acid synthetase activity. *Proc. Natl. Acad. Sci. USA*, 67:1315–1320.
30. Bonkowsky, H. L., Tschudy, D. P., Weinbach, F. C., Ebert, P. S., and Doherty, J. M. (1975): Porphyrin synthesis and mitochondrial respiration in acute intermittent porphyria: Studies using cultured human fibroblasts. *J. Lab. Clin. Med.*, 85:93–102.
31. Magnussen, C. R., Levine, J. B., Doherty, J. M., Cheesman, J. O., and Tschudy, D. P. (1974): A red cell enzyme method for the diagnosis of acute intermittent porphyria. *Blood*, 44:857–868.
32. Meyer, U. A. (1973): Clinical and biochemical studies of disordered heme biosynthesis. *Enzyme*, 16:334–342.
33. Meyer, U. A., Strand, L. J., Doss, M., Rees, A. C., and Marver, H. S. (1972): Intermittent acute porphyria—demonstration of a genetic defect in porphobilinogen metabolism. *N. Engl. J. Med.*, 286:1277–1282.
34. Sassa, S., Solish, G., and Levere, R. D. (1975): Studies in porphyria IV. Expression of the gene defect of acute intermittent porphyria in cultured human skin fibroblasts and amniotic cells: Prenatal diagnosis of the porphyric trait. *J. Exp. Med.*, 142:722–731.

35. Bonkowsky, H. L., Bloomer, J. R., Ebert, P. S., and Mahoney, M. J. (1975): Heme synthetase deficiency in human protoporphyria. Demonstration of the defect in liver and cultured skin fibroblasts. *J. Clin. Invest.*, 56:1139–1148.

36. Becker, D. M., Viljoen, J. D., Katz, J., and Kramer, S. (1976): Reduced ferrochelatase activity: A defect common to porphyria variegata and protoporphyria. *Br. J. Haematol.*, 36:171–179.

37. Bottomley, S. S., Tanaka, M., and Everett, M. A. (1975): Diminished erythroid ferrochelatase activity in protoporphyria. *J. Lab. Clin. Med.*, 86:126–131.

38. Brodie, M. J., Moore, M. R., Thompson, G. G., Goldberg, A., and Holti, G. (1977): Haem biosynthesis in peripheral blood in erythropoietic protoporphyria. *Clin. Exp. Dermatol.*, 2:351–388.

39. deGoeij, A. F. P. M., Christianse, K., and van Steveninck, I. (1975): Decreased haem synthetase activity in blood cells of patients with erythropoietic protoporphyria. *Eur. J. Clin. Invest.*, 5:397–400.

40. Elder, G. H., Evans, J. O., Thomas, N., Cox, R., Brodie, M. J., Moore, M. R., Goldberg, A., and Nicholson, D. C. (1976): The primary enzyme defect in hereditary coproporphyria. *Lancet*, 2:1217–1219.

41. Grandchamp, B., and Nordmann, Y. (1977): Decreased lymphocyte coproporphyrinogen III oxidase in hereditary coproporphyria. *Biochim. Biophys. Res. Commun.*, 74:1081–1095.

42. Elder, G. H., Lee, G. B., and Tovey, J. A. (1978): Decreased activity of hepatic uroporphyrinogen decarboxylase in sporadic porphyria cutanea tarda. *N. Engl. J. Med.*, 299:274–278.

43. Felsher, B. F., Norris, M. E., and Shih, J. C. (1978): Red-cell uroporphyrinogen decarboxylase activity in porphyria cutanea tarda and in other forms of porphyria. *N. Engl. J. Med.*, 299:1095–1098.

44. Brenner, D. A., and Bloomer, J. R. (1980): The enzymatic defect in variegate porphyria. Studies with human cultured skin fibroblasts. *N. Engl. J. Med.*, 302:765–769.

45. Waldo, E. D., and Tobias, H. (1973): Needle-like cytoplasmic inclusions in the liver in porphyria cutanea tarda. *Arch. Pathol.*, 96:368–371.

46. Bird, T. D., Hamernyik, P., Nutter, J. Y., and Labbe, R. F. (1979): Inherited deficiency of delta-aminolevulinic acid dehydratase. *Am. J. Hum. Genet.*, 31:662–668.

47. Doss, M., von Tiepermann, R., Schneider, J., and Schmid, H. (1979): New type of hepatic porphyria with porphobilinogen synthase defect and intermittent acute clinical manifestation. *Klin. Wochenschr.*, 57:1123–1127.

48. Dowdle, E. B., Mustard, P., and Eales, L. (1967): δ-Aminolaevulinic acid synthetase activity in normal and porphyric human livers. *S. Afr. Med. J.*, 41:1096–1098.

49. McIntyre, H., Pearson, A. J., Allan, D. J., Craske, S., West, G. M. L., Moore, M. R., Paxton, J., Beattie, A. D., and Goldberg, A. (1971): Hepatic δ-aminolaevulinic acid synthetase in an attack of hereditary coproporphyria and during remission. *Lancet*, 1:560–564.

50. Nakau, K., Wada, O., Kitamura, T., Vono, K., and Urata, G. (1966): Activity of amino-laevulinic acid synthetase in normal and porphyric human livers. *Nature*, 210:838–839.

51. Tschudy, D. P., Perlroth, M. G., Marver, H. S., Collins, A., Hunter, G., Jr., and Rechcigl, M., Jr. (1965): Acute intermittent porphyria: The first "overproduction disease" localized to a specific enzyme. *Proc. Natl. Acad. Sci.*, 53:841–847.

52. Kushner, J. P., Steinmuller, D. P., and Lee, G. R. (1975): The role of iron in the pathogenesis of porphyria cutanea tarda. II. Inhibition of uroporphyrinogen decarboxylase. *J. Clin. Invest.*, 56:661–667.

53. Eales, L. (1963): Porphyria as seen in Cape Town. A survey of 250 patients and some recent studies. *S. Afr. J. Lab. Clin. Med.*, 9:151–161.

54. Stein, J. A., and Tschudy, D. P. (1970): Acute intermittent porphyria. A clinical and biochemical study of 46 patients. *Medicine*, 49:1–16.

55. Sorensen, A. W. S., and With, T. K. (1971): Persistent pareses after porphyric attacks. *S. Afr. J. Lab. Clin. Med.*, 17:101–103.

56. Hellman, E. S., Tschudy, D. P., and Bartter, F. C. (1962): Abnormal electrolyte and water metabolism in acute intermittent porphyria. The transient inappropriate secretion of antidiuretic hormone. *Am. J. Med.*, 32:734–746.

57. Eales, L., and Dowdle, E. B. (1971): The acute porphyric attack I. The electrolyte disorder of the acute porphyric attack and the possible role of delta-aminolaevulic acid. *S. Afr. J. Lab. Clin. Med.*, 17:89–97.

58. Bloomer, J. R., Berk, P. D., Bonkowsky, H. L., Stein, J. A., Berlin, N. I., and Tschudy, D. P. (1971): Blood volume and bilirubin production in acute intermittent porphyria. *N. Engl. J. Med.*, 284:17–20.

59. Stanley, B. C., Neethling, A. C., Percy, V. A., and Carstens, H. (1975): Neurochemical aspects of porphyria. Studies on the possible neurotoxicity of delta-aminolaevulinic acid. *S. Afr. Med. J.*, 49:576–580.

60. Becker, D. M., Viljoen, J. D., and Kramer, S. (1971): The inhibition of red cell and brain ATPase by δ-aminolaevulinic acid. *Biochim. Biophys. Acta*, 225:26–34.

61. Brennan, M. J. W., and Cantrill, R. C. (1979): δ-Aminolaevulinic acid is a potent antagonist for GABA autoreceptors. *Nature*, 280:514–515.

62. Irvine, D. G., and Wetterberg, L. (1972): Kryptopyrrole-like substance in acute intermittent porphyria. *Lancet*, 2:1201.

63. Harber, L. C., and Bickers, D. R. (1975): The porphyrias: Basic science aspects of clinical diagnosis and management. In: *Year Book of Dermatology*, edited by F. D. Malkinson and R. W. Pearson, pp. 9–47. Yearbook Medical Publishers, Chicago.

64. Magnus, I. A., Porter, A. D., and Rimington (1959): The action spectrum for skin lesions in porphyria cutanea tarda. *Lancet*, 1:912–914.

65. Fleischer, A. S., Harber, L. C., Cook, J. S., and Baer, R. L. (1966): Mechanism of in vitro photohemolysis in erythropoietic protoporphyria (EPP). *J. Invest. Dermatol.*, 46:505–509.

66. Slater, T. F., and Riley, P. A. (1966): Photosensitization and lysosomal damage. *Nature*, 209:151–154.

67. Stein, J. A., Bloomer, J. R., Berk, P. D., Corcoran, P. L., and Tschudy, D. P. (1970): The kinetics of organic anion excretion by the liver in acute intermittent porphyria. *Clin. Sci.*, 38:677–686.

68. Haberman, H. F., Rosenberg, F., and Menon, I. A. (1975): Porphyria cutanea tarda: Comparison of cases precipitated by alcohol and estrogens. *Can. Med. Assoc. J.*, 113:653–655.

69. Kordac, V. (1972): Frequency and occurrence of hepatocellular carcinoma in patients with porphyria cutanea tarda in long-term follow-up. *Neoplasma*, 19:135–139.

70. Lundvall, O., Weinfield, A., and Lundin, P. (1970): Iron storage in porphyria cutanea tarda. *Acta Med. Scand.*, 188:37–58.

71. Uys, C. J., and Eales, L. (1968): The histopathology of the liver in acquired (symptomatic) porphyria. *S. Afr. J. Lab. Clin. Med.*, 9:190–197.

72. Bloomer, J. R. (1979): Pathogenesis and therapy of liver disease in protoporphyria. *Yale J. Biol. Med.*, 52:39–48.

73. Cripps, D. J., and Scheuer, P. J. (1965): Hepatobiliary changes in erythropoietic protoporphyria. *Arch. Pathol.*, 80:500–508.

74. DeLeo, V. A., Poh-Fitzpatrick, M., Mathews-Roth, M., and Harber, L. C. (1976): Erythropoietic protoporphyria. Ten years experience. *Am. J. Med.*, 60:8–22.

75. Eales, L. (1979): Porphyria and the dangerous life-threatening drugs. *S. Afr. Med. J.*, 59:914–917.

76. Bonkowsky, H. L., Tschudy, D. P., Collins, A., Doherty, J., Bossenmaier, I., Cardinal, R., and Watson, C. J. (1971): Repression of the overproduction of porphyrin precursors in acute intermittent porphyria by intravenous infusions of hematin. *Proc. Natl. Acad. Sci. USA*, 68:2725–2729.

77. Lamon, J. M., Frykholm, B. C., Hess, R. A., and Tschudy, D. P. (1979): Hematin therapy for acute porphyria. *Medicine*, 58:252–269.

78. Watson, C. J., Pierach, C. A., and Bossenmaier, I. (1978): Use of hematin in the acute attack of the "inducible" hepatic porphyrias. *Adv. Intern. Med.*, 23:126–137.

79. Lundvall, O. (1971): The effect of phlebotomy therapy in porphyria cutanea tarda. *Acta Med. Scand.*, 189:33–49.

80. Mathews-Roth, M. M., Pathak, M. A., Fitzpatrick, T. B., Harber, L. C., and Kass, E. H. (1970): Beta-carotene as a photoprotective agent in erythropoietic protoporphyria. *N. Engl. J. Med.*, 282:1231–1234.

81. Aziz, M. A., Schwartz, S., and Watson, C. J. (1964): Studies of coproporphyrin. VIII. Reinvestigation of the isomer distribu-

tion in jaundice and liver disease. *J. Lab. Clin. Med.*, 63: 596–604.

82. Doss, M. (1980): Pathobiochemical transition of secondary coproporphyrinuria to chronic hepatic porphyria in humans. *Klin. Wochenschr.*, 58:141–148.

83. Sutherland, D., and Watson, C. J. (1951): Studies of coproporphyrin. VI. The effect of alcohol on the per diem excretion and isomer distribution of the urinary coporporphyrins. *J. Lab. Clin. Med.*, 37:29–39.

84. Ben-Ezzer, J., Rimington, C., Shani, M., Seligsohn, V., Sheba, C., and Szeinberg, A. (1971): Abnormal excretion of the isomers of urinary coproporphyrin by patients with Dubin-Johnson syndrome in Israel. *Clin. Sci.*, 40:17–30.

85. Koskelo, P., Toironen, I., and Adelcreutz, H. (1967): Urinary coproporphyrin isomer distribution in the Dubin-Johnson syndrome. *Clin. Chem.*, 13:1006–1009.

86. Wolkoff, A. W., Cohen, L. E., and Arias, I. M. (1973): Inheritance of the Dubin-Johnson syndrome. *N. Engl. J. Med.*, 283:113–117.

87. Wolkoff, A. W., Wolpert, E., Pascasio, F. N., and Arias, I. M. (1976): Rotor's syndrome, a distinct inheritable pathophysiologic entity. *Am. J. Med.*, 60:173–179.

88. Kondo, T., Kuchiba, K., and Shimizu, Y. (1976): Coproporphyrin isomers in Dubin-Johnson syndrome. *Gastroenterology*, 70:1117–1120.

89. Bonkowsky, H. L., and Pomeroy, J. S. (1977): Human hepatic δ-aminolaevulinate synthase: Requirement of an exogenous system for succinyl-coenzyme A generation to demonstrate increased activity in cirrhotic and anti-convulsant-treated subjects. *Clin. Sci. J. Med.*, 52:509–521.

The Liver: Biology and Pathobiology, edited by
I. Arias, H. Popper, D. Schachter, and D. A. Schafritz.
Raven Press, New York © 1982.

Chapter 20

Vitamin A Metabolism

DeWitt S. Goodman

Vitamin A is a generic term used for all compounds that exhibit qualitatively the biological activity of retinol. The term retinoids has been adopted recently as a general term that includes both the natural forms of vitamin A and synthetic analogs, with or without biological activity, of retinol. Vitamin A is necessary for the support of growth, health, and life of higher animals. In the absence of vitamin A, animals will cease to grow and, in time, die. Vitamin A is essential for vision, reproduction, growth, the maintenance of differentiated epithelia, and mucus secretion. The exact nature of the role of vitamin A in these functions has not been defined at the molecular level, except for its well-documented role in vision (1).

The liver plays a major role in vitamin A metabolism. It is critically involved in the uptake, storage, and mobilization of vitamin A and in the regulation of plasma levels and of vitamin A delivery to peripheral target tissues. This chapter reviews our current knowledge about these and related aspects of vitamin A metabolism. Additional information and references can be obtained from recently published reviews on vitamin A (2,3), its plasma transport, and retinol-binding protein metabolism (4,5).

BIOSYNTHESIS AND INTESTINAL ABSORPTION OF VITAMIN A

The major natural sources of vitamin A in the diet are certain plant cartenoid pigments, such as β-carotene, and the long-chain retinyl esters found in animal tissues. β-carotene is converted to vitamin A primarily in the intestinal mucosa. The biosynthetic process involves two soluble enzymes: β-carotene-15,15'-dioxygenase and retinaldehyde reductase. The first catalyzes the cleavage of β-carotene at the central double bond by a dioxygenase mechanism to yield two molecules of retinaldehyde (6); the retinaldehyde then is reduced to retinol.

Dietary retinyl esters are hydrolyzed in the intestine, and the resulting retinol is absorbed into the mucosal cell. Retinol in the mucosal cell (newly absorbed or newly synthesized from carotene) is reesterified with long-chain, mainly saturated, fatty acids; the retinyl esters then are absorbed into the body, mainly in association with lymph chylomicrons. After entry into the vascular compartment, chylomicrons are metabolized by the lipolytic removal of much of the chylomicron triglyceride in extrahepatic tissues. The chylomicron remnant thus formed is a smaller and cholesterol-rich particle which contains essentially all the chylomicron retinyl esters and is removed from the circulation almost entirely by the liver (7).

HEPATIC UPTAKE AND STORAGE

After uptake of the chylomicron retinyl esters, hydrolysis and reesterification occur in the liver. The resulting retinyl esters (mainly retinyl palmitate) are largely stored in association with intracellular lipid droplets. Overall, hepatic retinyl esters normally represent most of the body stores of vitamin A, and 90% or more of the total body reserve of vitamin A is stored in the liver.

The liver is comprised of several different types of cells; it has been questioned which types are involved in vitamin A storage and other aspects of vitamin A metabolism. Several studies have shown that chylomicron remnants or their constituent lipids are taken up by parenchymal cells in the liver. Accordingly, chylomicron retinyl esters are also taken up (and then stored, after hydrolysis and retinol reesterification) by parenchymal cells. It has been shown that the Kupffer cells do not play an important role in the storage of vitamin A in the liver under normal conditions.

Another cell type that has been proposed as a storage site for vitamin A in the liver is the Ito cell (also referred to as fat-storing cells or lipocytes). These cells take up vitamin A into lipid droplets when the vitamin is administered in massive doses and in an unphysiological form (8). Chronic ingestion of large amounts of vitamin A may stimulate fibrogenesis by these cells and result in hepatic disorders (9). It is not clear whether or not Ito cells may be involved to any significant extent in the uptake or storage of vitamin A under physiological conditions. The available evidence suggests, instead, that the Ito cells may be involved in the hepatic pathology resulting from hypervitaminosis A. Available evidence indicates that the parenchymal cells contain most of the vitamin A stored in the liver under normal conditions.

RETINYL ESTER HYDROLYSIS AND VITAMIN A MOBILIZATION

Vitamin A is mobilized from hepatic retinyl ester stores as the free alcohol, retinol, bound to a specific plasma transport protein, retinol-binding protein (RBP). Thus retinyl ester hydrolysis occurs in the liver both during the hepatic uptake of chylomicron retinyl esters and prior to the mobilization of hepatic vitamin A stores.

Only limited information is available about the enzymatic hydrolysis of retinyl esters in liver. It has been shown recently (10) that retinyl palmitate hydrolase activity in rat liver requires a bile salt for stimulation and shows an unusual subcellular distribution, unlike that of known subcellular organelles and structures. Another unusual feature of this enzyme activity is its marked variability from rat to rat as assayed *in vitro*. Other studies have suggested that retinyl palmitate hydrolase has a high degree of hydrophobicity. Since this enzyme presumably acts at a lipid-water interface to hydrolyze retinyl esters stored in lipid droplets or present in the nonpolar core of a chylomicron

remnant, this hydrophobic property may have considerable physiological importance.

PLASMA TRANSPORT: RBP

Vitamin A is transported in plasma as retinol bound to RBP. This is the form in which vitamin A is transported from the liver to peripheral tissues (such as the eye, intestinal mucosa, gonads) to supply their metabolic needs. Since the initial isolation of human RBP in 1968 (11), extensive studies have provided information about the structure, metabolism, and biological roles of this protein. These studies have been reviewed recently (4,5,12). RBP is a single polypeptide chain with a molecular weight close to 20,000 α_1-mobility on electrophoresis, and a single binding site for one molecule of retinol. In plasma, most of the RBP normally circulates as the retinol-RBP complex (holo-RBP).

RBP interacts strongly with another protein, plasma prealbumin, and normally circulates as a 1:1 molar RBP-prealbumin complex. The usual level of RBP in plasma is about 40 to 50 μg/ml; that of prealbumin is about 200 to 300 μg/ml (13). In addition to its role in vitamin A transport, prealbumin plays a role in the binding and plasma transport of thyroid hormones. The formation of the RBP-prealbumin complex serves to reduce the glomerular filtration and renal catabolism of RBP.

Much is now known about the proteins and about the protein-protein and protein-ligand interactions involved in vitamin A transport. In particular, prealbumin is one of the most completely characterized human proteins. The prealbumin molecule is a stable tetramer, composed of four identical subunits with a molecular weight of 54,980. The complete amino acid sequence of prealbumin is known (14) and the full three-dimensional structure of the molecule has been determined by high resolution X-ray crystallography (15). Prealbumin appears to contain four binding sites for RBP, and each prealbumin subunit might contain one binding site for RBP.

Less detailed structural information is available about RBP. Studies employing circular dichroism and optical rotary dispersion have shown that human RBP appears to have a relatively high content of unordered conformation, a significant but small complement of β-conformation, and little or no α-helix. The RBP molecule contains no bound lipid (other than retinol) and no carbohydrate. The complete primary structure of human RBP has been reported (16). Figure 1 is a diagrammatic model for the RBP-prealbumin complex.

Many studies have explored the binding of a variety of retinoids and related compounds to apo-RBP (see ref. 12 for review and references). The structural features required for the binding of all-*trans*-retinol to

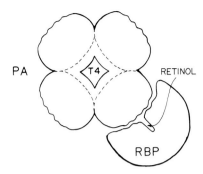

FIG. 1. Diagram for the RBP-prealbumin complex. Prealbumin (PA) is shown as a tetramer containing a central channel that is the site of thyroxine (T4) binding. The locations of the different binding sites suggest the known relationships between the several interactions: RBP and T4 bind at independent sites on prealbumin, whereas the binding of retinol to RBP is stabilized by formation of the protein-protein complex. (Reprinted from ref. 4, with permission.)

RBP appear to be fairly specific. A number of retinoids can bind to apo-RBP with varying degrees of effectiveness. Some of these (including allo-*trans*-retinoic acid) bind to RBP with an affinity similar to that of retinol. Compounds unrelated to vitamin A in structure bind minimally, or not at all, to RBP.

CLINICAL STUDIES ON RBP: LIVER AND KIDNEY DISEASES

RBP is synthesized and secreted by the liver and is largely catabolized in the kidneys. Accordingly, patients with hepatic or renal disease often show disordered metabolism of RBP. In patients with liver disease, the levels of vitamin A, RBP, and prealbumin were markedly decreased and were significantly correlated with each other over a wide range of concentrations (13). The reduced levels of RBP and prealbumin presumably reflected a reduced rate of synthesis of the proteins by the diseased liver. A series of patients with acute hepatitis were studied with serial samples; as the disease improved, the plasma concentrations of vitamin A, RBP, and prealbumin all increased. The RBP concentrations correlated negatively with the values of standard clinical tests of liver function. The levels of RBP and prealbumin appeared to be a valid index of the functional status of the liver. It has been reported that RBP is of value clinically in assessing the course of acute infectious hepatitis and, to a limited extent, in the differentiation of various forms of jaundice.

Patients with chronic liver disease may show impaired dark adaptation in association with low plasma levels of RBP and vitamin A (17). Thus such patients may manifest peripheral vitamin A deficiency symp-

toms secondary to their inability to mobilize vitamin A from the liver. These observations illustrate the key role played by RBP in controlling the delivery of vitamin A to extrahepatic tissues.

In patients with chronic renal disease, the level of RBP (and to a lesser extent of vitamin A) is highly elevated, while prealbumin remains normal (13). The elevated levels of RBP reflect the role of the kidney in RBP catabolism. RBP itself is small enough to be filtered by the renal glomeruli, whereas prealbumin and the RBP-prealbumin complex are not. Although little RBP is normally present in the free (uncomplexed) state, its glomerular filtration and renal metabolism are sufficiently large to constitute the major catabolic route for RBP.

Several studies have examined the plasma retinol transport system in patients with protein-calorie malnutrition. Such patients have decreased concentrations of plasma RBP, prealbumin, and vitamin A. Low intake of dietary protein and calories is frequently accompanied by an inadequate intake of vitamin A. Even in cases where there is adequate vitamin A intake, plasma RBP and vitamin A levels are low, reflecting a functional impairment in the hepatic release of vitamin A because of defective production of RBP in the liver.

RETINOL DELIVERY: RBP RECEPTORS

RBP is responsible for the delivery of retinol from the liver to the extrahepatic sites of action of the vitamin. Evidence indicates that this delivery process may involve cell surface receptors for RBP (see refs. 4 and 5 for references). Thus studies have suggested that there are specific cell surface receptors for RBP on monkey small intestine mucosal cells, bovine pigment epithelial cells, and chicken testicular cell membranes. In these studies, retinol appeared to be taken up (from holo-RBP) by the cells without a concomitant uptake of RBP. Retinol was not taken up by the pigment epithelial cells when it was presented nonspecifically bound to bovine serum albumin. Hence, RBP appears to deliver retinol to specific cell surface sites that "recognize" RBP and to release retinol at these locations. The retinol then enters the cell for subsequent metabolism and action. The apo-RBP does not appear to enter the cell but returns to the circulation, where it shows a reduced affinity for prealbumin and is selectively filtered by the renal glomeruli.

INTRACELLULAR RBP

After delivery of retinol and its uptake into the target cell, retinol may become associated with the intracellular binding protein for retinol (CRBP). It is now well established that a number of tissues of rats, humans, and other species contain soluble proteins with binding specificity for retinol (CRBP) or for retinoic acid (CRABP). These proteins have been purified from several tissues and partly characterized (see ref. 18 for a recent review). Both CRBP and CRABP have molecular weights close to 14,600 and single binding sites for one molecule of retinoid ligand. The intracellular binding proteins differ in a number of ways from plasma RBP and from each other in regard to binding specificity and immunoreactivity.

Interest in CRBP has been stimulated by reports suggesting a relationship between the binding affinity of the proteins for various vitamin A-related compounds and the biological activity of the compounds (18). Furthermore, a number of retinoids with anticarcinogenic activity can associate with the tissue binding proteins; it has been reported that binding ability tends to correlate with biological activity for given compounds (19).

CRBP has been purified from rat liver (20) as well as from other tissues; liver contains a significant concentration of CRBP but does not appear to contain CRABP. The function(s) of CRBP in the liver cell, however, has not been defined. It has been suggested that the intracellular binding proteins may play a direct role in the biological expression of vitamin A activity (e.g., analogous to steroid hormone receptors), and that CRBP may be involved in facilitating the specific interaction of retinol with binding sites for retinol in the cell nucleus. Another possibility is that CRBP serves in the liver cell as an intracellular transport protein, acting to transport retinol from one locus to another. Thus, for example, after hydrolysis of a molecule of retinyl palmitate, CRBP may transport the retinol to a newly synthesized molecule of RBP for secretion as the retinol-RBP complex. Future research is needed to explore these and other possibilities.

REGULATION OF RBP PRODUCTION AND SECRETION BY THE LIVER

Vitamin A mobilization from the liver and its delivery to peripheral tissues are highly regulated by factors that control the rates of RBP production and secretion by the liver. Studies have been conducted to attempt to elucidate the cellular and molecular mechanisms involved in the regulation of RBP production and secretion (see refs. 4 and 5 for reviews and references). These studies have employed the rat as an animal model and a sensitive and specific radioimmunoassay for rat RBP.

One factor that specifically regulates RBP secretion from the liver is the nutritional vitamin A status of the animal (21). Thus retinol deficiency specifically blocks the secretion of RBP from the liver, so that plasma RBP levels fall, and liver RBP levels rise. Conversely, repletion of vitamin A-deficient rats intravenously with retinol stimulates the rapid secretion of RBP from the expanded liver pool (in the deficient rat) into the plasma. This release of RBP is not blocked by inhibitors of protein synthesis, indicating that it comes from the expanded liver pool of RBP rather than from *de novo* protein synthesis.

The block in RBP secretion seen after vitamin A depletion is highly specific for RBP. Thus neither vitamin A depletion and deficiency nor retinol repletion of deficient rats significantly altered plasma levels of prealbumin. Secretion of RBP and prealbumin is an independently regulated process, with formation of the RBP-prealbumin complex occurring in plasma after secretion of the two proteins from the liver cell.

The roles of various subcellular organelles and structures in the secretion of RBP have been studied. RBP in the liver is found mainly associated with the liver microsomes and is particularly enriched in the rough microsomal fraction. The Golgi apparatus was found to contain a maximum of 23% of RBP in the liver in normal rats and a maximum of less than 10% of the expanded pool of liver RBP in vitamin A-deficient rats (22). Presumptive evidence that the microtubules are involved in the secretion of RBP has been obtained in studies with the drug colchicine. These recent studies suggest that the Golgi apparatus and secretory vesicles are involved in the pathway of RBP secretion from the liver but also demonstrate that the Golgi is not the major subcellular locus for RBP in either normal or vitamin A-deficient rats.

Two lines of differentiated rat hepatoma cells were found that synthesize RBP during culture *in vitro* (23). When the cells were incubated in a vitamin A-free serumless medium, a relatively large proportion of the RBP synthesized was retained within the cells. Addition of retinol to the medium (at levels of 0.1 or 1 μg/ml) stimulated the release of RBP from the cells into the medium and also increased the net synthesis of RBP. In contrast, retinol had no effect on either the synthesis or secretion of rat serum albumin by these cells. Thus these cell lines respond to vitamin A depletion and repletion in a manner similar to that of the intact rat liver cell *in vivo*.

More recent studies with glucocorticoid hormones demonstrated that these hormones markedly stimulate the net synthesis of RBP by rat hepatoma cells. When retinol and dexamethasone were added together to the incubation medium, the stimulatory effects were roughly additive. An optimal effect was obtained with approximately 5 to 10 $\times$ 10^{-9} M dexamethasone. In addition, studies with progesterone suggest that steroid hormone receptors are involved in the dexamethasone effect. The presence of dexamethasone did not alter the stimulatory effect of retinol on the secretion of RBP from the cells into the medium. Thus dexamethasone and retinol have distinctly separate effects on RBP metabolism by the liver cell.

Figure 2 summarizes the information available on vitamin A and RBP metabolism in the liver cell. While the rough endoplasmic reticulum appears to be a major subcellular location of RBP, we do not know the subcellular locus at which retinol normally interacts and forms a complex with RBP in the liver cell. The mechanism whereby this event (i.e., the formation of the retinol-RBP complex) regulates the secretion of RBP remains to be defined.

VITAMIN A AND GLYCOPROTEIN AND MEMBRANE METABOLISM

Vitamin A is necessary for the maintenance of normal differentiation and of mucus secretion of epithelial tissues. The biosynthesis of some glycoproteins is decreased in vitamin A deficiency and enhanced upon administration of excessive doses. It has been suggested that retinol or a derivative may serve as the lipid portion of a glycolipid intermediate involved in certain glycosylation reactions (see refs. 3,24,and 25 for reviews and references). Thus in this hypothesis, retinol is thought to function in a manner analogous to dolichol in specific glycosyl transfer reactions. It has been suggested that these particular glycosylation reactions may be involved in the biosynthesis of specific glycoproteins in vitamin A-requiring tissues. If this were true, then specific defects in glycoprotein synthesis would occur in vitamin A deficiency and might explain the range of abnormalities seen in vitamin A deficiency; glycoproteins are common constituents of membrane systems and are involved in a variety of biological functions.

Evidence has been reported that is consistent with this hypothesis. Retinyl phosphate, formed in liver and other tissues, has been identified as a constituent of mammalian membranes. Its glycosylated derivative, mannosyl retinyl phosphate, has also been shown to be formed both *in vivo* and *in vitro*. The enzyme system that forms mannosyl retinyl phosphate is located primarily in the rough endoplasmic reticulum of rat liver cells. Under appropriate conditions, glycosyl transfer can be demonstrated from the retinol glycolipid to membrane glycoproteins. It is not known whether this occurs *in vivo* under normal conditions.

The hypothesis that retinoid-containing glycoproteins are obligatory intermediates for specific glycosylation reactions is intriguing. At present, however, with the information available, the validity of this hypothesis remains to be established.

LIVER STORES AND VITAMIN A STATUS

In general, plasma levels of vitamin A tend to remain relatively constant for a given individual. The amount of vitamin A stored in the liver, however, can vary markedly, depending on nutritional vitamin A status. There is little or no correlation between plasma and liver levels of vitamin A. Since the liver is the main storage site for vitamin A, estimates of the vitamin A status of a population have been obtained by determining the vitamin A content of samples of liver obtained at autopsy. The results of such studies as carried out in the United States (26,27) and Canada (28) have shown a wide variation within a population and a significant number of persons with abnormally low levels. These studies have raised the question of the possible existence of significant nutritional inadequacies.

The assessment of vitamin A status from liver samples requires attention to the nature of the sample analyzed. Vitamin A is not homogeneously distributed in the liver. In a recent study, the distribution of vitamin A in human livers was examined in detail (29); concentrations varied tremendously throughout the liver, from values close to zero up to more than 400 μg/g. The distribution of values for any single liver showed, in addition to considerable dispersion, a significant skewing to the right. Mean vitamin A values of samples taken from the midcentral portion of the right lobe generally agreed within 15% with the overall mean values. It was concluded that with proper sam-

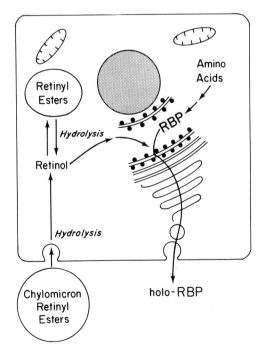

FIG. 2. Diagram summarizing the metabolism of vitamin A and RBP in the hepatocyte. (Reprinted from ref. 4, with permission.)

pling techniques, a single sample of liver may still serve as a useful indicator of the vitamin A status of an individual.

REFERENCES

1. Wald, G. (1968): Molecular basis of visual excitation. *Science,* 162:230–239.
2. Goodman, DeW. S. (1980): Vitamin A metabolism. *Fed. Proc.,* 39:2716–2722.
3. De Luca, L. M. (1978): Vitamin A. In: *Handbook of Lipid Research, Vol. 2,* edited by H. F. DeLuca, pp. 1–67. Plenum, New York.
4. Smith, J. E., and Goodman, DeW. S. (1979): Retinol-binding protein and the regulation of vitamin A transport. *Fed. Proc.,* 38:2504–2509.
5. Goodman, DeW. S. (1980): Plasma retinol-binding protein. *Ann. NY Acad. Sci.,* 348:378–390.
6. Goodman, DeW. S., and Olson, J. A. (1969): The conversion of all-trans β-carotene into retinal. In: *Methods in Enzymology, Vol. XV, Steroids and Terpenoids,* edited by R. B. Clayton, pp. 462–475. Academic Press, New York.
7. Goodman, DeW. S., Huang, H. S., and Shiratori, T. (1965): Tissue distribution and metabolism of newly absorbed vitamin A in the rat. *J. Lipid Res.,* 6:390–396.
8. Hirosawa, K., and Yamada, E. (1973): The localization of the vitamin A in the mouse liver as revealed by electron microscope radioautography. *J. Electron Microsc.,* 22:337–346.
9. Kent, G., Gay, S., Inouye, T., Bahu, R., Minick, O. T., and Popper, H. (1976): Vitamin A-containing lipocytes and formation of type III collagen in liver injury. *Proc. Natl. Acad. Sci. USA,* 73:3719–3722.
10. Harrison, E. H., Smith, J. E., and Goodman, DeW. S. (1979): Unusual properties of retinyl palmitate hydrolase activity in rat liver. *J. Lipid Res.,* 20:760–771.
11. Kanai, M., Raz, A., and Goodman, DeW. S. (1968): Retinol-binding protein: The transport protein for vitamin A in human plasma. *J. Clin. Invest.,* 47:2025–2044.
12. Goodman, DeW. S. (1976): Retinal-binding protein, prealbumin, and vitamin A transport. In: *Trace Components of Plasma: Isolation and Clinical Significance,* edited by G. A. Jamieson and T. J. Greenwalt, pp. 313–330. Alan R. Liss, New York.
13. Smith, F. R., and Goodman, DeW. S. (1971): The effect of diseases of the liver, thyroid, and kidneys on the transport of vitamin A in human plasma. *J. Clin. Invest.,* 50:2426–2436.
14. Kanda, Y., Goodman, DeW. S., Canfield, R. E., and Morgan, F. J. (1974): The amino acid sequence of human plasma prealbumin. *J. Biol. Chem.,* 249:6796–6805.
15. Blake, C. C. F., Geisow, M. J., Oatley, S. J., Rérat, B., and Rérat, C. (1978): Structure of prealbumin: Secondary, tertiary, and quarternary interactions determined by Fourier refinement at 1.8 Å. *J. Mol. Biol.,* 121:339–356.
16. Rask, L., Anundi, H., and Peterson, P. A. (1979): The primary structure of the human retinol-binding protein. *FEBS Lett.,* 104:55–58.
17. Patek, A. J., Jr., and Haig, C. (1939): The occurrence of abnormal dark adaptation and its relation to vitamin A metabolism in patients with cirrhosis of the liver. *J. Clin. Invest.,* 18:609–616.
18. Chytil, F., and Ong, D. E. (1979): Cellular retinol- and retinoic acid-binding proteins in vitamin A action. *Fed. Proc.,* 38:2510–2514.
19. Jetten, A. N., and Jetten, M. E. R. (1979): Possible role of retinoic acid binding protein in retinoid stimulation of embryonal carcinoma cell differentiation. *Nature,* 278:180–182.
20. Ong, D. E., and Chytil, F. (1978): Cellular retinol-binding protein from rat liver. Purification and characterization. *J. Biol. Chem.,* 253:828–832.
21. Muto, Y., Smith, J. E., Milch, P. O., and Goodman, DeW. S. (1972): Regulation of retinol-binding protein metabolism by vitamin A status in the rat. *J. Biol. Chem.,* 247:2542–2550.
22. Harrison, E. H., Smith, J. E., and Goodman, DeW. S. (1980): Effects of vitamin A deficiency on the levels and distribution of retinol-binding protein and marker enzymes in homogenates and Golgi-rich fractions of rat liver. *Biochim. Biophys. Acta,* 628:489–497.
23. Smith, J. E., Borek, C., and Goodman, DeW. S. (1978): Regulation of retinol-binding protein metabolism in cultured rat liver cell lines. *Cell,* 15:865–873.
24. De Luca, L. M. (1977): The direct involvement of vitamin A in glycosyl transfer reactions of mammalian membranes. *Vitam. Horm.,* 34:1–57.
25. De Luca, L. M., Bhat, P. V., Sasak, W., and Adamo, S. (1979): Biosynthesis of phosphoryl and glycosyl phosphoryl derivatives of vitamin A in biological membranes. *Fed. Proc.,* 38:2535–2539.
26. Underwood, B. A., Siegel, H., Weisell, R. C., and Dolinski, M. (1970): Liver stores of vitamin A in a normal population dying suddenly or rapidly from unnatural causes in New York City. *Am. J. Clin. Nutr.,* 23:1037–1042.
27. Mitchell, G. V., Young, M., and Seward, C. R. (1973): Vitamin A and carotene levels of a selected population in metropolitan Washington, D.C. *Am. J. Clin. Nutr.,* 26:992–997.
28. Hoppner, K., Phillips, W. E. J., Murray, T. K., and Campbell, J. S. (1968): Survey of liver vitamin A stores of Canadians. *Can. Med. Assoc. J.,* 99:983–986.
29. Olson, J. A., Gunning, D., and Tilton, R. (1979): The distribution of vitamin A in human liver. *Am. J. Clin. Nutr.,* 32:2500–2507.

The Liver: Biology and Pathobiology, edited by
I. Arias, H. Popper, D. Schachter, and D. A. Shafritz.
Raven Press, New York © 1982.

Chapter 21

Vitamin D Metabolism

John Edgar Smith

Several major advances have been made in the last 15 years in the understanding of the function and metabolism of vitamin D. Several excellent review articles describing these advances in detail have been published (1–3). The early work on vitamin D was thoroughly reviewed by Deuel (4).

Vitamin D plays an important role in the regulation of the dynamics of calcium and phosphorus metabolism. In particular, serum calcium level is maintained near 10 mg/100 ml with remarkable consistency, despite the extremely rapid flux of calcium in and out of the bloodstream. Vitamin D exerts its effects on the serum calcium and phosphorus levels by (a) mobilizing calcium and phosphorus from bone, (b) increasing the intestinal absorption of calcium and phosphorus, and (c) increasing calcium retention by the kidney.

While many forms of vitamin D exist, only two are of nutritional or biological significance: vitamin D_3 (cholecalciferol), which is derived from animal sources, and vitamin D_2 (ergocalciferol), which is prepared from the plant sterol ergosterol (see Fig. 1).

Vitamin D is unique among the vitamins in that the entire requirement can be met by a photolysis reaction in the skin as well as by dietary intake. Exposure of the skin to ultraviolet light can result in the conversion of 7-dehydrocholesterol to vitamin D_3 (5).

Newly absorbed dietary vitamin D enters the circulation as a component of the chylomicron (6). In contrast to vitamin A, where the retinyl esters are the predominant form in the chylomicron, the chylomicron vitamin D is principally in the form of the free alcohol (6). This suggests that vitamin D is likely to be a surface component of the chylomicron rather than a constituent of its hydrophobic core (like retinyl esters). Studies with vitamin A have shown that the retinyl esters remain with the chylomicron remnant and

are almost totally cleared from circulation by the liver. Similar studies have not been done with vitamin D. Since vitamin D may be largely a surface component, much of it may leave the chylomicron during the process of lipolysis. The amount of vitamin D thus stored in extrahepatic tissues may be considerable, since skeletal muscle and adipose tissue (which is active in the lipolysis of chylomicron triglyceride) have been shown to be the major sites of vitamin D reserves in both humans (7) and experimental animals (8).

The initial step in the activation of vitamin D occurs in the liver, where vitamin D_3 is converted to 25-hydroxycholecalciferol (25-OHD$_3$). 25-OHD$_3$ constitutes a major portion of the vitamin D activity that circulates in blood. Vitamin D and its metabolites circulate in serum bound to a specific transport protein, called the binding protein for vitamin D, or DBP, and its metabolites. Although 25-OHD$_3$ is two to five times more active (on a weight basis) than vitamin D_3, 25-OHD$_3$ at physiological levels does not directly stimulate the intestinal absorption of calcium or the mobilization of calcium from bone.

The active form of vitamin D is synthesized in the kidney by the conversion of 25-OHD to 1,25-dihydroxycholcalciferol [1,25(OH)$_2$D$_3$]. The production of 1,25(OH)$_2$D$_3$ is tightly regulated by the levels of phosphate and parathyroid hormone. Since the secretion of parathyroid hormone is regulated by the serum calcium level, the synthesis of 1,25(OH)$_2$D$_3$ and the serum calcium level are inversely correlated. When adequate levels of serum calcium and phosphate are present, 24(R),25-dihydroxycholecalciferol [24,25(OH)$_2$D$_3$] is the major metabolite of vitamin D formed in the kidney, rather than 1,25(OH)$_2$D$_3$. The function of 24,25(OH)$_2$D$_3$ is not yet understood.

While the role of vitamin D in the intestinal absorp-

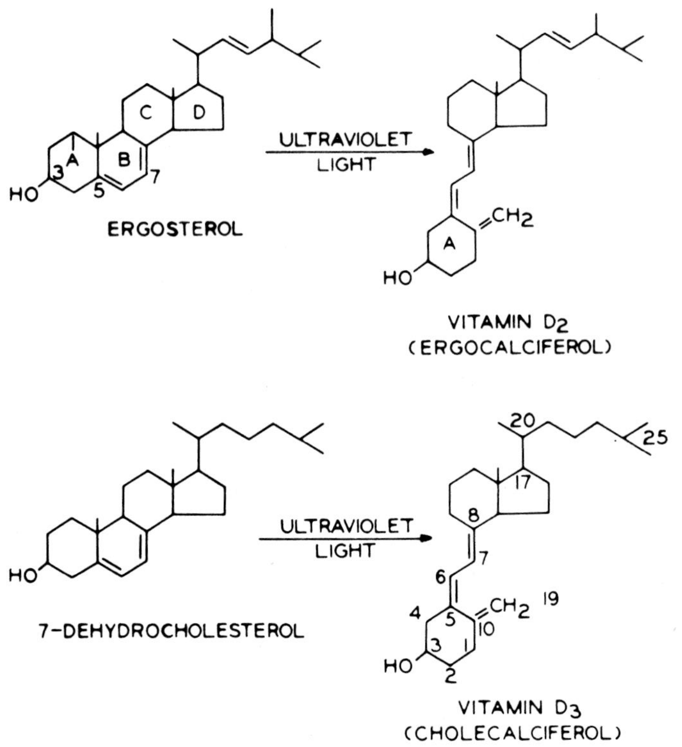

FIG. 1. Structures of vitamins D_2 and D_3 and their sterol precursors. (From ref. 1, by permission of *Nutrition Reviews.*)

tion of calcium has been the most extensively studied function of vitamin D and the vitamin is required to maintain a cellular transport mechanism for the cation, the mechanism by which $1,25(OH)_2D_3$ stimulates the absorption of calcium at a molecular level is not understood. $1,25(OH)_2D_3$ has been shown to induce the synthesis of a vitamin D-dependent calcium-binding protein in the intestine (9). However, this synthesis is not essential for $1,25(OH)_2D_3$ to stimulate the absorption of calcium; the function of the vitamin D-dependent calcium-binding protein remains to be defined.

ROLE OF THE LIVER IN VITAMIN D METABOLISM

The liver has two distinct functions in vitamin D metabolism: (a) conversion of vitamin D_3 to 25-OHD$_3$, and (b) synthesis of DBP. In addition, the liver may serve as a transient store for some vitamin D after its absorption. Unfortunately, no studies on vitamin D metabolism after absorption have been reported in which chylomicrons have been used as the injection vehicle. In the studies that have been conducted, vitamin D has been injected in a nonphysiological form, either as an ethanol solution or mixed in serum. Both these procedures result in an abnormal distribution of vitamin D among the serum proteins and thus do not yield physiologically valid information.

Both tracer and bioassay studies show that the liver contains a small store of vitamin D, but it is also clear

that the liver is not the major storage site for vitamin D (8). This contrasts markedly to the situation with vitamin A, where most of the vitamin is stored in the liver.

CONVERSION OF VITAMIN D_3 TO 25-OHD$_3$

The liver is the major site of the 25-hydroxylation of vitamin D. Although chick kidney and intestine have been reported to possess calciferol-25-hydroxylase activity, the significance of these tissues in the physiological 25-hydroxylation of vitamin D has been questioned (10). Hepatectomy virtually eliminates the ability of the rat to produce 25-OHD$_3$.

Studies with isolated liver cells have suggested that the hepatocyte is the cell responsible for the 25-hydroxylation of vitamin D. In these short-term incubations, production of 25-OHD$_3$ was not influenced by the deletion of either calcium or phosphate from the incubation medium. There is some controversy about the subcellular location of rat liver calciferol-25-hydroxylase. Studies conducted by DeLuca and his colleagues at Wisconsin (12) with physiological levels of vitamin D have suggested that calciferol-25-hydroxylase is a microsomal enzyme that depends on the addition of a cytosol fraction for the optimum production of 25-OHD$_3$. The cytosol fraction has been reported to both prevent the destruction of vitamin D_3 and stimulate the biosynthesis of 25-OHD$_3$. Several studies have suggested that the microsomal calciferol-25-hydroxylase is regulated to some extent by the vitamin D status of the rat. The K_m of

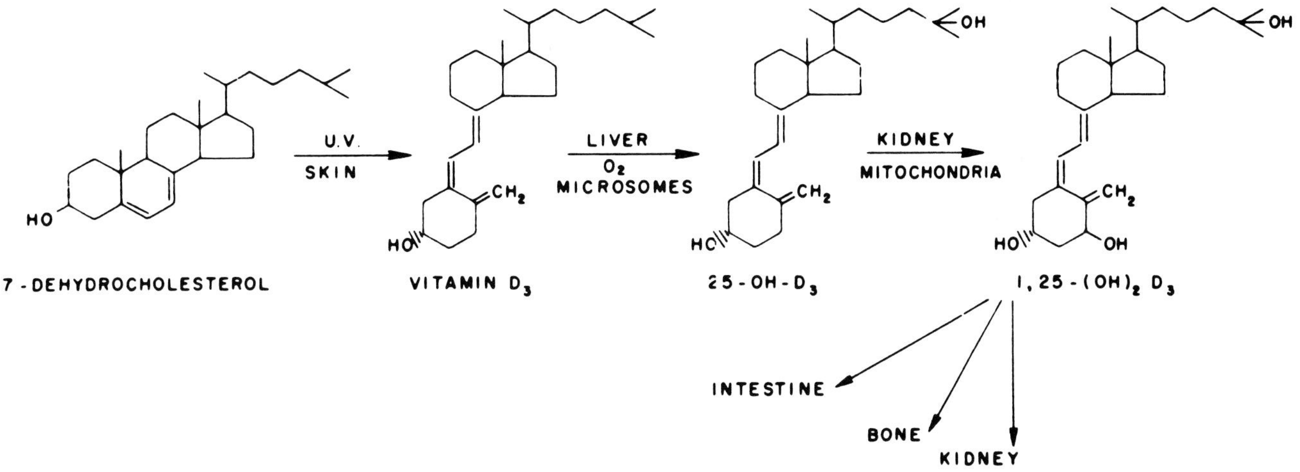

FIG. 2. Functional metabolism of vitamin D to activate target organs. (From ref. 1, by permission of *Nutrition Reviews.*)

calciferol-25-hydroxylase is significantly higher in animals with a normal vitamin D intake than in vitamin D-deficient animals (13). The mechanism by which the enzyme is regulated, however, is unclear.

Studies conducted with saturating levels of vitamin D_3 have demonstrated considerable calciferol-25-hydroxylase activity in an unwashed or crude mitochondrial fraction (14). This enzyme activity was thought to be associated with the outer mitochondrial membrane and to be distinctly different from the cholesterol-25-hydroxylase activity associated with the inner mitochondrial membrane. This enzyme was not regulated by the prior vitamin D status of the animal.

Both the microsomal and mitochondrial enzymes appear to be mixed function oxygenases that require molecular oxygen, NADPH, and cytochrome P-450 (14–17). The literature suggests that when vitamin D intake is in the normal range, the microsomal enzyme is the functional calciferol-25-hydroxylase, and the synthesis of 25-OHD$_3$ is regulated to some extent. In contrast, when massive doses of vitamin D are ingested, the mitochondrial enzyme, which is not regulated, appears to produce large amounts of 25-OHD$_3$, which circulate in the blood at several thousand times the normal level. These high levels, however, do not appear to influence the production of 1,25(OH)$_2$D$_3$. The kidney 1-hydroxylase enzyme is so well regulated that, despite the elevated 25-OHD$_3$ levels, the serum levels of 1,25(OH)$_2$D$_3$ remain in the normal range.

Although the levels of calciferol-25-hydroxylase may be slightly lowered in patients with hepatitis or cirrhosis, vitamin D deficiency symptoms do not appear as a result of a lack of calciferol-25-hydroxylase activity. On the other hand, it is not uncommon for these patients to have low serum levels of 25-OHD$_3$ and to develop osteomalacia. These low levels are related to a reduced ability of these patients to absorb vitamin D or to little exposure to sunlight, since the administration of 600 to 750 IU of vitamin D daily rapidly returns the serum levels of 25-OHD to normal (18).

PLASMA TRANSPORT OF VITAMIN D AND ITS METABOLITES

Vitamin D and all its common nonesterified metabolites circulate in plasma bound to a specific transport protein, DBP. The isolation of human DBP was independently reported in 1976 in three laboratories (19–21). Human DBP contains a single binding site for vitamin D and its metabolites, and estimates of its molecular weight range from 52,000 (21) to 59,000 (20). In normal humans, the plasma concentration of DBP ranges from 300 to 600 μg/ml. Only 2 to 3% of the DBP circulates with bound 25-OHD or vitamin D. Thus there is a large excess of DBP in plasma relative to the amount of vitamin D and its metabolites.

As suggested by Daiger et al. (22), DBP is identical with the group-specific component (Gc) protein of human plasma. Prior to the recognition of its transport function, Gc proteins were extensively studied as genetic marker proteins. Three common phenotypes (Gc 1-1, Gc 2-1, and Gc 2-2) of DBP have been found in varying proportions throughout the world. In addition, a large number of rare Gc phenotypes have also been observed. All the major genetic variants of DBP appear to have similar binding properties for vitamin D and its metabolites (23). DBP exhibited similar apparent association constants for 25-OHD$_3$ and 24,25(OH)$_2$D$_3$ ($\sim$ 1 to 2 $\times$ 10^8 M^{-1}). Lower affinities were found for 1,25(OH)$_2$D$_3$ ($\sim$ 1 $\times$ 10^7 M^{-1}) and for vitamin D$_3$ ($\sim$ 3 to 4 $\times$ 10^5 M^{-1}) in all the genetic variants studied (23).

The vitamin D transport system differs markedly from the well-characterized vitamin A transport system in that (a) vitamin D and all its metabolites are transported by the same protein; (b) DBP acquires its ligand (vitamin D and its metabolites) from several tissues in addition to liver; (c) most of the DBP circulates in the apo form (without vitamin D), and (d) the secretion of DBP is not regulated by vitamin D status.

All available evidence suggests that beyond the association of newly absorbed vitamin D with chylomicrons, the transport of vitamin D or its metabolites between tissues occurs with the compound bound to DBP. This includes (a) transport of newly synthesized vitamin D_3 from the skin (to the liver for 25-hydroxylation); (b) transport of 25-OHD$_3$ from the liver to the kidney (for 1-hydroxylation); (c) transport of 24,25(OH)$_2$D$_3$ from the kidney, and (d) transport of 1,25(OH)$_2$D$_3$ from the kidney to the various target tissues.

The liver is the only organ that has been demonstrated to synthesize DBP. During *in vitro* incubations with tissue slices, liver was the only tissue to incorporate radioactive amino acids into immunoprecipitable DBP (24). This conclusion has been further strengthened by clinical studies in patients with hepatitis and cirrhosis (18,25). In patients with liver disease, serum levels of DBP were significantly decreased. DBP levels correlated with serum albumin levels in these patients (18). Thus the low levels of DBP presumably reflect a reduced rate of protein synthesis by the diseased liver. Serum DBP levels were also negatively correlated with serum bilirubin levels. While DBP is particularly low in early phase hepatitis and cirrhosis ($\sim 60\%$ of normal), the levels are not low enough to impede the normal transport of vitamin D or its metabolites. This contrasts markedly to the vitamin A transport system, in which a reduction in retinol-binding protein production will produce vitamin A deficiency symptoms, despite normal vitamin A intake.

DBP has been detected in the cytosol fraction of all nucleated tissues (26). Recent studies have shown that cytosol DBP exists as a 1:1 molar complex with actin (27). Thus this observation accounts for the 5-6 S vitamin D binding protein detected in all nucleated tissues. DBP has been shown to depolymerize filamentous actin (F-actin) but will bind to the actin-deoxyribonuclease I complex without disrupting the complex. At present, it remains unclear if DBP is internalized during the delivery of vitamin D and its metabolites; the DBP-actin complex has some physiological role; or the cytoplasmic DBP simply represents a contamination of the cytosol fractions with serum.

REFERENCES

1. DeLuca, H. F. (1979): The vitamin D system in the regulation of calcium and phosphorus metabolism. *Nutr. Rev.*, 37:161–193.

2. DeLuca, H. F. (1980): Some new concepts emanating from a study of the metabolism and function of vitamin D. *Nutr. Rev.*, 38:169–182.

3. Haussler, M. R., and McCain, T. A. (1977): Basic and clinical concepts related to vitamin D metabolism and action. *N. Engl. J. Med.*, 297:974–983; 1041–1051.

4. Deuel, H. J., Jr. (1951, 1955, 1957): *The lipids. Their Chemistry and Biochemistry*. Volumes I, II, and III. Interscience, New York.

5. Holick, M. F., and Clark, M. B. (1978): The photobiogenesis and metabolism of vitamin D. *Fed. Proc.*, 37:2567–2574.

6. Schachter, D., Finkelstein, J. D., and Kowarski, S. (1964): Metabolism of vitamin D. I. Preparation of radioactive vitamin D and its intestinal absorption in the rat. *J. Clin. Invest.*, 43:787–796.

7. Mawer, E. B., Backhouse, J., Holman, C. A., Lumb, G. A., and Stanbury, S. W. (1972): The distribution and storage of vitamin D and its metabolites in human tissues. *Clin. Sci.*, 43:413–431.

8. Rosenstreich, S. J., Rich, C., and Volwiler, W. (1971): Deposition in and release of vitamin D_3 from body fat: Evidence for a storage site in the rat. *J. Clin. Invest.*, 50:679–687.

9. Spencer, R., Charman, M., Emtage, J. S., and Lawson, D. E. M. (1976): Production and properties of vitamin D-induced mRNA for chick calcium-binding protein. *Eur. J. Biochem.*, 71:399–409.

10. Olson, E. B., Jr., Knutson, J. D., Bhattacharyya, M. H., and DeLuca, H. F. (1976): The effect of hepatectomy on the synthesis of 25-hydroxyvitamin D_3. *J. Clin. Invest.*, 57:1213–1220.

11. Reitano, J. F., Reed, M. A., Rostron, P. L., Intenzo, C. M., and Capuzzi, D. M. (1977): In vitro metabolism of vitamin D_3 by isolated liver cells. *Mol. Cell. Biochem.*, 15:213–217.

12. Bhattacharyya, M. H., and DeLuca, H. F. (1974): Subcellular location of rat liver calciferol-25-hydroxylase. *Arch. Biochem. Biophys.*, 160:58–62.

13. Delvin, E. E., Arabian, A., and Glorieux, F. H. (1978): Kinetics of liver microsomal cholecalciferol 25-hydroxylase in vitamin D-depleted and -repleted rats. *Biochem. J.*, 172:417–422.

14. Bjorkhem, I., and Holmberg, I. (1978): Assay and properties of a mitochondrial 25-hydroxylase active on vitamin D_3. *J. Biol. Chem.*, 253:842–849.

15. Madhok, T. C., Schnoes, H. K., and deLuca, H. F. (1978): Incorporation of oxygen-18 into the 25-position of cholecalciferol by hepatic cholecalciferol 25-hydroxylase. *Biochem. J.*, 175:479–482.

16. Madhok, T. C., and DeLuca, H. F. (1979): Characteristics of the rat liver microsomal enzyme system converting cholecalciferol into 25-hydroxycholecalciferol. Evidence for the participation of cytochrome P-450. *Biochem. J.*, 184:491–499.

17. Pedersen, J. I., Holmberg, I., and Bjorkhem, I. (1979): Reconstitution of vitamin D_3 25-hydroxylase activity with a cytochrome P-340 preparation from rat liver mitochondria. *FEBS Lett.*, 98:394–398.

18. Imawari, M., Akanuma, Y., Itakura, H., Muto, Y., Kosaka, K., and Goodman, DeW. S. (1979): The effects of diseases of the liver on serum 25-hydroxyvitamin D and on the serum binding protein for vitamin D and its metabolites. *J. Lab. Clin. Med.*, 93:171–180.

19. Bouillon, R., Van Baelen, H., Rombauts, W., and De Moor, P. (1976): The purification and characterisation of the human-serum binding protein for the 25-hydroxycholecalciferol (Transcalciferin). Identity with group-specific component. *Eur. J. Biochem.*, 66:285–291.

20. Haddad, J. G., Jr., and Walgate, J. (1976): 25-hydroxy vitamin D transport in human plasma. Isolation and partial characterization of calcifidiol-binding protein. *J. Biol. Chem.*, 251:4803–4809.

21. Imawari, M., Kida, K., and Goodman, DeW. S. (1976): The transport of vitamin D and its 25-hydroxy metabolite in human plasma. Isolation and partial characterization of vitamin D and 25-hydroxy vitamin D binding protein. *J. Clin. Invest.*, 58:514–523.

22. Daiger, S. P., Schanfield, M. S., and Cavalli-Sforza, L. L.

(1975): Group-specific component (Gc) proteins bind vitamin D and 25-hydroxyvitamin D. *Proc. Natl. Acad. Sci. USA,* 72:2076–2080.

23. Kawakami, M., Imawari, M., and Goodman, DeW. S. (1979): Quantitative studies of the interaction of cholecalciferol (vitamin D₃) and its metabolites with different genetic variants of the serum binding protein for these sterols. *Biochem. J.,* 179:413–423.

24. Prunier, J. H., Bearn, A. G., and Cleve, H. (1964): Site of formation of the group-specific component and certain other serum proteins. *Proc. Soc. Exp. Biol. Med.,* 115:1005–1007.

25. Barragry, J. M., Corless, D., Auton, J., Carter, N. D., Long, R. G., Maxwell, J. D., and Switala, S. (1978): Plasma vitamin D-binding globulin in vitamin D deficiency, pregnancy and chronic liver disease. *Clin. Chim. Acta,* 87:359–365.

26. Cooke, N. E., Walgate, J., and Haddad, J. G., Jr. (1979): Human serum binding protein for vitamin D and its metabolites. II. Specific, high affinity association with a protein in nucleated tissue. *J. Biol. Chem.,* 254:5965–5971.

27. Van Baelen, H., Bouillon, R., and De Moor, P. (1980): Vitamin D-binding protein (Gc-globulin) binds actin. *J. Biol. Chem.,* 255:2270–2272.

The Liver: Biology and Pathobiology, edited by
I. Arias, H. Popper, D. Schachter, and D. A. Shafritz.
Raven Press, New York © 1982.

Chapter 22

Vitamin K

Paul A. Friedman

HISTORY

The discovery of the fat-soluble vitamin K was serendipitous. In 1929, while conducting studies of sterol metabolism, Henrik Dam (1) observed that chicks developed hemorrhages when fed fat-free diets. The blood of such animals showed delayed coagulation. Later it was shown that depressed levels of prothrombin (coagulation factor II) activity in the plasma led to hemorrhage. None of the established nutrients, including vitamins A, D, E, or ascorbic acid, could prevent the disease, and Dam designated the active principle in normal feed as vitamin K (for the German word *koagulation*). Furthermore, he showed that liver and leafy green vegetables were particularly abundant in the vitamin. Isolation of the active principle from alfalfa was followed by delineation of the structure of vitamin K_1 (phylloquinone):2-methyl-3-phytyl-1,4-naphthoquinone (Fig. 1). Soon thereafter, the structures of the animal K vitamins, the menaquinones, were described.

During these same years, a mysterious hemorrhagic disease, first reported by Schofield in 1922 (2), was observed in cattle; it was called "sweet clover disease" because only cattle that had foraged on improperly cured sweet clover developed hemorrhages, which were sometimes fatal. The hemorrhage was associated with depression of plasma prothrombin activity. Campbell and Link (3) later reported that the anticoagulant in spoiled clover is bishydroxycoumarin (Fig. 2), which is an antagonist to vitamin K. Used as rodenticides by virtue of their hemorrhagic effects

and later introduced to the clinic as anticoagulants, bishydroxycoumarin and the other 4-hydroxycoumarin drugs provided new tools to investigate the complexities of blood coagulation and the existence of vitamin K-dependent proteins other than prothrombin. Subsequently, three additional coagulation factors were discovered to be vitamin K dependent: (a) proconvertin (factor VII), (b) Stuart factor (factor X), and (c) Christmas factor (factor IX).

After more than 30 years of unsuccessful efforts to discern the function of vitamin K, several lines of evidence emerged in the 1960s and early 1970s suggesting that vitamin K is required for a posttranslational modification of a prothrombin precursor which results in conversion of the precursor to an active prothrombin. One series of studies showed that, when cows or humans are treated with 4-hydroxycoumarin anticoagulants, they secrete nonfunctional prothrombins into their plasmas which can be identified immunologically because of cross reaction with antibodies generated to their respective normal prothrombins. In fact, these plasmas, which possess only a small fraction of the normal complement of functional prothrombin, contained prothrombin immunogen in nearly normal concentration.

In other experiments, rats were made hypoprothrombinemic either by feeding them a vitamin K-deficient diet or by giving them a 4-hydroxycoumarin anticoagulant. The rats then received vitamin K parenterally. Subsequently, a curvilinear time course of the appearance of active prothrombin in plasma was observed. This finding is consistent with a pool of pre-

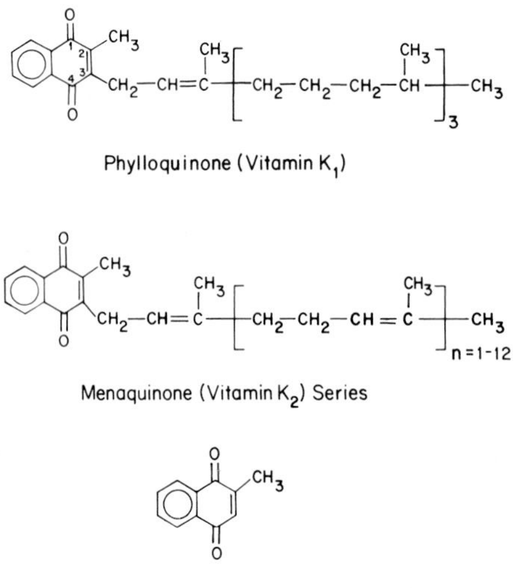

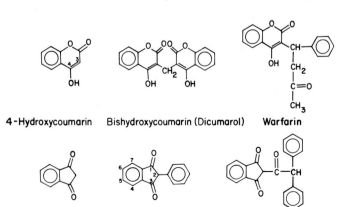

FIG. 1. Structures of various vitamins K.

cursor protein that could be converted to prothrombin. When the hypoprothrombinemic rats were given cycloheximide just prior to vitamin K, the prothrombin produced was not labeled with isotope when radioactive amino acids were administered at the same time as the vitamin. Plasma prothrombin had apparently been generated from an existing unlabeled precursor protein pool. Microsomes prepared from the livers of vitamin K-deficient rats contained material that was converted to thrombin by the proteases of certain venoms (such as that of the pit viper, *Echis carinatus*) but not by activated factor X (Xa), the physiologic activator.

Finally, it was shown that after incubation of these microsomes in the presence of vitamin K, much of the precursor was converted to a form that could be cleaved readily to thrombin by factor Xa. It should be emphasized that, unlike the human or cow, the vitamin K-deficient or anticoagulated rat retains most of its precursor in the hepatic endoplasmic reticulum rather than secreting it as a nonfunctional prothrombin.

Several laboratories independently purified large quantities of abnormal prothrombin from the plasma of cows which were anticoagulated with bishydroxy-

coumarin. A comparison of some of the characteristics of this molecule to those of normal bovine prothrombin is shown in Table 1. To ascertain the structural differences between normal and abnormal prothrombins, Stenflo and co-workers (4) isolated a tryptic peptide containing residues 4–10 of normal bovine prothrombin; this peptide was degraded further with aminopeptidase M and carboxypeptidase B. The resulting tetrapeptide (residues 6–9) possessed the sequence leucyl-glutamyl-glutamyl-valine by the standard Edman sequencing techniques. When exposed to an electrophoretic field, however, it had too much anodal mobility for its apparent amino acid composition. The tetrapeptide was examined by proton nuclear magnetic resonance spectroscopy and mass spectrometry; each "glutamyl" residue was shown to possess an extra carboxyl group situated on the gamma carbon atom. Thus the tetrapeptide possessed a heretofore unknown amino acid called γ-carboxyglutamic acid (γ-CGlu) (Fig. 3). The corresponding peptide of the prothrombin purified from the plasma of the anticoagulated cows had glutamyl residues in these positions. Shortly thereafter, both Nelsestuen and co-workers (5) and Magnusson and co-workers (6) reported the presence of γ-CGlu in prothrombin, thus confirming the observations of Stenflo et al. (4).

As a malonic acid derivative, γ-CGlu is labile to hot acid. It is converted by decarboxylation to glutamic acid during the acid hydrolysis routinely employed prior to amino acid analyses and in standard sequencing technique. It can be demonstrated directly, however, if alkaline hydrolysis is used prior to amino acid analysis.

These landmark studies, conducted 40 years after the discovery of vitamin K, confirmed that the function of the vitamin is to provide for posttranslational carboxylation of glutamyl residues in the prothrombin precursor as well as in precursors of other vitamin K-dependent proteins. After the discovery of γ-CGlu, sequencing of prothrombin revealed that γ-CGlu residues were located at positions 7, 8, 15, 17, 20, 21, 26, 27, 30, and 33 (Fig. 4). Thus the first 10 glutamyl resi-

4-Hydroxycoumarin   Bishydroxycoumarin (Dicumarol)   Warfarin

Indan-1,3-dione   Phenindione   Diphenadione

FIG. 2. Structures of several 4-hydroxycoumarin and indandione anticoagulants.

TABLE 1. *Some properties of normal and abnormal bovine prothrombins*

Property	Normal	Abnormal
Calcium binding	+	−
Barium adsorption	+	−
Activation by factor Xa	+	−
Activation by *E. carinatus* venom	+	+

dues in the N-terminal sequence of prothrombin are converted to γ-CGlu; of the 43 possible glutamyl residues in prothrombin, only these 10 are carboxylated. The mechanism of this specificity awaits clarification. The additional carboxyl groups of the γ-CGlu residues confer upon prothrombin the capacity to interact with phospholipid surfaces in the presence of calcium; this interaction accelerates the rate of cleavage of prothrombin to thrombin by factor Xa (Fig. 5).

THE VITAMIN K-DEPENDENT CARBOXYLATION REACTION

The normal *in vivo* function of vitamin K depends on a number of enzymatic activities (Fig. 6) which constitute a metabolic cycle for the vitamin. In this cycle, the vitamin first is reduced from its quinone to its hydroquinone form; the latter participates in the γ-glutamyl carboxylation reaction. During incubations of vitamin K with liver microsomes, a portion of vitamin K is converted to its 2,3-epoxide. While not proved, current evidence suggests strongly that this conversion is coupled to the carboxylation reaction. The epoxide is not active in the γ-carboxylation reaction; but another enzyme, vitamin K epoxide reductase, converts the epoxide back to the naphthoquinone so that the cycle can proceed anew. The levels of characterization of these various enzymes differ.

The enzyme catalyzing the reduction of vitamin K

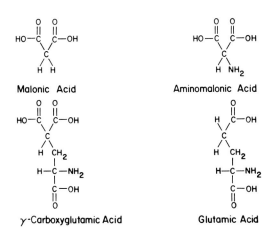

FIG. 3. Structures of γ-carboxyglutamic acid and related compounds.

naphthoquinone likely is identical or similar to the enzyme DT-diaphorase, also called NAD(P)H dehydrogenase or NAD(P)H-K oxidoreductase. The original designation, DT diaphorase, was applied because the enzyme catalyzes the oxidation of both NADH (DPNH) and NADPH (TPNH) in the presence of various organic dyes and quinones, including vitamins K. Electrons are accepted by the enzyme from either NADH or NADPH and then are transferred to the substrate (vitamin K):

$$NADH(NADPH) + E \rightarrow NAD^+ (NADP^+) + EH$$
$$EH + S \rightarrow E + SH$$

The diaphorase, which appears to be cytosolic or at most only loosely associated with membranes, has been purified to homogeneity. It has a molecular weight of 55,000 daltons and contains two nonidentical subunits of equal molecular weight plus one mole FAD per mole enzyme.

The enzyme that catalyzes the conversion of Glu residues in protein substrates to γ-CGlu residues (the vitamin K-dependent γ-glutamyl carboxylase) was first described by Suttie (7). It is an intrinsic membrane protein, located in the endoplasmic reticulum, and has not been purified extensively. As such, only its basic requirements are known. Either vitamin K naphthoquinone, a reduced pyridine nucleotide, and a vitamin K reductase (? DT diaphorase), or chemically prepared vitamin K hydroquinone are needed: additional requirements include molecular oxygen, an appropriate substrate, and either bicarbonate or CO_2. Neither biotin nor ATP appear to be involved.

In the rat liver, the activity of the enzyme (as well as the levels of endogenous substrates, such as prothrombin precursor) increases when the animals are fed a diet deficient in vitamin K and/or are given a 4-hydroxycoumarin anticoagulant. The enzyme can be solubilized in a variety of nonionic detergents and, in this form, will carboxylate, in addition to endogenous protein substrates, short Glu-containing peptide sequences of prothrombin (e.g., Phe-Leu-Glu-Glu-Leu) and even a substrate as simple as tBOC-glutamic acid α-benzoate.

More discriminating subcellular fractionation studies demonstrate that the rough endoplasmic reticulum is enriched markedly, not only in carboxylase activity, but also in epoxidase and epoxide reductase activities. Furthermore, since detergent-solubilized microsomes but not intact microsomes carboxylate the pentapeptide, Phe-Leu-Glu-Glu-Leu, and since the carboxylase in intact microsomes is relatively resistant to trypsin while that in detergent-solubilized microsomes is inhibited markedly, the transverse orientation of the carboxylase is such that its active site may be accessible only from the lumen of the endoplasmic reticulum.

1				5					10
Ala	Asn	Lys	Gly	Phe	Leu	γ-CGlu	γ-CGlu	Val	Arg
				15					20
Lys	Gly	Asn	Leu	γ-CGlu	Arg	γ-CGlu	Cys	Leu	γ-CGlu
				25					30
γ-CGlu	Pro	Cys	Ser	Arg	γ-CGlu	γ-CGlu	Ala	Phe	γ-CGlu
				35					
Ala	Leu	γ-CGlu	Ser	Leu	Ser	Ala	Thr		

FIG. 4. N-terminal sequence of bovine prothrombin.

Matschiner and co-workers (8) first described the existence of the 2,3-epoxide in liver and later demonstrated its *in vitro* formation in liver microsomes. Coupling of the vitamin K epoxidase activity to the carboxylase is suggested by a number of criteria: (a) basic requirements for both activities are similar; (b) both activities are proportional to the amount of prothrombin precursor present in liver; (c) inhibitors that block carboxylation (such as 2-chloro-3-phytyl-1,4-naphthoquinone or 2,3,5,6-tetrachloro-4-pyridinol) also block epoxidation; (d) tissues in which carboxylation has been detected are those in which epoxidase activity can be found; (e) only those vitamins K that support carboxylation have been shown to be converted to their respective epoxides by liver microsomes; (f) when carboxylation and epoxidation are measured in the same *in vitro* incubations, the stoichiometry approaches 1 at high bicarbonate concentrations. It is likely that it will be shown that each carboxylation event normally results in one epoxidation event.

The precise role of vitamin K in the carboxylation reaction needs clarification. Evidence suggests that the γ-glutamyl carboxylase catalyzes a reaction in which an oxygenated species of vitamin K, perhaps a 2- or 3-hydroperoxide, effects the cleavage of the γ-carbon-hydrogen bond of appropriate glutamyl residues and that, subsequent to the breaking of this bond,

a carboxylation normally occurs. Thus the vitamin, in a form activated by oxygen, is involved primarily with cleaving the γ-carbon-hydrogen bond. Evidence also suggests that either during or after this cleavage, the 2,3-epoxide of the vitamin is formed, regardless of whether or not a carboxylation ensues. The following is a generalized mechanistic scheme compatible with available data:

1. $KH_2 \rightarrow KH\cdot \overset{O_2}{\rightarrow} K[OO]$
2a. $K[OO] \rightarrow \rightarrow \rightarrow KO$ or
2b. $K[OO] \rightarrow \rightarrow \rightarrow KO$

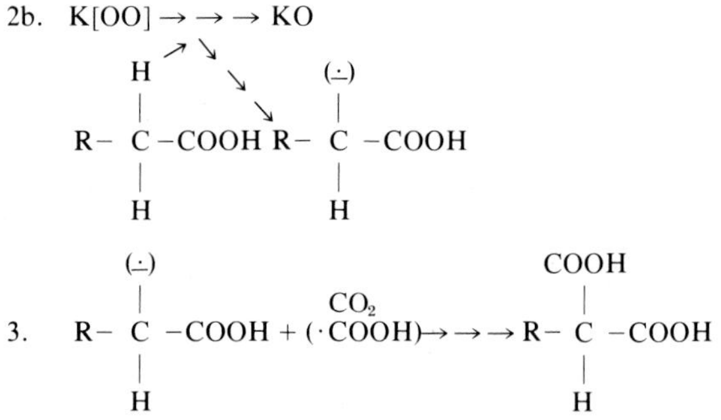

KH_2 = hydroquinone; $KH\cdot$ = semiquinone; $K[OO]$ = oxygenated intermediate (hydroperoxide or peroxy radical); KO = epoxide.

The data available do not distinguish between formation of a radical or carbanion at the γ-carbon of the glutamyl residue or the electronic nature of the attacking species. Although not depicted, it is also conceivable that the vitamin intermediate activates a heme

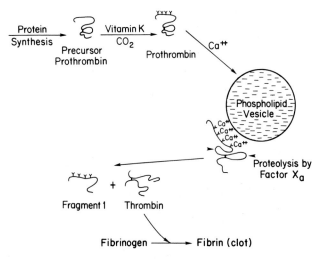

FIG. 5. Scheme of synthesis of an active prothrombin molecule and its proteolysis to thrombin by factor Xa.

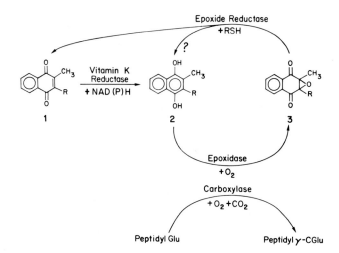

FIG. 6. Metabolic cycle for vitamin K and its coupling to γ-glutamyl carboxylation.

moiety or other reaction center, which in turn drives the carboxylation.

The final enzyme of the cycle shown in Fig. 6 reduces the vitamin K naphthoquinone 2,3-epoxide back to the naphthoquinone. This enzyme, the vitamin K epoxide reductase, also is located in the endoplasmic reticulum. It is dependent on sulfhydryl reagents for its *in vitro* function and is inhibited strongly by 4-hydroxycoumarin and indandione anticoagulants.

BIOSYNTHESIS AND PROCESSING OF PRECURSOR PROTHROMBINS

The ribonucleic acid messages for prothrombin and the three other vitamin K-dependent coagulation factors are translated on ribosomes of the hepatic rough endoplasmic reticulum. Since eventually these molecules are secreted from hepatocytes into the circulation, it is anticipated, although not proved, that they initially possess a secretory end piece which, as for other proteins to be secreted, directs them through the membrane of the rough endoplasmic reticulum to the interior of that organelle. Not only are they then modified by the vitamin K-dependent γ-glutamylcarboxylase but, since they are also glycoproteins, they are glycosylated prior to their secretion.

Studies with cultured hepatoma cells have shed light on the sequence of posttranslational events leading to the completion of the prothrombin molecule. These experiments, in which precursor prothrombins were followed from their translation until their secretion into the media as completed prothrombin, indicate that carboxylation occurs in the rough endoplasmic reticulum; the majority of glycosylation, as expected, occurs in the smooth endoplasmic reticulum as well as in the Golgi apparatus. Thus, since proteins to be secreted move from the rough to the smooth endoplasmic reticulum and then to the Golgi apparatus, carboxylation occurs prior to most glycosylation, although the degree of overlap between these two types of posttranslational modifications remains to be elucidated.

EFFECTS OF ANTICOAGULANTS

Oral anticoagulants, the 4-hydroxycoumarins and the indandiones, lower the functional plasma levels of coagulation factors II, VII, IX, and X. This results in a state of anticoagulation in which both the prothrombin time and the partial thromboplastin time are prolonged. As in the state of anticoagulation produced by a deficiency of vitamin K, this anticoagulant-induced decrease in human plasma levels of the functional coagulation factors is not accompanied by a decrease in the level of the respective antigens present in the

plasma; i.e., the abnormal coagulation factors, those not possessing γ-CGlu, circulate but are nonfunctional. This explanation is somewhat simplistic in that evidence from studies in both the cow and the human suggest that after clinically acceptable lowering of functional prothrombin levels (15 to 20% of normal), not only are there abnormal prothrombins in the plasma totally devoid of γ-CGlu but there also are multiple species of abnormal prothrombins that possess some but not all of the normal complement of γ-CGlu. The locations of the γ-CGlu on these partially carboxylated prothrombins are undetermined.

With respect to the mechanism of action of these anticoagulants, the most compelling evidence suggests that they act not by interference with the γ-glutamyl carboxylation reaction per se but rather by inhibition of the epoxide reductase, thereby preventing conversion of the inactive 2,3-epoxide form of the vitamin back to the active naphthoquinone. Strong evidence comes from *in vitro* assays of the several hepatic vitamin K-metabolizing enzymes from strains of rats resistant to the 4-hydroxycoumarins. When the sensitivities to the anticoagulants of the enzymes were studied and compared to the sensitivities of the same enzymes derived from the livers of rats sensitive to the anticoagulants, it was found that only the epoxide reductase manifested an intrinsic resistance to the oral anticoagulants (Table 2). Virtually complete inhibition of the epoxide reductase from sensitive animals occurs at micromolar concentrations of anticoagulant, while inhibition of this enzyme from resistant rats requires 50 times more drug. Inhibition of the carboxylase (and/or epoxidase) is seen only in the millimolar range. Fifty percent inhibition of the DT diaphorase occurs at 10^{-5} M concentration, but the enzymes derived from the livers of both sensitive and resistant rats are inhibited equally.

PHARMACOLOGY OF AND REQUIREMENTS FOR VITAMIN K IN THE HUMAN

Although mammals can prenylate the naphthoquinone ring system, they are incapable of synthesizing the ring itself and depend on dietary sources. Phyl-

TABLE 2. *Inhibition of enzymes by warfarin*

Enzyme	Sensitive rats	Resistant rats
DT diaphorase	10^{-5} M[a]	10^{-5} M
Carboxylase (and/or epoxidase)	10^{-3} M	10^{-3} M
Epoxide reductase	10^{-6} M	5×10^{-5} M

[a] Concentrations of warfarin producing approximately 50% inhibition of the respective enzyme in appropriate *in vitro* assays.

loquinone (vitamin K_1), found in plants, is an important source. It is the only natural vitamin K available for therapeutic use. In addition, menaquinones, synthesized by some strains of bacteria in the mammalian intestine, are absorbed and found in animal tissues. Among the large number of synthetic naphthoquinone derivatives that have vitamin K procoagulant activity, 2-methyl-1,4-naphthoquinone (vitamin K_3), commonly known as menadione, has been used therapeutically and is as active on a molar basis as phylloquinone.

The manner in which the fat-soluble vitamins K are transported from the intestine to critical organs, especially the liver, has not been delineated. The vitamin is present not only in liver but in most other tissues of the body and, in fact, probably is present in the largest amounts in skeletal muscle, although its function in that tissue and some others remains undefined. Human liver possesses a variety of K vitamins, including phylloquinone and menaquinones-7 to -11, with the principle vitamins being phylloquinone and menaquinone-7. Within the hepatocyte (and presumably other cell types), these vitamins are concentrated in membranes and are found not only in the endoplasmic reticulum but also in the mitochondrial and nuclear membranes.

Although there is no generally accepted figure for the minimum daily requirement of vitamin K for the human adult, it appears to be extremely small; that for phylloquinone is on the order of 0.03 μg/kg body weight. Requirements are almost always satisfied by the average diet; additional vitamin, synthesized by intestinal bacteria, is available to the host. The chief clinical manifestation of vitamin K deficiency is increased bleeding tendency resulting in ecchymosis, epistaxis, hematuria, gastrointestinal bleeding, postoperative hemorrhage, and, less commonly, intracranial hemorrhage.

Vitamin K is given in pharmacologic doses to counter the effects of excessive anticoagulation from either 4-hydroxycoumarins or indandiones. Since intestinal absorption is unreliable, replacement therapy with vitamin K should be with a derivative of phylloquinone administered parenterally. The synthetic provitamin, menadione, can be given orally. However, it can cause hemolytic anemia in the newborn as well as in individuals who are glucose-6-phosphate dehydrogenase deficient. In addition, since it is ineffective in the presence of the oral anticoagulants, it is used rarely.

While it is known that almost no unmetabolized vitamin K appears in bile or urine, the detailed catabolic fate of vitamin K is unknown. A metabolite common to both phylloquinone and the menaquinones is one in which the side chain has been shortened to seven carbon atoms with a terminal carboxylic acid. This metabolite ultimately is excreted as a glucuronide.

Little vitamin K is stored in the body. Under circumstances in which lack of bile interferes with vitamin K absorption, the limited stores of the vitamin in the liver are depleted gradually; hypoprothrombinemia develops slowly over a period of several weeks. Whether the stores in tissues other than liver are dissipated at a comparable rate is not known. For example, it would be possible for hypoprothrombinemia still to occur if these stores did turn over more slowly but were unavailable to the liver in sufficient concentrations because they only slowly escape these tissue stores and/or because the vitamin could be catabolized *in situ* to inactive forms.

VITAMIN K AND PATHOLOGIC CONDITIONS

Several categories of disease exist in which the normal vitamin K-dependent carboxylation of coagulation factor precursors fails to occur. In the malabsorption syndromes, malabsorption of fat and fat-soluble substances leads to a deficiency of vitamin K. The resulting prolonged prothrombin and partial thromboplastin times can be normalized if vitamin K is administered parenterally. This normalization is rapid, occurring over the course of several days. In chronic obstructive hepatic disease, lack of bile also results in malabsorption with insufficient absorption of vitamin K; here, too, parenteral administration of vitamin K will correct the prolonged clotting times. By contrast, hepatocellular disease, severe enough to prolong clotting times, does not respond to parenteral vitamin K with normalization of the prothrombin time. Occasionally, a patient with hepatocellular disease, such as an alcoholic, may manifest vitamin K deficiency and have a partial response to the administration of the vitamin; rarely will this bring the prothrombin time into the normal range.

Although uncommon, there are people who have been on marginal diets long enough to prolong their prothrombin times. Hypoprothrombinemia is especially likely to occur if these individuals also are given broad spectrum antibiotics, which decrease the level of gut flora and, thus, another source of vitamin K.

At present, there are no data comparing the levels of either plasma prothrombin antigen, the hepatic prothrombin precursors, or the enzymes critical to vitamin K function in different disease states. In particular, these data might be of diagnostic, therapeutic, or prognostic value in the various forms of hepatic dysfunction.

One interesting albeit rare adverse reaction to the parenteral administration of vitamin K consists of an indurated erythematous skin reaction at the injection

	1*				5						10					15					20					25
PROTHROMBIN	Ala	Asn	Lys	Gly		Phe	Leu	γ-CGlu	γ-CGlu	-	Val		Arg	Lys	Gly	Asn	Leu	γ-CGlu	Arg	γ-CGlu	Cys	Leu	γ-CGlu	γ-CGlu	Pro	Cys	Ser	Arg	γ-CGlu
FACTOR X	Ala	Asn	Ser	-		Phe	Leu	γ-CGlu	γ-CGlu	-	Val		Lys	Gln	Gly	Asn	Leu	γ-CGlu	Arg	γ-CGlu	Cys	Leu	γ-CGlu	γ-CGlu	Ala	Cys	Ser	Leu	γ-CGlu
PROTEIN C	Ala	Asn	Ser	-		Phe	Leu	γ-CGlu	γ-CGlu	-	Leu		Arg	Pro	Gly	Asn	Val	γ-CGlu	Arg	γ-CGlu	Cys	Ser	γ-CGlu	γ-CGlu	Val	Cys	?	Phe	γ-CGlu
FACTOR IX	Tyr	Asn	Ser	Gly		Lys	Leu	γ-CGlu	γ-CGlu	Phe	Val		Arg	-	Gly	Asn	Leu												
PROTEIN S	Ala	Asn	Thr	-		Leu	Leu	γ-CGlu	γ-CGlu	-	Thr		Lys	Lys	Gly	Asn	Leu												

				30						35				
PROTHROMBIN	γ-CGlu	Ala	Phe	γ-CGlu		Ala	Leu	γ-CGlu	Ser		Leu	Ser		Ala	Thr
FACTOR X	γ-CGlu	Ala	Arg	γ-CGlu		Val	Phe	γ-CGlu	Asp		Ala	γ-CGlu		Gln	Thr
PROTEIN C	γ-CGlu	Ala	Arg	γ-CGlu		Ile	Phe	?	Asn		Thr	?		?	Thr

*The numbering is that of prothrombin.

FIG. 7. Sequence homologies of some vitamin K-dependent plasma proteins.

site. This can develop when oil preparations of phylloquinone are given to individuals with hepatic dysfunction. The etiology of this reaction is unknown.

OTHER VITAMIN K-DEPENDENT PROTEINS AND CARBOXYLATING SYSTEMS

It is known that vitamin K-dependent proteins other than coagulation factors II, VII, IX, and X are synthesized and secreted into the plasma. In particular, proteins C and S are plasma proteins with amino terminal sequences homologous to those of the four vitamin K-dependent coagulation factors (Fig. 7). It seems likely that these two molecules also are synthesized and secreted by the liver. In addition to liver, the lung, spleen, kidney, pancreas, and placenta have been found to possess vitamin K-dependent γ-glutamyl carboxylating enzyme systems with endogenous substrates. The physiologic role of these systems remains to be established.

REFERENCES

1. Dam H. (1929): Cholesterinstoffwechsel in hühnereiern und huhnchen. *Biochem. Z.*, 215:475–492.
2. Schofield, F. W. (1924): Damaged sweet clover: Cause of a new disease in cattle simulating hemorrhagic septicemia and blackleg. *J. Am. Vet. Med. Assoc.*, 64:553–575.
3. Campbell, H. A., and Link, K. P. (1941): Studies on the hemorrhagic sweet clover disease. IV. The isolation and crystallization of the hemorrhagic agent. *J. Biol. Chem.*, 138:21–33.
4. Stenflo, J., Fernlund, P., Egan, W., and Roepstorff, P. (1974): Vitamin K dependent modifications of glutamic acid residues in prothrombin. *Proc. Natl. Acad. Sci. USA*, 71:2730–2733.
5. Nelsestuen, G. L., Zytkovicz, T. H., and Howard, J. B. (1974): The mode of action of vitamin K. Identification of γ-carboxyglutamic acid as a component of prothrombin. *J. Biol. Chem.*, 249:6347–6350.
6. Magnusson, S., Sottrup-Jensen, L., Peterson, T. E., Morris, H. R., and Dell, A. (1974): Primary structure of the vitamin K-dependent part of prothrombin. *FEBS Lett.*, 44:189–193.
7. Suttie, J. W. (1973): Mechanism of action of vitamin K: Demonstration of a liver precursor of prothrombin. *Science*, 179:192–194.
8. Matschiner, J. T., Bell, R. G., Amellotti, J. M., and Knauer, T. E. (1970): Isolation and characterization of a new metabolite of phylloquinone in the rat. *Biochim. Biophys Acta.*, 201:309–315.

The Liver: Biology and Pathobiology, edited by
I. Arias, H. Popper, D. Schachter, and D. A. Shafritz.
Raven Press, New York © 1982.

Chapter 23

The Liver in Relation to the B Vitamins

Darla E. Danford and Hamish N. Munro

Vitamins are organic substances that must be provided by the diet so that the tissues can make cofactors for metabolic processes. They differ from essential trace minerals, which are inorganic nutrients, and from the essential amino acids, which are organic constituents of the diet needed in much larger quantities. Chemically, the vitamins represent a variety of unrelated organic substances. When the vitamin occurs in more than one chemical form (e.g., pyridoxine, pyridoxal, pyridoxamine) or as a precursor (e.g., carotene for vitamin A), these analogs are commonly referred to as vitamers. The needs of people of different ages for each vitamin are suggested by the Recommended Dietary Allowances (RDA), of which the ninth edition has just appeared (1).

Following the discovery of the first vitamins early in this century, it soon became apparent that there were two main classes—fat-soluble and water-soluble—and that each class contained several active factors. The water-soluble vitamins include vitamin C and the vitamin B complex, which consists of seven active factors; thiamin (B$_1$), riboflavin (B$_2$), nicotinic acid, vitamin B$_6$, folic acid, cyanocobalamin (B$_{12}$), biotin, and pantothenic acid. These were grouped together because they occurred in high concentrations in certain foods, notably liver. Their continued classification together is justified by the similarity of their dietary sources and the consequent tendency for deficiency diseases to involve more than one member.

Three other compounds—choline, inositol, and para-aminobenzoic acid—have traditionally been included among the B complex vitamins. Since evidence of human dietary need for these is lacking (1), we do not consider them here.

Fat-soluble vitamins are mainly absorbed into the thoracic duct and bypass the liver. In contrast, the water-soluble B vitamins pass into the portal vein, presumably at higher concentrations than in the peripheral blood for some time after each meal, and thus are exposed to the actions of the liver. Some water-soluble vitamins are retained in large amounts by the liver, an organ that weighs about 2 kg in a 70-kg man. Table 1 shows that, by comparison with the RDA for adults, the concentration per kilogram liver is 5 to 100 times greater for riboflavin, nicotinic acid, B$_{12}$, folic acid, and pantothenic acid, whereas the liver concentrations per kilogram thiamin, B$_6$, and biotin are roughly equivalent to 1 day's needs of each vitamin. Preferential retention of some water-soluble vitamins in the liver is confirmed by the appreciably higher concentrations of riboflavin, B$_{12}$, folic acid, and pantothenic acid in the liver as compared to other tissues (Table 1). The storage forms of these vitamins, so far as they are known, are discussed below.

TABLE 1. *Daily recommended intakes and tissue and blood concentrations of B vitamins*

Tissue	Thiamin[b]	Riboflavin[b]	Nicotinic acid[b]	B_6[c]	B_{12}[d]	Folic acid[c]	Biotin[b]	Pantothenic acid[b]
Daily allowance for adults[a] (mg/day)								
Male	1.4	1.6	18	2.2	0.003	0.4	0.1–0.2	4–7
Female	1.0	1.2	13	2.0	0.003	0.4	0.1–0.2	4–7
Liver (mg/kg)	2.2	16	58	2.5	0.5	9.5	0.7	43
Heart (mg/kg)	3.6	8	41	0.8	—	1.0	0.2	16
Muscle (mg/kg)	1.2	2	47	0.9	0.008	0.8	0.004	12
Brain (mg/kg)	1.6	2.5	20	0.7	0.1	1.1	0.6	15
Kidney (mg/kg)	2.8	20	37	1.1	0.2	2.1	0.7	19
Whole blood[e] (mg/liter)	0.02–0.08	0.1–0.5	3–7	0.03–0.08	0.0002–0.0008	0.005–0.02	0.0002–0.0005	0.15–0.5

[a] RDA (1).
[b] Values for tissue concentrations from ref. 113.
[c] Values for tissue concentrations from ref. 114.
[d] Values for tissue concentrations from ref. 101.
[e] Values for whole blood or plasma for normal adults from ref. 17.

The metabolic significance of the B vitamins in the liver can be considered from several points of view. First, they are needed as cofactors in numerous enzyme-catalyzed reactions, some of which are illustrated in Fig. 1. Second, the liver is a common site of transformation of the vitamins to metabolites used either for storage (for example the polyglutamates of folic acid) or for the synthesis of active forms for export and use by other tissues (e.g., pyridoxal). Third, in some cases (B_{12}), the metabolically altered vitamin is recycled by biliary secretion and reabsorbed (enterohepatic circulation). Finally, the liver is the site of formation and secretion of carrier proteins for vitamins in the plasma (e.g., transcobalamin for B_{12}).

In cases of liver damage, metabolism of the water-soluble vitamins can be disordered, so that these various functions are impaired; thus liver damage can prevent vitamin B_6 from being transformed to pyridoxal phosphate and then secreted as pyridoxal into the blood for use by other tissues. Thus the nutritional state of other tissues is dependent on normal liver function. Russell (2) suggests that lack of secretion of transport proteins, as well as failure to synthesize and secrete active forms of the vitamins, can deprive other tissues of their vitamin needs, even when the diet provides adequate vitamin intake.

A considerable amount of information has been published on the liver content of various water-soluble vitamins in disease, notably alcohol-related liver damage. These changes are discussed under individual vitamins; nonetheless, the comprehensive survey by Baker and his colleagues (3) is worthy of note. They measured the levels of B vitamins at autopsy in the liver of alcoholics with fatty change or with overt cirrhosis and compared the results with liver of normal subjects obtained by liver biopsy or at autopsy. Their

data are expressed per milligram dry weight of liver, whereas Table 1 gives data for normal human liver B complex expressed in relation to wet weight. Even when allowance is made for this, the normal values do not always agree in Table 1 and Fig. 2. With respect to the pathological livers, their data (Fig. 2) show that livers with mild fatty degeneration had decreased levels of all B vitamins except pantothenic and folinic acids. In cases with more severe fatty liver, the magnitude of vitamin reduction was greater, the most depressed being biotin; folinic acid concentration remained unchanged. Liver specimens from cirrhotic patients showed no reduction in thiamin content, whereas nicotinic acid, folic acid, and vitamin B_{12} were markedly reduced in concentration. No differences in the levels of any B vitamin were found in vitamin-treated versus untreated alcoholic patients, suggesting that the primary cause of the low hepatic levels is incapacity of the damaged liver to retain the vitamin, and not dietary insufficiency. Interpretation of these data is complicated; in the case of cirrhosis, the normal hepatocyte population must have been replaced by fibrous tissue to an unrecorded extent. Nevertheless, the observation (Fig. 2) that some vitamins (e.g., thiamin, biotin) are less depressed in cirrhosis than in fatty liver suggests that many functional hepatocytes must have survived in the cirrhotic cases.

THIAMIN

It was shown at the end of the last century that beri-beri, a form of polyneuritis common in East Asian populations living on white rice, from which the vitamin-rich husk had been removed, could be cured by administering extracts of the rice husks. The active

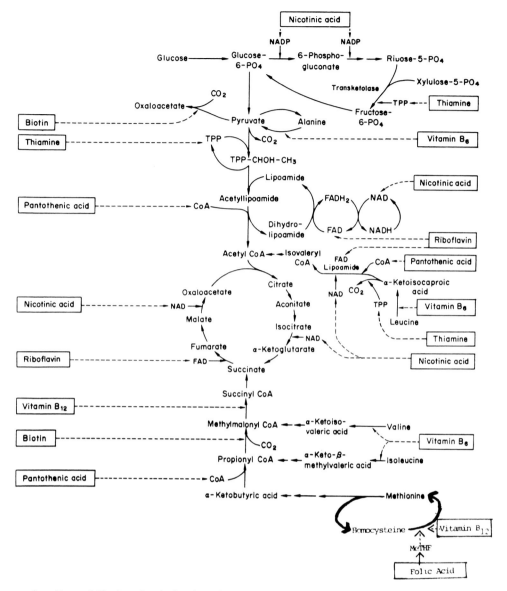

FIG. 1. Coenzyme function of B vitamin derivatives in some major pathways in the liver. (Adapted from ref. 4, with permission.)

factor, assigned the name vitamin B_1 to distinguish it from other B complex members, was finally isolated in 1926 and its structure determined in 1936. Thiamin (Fig. 3) consists of a pyrimidine nucleus linked to a thiazole ring. In the body, it occurs mainly as the pyrophosphate (Fig. 3) which functions in carbohydrate metabolism as a coenzyme in decarboxylation of α-keto acids, such as pyruvic and α-ketoglutaric acids, and in the hexose monophosphate shunt as a cofactor for transketolase. The former reactions are widespread in tissues, but transketolase occurs mainly in liver (5). Tissue thiamin occurs mostly as the thiamin pyrophosphate (80%), the mono- and triphosphates each accounting for about 10% of body thiamin (6,7). Table 1 shows that several organs as well as liver have high concentrations of thiamin.

Metabolism

The metabolic pathways of thiamin in the body are illustrated in Fig. 4. Thiamin is absorbed from the intestine by two processes, active and passive, depending on dose level (8). At low physiological doses, the mechanism is active and sodium dependent, whereas at high doses it enters by passive diffusion (6). Thiamin passes to the liver where it is phosphorylated to the pyrophosphate, of which 35% can be recovered from the mitochondria and 55% from cytosol (9). The liver appears to be the main site of thiamin phosphorylation in the body (10). Ferrari et al. (11) suggest that the liver may be the source of thiamine pyrophosphate for other tissues, such as brain. Finally, thiamin is catabolized to a variety of breakdown products; the major excre-

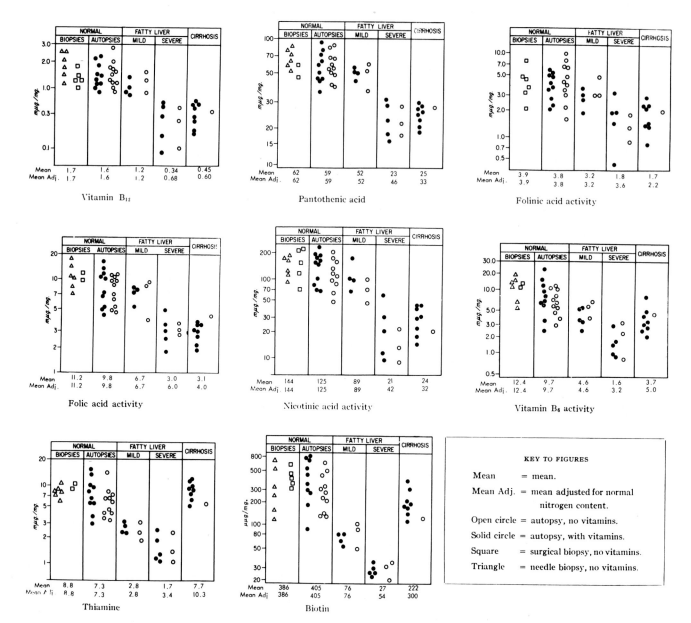

FIG. 2. Concentrations of B vitamins in the livers of normal subjects obtained by biopsy or at autopsy and from alcoholic subjects with mild or severe fatty liver infiltration, or with cirrhosis at autopsy. Some subjects were receiving supplements of vitamins. The data are expressed per miligram dry weight, and per milligram dry weight adjusted for *N* content. (Reproduced from ref. 3, with permission.)

tory products in the urine are pyrimidine carboxylic acid, thiazole acetic acid, and thiamin acetic acid (12).

Liver Function and Disease

Deficiency of thiamin results in reduced activity of the liver enzymes pyruvate decarboxylase and transketolase, but the levels of acetyl-CoA and ATP are little affected (13,14). Similarly, lack of dietary thiamin does not impair the capacity of the pentose phosphate cycle to function in the liver, although the regulatory enzymes decrease in concentration (15). Other nutritional factors affect liver thiamin levels. Neonatal rats

were found to have a low level of thiamin in the liver if the mother was receiving a deficient diet during pregnancy but not if deficiency in the mother rat was confined to the period before the onset of pregnancy (16), implying that there are no long-term stores of thiamin (Table 1).

In the United States, clinical thiamin deficiency usually is the result of alcoholism and can express itself as beri-beri, Wernicke encephalopathy, Korsakoff syndrome, or alcoholic polyneuritis (115). The degree of thiamin deprivation appears to determine the syndrome (4), severe deprivation resulting in encephalopathy and Korsakoff syndrome while less deficient

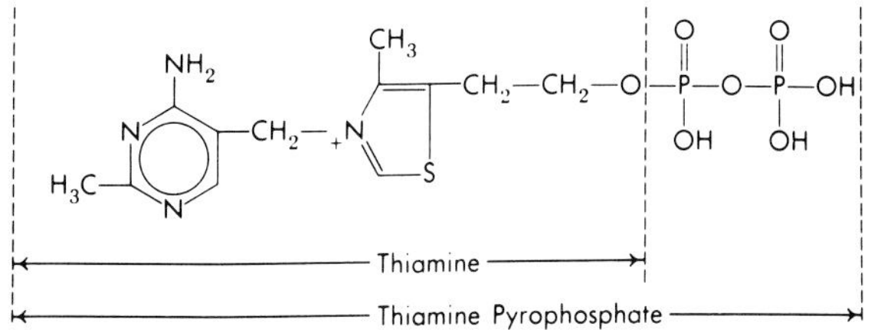

FIG. 3. Structures of thiamin and thiamin pyrophosphate. (Reproduced from ref. 4, with permission.)

subjects exhibit beri-beri, and relatively mild deficiency is expressed as polyneuritis. Details of these syndromes are given elsewhere (4).

In an extensive study, Baker et al. (3) showed that alcoholics with cirrhosis have no reduction in liver thiamin content, whereas those with fatty liver show a loss (Fig. 2). The effects of alcoholism on liver thiamin content are indirect and direct (116). Regarding the former mechanism, Leevy et al. (17) draw attention to the reduced gastrointestinal uptake of thiamin in subjects who are alcoholic with fatty or cirrhotic liver disease; intestinal transport fell from a V_{max} of 4.5 mg in normal subjects to 1 to 2 mg thiamin in alcoholic subjects not affected by overt cirrhosis. Other studies (18,19) demonstrate that thiamin absorption due to the active transport mechanism is responsive at low concentrations of the vitamin and is especially impaired by alcoholism. Within the liver, alcohol administration directly decreases phosphorylation to the active coenzyme thiamin pyrophosphate. Transketolase activity in the liver is also reduced by ethanol administration (20). Regarding the mechanism, the enzyme apoprotein of transketolase appears to be denatured and inactivated following ethanol administration to rats (20,21). Ethanol may promote thiamin release from the liver, thus contributing to the low level in that organ. This is evidenced by the release of thiamin and other water-soluble vitamins when rat liver is perfused with

ethanol (22). Finally, increases in plasma thiamin levels of cirrhotic cases following administration of thiamin are not necessarily accompanied by a rise in red cell transketolase activity (23).

The level of thiamin in plasma is grossly reduced in chronic liver disease. In hepatic failure, plasma thiamin concentration was reduced to 54% below normal, and in decompensated chronic liver disease to 65% (24). In a series of 24 patients with acute hepatocellular necrosis and halothane-associated hepatic necrosis, one-third showed thiamin deficiency as evidenced by reduced erythrocyte transketolase responding to *in vitro* stimulation by added thiamine pyrophosphate (TPP) (25). Since the liver of these cases could still convert administered thiamin to pyrophosphate, it was concluded that the defect in such cases of hepatic damage is not due to impaired hepatic phosphorylation. It is thus an open question whether severe liver disease deprives other tissues of their supply of thiamin pyrophosphate.

RIBOFLAVIN

Riboflavin was first recognized as a heat-stable growth factor for rats. When finally isolated in 1933, the growth factor had a yellow color, which led to its identification with the prosthetic group of the so-called "yellow" flavoprotein enzymes, which are involved in biological oxidations. The structure (Fig. 5) was elucidated in 1935 and was later shown to be a constituent of flavin mononucleotide (FMN) and flavin adenine dinucleotide (FAD), components of enzymes involved in oxidative systems related to electron transport.

Metabolism

The metabolic pathways of riboflavin in the body are illustrated in Fig. 6. Absorption of riboflavin occurs in

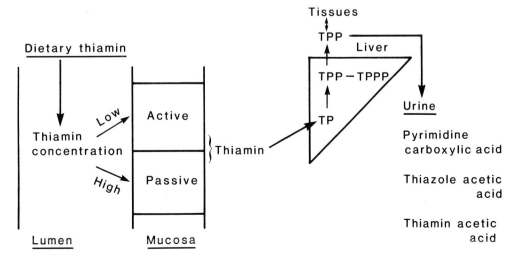

FIG. 4. Metabolism of thiamin. TP, thiamin monophosphate; TPP, thiamin pyrophosphate; TPPP, thiamin triphosphate.

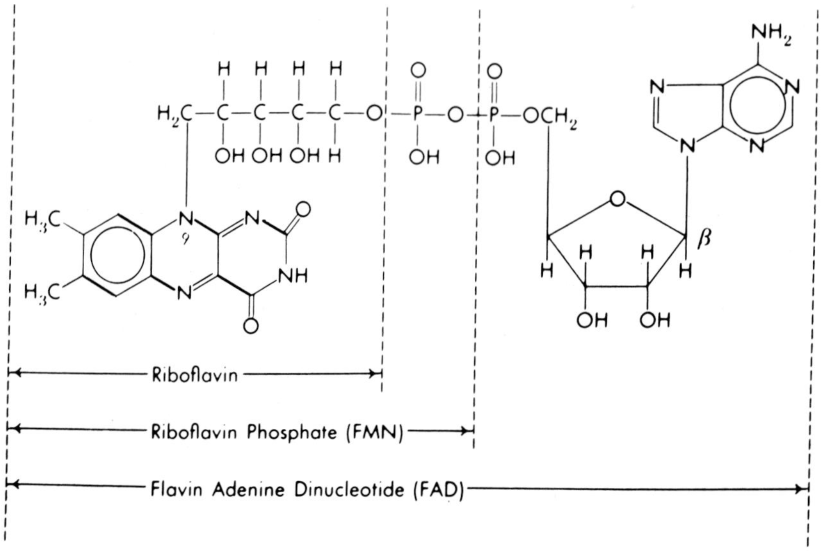

FIG. 5. Structures of riboflavin, FMN, and FAD. (Reproduced from ref. 4, with permission.)

the upper small intestine by a specialized active transport process. Some of the entering vitamin is phosphorylated to FMN by flavokinase in the mucosa and is converted to FAD in the liver (26,27). Both free and phosphorylated forms pass into the portal blood, where they bind to albumin and other plasma proteins (26). As Table 1 shows, the liver and kidney are the main storage sites (5), storage is not extensive and is easily depleted. The major intracellular forms in order of abundance are FAD, FMN, and free riboflavin (5). For example, in normally nourished rats, the concentrations per gram liver are 26 μg FAD, 5 μg FMN, and 0.7 μg free riboflavin (28). Animals fed large doses of riboflavin store mainly FAD in the liver (29). This may represent uptake by metabolic trapping of free riboflavin in other forms, similar to the case of vitamin B_6.

Some of the free riboflavin in the liver appears to be reexcreted via the bile and is subsequently reabsorbed, as evidenced by two peaks of urinary excretion following oral dosage of rats with riboflavin (30). Jusko and Levy (26), however, consider biliary recycling to be unimportant in man.

Liver Function and Disease

In rats deficient in riboflavin, hepatic concentrations of FAD are reported to be reduced to one-third the normal level (31), but the decrease is less than that of FMN, while flavokinase activity falls to half the normal level. In other tissues, riboflavin deficiency causes much smaller changes (32). Riboflavin deficiency in

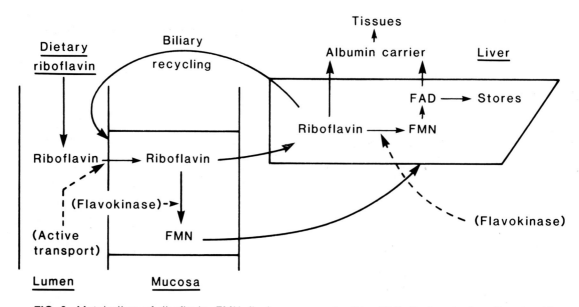

FIG. 6. Metabolism of riboflavin, FMN, flavin mononucleotide; FAD, flavin adenine dinucleotide.

mice results in loss of hepatic architecture, with enlargement and distortion of mitochondria (33), possibly due to defects in oxidative phosphorylation resulting from lack of flavoproteins (34). In deficiency, lipid metabolism becomes disordered, with accumulation of triglycerides in the liver (35) and subsequent reduced dehydrogenation of fatty acids with diminished levels of arachidonic, linoleic, and linolenic acids (36). Other metabolic effects of deficiency include increased conversion of tryptophan to xanthurenic acid (37), decreased activity of the flavin-dependent purine enzyme xanthine oxidase (28), impaired conversion of folic acid to 5-N-methyltetrahydrofolic acid (38), and decreased conversion of pyridoxine to pyridoxine phosphate (39). These effects of deficiency and their reversal by refeeding with riboflavin vary in magnitude from enzyme to enzyme. Bro-Rasmussen (40) has shown that negative nitrogen balance due to inadequate protein or energy intake, injury, or diabetic ketosis, reduces retention of riboflavin. Conversion of riboflavin to FMN and FAD is impaired by thyroid deficiency and is reversed by thyroid hormone administration, which acts on flavokinase activity (27,28). ACTH enhances synthesis of FMN in liver as well as in adrenal glands (41). In riboflavin deficiency in rats, there is a decrease in tissue epinephrine and norepinephrine (42). During pregnancy in rats, mitotic activity in the fetal liver is decreased when the dam is riboflavin-deficient (43). Finally, flavokinase is inhibited by such drugs as chlorpromazine and tricyclic antidepressants (4).

There is biochemical evidence of riboflavin deficiency in chronic alcoholism (44). The accumulation of liver fat in riboflavin deficiency resembles similar changes in chronic alcoholism. Stanko et al. (45) found that riboflavin administration to alcohol-fed rats reverses accumulation of free fatty acids and esterified fatty acids. Alcohol also has several effects on liver riboflavin content and metabolism seen with other B vitamins. Alcohol toxicity impedes conversion of free riboflavin to its active phosphorylated forms in the liver (5). Like other water-soluble vitamins, perfusion of rat liver with ethanol results in a large release of riboflavin (22). In human liver cirrhosis, decreased concentrations of riboflavin have been observed, mostly in necrotic regions (46). In a series of 140 cases of cirrhosis, there was a 6% reduction in plasma riboflavin concentration (17).

NICOTINIC ACID

Pellagra, a disease associated with dermatitis, gastrointestinal symptoms, and impaired mental function, was recognized in the 1920s to be caused by a dietary deficiency. It was only in 1937 that Elvehjem demonstrated that an analogous deficiency disease in dogs (black tongue) could be cured with nicotinic acid (niacin), and that pellagra of man was also treatable with this compound. The active compounds are nicotinic acid and its amide, nicotinamide; they are also named niacin and niacinamide. Nicotinic acid is also formed from tryptophan via quinolinic acid. Tissue levels of these coenzymes are determined by dietary content of nicotinic acid, nicotinamide, and tryptophan. The structures of nicotinic acid and its amide and of the coenzymes NAD and NADP are shown in Fig. 7. These coenzymes function in tissue respiration, where they serve in dehydrogenation reactions and are reoxidized by the flavoprotein system. Wiss and Weber (5) term them "mobile coenzymes" because of their loose association with the dehydrogenases.

Metabolism

Free nicotinic acid and its amide are rapidly absorbed (47). Biosynthesis of the pyridine nucleotides by the Preiss-Handler pathway (48) involves phosphoribosyl pyrophosphate, ATP, and glutamine. The preferred substrate for coenzyme biosynthesis is nicotinic acid in the liver, kidney, and brain, but nicotinamide in some other tissues (5).

Liver Function and Disease

The turnover time of nicotinic acid in mouse liver is about 4 days (49). The main pathway of breakdown involves formation of N-methyl-4-pyridine-3-carboxamide. In addition, nicotinic acid forms nicotinuric acid with glycine by peptide bond formation. These compounds are excreted in the urine.

The liver of man contains about 60 mg nicotinic acid per kilogram wet weight (Table 1), which is not much greater than the concentration in many other tissues (5) and is presumably related to the intensity of energy release in the various tissues. It can be concluded that the liver has no special stores of nicotinic acid or its derivatives. Bro-Rasmussen (40) has shown that factors causing a negative nitrogen balance result in an outpouring of nicotinic acid in the urine.

In alcoholism, mild fatty infiltration of the liver causes a reduction in liver nicotinic acid concentration of 34%; in severe fatty infiltration, this increases to 71% (3) (Fig. 2). In cirrhosis, total nicotinic acid content in the liver can fall as much as 80% (3,17). In addition, nicotinic acid but not nicotinamide has long been known to depress blood lipids. Baker et al (50) have shown that the increase in liver lipid content caused by ethanol administration can be abolished by nicotinic acid treatment. This effect is attributed to inhibition of peripheral release of free fatty acid and direct inhibitory action of nicotinic acid on liver alcohol dehydrogenase, thus preventing the shift in NAD/

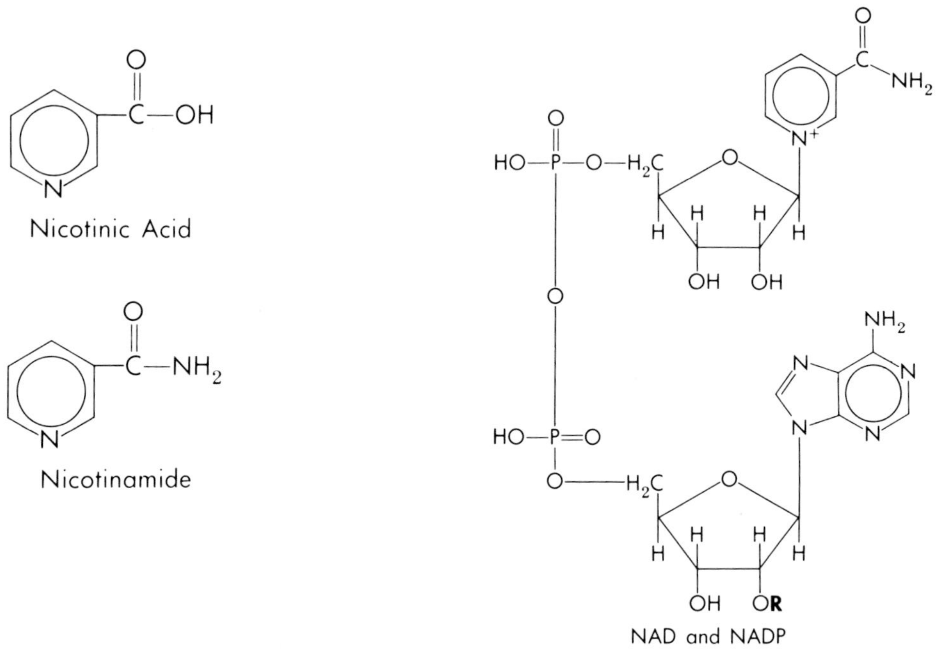

FIG. 7. Structures of nicotinic acid, nicotinamide, NAD, and NADP. (Reproduced from ref. 4, with permission.)

NADH ratio produced by ethanol conversion to acetaldehyde. In hepatic failure, the nicotinic acid blood level has been found to be either raised or reduced when compared with controls (24).

VITAMIN B₆

Vitamin B₆ was first recognized as a factor needed to prevent dermatitis of nutritional origin in rats. It was isolated in 1938, and its chemical structure was elucidated the following year. Vitamin B₆ occurs in three forms (Fig. 8): pyridoxine (PN), pyridoxal (PL), and pyridoxamine (PM) (51). All three can exist as phosphorylated derivatives formed by pyridoxal kinase, namely, pyridoxine phosphate (PNP), pyridoxal phosphate (PLP), and pyridoxamine phosphate (PMP). Only PLP, however, can serve all the many coenzyme functions associated with vitamin B₆. Recent research on vitamin B₆ is summarized elsewhere (52).

Metabolism

Vitamin B₆ in coenzyme (phosphorylated) form takes part in reactions mostly associated with protein metabolism. These reactions include transamination, decarboxylation, and deamination, in which pyridoxal phosphate functions by a Schiff base mechanism. It has also been claimed (53) that PLP regulates binding of glucocorticoids to nuclei, but the physiological significance of this action of PLP is disputed (54).

Following ingestion, the B₆ vitamins are absorbed into the portal blood (Fig. 9)). Using isolated, vascu-

larly perfused rat small intestine, Mehansho and colleagues (55) have shown that PL is more rapidly absorbed than PN or PM. Although some PL becomes phosphorylated in the mucosa to PLP and PN to PNP, the main products entering the portal blood are PL and PN. The subsequent metabolism of B₆ vitamins in the portal blood has been examined (56) using perfused rat liver. When PN was added to the perfusate, it was rapidly taken up by the liver. The concentration of free PN in the liver, however, failed to attain that in the perfusate. Instead, much PN entering the liver cells was rapidly transformed to PNP, PLP, and PMP. This metabolic trapping was shown to be the major factor in PN uptake and retention by the liver, since inhibition of phosphorylation greatly retarded PN entry into the liver.

These investigators (56–58) further showed that PNP formed in the liver is converted to PLP by the action of pyridoxine phosphate oxidase, an enzyme absent from intestinal mucosa (57) and muscle (56) and showing only slight activity in kidney (58). Some of the liver PLP was dephosphorylated to PL and released into the blood, while another portion became PMP. Figure 9 shows how this active transformation of PN to PLP and release as PL appears to be the major source of PL (and thus of the coenzyme PLP) for some other rat tissues, notably muscle and erythrocytes. For intestine, dietary PL is likely to be a major source for the mucosal cell. The role of the liver as a main source of plasma PL and PLP is confirmed by the work of Lumeng et al. (59), who showed a fall in plasma levels of PL when the liver was removed from dogs.

Shane (60) reviewed data in man for plasma levels

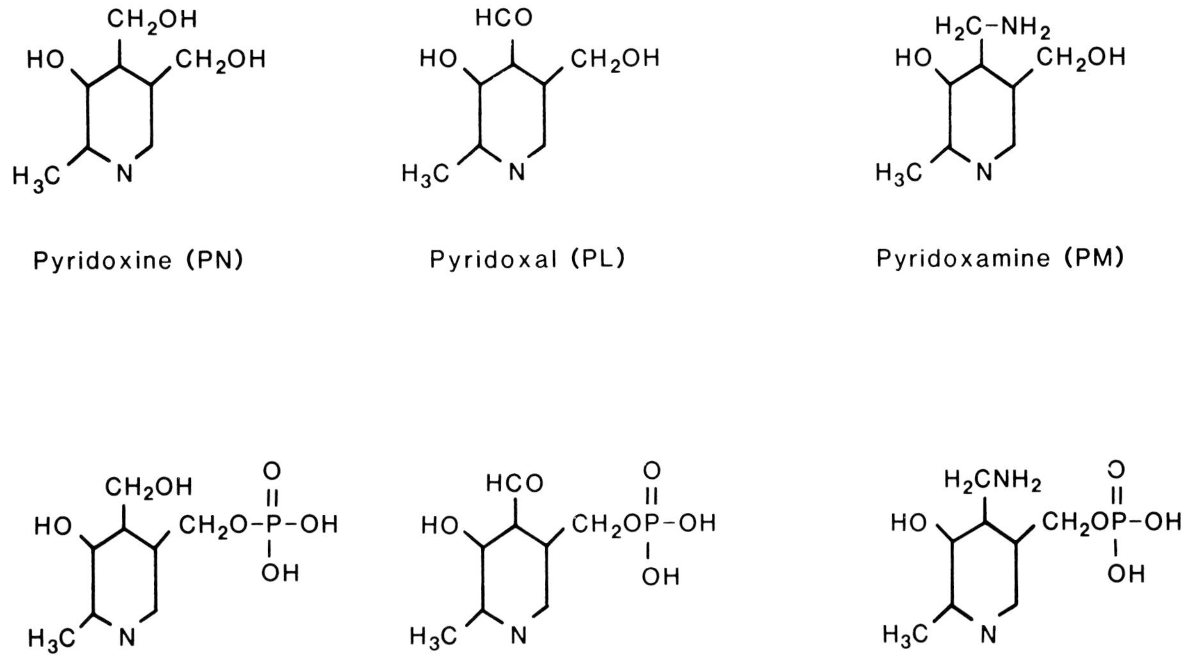

CH₂OH ... Pyridoxine (PN)

Pyridoxal (PL)

Pyridoxamine (PM)

Pyridoxine phosphate (PNP)

Pyridoxal phosphate (PLP)

Pyridoxamine phosphate (PMP)

FIG. 8. Structures of B₆ vitamers.

and showed that concentrations of the B₆ vitamers (grams per milliliter) are: PLP, 13.5; PNP, 0; PMP, 20.0 (9.3 in women); PL, 0.8; PN, 0; and PM, 24.7. This implies that the phosphorylated forms (PLP, PMP) are the major plasma vitamers, where they are bound to albumin in plasma. This appears to be in conflict with Fig. 9; however, entry into tissues involves the free forms (PL) rather than the phosphorylated derivatives. Mehansho et al. (56) speculate that

the low level of plasma PL is due to this extensive tissue uptake, whereas the high level of PLP represents albumin binding with retarded uptake.

Liver Function and Disease

The main forms of B₆ vitamers in normal liver are PLP and PMP (61). The liver level of B₆ vitamers is considerably reduced in cirrhosis (3,17) (Fig. 2). Since

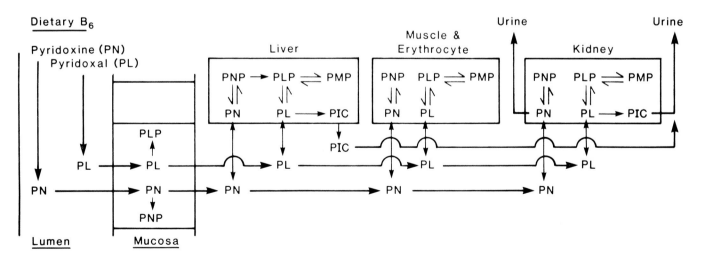

FIG. 9. Metabolism of vitamin B₆. Note the presence of the enzyme pyridoxine phosphate oxidase only in the liver, which allows that organ to be the major site in the body for converting pyridoxine to pyridoxal, thus ensuring availability of pyridoxal to other tissues. Note that PLP is the main form in plasma. Mehansho et al. (56) speculate that this may be because PL is more readily taken up by tissues. PN, pyridoxine; PNP, pyridoxine phosphate; PL, pyridoxal; PLP, pyridoxal phosphate; PMP, pyridoxamine phosphate; PIC, pyridoxic acid. (Adapted from data from refs. 56–58.)

the liver plays a dominant role in transforming PN to PL and PLP (Fig. 9), it is not surprising that injected doses of PN raise plasma PL and PLP levels in normal human subjects but often fail to do so in cases of liver damage (Fig. 10) (62). Spannuth et al. (62) have found accelerated removal of PLP from the plasma of patients with liver damage and attribute the low plasma PLP levels to this factor. Some authors (63) consider that accelerated degradation occurs in the diseased liver itself.

It has been claimed that B_6 undernutrition, as measured by B_6 or PLP levels in plasma, can affect as many as 30 to 50% of alcoholics without liver disease and 80 to 100% of those with liver damage (62,64). Leevy et al. (17), however, found depressed levels of B_6 in the plasma in only 50% of their series of cirrhotic cases. In another series, 87% of patients with decompensated chronic liver cirrhosis showed a reduction of circulating PLP, whereas in fulminating liver disease the plasma changes were independently variable (24, 117). The occurrence of high levels of plasma PLP in some cases of liver disease makes this an unreliable indicator of vitamin B_6 status (24). Since albumin is the major B_6-binding protein in plasma (65), it is possible that the low vitamin levels in the plasma of cirrhotic subjects may partially result from reduced plasma albumin concentrations (61). The mechanism for increased degradation of PLP in liver disease remains unknown (63,117).

FOLIC ACID

Folic acid was isolated as a bacterial growth factor in 1943 from various sources, including liver. Because it was effective in preventing a specific anemia of chicks and monkeys, it was at first thought to be the antipernicious anemia factor, which was later identified as vitamin B_{12}. Folic acid (Fig. 11) consists of a pteridine ring system linked to para-aminobenzoic acid, which is linked in turn to a glutamic acid residue ($PteGlu_1$) or to several such residues (up to eight) ($PteGlu_8$, polyglutamates), the latter being the form predominating in foods and tissues. The active coenzyme form is the reduced methylated product, 5-methyltetrahydrofolic acid (CH_3THF).

In this section, we examine the absorption and metabolism of folic acid in relation to the liver in health and disease. Further information can be obtained from a recent symposium (66) and from an excellent account of folate metabolism in liver disease (67).

Metabolism

The main metabolic pathways involving folic acid coenzymes include synthesis of the purine ring, thymidylic acid, and metabolism of serine, glycine, histidine, and methionine, in all of which it functions in one-carbon reactions. Figure 12 summarizes the metabolism of ingested folic acid (68,69), which first undergoes loss of polyglutamate residues through the action of a conjugase, an enzyme present in the brush border and cytoplasm of the intestinal mucosal cell. Some of the $PteGlu_1$ so formed is then reduced and methylated by the mucosal cell to the active form CH_3THF, which then enters the portal circulation. The remainder of the absorbed folate is transported as unchanged $PteGlu_1$. In plasma, folates circulate in the free form and in two bound forms, one loosely bound

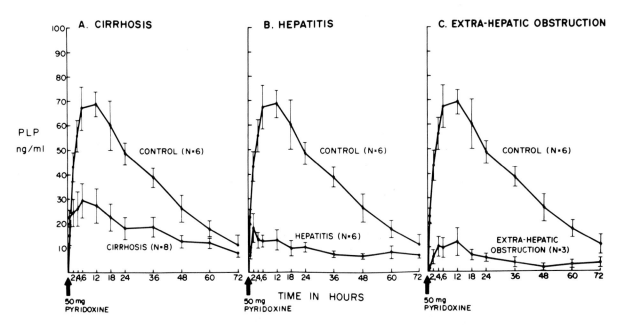

FIG. 10. Plasma PLP levels following intravenous administration of 50 mg pyridoxine to control subjects and to patients with various types of liver disease. (Reproduced from ref. 62, with permission.)

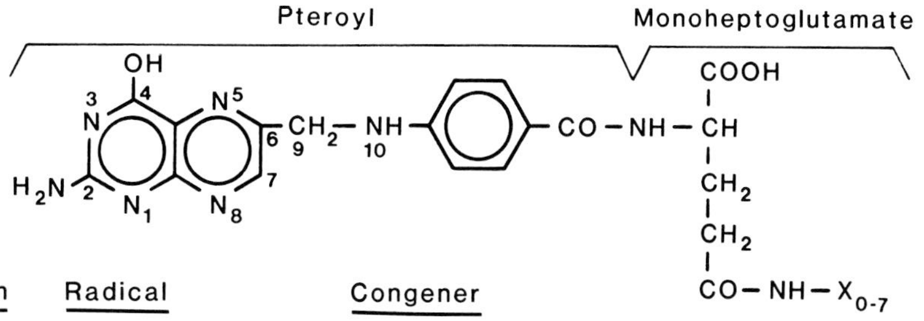

Pteroyl Monoheptoglutamate

Position	Radical	Congener	
N^5	$-CH_3$	$CH_3H_4PteGlu$	Methyltetrahydrofolate
N^5	$-CHO$	$5-CHOH_4PteGlu$	Folinic acid (Citrovorum Factor)
N^{10}	$-CHO$	$10-CHOH_4PteGlu$	10-Formyltetrahydrofolate
N^{5-10}	$-CH-$	$5,10-CHH_4PteGlu$	5,10-Methenyltetrahydrofolate
N^{5-10}	$-CH_2-$	$5,10-CH_2H_4PteGlu$	5,10-Methylenetetrahydrofolate
N^5	$-CHNH$	$CHNHH_4PteGlu$	Formiminotetrahydrofolate
N^{10}	$-CH_2OH$	$CH_2OHH_4PteGlu$	Hydroxymethyltetrahydrofolate

FIG. 11. Structure of folic acid and its polyglutamates. (Reproduced from ref. 68, with permission.)

to plasma proteins, the other firmly attached to high-affinity carriers (70). The folates appear to be taken up by tissues, including liver, by an energy-dependent, carrier-mediated transport mechanism (70). Recent evidence (71,72) suggests that PteGlu₁ in circulation is avidly taken up by the liver, where it is rapidly reduced to tetrahydrofolic acid and methylated to form CH₃THF, which then either enters the liver pool of polyglutamates or is excreted in the bile. Methylated reduced folate (CH₃THF) already present in the plasma is taken up more slowly by the liver (70) and thereafter is extensively excreted in the bile. The biliary CH₃THF from either source thus reenters the gut and recycles back into the plasma (72). The slower hepatic uptake of this form of folate probably has the advantage that less is retained by the liver and more is available to the peripheral tissues, which take up the

CH₃THF form preferentially (70). These changes have been quantitated in a recent rat study (73), in which ³H-folic acid and ¹⁴CH₃-THF were administered intravenously and were found to have a similar clearance (10 to 15 min) from the serum. Labeled CH₃THF was almost completely reexcreted in the bile, whereas only 80% of the folic acid was eliminated by this route, all as CH₃THF monoglutamate. Of the amount retained in the liver, only 4% was recovered as the monoglutamate; the remainder was polyglutamate (73). In folate deficiency in rats, conversion to the polyglutamate form and its clearance in bile is diminished (72).

Estimates of liver stores are only approximate (Table 1). The total body content of folic acid is said to be 5 to 10 mg (70), while Hoppner and Lampi (74) observed a mean level of 7.8 ± 2.3 mg/kg liver in a

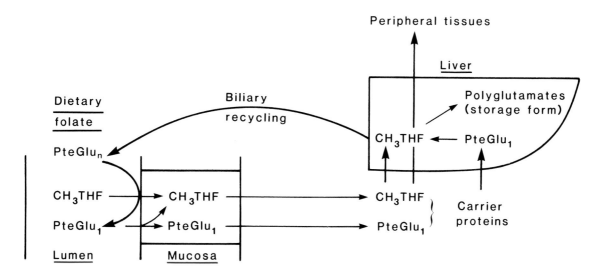

FIG. 12. Metabolism of folates. PteGlu₁, pteroylmonoglutamate; CH₃THF, methyltetrahydrofolic acid.

series of accidental deaths. Mean values for patients dying from various diseases (coronary disease, cancer) were not appreciably lower. Red cell folate levels are said to correlate well with liver stores (75). In the rat, liver folate content is influenced considerably by folate intake (76). Available folate is also altered by drugs that affect its absorption and conversion to CH_3THF (azulfdine, dilantin, primidine, barbiturates, oral contraceptives, ethanol, cycloserine) and by inhibitors of dihydrofolate reductase (methotrexate, pyrimethamine, triamterine). It can be expected that these also lower the liver stores of folate (77,118).

Liver Function and Disease

Halsted (67,119) has provided excellent surveys of folate metabolism in liver disease. In alcoholism, folate deficiency is probably caused by impaired uptake by the intestine as well as less storage in the damaged liver (67,68). In cirrhotic cases, Leevy et al. (17) observed a 60% reduction in total liver folate content; administration of folate resulted in deposition in the liver of only one-tenth the amount achieved by normal subjects. This agrees with evidence (3) that vitamin administration does not generally raise the reduced levels in the liver of alcoholics (Fig. 2). Chronic administration of ethanol in man resulted in reduced uptake of labeled folic acid by the liver (78). Other kinetic studies (79–81) in humans and animals, however, failed to confirm that alcohol has any effect on the uptake, storage, reduction, or methylation of labeled folate. Brown et al. (79) reported that polyglutamate synthesis is diminished in alcohol-fed rats. Monkeys fed ethanol chronically also fail to form polyglutamates in the liver and excrete large amounts of folates in the urine (82), an observation also made on human subjects receiving ethanol (83). Horne (84) reported that ethanol *in vitro* results in an apparent increase of polyglutamates in freshly isolated hepatocytes. The cumulated data remain unclear as to whether ethanol increases or decreases polyglutamates in the liver. Alcoholic cirrhotics can develop megaloblastic anemia due to folate deficiency (85). Inadequate retention in the liver and low dietary intake of folate contribute to this picture. Healthy subjects receiving a folate-free diet develop megaloblastic anemia after about 22 weeks (86), whereas chronic alcoholics show a similar hematological picture within 5 to 10 weeks (87,88).

Failure of the liver to store folic acid may be associated with reduced capacity to form polyglutamates and may represent insufficient recycling of folic acid because of interference by ethanol with mucosal uptake of folates entering the intestine from the bile. In view of these aberrations in folate metabolism associated with alcoholic liver damage, it is not surprising that folate deficiency is a common feature of cirrhosis.

Other hepatic diseases are associated with disordered folate metabolism. The onset of viral hepatitis results in an increased excretion of urinary folate (89,90), presumably because of release of stored folates from the liver with overloading of the capacity of the plasma to bind them. In chronic hepatitis and nonalcoholic cirrhosis, low folates have been recorded in one series of cases (75) but not in two others (91,92).

An interrelationship of folate sufficiency to liver repair has been suggested. The course of the disease was reduced by folic acid and viamin B_{12} administration in cases of acute viral hepatitis (93) and alcoholic cirrhosis (17). Leevy (94) found that folic acid administration increased liver DNA synthesis. Rats that were folate-deficient responded poorly to carbon tetrachloride liver injury and were protected by folate administration (95). Finally, enhanced polyglutamate formation from tetrahydrofolate in regenerating rat liver (96) may indicate that this form of folic acid is therapeutically preferable.

VITAMIN B_{12}

The observation in 1926 that liver extracts cure pernicious (megaloblastic) anemia was followed in 1948 by isolation of the active factor and its subsequent structural analysis. It consists (Fig. 13) of a corrin nucleus linked through aminopropanol to a nucleotide containing the base dimethylbenzimidazole. An atom of cobalt present in the corrin ring system is also linked to the benzimidazole through a bridge. To this cobalt atom can be attached cyanide (vitamin B_{12}, cyanocobalamin); but in the active form (coenzyme B_{12}), the substituent is 5-deoxyadenosine. Coenzyme B_{12} is involved in a series of reactions, including conversion of methylmalonate to succinate, the maintenance of sulfhydryl groups in the reduced form, and the formation of methionine from homocysteine. The latter reaction links vitamin B_{12} to folic acid (Fig. 1).

Metabolism

The metabolic pathways of vitamin B_{12} are illustrated in Fig. 14. Dietary B_{12} is provided by animal tissues, where it is attached to the protein in coenzyme form. Absorption is dependent on the gastric intrinsic factor of Castle, following digestive liberation of vitamin B_{12} from proteins to which it is bound. The vitamin B_{12}-intrinsic factor complex binds to the ileal mucosa, where it is absorbed by attachment of the complex to specific receptors on the absorptive surface of the ileum, transfer of the vitamin across the epithelial absorptive cell (enterocyte) to the portal plasma, and release of the vitamin from the cobalamin-intrinsic factor

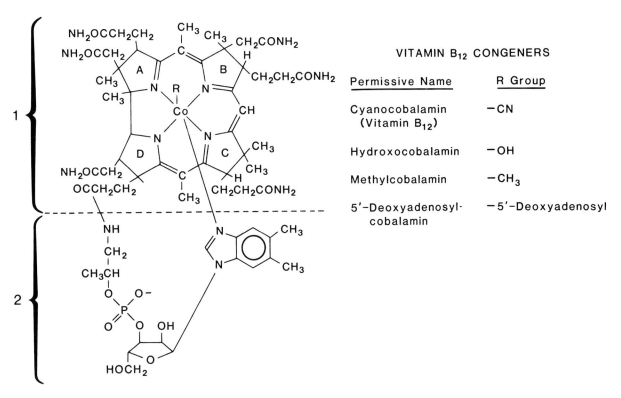

VITAMIN B₁₂ CONGENERS

Permissive Name	R Group
Cyanocobalamin (Vitamin B₁₂)	−CN
Hydroxocobalamin	−OH
Methylcobalamin	−CH₃
5′-Deoxyadenosyl-cobalamin	−5′-Deoxyadenosyl

FIG. 13. Structure of vitamin B₁₂. (Reproduced from ref. 68, with permission.)

complex (97). When cobalamin enters the portal blood, it is no longer bound to intrinsic factor but to specific transport proteins, namely, transcobalamins (98). In the plasma, B₁₂ binds to three proteins, the chief one being transcobalamin II, the other two mainly serving as a reserve store.

Stores in the body range from 1 to 10 mg, of which 50 to 90% is present in the liver; the liver of a healthy person contains about 1 mg 5-deoxyadenosylcobala-min (approximately one-fifth to one-half of total body cobalamin). Hydroxycobalamin accounts for 20 to 30% and methylcobalamin for 1 to 5% of total cobala-min in the liver (99); the latter is the predominant form in blood. Since the RDA of vitamin B₁₂ (1) is only 3 μg daily, normal liver stores can maintain the subject for several years. Neurological evidence of vitamin B₁₂ deficiency occurs when the stores are reduced below 0.1 mg and the plasma level falls below 100 pg/ml. The

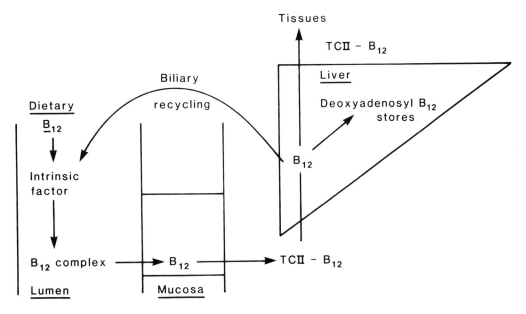

FIG. 14. Metabolism of vitamin B₁₂.

stored form of vitamin B_{12} is the coenzyme 5-deoxy-adenosylcobalamin, the form to which injected cyano-cobalamin and hydroxycobalamin are mainly converted (100). It is said to be most abundant in microsomes (5). Total cobalamin content of organs (Table 1) varies widely (101). In adult man, the liver contains more total cobalamin (primarily as 5-deoxyadenosylcobala-min) than any other organ, the major part occurring in mitochondria (5,99). Recent findings of high levels of cobalamin-dependent enzymes in the liver (99) suggest that the liver may have more than a storage function for the vitamin.

Finally, vitamin B_{12} is significantly excreted in the bile (0.5 to 5 μg daily) and is 65 to 75% reabsorbed (102). In pernicious anemia, due to lack of the intrinsic (absorption) factor, this recycling mechanism is defective, and liver stores become depleted. Absorption of vitamin B_{12} can be inhibited by ethanol, neomycin, and para-aminosalicylic acid (77).

Liver Function and Disease

Storage of vitamin B_{12} in the liver is affected by intake of ethanol. Chronic liver damage due to ethanol varies in its action (Fig. 2). If accompanied by mild fatty changes in the liver, only a slight reduction in liver B_{12} concentration occurred, but severe fatty change and cirrhosis caused an extensive reduction (3). In vitamin B_{12} deficiency, liver stores of folate can be decreased, without significant reduction in plasma folate levels (103).

The relationship of liver B_{12} and plasma B_{12} concentrations in disease has been extensively studied. The general picture is that acute liver damage causes release of B_{12} into the plasma, some bound to serum proteins, some remaining free. For example, perfusion of rat livers with ethanol (22) results in rapid release of vitamin B_{12} and an increase in serum B_{12} levels. Similarly, in experimental liver damage in rats due to carbon tetrachloride, the increased vitamin B_{12} content of serum is proportional to the degree of liver damage (5). Various liver diseases (viral hepatitis, cirrhosis, malignancy, hypersplenism, obstructive jaundice) also result in reduction in liver B_{12} content, accompanied by an increase in plasma concentration (5,99), which is a result of necrosis of liver with release of B_{12} (104). Excessive levels of total vitamin B_{12} are also reported in serum, mostly in free form, in viral hepatitis and cirrhosis (5). In other cases of cirrhosis, gross reductions in plasma B_{12} content have been observed (17). These discrepancies may be explained by differences in plasma-protein binding of B_{12} (104). Davis et al (105) report that patients with acute hepatitis and jaundice have low levels of vitamin B_{12} binding capacity, possibly associated with hyperbilirubinemia. Patients with acute hepatitis and necrosis have high levels of *free* plasma B_{12}, whereas in chronic liver disease, the *bound* form rises (104).

Plasma B_{12} has been extensively studied. In healthy adults, methylcobalamin is the major cobalamin and usually accounts for 60 to 80% of total plasma cobalamin (70). Smaller amounts of 5-deoxyadenosylcobalamin and hydroxycobalamin are also present. In leukemia and liver disease (acute and chronic hepatitis, cirrhosis, hepatoma), increases in plasma transcobalamin concentrations, particularly transcobalamin I (TCI), result in concomitant increases in plasma cobalamins (99). An additional factor may be the release of 5-deoxyadenosylcobalamin from damaged hepatic cells into the blood leading to a disproportionate increase in plasma 5-deoxyadenosylcobalamin (99).

PANTOTHENIC ACID

Pantothenic acid was first identified in 1933 as a factor associated with growth of yeast cells. It was later shown that, in chicks, lack of the same factor gave rise to dermatitis. The factor was isolated and named pantothenic acid because of its widespread distribution. It consists chemically of β-alanine joined to pantoic acid (Fig. 15). It is used in the body as the basis of coenzyme A which participates in the metabolism of acetate (Fig. 1).

Metabolism

Pantothenic acid is readily absorbed from the small intestine, not metabolized to a significant extent, and largely excreted in the urine. In the liver, it is present in the bound form of coenzyme A, notably in mitochondria (5). Table 1 shows that the concentration of pantothenic acid is several times greater than that found in other tissues. In agreement with this evidence of hepatic storage, liver is more affected by variations in dietary intake than are other organs. In pantothenic acid deficiency in rats, the mitochondria of the liver show abnormalities. Hurley (106) examined pregnant rats and found that fetal death occurred when the level of pantothenate in the maternal liver fell to 40% below normal levels.

Liver Function and Disease

Spontaneous gross deficiency of pantothenic acid has not been described in man, although some symptoms have been thought to relate to deficiency of the vitamin. Coenzyme A levels in the liver of man are reduced by chronic ethanol intake with fatty change, but less so than by cirrhosis (Fig. 2). Plasma levels of pantothenic acid in liver disease are variable. In cirrhosis, Leevy et al. (17) note low plasma levels of

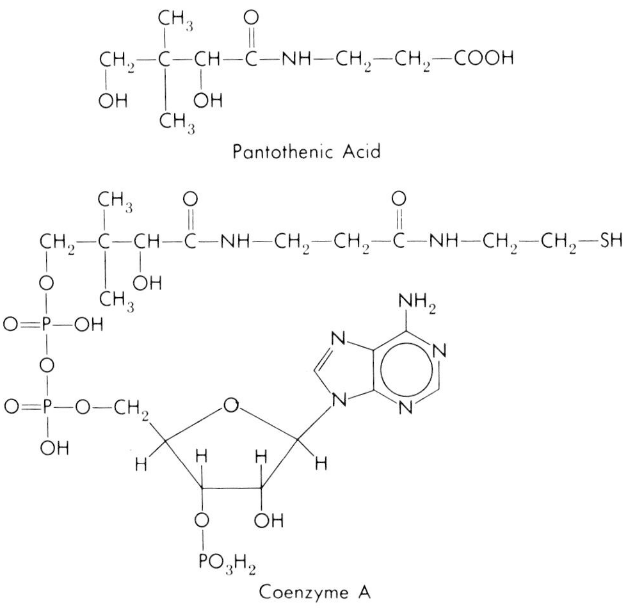

FIG. 15. Structure of pantothenic acid and coenzyme A. (Reproduced from ref. 4, with permission.)

pantothenic acid, whereas in another series of patients with acute fatty infiltration of liver due to alcohol, plasma pantothenic acid levels increased (3). Leevy et al. (107) found that low levels of pantothenic acid were uncommon in 172 alcoholic patients. On the other hand, 20% of patients with cirrhosis, 15% with fatty liver, and 12% with normal liver function had decreased blood levels of pantothenic acid.

BIOTIN

Biotin deficiency is known to cause dermatitis in laboratory animals, notably those receiving raw egg white, which contains a protein (avidin) that binds the vitamin. The structure of biotin is shown in Fig. 16. As shown in Fig. 1, biotin functions in CO_2 fixation and decarboxylation reactions (108).

Metabolism

Biotin is rapidly absorbed from the intestine and is readily excreted in the urine as intact biotin and as biotin sulfoxide and *bis*-norbiotin (108).

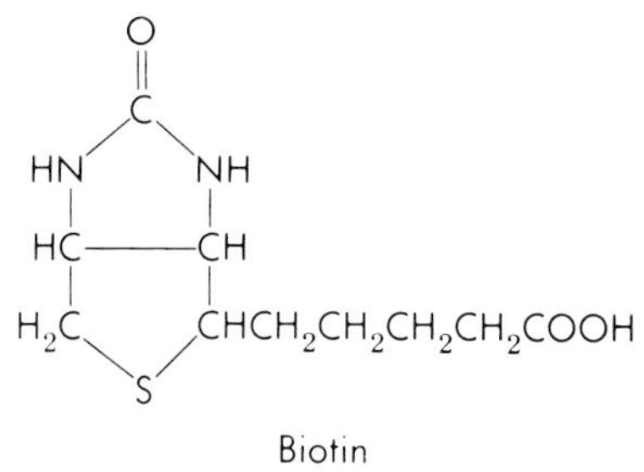

FIG. 16. Structure of biotin. (Reproduced from ref. 4, with permission.)

Liver Function and Disease

The concentration of biotin in the liver is higher than in other organs (Table 1); within the liver, 90% is bound to protein (109). In chicks, biotin deficiency reduces the proportion of ribosomes attached to the rough endoplasmic reticulum. This correlates with the known reduction in liver protein synthesis in deficiency (110). Sorrell et al. (22) perfused the liver of normal and alcohol-fed rats and showed that, in contrast to other vitamins, ethanol did not cause general release of the vitamin from the liver.

In cirrhosis, Baker et al. (3) showed that even mild fatty infiltration of the liver reduced liver biotin levels; the change in frank cirrhosis was much less (Fig. 2).

CONCLUSION

The literature on the metabolism of the B complex vitamins emphasizes the important role of the liver, which often contains higher concentrations of the vitamin. It remains uncertain whether this represents a true store, as in the case of vitamin A, or whether it is attributable to an unusually high metabolic need for the vitamin by the liver.

An important feature of the liver is its function in the synthesis of active forms of B vitamins for use by other tissues (e.g., thiamin pyrophosphate, pyridoxal phosphate, possibly methyltetrahydrofolic acid, and methylcobalamin). This makes other tissues dependent on liver function for their supply of active vitamins and thus liable to deficiency in cases of liver damage, even when supplementary vitamins are given. Thus vitamin therapy for liver disease should be given as the metabolically active forms of each vitamin.

Finally, a number of vitamins are transported by plasma proteins, most of which are synthesized and secreted by the liver. The plasma levels of these are affected to various extents by protein deficiency, as reported by Shetty et al. (111). There is little information, however, about the effects of protein malnutrition on the levels of individual transport-proteins for the B vitamins. Since a major function of such transport proteins is to prevent excessive urinary losses of the vitamin, a reduction in level can result in less efficient utilization of the dietary intake of the vitamin. In some cases, the transport proteins can bind to specific receptors on tissues. Thus transcobalamin II binds to receptors on bone marrow cells and delivers vitamin B_{12}. Cases of congenital deficiency of this transport protein require enormous doses of vitamin B_{12} to survive (112).

These observations emphasize the interaction of the liver with other tissues in ensuring distribution of the water-soluble B vitamins and their active derivatives. A better understanding of the role of the liver is likely to result in improved therapy with active forms of vitamins in patients with liver disease.

REFERENCES

1. Food and Nutrition Board (1980): *Recommended Dietary Allowances.* National Academy of Sciences, Washington, D.C.
2. Russell, R. M. (1979): Vitamin and mineral supplements in the management of liver disease. *Med. Clin. North Am.,* 63:537–544.
3. Baker, H., Frank, O., Ziffer, H., Goldfarb, S., Leevy, C. M., and Sobotka, H. (1964): Effect of hepatic disease on liver B-complex vitamin titers. *Am. J. Clin. Nutr.,* 14:1–6.
4. Danford, D. E., and Munro, H. N. (1980): The water-soluble vitamins: The vitamin B-complex and ascorbic acid. In: *The Pharmacological Basis of Therapeutics,* sixth edition, edited by L. S. Goodman and A. Gillman, pp. 1560–1582. Macmillan, New York.
5. Wiss, O., and Weber, F. (1964): The liver and vitamins. In: *The Liver: Morphology, Biochemistry, Physiology, Vol. II.,* edited by C. H. Rouiller, pp. 145-162. Academic Press, New York.
6. Moran, J. R., and Greene, H. I. (1969): The B vitamins and vitamin C in human nutrition. I. General considerations and "Obligatory" B vitamins. *Am. J. Dis. Child,* 133:192–199.
7. Tanphaichitr, V. (1976): Thiamin. In: *Present Knowledge in Nutrition,* edited by Hegsted, D. M., Chichester, C. O., Darby, W. J., McKnutt, K. W., Stalvey, R. M., and Stotz, E. H., pp. 141–148. Nutrition Foundation, New York.
8. Rindi, G., and Ventura U. (1972): Thiamine intestinal transport. *Physiol. Rev.,* 52:821–827.
9. Dianzani, M. U., and Dianzani Mor, M. A. (1957): Displacement of thiamine pyrophosphate from swollen mitochondria. *Biochim. Biophys. Acta,* 24:564–568.
10. Westenbrink, H. G. (1960): Biochemical features of thiamine metabolism. *Proc. Intern. Congr. Biochem., 4th Congr., Vienna, 1958,* 11:73–85.
11. Ferrari, G., Cappelli, V., and Ceriani, T. (1976): Liver and brain thiamin depletion and neurologic signs in pigeon athiaminosis. *Int. J. Vitam. Nutr. Res.,* 46:303–309.
12. Anonymous (1971): Catabolites of thiamin from the rat. *Nutr. Rev.,* 29:119–121.
13. Holowach, J., Kauffman F., Ikossi, M., Thomas, C., and McDougal, D. (1968): The effects of a thiamine antagonist, pyrithiamine, on levels of selected metabolic intermediates and on activities of thiamine-dependent enzymes in brain and liver. *J. Neurochem.,* 15:621–631.
14. Schenker, S., Chen, D., Speeg, V., Walker, C., and McCandless, D. (1971): Hepatic metabolism and transport in thiamine deficiency. *Dig. Dis.,* 16:255–264.
15. McCandless, D. W., Cassidy, C. E., and Curley, A. D. (1975): Thiamine deficiency and the hepatic pentose phosphate cycle. *Biochem. Med.,* 14:384–390.
16. Brown, M. L., and Snodgrass, C. H. (1965): Effect of dietary level of thiamine on reproduction in the rat. *J. Nutr.,* 85:102–106.
17. Leevy, C. M., Thompson, A., and Baker, H. (1970): Vitamins and liver injury. *Am. J. Clin. Nutr.,* 23:493–499.
18. Hoyumpa, A. M., Green K. J., Schenker, S., and Wilson, S. A. (1975): Thiamine transport across the rat intestine: II. Effects of ethanol. *J. Lab. Clin. Med.,* 86:803–813.
19. Hoyumpa, A. M., Jr., Nichols, S., Henderson, G. T., and Schenker, S. (1978): Intestinal thiamine transport: Effect of chronic ethanol administration in rats. *Am. J. Clin. Nutr.,* 31:938–945.
20. Abe, T. (1977): Effect of ethanol administration on thiamine metabolism and transketolase activity in rats. *Int. J. Vitam. Nutr. Res.,* 47:307–314.
21. Fennelly, J. J., Baker, H., Frank, O., and Leevy, C. M. (1963): Deficiency of thiamine pyrophosphate apoenzyme in liver disease. *Clin. Res.,* 11:182.
22. Sorrell, M. F., Baker, H., Barak, A. J., and Frank, O. (1974):

Release by ethanol of vitamins into rat liver perfusates. *Am. J. Clin. Nutr.,* 27:743–745.
23. Fennelly, J., Frank, O, Baker, H., and Leevy, C. M. (1967): Red blood cell-transketolase activity in malnourished alcoholics with cirrhosis. *Am. J. Clin. Nutr.,* 20:946–949.
24. Rossouw, J. E., Labadarios, D., Davis, M., and Williams, R. (1978): Water-soluble vitamins in severe liver disease. *S. Afr. Med. J.,* 54:183–186.
25. Labadarios, D., Rossouw, J. E., McConnell, J. B., Davis, R. L., and Williams, R. (1977): Thiamine deficiency in fulminant hepatic failure and effects of supplementation. *Int. J. Vitam. Nutr. Res.,* 47:17–22.
26. Jusko, W. J., and Levy, G. (1975): Absorption, protein binding, and elimination of riboflavin. In: *Riboflavin,* edited by R. S. Rivlin, pp. 99–152. Plenum, New York.
27. Rivlin, R. S. (1979): Hormones, drugs and riboflavin. *Nutr. Rev.,* 37:241–246.
28. Rivlin, R. S. (1970): Regulation of flavoprotein enzymes in hypothyroidism and in riboflavin deficiency. *Adv. Enz. Regul.* 8:239–250.
29. McCormick, D. B. (1976): Riboflavin. In: *Present Knowledge in Nutrition,* edited by D. M. Hegsted, Chichester, C. O., Darby, W. J., McKnutt, K. W., Stalvey, R. M., and Stotz, E. H., pp. 131–140. Nutrition Foundation, New York.
30. Jusko, W. J., and Levy, G. (1967): Absorption, metabolism, and excretion of riboflavin 5-phosphate in man. *J. Pharm. Sci.,* 56:58–62.
31. Fass, S., and Rivlin, R. S. (1969): Regulation of riboflavin-metabolizing enzymes in riboflavin deficiency. *Am. J. Physiol.,* 217:988–991.
32. Rivlin, R. S. (1970): Riboflavin metabolism. *N. Engl. J. Med.,* 283:463–472.
33. Tandler, B., Erlandson, R. A., and Wynder, E. L. (1968): Riboflavin and mouse hepatic cell structure and function I. Ultrastructural alterations in simple deficiency. *Am. J. Pathol.* 52:69–95.
34. Burch, H. B., Hunter, F. E., Jr., Combs, A. M., and Schutz, B. A. (1960): Oxidative enzymes and phosphorylation in hepatic mitochondria from riboflavin-deficient rats. *J. Biol. Chem.,* 235:1540–1544.
35. Sugioka, G., Porta, E. A., Corey, P. N., and Hartroft, W. S. (1969): The liver of rats fed riboflavin deficient diets at two levels of protein. *Am. J. Pathol.,* 54:1–19.
36. Mookerjea, S., and Hawkins, W. W. (1960): Some anabolic aspects of protein metabolism in riboflavin deficiency in the rat. *Br. J. Nutr.,* 14:231–238.
37. Mason, M. (1953): The metabolism of tryptophan in riboflavin-deficient rats. *J. Biol. Chem.,* 201:513–518.
38. Honda, Y. (1968): Folate derivatives in the liver of riboflavin-deficient rats. *Tohoku J. Exp. Med.,* 95:79–86.
39. Lakshuni, A. V., and Bamji, M. S. (1976): Regulation of blood pyridoxal phosphate in riboflavin deficiency in men. *Nutr. Metab.,* 20:228–233.
40. Bro-Rasmussen, F. (1958): The riboflavin requirement of animals and man and associated metabolic relations. Part II. Relation of requirement to the metabolism of protein and energy. *Nutr. Abstr. Rev.,* 28:369–386.
41. Fazekas, A. G., and Sandor, T. (1971): The *in vivo* effect of adrenocorticotropin on the biosynthesis of flavin nucleotides in rat liver and kidney. *Can. J. Biochem.,* 49:987–989.
42. Sourkes, T. L., Murphy, G. F., and Woodford, V. R. (1960): Effects of deficiencies of pyridoxine, riboflavin and thiamine upon the catecholamine content of rat tissues. *J. Nutr.,* 72:145–152.
43. Miller, Z., Poncet, I., and Lakacs, E. (1962): Biochemical studies on experimental congential malformations: Flavin nucleotides and folic acid in fetuses and livers from normal and riboflavin-deficient rats. *J. Biol. Chem.,* 237:968–973.
44. Rosenthal, W. S., Adham, N. F., Lopez R., and Cooperman, J. M. (1973): Riboflavin deficiency in complicated chronic alcoholism. *Am. J. Clin. Nutr.,* 26:858–860.
45. Stanko, R. T., Medelow, H., Shinozuka, H., and Abidi, S. A. (1978): Prevention of alcohol-induced fatty liver by natural metabolites and riboflavin. *J. Lab. Clin. Med.,* 91:228–235.

46. Chen, C., and Liao, T. (1960): Histochemical study on riboflavin. *J. Vitam. (Osaka)*, 6:171–195.

47. Henderson, L. M., and Gross, C. J. (1979): Metabolism of niacin and niacinamide in perfused rat intestine. *J. Nutr.*, 109:654–662.

48. Preiss, J., and Handler, P. (1958): Biosynthesis of diphosphopyridine nucleotide. II. Enzymatic aspects. *J. Biol. Chem.*, 233:493–500.

49. Roth, L. J., Leifer, E., Hogness, J. R., and Langham, W. H., (1948): Studies on the metabolism of radioactive nicotinic acid and nicotinamide in mice. *J. Biol. Chem.*, 176:249–257.

50. Baker, H., Frank, O., and Sorrell, M. F. (1976): Nicotinic acid and alcoholism. *Bibl. Nutr. Dieta*, 24:32–39.

51. Brin, M. (1978): Vitamin B_6: Chemistry, absorption, metabolism, catabolism, and toxicity. In: *Human Vitamin B_6 Requirements*, pp. 1–20. National Academy of Sciences, Washington, D.C.

52. Food and Nutrition Board (1978): *Human Vitamin B_6 Requirements.* National Academy of Sciences, Washington, D.C.

53. DiSorbo, D. M., Phelps, D. S., Ohl, U. S., and Litwack, G. (1980): Pyridoxine deficiency influences the behavior of the glucocorticoid-receptor complex. *J. Biol. Chem.*, 255: 3866–3870.

54. Müller, R. E., Traish, A., and Wotiz, H. H. (1980): Effects of pyridoxal 5′-phosphate on uterine estrogen receptor. I. Inhibition of nuclear binding in cell-free system and intact uterus. *J. Biol. Chem.*, 255:4062–4067.

55. Mehansho, H., Hamm, M. W., and Henderson, L. M. (1979): Transport and metabolism of pyridoxal and pyridoxal phosphate in the small intestine of the rat. *J. Nutr.*, 109:1542–1551.

56. Mehansho, H., Buss, D. D., Hamm, M. W., and Henderson, L. M. (1980): Transport and metabolism of pyridoxine in rat liver. *Biochim. Biophys. Acta*, 631:112–123.

57. Buss, D. D., Hamm, M. W., Mehansho, H., and Henderson, L. M. (1980): Transport and metabolism of pyridoxine in the perfused small intestine and the hind limb of the rat. *J. Nutr.*, 110:1655–1663.

58. Hamm, M. W., Mehansho, H., and Henderson, L. M. (1980): Management of pyridoxine and pyridoxal in the isolated kidney of the rat. *J. Nutr.*, 110:1597–1609.

59. Lumeng, L., Brashear, R. E., and Li, T. K. (1974): Pyridoxal 5-phosphate in plasma: Source, protein-binding, and cellular transport. *J. Lab. Clin.*, 84:334–343.

60. Shane, B. (1978): Vitamin B_6 and blood. In: *Human Vitamin B_6 Requirements*, pp. 111–128. National Academy of Sciences, Washington, D.C.

61. Lyon, J. B., Bain, J. A., and Williams, H. L. (1962): The distribution of vitamin B_6 in the tissues of two inbred strains of mice fed complete and vitamin B_6-deficient rations. *J. Biol. Chem.*, 237:1989–1991.

62. Spannuth, C. L., Mitchell, D., Stone, W. J., Schenker, S., and Wagner, C. (1978): Vitamin B_6 nutriture in patients with uremia and with liver disease. In: *Human Vitamin B_6 Requirements*, edited by Food and Nutrition Board, pp. 180–192. National Academy of Sciences, Washington, D.C.

63. Mitchell, D., Wagner, C., Stone, W. J., Wilkinson, G., and Schenker, S. (1976): Abnormal regulation of plasma pyridoxal 5-phosphate in patients with liver disease. *Gastroenterology*, 71:1043–1049.

64. Leevy, C. M., Baker, H., Ten Hove, W., Frank, O., and Cherrick, G. R. (1965): B-complex vitamins in liver disease of the alcoholic. *Am. J. Clin. Nutr.*, 16:339–346.

65. Anderson, B. B., Newmark, P. A., Rawlins, M., and Green, R. (1974): Plasma binding of vitamin B_6 compounds. *Nature*, 250:502–504.

66. Food and Nutrition Board (1977): *Folic Acid: Biochemistry and Physiology in Relation to the Human Nutrition Requirement.* National Academy of Sciences, Washington, D.C.

67. Halsted, C. H., and Tamura, T. (1979): Folate deficiency in liver disease. In: *Problems in Liver Diseases*, edited by C. S. Davidson, pp. 91–100. Stratton, New York.

68. Hillman, R. S. (1980): Vitamin B_{12}, folic acid, and the treatment of megaloblastic anemias. In: *The Pharmacological Basis of Therapeutics*, edited by A. G. Gilman, L. S. Goodman, and A. Gilman, pp. 1331–1346. Macmillan, New York.

69. Rosenberg, I. H. (1977): Role of intestinal conjugase in the control of the absorption of polyglutamyl folates. In: *Folic Acid: Biochemistry and Physiology in Relation to the Human Nutrition Requirement*, pp. 136–146. National Academy of Sciences, Washington, D.C.

70. Herbert, V., Colman, N., and Jacob, E. (1980): Folic acid and vitamin B_{12}. In: *Modern Nutrition in Health and Disease*, edited by R. S. Goodhart and M. E. Shils, pp. 229–259. Lea & Febiger, Philadelphia.

71. Kiil, J., Jagerstad, M., and Elsborg, L. (1979): The role of liver passage for conversion of pteroylmonoglutamate and pteroyltriglutamate to active folate coenzyme. *Int. J. Vitam. Nutr. Res.*, 49:296–306.

72. Steinberg, S. E., Campbell, C. L., and Hillman, R. S. (1979): Kinetics of the normal folate enterohepatic cycle. *J. Clin. Invest.*, 64:83–88.

73. Hillman, R. S., McGuffin R., and Campbell, C. (1977): Alcohol interference with the folate enterhepatic cycle. *Trans. Assoc. Am. Physicians*, 90:145–156.

74. Hoppner, K., and Lampi, B. (1980): Folate levels in human liver from autopsies in Canada. *Am. J. Clin. Nutr.*, 33:862–864.

75. Wu, A., Chanarin L., Slavin, G., and Levi, A. J. (1975): Folate deficiency in the alcoholic—its relationship to clinical and haematological abnormalities, liver disease and folate stores. *Br. J. Haematol.*, 29:469–478.

76. Richardson, R. E., Healy, M. J., and Nixon, P. F. (1979): Folates of rat tissue: Bioassay of tissue foly/polyglutamates and a relationship of liver foly/polyglutamates to nutritional folate sufficiency. *Biochim. Biophys. Acta*, 585:128–133.

77. Waxman, S., Corcino, J. J., and Herbert, V. (1970): Drugs, toxins and dietary amino acids affecting vitamin B_{12} or folic acid absorption or utilization. *Am. J. Med.*, 48:599–608.

78. Cherrick, G. R., Baker H., Frank, O., and Leevy, C. M. (1965): Observations on hepatic avidity for folate in Laennec's cirrhosis. *J. Lab. Clin. Med.*, 66:446–451.

79. Brown, J. P., Davidson, G. E., Scott, J. M., and Weir, J. (1973): Effect of diphenylhydantoin and ethanol feeding on the synthesis of rat liver folates from exogenous pteroylglutamate [³H]. *Biochem. Pharmacol.*, 22:3287–3289.

80. Lane, P., Goff, R., McGuffin, R., Eichner, R., and Hillman, R. S. (1976): Folic acid metabolism in normal, folate deficient and alcoholic man. *Br. J. Haematol.*, 34:489–500.

81. McGuffin, R., Goff, P., and Hillman, R. S. (1975): The effect of diet and alcohol on the development of folate deficiency in the rat. *Br. J. Haematol.*, 31:185–192.

82. Tamura, T., Watson, J. E., Romero, J. J., and Halsted, C. H. (1978): Effect of alcoholism on hepatic folate metabolism. *Clin. Res.*, 26:327A.

83. Russell, R. M., et al. (1982): Diminished turnover and increased urinary excretion of folic acid due to ethanol ingestion. *J. Lab. Clin. Med.* (in press).

84. Horne, D. W., Briggs, W. T., and Wagner, C. (1978): Ethanol stimulates 5-methyl-tetrahydrofolate accumulation in isolated rat liver cells. *Biochem. Pharmacol.*, 27:2069–2074.

85. Hillman, R. S. (1975): Alcohol and hematopoiesis. *Ann. NY Acad. Sci.*, 252:297–306.

86. Herbert, V. (1962): Experimental nutritional folate deficiency in man. *Trans. Assoc. Am. Physicians*, 75:307–320.

87. Eishner, E. R., and Hillman R. S. (1971): The evolution of anemia in alcoholic patients. *Am. J. Med.*, 50:218–232.

88. Halsted, C. H., Robles, E. A., and Mezey, E. (1973): Intestinal malabsorption in folate-deficient alcoholics. *Gastroenterology*, 64:526–532.

89. Retief, F. P., and Huskisson, Y. J. (1969): Serum and urinary folate in liver disease. *Br. Med. J.*, 2:150–153.

90. Tamura, T., and Stokstad, E. L. R. (1977): Increased folate excretion in acute hepatitis. *Am. J. Clin. Nutr.*, 30:1378–1379.

91. Kimber, C., Deller, D. J., Ibbotson, R. N., and Lander, H. (1965): The mechanism of anaemia in chronic liver disease. *Q. J. Med.*, 133:33–64.

92. Klipstein, F. A., and Lindenbaum, J. (1965): Folate deficiency in chronic liver disease. *Blood*, 25:443–456.

93. Campbell, R. E., and Pruitt, F. W. (1955): The effect of vitamin B_{12} and folic acid in the treatment of viral hepatitis. *Am. J. Med. Sci.*, 229:8–15.

94. Leevy, C. M. (1966): Abnormalities of hepatic DNA synthesis in man. *Medicine*, 45:423–433.

95. Leevy, C. M., LenHove, W., Frank, O., and Baker, H. (1964): Folic acid deficiency and hepatic DNA synthesis. *Proc. Soc. Exp. Biol. Med.*, 117:746–748.

96. Marchetti, M., Tolomelli, B., Formiggini, G., and Bovina, C. (1980): Distribution of pteroylglutamates in rat liver during regeneration after partial hepatectomy. *Biochem. J.*, 188:553–556.

97. Retief, F. P., Gottlieb, C. W., and Herbert, V. (1966): Mechanism of vitamin B_{12} uptake by erythrocytes. *J. Clin. Invest.*, 45:1907–1915.

98. Ellenbogen, L. (1975): Absorption and transport of cobalamin. Intrinsic factor and the transcobalamins. In: *Cobalamin Biochemistry and Pathophysiology*, edited by B. M. Babior, pp. 215–286. Wiley, New York.

99. Linnell, J. (1975): The fate of cobalamins *in vivo*. In: *Cobalamin Biochemistry and Pathophysiology*, edited by B. M. Babior, pp. 287–333. Wiley, New York.

100. Toohey, J. I., and Barker, H. A. (1961): Isolation of coenzyme B_{12} from liver. *J. Biol. Chem.*, 236:560–563.

101. Girdwood, R. H. (1952): The occurrence of growth factors for *Lactobacillus leichmannii*, *Streptococcus faecalis* and *leuconostoc citrovorum* in the tissues of pernicious anaemia patients and controls. *Biochem. J.*, 52:58–63.

102. Gräsbeck, R., Myberg, W., and Reizenstein, P. G. (1958): Biliary and fecal vitamin B_{12} excretion in man. An isotope study. *Proc. Soc. Exp. Biol. Med.*, 97:780–784.

103. Tisman, G., and Herbert, V. (1973): B-12 dependence of cell uptake of serum folate: An explanation for high serum folate and cell folate depletion in B-12 deficiency. *Blood*, 41:465–469.

104. Jones, P. N., Mills E. H., and Capps, R. B. (1957): The effect of liver on serum vitamin B_{12} concentrations. *J. Lab. Clin. Med.*, 49:910–922.

105. Davis, R. L., Duvall, R. C., and Chow, B. F. (1957): Serum vitamin B_{12} level and binding substance of tuberculosis patients with and without liver disease. *J. Lab. Clin. Med.*, 49:422–428.

106. Hurley, L. S. (1980): Water-soluble vitamins In: *Developmental Nutrition*, pp. 143–167. Prentice-Hall, Englewood Cliffs, New Jersey.

107. Leevy, C. M., George, W. S., Ziffer, H., and Baker, H. (1960): Pantothenic acid, fatty liver and alcoholism. *J. Clin. Invest.*, 39:1005.

108. Appel, J. A., and Briggs, G. M. (1980): Biotin. In: *Modern Nutrition in Health and Disease*, edited by R. S. Goodhart and M. E. Shils, pp. 274–279. Lea & Febiger, Philadelphia.

109. Semenza, G., Prestidge, L. S., Menard-Jeker, D., and Bettex-Galland, M. (1959): Oxalacetate-carboxylase and biotin. *Helv. Chim. Acta*, 42:669–678.

110. Frigg, M., and Rohr, H. P. (1978): Stereological composition of the liver of biotin deficient and control chicks. *Int. J. Vitam. Nutr. Res.*, 48:348–350.

111. Shetty, P. S., Jung, R. T., Watrasiewicz, K. E., and James, W. P. T. (1979): Rapid-turnover transport proteins: An index of subclinical protein-energy malnutrition. *Lancet*, 2:230–232.

112. Hakami, N., Neiman, P. E., Carnellos, P. E., and Lazerson, J. (1972): Neonatal megaloblastic anemia due to inherited transobalamin II deficiency in two siblings. *N. Engl. J. Med.*, 285:1163–1170.

113. Spector, W. S. (editor) (1956): In: *Handbook of Biological Data*, pp. 1–584. Saunders, Philadelphia.

114. Williams, R. J. (1943): The significance of the vitamin content of tissues. *Vitam. Horm.*, 1:229–247.

115. Schenker, S., Henderson, G. I., Hoyumpa, A. M., and McCandless, D. W. (1980): Hepatic and Wernicke's encephalopathies: current concepts of pathogenesis. *Am. J. Clin. Nutr.*, 33:2719–2726.

116. Hoyumpa, A. M. (1980): Mechanisms of thiamin deficiency in chronic alcoholism. *Am. J. Clin. Nutr.*, 33:2750–2761.

117. Mezey, E. (1980): Alcoholic liver disease: Roles of alcohol and malnutrition. *Am. J. Clin. Nutr.*, 33:2709–2718.

118. Selhub, J., Dhar, G. J., and Rosenberg, I. H. (1978): Inhibition of folate enzymes by sulfasalazine. *J. Clin. Invest.*, 61:221–224.

119. Halsted, C. H. (1980): Folate deficiency in alcoholism. *Am. J. Clin. Nutr.*, 33:2736–2740.

The Liver: Biology and Pathobiology, edited by
I. Arias, H. Popper, D. Schachter, and D. A. Shafritz.
Raven Press, New York © 1982.

Chapter 24

Pathobiology of Metals

Irmin Sternlieb

Iron, copper, zinc, manganese, selenium, and cobalt are essential for normal liver function. Their importance derives from the fact that these metals form prosthetic groups of certain enzymes or serve as cofactors for enzyme activation. Examples for the former are cytochrome oxidase, an enzyme that contains iron and copper, alcohol dehydrogenase, which contains zinc, and pyruvate carboxylase, which contains manganese. Manganese is also required for the activation of mevalonic kinase, which catalyzes the conversion of mevalonic acid to squalene, a major precursor of hepatic cholesterol. Average balanced diets supply adequate amounts of these metals relative to body needs, so that nutritional deficiencies rarely occur unless reduced absorption, impaired transport across the intestinal mucosa, or pathologic losses of the metal take place. Even under adverse conditions, however, the liver has a remarkable capacity for conservation, so that hepatic dysfunction due to deficiency of any of these metals is unknown. In contrast, accumulation of excess iron or copper may be injurious to the liver and other organs, albeit resulting in different defects and displaying different pathologic features. In this chapter, we deal specifically with liver diseases related to the essential metals copper and zinc and the nonessential metal arsenic.

COPPER

Absorption and Storage

Approximately half of the 2 to 5 mg dietary copper ingested daily is absorbed from the upper small intes-

tine. The remainder is excreted directly in the feces (1). Although the form and mechanism by which copper is absorbed by the intestine are unknown, it has been established that a cytosolic protein having the characteristics of metallothionein binds the copper that has entered the epithelial cells (2). Transport from intestinal cells into the portal circulation is under control of an inherited, X-linked mechanism which is absent in infants with Menkes' kinky or steely hair disease (3,4). Absorption of copper also may be impaired when the intestinal absorptive surface is reduced by severe, diffuse diseases, such as celiac sprue, lymphosarcoma, or scleroderma, or because of malnutrition (1). A schematic diagram illustrating the essential features of copper ingestion and transport to and from the liver is shown in Fig. 1.

A portion of absorbed copper is transported in plasma loosely bound to albumin and perhaps to amino acids or peptides (5,6). This fraction of the circulating copper constitutes about 5 to 10% of the total amount of copper present in human plasma. It is promptly cleared by the liver, where there is a highly efficient membrane recognition system for albumin-bound copper. This is evident from radiocopper studies demonstrating that the liver takes up 60 to 90% of the absorbed copper within a few hours (7). Initially, the deposited copper binds predominantly to a low molecular thiol-rich cytosolic protein (2,8) and, to a lesser extent and more slowly, to a larger protein, hepatocuprein or superoxide dismutase (9,10). These two proteins account for the binding of about 80% of the copper content of normal human liver. The remainder is incorpo-

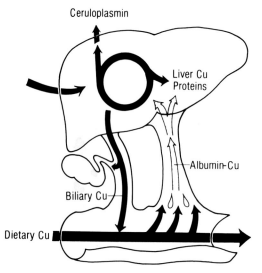

FIG. 1. Metabolic pathways of orally ingested copper.

rated into specific copper proteins such as cytochrome c oxidase, mitochondrial monoamine oxidase, and ceruloplasmin, or is taken up by lysosomes before excretion into the bile (Fig. 2) (7,11,12).

Mobilization of copper from hepatocytes takes place via two main routes. About 0.5 mg/day freshly deposited copper is incorporated into ceruloplasmin during hepatic synthesis and is released into the bloodstream (6). More important in maintaining the constancy of hepatic concentration in the normal human adult, however, is the bile, which mobilizes approximately 1.5 mg/day copper (11,13), while the urine accounts for merely 0.03 mg. Biliary copper seems to originate from hepatocellular lysosomes, but the site at which it is bound to a carrier which inhibits its reabsorption from the intestine is uncertain. Kupffer cells do not appear to play a role in hepatic copper metabolism.

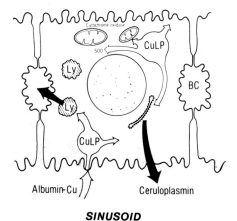

SINUSOID

FIG. 2. Details of metabolic pathways and copper utilization in hepatocytes. BC, bile canaliculus; CuLP, cytosolic low molecular weight copper-binding protein; Ly, lysosome; SOD, cytosolic superoxide dismutase (hepatocuprein).

Proteins

Two low molecular weight copper-binding proteins, L-6-D (Cu-LP) (8) and metallothionein (2,14−16) with molecular weights of 10,000 and 6,000 daltons, respectively, have been studied extensively. Both these proteins have high sulfhydryl contents, but their capacities for copper differ. Human cytosolic metallothionein contains 0.3 g atoms copper and about 3 g atoms zinc (14). On the other hand, L-6-D, comprising about 2 mg/g wet human liver, contains up to 3% copper and little zinc (8). The two proteins differ also with respect to their cysteine content, which is considerably more abundant in metallothionein. A different metallothionein, which binds 2.5 g atoms copper and less than half the amount of zinc of the cytosolic sulfhydryl-rich protein, was isolated from the particulate, presumably lysosomal, fraction of human neonatal liver (17). This form of metallothionein probably is identical with the hepatomitochondrocuprein, found earlier in the liver of neonates and patients with Wilson's disease (16).

Superoxide dismutase (cytocuprein or hepatocuprein) is a light blue-green, copper and zinc-containing metalloprotein of MW 33,600 (9,10). It is present in cytosol and in the intermembraneous space of mitochondria. It catalyzes dismutation of the superoxide anion into hydrogen peroxide and oxygen and may scavenge oxygen atoms in certain reactions. Superoxide dismutase may prevent injury to hepatocytic components from superoxide radicals generated by aerobic metabolic reactions.

Mitochondrial monoamine oxidase, present in liver mitochondria, forms hydrogen peroxide enzymatically and ammonia and aldehydes from several monoamines, epinephrine, and serotonin through oxidative deamination.

Cytochrome c oxidase, or ferrocytochrome c oxygen oxidoreductase, is the major component of the inner mitochondrial membranes and serves as the terminal enzyme in the respiratory chain. It has a molecular weight of ∼270,000 daltons and contains prosthetic heme molecules and copper atoms, both of which are essential to the enzymatic activity of the protein and its role in normal iron metabolism.

Ceruloplasmin (ferroxidase I) is a blue glycoprotein, which is synthesized by the liver and secreted into the plasma. It has a molecular weight of 130,000 daltons and contains 6 atoms of copper and 8% of carbohydrate (6). It catalyzes the oxidation of several polyamines, catecholamines, and polyphenols, particularly paraphenylenediamine, and Fe^{2+} to Fe^{3+}. The last reaction may facilitate the binding of iron to transferrin, since this requires uptake of ferric iron. Histaminase activity has also been attributed to ceruloplasmin. The physiologic significance of these activities (all of which, with the exception of feroxidase activity, have been observed only *in vitro*) is obscure. The 8 to 10 oligosaccharide chains of ceruloplasmin are composed principally of glucosamine, mannose, and galactose, with most, if not all, chains terminated by a sialic acid residue. The presence of sialic acid appears to be essential to the survival of ceruloplasmin in the circulation (6).

Ceruloplasmin is normally present in plasma at concentrations between 20 and 45 mg/dl. Its concentration is lowered in 95% of the patients with Wilson's disease and in untreated Menkes' disease. As an isolated finding, however, deficiency of serum ceruloplasmin does not necessarily indicate disease, because the normal neonate and 10% of healthy heterozygous carriers of a single Wilson's disease gene have lowered concentrations of ceruloplasmin. Occasionally, reduced concentration of ceruloplasmin is found in severe hepatic necrosis or as consequences of urinary or gastrointestinal protein loss. The opposite—namely, increases above the upper limits of the normal range (40mg/dl)—occur late in pregnancy, in a number of acute and chronic diseases, and during the administration of estrogens or their analogs. Molecular heterogeneity of ceruloplasmin, both genetic and acquired, has been reported.

Deficiency

When the supply of copper is severely curtailed, e.g., in infants with Menkes' kinky or steely hair disease, cytochrome content of the liver and serum ceruloplasmin concentrations are reduced without identifiable structural change (3,4). Experimentally, however, copper deficiency in rats leads to enlargement and alteration in the shape of hepatocellular mitochondria, as well as to depletion of cytochrome c oxidase.

Toxicosis

Numerous metabolic functions are affected when the liver is exposed experimentally to excess copper (7,18). If this surfeit cannot be disposed of readily, inhibition of mitochondrial respiration, inhibition of 26-hydroxylation of cholesterol, reduction of RNA polymerase activity, changes in certain microsomal enzyme activities, induction of lysosomes, and the release of lysosomal enzymes into the cytosol have been observed. Also, the plasma membrane may be altered through the displacement of components normally bound at negative sites, thus diminishing its ability to form a barrier to the diffusion of small molecules and ions. Some cytosolic components are also susceptible to the effects of copper because of their high content of

sulfhydryl groups. For example, polymerization of tubulin may be blocked, and microtubules may be degraded in the presence of excess copper. Such pertubations, in turn, may affect spindle formation, nuclear functions, and export of proteins and triglycerides from hepatocytes. Excess copper may also deplete cellular gluthathione reserves, destabilize nuclear DNA, and labilize lysosomal membranes. Although the actual importance of these disturbances cannot be evaluated, each may cause or contribute to cell death. Based on observations of patterns of evolution of liver injury in patients with Wilson's disease (19–21) and in Bedlington terriers, copper may play a direct or indirect role in hepatic fibrogenesis.

Wilson's Disease

Within 1 year after the description of hepatolenticular degeneration (Wilson's disease), there were hints relating copper to this entity. Forty years passed, however, before sufficient evidence established unequivocally that copper was an etiologic factor, and that the liver was invariably affected in this disorder. These discoveries in turn led to the development of rational therapy (22) capable of reversing the inexorably progressive course and even preventing the appearance of clinical disease (23). Despite these remarkable advances, the precise mechanism by which the liver accumulates copper is still unknown. The following hypotheses regarding the pathogenesis of copper accumulation in patients with Wilson's disease have been proposed:

1. An increased net absorption of dietary copper as the cause for copper overload was suggested by positive copper balance studies. Apart from the inability of such studies to discriminate between overabsorption and diminished excretion, the increments that were reported would result in far greater accumulation of copper than actually observed. Obviously, these studies were inaccurate. On the other hand, when double isotope (^{64}Cu and ^{67}Cu) studies were performed, or when the height of the initial peak of plasma radioactivity following an oral test dose of radiocopper was used as a gross measure of absorption, no significant difference between normal subjects, heterozygotes, and patients with Wilson's disease were detected (1). Consequently, these observations do not support overabsorption as a significant factor in the accumulation of copper in Wilson's disease.

2. Absent, diminished, or altered synthesis and secretion of ceruloplasmin, with consequent reduced mobilization of hepatic copper, provides a rational basis for the retention of excessive amounts of copper. A lack of correlation between these two most characteristic biochemical abnormalities, as well as the oc-

currence of serum ceruloplasmin deficiency in some heterozygous carriers of a single Wilson's disease gene, unaccompanied by elevation of the hepatic copper concentration, argues against the assumption that ceruloplasmin plays a central role in maintaining copper balance.

3. Increased binding and uptake of copper by an abnormal cytosolic metallothionein with a higher affinity for copper was considered to be the principal defect of Wilson's disease (2). Apart from objections to the interpretation of the data, this conclusion is inconsistent with the finding that uptake of radiocopper by the liver of patients with Wilson's disease is less than that of normal subjects.

4. A decreased excretion of biliary copper by patients with Wilson's disease compared to normal subjects was established in several laboratories (7,11,12). Although the nature of this defect is unknown, it seems to be localized to hepatocellular lysosomes (24). This conclusion is based on observations of identical specific activities of radiocopper in the bile and in the lysosomal fraction of a liver homogenate obtained from a patient with Wilson's disease, whereas the specific activities of the isotope in other subcellular fractions differed widely from that of the bile (25).

Taken individually, many of the structural changes observed in the liver of patients with Wilson's disease are similar to those seen in other forms of liver injury. Thus, for instance, the histologic picture of steatosis characteristic of the early stages of copper-induced hepatic toxicosis can be easily confused with that of alcoholic fatty liver. Yet the experienced observer may be alerted to a different etiology by some distinctive features: (a) the lipid droplets in hepatocytes are usually smaller; (b) there may be conspicuous glycogen-filled hepatocellular nuclei in the periportal areas; and (c) pathognomonic hepatocellular mitochondria or, occasionally, abnormal enlarged peroxisomes are seen in electron micrographs (20,26,27). Clearly, the mechanism that causes retention of triglycerides by hepatocytes and the pronounced cytopathologic changes during the early stages of Wilson disease differs from that of other forms of metabolic injury. Furthermore, the progression from a fatty liver to either chronic active hepatitis (28) or, insidiously, to micro- and macronodular cirrhosis when mitochondrial lesions are minimal is distinctive. The transition from the early phase, when cytopathologic features predominate, to the scarred cirrhotic liver is accompanied by changes in the diffusely cytoplasmic distribution of copper to sequestration in lysosomes (30). The factors that cause this transition are unknown, although its frequent occurrence during adolescence suggests that age-related factors (possibly hormonal) may influence the development of the

lysosomal copper sequestering and thereby determine the evolution of the hepatic lesion. Coincidentally, there is release of some excess copper from the liver with accumulation of copper in other tissues, particularly in brain, kidney, and corneas, and an elevation of the nonceruloplasmin-bound fraction of plasma copper.

Although this schema (Figs. 1 and 2) seems to accommodate the majority of patients with Wilson's disease (22,25,31), it fails to deal with at least two puzzling situations. The first is fulminant, submassive hepatic necrosis, often associated with Mallory bodies and hemolysis that develop suddenly and without an identifiable extraneous cause in some patients. The second is the inexplicable delay in the progression from hepatic steatosis to cirrhosis in rare patients who maintain the "juvenile pattern" of steatosis, characterized by elevation of hepatic copper concentration but no symptoms of Wilson's disease for decades or longer.

Despite these gaps in our understanding of the factors that modulate expression of copper toxicosis, it appears that the lysosome plays a pivotal role by sequestering copper and thus protecting the hepatocytes from its toxic effects. It is unclear, however, why this protective effect of the lysosomes is not evident in young patients, why it is delayed or activated only at a more advanced stage of the disease, and what determines the capacity of the lysosome to sequester copper; nor do we know whether copper released from lysosomes is directly toxic or fibrogenic.

Clinical Manifestations

During the early stages of Wilson's disease, the liver binds 30 to 50 times its normal concentration of copper with little if any overt clinical manifestations. Symptoms of liver disease never appear before 6 years of age. In untreated patients, neurologic effects generally occur later in adolescence. The age of onset of clinical disease varies from patient to patient. In addition to hepatic, neurologic, or psychiatric disorders, Wilson's disease may manifest itself in (a) Kayser-Fleischer rings and sunflower cataracts, (b) renal abnormalities, including hematuria, proteinuria, aminoaciduria, uricosuria, phosphaturia, and acidification defects, (c) hematologic disturbances, including anemia, leukopenia, thrombocytopenia, and clotting disturbances, (d) endocrine dysfunctions, such as amenorrhea, miscarriage, gynecomastia, and delayed puberty, (e) osseous and articular abnormalities, and (f) skin and nailbed pigmentation. Some of these abnormalities are primary; some, such as the endocrine disturbances, are secondary to liver dysfunction in hormone metabolism.

Manifestations of liver disease may include weakness, lassitude, jaundice, upper abdominal pain, spider angiomas, fever, splenomegaly, hypersplenism, ascites, portal hypertension, hematemesis, a tendency toward bruising, and spontaneous bacterial peritonitis. Hepatic insufficiency, particularly if complicated by hemolysis, may mimic the clinical picture of fulminant hepatitis and lead to death within weeks or months (25,32,33).

The hepatic manifestations of Wilson's disease are nonspecific and can be easily confused with those of acute viral hepatitis, infectious mononucleosis, chronic active hepatitis, juvenile cirrhosis, cryptogenic or alcoholic cirrhosis, and idiopathic thrombocytopenic purpura. By the time patients develop neurologic manifestations, cirrhosis with fine fibrotic bands separating nodules of different sizes is invariably present (25).

A comparison of several features of Wilson's disease with those of hemochromatosis underscores the remarkable differences between these metal storage diseases (Table 1).

In addition to this clearly inherited form of copper toxicosis of the liver, several other diseases are associated with retention of copper in hepatocytes secondary to cholestasis, inhalation of copper salts, or undetermined mechanisms. Two- or three fold elevations of hepatic copper concentration are present nonspecifically in various forms of liver disease, including chronic active hepatitis (34,35). These increases are probably without pathologic significance.

Cholestatic Syndromes and Primary Biliary Cirrhosis

Intra- or extrahepatic disturbances in the secretion of bile—the major route of excretion of copper from the body—result in the retention of copper by the liver. In these instances, the pathologic process precedes the accumulation of copper, and the latter progresses with the duration of cholestasis or with the stage of primary biliary cirrhosis (PBC). Both "copper-associated protein" (36) and copper itself can be demonstrated by the use of Shikata's orcein, rhodanine, rubeanic acid, and Timm's stains. These materials accumulate in granules around portal tracts undergoing scarring and occasionally in the cytoplasm of the periportal or peripherally located hepatocytes of most lobules and nodules (30). It is still uncertain whether this copper excess is harmful. Despite hepatic copper concentrations that equal those seen in Wilson's disease, copper does not affect the central nervous system of patients with PBC (15,30,37,38). Hypercupriuria or Kayser-Fleischer rings can occur in PBC and in other cholestatic syndromes and may raise diagnostic problems, but the presence of clinical, laboratory, and histologic features of cholestasis, normal or elevated ceruloplasmin concentration in the serum of these patients, and the topographic distribution of copper in the liver rule out the diagnosis of Wilson's disease.

Indian childhood cirrhosis (ICC) is a severe, progressive, and fatal disease of unknown etiology affecting children ages 1 to 3 years. The histologic picture varies from one resembling a subacute stage of viral hepatitis, to micronodular cirrhosis or fulminant massive necrosis with some hepatocytes containing Mallory's hyalin. Once hepatic insufficiency and ascites appear, death is inevitable. The entity is distinguished by its age of onset and its restriction to the Asian subcontinent. It is not Wilson's disease, since patients with ICC uniformly have normal concentrations of ceruloplasmin in their serum. Furthermore, Kayser-Fleischer rings or neurologic lesions have not been described in this disease. The finding of orcein- or

TABLE 1. *Comparison of certain features of Wilson's disease and hemochromatosis*

Characteristic	Wilson's disease	Hemochromatosis
Inheritance	Recessive (not HLA linked)	Recessive (HLA linked)
Metabolic defect	Decreased biliary excretion of copper	Increased intestinal absorption of iron
Clinical onset	Childhood, early adulthood	Late adulthood
Primary target cell	Hepatocyte	Hepatocyte
Hepatocellular metal-storing protein	Cytosolic copper binding: early; lysosomal Cu-associated protein: late	Cytosolic and lysosomal ferritin; hemosiderin
Evolution of histopathology	Steatosis→fibrosis→ (chronic active hepatitis) →multilobular cirrhosis	Periportal fibrosis→perilobular fibrosis→mono- and multilobular cirrhosis
Diagnostic plasma protein abnormality	Ceruloplasmin reduced	Ferritin increased
Incidence of hepatocellular carcinoma	Very low	High
Organs involved secondarily	Brain, eyes, kidneys	Heart, pancreas, joints

rhodanine-stained hepatocytic granules indicating copper-associated protein and copper, respectively, as well as determinations of hepatic copper concentrations, established that this disease was associated with an enormous hepatic copper overload (39,40). Even though some cholestasis is present in these specimens, it is not sufficient to account for the extent of copper retention. Moreover, the stage of disease during which copper is deposited has not been determined, since most specimens available for study were from patients with advanced disease.

Liver Disease in Vineyard Sprayers

Although liver disease due to oral ingestion of excess copper has not been noted even in miners working and eating in atmospheres heavily contaminated with copper, a peculiar liver disease characterized by swelling and proliferation of Kupffer cells, histiocytic and sarcoid-like granulomata, fibrosis, proliferation of sinusoidal lining cells, micronodular cirrhosis, angiosarcoma, and idiopathic portal hypertension has been reported in a few workers exposed to Bordeaux mixture sprays, which contain copper sulfate. It is unclear why this entity has been encountered only in Portugal, and whether the development of these lesions is related to the chemical form or to the route of entry of copper into the body (41).

Therapy of Hepatic Copper Overload

The effect of copper-chelating therapy in patients with Wilson's disease provides compelling evidence for the injurious role of excess copper on the liver. D-Penicillamine (0.75 to 2 g) is the drug of choice for the treatment of Wilson's disease at any stage. The earlier this therapy is instituted, the better the results, particularly for asymptomatic patients who are being treated prophylactically. Moreover, morphologic abnormalities of hepatocytes, including mitochondrial alterations, seen in pretreatment biopsy samples disappear with D-Penicillamine administration. Most clinical manifestations of hepatic dysfunction improve on a long-term "decopperizing" regimen: ascites and jaundice disappear, and serum albumin and aminotransferase concentrations return to normal levels, as does gonadal function. However, portal hypertension, cirrhosis, distended esophageal varices, splenomegaly, and hypersplenism often remain unchanged (22,25).

In contrast with the established role of chelation therapy for Wilson's disease, preliminary results of D-penicillamine therapy of PBC are encouraging but not conclusive. Liver copper concentrations fall, and serum aminotransferase levels are significantly reduced compared with those in placebo-treated patients. Although these beneficial effects may be due to removal of copper, D-penicillamine is also known to affect the immune system and reduce circulating immune complexes, which may be the reason for clinical amelioration.

Animal Models of Hepatic Copper Toxicosis

Prolonged oral or parenteral administration of copper salts to experimental animals failed to produce hepatic lesions similar to those seen in Wilson's disease. Nonetheless, the accumulation of copper is associated with injury to the liver in several animal species (18,42). Sheep grazing on pastures enriched with copper and poor in molybdenum may accumulate excess hepatic copper. This in turn causes necrosis and portal fibrosis and a clinical disorder manifested by weakness, trembling, anorexia, and ultimately hemolysis. This last feature bears a striking resemblance to the hemolytic episodes experienced by some patients with Wilson's disease (25,32).

A closer similarity between human Wilson disease and an animal disorder has emerged from the study of certain Bedlington terriers with a genetic disorder associated with accumulations as high as 10 mg copper/g liver (19,21,43). The striking morphologic feature of this disorder is the presence of dense, copper-containing lysosomal granules in hepatocytes. As the concentration of copper increases with time, there is progression from focal and chronic active hepatitis to micro- and macronodular cirrhosis. Fatal hemolysis occurs in some of these dogs relatively early in life, while late manifestations of hepatic insufficiency develop in others. Of note is the striking similarity in the ability of the canine and advanced Wilsonian hepatic lysosomal granules to sequester copper. There is also similarity in some clinical and histologic features, although neither the concentration of serum ceruloplasmin nor any copper-induced lesion of the brain, kidney, or cornea was seen in the mutant dogs. Nonetheless, important concepts in our understanding of inherited defects in copper metabolism should emerge from the study of these animals.

ZINC

Absorption and Storage

The recommended dietary intake of 15 mg zinc for a normal adult represents a somewhat higher proportion of the total body stores (2 to 3 g) of this metal as compared to copper (18,44). Most of the zinc is ingested with dietary protein and is absorbed from the upper small intestine. Binding of zinc to the same metallothionein that binds copper is suggested by competition for absorption between these two metals if an excess of either is administered. Once dietary zinc is taken up by the intestinal epithelial cells, a portion is rapidly transported to the plasma, where it is associated with albumin, alpha₂-macroglobulin, transferrin, and amino acids. Unlike copper, of which at most 5 to 10% is loosely bound to albumin, as much as two-thirds of the 100 mcg zinc present in plasma is bound to this protein and to amino acids. Roughly 3% of total body zinc is stored in the liver, and some is bound to specific zinc proteins.

Intake of zinc may vary considerably, and interference of absorption may occur because of other nutrients (e.g., phytate) or because of an inherited defect that causes acrodermatitis enteropathica in children. Except for this latter disorder, clinically manifest zinc deficiency (hypogonadal dwarfism, hypogeusia, skin disorders) is rare and can be explained by dietary perversion (geophagia), severe malabsorption, or parenteral hyperalimentation without zinc supplements (44). Zinc deficiency has been implicated in defective mobilization of vitamin A from the liver (45).

Hepatic Zinc Proteins

Alcohol dehydrogenase (ADH) is a well-characterized microsomal enzyme which catalyzes the oxidation of ethanol, methanol, ethylene glycol, vitamin A alcohol, and certain sterols, using NAD as a cofactor. ADH has a molecular weight of 87,000 and 4 g atoms zinc. Its content is decreased in livers of alcoholic patients. Superoxide dismutase (hepatocuprein) is a zinc- and copper-containing enzyme listed in the previous section.

Pathologic Conditions

No liver disease is caused by either deficiency or excess storage of hepatic zinc. In patients with alcoholic liver disease, viral hepatitis, or other forms of liver disease, however, the concentrations of zinc in liver and plasma are often decreased (44). Concomitantly, there may be increased excretion of urinary zinc, which may contribute to the decrease in plasma zinc. This probably is not the only factor determining this abnormality, since similar low plasma values are encountered in patients with intestinal malabsorption and hypoalbuminemia but with zincuria (45). Except for these biochemical abnormalities, which some authors have related to the hypogeusia and anosmia experienced by some patients with liver disease, no pathologic lesion of the liver can be etiologically related to zinc.

ARSENIC

Chronic ingestion of medicinal arsenic, previously used for the treatment of psoriasis, may cause noncir-

rhotic portal fibrosis and portal hypertension. Occasionally, cirrhosis, angiosarcoma, or hepatocellular carcinoma is seen in association with chronic arsenicism years after discontinuation of the toxin. Arsenic should be suspected whenever patients with chronic liver disease present with hyperkeratosis of palms and soles or have cancers in unexposed areas of the skin (46). Arsenic-induced liver disease demonstrates complications of portal hypertension, hepatic insufficiency, or neoplasia. Elevated hepatic arsenic concentrations are also found in autopsy specimens obtained from patients with ICC (47), raising the possibility that more than one toxic metal, i.e., arsenic and copper, may be involved in the pathogenesis of this puzzling disorder.

ACKNOWLEDGMENTS

The original work included in this chapter was supported in part by grants from the National Institute of Arthritis, Metabolism and Digestive Diseases (AM-17702) and the General Clinical Research Center (5 M01 RR-50) and by the Foundation for the Study of Wilson's Disease, Inc.

REFERENCES

1. Sternlieb, I. (1967): Gastrointestinal copper absorption in man. *Gastroenterology*, 52:1038–1041.
2. Evans, G. W. (1973): Copper homeostasis in the mammalian system. *Physiol. Rev.*, 53:535–570.
3. Danks, D. M. (1977): Copper transport and utilization in Menkes' syndrome and in mottled mice. *Inorg. Persp. Biol. Med.*, 1:73–100.
4. French, J. H. (1977): X-chromosome linked copper malabsorption (X-cLCM). In: *Handbook of Clinical Neurology*, edited by P. J. Vinken, G. W. Bruyn, and H. L. Klawans, pp. 279-304. North Holland, New York.
5. Sass-Kortsak, A., and Bearn, A. G. (1978): Hereditary disorders of copper metabolism. In: *The Metabolic Basis of Inherited Disease*, 4th edition, edited by J. B. Stanbury, J. B. Wyngaarden, and D. S. Fredrickson, pp. 1098–1126. McGraw-Hill, New York.
6. Scheinberg, I. H., and Morell, A. G. (1973): Ceruloplasmin. In: *Inorganic Biochemistry, Vol. 1*, edited by G. L. Eichhorn, pp. 306-319. Elsevier, New York.
7. Sternlieb, I. (1980): Copper and the liver. *Gastroenterology*, 78:1615–1628.
8. Morell, A. G., Shapiro, J. R., and Scheinberg, I. H. (1961): Copper binding protein from human liver. In: *Wilson's Disease: Some Current Concepts*, edited by J. M. Walshe and J. N. Cumings, pp. 36–41. Charles C Thomas, Springfield, Illinois.
9. Carrico, R. J., and Deutsch, H. F. (1969): Isolation of human hepatocuprein and cerebrocuprein. Their identity with erythrocuprein. *J. Biol. Chem.*, 244:6087–6093.
10. Fridovich, I. (1974): Superoxide dismutases. *Adv. Enzymol.*, 41:35–97.
11. Frommer, D. J. (1974): Defective biliary excretion of copper in Wilson's disease. *Gut*, 15:125–129.
12. O'Reilly, S., Weber, P. M., Oswald, M., and Shipley, L. (1971): Abnormalities of the physiology of copper in Wilson's disease. III. The excretion of copper. *Arch. Neurol.*, 25:28–32.
13. van Berge Henegouwen, G. P., Tangedahl, T. N., Hofmann, A. E., Northfield, T. C., LaRusso, N. F., and McCall, J. T. (1977): Biliary secretion of copper in healthy man. Quantitation by an intestinal perfusion technique. *Gastroenterology*, 72: 1228–1231.

14. Kagi, J. H. R., Kojima, Y., Berger, C., Kissling, M. M., Lerch, K., and Vašak, M. (1979): Metallothionein: Structure and evolution. In *Metalloproteins*, edited by U. Weser, pp. 194–206. Georg Thieme, Stuttgart.

15. Owen, C. A., Jr., Dickson, R. E., Goldstein, N. P., Baggenstoss, A. H., and McCall, J. T. (1977): Hepatic subcellular distribution of copper in primary biliary cirrhosis. Comparison with other hyperhepatocupric states and review of the literature. *Mayo Clin. Proc.*, 52:73–80.

16. Porter H. (1968): Copper proteins in brain and liver in normal subjects and in cases of Wilson's disease. In: *Wilson's Disease—Birth Defects Original Article Series. Vol. 4, No. 2,* edited by D. Bergsma, I. H. Scheinberg, and I. Sternlieb, pp. 23–28. National Foundation, March of Dimes, New York.

17. Ryden, L., and Deutsch, H. F. (1978): Preparation and properties of the major copper-binding component in human fetal liver. *J. Biol. Chem.*, 253:519–524.

18. Bremner, I. (1974): Heavy metal toxicities. *Q. Rev. Biophys.*, 7:75–124.

19. Ludwig, J., Owen, C. A., Jr., Barham, S. S., McCall, J. T., and Hardy, R. M. (1980): The liver in the inherited copper disease of Bedlington terriers. *Lab. Invest.*, 43:82–87.

20. Sternlieb, I. (1972): Evolution of the hepatic lesion in Wilson's disease (hepatolenticular degeneration). In: *Progress in Liver Diseases, Vol. 4,* edited by H. Popper and F. Schaffner, pp. 511–525. Grune & Stratton, New York.

21. Twedt, D. C., Sternlieb, I., and Gilbertson, S. R. (1979): Clinical, morphologic, and chemical studies on copper toxicosis of Bedlington terriers. *J. Am. Vet. Med. Assoc.*, 175:269–275.

22. Walshe, J. M. (1976): Wilson's disease (hepatolenticular degeneration). In: *Handbook of Clinical Neurology, Vol. 27,* edited by P. J. Vinken and H. L. Klaven, pp. 379–414. Elsevier, New York.

23. Sternlieb, I., and Scheinberg, I. H. (1968): Prevention of Wilson's disease in asymptomatic patients. *N. Engl. J. Med.*, 278:352–359.

24. Sternlieb, I., and Goldfischer, S. (1976): Heavy metals and lysosomes. In: *Lysosomes in Biology and Pathology, Vol. 5,* edited by J. T. Dingle and R. T. Dean, pp. 185–200. Elsevier, New York.

25. Sternlieb, I., and Scheinberg, I. H. (1979): Wilson's disease. In: *Liver and Biliary Disease,* edited by R. Wright, K. G. M. M. Alberti, S. Karran, and G. H. Millward-Sadler, pp. 774–787. Saunders, London.

26. Sternlieb, I. (1979): Electron microscopy of mitochondria and peroxisomes of human hepatocytes. In: *Progress in Liver Diseases, Vol. 6,* edited by H. Popper and F. Schaffner, pp. 81–104. Grune & Stratton, New York.

27. Stromeyer, F. W., and Ishak, K. G. (1980): Histology of the liver in Wilson's disease. *Am. J. Clin. Pathol.*, 73:12–24.

28. Sternlieb, I., and Scheinberg, I. H. (1972): Chronic hepatitis as a first manifestation of Wilson's disease. *Ann. Intern. Med.*, 76:59–64.

29. Scott, J., Gollan, J. L., Samourian, S., and Sherlock, S. (1978): Wilson's disease presenting as chronic active hepatitis. *Gastroenterology*, 74:645–651.

30. Goldfischer, S., Popper, H., and Sternlieb, I. (1980): The significance of bariations in the distribution of copper in liver disease. *Am. J. Pathol.*, 99:715–730.

31. Strickland, G. T., Frommer, D., Leu, M. L., Pollard, R., Sherlock, S., and Cumings, J. N. (1973): Wilson's disease in the United Kingdom and Taiwan. *Q. J. Med.*, 62:619–638.

32. Deiss, A., Lee, G. R., and Cartwright, G. E. (1970): Hemolytic anemia in Wilson's disease. *Ann. Intern Med.*, 73:413–418.

33. Sternlieb, I. (1978): Diagnosis of Wilson's disease. *Gastroenterology*, 74:787–789.

34. Gubler, C. J., Brown, H., Markowitz, H., Cartwright, G. E., and Wintrobe, M. M. (1957): Studies on copper metabolism XXIII. Portal (Laennec's) cirrhosis of the liver. *J. Clin. Invest.*, 36:1208–1216.

35. Smallwood, R. A. (1978): Other liver diseases associated with increased liver copper concentration. In: *Metals and the Liver,* edited by L. W. Powell, pp. 313–330. Marcel Dekker, New York.

36. Sipponen, P. (1976): Orcein positive hepatocellular material in long-standing biliary diseases. I. Histochemical characteristics. *Scand. J. Gastroenterol.*, 11:545–552.

37. Benson, G. D. (1979): Hepatic copper accumulation in primary biliary cirrhosis. *Yale J. Biol. Med.*, 52:83–88.

38. Fleming, C. R., Dickson, E. R., Baggenstoss, A. H., and McCall, J. T. (1974): Copper and primary biliary cirrhosis. *Gastroenterology*, 67:1182–1187.

39. Popper, H., Goldfischer, S., Sternlieb, I., Nayak, N. C., and Madhavan, T. V. (1979): Cytoplasmic copper and its toxic effects. Studies in Indian childhood cirrhosis. *Lancet,* i:1205–1208.

40. Tanner, M. S., Portmann, B., Mowat, A. P. Williams, R., Pandit, A. N., Mills, C. F., and Bremner, M. N. (1979): Increased hepatic copper concentration in Indian childhood cirrhosis. *Lancet,* i:1203–1204.

41. Pimentel, J. C., and Menezes, A. P. (1975): Liver granulomas containing copper in vineyard sprayer's lung. A new etiology of hepatic granulomatosis. *Am. Rev. Resp. Dis.*, 111:189–195.

42. Ishmael, J., Gopinath, C., and Howell, J. M. (1971): Experimental chronic copper toxicity in sheep. Histological and histochemical changes during the development of lesions in the liver. *Res. Vet. Sci.*, 12:358–366.

43. Johnson, G. F., Sternlieb, I., Twedt, D. C., Grushoff, P. S., and Scheinberg, I. H. (1981): Inheritance of the copper toxicosis of Bedlington terriers. *Am. J. Vet. Res.* 41:1865–1866.

44. Prasad, A. S. (editor) (1976): *Trace Elements in Human Health and Disease.* Academic Press, New York.

45. Walker, B. E., Dawson, J. B., Kelleher, J., and Losowsky, N. S. (1973): Plasma and urinary zinc in patients with malabsorption syndromes or hepatic cirrhosis. *Gut,* 14:943–948.

46. Cowlishaw, J. L., Pollard, E. J., Cowen, A. E., and Powell, L. W. (1979): Liver disease associated with chronic arsenic ingestion. *Aust. N.Z. J. Med.*, 9:310–313.

47. Datta, D. V., Sahni, M. M., Narang, A. P. S., Sharma, J. P., Dang, H. S., Walia, B. N. S., and Somasundram, S. (1978): Arsenic and copper levels in Indian childhood cirrhosis. *Proc. Ind. Soc. Gastroenterol. Falk Hepatology,* X:227 (*Abstr.*).

The Liver: Biology and Pathobiology, edited by
I. Arias, H. Popper, D. Schachter, and D. A. Shafritz.
Raven Press, New York © 1982.

Chapter 25

The Liver and Iron

Stephen P. Young and Philip Aisen

ROLE OF THE LIVER IN IRON METABOLISM

In keeping with its essential role in a wide variety of biochemical reactions, iron is extremely well conserved in man. Daily loss is normally limited to 1 mg in the normal adult male (1), representing about 0.02% of total body iron, and is balanced by absorption of iron from the gut. The liver plays a dual role in this conservation.

The Kupffer cell, as part of the reticuloendothelial system, is involved in the recycling of iron from senescent erythrocytes, especially in pathological states, and thus helps maintain a steady-state supply of iron for the biosynthesis of hemoglobin and other iron proteins. When confronted by situations of iron deficiency or iron excess, the storage reserve of hepatocytes acts as a buffer for an element without which life is inconceivable but which in excess is a threat to life.

Storage of Iron

Hepatocytes

In man, less than 10% of iron turnover in plasma represents exchange of iron between transferrin and the iron stores of the hepatocytes (2). About 0.4 g iron, chiefly as ferritin, is present in these hepatic stores (3,4). Although the control of iron uptake into and release from the iron store is not well understood at the

molecular level, the main factor probably is the serum iron concentration. This in turn is a function of the rate of use of iron for synthesis of hemoglobin and other iron proteins, release of iron from the reticuloendothelial system, and absorption from the lumen of the gut.

Using the perfused rat liver, it has been shown that the total iron concentration in the perfusate controls net uptake of iron into the liver (5), while with cultured isolated hepatocytes (6) and whole animals (7), saturation of transferrin determines uptake by the liver. Iron from diferric transferrin may be particularly well sequestered by hepatocytes, although many other tissues also take up iron from transferrin at a rate that increases as the protein approaches saturation (8). Clearly, therefore, either transferrin saturation or serum iron concentration, or both, regulate uptake of iron by the liver. Cellular factors undoubtedly are operating as well, but these have not been studied in depth. In contrast to the essentially unidirectional uptake by erythroid cells, transfer of iron between transferrin and the hepatocyte is a two-way process; thus net retention depends on flow in each direction.

We have shown recently (9) that iron uptake and release by isolated rat hepatocytes can occur simultaneously. The rate of release appears to be constant as long as a minimum concentration of apotransferrin is present in the medium. The rate of uptake, on the other hand, increases with higher concentrations of diferric transferrin. If *in vitro* observations with isolated hepatocytes apply to the intact organism, high serum iron concentration would promote uptake over release; at lower serum iron concentrations, release would exceed uptake, representing a net efflux of iron from the stores. Whether iron from diferric or monoferric transferrin iron is taken up preferentially or whether one or the other of the two sites of transferrin is a better donor of iron for the hepatocyte remain problems for further investigation.

Kupffer Cells

Until recently, it was thought that the Kupffer cells and the rest of the reticuloendothelial system were the main sites of long-term storage of iron (10). It now appears, however, that the hepatocytes perform this function. Little ferritin or nonheme iron is to be found in the Kupffer cells of the normal rat (11). Injection of iron dextran or hemoglobin in large doses increases the so-called nonheme but not the ferritin iron in these cells (11). About 85% of the iron of heat-damaged erythrocytes can be captured by the human reticuloendothelial system and returned to circulating erythrocytes within 12 days, the remainder presumably exchanging with parenchymal iron stores and other nonhemoglobin iron-containing compartments (12). How this recycling varies with iron status is not known.

Red Blood Cell Breakdown

Most iron transfer across the Kupffer cell membrane is an efflux of iron from catabolized erythrocytes to serum transferrin. Nevertheless, isolated Kupffer cells are reported to be capable of taking up iron from transferrin (13). This uptake is much slower than uptake into hepatocytes, perhaps explaining why only an insignificant removal of iron-59 from transferrin by reticuloendothelial cells *in vivo* is seen (14). Administration of iron-59-labeled heat-damaged erythrocytes to normal rats leads to exclusive labeling of reticuloendothelial cells with the same proportion of radioactivity in the liver as in the spleen (15). Radioactivity in the spleen decreases more rapidly than in the liver, suggesting either preferential release of iron by the spleen or redistribution of iron to the hepatic iron stores. Recirculation of iron from the reticuloendothelial cells to the hepatocytes is diminished in bled animals when the demand of the bone marrow for iron is stimulated but is increased when erythropoiesis is suppressed by hypertransfusion (14). Experiments with normal human subjects suggest that the spleen preferentially removes erythrocytes with slight damage, the Kupffer cells becoming more important as the degree of damage to the erythrocytes increases (16). The narrowness of the splenic sinusoids may make them better filters for minimally altered erythrocytes.

CELLULAR ASPECTS OF IRON METABOLISM

Hepatocytes

Membrane Involvement

The uptake of iron into the reticulocyte involves the binding of iron-laden transferrin to a cell surface receptor, followed by removal of iron by the cell and release of the iron-depleted but otherwise intact protein (17, Fig. 1). The presence of transferrin receptors on erythroid cells (17), B and T lymphoblastoid cells (18), placental trophoblasts (19), and many types of cultured human cells (20) suggests the ubiquity of transferrin receptors and that they are required to allow the uptake of iron from transferrin into these cells. The hepatocyte is no exception to this rule, since the isolated rat hepatocyte appears to have about 37,000 high-affinity receptors for diferric transferrin. The apparent association constant for the binding of transferrin by its hepatocyte receptor is 1.6×10^7 liters/mole^{-1} (9). As this association constant is similar to that reported for the binding of transferrin to the isolated rabbit reticulocyte transferrin receptor (21), the relative uptake of iron from transferrin by different cells probably is not determined by differences in the affinity of their receptors for transferrin. More likely, the uptake is determined by the absolute number of receptors. Red blood cell precursors, with a large requirement for iron, have from 100,000 (21) to 7 million (22) transferrin receptors per cell, whereas B and T lymphoblastoid cells (18) and hepatocytes (9), each with a relatively modest demand for iron, have only 30,000 and 37,000 transferrin receptors, respectively.

Release of iron from hepatocytes to apotransferrin has been demonstrated with the perfused rat liver (23) and with suspensions of isolated hepatocytes (9). In

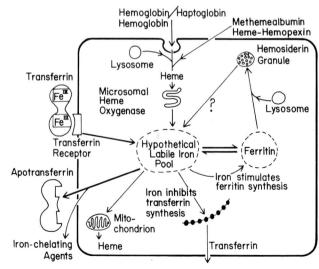

FIG. 1. Schema of the possible pathways followed by iron in the hepatocyte.

neither system could release of iron be increased above a basal level by increasing the apotransferrin concentration, perhaps indicating that the rate of release is predominantly modulated by intracellular factors.

The mechanism of release of iron from transferrin to cells is unknown. Since transferrin has a serum half-life of 7 to 8 days (30), many times longer than the 1 to 2 hr half-life of serum iron (24), degradation of the protein is not required for release of iron. It has been suggested that transferrin is internalized by pinocytosis before its iron is made available to cells (25). This mechanism is similar to that suggested for the internalization of many extracellular proteins, as has been pointed out in a recent review (26); most of the other proteins cited in this review were destined for lysosomal destruction, in contrast to transferrin, which escapes intact from reticulocytes and presumably from other cell types as well. Analysis of data on the uptake of iron by hepatocytes (9) indicates that each transferrin receptor handles at least two iron atoms each minute. It is unclear whether this is sufficient time for internalization, release of iron, and extrusion of the iron-depleted protein to occur. Alternatively, iron may be released at or near the cell membrane by an unknown mechanism, followed by transmembrane transport of the iron.

Once the iron has been captured by the cell, it probably enters a transient, low molecular weight cytosolic iron pool (27). Iron from this pool is then available for rerelease to the plasma, incorporation into iron proteins synthesized by the liver, principally cytochrome P_{450}, or storage in ferritin.

Lysosomes

Although transferrin probably is the major source of iron for hepatocytes, these cells also derive iron from the uptake of heme-hemopexin (28), hemoglobin-haptoglobin (28,29), methemalbumin, and free plasma hemoglobin (29). Heme is dissociated from albumin and probably transferred to hemopexin before being taken up by the liver (30,31). The other heme complexes are taken up *in toto* (30,32). After entry into the cells, hemoglobin appears largely in phagosomes, which then fuse with primary lysosomes for digestion of the protein (33). Free heme, in contrast, accumulates in the microsomal fraction (34), where the enzyme system responsible for the oxidation of heme and the release of the iron is located (35). It is likely, therefore, that heme is released from hemoglobin after lysosomal degradation of the protein and then transferred to the smooth endoplasmic reticulum for removal of the iron. Much of the iron released in this process is subsequently found in the cytosolic ferritin of the hepatocytes (33).

Heme Synthesis

Much of the information on the incorporation of iron into heme has been gained using isolated liver mitochondria. The mechanisms deduced are applicable for the process in erythrocyte precursors as well. Iron from a variety of low molecular weight complexes and ferritin can be used by mitochondria (36). If iron is presented as Fe(III), it first binds to ligands on the outer phase of the inner mitochondria membrane (36). Reduction to Fe(II) then occurs, followed by ATP-dependent transport across the inner membrane. The metal is then bound, as Fe(II), to a high molecular weight component (37). The transmembrane transport of Fe(II) has many of the characteristics of calcium transport; in fact, it is competitively inhibited by the presence of Ca^{2+} (38). Ferrochelatase, an enzyme associated with the inner mitochondrial membrane, appears to insert the Fe(II) into protoporphyrin (39). The resulting heme may remain in the mitochondria or be exported for binding to cytosolic proteins (40). The primary source of iron for the mitochondria is probably the so-called labile pool of low molecular weight complexes of the cytosol, which in turn is in equilibrium with ferritin iron and iron introduced into the cell from transferrin (27).

Kupffer Cells

Increased rigidity of senescent or damaged red blood cells, perhaps a secondary effect of the loss of sulfhydryl groups, may be the signal that initiates their removal by the reticuloendothelial system (41, Fig. 2). Experimentally, coating cells with antibody or denaturing them with heat is commonly used to produce cells readily removed by phagocytic cells *in vivo* or in isolated cultures. Sheep red cells coated with antibody are readily recognized and engulfed by isolated Kupffer cells in tissue cultures. When phagocytosis was observed using time-lapsed photography, each Kupffer cell interiorized five to six red cells per minute for the 8 min it was observed (42). Using ^{51}Cr-labeled red cells, internalization was shown to reach a peak after 1 hr; after 4 to 5 hr, the internalized red blood cells started to disappear; by 17 hr (overnight culture), the internal radioactivity approached background levels. Complete recovery of the erythrophagocytic activity was achieved after 40 hr in culture (43).

These results imply that each Kupffer cell is capable of processing at least 40 to 50 antibody-coated red cells in a period of about 40 hr. Although the process of recognition of damaged red blood cells is presumably different to that for antibody-coated cells, the internal processing is probably similar. This large capacity for red blood cell destruction implies a huge reserve capacity over that which is needed for physiological

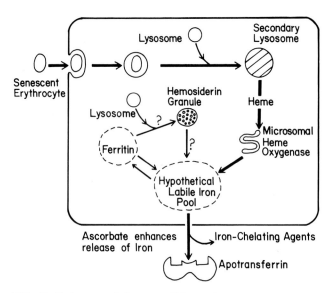

FIG. 2. Schema of the possible pathways followed by iron in the Kupffer cell.

breakdown of red blood cells. After splenectomy, the lifetime of circulating red cells is not prolonged (44), indicating that the remaining reticuloendothelial system has the capacity to deal normally with senescent erythrocytes.

The intracellular degradation of engulfed erythrocytes by phagocytes resembles the process used by hepatocytes to degrade free hemoglobin. The cells are digested in secondary lysosomes, the heme released, and the iron freed from the heme by the microsomal heme oxygenase (33). This enzyme can be induced in Kupffer cells by damaged erythrocytes and in hepatocytes by free hemoglobin, with the maximum level occurring 8 to 12 hr after administration (33). Much of the iron freed from the senescent red cells is immediately returned to the plasma transferrin (12), but some may be retained by the Kupffer cells to be incorporated into ferritin or hemosiderin (45).

REGULATION OF FERRITIN SYNTHESIS AND TURNOVER

Structure and Function of Ferritin

Widely distributed throughout nature, ferritin has been identified in plants, microorganisms, and higher organisms (46). It consists of a roughly spherical hollow protein shell, within which iron is stored in a microcrystalline core of polymeric ferric oxyhydroxide phosphate (47,48). The average iron content of rat liver ferritin molecules is 3,000 atoms (49), but up to about 4,500 atoms can be included in the protein shell. In this fully loaded state, iron represents about 26% of the dry molecular mass (46).

The protein has a molecular weight of about 450,000

and consists of 24 subunits (50). As revealed by high resolution X-ray crystallography, the subunits approximate cylinders with a length of about 55 Å and diameter of about 27 Å. Four long α-helices, with nearly parallel axes, make up most of the cylinder length. The packing of subunits into the quarternary structure suggests the formation of stable dimers as intermediates in self-assembly (51). Six symmetry-related channels, running through the protein (51,52), are thought to allow small molecules access to the core (53), thus providing conduits for iron deposition and release.

Although still contested (54), the evidence for the existence of two types of ferritin subunits, of molecular weights 19,000 and 21,000, respectively, is strong (55). It has been suggested that one is produced from the other by posttranslational processing or as an artifact of isolation procedures (54); simultaneous synthesis of the acidic, heavier subunit (H), characteristic of heart ferritin, and the basic, lighter subunit (L), predominating in liver, in a cell-free heterologous system (56), together with the different organ-specific distributions of the two types (57), have led to a widespread conviction that these subunits are real. To account for the heterogeneity of tissue ferritin, it has been suggested that H subunits abound when iron is abundant, while L subunits predominate when the metal is scarce; what ferritin there is exists largely as the apoprotein (58). However, the variation of subunit types in ferritins of varying iron content is not systematic and reflects also tissue of origin (59); thus further experiments are needed to define the differences (if any) in the functional roles of the isoferritins. Interestingly and inexplicably, serum ferritin, levels of which reflect overall iron status, is predominantly iron free and composed of L subunits (58).

Synthesis of Ferritin Subunits

The bulk of ferritin synthesis in the liver is thought to occur on free polyribosomes of hepatocytes, in contrast to the synthesis of the export protein albumin, which is produced on membrane-bound polyribosomes (60). In keeping with its role as an iron store, the rate of ferritin synthesis is sensitive to the presence of iron.

Effect of Iron on Ferritin Synthesis

When rats are treated with iron, ferritin synthetic capacity increases fourfold in free polyribosomes but remains unchanged in membrane-associated polyribosomes (60); this may account for the increase in ferritin synthesis provoked by iron. When ferritin synthesis is stimulated with iron, the rate of ^{14}C-leucine incorporation into the protein reaches a maximum after 5 hr (61), with radioactive ferritin continuing to accumulate for up to 12 hr. Radioactivity is first detectable in apoferritin but then gradually accumulates in iron-containing protein as iron loading proceeds (61). Pretreatment of liver with actinomycin D, which suppresses mRNA formation, fails to impede the inducing effect of iron (62). In this instance, however, iron still causes a twofold increase in the number of ferritin-synthesizing polyribosomes and a threefold increase in the ferritin-mRNA extractable from the free ribosome fraction (60,63). To explain these observations, it has been postulated (64) that an influx of iron into the cell causes the assembly of holoferritin from ferritin subunits which were initially bound to the free mRNA. The removal of the protein subunits frees the mRNA to combine with ribosomes and to proceed with ferritin biosynthesis.

Incorporation of Iron into Ferritin

Newly synthesized ferritin subunits probably are assembled into apoferritin, which then incorporates iron (61). Nucleation centers within the protein may be necessary for the polymeric iron core to form. It is widely assumed that these centers promote the oxidation of Fe^{2+} to Fe^{3+}, which then hydrolyzes to form the polymeric $(Fe \cdot O \cdot OH)_x$. The nature of the sites where oxidation occurs is not known, but chemical modification studies implicate carboxylic acid residues (65). Once polymerization of the iron core has commenced, the growing polymer itself may provide the requisite sites for the oxidation of the iron (66). Alternatively, oxidation may take place continuously within or near the channels themselves (67), with the resulting Fe^{3+} then transported to the core.

Because of the small diameter of the channels, the size of the iron complexes that may enter or leave the core is restricted (53). Therefore, much interest has centered on the search for a low molecular weight complex of iron in transit in the cytosol of liver cells. The size of this labile pool may help determine the rate of ferritin synthesis, since iron stimulates ferritin synthesis.

Iron Release From Ferritin

In the hepatocyte, the so-called labile pool of low molecular weight iron complex(es) is thought to be intermediate between ferritin and plasma transferrin (68). In the Kupffer cell, this pool may be the conduit between microsomal heme oxygenase, where heme is degraded, and plasma transferrin (15). When plasma iron is low, iron probably shifts from the labile intracellular pool of the hepatocyte to transferrin and is then replaced by iron mobilized from ferritin (69).

The mobilization of iron from ferritin is thought to involve a reduction of iron to Fe(II), since reductants, such as ascorbic acid, enhance mobilization of iron *in vitro* (70). The most effective reductants are $FMNH_2$, $FADH_2$, and reduced riboflavin, the efficiency of each varying inversely with its molecular size and, possibly, with its ability to diffuse through the pores of the ferritin protein shell (70). The maximum rate of release of iron induced by reduced riboflavin is about 42 atoms per minute per molecule ferritin (70). At this rate, the average load of a ferritin molecule *in vivo*, 1,200 iron atoms, could be mobilized in less than 1 hr. This is sufficiently fast for the reductive mechanism to operate *in vivo*. The pathways along which the released iron crosses the cell membrane to serum transferrin are unknown. Since the rate of release from normal rat hepatocytes cannot be enhanced by increasing the extracellular apotransferrin concentration (9), the transport of the iron across the cell membrane may be the rate-limiting step of the release process. The involvement of ceruloplasmin in the release process has been suggested, perhaps by a mechanism involving the ability of the protein to catalyze the oxidation of Fe(II) to Fe(III) and so facilitate the binding of released iron by transferrin (71). Increases in ceruloplasmin concentration do not enhance the rate of release, however, again suggesting that the actual transmembrane transport process may be the rate-limiting step.

Degradation and Turnover of Ferritin

The half-life of hepatic ferritin in male rats is approximately 58 hr (72). As with other intracellular proteins, degradation of ferritin probably occurs in the lysosomal system after autophagocytosis of cell contents (73). Partial degradation of ferritin protein may lead to the production of intralysosomal hemosiderin (73), an ill-defined entity perhaps consisting of clumps of ferritin cores with varying amounts of protein, lipids, and sugar (74). Hemosiderin may be a normal product of cell ferritin turnover, representing much of the nonheme, nonferritin iron ordinarily found in rat hepatocytes (11). Much of the iron in the Kupffer cell, probably derived largely from red blood cells (14), is also present in a nonheme, nonferritin fraction. Relatively little ferritin is present in Kupffer cells even in iron overload (11). The low pH of the interior of the lysosomes might facilitate the solubilization of iron to allow rapid release to the cytosol of the metal from catabolized ferritin.

TRANSFERRIN SYNTHESIS

The transferrin molecule consists of a single polypeptide chain on which are disposed two similar, but not identical, iron-binding sites. Like ferritin synthesis, the synthesis of serum transferrin is influenced by iron load; with transferrin, however, the synthetic rate has an inverse relationship to the iron load (75,76). Thus in iron deficiency, serum transferrin concentrations may rise, possibly serving to promote iron absorption from the gut. The liver is the major site of transferrin synthesis (77). It appears that the size of the ferritin iron store is involved in the regulation of transferrin synthesis (78).

When newly hatched chicks are raised on an iron-deficient diet, circulating transferrin levels are increased two- to fourfold over that in normal chicks, reflecting a correspondingly increased rate of synthesis in the liver (79). Levels of transferrin mRNA are increased two- to threefold with more than 80% of the transferrin mRNA associated with polyribosomes, suggesting that the induction of transferrin synthesis is regulated directly by an increase in transferrin mRNA. Synthesis of transferrin and its mRNA return to normal after administration of iron-containing ferritin. Evidence suggests that transferrin is synthesized, bearing at its N-terminus a 20-amino acid leader which is cleaved during export of the protein from the cell (80). Only one transferrin gene per haploid complement is found in chicken liver and chicken oviduct, with similar nontranscribed introns in both tissues. Control of transferrin synthesis presumably involves only the rate of transcription of this one gene (81). Interestingly, synthesis of ovotransferrin (conalbumin) by oviduct is responsive to stimulation by progesterone but, in contrast to what obtains in the liver, is insensitive to iron (81). Serum transferrin and ovotransferrin in the chicken differ only in their carbohydrate moieties (82), presumably as a consequence of differences in posttranslational modification (83).

PATHOLOGY OF HEPATIC IRON METABOLISM

Iron Overload

Mechanisms of Toxicity

The liver is particularly vulnerable in disorders characterized by iron overload; liver disease is an important cause of morbidity and mortality in such states. Because free iron is toxic, elaborate transport and storage processes exist in most organisms to minimize the amount of nonprotein-bound iron. When the capacity of these systems is exceeded, toxicity supervenes. The precise mechanisms underlying the noxious effects of iron are still in doubt. Because iron may catalyze the production of free radicals *in vitro* (84), these reactive intermediates have been implicated in the pathogenesis of iron toxicity, although little direct evidence supports their role *in vivo*. Iron may

react with reducing agents and oxygen to form the superoxide radical anion, O_2^-, which may lead in turn to the production of the hydroxy radical, OH·, a highly reactive and destructive entity. The iron-catalyzed peroxidation of unsaturated fatty acids in the presence of ascorbic acid is thought to occur via a free radical intermediate (85). Patients with β-thalassemia, hemoglobin Koln, and sickle cell disease have been shown to have red cells susceptible to membrane lipid peroxidation (86), perhaps because precipitated hemoglobin within the cells also catalyzes the peroxidation reaction (87). Damage to nucleic acids caused by free radicals induced by iron overload may be a cofactor or even a major cause of proliferative disease (84). There is little direct evidence, however, for increased occurrence of carcinoma in iron-overloaded patients, except insofar as the concomitant cirrhosis is associated with increased incidence of hepatoma (88).

Hemochromatosis

In primary idiopathic hemochromatosis, an intrinsic, probably familial, abnormality apparently inherited in an autosomal recessive manner (89) leads to an increased absorption of iron in otherwise hematologically normal subjects. Absorption of iron appears to vary inversely with body iron load, decreasing as iron accumulates but increasing again if iron stores are depleted by venesection (90). Iron absorption studies are often based on appearance of orally administered radioiron in the hemoglobin of circulating red cells. Such studies may not be straightforward in interpretation, since hepatic retention of iron, and hence availability of iron to the erythron, may depend on transferrin saturation (91).

Patients with hemochromatosis who are reaccumulating iron following venesection display normal levels of serum ferritin but high concentration of serum iron and a greatly increased intracellular low molecular weight hepatic iron pool (92). One explanation may be that a defect in the regulation of ferritin synthesis promotes an imbalance between the labile iron pool and ferritin. This could be explained by a defect in regulation of ferritin synthesis. In the small intestinal epithelium, this might lead to enlargement of the chelatable iron pool, from which iron could then be available for absorption in excessive amounts (92). If, as has been suggested (93), the rate-limiting step in normal iron absorption is discharge of iron from mucosal cell to the circulation, rather than transfer of iron across the brush border, the relatively labile iron of the chelatable pool might be more readily available than ferritin-bound iron to transferrin. Other workers (94,95), however, have adduced evidence that mucosal uptake of iron may also be a rate-limiting process. Thus both mucosal iron uptake and discharge of the metal to the circulation should be considered in the pathogenesis of idiopathic hemochromatosis.

The iron deposited in the liver is mostly derived from transferrin. Thus if the metabolic fault in hemochromatosis lies in an increased rate of absorption, the liver may receive a major burden of iron since its blood flows directly from the gut via the portal vein. The primary site of iron deposition is the parenchyme of the liver (96); iron accumulation in the reticuloendothelial cell may be only secondary, caused by the inability of serum transferrin, which is usually fully saturated in hemochromatosis (92), to accept iron at a normal rate from these cells.

An increased incidence of hepatoma has been reported by several (68,98) but not all (97) observers. Whether this is a direct consequence of iron toxicity or simply reflects the relatively indolent nature of the cirrhosis and hence a prolonged risk of hepatoma is not clear. An increase in frequency of cancer at sites other than the liver has also been observed in patients with hemochromatosis (98).

Alcoholic Cirrhosis and Porphyria Cutanea Tarda

Hepatic iron overload in alcoholic cirrhosis of the liver is frequently encountered and is occasionally so severe as to mimic primary hemochromatosis (99). Most alcoholic patients show only mild degrees of hepatic siderosis, however, and the incidence of histologically severe siderosis in British patients is reported to be no greater than 7% (100).

The mechanisms driving hepatic accumulation of iron in cirrhosis are not understood. Subjects with alcoholic and cryptogenic cirrhosis display increased absorption of iron derived from ferrous sulfate or hemoglobin (99). It has been suggested that impaired pancreatic function removes the inhibitory effect of pancreatic juice on iron absorption, but this effect has not been consistently observed (101). Abstaining alcoholic patients exhibit normal or even decreased absorption of iron (101). Some but not all alcoholic beverages contain appreciable quantities of iron, possibly in a readily absorbable form (102).

Acute or chronic hemolysis may also dispose toward increased absorption of iron in patients with cirrhosis (99). An abnormal heterogeneity of serum transferrin has been reported to be a sensitive indicator of prolonged alcohol ingestion (103), but it is not evident that this bears any relation to the mechanisms of hepatic iron accumulation in chronic alcoholism.

Most patients with porphyria cutanea tarda, regardless of the coexistence of alcoholism, have appreciable hepatic siderosis, often accompanied by elevated serum iron levels (104). Although iron overload is a characteristic of the disease, there are serious questions about whether it is a cause or an effect of the porphyric state. It has been suggested that ferrous iron enhances porphyrin synthesis (105). The beneficial effect of phlebotomy in porphyria cutanea tarda is usually ascribed to depletion of excessive hepatic iron.

Transfusional and Dietary Overload

In β-thalassemia major, an abnormality of hemoglobin synthesis, leads to severe anemia and, if not treated, death. Treatment consists of regular transfusions of red cells. Approximately 2 pints each 6 weeks are necessary to keep hemoglobin levels sufficiently high for normal development and growth of the affected infants (106). At this rate of transfusion, subjects accumulate iron at the rate of 4 g/year. By the time patients achieve the age of 20 years, 75 to 100 g iron have been taken in. Unless attempts are made to remove this iron, or at least stem the accumulation, iron poisoning is inevitable and relentless.

Since the source of iron in such cases is effete red cells, iron overload is predominantly in the reticuloendothelial cells (107), and splenomegaly and hepatomegaly regularly occur (108). Perhaps consequent to the defect in erythropoiesis and the high levels of serum iron, release of iron from the reticuloendothelial cells is inhibited; thus accumulation of iron in hepatocytes ultimately follows the overload of Kupffer cells (109). Hepatic accumulation of iron in β-thalassemia major is also aggravated by enhanced absorption of iron from the gut due to the anemia or other mechanisms, although gross overabsorption may be suppressed by transfusion (110). Lysosomes in Kupffer cells become engorged with heavy deposits of hemosiderin and ferritin. Parenchymal cells accumulate iron largely in ferritin, seen in both cytosol and lysosomes, until the load is so great that the capacity of the cells to synthesize ferritin may be exceeded, when hemosiderin also starts to pile up (46). Iron loading of lysosomes may lead to their disruption, with the consequent release of proteolytic enzymes and hemosiderin into the cytosol (111) and thus to cell damage.

In some cases of transfusion-treated thalassemia, the burden of serum iron may exceed the binding capacity of transferrin. A nonspecific fraction of serum iron, bound neither to transferrin, ferritin, nor hemoglobin, is then observed (112). Such iron is more reactive than transferrin-bound iron and may contribute to the toxic effects of iron in transfusional siderosis and perhaps other disorders of iron overload.

Conditions of excessive absorption of dietary iron are not widely observed, but a fairly high incidence is seen among South African blacks. This has been ascribed to the widespread use of iron in cooking pots and in vessels for brewing homemade beer (113). Surprisingly, the deposition of iron in South African siderosis is largely reticuloendothelial, whereas it would be expected that iron absorbed from the gut via transferrin would be found in the hepatocytes. This anomaly can be explained by the high incidence of concurrent ascorbate deficiency, possibly a result of iron-catalyzed oxidation of dietary ascorbate (114), a reaction known to occur *in vitro* (88). Ascorbate is necessary for the release from reticuloendothelial cells of the iron in catabolized red cells (115); administration of ascorbate allows the transfer of iron from the reticuloendothelial cells to hepatocytes.

Atransferrinemia

The rare disorder atransferrinemia is characterized by almost complete absence of serum transferrin due to a genetic defect in its synthesis. In one 8-year-old girl, serum iron was 14 to 20 μg/100 ml and iron binding capacity was 20 to 33 μg/ml (116). Radioactive iron, injected after incubation with the patient's plasma, showed a half-life of 5 min (normally about 90 min). Only 12% of the injected radioiron was utilized for hemoglobin synthesis in a period of 8 days, whereas normally approximately 85% would have been utilized. Most of the radioiron was localized in the liver, which can take up iron even though rerelease is very slow. Severe iron loading of all organs was shown at autopsy after the patient died of circulatory failure. In another subject, infusion of transferrin led to increase in red cell production (117), as would be expected from the essential role of transferrin in providing iron for the biosynthesis of hemoglobin.

Zellweger Syndrome

Zellweger syndrome, once thought to be synonymous with idiopathic hemochromatosis, is seen in infants and is usually fatal by the age of 6 months. It is characterized by widespread deposits of iron in all organs, but especially the liver, in contrast to idiopathic hemochromatosis, in which iron loading is, at least initially, predominant in the parenchymal cells of the liver (96). The hallmark of the condition is the absence of demonstrable peroxisomes in hepatocytes (118, 119). It has been suggested that the primary defect is in energy metabolism of mitochondria (120). Mobilization of iron from ferritin and hemosiderin is energy dependent and may also require a supply of reducing equivalents from mitochondria (121). A generalized mitochondrial disorder might lead to inability to mobilize iron from stores in all cells, with resultant build-up of iron deposits.

Chelation Therapy and Intracellular Iron Metabolism

As there is no abnormality of erythropoiesis in primary hemochromatosis, simple venesection is effective in mobilizing iron from hepatic stores by stimulating erythropoiesis. Absorption of iron increases as iron stores are depleted (91), however, so that repeated phlebotomy every 3 to 4 months is required to keep iron stores within the normal range (122). Phlebotomy also may be useful in reducing the hepatic burden of iron in selected cases of dyserythropoietic or sideroblastic anemia, in which there is marked elevation of hepatic iron in the absence of severe anemia (123).

Transfusional siderosis, as in thalassemia, can be treated only by iron chelation therapy to remove accumulated iron. The most successful regimen entails slow infusions of the chelating agent, desferrioxamine, together with supplemental ascorbic acid (124). The ascorbate is thought to increase the rate of mobilization of iron from the reticuloendothelial cells (115), perhaps by facilitating reduction of Fe(III) to Fe(II) to replenish the low molecular weight intracellular iron pool thought to be the primary source from which iron is chelated by desferrioxamine (125). Ascorbate may aggravate cardiac damage in iron-overloaded patients, however, perhaps by mobilizing iron from nontoxic stores to parenchymal cells or by enhancing lipid peroxidation in membranes of cells and their organelles (126).

The main problem with desferrioxamine is that it is rapidly cleared from plasma (127,128); thus continuous slow infusion is necessary to keep an adequate concentration for chelating iron, which is mobilizable from stores at only a limited rate. In experiments in which hepatocytes were selectively labeled with iron-59 bound to transferrin, and reticuloendothelial cells were labeled with denatured red blood cells containing iron-59, both types of cells could provide iron for chelation by desferrioxamine (125). The chelator probably does not sequester iron directly from the iron stores but rather from the so-called labile pool where the metal is in transit between ferritin or hemosiderin in the cell and transferrin in serum. The chemical nature of this pool is not known, but it seems to be a heterogeneous mixture of low molecular weight compounds. Since citrate, sugars, amino acids, and nucleotides may all function as intermediates in iron exchange between ferritin and transferrin (129), it has been suggested that such complexes may be involved in the labile iron pool *in vivo* (28).

The absence of high affinity receptors for apotransferrin on hepatocytes (138) suggests that chelating agents may compete with apotransferrin at the circulatory side of the cell membrane for iron being released from the cells. Since the affinity of desferrioxamine for iron is even higher than that of transferrin (127), it could compete effectively with the protein in iron overload, when much of the transferrin is saturated with iron.

Entrapment of desferrioxamine in liposomes (lipid vesicles) has been shown to greatly enhance its iron chelating efficacy in mice (130), perhaps by preventing the rapid excretion of the drug or by introducing it directly into the lysosomal system by phagocytosis.

Iron Deficiency States

The relatively large stores of iron in the liver require that substantial blood losses occur before iron deficiency and anemia develop. In man, mobilization of the 400 mg iron in the hepatic store will provide sufficient iron for the synthesis of red cells for about 1 liter of blood. The ferritin content of liver decreases rapidly after acute blood loss as iron is mobilized and the synthesis of apoferritin is correspondingly decreased (131,132). The erythropoietic marrow appears to have priority for the supply of iron, so that biochemical changes in other tissues sometimes precede the onset of anemia in iron-deficient states (4).

The effects of iron deficiency reflect the rate of growth or turnover of a particular tissue. For instance, severe depletion of hemoproteins has been observed in rapidly growing skeletal muscle and in intestinal mucosa, which normally turns over rapidly (133). Mitochondrial cytochromes c and a were diminished in liver after young rats had been fed an iron-deficient diet for 3 weeks. In contrast, microsomal P-450 declined after only 8 weeks on the same diet, and microsomal cytochrome b_5 did not change even after this period (134). Levels of cytochrome P-450 responded normally to phenobarbital treatment with a fourfold increase, indicating that this protein has a high priority for iron even in iron deficiency (134).

Other effects of iron deficiency in the liver include decreases in DNA synthesis (135), monoamine oxidase activity (136), glucose-6-phosphate dehydrogenase activity, 6-phosphogluconate dehydrogenase activity (137), lipogenesis (138), and porphyrin synthesis (139). Interestingly, the iron-bearing enzymes catalase (140) aconitase (141), and succinate dehydrogenase (142) in rat liver are not affected by iron depletion, and no clear causal relationship has been established between the biochemical abnormalities of iron deficiency and the functional disturbances often observed (134).

REFERENCES

1. Green, R., Charlton, R., Seftel, M., Bothwell, T., Mayet, F., Adams, B., Finch, C., and Layrisse, M. (1968): Body iron excretion in man. *Am. J. Med.*, 45:336–353.
2. Pollycove, M., and Mortimer, R. (1961): The quantitative determination of iron kinetics and hemoglobin synthesis in human subjects. *J. Clin. Invest.*, 40:753–782.
3. Chang, L. L. (1973): Tissue storage iron in Singapore. *Am. J. Clin. Nutr.*, 26:952–957.
4. Jacobs, A., and Worwood, M. (1978): Normal iron metabolism. In: *Metals and the Liver*, edited by L. W. Powell, pp. 3–51. Dekker, New York.
5. Zimelman, A. P., Zimmerman, H. J., McLean, R., and Weintraub, L. R. (1977): Effect of iron saturation of transferrin on hepatic iron uptake: An *in vitro* study. *Gastroenterology*, 72:129–131.
6. Beamish, M. R., Keay, L., Okigaki, T., and Brown, E. B. (1975): Uptake of transferrin-bound iron by rat cells in tissue culture. *Br. J. Haematol.*, 31:479–491.
7. Fletcher, J. (1971): The plasma clearance and liver uptake of iron from transferrin of low and high iron saturation. *Clin. Sci.*, 41:395–402.
8. Christensen, A. C., Huebers, H., and Finch, C. A. (1978): Effect of transferrin saturation on iron delivery in rats. *Am. J. Physiol.*, 235:R18–22.
9. Young, S. P., and Aisen, P. (1980): The interaction of transferrin with isolated hepatocytes. *Biochim. Biophys. Acta*, 633:145–153.
10. Lynch, S. R., Lipschitz, D. A., Bothwell, T. H., and Charlton, R. W. (1974): Iron and the reticuloendothelial system. In: *Iron in Biochemistry and Medicine*, edited by A. Jacobs and R. Worwood, pp. 563–587. Academic Press, London.
11. Van Wyck, C. P., Linder-Horowitz, M., and Munro, H. N. (1971): The effect of iron loading on non-heme iron compounds in different liver cell populations. *J. Biol. Chem.*, 246:1025–1031.
12. Noyes, W. D., Bothwell, T. H., and Finch, C. A. (1960): The role of the reticuloendothelial cell in iron metabolism. *Br. J. Haematol.*, 6:43–55.
13. Verhoef, N. J., Kottenhagen, M. J., Mulder, H. J. M., Noordeloos, P. J., and Leijnse, B. (1978): Functional heterogeneity of transferrin-bound iron. *Acta Haematol.*, 60:210–226.
14. Hershko, C., Cook, J. D., and Finch, C. A. (1973): Storage iron kinetics: III. Study of desferrioxamine action by selective radioiron labels of reticuloendothelial and parenchymal cells. *J. Lab. Clin. Med.*, 81:876–886.
15. Lipschitz, D. A., Simon, M. O., Lynch, S. R., Dugard, J., Bothwell, T. H., and Charlton, R. W. (1971): Some factors affecting the release of iron from reticuloendothelial cells. *Br. J. Haematol.*, 21:289–303.
16. Jacob, H. S., and Jandl, J. H. (1962): Effects of sulfhydryl inhibition on red blood cells. II. Studies in vivo. *J. Clin. Invest.*, 41:1514–1523.
17. Jandl, J. H., and Katz, J. H. (1963): The plasma-to-cell cycle of transferrin. *J. Clin. Invest.*, 42:314–326.
18. Larrick, J. W., and Cresswell, P. (1979): Transferrin receptors on human B and T lymphoblastoid cell lines. *Biochim. Biophys. Acta*, 583:483–490.
19. Galbraith, G. M. P., Galbraith, R. M., Temple, A., and Faulk, W. P. (1980): Demonstration of transferrin receptors on human placental trophoblasts. *Blood*, 55:240–242.
20. Galbraith, G. M. P., Galbraith, R. M., and Faulk, W. P. (1980): Transferrin binding to human lymphoblastoid cell lines and other transformed cells. *Cell. Immunol.*, 49:215–222.
21. Van Bockxmeer, F. M., Yates, G. K., and Morgan, E. H. (1978): Interaction of transferrin with solubilized receptors from reticulocytes. *Eur. J. Biochem.*, 92:147–154.
22. Nunez, M. T., Glass, J., Fischer, S., Lavidor, L. M., Lenk, E. M., and Robinson, S. H. (1977): Transferrin receptors in developing murine erythroid cells. *Br. J. Haematol.*, 36:519–526.
23. Baker, E., Morton, A. G., and Tavill, A. S. (1975): The effect of transferrin on iron release from the perfused rat liver. In: *Proteins of Iron Storage and Transport in Biochemistry and Medicine*, edited by R. R. Crichton, pp. 173–180. North Holland, Amsterdam.
24. Katz, J. H. (1961): Iron and protein kinetics studied by means of doubly labeled human crystalline transferrin. *J. Clin. Invest.*, 40:2143–2151.
25. Hemmalplardh, D., Kailis, S. G., and Morgan, E. H. (1974): The effect of inhibitors of microtubule and microfilament function on transferrin and iron uptake by rabbit reticulocytes and bone marrow. *Br. J. Haematol.*, 28:53–65.
26. Goldstein, J. L., Anderson, R. G. W., and Brown, M. S. (1979): Coated pits, coated vesicles and receptor-mediated endocytosis. *Nature*, 279:679–685.
27. Jacobs, A. (1977): Low molecular weight intracellular iron transport compounds. *Blood*, 50:433–439.
28. Hershko, C., Cook, J. D., and Finch, C. A. (1972): Storage

iron kinetics. II. The uptake of hemoglobin iron by hepatic parenchymal cells. *J. Lab. Clin. Med.*, 80:624–634.

29. Bissel, D. M., Hammaker, L., and Schmid, R. (1972): Hemoglobin and erythrocyte catabolism in rat liver: The separate roles of parenchymal and sinusoidal cells. *Blood*, 40:812–822.

30. Liem, H. L. (1974): Hepatic uptake of heme and hemopexin but not albumin. *Biochim. Biophys. Acta*, 343:546–550.

31. Sears, D. A. (1970): Disposal of plasma heme in normal man and patients with intravascular hemolysis. *J. Clin. Invest.*, 49:5–14.

32. Freeman, T. (1964): Haptoglobin metabolism in relation to red cell destruction. *Protides Biol. Fluids*, 12:344–352.

33. Kornfeld, S., Chipman, B., and Brown, E. B. (1969): Intracellular catabolism of hemoglobin and iron dextran by the rat liver. *J. Lab. Clin. Med.*, 73:181–193.

34. Marver, H. S. (1969): The role of heme in the synthesis and repression of microsomal proteins. In: *Microsomes and Drug Oxidation*, edited by J. R. Gillette, A. H. Conney, G. J. Cosmides, R. W. Estabrook, J. R. Foots, and G. J. Mannering, pp. 495–511. Academic Press, New York.

35. Tenhunen, R., Marver, H. S., and Schmid, R. (1968): The enzymatic conversion of heme to bilirubin by microsomal heme-oxygenase. *Proc. Natl. Acad. Sci. USA*, 61:748–755.

36. Flatmark, T., and Romslo, I. (1977): Iron transporting system of mitochondria. In: *Advances in Chemistry Series No. 162 Bioinorganic Chemistry-II*, edited by K. N. Raymond, pp. 78–92. American Chemical Society, Washington, D.C.

37. Flatmark, T., and Romslo, I. (1975): Energy-dependent accumulation of iron by isolated rat liver mitochondria: Requirement for reducing equivalents and evidence for a unidirectional flux of Fe(II) across the inner membrane. *J. Biol. Chem.*, 250:6433–6438.

38. Romslo, I., and Flatmark, T. (1973): Energy-dependent accumulation of iron by isolated rat liver mitochondria. II. Relationship to the active transport of Ca^{2+}. *Biochim. Biophys. Acta*, 325:38–46.

39. Koller, M. E., Romslo, I., and Flatmark, T. (1976): Studies on the ferrochelatase activity of isolated rat liver mitochondria with special reference to the effect of oxidizable substrates and oxygen concentration. *Biochim. Biophys. Acta*, 449:480–490.

40. Yoda, B., and Israel, L. G. (1972): Transfer of heme from mitochondria in rat liver cells. *Can. J. Biochem.*, 50:633–637.

41. Bunn, H. F. (1972): Erythrocyte destruction and hemoglobin catabolism. *Semin. Hematol.*, 9:3–17.

42. Munthe-Kaas, A. C., Kaplan, G., and Seljeld, R. (1976): On the mechanism of internalisation of opsonized particles by rat Kupffer cells in vitro. *Exp. Cell Res.*, 103:201–212.

43. Munthe-Kaas, A. C. (1976): Phagocytosis in rat Kupffer cells in vitro. *Exp. Cell Res.*, 99:319–327.

44. Gervitz, N. R., Nathan, D. G., and Berlin, N. I. (1962): Erythrokinetic studies in primary hypersplenism and pancytopenia. *Am. J. Med.*, 32:148–152.

45. Iancu, T. C., Neustein, H. B., and Landing, B. H. (1977): The liver in thalassemia major: Ultrastructural observations. In: *Ciba Symposium No. 51 (New Series): Iron Metabolism*, pp. 293–309. Elsevier, Amsterdam.

46. Richter, G. W. (1978): The iron-loaded cell—The cytopathology of iron storage. *Am. J. Pathol.*, 91:362–404.

47. Harrison, P. M., Fischbach, F. A., Hoy, T. G., and Haggis, G. H. (1967): Ferric oxyhydroxide core of ferritin. *Nature*, 216:1188–1190.

48. Granick, S. (1946): Ferritin: Its properties and significance for iron metabolism. *Chem. Rev.*, 38:379–403.

49. Linder, M. C., and Munro, H. N. (1972): Assay of tissue ferritin. *Anal. Biochem.*, 48:266–278.

50. Bryce, C. F. A., and Crichton, R. R. (1971): The subunit structure of horse spleen ferritin. I. The molecular weight of the subunit. *J. Biol. Chem.*, 246:4198–4205.

51. Banyard, S. H., Stammers, D. K., and Harrison, P. M. (1978): Electron density map of apoferritin at 2·8-Å resolution. *Nature*, 271:282–284.

52. Hoare, R. J., Harrison, P. M., and Hoy, T. G. (1975): Structure of horse spleen apoferritin at 6Å resolution. *Nature*, 255:653–654.

53. Fish, W. W. (1976): Ferritin structure: Possible models for apoferritin subunit arrangement. *J. Theor. Biol.*, 60:385–392.

54. Bryce, C. F. A., Magnusson, C. G. M., and Crichton, R. R. (1978): A reappraisal of the electrophoretic patterns obtained from ferritin and apoferritin in the presence of denaturants. *FEBS Lett.*, 96:257–262.

55. Drysdale, J. W., Adelman, T. G., Arosio, P., Casareale, D., Fitzpatrick, J., Hazard, J. T., and Yokota, M. (1977): Human isoferritins in normal and disease states. *Semin. Hematol.*, 14:71–88.

56. Arosio, P., Adelman, T. G., and Drysdale, J. W. (1978): On ferritin heterogeneity. Further evidence for heteropolymers. *J. Biol. Chem.*, 253:4451–4458.

57. Drysdale, J. W. (1977): Ferritin phenotypes: Structure and metabolism. In: *Ciba Symposium No. 51 (New Series): Iron Metabolism*, pp. 41–57. Elsevier, Amsterdam.

58. Arosio, P., Yokota, M., and Drysdale, J. W. (1977): Characterization of serum ferritin in iron overload: possible identity to natural apoferritin. *Br. J. Haematol.*, 36:201–209.

59. Ishitani, K., Listowsky, I., Hazard, J. T., and Drysdale, J. W. (1975): Differences in subunit composition and iron content of isoferritins. *J. Biol. Chem.*, 250:5446–5449.

60. Zähringer, J., Baliga, B. S., Drake, R. L., and Munro, H. N. (1977): Distribution of ferritin mRNA and albumin mRNA between free and membrane-bound rat liver polysomes. *Biochim. Biophys. Acta*, 474:234–244.

61. Drysdale, J. W., and Munro, H. N. (1966): Regulation of synthesis and turnover of ferritin in rat liver. *J. Biol. Chem.*, 241:3630–3637.

62. Drysdale, J. W., and Munro, H. N. (1965): Failure of actinomycin to prevent induction of liver apoferritin after iron administration. *Biochim. Biophys. Acta*, 103:185–188.

63. Zähringer, J., Konijn, A. M., Baliga, B. S., and Munro, H. N. (1975): Mechanism of iron induction of ferritin synthesis. *Biochem. Biophys. Res. Commun.*, 65:583–590.

64. Zähringer, J., Baliga, B. S., and Munro, H. N. (1976): Novel mechanism for translational control in regulation of ferritin synthesis by iron. *Proc. Natl. Acad. Sci. USA*, 73:857–861.

65. Wetz, K., and Crichton, R. R. (1976): Chemical modification as a probe of the topography and reactivity of horse-spleen apoferritin. *Eur. J. Biochem.*, 61:545–550.

66. Macara, I. G., Hoy, T. G., and Harrison, P. M. (1972): The formation of ferritin from apoferritin. Kinetics and mechanism of iron uptake. *Biochem. J.*, 126:151–162.

67. Crichton, R. R., Collet-Cassart, D., Ponce-Ortiz, Y., Wauters, M., Roman, F., and Paques, E. (1977): Ferritin: Comparative structural studies, iron deposition and mobilisation. In: *Proteins of Iron Metabolism*, edited by E. B. Brown, P. Aisen, R. R. Crichton, and J. Fielding. pp. 13–33. Grune & Stratton, New York.

68. White, G. P., Bailey-Wood, R., and Jacobs, A. (1976): The effect of chelating agents on cellular iron metabolism. *Clin. Sci. Mol. Med.*, 50:145–152.

69. White, G. P., Jacobs, A., Grady, R. W., and Cerami, A. (1976): The effect of chelating agents on iron mobilization in Chang cell cultures. *Blood*, 48:923–929.

70. Sirivach, S., Frieden, E., and Osaki, S. (1974): The release of iron from horse spleen ferritin by reducing flavins. *Biochem. J.*, 143:311–315.

71. Williams, D. M., Lee, G. R., and Cartwright, G. E. (1974): Ferroxidase activity of rat ceruloplasmin. *Am. J. Physiol.*, 227:1094–1097.

72. Linder, M. C., Moor, J. R., Scott, L. E., and Munro, H. N. (1973): Mechanism of sex difference in rat tissue iron stores. *Biochim. Biophys. Acta*, 297:70–80.

73. Trump, B. F., Valigorsky, J. M., Arstila, A. V., Mergner, W. J., and Kinney, T. D. (1973): The relationship of intracellular pathways of iron metabolism to cellular iron overload and the iron storage diseases. *Am. J. Pathol.*, 72:295–324.

74. Ludewig, S., and Franz, S. W. (1970): Hemosiderin V. The occurrence of heme and lipids in hemosiderin. *Arch. Biochem. Biophys.*, 138:397–407.

75. Lane, R. S. (1966): Changes in plasma transferrin levels fol-

lowing the administration of iron. *Br. J. Haematol.*, 12:249–258.

76. Weinfeld, A. (1964): Storage iron in man. *Acta Med. Scand.* [*Suppl. 427*], 177:1–55.

77. Morgan, E. H. (1969): Factors affecting the synthesis of transferrin by rat tissue slices. *J. Biol. Chem.*, 244:4193–4199.

78. Morton, A. G., and Tavill, A. S. (1977): The role of iron in the regulation of hepatic transferrin synthesis. *Br. J. Haematol.*, 36:383–394.

79. McKnight, G. S., Lee, D. C., Hemmaplardh, D., Finch, C. A., and Palmiter, R. D. (1980): Transferrin gene expression. Effects of nutritional iron deficiency. *J. Biol. Chem.*, 255:144–147.

80. Schreiber, G., Dryburgh, H., Millership, A., Matsuda, Y., Inglis, A., Phillips, J., Edwards, K., and Maggs, J. (1979): The synthesis and secretion of rat transferrin. *J. Biol. Chem.*, 254:12013–12019.

81. McKnight, G. S., Lee, D. C., and Palmiter, R. D. (1980): The chicken transferrin gene. Restriction endonuclease analysis of gene sequences in liver and oviduct DNA. *J. Biol. Chem.*, 255:1442–1450.

82. Graham, I., and Williams, J. (1975): A comparison of glycopeptides from the transferrins of several species. *Biochem. J.*, 145:263–279.

83. Lee, D. C., McKnight, G. S., and Palmiter, R. D. (1978): The action of estrogen and progesterone on the expression of the transferrin gene. A comparison of the response in chick liver and oviduct. *J. Biol. Chem.*, 253:3494–3503.

84. Willson, R. L. (1977): Iron, zinc, free radicals and oxygen in tissue disorders and cancer control. In: *Ciba Symposium 51 (New Series): Iron Metabolism*, pp. 331–349. Elsevier, Amsterdam.

85. Wills, E. D. (1965): Mechanisms of lipid peroxide formation in tissue. Role of metals and haematin proteins in the catalysis of the oxidation of unsaturated fatty acids. *Biochim. Biophys. Acta*, 98:238–251.

86. Stocks, J., Offerman, E. L., Modell, O. B., and Dormandy, T. L. (1972): The susceptibility to autoxidation of human red cell lipids in health and disease. *Br. J. Haematol.*, 23:713–724.

87. Carrell, R. W., Winterbourn, C. C., and Rachmilewitz, E. A. (1975): Activated oxygen and haemolysis. *Br. J. Haematol.*, 30:259–264.

88. Walker, R. J., and Williams, R. (1974): Haemochromatosis and iron overload. In: *Iron in Biochemistry and Medicine*, edited by A. Jacobs and M. Worwood, pp. 589–612. Academic Press, London.

89. Williams, R., Pitcher, C. S., Parsonson, A., and Williams, H. S. (1965): Iron absorption in the relatives of patients with idiopathic haemochromatosis. *Lancet*, 1:1243–1246.

90. Wheby, M. S., and Umpierre, G. (1964): Effect of transferrin on iron absorption in man. *N. Engl. J. Med.*, 271:1391–1395.

91. Williams, R., Manenti, F., Williams, H. S., and Pitcher, C. S. (1966): Iron absorption in idiopathic haemochromatosis before, during and after venesection therapy. *Br. Med. J.*, 2:78–81.

92. Beamish, M. R., Walker, R., Miller, F., Worwood, M., Jacobs, A., Williams, R., and Corrigall, A. (1974): Transferrin iron, chelatable iron and ferritin in idiopathic haemochromatosis. *Br. J. Haematol.*, 27:219–228.

93. Cavill, I., Worwood, M., and Jacobs, A. (1975): Internal regulation of iron absorption. *Nature*, 256:328–329.

94. Marx, J. J. M. (1979): Mucosal uptake, mucosal transfer and retention of iron, measured by whole-body counting. *Scand. J. Haematol.*, 23:293–302.

95. Cox, T. M., and Peters, T. J. (1980): Cellular mechanisms in the regulation of iron absorption by the human intestine: Studies in patients with iron deficiency before and after treatment. *Br. J. Haematol.*, 44:75–86.

96. Brink, B., Disler, P., Lynch, S., Jacobs, P., Charlton, R., and Bothwell, T. (1976): Patterns of iron storage in dietary iron overload and idiopathic hemochromatosis. *J. Lab. Clin. Med.*, 88:725–731.

97. MacSween, R. N. M. (1974): A clinicopathological review of 100 cases of primary malignant tumors of the liver. *J. Clin. Pathol.*, 27:669–682.

98. Bomford, A., and Williams, R. (1976): Long-term results of venesection therapy in idiopathic haemochromatosis. *Q. J. Med.*, 45:611–623.

99. Callender, S. T., and Malpas, J. S. (1963): Absorption of iron in cirrhosis of liver. *Br. Med. J.*, 5371:1516–1518.

100. Jakobvits, A. W., Morgan, M. Y., and Sherlock, S. (1979): Hepatic siderosis in alcoholics. *Dig. Dis. Sci.*, 24:305–310.

101. Celadar, A., Rudolf, H., Herreros, V., and Donath, A. (1978): Inorganic iron absorption in subjects with iron deficiency anemia, achylia gastrica and alcoholic cirrhosis using a whole-body counter. *Acta Haematol.*, 60:182–192.

102. Charlton, R. W., Jacobs, P., Seftel, H., and Bothwell, T. H. (1964): Effect of alcohol on iron absorption. *Br. Med. J.*, 2:1427–1429.

103. Stibler, H., Borg, S., and Allgulander, C. (1979): Clinical significance of abnormal heterogeneity of transferrin in relation to alcohol consumption. *Acta Med. Scand.*, 206:275–281.

104. Grossman, M. E., Bickers, D. R., Poh-Fitzpatrick, M. B., Deleo, V. A., and Harber, L. C. (1979): Porphyria cutanea tarda. Clinical features and laboratory findings in 40 patients. *Am. J. Med.*, 67:277–286.

105. Kushner, J. P., Lee, G. R., and Nacht, S. (1972): The role of iron in the pathogenesis of porphyria cutanea tarda. *J. Clin. Invest.*, 51:3044–3051.

106. Modell, C. B. (1975): Transfusional haemochromatosis. In: *Iron Metabolism and Its Disorders. Workshop Conferences Hoechst Vol. 3*, pp. 230–240, edited by H. Kief. Excerpta Medica, Amsterdam.

107. Oliver, R. A. M. (1959): Siderosis following transfusions of blood. *J. Pathol. Bacteriol.*, 77:171–194.

108. Hammond, D., Sturgeon, P., Bergren, W., and Caviles, A. (1964): Definition of Cooley's trait or thalassemia minor: Classical, clinical and routine laboratory hematology. *Ann. NY Acad. Sci.*, 119:372–389.

109. Finch, S. C., and Finch, C. A. (1955): Idiopathic hemochromatosis, an iron storage disease. *Medicine*, 34:381–430.

110. Erlandson, M. E., Walden, B., Stern, G., Hilgartner, M. W., Wehman, J., and Smith, C. H. (1962): Studies on congenital hemolytic syndromes. IV. Gastrointestinal absorption of iron. *Blood*, 19:359–378.

111. Peters, T. J., Selden, C., and Seymour, C. A. (1977): Lysosomal disruption in the pathogenesis of hepatic damage in primary and secondary haemochromatosis. In: *Ciba Symposium 51 (New Series): Iron Metabolism*, pp. 317–325. Elsevier, Amsterdam.

112. Graham, G., Bates, G. W., Rachmilewitz, E. A., and Hershko, C. (1979): Nonspecific serum iron in thalassemia: Quantitation and chemical reactivity. *Am. J. Hematol.*, 6:207–217.

113. Charlton, R. W., and Bothwell, T. H. (1966): Hemochromatosis: Dietary and genetic aspects. *Prog. Hematol.*, 5:298–323.

114. Lynch, S. R., Seftel, H. C., Torrance, J. D., Charlton, R. W., and Bothwell, T. H. (1967): Accelerated oxidative catabolism of ascorbic acid in siderotic Bantu. *Am. J. Clin. Nutr.*, 20:641–647.

115. Lipschitz, D. A., Bothwell, T. H., Seftel, H. C., Wapnick, A. A., and Charlton, R. W. (1971): The role of ascorbic acid in the metabolism of storage iron. *Br. J. Haematol.*, 20:155–163.

116. Heilmeyer, L., Keller, W., Vivell, O., Keiderling, W., Betke, K., Wöhler, F., and Schultze, H. E. (1961): Kongenitale Attransferrinämie bei einem sieben Jahre alten Kind. *Dtsch. Med. Wochenschr.*, 86:1745–1751.

117. Goya, N., Miyazaki, S., Kodate, S., and Ushio, B. (1972): A family of congenital atransferrinemia. *Blood*, 40:239–245.

118. Goldfischer, S. (1979): Peroxisomes in disease. *J. Histochem. Cytochem.*, 27:1371–1373.

119. Pfeifer, U., and Sandhage, K. (1979): Licht-und elektronenmikroskopische laberbefunde beim cerebo-hepato-ranalen syndrom nach Zellweger (peroxisomen-defizienz). *Virchows. Arch. [Pathol. Anat.]*, 384:269–284.

120. Goldfischer, S., Moore, C. L., Johnson, A. B., Spiro, A. J., Valsamis, M. P., Wisniewski, H. K., Ritch, R. H., Norton, W. T., Rapin, I., and Gartner, L. M. (1973): Peroxisomal and

mitochondrial defects in the cerebro-hepato-renal syndrome. *Science,* 182:62–64.

121. Ulvik, R., and Romslo, I. (1978): Studies on the utilization of ferritin iron in the ferrochelatase reaction of isolated rat liver mitochondria. *Biochim. Biophys. Acta,* 541:251–262.

122. Powell, L. W., Bassett, M. L., and Halliday, J. W. (1980): Hemochromatosis: 1980 update. *Gastroenterology,* 78:374–381.

123. Marx, J. J. M. (1980): *(Personal communication).*

124. Propper, R. D., Cooper, B., Rufo, R. R., Nienhuis, A. W., Anderson, W. F., Bunn, H. F., Rosenthal, A., and Nathan, D. G. (1977): Continuous subcutaneous administration of desferrioxamine in patients with iron overload. *N. Engl. J. Med.,* 297:418–423.

125. Lipschitz, D. A., Dugard, J., Simon, M. O., Bothwell, T. H., and Charlton, R. W. (1971): The site of action of desferrioxamine. *Br. J. Haematol.,* 20:395–404.

126. Nienhuis, A. W., Griffith, P., Strawczynski, H., Henry, W., Borer, J., Leon, M., and Anderson, W. F. (1980): Evaluation of cardiac function in patients with thalassemia major. *Ann. NY Acad. Sci.,* 344:384–396.

127. Keberle, H. (1964): The biochemistry of desferrioxamine and its relation to iron metabolism. *Ann. NY Acad. Sci.,* 119: 758–768.

128. Summers, M. R., Jacobs, A., Tudway, D., Perera, P., and Ricketts, C. (1979): Studies in desferrioxamine and ferrioxamine metabolism in normal and iron-loaded subjects. *Br. J. Haematol.,* 42:547–556.

129. Miller, J. P. G., and Perkins, D. J. (1969): Model experiments for the study of iron transfer from transferrin to ferritin. *Eur. J. Biochem.,* 10:146–151.

130. Young, S. P., Baker, E., and Huehns, E. R. (1979): Liposome-entrapped desferrioxamine and iron-transporting ionophores: a new approach to iron-chelation therapy. *Br. J. Haematol.,* 41:357–363.

131. Millar, J. A., Cumming, R. L. C., Smith, J. A., and Goldberg, A. (1970): Effect of actinomycin D, cycloheximide, and acute blood loss on ferritin synthesis in rat liver. *Biochem. J.,* 119:643–649.

132. Munro, H. N., and Drysdale, J. W. (1970): Role of iron in the regulation of ferritin metabolism. *Fed. Proc.,* 29:1469–1473.

133. Dallman, P. R., and Schwartz, H. C. (1965): Distribution of cytochrome c and myoglobin in rats with dietary iron deficiency. *Pediatrics,* 35:677–686.

134. Dallman, P. R., Beutler, E., and Finch, C. A. (1978): Effects of iron deficiency exclusive of anaemia. *Br. J. Haematol.,* 40:179–184.

135. Siimes, M. A., and Dallman, P. R. (1974): Iron deficiency: Impaired liver growth and DNA synthesis in the rat. *Br. J. Haematol.,* 28:457–462.

136. Youdim, M. B. H., and Green, A. R. (1977): Biogenic monoamine metabolism and functional activity in iron-deficient rats: behavioral correlates. In: *Ciba Symposium 51 (New Series): Iron Metabolism,* pp. 201–221. Elsevier, Amsterdam.

137. Bailey-Wood, R., Blayney, L. M., Muir, J. R., and Jacobs, A. (1975): The effects of iron deficiency on rat liver enzymes. *Br. J. Exp. Pathol.,* 56:193–198.

138. Amine, E. K., Desilets, E. J., and Hegsted, D. M. (1976): Effect of dietary fats on lipogenesis in iron deficiency anemic chicks and rats. *J. Nutr.,* 106:405–411.

139. Sharma, D. C. (1973): Aberration of porphyrin metabolism in iron-deficient anaemic rats. *Biochem. J.,* 134:821–823.

140. Cusack, R. P., and Brown, W. D. (1965): Iron deficiency in rats: Changes in body and organ weights, plasma proteins, hemoglobins and catalase. *J. Nutr.,* 86:383–393.

141. Beutler, E. (1959): Iron enzymes in iron deficiency: VI. Aconitase activity and citrate metabolism. *J. Clin. Invest.,* 38:1605–1616.

142. Beutler, E., and Blaisdell, R. F. (1960): Iron enzymes in iron deficiency: V. Succinate dehydrogenase in rat liver, kidney and heart. *Blood,* 15:30–35.

143. Taqui-Khan, M. M., and Martell, A. E. (1967): Metal ion and metal chelate catalyzed oxidation of ascorbic acid by molecular oxygen. I. Cupric and ferric ion catalyzed oxidation. *J. Am. Chem. Soc.,* 89:4176–4185.

144. Young, S. P., and Aisen, P. (1981): Transferrin receptors and the uptake and release of iron by isolated hepatocytes. *Hepatology,* 1:114–119.

Section II

The Cells

B. Bile Secretion

The following section describes the functional interrelationships among the hepatic secretion of bile, the metabolism and physiology of the bile salts, and the overall pathway subsuming these processes: the enterohepatic circulation. While biliary secretion is an essential route for the flow of a variety of substances, including lipids, bile pigments, vitamins, drugs, and drug metabolites, the attention of the clinician and physiologist is justifiably drawn to the bile salts themselves, the constituents of the bile that provide the amphipathic detergent molecules necessary for lipid digestion and absorption in the aqueous milieu of the intestinal lumen. The primary secretory mechanism for the elaboration of bile derives its driving force, at least in part, from the active transport, i.e., pumping, of bile salts across the hepatocyte from the sinusoidal surface to the canalicular lumen. At the same time, the secretion of bile is an essential intermediate step of the enterohepatic circulation, which ensures the availability of bile salts in excess of their critical micellar concentrations in the lumen of the small intestine.

One cannot contemplate this beautifully integrated homeostatic system in man without wondering about its evolutionary development. Almost 45 years ago, Sobotka (1) summarized many of the important issues in a prescient sentence:

> A future comparative biochemistry will be called upon to explain the phylogenetic parallelism and simultaneity of the secretion of bile acids with a calcified skeleton, and perhaps connect them with the need for exogenous antirachitic factors, the development of parathyroid glands, and the beginning of a special cholesterol metabolism based on its endogenous synthesis, and correlate these steps in biochemical evolution even with remoter points such as the increased resistance to lead poisoning or susceptibility to certain tumorous growths.

The challenge posed by the author has not been answered, nor are we in a position to offer unequivocal explanations. Nonetheless, it is heuristic to pose some generalities that may help provide an evolutionary backdrop to the material of the following chapters.

It is striking that the evolution of a well-developed capacity to synthesize cholesterol endogenously, to convert cholesterol to bile salts, and to secrete bile salts via a distinct organ, the liver, are all associated with the transition in evolution from invertebrate to vertebrate forms. The possibility exists, therefore, that one of the natural selection forces which led to the enterohepatic circulation originated from the need to assure sufficient intestinal absorption of calcium and phosphate for calcification of the skeleton and, thereby, for locomotion, "fight or flight." Clinicians in particular are well aware that interruption of the enterohepatic circulation of the bile salts leads to malapsorption of vitamin D and thereby to decalcification of the bones. As Sobotka (1) predicted, vitamin D sterols and the parathyroid glands are involved in this gut-bone interrelationship.

In the 45 years since publication of Sobotka's monograph (1), animal experiments have established that exogenous vitamin D is activated via hydroxylation in the liver and kidney and that the active metabolites function to maintain separate ion pumps for the absorption of calcium and phosphate, respectively, in the mucosa of the small intestine. Moreover, parathyroid hormone stimulates the hydroxylation of vitamin D metabolites in the kidney and thus modulates the activation of the sterol vitamin. The biochemical and physiological evidence available today is in accord with the hypothesis that the enterohepatic circulation of the bile salts, and the processes of bile secretion and bile salt synthesis, evolved to meet the needs of the organisms for skeletal calcification and efficient locomotion.

The scholarly studies of Haslewood (2–4) on the evolutionary implications of bile salt differences in various species are also in accord with the foregoing suggestion. The author suggests that an evolutionary progression of the bile salt structure has taken place and that "the evolutionary course has evidently been: C_{27} (and C_{26}) alcohols (sulphates) $\rightarrow$ C_{27} acids (taurine conjugates) $\rightarrow$ C_{24} acids (taurine conjugates) $\rightarrow$ C_{24} acids (glycine conjugates)" (4). The structures referred to occur primarily in vertebrates and represent derivatives of cholesterol or other sterols. Indeed, "the most obviously 'modern' vertebrates (most bony fish, snakes, birds, mammals) have C_{24} bile acids" (2). Evolution of these "modern" bile acids evidently depended on the absence of a methyl or ethyl group on the C_{24} of the cholesterol side chain. This permitted β-oxidation to take place with the formation of the C_{24} bile acids typical of the "higher" vertebrates. An additional factor in bile salt structure is evidently the nature of the diet. Thus carnivores tend to have taurine conjugates and trihydroxy acids; herbivores have dihydroxy acids, which are often conjugated with glycine; and man and other omnivores have both types (2).

The evolutionary picture, as fragmentary and incomplete as it is, prepares us for the close metabolic and physiological interrelationships of cholesterol metabolism; bile salt formation, action and transport; the hepatic secretory mechanism for the elaboration of bile; and the general enterohepatic circulation.

These topics are described in detail in the ensuing chapters, and the attentive reader will find additional observations that can be interrelated by the perspective of evolutionary development.

REFERENCES

1. Sobotka, H. (1937): *Physiological Chemistry of Bile*. Williams & Wilkins, Baltimore.
2. Haslewood, G. A. D., (1959): In: *Ciba Foundation Symposium on the Biosynthesis of Terpenes and Sterols*. edited by G. E. W. Wolstenhome and M. O'Connor, pp. 206–216. Little, Brown, Boston.
3. Haslewood, G. A. D. (1962): In: *Comparative Biochemistry, Volume III*, edited by M. Florkin and H. S. Mason, pp. 205–229. Academic Press, New York.
4. Haslewood, G. A. D., *Bile Salts*. Methuen and Co., London.

The Liver: Biology and Pathobiology, edited by
I. Arias, H. Popper, D. Schachter, and D. A. Shafritz.
Raven Press, New York © 1982.

Chapter 26

Bile Flow

Serge Erlinger

Bile is the exocrine secretion of the liver. Like most other exocrine secretions, it is an aqueous solution of organic and inorganic compounds. Bile acids, bile pigments, cholesterol, and phospholipids are the major organic compounds. Bile also contains small amounts of proteins. Because of the peculiar aggregation properties of the bile acids, which readily form micelles at physiologic concentrations, bile is more complex than most other secretions, especially in regard to the osmotic properties of its constituents. This chapter focuses on the mechanisms of bile flow. Bile formed by the hepatocytes is secreted in the bile canaliculi and then modified during its passage in the bile ductules and ducts. Since direct sampling of canalicular bile is not possible at present, most conclusions regarding canalicular bile formation are derived from indirect evidence and must be regarded as hypothetical. Nevertheless, an attempt is made to summarize the available experimental data and to discuss the current theories of bile formation. Emphasis is placed on recent developments; detailed references to the older literature may be found in several comprehensive reviews (1–3).

BILE COMPOSITION

Concentration of Biliary Electrolytes and Their Plasma Concentration

In general, inorganic electrolytes are present in common duct bile at concentrations closely reflecting those in plasma (4). Whether this is true of canalicular bile is not known. The range of reported values is shown in Table 1. Bile concentrations of sodium, potassium, calcium, and bicarbonate may be appreciably higher than in plasma, while chloride level may be lower. These differences could be due to one or more of the following phenomena: (a) the formation by the bile acids of polymolecular aggregates (or micelles) (5), which have low osmotic activity, (b) differences in electrical potential between the biliary lumen and the extracellular fluid, (c) variable repartition of different electrolytes due to the Donnan distribution, and (d) possible active transport of inorganic ions.

The predominant biliary cation is sodium, which is present in normal human bile in concentrations ranging

Table 1. *Flow and electrolyte concentrations of hepatic bile*

Species	Flow (μl·min^{-1} kg^{-1})	Na$^+$	K$^+$	Ca^{2+}	Mg^{2+}	Cl$^-$	HCO$_3^-$	Bile acids (mM)	References
				(mEq/liter)					
Man	1.5–15.4	132–165	4.2–5.6	1.2–4.8	1.4–3.0	96–126	17–55	3–45	6–8,10,11,
Dog	10	141–230	4.5–11.9	3.1–13.8	2.2–5.5	31–107	14–61	16–187	14,117
Sheep	9.4	159.6	5.3	—	—	95	21.2	42.5	181
Rabbit	90	148–156	3.6–6.7	2.7–6.7	0.3–0.7	77–99	40–63	6–24	73,241,247
Rat	30–150	157–166	5.8–6.4	—	—	94–98	22–26	8–25	115,164
Guinea pig	115.9	175	6.3	—	—	69	49–65	—	181

Numbers indicate range or means of published values.

from 145 to 165 mEq/liter (6–8). Lower concentrations prevail when substances such as dehydrocholate, phenol red, or polyethylene glycol-1500, whose micelle-forming capacity is inferior to that of the natural bile acids, are excreted in the bile (9). Micelle formation probably also explains why, under physiologic conditions, fluctuations in biliary bile acid concentration are accompanied by equivalent fluctuations in biliary sodium concentration (10,11). Sodium concentrations of up to 340 mEq/liter have been seen in concentrated gall bladder bile of rabbits (12,13) and concentrations of up to 240 mEq/liter in the hepatic bile of cholecystectomized dogs (11,14). Variations of bile potassium levels are usually parallel to those of sodium.

The concentration of calcium in bile, especially gall bladder bile, may be even higher, in comparison with its plasma concentration, than is the case with sodium and potassium (15,16). The electronegativity of the gallbladder lumen (12) may predispose to higher concentrations of divalent than monovalent cations.

The concentration of bicarbonate in bile is often higher than in plasma (6,7,14), especially in rabbits (241) and guinea pigs (18), whereas the concentration of chloride is generally similar to, or even lower than, that prevailing in plasma (6,7,10). The reason for these observations is not known, but a bicarbonate-transporting mechanism has been suggested. One result of these variations is that the pH of bile, although generally alkaline, also varies (11,14). Bicarbonate concentration in bile in dog and in man is higher than in plasma after administration of the hormone secretin.

Bile Acids: Major Organic Solutes in Bile

The main organic compounds of bile are the conjugated bile acids, phospholipids, cholesterol, and the bile pigments. Proteins are present at very low concentrations. Metabolites of various endogenous compounds (chiefly hormones) may also be found. Bile acid concentration in human hepatic bile ranges from 2 to 45 mM (7). Bile acids are mostly present as glycine and taurine conjugates, with a pK well below the physiologic range of biliary pH, and therefore are present as anions (referred to as bile salts) rather than undissociated bile acids.

Bile acids and salts are amphipathic molecules which form micelles (or polymolecular aggregates) above a critical micellar concentration (5,19). The concentration of bile acids in human hepatic and gall bladder bile is usually well above the critical micellar concentration, so that bile acids are mostly in the micellar form in normal bile, as well as in the duodenal and jejunal lumen. The major bile acids of man are conjugates of the primary (cholic and chenodeoxycholic) and secondary (deoxycholic and, to a lesser extent, lithocholic) bile acids.

Phospholipid and cholesterol concentrations of human hepatic bile range from 25 to 810 and from 60 to 320 mg/100 ml or 0.3 to 11 and 1.6 to 8.3 mM, respectively (7). In gall bladder bile, the concentrations of nonabsorbable constituents (bile acids, phospholipids, cholesterol) are appreciably higher, owing to reabsorption of water (and inorganic electrolytes) by the gall bladder. Theoretically, however, the molar percentage of each of these compounds in gall bladder bile relative to the total biliary lipid concentration should remain unchanged as compared to hepatic bile, although deviations may be observed (20). The secretion into bile of cholesterol and phospholipid is intimately dependent on bile acid secretion in animals and in man. Bile acids are a major determinant of phospholipid and cholesterol solubilization in bile. This process probably occurs through mixed micellar formation, a phenomenon that explains why biliary phospholipid and cholesterol concentrations far exceed the maximal solubility of these compounds in a simple aqueous solution. Cholesterol concentration in human bile frequently exceeds the maximal cholesterol-solubilizing capacity; this may lead to cholesterol precipitation and cholesterol gallstone formation.

Bile pigments are present in human hepatic and gall bladder bile at concentrations averaging, respectively, 0.8 and 3.2 mM (0.5 and 2 g/liter) (21). The origin, nature, mechanisms of secretion, and fate of bile pigments are discussed elsewhere in this volume. The solubility of the various bile pigments and its relationship to pigment gallstone formation are discussed by Soloway et al. (21).

Protein concentrations in bile are low, of the order of 60 to 400 mg/liter in canine bile and 300 to 3,000 mg/liter in human bile (7,22–24). Serum albumin is the most abundant and is derived from the plasma pool (23,25,26). Other bile proteins probably originate from plasma (27), and their concentration appears to be inversely related to their molecular weight (25,26). Bile also contains a variety of lysosomal enzymes, probably excreted via hepatocyte exocytosis independently of bile acid secretion (28), as well as many plasma membrane ectoenzymes (29,30).

Osmolality

Bile osmolality, as measured by freezing point depression, is usually approximately 300 mOsm/kg (11,31–33); it varies in parallel to plasma osmolality (32). Slight deviation from isotonicity has been observed in dogs. Bile tends to be hypotonic during high bile acid infusions, whereas it tends to be hypertonic during secretin administration (14,34). The significance of these deviations has not been fully elucidated but may be related, in part, to the nonideal osmotic behavior of the bile acids (34).

Total ion concentration (especially cation concentration) may be much higher in bile than in plasma (11) despite the isotonicity of bile. Total osmotic activity is accounted for only by the inorganic electrolytes, ignoring the bile salt anions (11). It is generally assumed that bile acids, because they are in micellar form, have little or no osmotic activity, and that the osmolality of bile is attributable mostly to the osmotic activity of the inorganic ions.

BILE FLOW: GENERAL PRINCIPLES

Osmotic Filtration: Major Mechanism of Bile Flow

Absorption and secretion of fluid in living organisms result from net movement of water. Active transport of water has never been observed in a living organism, and the water potential is identical inside and outside the living mammalian cell (35). Therefore, the driving force for water transport across epithelia must come from hydrostatic or osmotic pressure.

Hydrostatic filtration is unlikely to be the initiating event in bile flow. In the isolated perfused rat liver,

bile can be secreted at pressures exceeding the perfusion pressure (36,37); in the intact animal, maximum biliary pressure (or maximum secretory pressure) is invariably greater than sinusoidal (or portal) pressure (38–43). Under experimental or pathologic conditions, however, variations in hydrostatic pressure may affect bile formation. Excessive output of bile has been observed in cirrhosis and attributed, at least in part, to increased hepatic venous pressure (44). Acute increase in hepatic venous pressure in dogs, on the other hand, may reduce bile flow (14). Partial obstruction of the suprahepatic portion of the inferior vena cava has been reported to increase bile flow (45) or to have no effect (46).

Osmotic filtration is widely assumed to be the major flow-generating mechanism. The mechanisms of osmotic water flow across epithelia have been studied extensively in absorptive epithelia, such as the gall bladder and intestine. Current concepts of osmotic absorption of water are derived from the models of Curran (47) and Diamond (48–51), in which the active transport of a solute is coupled to water transport until osmotic equilibration is achieved. Such models have been postulated to apply also to secretory epithelia (52), although some of their features are still under active study (53). Prerequisites are: (a) a lumen closed at one end and provided with a high surface-volume ratio, and (b) active (energy-dependent) transport of one or several solutes. The bile canalicular network satisfies the first of these conditions. As for the second, the solutes in question could be either nonreabsorbable solutes that induce choleresis analogous to osmotic diuresis, or solutes of lower molecular weight that induce choleresis by establishing a local osmotic gradient. The site of the establishment of local osmotic gradients, if any, within the liver parenchyma has not been established. The intercellular spaces (54), as in the gall bladder (51), the canalicular lumen itself, or the spaces separating canalicular microvilli (55), as proposed in other secretory epithelia (52), are possible candidates. Appropriate solutes are considered below.

The anatomic sites of fluid movement in the biliary system are bile canaliculi, ductules, ducts, and gall bladder. Water movement of canalicular origin can be distinguished from movement of water of ductal or ductular origin by measurement of biliary clearance of inert solutes. More detailed analysis must await the development of more refined techniques, such as micropuncture. Water transport in the gall bladder has been studied elsewhere (48,56,57).

EXPERIMENTAL SYSTEMS AND METHODS

Systems for the Study of Bile Secretion

The simplest experimental preparation for studying bile formation is the total biliary fistula. Its major disadvantage is the total interruption of the enterohepatic circulation and the consequent depletion of the natural bile acids. This is usually overcome by constant intravenous or intraduodenal administration of exogenous bile acids at controlled rates. The partial biliary fistula allows controlled interruption of the enterohepatic circulation. After collection of a known quantity of bile, bile is returned to the stomach or duodenum, thus replenishing the pool of natural bile acids (58). The isolated perfused liver preparation is useful for observing the effects of single factors or of drugs with a toxic systemic action. Finally, isolated or cultured liver cells (59–62) may be used for transport studies (63–65). These techniques indicate that, in interpreting the results of an experiment, it is necessary to consider the species of animal and the experimental preparation used.

Canalicular Bile Flow Estimated Indirectly by Biliary Clearance of Nonmetabolized Solutes

Canalicular bile flow may be estimated by measuring the biliary clearance of nonmetabolized solutes, which enter the canalicular bile by passive processes (66) and are neither secreted nor reabsorbed by the ductules or the ducts. This method is analogous to measurement of glomerular filtration rate by urinary clearance of substances that do not cross the renal tubular epithelium. The theoretical basis of the method and some of its limitations are discussed by Forker (18,67–69) and Wheeler et al. (70); the relationship between the biliary clearance of such a solute and canalicular bile flow is shown in Fig. 1.

In brief, when such a solute is administered in the systemic circulation, its excretion rate in bile during a steady state should depend on the permeability of the epithelium and on bile flow. The biliary clearance (C) is calculated as: $C = F \times [B]/[P]$, where F is bile flow and [B] and [P] the biliary and plasma concentrations of the solute. The technique implies that the selected solute is unable to cross the ductular epithelium, and that its permeability in the canaliculi is high enough so that diffusion equilibrium is achieved at the highest rates of canalicular bile flow. Neither of these assumptions is presently accessible to direct experimental testing. An operational test of adequate canalicular permeability, however, is the finding that increments in bile flow produced by bile acid infusions (which are presumably of canalicular origin) are accompanied by parallel increases in clearance. Erythritol (MW 122) meets this requirement in dogs (70), hamsters (71), rats (72), rabbits (73), monkeys (74), and man (75). Mannitol (MW 182) appears to equilibrate in canalicular bile in dogs (70), but not in hamsters (71), rabbits (73), or man (76). Passage of both solutes in the canaliculi is restricted in guinea pigs (18).

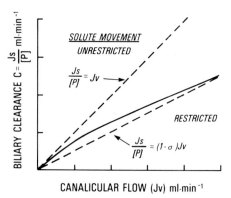

FIG. 1. Relationship between the clearance (C) of a nonmetabolized solute and canalicular bile flow (Jv). Flux of a nonmetabolized solute (such as erythritol) (Js) occurs by a combination of diffusion and bulk flow. When equilibrium is achieved between plasma and bile (no restriction to solute movement), solute clearance is equal to canalicular flow (*upper dashed line*). If there is restriction to solute movement, the reflection coefficient (σ) is greater than 0, and solute clearance will tend toward a fraction of solvent flux (*lower dashed line*). [P], plasma concentration. Note that Js = bile flow × biliary concentration of the solute. (After ref. 70.)

The assumption that these solutes are unable to cross the bile ductular or ductal epithelium is tested, again operationally, by the finding that their clearance is unaltered by secretin choleresis (18,70). It has been suggested that secretin acts at a site distal to the canaliculus and impermeable to the solutes, supposedly the bile ductules or ducts. Because secretin does not enhance choleresis in rabbits or rats, however, the assumption cannot be tested in these species. Moreover, experiments in dogs have shown an increase in the biliary clearances of erythritol and mannitol during secretin choleresis (77,77a). This observation could be explained by either stimulation of canalicular secretion by the hormone or by permeability of the bile ductules or ducts to erythritol and mannitol. Finally, it is impossible with this method to determine whether secretin choleresis originates in the small periportal bile ductules or in the larger bile ducts.

How do erythritol and mannitol pass from the sinusoids into the canalicular bile? The predominant mode of transit is thought to be by osmotic filtration through the sinusoidal membrane, the hepatocyte, and the canalicular membrane (Fig. 2). Two findings suggest that the sinusoidal membrane is permeable to these solutes, and that they rapidly penetrate the totality of the hepatocyte: (a) the equilibrium between plasma and hepatic concentrations of 5- or 6-carbon sugars and polyalcohols is rapidly established in the steady state (66,78,79); and (b) the hepatic venous dilution curve of erythritol after a single intraportal injection is superimposable upon that of water (80). If this is so, their entry into bile depends on their passage through the canalicular membrane. The following ob-

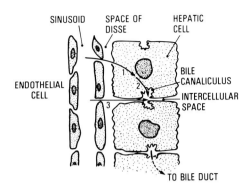

FIG. 2. Antomic pathways for entry of solutes from blood to bile. Solutes can enter bile through the transcellular pathway after uptake and transport by the hepatocyte (*1*) and secretion by the canalicular membrane (*2*), or through the paracellular pathway via the intercellular junctions (*3*).

servations suggest the possibility of a paracellular pathway (Fig. 2): (a) The bile-to-plasma concentration ratios of relatively larger solutes, such as inulin (MW 5,000), sucrose (MW 342), or polyethylene glycol-4000, stabilize well before the hepatocyte-to-plasma concentration ratios (68,81); and (b) the appearance in bile of ferrocyanide (MW 484, hydrated form) is very rapid (82).

This alternative route of entry should not preclude the use of such solutes as indicators of canalicular flow, provided a parallel increase in bile flow and solute clearance is clearly demonstrated during bile acid-induced choleresis. Finally, it has been shown that the biliary clearances of charged solutes (such as ferrocyanide and carboxylinulin) are consistently lower than those of uncharged solutes of comparable molecular size, an observation suggesting that the pathway of entry into bile includes a barrier that selectively restricts passive anionic movement (82).

Solutes, such as sucrose and inulin, also enter canalicular bile; however, their bile-to-plasma concentration ratio in the rat is approximately 0.15 to 0.20 and 0.05 to 0.10, respectively (66,68). This is due to restriction of movement across the pathway which permits their entry into canalicular bile. Consequently, their biliary clearance does not estimate canalicular bile flow; they may be used to estimate qualitatively changes in the permeability of the biliary system (83).

CANALICULAR (HEPATOCYTIC) BILE FLOW

One- and Two-Component Theories

Canalicular bile formation is regarded as an osmotic water flow in response to active solute transport. Because of the excellent correlation between bile flow and bile acid output in bile, bile acids are considered to be one of the solutes generating bile flow: the term bile

acid-dependent flow is widely used to describe this fraction of bile flow; some consider that bile acids may account for all canalicular bile flow (84). The latter view may be referred to as a one-component theory of canalicular bile flow (Fig. 3). Under several circumstances, however, canalicular flow may be generated at low bile acid outputs, in the absence of bile acids, or in addition to the bile acid-dependent flow. This is usually designated as the bile acid-independent flow (1,2,84); this view may be referred to as a two-component theory of canalicular bile flow (Fig. 3). Although most of the evidence supports the two-component theory, direct proof is still lacking.

Bile Acid-Dependent Flow Generated by Biliary Secretion of Bile Acids

Bile Acids Taken Up and Secreted by Two Successive Membrane Transport Processes

The mechanisms for the uptake of bile acids into the hepatocytes, their intracellular transport, and their secretion into bile are incompletely understood (85). The liver has a high extraction efficiency for bile acids (86). The uptake of bile acids by the liver cells meets the criteria of a carrier-mediated process. As illustrated in Fig. 4, it appears to be saturable, as shown by an indicator dilution technique in the intact dog (87,88) and in the *in situ* perfused rat liver (89,90) and by studies with isolated liver cells (63,64). It exhibits sodium dependence, both in the isolated perfused rat liver (90,91)

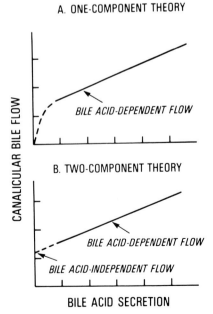

FIG. 3. Canalicular (hepatocytic) bile flow: one-component (**A**) and two-component (**B**) theories. **A:** Bile acids account for all canalicular bile flow. **B:** A fraction of canalicular bile flow is secreted in the absence of bile acids (bile acid-independent flow).

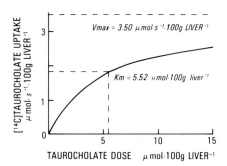

FIG. 4. Hepatic uptake of taurocholate in the dog. Uptake of taurocholate was measured by the indicator dilution techique in anesthetized dogs, using albumin as an extracellular reference. The initial velocity of uptake (ordinate) increased in a nonlinear way with increasing doses, consistent with Michaelis-Menten kinetics. (From ref. 87.)

and in isolated liver cells (64). Competitive inhibition may be shown when two bile acids are given simultaneously but not with other organic anions, such an indocyanine green (92). The exact nature of the postulated carrier system is not known. A bile-acid receptor, however, probably a protein, has been characterized in the liver cell plasma membrane (93,94) and may serve as initial interaction in the bile acid translocation across the membrane. The maximal capacity for uptake (about 3.5 to 4.5 μmoles·s^{-1}·100 g liver^{-1}) is approximately 10 times greater than the maximal capacity for bromosulfophthalein (BSP) uptake (95). It also greatly exceeds the maximal capacity for biliary excretion so that, under normal bile acid loads, transport takes place far from saturation. The strong sodium-dependence of the uptake suggests that the process is a secondary active, sodium-bile cotransport (symport) system energized by the sodium gradient.

Little is known about intracellular transport from the sinusoidal to the canalicular pole of the hepatocyte. Bile acids have little affinity for the Y (ligandin) or Z proteins (96–98), which bind a variety of other organic anions, including BSP and iodinated contrast agents. Cytoplasmic bile acid-binding proteins, which have been detected and partially purified (99,100), may play a role in transport. One exhibits glutathione-transferase activity and could be identical to ligandin (100). During this phase of hepatic transport, unconjugated bile acids are conjugated to taurine and glycine. Keto-bile acids also can be hydroxylated (101–103).

The secretion of bile acids into bile probably takes place through another carrier-mediated process. Bile acids are secreted against a concentration gradient. Their biliary concentration (10 to 100 mM) is 100 to 1,000 times higher than their plasma concentration in systemic or portal blood, suggesting an active process. Secretion into bile is saturable, with a maximal capacity of 8 to 8.5 μmoles·min^{-1}·kg^{-1} in dogs (104), 14

μmoles·min^{-1}·kg^{-1} in sheep (105), and 10 to 12 μmoles·min^{-1}·kg^{-1} in rats (106). Three lines of evidence suggest that the hepatic secretory mechanism for bile acids is not the same as that for other organic anions excreted in the bile, particularly bilirubin, BSP, and iodinated contrast agents. The Tm for bile acids is five to 10 times higher than that of BSP (107). Bile acids and BSP do not compete for biliary excretion. On the contrary, administration of bile acids increases the apparent Tm for BSP (108–111); the mechanism of this effect is examined below. In mutant Corriedale sheep, which have an inherited defect in biliary excretion of organic anions that is closely related to the Dubin-Johnson syndrome in man, maximal biliary excretion of BSP was low, whereas that of bile acids was normal (105).

As shown for galactose (112), a lobular concentration gradient (periportal > centrilobular) for bile acids has been demonstrated (113). Morphologic studies have also shown a gradient in canalicular diameter (114), suggesting that under physiologic conditions, the bulk of bile acid secretion (and hence of the bile acid-dependent flow) occurs in the periportal region.

Because of their efficient hepatic transport and their enterohepatic circulation, bile acids are secreted into bile in considerable amounts. With a synthetic rate of approximately 600 mg/day, the liver is able to maintain a bile acid pool of 2 to 3 g and to secrete into bile 20 to 30 g/day of bile acids.

Canalicular Bile Flow Linearly Related to Bile Acid Secretion Rate

Bile acids stimulate bile production in many species. An apparently linear relationship between bile acid secretion rates and bile flow has been demonstrated in the dog (14), rabbit (73), rat and isolated rat liver (72,115,116), rhesus monkey (58,74), and man (75,117, 118). Bile acid-induced choleresis is presumably of canalicular origin; it is accompanied by a parallel increase in erythritol clearance (18,67,70). A linear relationship is found between bile acid secretion rate and erythritol or mannitol clearance in both animals (70,72) and man (75,76,119). This relationship in man is shown schematically in Fig. 5.

The hypothesis that bile acids increase bile flow because they provide an osmotic driving force for filtration of water and electrolytes was first proposed by Sperber (9,120). The reduction in bile flow and electrolyte excretion without reduction in bile acid secretion that has been recorded after intravenous injections of hypertonic solutions (31) could be due to a fall in this osmotic gradient. The observation that other osmotically active compounds (organic anions other than bile acids, and nonanionic substances) that also appear in bile at high concentrations also have a

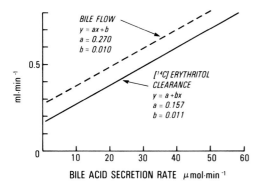

FIG. 5. Relationship between bile acid secretion rate (abcissa) and bile flow (*dashed line*) and erythritol clearance (*solid line*) (ordinate). The relationship is linear in both cases. The slope is similar and is thought to estimate the osmotic activity of the bile acids. When extrapolated to a zero bile acid secretion, the line for erythritol clearance is assumed to estimate the canalicular bile acid-independent secretion, while the line for bile flow is assumed to estimate total (canalicular and ductal/ductular) bile acid-independent flow. (From ref. 75.)

choleretic action proportional to the osmotic load supports this hypothesis.

Since bile acids are in the micellar form, most of the osmotic activity must be accounted for by their accompanying counter-ions. The slope of the line that relates bile flow to bile acid secretion (which is an operational estimate of the osmotic effect of bile acids) varies from species to species. Expressed in microliters bile per micromole bile acid secreted, it is approximately 8 in the dog (14,70), 13 in the rhesus monkey (58), 15 in the rat (115), and 30 in the rabbit (73). The smallest of these volumes is far larger than the amount of water that would be expected if bile acids alone were secreted in an isotonic solution. The reasonable conclusion is that bile acid-dependent bile flow includes substantial amounts of other osmotically active solutes, probably driven by passive diffusion and solvent drag. The magnitude of these processes depends on the permeability characteristics of the canaliculus and may differ from species to species.

An alternative explanation of bile acid-dependent bile flow is that the choleretic effect of bile acids could be due, at least in part, to their regulation of the activity of other solute pumps (1,103). This hypothesis is supported by several pieces of suggestive evidence: (a) In some species, dehydrocholate produces a higher flow than do other bile acids (9,101). This difference traditionally is attributed to this compound and its metabolites having less tendency to micelle formation than the natural bile acids (9,120,121). During dehydrocholate choleresis, however, bile flow reached a maximum well after the bulk of the bile acid load had been secreted into bile (21), an observation not easily explained by the osmotic theory, which predicts simultaneity between the excretion of the osmotic load

and the choleresis. (b) Experiments in rats with ursodeoxycholate and 7-ketolithocholate (its precursor during synthesis from chenodeoxycholic acid) have shown that the choleretic effect of these compounds was much greater than that of taurocholate and deviated from the expected linearity (122). (c) In the rhesus monkey, erythritol clearance was greater per mole of secreted taurocholate when the bile acid was infused at a high rate than when infused at a low rate (123). Analysis of the data showed that this could be due to enhancement of the bile acid-independent flow. (d) In the dog, bile flow associated with unconjugated cholate secretion is much higher than that associated with taurocholate secretion at the same rate (104); the "extra" bile flow is not related to a higher osmotic activity of the unconjugated bile acid (104). It could again be due to stimulation of fluid secretion other than by the osmotic effect of cholate. Alternatively, it could be due to a change in permeability at the site of bile acid-dependent bile formation. (e) In rats with selective biliary obstruction, an increase in bile acid flux through the nonobstructed liver together with a disproportionate increase in bile flow have been reported (123a). These observations suggest that bile acids may stimulate inorganic ion transport. Sodium transport mediated by the sodium, potassium-activated adenosine triphosphatase (Na$^+$,K$^+$-ATPase), whose role is discussed later in this chapter, might be one of the candidates for such an activation. In rats with selective biliary obstruction (123a), the activity of this enzyme in liver plasma membranes was increased. Alternatively, bicarbonate transport may be stimulated, as observed with ursodeoxycholate and 7-ketolithocholate (122).

Pathway of Fluid Movement: Transcellular or Paracellular?

The pathway of fluid transport during bile acid-induced choleresis is unclear. Since bile acids are transported through the canalicular membrane of the hepatocyte, it is often stated that the osmotic water flow in response to this transport also occurs through the canalicular membrane (Fig. 6). The ionic composition of bile closely resembles that of the extracellular fluid. It is necessary, therefore, to postulate either an ionic equilibration downstream along the biliary channels or a paracellular fluid pathway from the intercellular space into the bile canaliculi. Evidence that solutes, such as inulin, sucrose, polyethylene glycol, or ferrocyanide, may gain access to canalicular bile through this pathway has already been presented. Experiments with dehydrocholate and taurodehydrocholate have demonstrated a progressive increase in the bile-to-plasma concentration ratio of sucrose, a penetration of ionic lanthanum into the tight junctions,

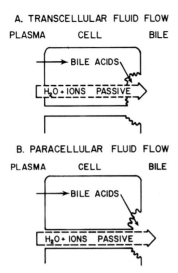

FIG. 6. Possible pathways of bile acid-induced water flow. Water flow in response to bile acid secretion may occur through the cell **(A)** or through the intercellular spaces and tight junctions **(B)**.

and an increase in the number of intercellular "blisters" (54). These observations have suggested that the paracellular pathway may be an important site for bile acid-induced water and solute movement into bile (Fig. 6). Such a hypothesis requires that the tight junctions between liver cells be relatively "leaky." Indirect morphologic evidence suggests that this could be the case (124), but this question clearly requires further evaluation.

In summary, bile acid-dependent canalicular bile flow probably is related to the osmotic activity of bile acids or of their associated counter-ions. In addition, there is suggestive evidence that some bile acids, such as dehydrocholate, ursodeoxycholate, or others, may increase canalicular bile flow in certain species, by stimulating inorganic ion transport. Bile acid-induced water and solute movement into bile may take place, at least in part, through the paracellular (tight junction) pathway.

Exogenous Compounds may have a Bile Acid-Like Choleretic Effect

Organic anions include BSP, fluorescein, indocyanine green, ioglycamide, iodipamide, phenol red, phloridzin, and rose bengal, all of which are secreted into the bile. In general, they increase bile flow in proportion to their secretion rate into bile. The choleresis is thought to depend on an osmotic mechanism similar to that of bile acid choleresis (9,125,126). However, marked species differences are observed with respect to the effect of these compounds on bile flow.

In a study in dogs, the choleretic response to infusions of BSP, ioglycamide, and taurocholate was pro-

portional to biliary output. The volume of water secreted per micromole of the three compounds was 9.2, 11.9, and 7.3 μliters, respectively (126). The greater choleretic potency of BSP and ioglycamide as compared to taurocholate could be explained by a higher osmotic activity. This is even more marked with iodipamide, which "obligates" 22 μliters bile per μmole (127); yet its osmotic activity in bile (1.5 mOsm/mmole) is only twice as great as that of taurocholate (0.8 mOsm/mmole). The reason for the apparent "extra" water is not clear. It could be due to stimulation of an inorganic solute pump, modifications of canalicular permeability, generation of an electrical potential with subsequent passive movement of ions, or a combination of these mechanisms.

Increased bile flow has been induced by fluorescein in the rat, by phenol red in the chicken, and by phloridzin in the chicken and dog (9). Rose bengal increased bile flow in dogs but reduced it in rabbits (128). In contrast to its choleretic action in the dog, BSP has been shown to reduce bile flow in the rat (109,129–131). Anticholeresis in the rat by indocyanine green has also been reported (129,132); the mechanism is examined below.

Bilirubin in physiologic doses does not cause choleresis (133), possibly because the osmotic load is low and/or because of the incorporation of bilirubin into micelles, with loss of osmotic activity. Choleresis after infusion of bilirubin in quantities close to its Tm has been recorded (134). Reproduction of this experiment by us showed the choleretic response to be transitory and followed by a decreased flow.

Organic cations are also excreted into bile (135,136). Their transport process appears to be different from that which secretes organic anions. No effect on choleresis has been documented.

Many substances other than organic anions or cations are excreted into bile and increase choleresis. Although they include compounds as chemically disparate as polyethylene glycol 1500 (271) and ferrioxamine derivatives (137,138), they may be grouped into two categories: (a) neutral substances excreted into bile in the form of metabolites, chiefly glucuronides, for example, 4-methylumbelliferone (139–141) and probably many of the commercial choleretics, and (b) neutral substances excreted into bile unconverted into anionic compounds. For some, such as the ferrioxamine derivatives (138), a correlation has been found between bile flow and the biliary output of the substance, suggesting that these compounds also increase bile flow by an osmotic mechanism.

Bile Acids Enhance Biliary Transport Capacity of Other Organic Anions

Bile acid administration is usually associated with an increase in the transport maximum (Tm) into bile of organic anions, such as BSP (105,108–111,142), indocyanine green (143), iopanoic acid (144,145), and ampicillin (146). The following may explain such an effect: (a) a role of bile flow, (b) sequestration of the agent in micelles formed by the bile acid, (c) a direct effect of the bile acid on the organic anion carrier or (d) recruitment of transporting hepatocytes under the influence of the bile acid. There is good evidence that the increase in Tm is not related to the increase in flow. Canalicular choleresis induced by agents other than bile acids, such as theophylline (147,148), 4-methylumbelliferone (148), and the bicyclic organic anion SC 2644 (144, 149), has no influence on the Tm of BSP or iopanoic acid. Incorporation into mixed micelles has been shown to occur *in vitro* (150,151) and could serve as a micellar "sink" (150). No correlation has been found *in vivo* however, between incorporation into micelles and the effect of several bile acids on the Tm of various compounds (151). Moreover, dehydrocholate and its metabolites, which have little or no micelle-forming capacity, increase BSP Tm to the same extent as micelle-forming bile acids (109,142,150,152). In contrast, glycodihydrofusidate, a steroid compound that forms mixed micelles *in vitro* and is excreted into bile, did not increase BSP Tm in the hamster (153). It is more likely, therefore, that bile acids increase the biliary Tm of other organic anions by a direct action on the transport system of these agents. The theoretical possibilities are: (a) the active transport of bile acids provides the driving force for other organic anions by a cotransport system; (b) bile acids modify, possibly in an allosteric way, the carrier of the other organic anions (154); and (c) bile acids increase, by a recruitment process, the number of hepatocytes available for transport. On the basis of available kinetic data, it is not yet possible to distinguish among these possibilities.

Monohydroxylated Bile Acids have a Cholestatic Effect

Administration of taurolithocholate or taurocholenate to rats and hamsters decreases bile flow and bile acid secretion and leads to the electron microscope changes of cholestasis (155,156). The diminution of bile flow can be prevented or corrected by administration of taurocholate or taurochenodeoxycholate. Although the mechanism is poorly understood, several possibilities have been proposed: (a) precipitation of taurolithocholate in the canaliculi (because of its low water solubility) with resultant canalicular obstruction (157); (b) decrease in bile acid-independent flow, as suggested in the hamster (158); and (c) toxic effect of bile acid on membrane structure, as suggested by scanning electron microscope observations (159). Cholestasis may be induced by other bile acids, such as chenodeoxycholic acid in the rat (160,161) or even

taurocholate when given at rates above its biliary Tm (162).

Some of the anionic dyes used for investigation of liver function are anticholeretic when given in high doses. Bile flow in rabbits is lowered by the phthalein dye, rose bengal (128); BSP and indocyanine green have been shown to reduce bile flow in the rat (109,129,130,131,132). These effects have been attributed, at least in part, to inhibition of bile acid-independent bile formation (128,132).

Bile Acid-Independent Flow as a Result of Inorganic Ion Transport

Evidence and Estimation

In all animal species studied, plots of bile acid secretion rates against bile flow (14,58,72,75,115–118) and against erythritol or mannitol clearance (70,73–76,115,116,119) yield a positive intercept upon extrapolation to the flow axis (Figs. 5 and 7). The extrapolated value of erythritol clearance at zero bile acid secretion is generally regarded as estimating the bile acid-independent fraction of canalicular bile. Its actual amount differs from species to species: it was ~5 $\mu l \cdot min^{-1} \cdot kg$ body weight^{-1} in dogs (70), 70 in rats (115), 60 in rabbits (73), 7 in the rhesus monkey (74), and 1.5 to 2 in man (75,76,119).

This procedure, however, rests on the assumption that the osmotic activity of bile acids does not increase when their concentration falls below the critical micellar concentration. Testing this assumption requires examination of the relationship between bile flow and bile acid secretion at low bile acid concentrations and secretion rates. In the isolated perfused rat liver, linearity seems to extend into the critical range (72,116), and the intercept measured in this prepara-

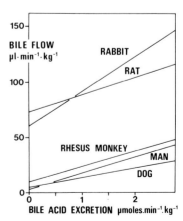

FIG. 7. Relationship between bile flow and bile acid secretion in various animal species. Note that extrapolation to a zero bile acid secretion yields a positive intercept. The magnitude of this intercept is higher in rats and rabbits than in the three other species.

tion agrees with the value calculated by extrapolation. In the rat *in vivo*, however, careful analysis of this relationship has shown a variation of the slope with bile acid concentration (163). The slope decreased from 90 μl bile/μmole bile acid at concentrations below 10 mM, to 12 at concentrations between 30 and 45 mM. This suggests that quantitation of the bile acid-independent flow by the extrapolation procedure may be subject to error. Moreover, by making several postulates concerning the permeability of the canaliculus, it may be that, at low bile acid secretion rates, the relationship between canalicular bile flow and bile acid secretion extrapolates to the origin, and that bile acids alone account for all canalicular bile flow under physiologic conditions (84).

Evidence for canalicular flow-generating mechanisms independent of bile acid secretion also, and more convincingly, comes from the study of drugs that increase in parallel bile flow and erythritol clearance, without modifying bile acid secretion rate, such as phenobarbital and other barbiturates (115,164,165), theophylline (166) and glucagon (167), hydrocortisone (168,169), and SC 2644 (170) (see below). With the possible exception of hydrocortisone, neither these drugs themselves nor their metabolites are excreted into bile in sufficient amounts to provide an osmotic driving force. They do not increase either the osmotic activity of the bile acids, as estimated by the slope of the bile flow-bile acid secretion plot (115,164,165), or the permeability of the canalicular membrane or tight junction to water and ions, as estimated by the bile-to-plasma concentration ratio of sucrose (170). The most reasonable hypothesis to explain the effect of these compounds on bile flow is that they stimulate the transport into bile of some other solute (or solutes), probably inorganic electrolytes. Sodium transport linked to Na$^+$,K$^+$—ATPase (72,73,171) and, more recently, bicarbonate transport (172) have been implicated as possible mediators.

Possible Role of Sodium Transport

Active sodium transport occurs through most cell plasma membranes; it is associated with a membrane-bound enzyme, Na$^+$,K$^+$-ATPase (173,174). In isolated cells, extrusion of sodium is coupled with entry of potassium and does not generate osmotic water flow. In transporting epithelia, however, the Na$^+$,K$^+$-ATPase has been implicated in various secretions and is thought to generate water flow by local osmosis. Hepatocyte plasma membranes (175,176) have been shown to contain Na$^+$,K$^+$-ATPase. In various situations, a correlation has been found between Na$^+$,K$^+$-ATPase activity in liver plasma membranes and bile flow (Fig. 8). Several lines of evidence suggest that it is implicated in the generation of bile flow.

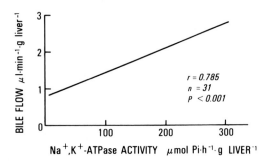

FIG. 8. Relationship between Na$^+$,K$^+$-ATPase activity in liver plasma membranes and bile flow. Liver plasma membranes were obtained from normal rats and rats treated with phenobarbital, estrogen, and methylcholantrene. Note that enzyme activity and bile flow are expressed per gram liver. (From ref. 186.)

Inhibitors of sodium transport

Three inhibitors of sodium transport (ouabain, ethacrynic acid, and amiloride) diminished or suppressed the bile acid-independent flow when injected into the portal vein of anesthetized rabbits (73,171). Scillaren had the same effect in the isolated perfused liver (72). Interpretation of *in vivo* experiments with these agents, however, may be difficult, since ouabain (177) and ethacrynic acid metabolites (178,179) are excreted into bile by concentrative processes and may produce an osmotic choleresis. This choleresis may mask, in part or totally, their possible inhibitory effects. Indeed, in subsequent experiments, both ouabain and ethacrynic acid induced choleresis in various species (178–181). With ethacrynic acid, a linear relationship was seen between drug excretion and erythritol clearance (177). Thus the observed effect of these agents in any given experimental situation probably depends on the relative contribution of the inhibitory and osmotic effects. Alternatively, it has been suggested that ouabain and sodium may be cotransported into the hepatocyte, and that the secondary extrusion of sodium into the bile canaliculi may account for the choleretic effect (182).

Estrogen

Although cholestasis has been observed in both rats and man after treatment with estrogens, the mechanism is not fully understood. It has been shown with ethynylestradiol in rats that the decrease in bile flow was due mostly to a decrease in the bile acid-independent flow (183), although a diminution of the bile acid Tm and a moderate diminution of bile acid secretion were also observed. An inhibition of Na$^+$,K$^+$-ATPase activity in liver plasma membranes *in vitro* has been reported (183); steroids, having no effect on Na$^+$,K$^+$-ATPase, had no effect on bile flow (184). Subsequent experiments *in vivo* with estrogen-treated rats have shown a parallel decrease in Na$^+$,K$^+$-

ATPase activity in liver cell plasma membranes and in bile acid-independent bile flow (185,186).

A decrease in bile acid-independent bile flow and Na^+,K^+-ATPase activity has also been reported during pregnancy (187). The mechanism of the decrease in enzyme activity could be an alteration of the lipid composition of the membrane (185). These observations suggest that estrogen-induced cholestasis could be initiated by a failure of the sodium pump. In estrone-treated rats, increases have been reported in the bile-to-plasma concentration ratio of sucrose and in sucrose biliary clearance (83). This suggests that the decreased flow could be due, at least in part, to an increased permeability of the biliary system, leading to an increased "back-diffusion" of bile. These two proposed mechanisms are not mutually exclusive. It should be noted, however, that an increased permeability may also be observed during bile acid-induced choleresis (54). Its contribution to cholestasis, although still a possibility, requires further evaluation.

Phenobarbital

Administration of phenobarbital to rats for 3 or 4 days results in an increase in bile flow due solely to an increase in the bile acid-independent flow, with no change in bile acid secretion (115,164,165) or in the relative outputs of individual bile acids (165). When given to rats for 7 days (188) or to rhesus monkeys for 14 days (189), phenobarbital stimulates bile acid secretion. Again, studies *in vivo* in phenobarbital-treated rats have shown parallel increases in bile flow and Na^+,K^+-ATPase activity in liver cell plasma membranes (186,186a), although other experiments have not detected any effect of phenobarbital on the activity of the enzyme (190–192). Failure to detect an increase in the specific activity of the Na^+,K^+-ATPase (i.e., activity per gram liver or per milligram protein) does not rule out a role of the enzyme; since liver weight is increased, total liver enzyme activity is increased. (In the same way, bile flow per gram liver is not increased, while total bile flow is increased.) The increase in activity is suppressed by inhibitors of protein synthesis, suggesting that it is attributable to enhanced synthesis.

Phenobarbital has a number of other effects on the liver and on biliary function (193): (a) it decreases serum bilirubin concentrations in patients with familial nonhemolytic hyperbilirubinemia; (b) it may improve cholestasis, especially in children; and (c) it enhances the biliary clearance and elimination of certain dyes. The relationship of these effects to the stimulation of bile flow is, at present, unclear. It is apparent, however, that the effect on bile flow is not strongly related to the induction of microsomal drug-metabolizing enzymes: (a) other microsomal enzyme inducers do not affect bile flow (164); (b) pentobarbital may increase bile flow without producing any detectable microsomal

enzyme induction (194); and (c) inhibition of microsomal enzyme induction by SKF-525 A or cobaltous chloride does not suppress the effect of phenobarbital on bile flow (195).

Thyroid Hormones

Bile flow in hypothyroid rats is reduced (196) because of a decrease in bile acid-independent bile flow (197); a parallel decrease in Na^+,K^+-ATPase activity in liver plasma membranes is observed (197). Administration of L-thyroxine restores both bile flow and Na^+,K^+-ATPase to normal. Animals made hyperthyroid by administration of L-3,5,3'-triiodothyronine have an increased bile acid-independent flow (as well as an increase in bile acid secretion) and a parallel increase in plasma membrane Na^+,K^+-ATPase activity (197).

Chlorpromazine

Chlorpromazine hydrochloride infused intravenously in pharmacologic doses in the rhesus monkey induces a dose-dependent inhibition of the bile acid-independent flow (198); it also inhibits both Mg^{2+} and Na^+,K^+-ATPase in liver plasma membranes in a dose-dependent fashion (199). The inhibition is reduced by glutathione and enhanced when chlorpromazine semiquinone free radical formation is increased, observations which may explain in part the irregular appearance of chlorpromazine-induced cholestasis in man.

Location of sodium transport

The localization of transport Na^+,K^+-ATPase on the hepatocyte plasma membrane is not firmly established. A simple view for sodium pumping into the canalicular lumen would require the enzyme to be located on the canalicular ("mucosal") site of the membrane, facing secretion. In most epithelia involved in either absorption or secretion, however, the enzyme appears to be situated on the basolateral ("serosal") site of the epithelial cell (200–203), regardless of the polarity of salt transport by the system. The only exception to this rule is the choroid plexus (200).

Cytochemical studies have also suggested a basolateral site (i.e., sinusoidal and intercellular) of the hepatocyte Na^+,K^+-ATPase (17,204). This localization is paradoxical because the enzyme is oriented in the wrong direction to transport sodium into the canalicular lumen; however, this apparent paradox extends to many secretory organs, in particular osmoregulatory organs with high Na^+,K^+-ATPase activity (200–203, 205,206). A Na^+,K^+-ATPase orientation opposite to the direction of net electrolyte and water secretion is consistent with a role of this enzyme in bile formation. The mechanism of coupling of enzyme to net electrolyte and water transport into bile remains to be elucidated. Among the theoretical possibilities are: (a) secondary transport of other electrolytes along the electrical gradient created by sodium extrusion, and (b) establishment of a standing gradient within the intercellular space, followed by an osmotic flow through the relatively leaky junctional complexes. This view is consistent with the recent biochemical localization of Na^+,K^+-ATPase activity to intercellular hepatocyte membranes (207). Neither of these possibilities has yet been tested directly, however, although a paracellular sodium movement from the sinusoids to the canalicular lumen has been suggested (182, 208).

Attempts have been made to localize sites of origin of the bile acid-independent flow within the hepatic lobule. After selective destruction of centrilobular hepatocytes by bromobenzene, canalicular bile flow decreased with no change in bile acid secretion (209). This suggests that centrilobular hepatocytes contribute predominantly to the secretion of the bile acid-independent fraction at physiologic bile acid loads, while periportal hepatocytes may contribute predominantly to bile acid-dependent bile formation.

Other Possible Mechanisms

Bicarbonate transport

In the isolated perfused rat liver, perfusion with a bicarbonate-free solution reduced the bile-acid independent flow by 50% (172). Under this condition, bicarbonate secretion was nearly eliminated, while sodium secretion was markedly reduced. In contrast, administration of SC-2644 to dogs increased canalicular bile flow and bicarbonate concentration in bile (210). These observations lead to the suggestion that a bicarbonate transport mechanism may have a role in the elaboration of the bile acid-independent flow. Ursodeoxycholate and 7-ketolithocholate increase bicarbonate secretion as well as canalicular bile flow, an effect possibly related to stimulation of the bicarbonate transport system by these bile acids. The cellular mechanism remains to be elucidated. Attempts to demonstrate a bicarbonate-sensitive ATPase in liver cell plasma membranes have been unsuccessful (172,211).

Effect of other pharmacologic agents

Cyclic 3',5'-adenosine monophosphate (cAMP) is known to increase sodium transport. It stimulates choleresis in dogs by increasing the bile acid-independent flow (212). Theophylline and glucagon, which both increase the intracellular concentration of cAMP, also increase bile flow in the dog and man (125,166,167,212–215). This has led to the suggestion that cAMP could play a role in bile formation, perhaps by regulating electrolyte transport. In a systematic study of liver cAMP in rats and dogs, however, no correlation could be found between cAMP content and choleresis during theophylline, methylisobutylxanthine, dibutyryl cAMP, or glucagon administration (216). The role of the cAMP system in bile formation, therefore, is still uncertain. Its role in secretin-induced choleresis has also been claimed (217). Prostaglandins A_1, E_1, and E_2 increase bile flow in dogs, rats, and cats (218a,219,220). This effect in the rat is attributable to stimulation of bile acid-independent bile formation (220); in the cat, available data suggest an inhibition of fluid reabsorption by the bile ducts (219). The cellular mechanisms are not known. Salicylates are choleretics in dogs and rats (221–224) also by stimulation of bile acid-independent flow (223). Their mechanism of action likewise is unknown.

In summary, flow-generating mechanisms that cannot be attributed to the active transport of bile acids are present in the canaliculi. Flow due to these mechanisms is generally referred to as bile acid-independent canalicular bile flow. Strongly suggestive evidence has accumulated in favor of a role of Na^+,K^+-ATPase-mediated sodium transport. The mechanism of coupling of the enzyme with solute and fluid transport has not been elucidated. Bicarbonate transport, although less clearly characterized, may also play a role.

Possible Role in Bile Formation of Microfilaments and Microtubules

Cytoskeletal and contractile organelles in hepatocytes include (225): (a) microtubules, (b) thick myosin filaments, (c) intermediate (keratin) filaments, and (d) thin actin microfilaments. Available data suggest a role of these organelles in the maintenance of cell shape, cell motility, and various secretions, including protein and lipoprotein secretion by the hepatocytes into the plasma. It is hypothesized that microfilaments and microtubules may have a role in bile formation, and that dysfunction of these organelles may lead to cholestasis.

The role of microfilaments has been studied using cytochalasin B (which disrupts microfilaments) and phalloidin (which induces an irreversible polymerization of monomeric actin into microfilaments in the hepatocytes). Both cytochalasin (226) and phalloidin (227,228) decrease bile flow in the rat. The effect of cytochalasin was immediate, while the effect of phalloidin was detectable after 1 day of treatment and increased with time (227). Electron microscopy and morphometric analysis showed that phalloidin induced a marked increase in the thickness of the pericanalicular microfilamentous network (227,229), and that this effect was parallel in time to the decrease in bile flow (227). Phalloidin also decreased bile acid secretion into bile and delayed [³H]taurocholate disappearance from plasma after a single injection (230). These observations indicate an effect of phalloidin on bile acid transport by the liver. Finally, phalloidin increased the bile-to-plasma concentration ratio of [¹⁴C]sucrose, suggesting an increased "permeability" of the biliary system and decreased cholesterol secretion into bile (231). These findings provide strong circumstantial evidence that microfilament alterations may impair hepatic excretory function and lead to cholestasis.

The role of microtubules has been studied with agents that interfere with the structure of these organelles, colchicine and vinblastin. Conflicting reports on the effect of these agents on bile flow have appeared. No effect of colchicine in bile flow and biliary lipids in the rat was reported by Stein et al. (232), while a decrease in bile flow and biliary phospholipid secretion was observed by Gregory et al. (233) in the isolated rat liver. We have found in the intact rat that colchicine had no effect on basal, unstimulated bile flow but markedly decreased bile flow and bile acid secretion induced by a taurocholate load (230). It also delayed [³H]taurocholate disappearance from plasma. These observations suggest that microtubule dysfunction may lead to an impairment of hepatic excretory function, especially of bile acid transport after a load.

Although these studies suggest a role of cytoskeletal and contractile proteins in the secretion of bile, the results should be interpreted with care, because the effects of the agents used may not be specific. In particular, cytochalasin B, colchicine, and phalloidin also have effects on the plasma membrane.

Relevance of these findings to human pathology also remains to be established. It has been shown that norethandrolone, an agent that induces cholestasis in man, induces changes in the rat liver similar to those observed with cytochalasin B (234). An increase in the number of hepatocyte microfilaments and in the apparent density of the filamentous network around bile canaliculi have been observed in various types of human cholestasis (235). These observations suggest that microfilament alterations may play a role in human cholestasis.

BILE DUCTS: SECRETORY AND ABSORPTIVE ACTIVITY

Secretion (Ductular/Ductal Bile Acid-Independent Flow)

The earliest indication that secretion may occur in the bile ductules and ducts was obtained in isolated segments of canine bile duct (236). It has been confirmed by studies using the hormone secretin, which has long been known to possess choleretic activity (237), and by observing secretion in isolated segments of bile duct (238–240).

The choleretic action of secretin has been demonstrated in cats (241), dogs (11,14,214,242), guinea pigs (67), rhesus monkeys (74), baboons (217), man (8,94, 243), and the isolated perfused pig liver (244). It does not appear to occur in the rabbit (241) or the rat (245), although increased bile flow rates have been reported after infusion of secretin into the hepatic arterial circulation of the rat (246) or after intravenous injections in rabbits (247).

Secretin choleresis is generally accompanied by changes in bile composition, chiefly, a rise in bicarbonate (and pH) and a fall in bile acids (11,14,241). Bicarbonate and chloride concentrations of about 120 and 50 mEq/liter, respectively, were found in the secretin-stimulated bile fraction from the perfused pig liver (248). Intraduodenal infusion of hydrochloric acid in dogs induces the same choleretic response as exogenous secretin (14), an effect probably due to endogenous secretin release, which is thought to be responsible for spontaneous variations of "basal" bile flow in dogs and is blocked by administration of pipenzolate methylbromide, an anticholinergic drug (11).

Several lines of evidence support the view that secretin acts chiefly on the duct system and not on the hepatocyte: (a) The choleretic response to secretin was greater when it was infused into the hepatic artery (which provides the main blood supply to the bile ducts) than into the portal system (249). (b) The biliary "wash-out volume" during constant-rate BSP infusion was less during secretin choleresis than during bile acid choleresis, a finding which suggests that secretin acts distal to the canaliculi (249). (c) Biliary clearances of erythritol and mannitol are increased during bile acid choleresis and not during secretin choleresis, as discussed above (18,70).

Isolated segments of bile duct of rabbit secreted electrolyte solutions isotonic with plasma *in vivo* (238) and *in vitro* (230); the secretion was inhibited by 2,4-dinitrophenol (230). An isolated segment of canine bile duct likewise secreted 0.55 to 0.81 ml/hr of an electrolyte solution (240). Secretin is the only hormone or agent known to stimulate bile duct activity. Gastrin also increased choleresis in dogs (250,251), although pentagastrin has no effect (218). Gastrin choleresis is associated with an increase in concentration and output of bicarbonate (251). Study of an isolated segment of dog bile duct after intravenous administration of synthetic gastrin suggested that the site of action of gastrin on bile flow may be the bile ducts (240).

The secretory activity of the bile ductules and ducts may explain the choleresis that occurs in certain diseases. Elevated bile flows have been recorded in patients with cirrhosis or other chronic liver diseases associated with ductular proliferation (44,252). An increased response to secretin in these patients suggests a ductular/ductal origin for the increased bile flow (253). High bile flows have also been reported in patients with congenital dilation of the intrahepatic biliary tree (254,255). An augmented surface of the biliary epithelium is common to these conditions. Ductular cell proliferation induced experimentally by α-naphthylisothiocyanate and by ethionine is also associated with raised bile flow and increased capacity of the biliary tree (256–258).

Reabsorption

Bile ductules and/or ducts are capable of a reabsorptive function. This was suggested by study of bile composition in cholecystectomized dogs (11). Bile stored in the common bile duct of fasting animals was similar in composition to typical gall bladder bile. Bile-to-plasma concentration ratios above unity in the steady state found for mannitol in the dog (70), erythritol in the rabbit (73), occasionally mannitol or erythritol in the rat (66,197), and erythritol in the rhesus monkey (74) strongly suggest water reabsorption in the ductal/ductular system, since neither of these solutes is thought to be transported by carrier-mediated or active concentrative processes. Evidence that the bile ducts may absorb glucose and 3-0-methylglucose has also been reported (259). Structural evidence that absorption can take place in human bile ductules has been obtained in cholestasis from various causes (260). The relative importance of these two processes—secretion and absorption—probably varies during the day in the normal individual but has not been precisely quantitated.

OTHER FACTORS

Insulin and Vagal Stimulation

Insulin increases bile flow and, more specifically, the canalicular bile acid-independent fraction (261–264). The mechanism is unknown. It does not seem to be mediated by hypoglycemia and vagus nerve stimulation. In the dog, truncal vagotomy has variable effects on insulin-induced choleresis (262,265,266), while in the rat, 2-deoxy-D-glucose and acetylcholine, two vagal stimulants, have no effect on bile flow (267).

Vascular Factors

Bile flow was largely unaffected by variations in blood flow rates in the isolated perfused rat liver (36,37). A small decrease in bile acid-independent bile formation has been recorded, however, in the isolated rat liver perfused at a low rate (268), possibly as a

consequence of regional alterations of perfusion. End-to-side portacaval anastomis and arterialization of the portal circulation were without effect on bile flow in dogs (269); end-to-side portacaval shunt in rats caused a reduction of the canalicular bile acid-independent bile flow (270,271) together with a reduction in liver weight. Pronounced decrease in bile flow has been recorded as resulting from acute hepatic ischemia (36,272) and also from acute increase in hepatic venous pressure (273).

Ethanol

Acute ethanol administration in the isolated rat liver impaired bile flow and excretion of BSP and indocyanine green (274). In contrast, chronic ethanol feeding to rats in vivo was associated with a moderate increase in canalicular bile flow and bile acid excretion.

Other Drugs

Diuretics other than amiloride and ethacrynic acid have variable effects on bile flow. Spironolactone increases canalicular bile acid-independent bile formation (275), an effect which resembles that of phenobarbital and is likewise associated with an increase in liver weight. Furosemide may decrease or increase bile flow (276,277).

Carbonic anhydrase inhibitors cause a rise in biliary chloride concentration in dogs and man (8,11,83,278, 279). Their effect on bile flow is controversial.

Various hypolipidemic drugs (280–282) have been shown to increase bile flow; the choleresis is bile acid independent and associated with increased liver weight.

BILIARY SECRETION IN MAN

The existence of the processes described above is mostly inferred from studies of different animal species. Available data, however, suggest that similar processes may operate in man. As mentioned, there is a linear relationship between bile flow and bile acid secretion and between erythritol (or mannitol) clearance and bile acid secretion (75,76,119). A mean of 11 μl canalicular bile is secreted per micromole bile acid. In the presence of an intact enterohepatic circulation, a mean of approximately 15 μmoles bile acid is secreted per minute, giving a mean bile acid-dependent flow of 0.15 to 0.16 ml/min. The estimated canalicular bile acid-independent flow is 0.16 to 0.17 ml/min, and the estimated ductular/ductal secretion is about 0.11 ml/min. These studies point to a daily production of bile of approximately 600 ml. Similar values have been obtained in patients with T-tubes in the common bile duct (7,8). Under physiologic conditions, however, the volume of bile reaching the duodenum depends on (a) the production of hepatocyte bile, which itself depends in part on the rate at which the bile acid pool circulates within the enterohepatic circulation, (b) reabsorption in the gall bladder and bile ducts, and (c) secretion in the ductules or ducts, which depends on endogenous secretin.

SUMMARY

Bile is an isotonic aqueous solution of bile acids, cholesterol, phospholipids, bile pigments, and inorganic electrolytes. It is secreted by the hepatocytes into the bile canaliculi and modified in the bile ductules or ducts. According to current prevailing theories, three main processes have been postulated in bile flow: (a) Concentrative secretion of bile acids by the hepatocytes is responsible for the bile acid-dependent fraction of canalicular bile flow. Coupling between water flow and bile acid secretion probably is affected mostly through an osmotic mechanism. Since the osmotic activity of the bile acid anions is reduced by their aggregation into micelles, the major component of the osmotic gradient is probably provided by counter-ions. There is suggestive evidence that water flows through the intercellular junctions. The bile acid-dependent fraction accounts for 30 to 60% of spontaneous basal bile flow. (b) A canalicular bile acid-independent secretion is probably driven by Na^+,K^+-ATPase-mediated sodium transport (and possibly other inorganic ion pumps) and stimulated by phenobarbital. It has been suggested that bile acids may also have some influence on this fraction of bile flow. It represents 30 to 60% of basal bile flow. (c) Reabsorption and/or secretion of fluid and inorganic electrolytes occurs by the ductules or ducts. Secretion occurs chiefly in response to secretin and represents 30% of basal bile flow. Normal canalicular bile flow may also depend on the integrity of intracellular organelles, mainly pericanalicular microfilaments and, possibly, microtubules.

REFERENCES

1. Erlinger, S., and Dhumeaux, D. (1974): Mechanisms and control of secretion of bile water and electrolytes. *Gastroenterology*, 66:281–304.
2. Forker, E. L. (1977): Mechanisms of hepatic bile formation. *Ann. Rev. Physiol.*, 39:323–347.
3. Wheeler, H. O. (1968): Water and electrolytes in bile, In: *Handbook of Physiology, Section 6, Alimentary Canal, Vol. 5*, edited by C. F. Code, pp. 2409–2431. Am. Physiol. Soc., Washington.
4. Brauer, R. W. (1959): Mechanisms of bile secretion. *JAMA*, 169:1462–1466.
5. Carey, M. C., and Small, D. M. (1972): Micelle formation by bile salts. Physical-chemical and thermodynamic considerations. *Arch. Intern. Med.*, 130:506–527.
6. Fink, S. (1956): Studies on hepatic bile obtained from a patient with an external biliary fistula; its composition and changes after diamox administration. *N. Engl. J. Med.*, 254:258–262.
7. Thureborn, E. (1962): Human hepatic bile. Composition changes due to altered enterophepatic circulation. *Acta Chir. Scand. [Suppl.]* 303:1–63.
8. Waitman, A. M., Dyck, W. P., and Janowitz, H. D. (1969): Effect of secretin and acetazolamide on the volume and electrolyte composition of hepatic bile in man. *Gastroenterology*, 56:286–294.
9. Sperber, I. (1965): Biliary secretion of organic anions and its influence on bile flow. In: *The Biliary System*, edited by W. Taylor, pp. 457–467. Blackwell, Oxford.
10. Johnston, C. G., Riegel, C., and Ravdin, I. S. (1932): Studies of gall-bladder function. VII. The anion-cation content of hepatic and gall-bladder bile. *Am. J. Physiol.*, 100:317–327.
11. Wheeler, H. O., and Ramos, O. L. (1960): Determinants of the flow and composition of bile in the unanesthetized dog during constant infusions of sodium taurocholate. *J. Clin. Invest.*, 39:161–170.
12. Dietschy, J. M., and Moore, E. W. (1964): Diffusion potentials and potassium distribution across the gallbladder wall. *J. Clin. Invest.*, 43:1551–1560.
13. Moore, E. W., and Dietschy, J. M. (1964): Na and K activity coefficients in bile and bile salts determined by glass electrodes. *Am. J. Physiol.*, 206:1111–1117.
14. Preisig, R., Cooper, H. L., and Wheeler, H. O. (1962): The relationship between taurocholate secretion rate and bile production in the unanesthetized dog during cholinergic blockade and during secretin administration. *J. Clin. Invest.*, 41:1152–1162.
15. Briscoe, A. M., and Ragan, C. (1965): Bile and endogenous fecal calcium in man. *Am. J. Clin. Nutr.*, 16:281–286.
16. Burnett, W. (1965): The pathogenesis of gall stones. In: *The Biliary System*, edited by W. Taylor, pp. 601–618. Blackwell, Oxford.
17. Blitzer, B. L., and Boyer, J. L. (1978): Cytochemical localization of Na^+,K^+-ATPase in the rat hepatocyte. *J. Clin. Invest.*, 62:1104–1108.
18. Forker, E. L. (1967): Two sites of bile formation as determined by mannitol and erythritol clearance in the guinea pig. *J. Clin. Invest.*, 46:1189–1195.
19. Hofmann, A. F., and Small, D. M. (1967): Detergent properties of bile salts: Correlation with physiological function. *Ann. Rev. Med.*, 18:333–376.
20. Small, D. M., and Rapo, S. (1970): Source of abnormal bile in patients with cholesterol gallstones. *N. Engl. J. Med.*, 283:53–57.
21. Soloway, R. D., Trotman, B. W., and Ostrow, J. D. (1977): Pigment gallstones. *Gastroenterology*, 72:162–182.
22. Hardwicke, J., Rankin, G., Baker, K. J., and Preisig, R. (1964): The loss of protein in human and canine hepatic bile. *Clin. Sci.*, 26:509–517.
23. Rosenthal, W. S., Kubo, K., Dolinski, M., Marino, J., Mersheimer, W. L., and Glass, G. B. J. (1965): The passage of serum albumin into bile in man. *Am. J. Dig. Dis.*, 10:271–283.
24. Russell, I. S., Fleck A., and Burnett, W. (1964): The protein content of human bile. *Clin. Chim. Acta*, 10:210–213.
25. Dive, C., and Heremans, J. F. (1974): Nature and origin of the proteins of bile. I. A comparative analysis of serum and bile proteins in man. *Eur. J. Clin. Invest.*, 4:235–239.
26. Dive, C., Nadalini, R. A., Vaerman, J. P., and Heremans, J. F. (1974): Origin and nature of the proteins of bile. II. A comparative analysis of serum, hepatic lymph and bile proteins in the dog. *Eur. J. Clin. Invest.*, 4:241–246.
27. Mullock, B. M., Dobrota, M., and Hinton, R. H. (1978): Sources of proteins of rat bile. *Biochim. Biophys. Acta*, 543:497–507.
28. La Russo, N. F., and Fowler, S. (1979): Coordinate secretion of acid hydrolases in rat bile. Hepatocyte exocytosis of lysosomal protein? *J. Clin. Invest.*, 64:948–954.

29. Coleman, R., Iqbal, S., Godfrey, P. P., and Billington, D. (1979): Membranes and bile formation. Composition of several mammalian biles and their membrane damaging properties. *Biochem. J.*, 178:201–208.

30. Holdsworth, G., and Coleman, R. (1975): Enzyme profiles of mammalian bile. *Biochim. Biophys. Acta*, 389:47–50.

31. Chenderovitch, J., Phocas, E., and Rautureau, M. (1963): Effects of hypertonic solutions on bile formation. *Am. J. Physiol.*, 205:863–867.

32. Gilman, A., and Cowgill, G. R. (1933): Osmotic relations between blood and body fluids. IV. Pancreatic juice, bile and lymph. *Am. J. Physiol.*, 104:476–479.

33. Sobotka, H. (1937): *Physiological Chemistry of the Bile.* Williams & Wilkins, Baltimore.

34. Hardison, W. G. M., and Norman, J. C. (1969): Effect of secretin on bile osmolality. *J. Lab. Clin. Med.*, 73:34–41.

35. Maffly, R. H., and Leaf, A. (1959): The potential of water in mammalian tissues. *J. Gen. Physiol.*, 42:1257–1275.

36. Brauer, R. W., (1965): Hepatic blood supply and the secretion of bile. In: *The Biliary System,* edited by W. Taylor, pp. 41–67. Blackwell, Oxford.

37. Brauer, R. W., Leong, G. F., and Holloway, R. J. (1954): Mechanics of bile secretion. Effect of perfusion pressure and temperature on bile flow and bile secretion pressure. *Am. J. Physiol.*, 177:103–119.

38. Barber-Riley, G. (1963): Rat biliary tree during short periods of obstruction of common duct. *Am. J. Physiol.*, 205:1127–1131.

39. Barber-Riley, G. (1964): The rate of biliary secretion during flow up vertical cannulas of different bore. *Experientia*, 20:639–640.

40. Debray, C., and Besançon, F. (1961): Le débit et la pression au cours de l'obstruction biliaire graduée chez le rat. *Rev. Int. Hepat.*, 11:49–68.

41. Richards, T. G., and Thomson, J. Y. (1961): The secretion of bile against pressure. *Gastroenterology*, 40:705–707.

42. Shorter, R. G., Bollman, J. L., and Baggenstoss, A. H. (1959): Pressures in the common hepatic duct of the rat. *Proc. Soc. Exp. Biol. Med.*, 102:682–686.

43. Strasberg, S. M., Dorn, B. C., Redinger, R. N., Small, D. M., and Egdahl, R. H. (1971): Effects of alterations of biliary pressure on bile composition—a method for study: Primate biliary physiology V. *Gastroenterology*, 61:357–362.

44. Lenthall, J., Reynolds, T. B., and Donovan, A. J. (1970): Excessive output of bile in chronic hepatic disease. *Surg. Gynecol. Obstet.*, 130:243–253.

45. Donovan, A. J., Child, M. A., and Masto, A. S. (1972): The effect of hepatic venous obstruction on the rate of flow of bile. *Surg. Gynecol. Obstet.*, 134:89–93.

46. Sadiz, S., Rao, S. P., and Enquist, I. F. (1972): Hepatic congestion and bile secretion. *Arch. Surg.*, 105:749–751.

47. Curran, P. F., and McIntosh, J. R. (1962): A model system for biological water transport. *Nature*, 193:347–348.

48. Diamond, J. M. (1962): The reabsorptive function of the gallbladder. *J. Physiol. (Lond.)*, 161:442–473.

49. Diamond, J. M., and Bossert, W. H. (1967): Standing gradient osmotic flow. A mechanism for coupling of water and solute transport in epithelia. *J. Gen. Physiol.*, 50:2061–2083.

50. Diamond, J. M., and Tormey, J. McD. (1966): Studies on the structural basis of water transport across epithelial membranes. *Fed. Proc.*, 25:1458–1463.

51. Diamond, J. M., and Tormey, J. McD. (1966): Role of long extracellular channels in fluid transport across epithelia. *Nature*, 210:817–820.

52. Oschman, J. L., and Berridge, M. J. (1971): The structural basis of fluid secretion. *Fed. Proc.*, 30:49–56.

53. Schafer, J. A. (1979): Water transport in epithelia. *Fed. Proc.*, 38:119–160.

54. Layden, T. J., Elias, E., and Boyer, J. L. (1978): Bile formation in the rat. The role of the paracellular shunt pathway. *J. Clin. Invest.*, 62:1375–1385.

55. Erlinger, S. (1978): Cholestasis: Pump failure, microvilli defect or both? *Lancet*, 1:533–534.

56. Diamond, J. M. (1962): The mechanism of water transport by the gall-bladder. *J. Physiol. (Lond.)*, 161:503–527.

57. Whitlock, R. T., and Wheeler, H. O. (1964): Coupled transport of solute and water across rabbit gallbladder epithelium. *J. Clin. Invest.*, 43:2249–2265.

58. Dowling, R. H., Mack, E., Picott, J., Berger, J., and Small, D. M. (1968): Experimental model for the study of the enterohepatic circulation of bile in rhesus monkeys. *J. Lab. Clin. Med.*, 72:169–176.

59. Berry, M. N., and Friend, D. S. (1969): High-yield preparation of isolated rat liver parenchymal cells. A biochemical and fine structural study. *J. Cell Biol.*, 43:506–520.

60. Bissel, D. M., (1976): Study of hepatocyte function in cell culture. In: *Progress in Liver Diseases, Vol. V.,* edited by H. Popper and F. Schaffner, pp. 69–82. Grune & Stratton, New York.

61. Seglen, P. O. (1972): Preparation of rat liver cells. I. Effect of Ca^{2+} on enzymatic dispersion of isolated, perfused liver. *Exp. Cell. Res.*, 74:450–454.

62. Wanson, J. C., Bernaert, D., and May, C. (1979): Morphology and functional properties of isolated and cultured hepatocytes. In: *Progress in Liver Diseases, Vol. IV,* edited by H. Popper and F. Schaffner, pp. 1–22. Grune & Stratton, New York.

63. Anwer, M. S., Kroker, R., and Hegner, D. (1976): Cholic acid uptake into isolated rat hepatocytes. *Hoppe Seylers Z. Physiol. Chem.*, 357:1477–1486.

64. Schwarz, L. R., Burr, R., Schwenk, M., Pfaff, E., and Greim, H. (1975): Uptake of taurocholic acid into isolated rat-liver cells. *Eur. J. Biochem.*, 55:617–623.

65. Schwenk, M., Burr, R., Schwarz, L., and Pfaff, E. (1976): Uptake of bromosulfophthalein by isolated liver cells. *Eur. J. Biochem.*, 64:189–197.

66. Schanker, L. S., and Hogben, C. A. M. (1961): Biliary excretion of inulin, sucrose, and mannitol: Analysis of bile formation. *Am. J. Physiol.*, 200:1087–1090.

67. Forker, E. L. (1968): Bile formation in guinea pigs: Analysis with inert solutes of graded molecular radius. *Am. J. Physiol.*, 215:56–62.

68. Forker, E. L. (1970): Hepatocellular uptake of inulin, sucrose and mannitol in rats. *Am. J. Physiol.*, 219:1568–1573.

69. Forker, E. L., Hicklin, T., and Sornson, H. (1967): The clearance of mannitol and erythritol in rat bile. *Proc. Soc. Exp. Biol. Med.*, 126:115–119.

70. Wheeler, H. O., Ross, E. D., and Bradley, S. E. (1968): Canalicular bile production in dogs. *Am. J. Physiol.*, 214:866–874.

71. Sarfeh, I. J., Beeler, D. A., Treble, D. H., and Balint, J. A. (1974): Studies of the hepatic excretory defects in essential fatty acid deficiency. Their possible relationship to the genesis of cholesterol gallstones. *J. Clin. Invest.*, 53:423–430.

72. Boyer, J. L. (1971): Bile formation in the isolated perfused rat liver. *Am. J. Physiol.*, 221:1156–1163.

73. Erlinger, S., Dhumeaux, D., Berthelot, P., and Dumont, M. (1970): Effect of inhibitors of sodium transport on bile formation in the rabbit. *Am. J. Physiol.*, 219:416–422.

74. Strasberg, S. M., Ilson, R. G., Siminovitch, K. A., Brenner, D., and Palaheimo, J. E. (1975): Analysis of the components of bile flow in the rhesus monkey. *Am. J. Physiol.*, 228:115–121.

75. Prandi, D., Erlinger, S., Glasinović, J. C., and Dumont, M. (1975): Canalicular bile production in man. *Eur. J. Clin. Invest.*, 5:1–6.

76. Boyer, J. L., and Bloomer, J. R. (1974): Canalicular bile secretion in man. Studies utilizing the biliary clearance of [14C] mannitol. *J. Clin. Invest.*, 54:773–781.

77. Barnhart, J. L., and Combes, B. (1978): Erythritol and mannitol clearances with taurocholate and secretin-induced cholereses. *Am. J. Physiol.*, 234:E146–E156.

77a. Nicholls, R. J. (1979): Biliary mannitol clearance and bile salt output before and during secretin choleresis in the dog. *Gastroenterology*, 76:983–987.

78. Cahill, G. F., Jr., Ashmore, J., Earle, A. S., and Zottu, S. (1958): Glucose penetration into liver. *Am. J. Physiol.*, 192:491–496.

79. Sacks, J., and Bakshy, S. (1957): Insulin and tissue distribution of pentose in nephrectomized cats. *Am. J. Physiol.*, 189:339–342.

80. Glasinović, J. C., Dumont, M., Duval, M., and Erlinger, S. (1975): Hepatocellular uptake of erythritol, mannitol and sucrose in the dog. *Am. J. Physiol.*, 229:1455–1460.

81. Dillon, L., Kok, E., Wachtel, N., and Javitt, N. B. (1978): Hepatic bile formation: Modifications of concepts of canalicular water flow. *Gastroenterology*, 75:961A (Abstr.).

82. Bradley, S. E., and Herz, R. (1978): Permselectivity of biliary canalicular membrane in rats: Clearance probe analysis. *Am. J. Physiol.*, 235:E570–E576.

83. Forker, E. L. (1969): The effect of estrogen on bile formation in the rat. *J. Clin. Invest.*, 48:654–663.

84. Javitt, N. B. (1976): Hepatic bile formation. *N. Engl. J. Med.*, 295:1464–1469, 1511–1516.

85. Erlinger, S., Glasinović, J. C., Poupon, R., and Dumont, M. (1976): Hepatic transport of bile acids, In: *The Hepatobiliary System*, edited by W. Taylor, pp. 433–447. Plenum, New York.

86. O'Maille, E. R. L., Richards, T. G., and Short, A. H. (1967): The influence of conjugation of cholic acid on its uptake and secretion: Hepatic extraction of taurocholate and cholate in the dog. *J. Physiol. (Lond.)*, 189:337–350.

87. Glasinović, J. C., Dumont, M., Duval, M., and Erlinger, S. (1975): Hepatocellular uptake of taurocholate in the dog. *J. Clin. Invest.*, 55:419–426.

88. Glasinović, J. C., Dumont, M., Duval, M., and Erlinger, S. (1975): Hepatocellular uptake of bile acids in the dog: Evidence for a common carrier-mediated transport system. An indicator dilution study. *Gastroenterology*, 69:973–981.

89. Reichen, J., and Paumgartner, G. (1975): Kinetics of taurocholate uptake by the perfused rat liver. *Gastroenterology*, 68:132–136.

90. Reichen, J., and Paumgartner, G. (1976): Uptake of bile acids by the perfused rat liver. *Am. J. Physiol.*, 231:734–742.

91. Dietmaier, A., Gasser, R., Graf, J., and Peterlik, M. (1976): Investigations on the sodium dependence of bile acid fluxes in the isolated perfused rat liver. *Biochim. Biophys. Acta*, 443:81–91.

92. Paumgartner, G., and Reichen, J. (1975): Different pathways for hepatic uptake of taurocholate and indocyanine green. *Experientia*, 31:306–307.

93. Accatino, L., and Simon, F. R. (1976): Identification and characterization of a bile acid receptor in isolated liver surface membranes. *J. Clin. Invest.*, 56:496–508.

94. Gonzalez, M. C., Sutherland, E., and Simon, F. R. (1979): Regulation of hepatic transport of bile salts. Effect of protein synthesis inhibition on excretion of bile salts and their binding to liver surface membrane fractions. *J. Clin. Invest.*, 63:684–694.

95. Goresky, C. A. (1965): The hepatic uptake and excretion of sulfobromophthalein and bilirubin. *Can. Med. Assoc. J.*, 92:851–857.

96. Arias, I. M., Fleischner, G., Listowski, I., Bhrgava, M., Kamisaka, K., and Gatmaitan, Z. (1977): Ligandin: Structure and function. In: *Liver and Bile*, edited by L. Bianchi, W. Gerok, and K. Sickinger, pp. 157–166. MTP Press, Lancaster.

97. Levi, A. J., Gatmaitan, Z., and Arias, I. M. (1969): Two hepatic cytoplasmic protein fractions, Y and Z, and their possible role in the hepatic uptake of bilirubin, sulfobromophthalein, and other anions. *J. Clin. Invest.*, 48:2156–2167.

98. Reyes, H., Levi, A. J., Gatmaitan, Z., and Arias, I. M. (1971): Studies of Y and Z, two hepatic cytoplasmic organic anion-binding proteins: Effect of drugs, chemicals, hormones, and cholestasis. *J. Clin. Invest.*, 50:2242–2252.

99. Strange, R. C., Cramb, R., Hayes, J. D., and Percy-Robb, I. W. (1977): Partial purification of two lithocholic acid-binding proteins from rat liver 100,000g supernatants. *Biochem. J.*, 165:425–429.

100. Strange, R. C., Nimmo, I. A., and Percy-Robb, I. W. (1977): Binding of bile acids by 100,000g supernatants of rat liver. *Biochem. J.*, 162:659–664.

101. Desjeux, J. F., Dumont, M., and Erlinger, S. (1973): Métabolisme et influence sur la sécrétion biliaire du dehydrocholate chez le chien. *Biol. Gastroenterol. (Paris)*, 6:9–18.

102. Hardison, W. G. M. (1971): Metabolism of sodium dehydro-

103. Soloway, R. D., Hofmann, A. F., Thomas, P. J., Schoenfield, L. J., and Klein, P. D. (1973): Triketocholanoic (dehydrocholic) acid. Hepatic metabolism and effect on bile flow and biliary lipid secretion in man. *J. Clin. Invest.*, 52:715–724.

104. O'Maille, E. R. L., Richards, T. G., and Short, A. H. (1965): Acute taurine depletion and maximal rates of hepatic conjugation and secretion of cholic acid in the dog. *J. Physiol. (Lond.)*, 180:67–79.

105. Alpert, S., Mosher, M., Shanske, A., and Arias, I. M. (1969): Multiplicity of hepatic excretory mechanisms for organic anions. *J. Gen. Physiol.*, 53:238–247.

106. Adler, R. D., Wannagat, F. J., and Ockner, R. D. (1977): Bile secretion in selective biliary obstruction: Adaptation of taurocholate transport maximum to increased secretory load in the rat. *Gastroenterology*, 73:129–136.

107. Wheeler, H. O., Meltzer, J. I., and Bradley, S. E. (1960): Biliary transport and hepatic storage of sulfobromophthalein sodium in the unanesthetized dog, in normal man, and in patients with hepatic disease. *J. Clin. Invest.*, 39:1131–1141.

108. Boyer, J. L., Scheig, R. L., and Klatskin, G. (1970): The effect of sodium taurocholate on the hepatic metabolism of sulfobromphthalein sodium (BSP): The role of bile flow. *J. Clin. Invest.*, 49:206-215.

109. Dhumeaux, D., Berthelot, P., Préaux, A. M., Erlinger, S., and Fauvert, R. (1970): A critical study of the concept of maximal biliary transport of sulformophthalein (BSP) in the Wistar rat. *Rev. Eur. Etud. Clin. Biol.*, 15:279–286.

110. Gronwall, R., and Cornelius, C. E. (1970): Maximal biliary excretion of sulfobromophthalein sodium in sheep. *Am. J. Dig. Dis.*, 15:37–47.

111. O'Maille, E. R. L., Richards, T. G., and Short, A. H. (1966): Factors determining the maximal rate of organic anion secretion by the liver and further evidence on the hepatic site of action of the hormone secretin. *J. Physiol. (Lond.)*, 186:424–438.

112. Goresky, C. A., Bach, G. G., and Nadeau, B. E. (1973): On the uptake of materials by the intact liver. The transport and net removal of galactose. *J. Clin. Invest.*, 52:991–1009.

113. Jones, A. L., Hradek, G. T., Renston, R. H., Wong, K. Y., Karlaganis, G., and Paumgartner, G. (1980): Autoradiographic evidence for hepatic lobular concentration gradient of bile acid derivative. *Am. J. Physiol.*, 238:G233–G237.

114. Layden, T. J., and Boyer, J. L. (1978): Influence of bile acids on bile canalicular membrane morphology and the lobular gradient in canalicular size. *Lab. Invest.*, 39:110–119.

115. Berthelot, P., Erlinger, S., Dhumeaux, D., and Préaux, A. M. (1970): Mechanism of phenobarbital-induced hypercholeresis in the rat. *Am. J. Physiol.*, 219:809–813.

116. Boyer, J. L., and Klatskin, G. (1970): Canalicular bile flow and bile secretory pressure: Evidence for a non-bile salt dependent fraction in the isolated perfused rat liver. *Gastroenterology*, 59:853–859.

117. Preisig, R., Bucher, H., Stirnemann, H., and Tauber, J. (1969): Postoperative choleresis following bile duct obstruction in man. *Rev. Fr. Etud. Clin. Biol.*, 14:151–158.

118. Scherstén, T., Nilson, J., Cahlin E., Filipson, M., and Brodin-Person (1971): Relationship between the biliary excretion of bile acids and the excretion of water, lecithin and cholesterol in man. *Eur. J. Clin. Invest.* 1:242–247.

119. Linblad, L., and Scherstén, T. (1976): Influence of cholic and chenodeoxycholic acid on canalicular bile flow in man. *Gastroenterology*, 70:1121–1124.

120. Sperber, I. (1959): Secretion of organic anions in the formation of urine and bile. *Pharmacol. Rev.*, 11:109–134.

121. O'Maille, E. R. L., and Richards, T. G. (1976): The secretory characteristics of dehydrocholate in the dog: Comparison with the natural bile salts. *J. Physiol. (Lond.)*, 261:337–357.

122. Dumont, M., Uchman, S., and Erlinger, S. (1981): Hypercholeresis induced by ursodeoxycholic acid and 7-ketolithocholic acid in the rat. Possible role of bicarbonate transport. *Gastroenterology*, 79:82–89.

123. Baker, A. L., Wood, R. A. B., Moossa, A. R., and Boyer,

J. L. (1979): Sodium taurocholate modifies the bile acid-independent fraction of canalicular bile flow in the rhesus monkey. *J. Clin. Invest.* 64:312–320.

123a. Wannagat, F. J., Adler, R. D., and Ockner, R. K. (1978): Bile acid-induced increase in bile acid-independent flow and plasma membrane Na,K ATPase activity in rat liver. *J. Clin. Invest.,* 61:297–307.

124. Friend, D. S., and Gilula, N. B. (1972): Variations in tight and gap junctions in mammalian tissues. *J. Cell Biol.,* 53:758–776.

125. Dyck, W. P., and Janowitz, H. D. (1971): Effect of glucagon on hepatic bile secretion in man. *Gastroenterology,* 60:400–404.

126. Hoenig, V., and Preisig, R. (1973): Organic-anionic choleresis in the dog: Comparative effects of bromsulfalein, ioglycamide and taurocholate. *Biomedicine,* 18:23–30.

127. Feld, G. K., Loeb, P. M., Berk, R. N., and Wheeler, H. O. (1975): The choleretic effect of iodipamide. *J. Clin. Invest.,* 55:528–535.

128. Dhumeaux, D., Erlinger, S., Benhamou, J. P., and Fauvert, R. (1970): Effect of rose bengal on bile secretion in the rabbit: Inhibition of a bile-salt independent fraction. *Gut,* 11:134–140.

129. Groszmann, R. J., Kotelanski, B., Kendler, J., and Zimmerman, H. J. (1969): Effect of sulfobromophthalein and indocyanine green on bile excretion. *Proc. Soc. Exp. Biol. Med.,* 132:712–714.

130. Priestly, B. G., and Plaa, G. L. (1970): Reduced bile flow after sulfobromophthalein administration in the rat. *Proc. Soc. Exp. Biol. Med.,* 135:373–376.

131. Schulze, P. J., and Czok, G. (1975): Reduced bile flow in rats during sulfobromophthalein infusion. *Toxicol. Appl. Pharmacol.,* 32:213–224.

132. Horak, W., Grabner, G., and Paumgartner, G. (1973): Inhibition of bile salt-independent bile formation by indocyanine green. *Gastroenterology,* 64:1005–1012.

133. Takane, S. (1932): Uber den einfluss verschiedener narkosemittel auf die leberfunktion. Experimentelle untersuchungen mit bilirubin und kongorot. *Arch. Klin. Chir.,* 170:672–695.

134. Whelan, G., and Combes, B. (1971): Depression of biliary excretion of infused bilirubin in rats and guinea-pigs by bile. *Am. J. Physiol.,* 220:683–687.

135. Hunter, A., and Klaassen, C. D. (1972): Species differences in the plasma disappearance and biliary excretion of procaine amide ethobromide. *Proc. Soc. Exp. Biol. Med.,* 139:1445–1453.

136. Schanker, L. S., and Solomon, H. M. (1963): Active transport of quaternary ammonium compounds into bile. *Am. J. Physiol.,* 204:829–832.

137. Meyer-Brunot, H. G., and Keberle, H. (1971): Biliary excretion of ferrioxamines of varying liposolubility in perfused rat liver. *Am. J. Physiol.,* 214:1193–1200.

138. Meyer-Brunot, H. G., and Keberle, H. (1971): What role do choleretic agents play in bile formation? *Digestion,* 4:166 (Abstr.).

139. Fontaine, L. M., Belleville, J. C., Lechevin, J. C., and Tete, R. (1968): Etude du métabolisme de la méthyl-4-ombelliferone sur l'animal et chez l'homme. *Therapie,* 23:373–382.

140. Fontaine, L., Grand, M., Molho, D., Chabert, J., and Boschetti, E. (1968): Activités cholérétique et spasmolytique; pharmacologie générale de la méthyl-4-ombelliférone. *Therapie,* 23:51–62.

141. Kroker, R., Anwer, M. S., and Hegner, D. (1977): Characterization of methylumbelliferone (Mendiaxon®)-induced choleresis in the isolated perfused rat liver. *Acta Hepatogastroenterol.,* 24:348–354.

142. Ritt, D. J., and Combes, B. (1967): Enhancement of apparent excretory maximum of sulfobromophthalein sodium (BSP) by taurocholate and dehydrocholate. *J. Clin. Invest.,* 46:1108–1109 (Abstr.).

143. Vonk, R. J., van der Veen, H., Prop, G., and Meijer, D. K. (1974): The influence of taurocholate and dehydrocholate choleresis on plasma disappearance and biliary excretion of indocyanine green in the rat. *Naunyn Schmiedebergs Arch. Pharmacol.,* 282:401–410.

144. Berk, R. N., Golberger, L. E., and Loeb, P. M. (1974): The role of bile salts in the hepatic excretion of iopanoic acid. *Invest. Radiol.,* 9:7–15.

145. Nelson, J. A., Staubus, A. E., and Riegelman, S., (1975): Saturation kinetics of iopanoate in the dog. *Invest. Radiol.,* 10:371–377.

146. Mandiola, S., Johnson, B. L., Winters, R. E., and Longmire, W. P. (1972): Biliary excretion of ampicillin in the anesthetized dog. I. Effect of serum ampicillin concentration, taurocholate infusion rate, biliary secretion pressure, and secretin infusion. *Surgery,* 71:664–674.

147. Barnhart, J. L., and Combes, B. (1974): Effect of theophylline on hepatic excretory function. *Am. J. Physiol.,* 227:194–199.

148. Erlinger, S., and Dumont, M. (1973): Influence of canalicular bile flow on sulfobromophthalein transport maximum in bile in the dog. In: *The Liver. Quantitative Aspects of Structure and Function,* edited by G. Paumgartner and R. Preisig, pp. 306–313. Karger, Basel.

149. Gibson, G. E., and Forker, E. L. (1974): Canalicular bile flow and bromsulfophthalein transport maximum: The effect of a bile salt-independent choleretic, SC 2644. *Gastroenterology,* 66:1046–1053.

150. Scharschmidt, B. F., and Schmid, R. (1978): The micellar sink. A quantitative assessment of the association of organic anions with mixed micelles and other macromolecular aggregates in rat bile. *J. Clin. Invest.,* 62:1122–1131.

151. Vonk, R. J., Jekel, P., and Meijer, D. K. F. (1975): Choleresis and hepatic transport mechanisms. II. Influence of bile salt choleresis and biliary micelle binding on biliary excretion of various organic anions. *Naunyn Schmiedebergs Arch. Pharmacol.,* 290:375–387.

152. Binet, S., Delage, Y., and Erlinger, S. (1979): Influence of taurocholate, taurochenodeoxycholate, and taurodehydrocholate on sulfobromphthalein transport into bile. *Am. J. Physiol.,* 236:E10–E14.

153. Delage, Y., Dumont, M., and Erlinger, S. (1976): Effect of glycodihydrofusidate on sulfobromophthalein transport maximum in the hamster. *Am. J. Physiol.,* 231:1875–1878.

154. Forker, E. L., and Gibson, G. (1973): Interaction between sulfobromophthalein (BSP) and taurocholate. The kinetics of transport from liver cells to bile in rats. In: *The Liver. Quantitative Aspects of Structure and Function,* edited by G. Paumgartner and R. Preisig, pp. 326–335. Karger, Basel.

155. Javitt, N. B., and Emerman, S. (1968): Effect of sodium taurolithocholate on bile flow and bile acid excretion. *J. Clin. Invest.,* 67:1002–1014.

156. Schaffner, F., and Javitt, N. B. (1966): Morphologic changes in hamster liver during intrahepatic cholestasis induced by taurolithocholate. *Lab. Invest.,* 15:1783–1792.

157. Javitt, N. B. (1975): Current status of cholestasis induced by monohydroxylated bile acids. In: *Jaundice,* edited by C. A. Goresky and M. M. Fisher, pp. 401–409. Plenum, New York.

158. King, J. E., and Schoenfield, L. J. (1971): Cholestasis induced by sodium taurolithocholate in isolated hamster liver. *J. Clin. Invest.,* 50:2305–2312.

159. Layden, T. J., Schwarz, J., and Boyer, J. L. (1975): Scanning electron microscopy of the rat liver. Studies of the effect of taurolithocholate and other models of cholestasis. *Gastroenterology,* 69:726–738.

160. Miyai, K., and Fisher, M. M. (1971): The hepatotoxicity of chenodeoxycholic acid. *Gastroenterology,* 60:189 (Abstr.).

161. Miyai, K., Price, V. M., and Fisher, M. M. (1971): Bile acid metabolism in mammals. Ultrastructural studies on the intrahepatic cholestasis induced by lithocholic and chenodeoxycholic acids in the rat. *Lab. Invest.,* 24:292–302.

162. Schwarz, H. P., Herz, R., Sauter, K., and Paumgartner, G. (1973): Taurocholate-induced anticholeresis in the rat. *Eur. J. Clin. Invest.* 3:268 (Abstr.).

163. Balabaud, C., Kron, K. A., and Gumucio, J. J. (1977): The assessment of the bile salt-non-dependent fraction of canalicular bile water in the rat. *J. Lab. Clin. Med.,* 89:393–399.

164. Klaassen, C. D. (1971): Studies on the increased biliary flow produced by phenobarbital in rats. *J. Pharmacol. Exp. Ther.,* 176:743–751.

165. Paumgartner, G., Horak, W., Probst, P., and Grabner, G.

(1971): Effect of phenobarbital on bile flow and bile salt excretion in the rat. *Naunyn Schmiedebergs Arch. Pharmacol.*, 270:98–101.

166. Erlinger, S., and Dumont, M. (1973): Influence of theophylline on bile formation in the dog. *Biomedicine*, 19:27–32.

167. Khedis, A., Dumont, M., Duval, M., and Erlinger, S. (1974): Influence of glucagon on canalicular bile production in the dog. *Biomedicine*, 21:176–181.

168. Dumont, M., and Erlinger, S. (1973): Influence of hydrocortisone on bile formation in the rat. *Biol. Gastroenterol. (Paris)*, 6:197–203.

169. Macarol, V., Morris, T. Q., Baker, K. J., and Bradley, S. E. (1970): Hydrocortisone choleresis in the dog. *J. Clin. Invest.*, 49:1714–1723.

170. Wheeler, H. O., and King, K. K. (1973): Biliary excretion of lecithin and cholesterol in the dog. *J. Clin. Invest.*, 51:1337–1350.

171. Erlinger, S., Dumont, M., and Benhamou, J. P. (1969): Effect of inhibitors of sodium transport on bile formation in the rabbit. *Nature*, 223:1276–1277.

172. Hardison, W. G. M., and Wood, C. A. (1978): Importance of bicarbonate in bile salt independent fraction of bile flow. *Am. J. Physiol.*, 235:E158-E164.

173. Schwartz, A., Lindenmayer, G. E., and Allen, J. C. (1975): The sodium-potassium adenosine triphosphatase: Pharmacological, physiological and biochemical aspects. *Pharmacol. Rev.*, 27:3–134.

174. Skou, J. C. (1965): Enzymatic basis for active transport of Na+ and K+ across cell membrane. *Physiol. Rev.*, 45:596–617.

175. Boyer, J. L., and Reno, D. (1975): Properties of (Na+ + K+)-activated ATPase in rat liver plasma membranes enriched with bile canaliculi. *Biochim. Biophys. Acta*, 401:59–72.

176. Emmelot, P., Bos, C. J., Benedetti, E. L., and Rumke, P. (1964): Studies on plasma membranes. I. Chemical composition and enzyme content of plasma membranes isolated from rat liver. *Biochim. Biophys. Acta*, 90:126–145.

177. Kupferberg, H. J., and Schanker, L. S. (1968): Biliary secretion of ouabain-³H and its uptake by liver slices in the rat. *Am. J. Physiol.*, 214:1048–1053.

178. Chenderovitch, J., Raizman, A., and Infante, R., (1975): Mechanism of ethacrynic acid-induced choleresis in the rat. *Am. J. Physiol.*, 229:1180–1187.

179. Klaassen, C. D., and Fitzgerald, T. J. (1974): Metabolism and biliary excretion of ethacrynic acid. *J. Pharmacol. Exp. Ther.* 191:548–556.

180. Graf, J., Korn, P., and Peterlik, M. (1972): Choleretic effects of ouabain and ethracrynic acid in the isolated perfused rat liver. *Naunyn Schmiedebergs Arch. Pharmacol.*, 272:230–233.

181. Shaw, H., Caple, I., and Heath, T. (1972): Effect of ethacrynic acid on bile formation in sheep, dogs, rats, guinea-pigs and rabbits. *J. Pharmacol. Exp. Ther.*, 182:27–33.

182. Graf, J., and Peterlik, M. (1976): Ouabain-mediated sodium uptake and bile formation by isolated perfused rat liver . *Am. J. Physiol.*, 230:876–885.

183. Gumucio, J. J., and Valdivieso, V. D. (1971): Studies on the mechanism of ethynylestradiol impairment of bile flow in the rat. *Gastroenterology*, 61:339–344.

184. Heikel, T. A. J., and Lathe, G. H. (1970): The effect of 17α-ethinyl-substituted steroids on adenosine triphosphatases of rat liver plasma membrane. *Biochem. J.*, 118:187–189.

185. Davis, R. A., Kern, F., Jr., Showalter, R., Sutherland, E., Sinensky, M., and Simon, F. R. (1978): Alterations of hepatic Na+,K+-ATPase and bile flow by estrogen: Effects on liver surface membrane lipid structure and function. *Proc. Natl. Acad. Sci. USA*, 75:4130–4134.

186. Reichen, J., and Paumgartner, G. (1977): Relationship between bile flow and Na+,K+-adenosinetriphosphatase in liver plasma membranes enriched in bile canaliculi. *J. Clin. Invest.*, 60:429–434.

186a. Simon, F. R., Sutherland, E., and Accatino, L. (1977): Stimulation of hepatic sodium and potassium-activated adenosine triphosphatase activity by phenobarbital. Its possible role in regulation of bile flow. *J. Clin. Invest.*, 59:849–861.

187. Reyes, H., and Kern, F., Jr. (1979): Effect of pregnancy on bile flow and biliary lipids in the hamster. *Gastroenterology*, 76:144–150.

188. Gumucio, J. J., Accatino, L., Macho, A. M., and Contreras, A. (1973): Effect of phenobarbital on the ethynyl estradiol-induced cholestasis in the rat. *Gastroenterology*, 65:651–657.

189. Redinger, R. N., and Small, D. M. (1973): Primate biliary physiology. VIII. The effect of phenobarbital upon bile salt synthesis and pool size, biliary lipid secretion and bile composition. *J. Clin. Invest.*, 52:161–172.

190. Boyer, J. L., Reno, D., and Layden, T. (1976): Bile canalicular membrane Na+,K+-ATPase. The relationship of enzyme activity to the secretion of bile salt independent canalicular flow. In: *Diseases of the Liver and Biliary Tract*, edited by C. M. Leevy, pp. 108–112. Karger, Basel.

191. Keefe, E. B., Scharschmidt, B. F., Blankenship, N. M., and Ockner, R. K. (1979): Studies on relationships among bile flow, liver plasma membrane NaK-ATPase, and membrane microviscosity in the rat. *J. Clin. Invest.*, 64:1590–1598.

192. Laperche, Y., Launay, A., Oudéa, P., Doulin, A., and Baraud, J. (1972): Effects of phenobarbital and rose bengal on the ATPases of plasma membranes of rat and rabbit liver. *Gut*, 13:920–925.

193. Capron, J. P., and Erlinger, S. (1975): Barbiturates and biliary function. *Digestion*, 12:43–56.

194. Capron, J. P., Dumont, M., Feldmann, G., and Erlinger, S., (1977): Barbiturate-induced choleresis: Possible independence from microsomal enzyme induction. *Digestion*, 15:556–565.

195. Chivrac, D., Dumont, M., and Erlinger, S. (1978): Lack of parallelism between microsomal enzyme induction and phenobarbital-induced hypercholeresis in the rat. *Digestion*, 17:516–525.

196. Gartner, L. M., and Arias, I. M. (1972): Hormonal control of hepatic bilirubin transport and conjugation. *Am. J. Physiol.*, 222:1091–1099.

197. Layden, T. J., and Boyer, J. L. (1976): The effect of thyroid hormone on bile salt-independent bile flow and Na+,K+-ATPase activity in liver plasma membranes enriched in bile canaliculi. *J. Clin. Invest.*, 57:1009–1018.

198. Ros, E., and Carey, M. C. (1972): Effects of chlorpromazine hydrochloride on bile flow, bile salt synthesis, and biliary lipid secretion in the primate. In: *Bile Acid Metabolism in Health and Disease*, edited by G. Paumgarther and A. Stiehl, pp. 219–227. MTP Press, Lancaster.

199. Samuels, A. M., and Carey, M. C. (1978): Effects of chlorpromazine hydrochloride and its metabolites on Mg²⁺ and Na+,K+-ATPase activities of canalicular-enriched liver plasma membranes. *Gastroenterology*, 74:1183–1190.

200. Dibona, D. R., and Mills, J. W. (1979): Distribution of Na+-pump sites in transporting epithelia. *Fed. Proc.*, 38:134–143.

201. Ernst, S. A. (1972): Transport adenosine triphosphatase cytochemistry. II. Cytochemical localization of ouabain-sensitive, potassium-dependent phosphatase activity in the secretory epithelium of the avian salt gland. *J. Histochem. Cytochem.*, 20:23–38.

202. Ernst, S. A., and Mills, J. W. (1977): Basolateral plasma membrane localization of ouabain-sensitive sodium transport sites in the secretory epithelium of the avian salt gland. *J. Cell Biol.*, 75:74–94.

203. Quinton, P. M., and Tormey, J. M. (1976): Localization of Na+,K+-ATPase sites in the secretory and reabsorptive epithelia of perfused eccrine sweat glands; a question to the role of the enzyme in secretion. *J. Membrane Biol.*, 29:383–399.

204. Latham, P. S., and Kashgarian, M. (1979): The ultrastructural localization of transport ATPase in the rat liver at non-bile canalicular plasma membranes. *Gastroenterology*, 76:988–996.

205. Eveloff, J., Karnaky, K. J., Jr., Silva, P., Epstein, F. H., and Kinter, W. B. (1979): Elasmobranch rectal gland cell. Autoradiographic localization of [³H]ouabain-sensitive Na, K-ATPase in rectal gland of dogfish, *squalus acanthias*. *J. Cell Biol.*, 83:16–32.

206. Karnaky, K. J., Jr., Kinter, L. B., Kinter, W. B., and Stirling, C. E. (1976): Teleost chloride cell. II. Autoradiographic localization of gill Na, K-ATPase in killifish *Fundulus hetero-*

clitus adapted to low and high salinity environments. *J. Cell Biol.*, 70:157–177.

207. Poupon, R. E., and Evans, W. H. (1979): Biochemical evidence that Na⁺,K⁺-ATPase is located at the lateral region of the hepatocyte surface membrane. *FEBS Lett.*, 108:374–378.

208. Boyer, J. L. (1980): Newer concepts of mechanisms of hepatocytic bile formation. *Physiol. Rev.*, 60:303–326.

209. Gumucio, J. J., Balabaud, C., Miller, D. L., DeMason, L. J., Appelman, H. D., Stoecker, T. J., and Franzblau, D. R. (1978): Bile secretion and liver cell heterogeneity in the rat. *J. Lab. Clin. Med.*, 91:350–362.

210. Barnhart, J. L., and Combes, B. (1978): Characterization of SC 2644-induced choleresis in the dog. Evidence for canalicular bicarbonate secretion. *J. Pharmacol. Exp. Ther.*, 206:190–197.

211. Izutsu, K. T., Siegel, I. A., and Smuckler, E. A. (1978): HCO₃⁻-ATPase activity distribution in rat liver cell fractions prepared by zonal centrifugation. *Experientia*, 34:731–733.

212. Morris, T. Q. (1972): Choleretic responses to cyclic AMP and theophylline in the dog. *Gastroenterology*, 62:187 (Abstr.).

213. Barnhart, J. L., and Combes, B. (1975): Characteristics common to choleretic increments of bile induced by theophylline, glucagon and SQ-20009 in the dog. *Proc. Soc. Exp. Biol. Med.*, 150:591–596.

214. Jones, R. S., Geist, R. E., and Hall, A. D. (1971): The choleretic effects of glucagon and secretin in the dog. *Gastroenterology*, 60:64–68.

215. Morris, T. Q., Sardi, G. F., and Bradley, S. E. (1967): Character of glucagon-induced choleresis. *Fed. Proc.*, 26:774 (Abstr.).

216. Poupon, R. E., Dol, M. L., Dumont, M., and Erlinger, S. (1978): Evidence against a physiological role of cAMP in choleresis in dogs and rats. *Biochem. Pharmacol.*, 27:2413–2416.

217. Levine, R. A., and Hall, R. C. (1976): Cyclic AMP in secretin choleresis. Evidence for a regulatory role in man and baboons but not in dogs. *Gastroenterology*, 70:537–546.

218. Kaminski, D. L., Rose, R. C., and Nahrwold, D. L. (1973): Effect of pentagastrin on canine bile flow. *Gastroenterology*, 64:630–633.

218a. Kaminski, D. L., Ruwart, M., and William, V. L. (1975): The effect of prostaglandin A₁ and E₁ on canine hepatic bile flow. *J. Surg. Res.*, 18:391–397.

219. Krarup, N., Larsen, J. A., and Munck, A. (1976): Secretin-like choleretic effect of prostaglandins E₁ and E₂ in cats. *J. Physiol. (Lond.)*, 254:813–820.

220. Lauterburg, B., Paumgartner, G., and Preisig, R. (1975): Prostaglandin-induced choleresis in the rat. *Experientia*, 31:1191–1193.

221. Bullock, G. R., Delaney, V. B., Sawyer, B. C., and Slater, T. F. (1970): Biochemical changes in rat liver resulting from parenteral administration of a large dose of sodium salicylate. *Biochem. Pharmacol.*, 19:245–253.

222. Buttar, H. S., Coldwell, B. B., and Thomas, B. H. (1973): The effect of salicylate on the biliary excretion of ¹⁶C-bishydroxycoumarin in rat. *Br. J. Pharmacol.*, 48:278–287.

223. Erlinger, S., Bienfait, D., Poupon, R., Dumont, M., and Duval, M. (1975): Effect of lysine acetylsalicylate on biliary lipid secretion in dogs. *Clin. Sci. Mol. Med.*, 49:253–256.

224. Rutishauser, S. C. B., and Stone, S. L. (1975): The effect of sodium salicylate on bile secretion in the dog. *J. Physiol. (Lond.)*, 245:549–565.

225. Fisher, M. M., and Phillips, M. J. (1979): Cytoskeleton of the hepatocyte. In: *Progress in Liver Diseases, Vol. VI*, edited by H. Popper and F. Schaffner, pp. 105–121. Grune & Stratton, New York.

226. Phillips, M. J., Oda, M., Mak, E., Fisher, M. M., and Jeejeebhoy, K. N. (1975): Microfilament dysfunction as a possible cause of intrahepatic cholestasis. *Gastroenterology*, 69:48–58.

227. Dubin, M., Maurice, M., Feldmann, G., and Erlinger, S. (1978): Phalloidin-induced cholestasis in the rat: Relation to changes of microfilaments. *Gastroenterology*, 75:450–455.

228. Tuchweber, B., and Gabbiani, G. (1976): Phalloidin-induced

hyperplasia of actin microfilaments in rat hepatocytes, In: *The Liver, Quantitative Aspects of Structure and Function*, edited by R. Preisig, J. Bircher, and G. Paumgartner, pp. 84–90. Cantor, Aulendorf.

229. Gabbiani, G., Montesano, R., Tuchweber, B., Salas, M., and Orci, L. (1975): Phalloidin-induced hyperplasia of actin filaments in rat hepatocytes. *Lab. Invest.*, 33:562–569.

230. Dubin, M., Maurice, M., Feldmann, G., and Erlinger, S. (1981): Influence of colchicine and phalloidin on bile secretion and hepatic ultrastructure in the rat. Possible interaction between microtubules and microfilaments. *Gastroenterology*, 79:646–654.

231. Dubin, M., and Erlinger, S. (1981): Effect of phalloidin on biliary lipid secretion in rats. *Clin. Sci.* 58:545–548.

232. Stein, O., Sanger, L., and Stein, Y. (1974): Colchicine-induced inhibition of lipoprotein and protein secretion into the serum and lack of interference with secretion of biliary phospholipids and cholesterol by rat liver in vivo. *J. Cell Biol.* 62:90–103.

233. Gregory, D. H., Vlahcevic, Z. R., Prugh, M. F., and Swell, L. (1978): Mechanism of secretion of biliary lipids: Role of a microtubular system in hepatocellular transport of biliary lipids in the rat. *Gastroenterology*, 74:93–100.

234. Phillips, M. J., Oda, M., and Funatsu, K. (1978): Evidence for microfilament involvement in norenthandrolone-induced intrahepatic cholestasis. *Am. J. Pathol.*, 93:729–744.

235. Adler, M., Chung, K. W., and Schaffner, F. (1980): Pericanalicular hepatocytic and bile ductular microfilaments in cholestasis in man. *Am. J. Pathol.*, 98:603–616.

236. Rous, P., and McMaster, P. D. (1921): Physiological causes for the varied character of stasis bile. *J. Exp. Med.*, 34:75–96.

237. Bayliss, W. M., and Starling, E. H. (1902): The mechanism of pancreatic secretion. *J. Physiol. (Lond.)*, 28:325–353.

238. Chenderovitch, J. (1971): Transports d'eau et d'electrolytes dans le cholédoque du lapin "in vivo." *Rev. Eur. Etud. Clin. Biol.*, 16:591–595.

239. Chenderovitch, J. (1972): Secretory function of the rabbit common bile duct. *Am. J. Physiol.*, 223:695–706.

240. Nahrwold, D. L., and Shariatzedeh, A. N. (1971): Role of the common bile duct in formation of bile and in gastrin-induced choleresis. *Surgery*, 70:147–153.

241. Scratcherd, T. (1965): Electrolyte composition and control of biliary secretion in the cat and rabbit. In: *The Biliary System*, edited by W. Taylor, pp. 515–529. Blackwell, Oxford.

242. Jones, R. S., and Grossman, M. I. (1969): Choleretic effects of secretin and histamine in the dog. *Am. J. Physiol.*, 217:532–535.

243. Grossman, M. I., Janowitz, H. D., and Ralston, H. (1969): The effect of secretin on bile formation in man. *Gastroenterology*, 12:133–138.

244. Hardison, W. G. M., and Norman, J. C. (1967): Effect of bile salt and secretin upon bile flow from the isolated perfused pig liver. *Gastroenterology*, 53:412–417.

245. Debray, C., Vaille, C., Rozé, C., De La Tour, J., and Souchard, M. (1962): Action des sécrétines du commerce sur la sécrétion pancréatique externe du rat. *J. Physiol. (Paris)*, 54:549–577.

245a. Ashworth, C. T., and Sanders, E. (1960): Anatomic pathway of bile formation. *Am. J. Pathol.*, 37:343–355.

246. Back, D. J., and Calvey, T. N. (1971): Infusion of secretin into the hepatic arterial circulation of the rat. *J. Physiol. (Lond.)*, 219:14P.

247. Esteller, A., Lopez, M. A., and Murillo, A. (1977): The effect of secretin and cholecystokinin-pancreozymin on the secretion of bile in the anesthetized rabbit. *Q. J. Exp. Physiol.*, 62:353–359.

248. Hardison, W. G. M., and Norman, J. C. (1968): Electrolyte composition of the secretin fraction of bile from the perfused pig liver. *Am. J. Physiol.*, 214:758–763.

249. Wheeler, H. O., and Mancusi-Ungaro, P. L. (1966): Role of bile ducts during secretin choleresis in dogs. *Am. J. Physiol.*, 210:1153–1159.

250. Jones, R. S., and Grossman, M. I. (1970): Choleretic effects of cholecystokinin, gastrin II and caerulein in the dog. *Am. J. Physiol.*, 219:1016–1018.

251. Zaterka, S., and Grossman, M. I. (1966): The effect of gastrin and histamine on secretion of bile. *Gastroenterology,* 50:500–505.

252. Caroli, J., and Tanasoglu, Y. (1953): Le temps d'apparition de la bromesulfonephtaléine dans la bile. Nouveau test pour le diagnostic des ictères incomplets par rétention et des blocages anictériques de la voie biliaire principale. *Sem. Hop. Paris,* 29:591–606.

253. Bode, C., Zelder, O., Goebell, H., and Neuberger, H. O. (1972): Choleresis induced by secretin: Distinctly increased response in cirrhotics. *Scand. J. Gastroenterol.,* 7:697–699.

254. Erlinger, S., Sakellaridis, D., Maillard, J. N., and Benhamou, J. P. (1969): Les formes angiocholitiques de la fibrose hépatique congénitale. *Presse Med.,* 77:1189–1191.

255. Turnberg, L. A., Jones, E. A., and Sherlock, S. (1968): Biliary secretion in a patient with cystic duct dilatation of the intrahepatic biliary tree. *Gastroenterology,* 54:1155–1161.

256. Barber-Riley, G. (1968): Biliary capacity in rats following ethionine ingestion. *Am. J. Physiol.,* 214:133–138.

257. Goldfarb, S., Singer, E. J., and Popper, H. (1963): Biliary ductules and bile secretion. *J. Lab. Clin. Med.,* 62:608–615.

258. Popper, H. (1961): Roles of the bile ductules in bile formation. *Am. J. Med. Sci.* 242:519.

259. Guzelian, P., and Boyer, J. L. (1974): Glucose reabsorption from bile. Evidence for a biliohepatic circulation. *J. Clin. Invest.,* 53:526–535.

260. Sasaki, H., Schaffner, F., and Popper, H. (1967): Bile ductules in cholestasis: Morphologic evidence for secretion and absorption in man. *Lab. Invest.,* 16:84–95.

261. Baldwin, J., Heer, F. W., Albo, R., Peloso, O., Ruby, L., and Silen, W. (1966): Effect of vagus nerve stimulation on hepatic secretion of bile in human subjects. *Am. J. Surg.,* 111:66–69.

262. Fritz, M. E., and Brooks, F. P. (1963): Control of bile flow in the cholecystectomized dog. *Am. J. Physiol.,* 204:825–828.

263. Jones, R. S. (1976): Effect of insulin on canalicular bile formation. *Am. J. Physiol.,* 231:40–43.

264. Rozé, C., and Feldmann, D. (1971): Stimulation par l'insuline d'une fraction de la cholérèse indépendante des sels biliaires chez le rat. *C.R. Acad. Sci. (Paris),* 273:887–890.

265. Geist, R. E., and Jones, R. S. (1971): Effect of selective and truncal vagotomy on insulin-stimulated bile secretion in dogs. *Gastroenterology,* 60:566–567.

266. Jones, R. S., and Smith, B. M. (1977): The effect of truncal vagotomy on taurocholate choleresis and secretin choleresis. *J. Surg. Res.,* 23:149–154.

267. Debray, C., De La Tour, J., Rozé, C., Souchard, M., and Vaille, C. (1974): Independence from vagal control of biliary secretion in the rat. *Digestion,* 10:413–422.

268. Tavoloni, N., Reed, J. S., and Boyer, J. L. (1978): Hemodynamic effects on determinants of bile secretion in isolated rat liver. *Am. J. Physiol.,* 234:E584–E592.

269. Fisher, B., Lee, S. H., and Fedor, E. J. (1958): Effect of permanent alteration of hepatic blood flow upon biliary secretion. *Arch. Surg.,* 76:41–45.

270. Herz, R., Paumgartner, G., and Preisig, R. (1974): Bile salt metabolism and bile formation in the rat with a portacaval shunt. *Eur. J. Clin. Invest.,* 4:223–228.

271. Prandi, D., Dumont, M., and Erlinger, S. (1974): Influence of portacaval shunt on bile formation in the rat. *Eur. J. Clin. Invest.,* 4:197–200.

272. Engstrand, L. (1949): Bile secretion and hepatic nitrogen metabolism in relation to variations of blood and oxygen supply to the liver. *Acta. Chir. Scand. [suppl.],* 146:1–190.

273. Preisig, R., Bircher, H., and Paumgartner, G. (1972): Physiologic and pathophysiologic aspects of the hepatic hemodynamics. In: *Progress in Liver Diseases, Vol. 4,* edited by H. Popper and F. Schaffner, pp. 201–216. Grune & Stratton, New York.

274. Kotelanski, B., Groszmann, R. J., and Kendler, J. (1969): Effect of ethanol on sulfobromophthalein and indocyanine green metabolism in isolated perfused rat liver. *Proc. Soc. Exp. Biol. Med.,* 132:715–721.

275. Zsigmond, G., and Solymoss, B. (1972): Effect of spironolactone, pregnenolone-16-carbonitrile and cortisol on the metabolism and biliary excretion of sulfobromophthalein and phenol-3, 6-dibromphthalein disulfonate in rats. *J. Pharmacol. Exp. Ther.,* 183:499–507.

276. Di Padova, C., Zuin, M., Bellomi, M., and Podda, M. (1978): Choleretic and anticholeretic effects of furosemide in the rat. *Ital. J. Gastroenterol.,* 10:92–96.

277. Siro-Brigiani, G., Campese, V. M., and Antoncecci, E. (1970): Azione coleretica del furosemide e della teofillina nel ratto. *Boll. Soc. Ital. Biol. Sper.,* 46:607–608.

278. Maren, T. H., Ellison, A. C., Fellner, S. K., and Graham, W. B. (1966): A study of hepatic carbonic anhydrase. *Mol. Pharmacol.,* 2:144–157.

279. Pak. B. H., Hong, S. S., Pak, H. K., and Hong, S. K. (1966): Effect of acetazolamide and acid-base changes on biliary and pancreatic secretion. *Am. J. Physiol.,* 210:624–628.

280. Levine, W. G., Braunstein, I. R., and Meijer, D. K. F. (1975): Effect of nafenopin (SU-13,437) on liver function. Mechanism of choleretic effect. *Naunyn Schmiedebergs Arch. Pharmacol.,* 290:221–234.

281. Rozé, C., Cuchet, P., Souchard, M., Vaille, C., and Debray, C. (1977): The effects of tiadenol, clofibrate and clofibride on bile composition in the rat. *Eur. J. Pharmacol.,* 43:57–64.

282. Rozé, C., Debray, C., Vaille, C., and Souchard, M. (1972): Hypercholérèse induite et excretion des sels biliaires après traitement par le clofibrate. *C.R. Acad. Sci. (Paris),* 274:3472–3475.

The Liver: Biology and Pathobiology, edited by
I. Arias, H. Popper, D. Schachter, and D. A. Shafritz.
Raven Press, New York © 1982.

Chapter 27

The Enterohepatic Circulation*

Martin C. Carey

In its role as an exocrine gland, the liver secretes
bile, a solution of detergent-like molecules called bile
salts whose target organs are the lumen of the biliary
tree and gut. Here they perform a number of important
solubilization, transport, and regulatory functions.
From the gut lumen, they are avidly absorbed and returned to the liver in the portal blood. The secondary
target organs for returning bile salts are the parenchymal cells of the liver. Here they regulate intracellular
lipid metabolism, solubilize and/or disperse a number
of intracellular membrane lipids, and transport them
into bile. Since the topographical localization of this
continuous flow of bile salt molecules is essentially
limited to the hepatocyte, biliary tree, intestine, enterocyte, and portal blood, it is aptly called the enterohepatic circulation. Not only does this ecological
device enable the organism to reutilize a physiologically valuable detergent-like molecule many times
over, but the regulatory functions of recycling bile
salts within this circulation facilitate continuous homeostatic control over diverse metabolic events.
These include the synthesis and mass transfer of a variety of lipids within the hepatocyte-enterocyte axis
and both fluid and electrolyte movements within the
biliary tree, small intestine, and colon. Finally, the obligatory "leak" of bile salts from the enterohepatic
circulation principally by excretion in the feces serves
as the primary quantitative mechanism by which the
organism loses cholesterol. Hence bile salts in their
enterohepatic circulation play a role in lipid mass
transfer and removal of unwanted molecules analo-

---

* This work is dedicated to my father J. J. (Jack) Carey on the
occasion of his 75th birthday.

gous to the role played by hemoglobin and the circulation of the blood in the mass transfer of O_2 and CO_2.

This chapter reviews current concepts of the enterohepatic circulation of bile salts in man. The diverse roles played by bile salts in this circulation are discussed from a perspective of their molecular and biological properties. An attempt is made to demonstrate how the interplay of the distinct biophysical properties of bile salts and the physiochemical environment of different anatomic locations of the enterohepatic circulation facilitate their unique biological functions. Further details, including clinical aspects of the enterohepatic circulation, are found in several excellent reviews and monographs (1–9).

PARTICIPANTS

The relative proportions of the major solutes of bile are shown in Fig. 1. The bile salts are a family of molecules that are the soluble sodium and potassium salts of hydroxyl-substituted cholanic acids (Table 1). In addition to bile salts, bile contains phospholipids (principally lecithin), unesterified cholesterol, bile pigments, and a mixture of proteins. However, a host of other endogenous substances may be secreted in bile and undergo enterohepatic cycling (5,6,10,11). These include the bacterial reduction products of bilirubin; lipovitamins, particularly the biologically active forms of vitamin D_2; water-soluble vitamins, particularly vitamin B_{12}; folic acid and pyridoxine, and many estrogenic steroids. Several exogenous substances also undergo some degree of enterohepatic cycling. These include commonly used drugs, such as indomethacin, cardiac glycosides, chlorpromazine, antibiotics, cholephilic dyes, and radiocontrast media. Only the enterohepatic circulation of bile salts is unique, however, in its physiological importance and

efficiency. In fact, since the active transport of bile salts from liver cell to bile and from ileal enterocytes to the portal blood constitutes the major metabolic driving force for solute and water movement within the enterohepatic circulation, the degree of enterohepatic cycling of other lipophilic and hydrophilic materials is critically dependent on bile salt movement within this circulation.

BIOLOGICAL PERSPECTIVE

The bile salts (Fig. 2) participating in the enterohepatic circulation are a family of molecules ultimately derived from the hepatic catabolism of cholesterol (12,13). In man, two bile salts, termed primary bile salts, are formed from cholesterol in the liver. They are cholic acid [1], a trihydroxy bile acid (Table 1), and chenodeoxycholic acid, a dihydroxy bile acid (Table 1). By the action of intestinal bacteria, secondary bile acids are formed from primary bile acids. The major reaction of physiological significance is 7α-dehydroxylation of primary bile salts to give deoxycholic acid from cholic and lithocholic acid from chenodeoxycholic acid (Table 1). A third important secondary bile salt, 7-oxo-lithocholic acid, is formed by 7α-dehydrogenation of chenodeoxycholic acid (16–19). Tertiary bile acids are formed in the liver and by intestinal bacteria from secondary bile acids (Fig. 2; Table 1). The major reactions are hepatic sulfation of lithocholate (20,21) and hepatic (22) or bacterial reduction (17–19) of 7-oxo-lithocholic acid to chenodeoxycholic (mainly in the liver) or to its 7β-epimer ursodeoxycholic acid (mainly by intestinal bacteria). As glycine and taurine

---

[1] The nomenclature bile acid and bile salt are used interchangeably in this review. The reader should bear in mind that the physicochemical properties of the undissociated (acid) and ionized (anionic) forms of these amphiphiles differ (14,15).

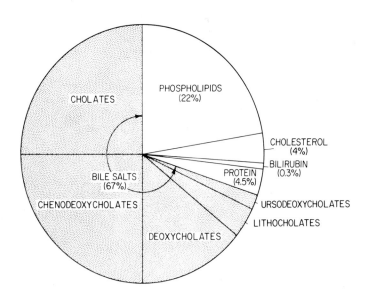

FIG. 1. Typical solute composition of hepatic and gallbladder bile in man.

TABLE 1. *Biliary bile salt composition in man[a]*

| Bile salt | | Percent in bile | | Percent of total | |
Trivial name	Systematic name	Taurine conjugates	Glycine conjugates	Sulfated	Glucuronidated
Common					
CHOLATE	$3\alpha,7\alpha, 12\alpha$-trihydroxy-$5\beta$-cholanoate	12	23	0.1%	0.1%
CHENODEOXYCHOLATE (CHENIC)	$3\alpha,7\alpha$-dihydroxy-5β-cholanoate	12	23	0.2%	0.1%
DEOXYCHOLATE	$3\alpha,12\alpha$-dihydroxy-5β-cholanoate	8	16	n.d.[b]	n.d.
URSODEOXYCHOLATE[c] (URSIC)	$3\alpha,7\beta$-dihydroxy-5β-cholanoate	tr[d] $\to$ 2	tr $\to$ 5	n.d.	n.d.
LITHOCHOLATE	3α-monohydroxy-5β-cholanoate	1 $\to$ 2	3 $\to$ 4	60–80%	tr.
Uncommon					
ISOCHENODEOXYCHOLATE	$3\beta,7\alpha$-dihydroxy-5β-cholanoate	tr $\to$ 1.0		n.d.	n.d.
7-OXO-LITHOCHOLATE	3α-monohydroxy,7-oxo-5β-cholanoate	tr $\to$ .3		n.d.	n.d.
12-OXO-LITHOCHOLATE	3α-monohydroxy,12-oxo-5β-cholanoate	tr $\to$ .4		n.d.	n.d.
12-OXO-CHENODEOXYCHOLATE	$3\alpha,7\alpha$-dihydroxy,12-oxo-5β-cholanoate	<.1		n.d.	n.d.
7-OXO-DEOXYCHOLATE	$3\alpha,12\alpha$-dihydroxy,7-oxo-5β-cholanoate	<.1		n.d.	n.d.
—	3-oxo,12α-monohydroxy-5β-cholanoate	<.1		n.d.	n.d.
—	3-oxo,7α-monohydroxy-5β-cholanoate	<.1		n.d.	n.d.
—	3β-monohydroxy-delta-5-cholenoate	tr		n.d.	n.d.

[a] Adapted from refs. 1, 173, 205.
[b] n.d. = not determined.
[c] In some healthy subjects, ursodeoxycholate levels can be as high as 30%.
[d] tr = trace.

conjugates, this complex family of molecules exists in soluble form in the biliary tree and intestine where they cooperate and share physical properties. Within the other anatomic sites of the enterohepatic circulation, individual bile salts exhibit specific metabolic activities.

One of the functions of the enterohepatic circulation is a means for the adult organism to eliminate excess cholesterol. Cholesterol is synthesized in all cells of vertebrates and is vital for their function and growth. Excessive synthesis and retention of cholesterol may be lethal and characterizes the lesions of atherosclerosis and most gall stones (23). Bile secretion provides the only significant mechanism for its removal; not only are cholesterol molecules converted to bile salts continually to balance fecal loss, but conjugated bile salts, by their detergent action, solubilize cholesterol in macromolecular aggregates called mixed micelles (24,25). These mixed micelles promote excretion of cholesterol from the liver and its eventual loss in the feces. Hence the overflow of steroids from the enterohepatic circulation provides a means of elimination

of cholesterol as both precursor and metabolic products. Moreover, intestinal conservation of bile salt molecules permits them to mediate continuously hepatic cholesterol excretion by recycling repeatedly through the parenchymal cells of the liver. Furthermore, by their extra- and intracellular control of the mass transfer of cholesterol through enterocyte and hepatocyte, bile salts indirectly regulate cholesterol synthesis in these organs (26).

Bile salts serve an equally important transport role in the efficient absorption of dietary fat from the gut lumen (27,28). Bile salt molecules, acting together with biliary lecithin and cholesterol, serve colloidal and transport roles. Upon dilution in the intestinal lumen, portions of the three biliary lipids adsorb to the interface of fat (triglyceride) globules and provide stable emulsification (28). Pancreatic lipolysis of lecithin and triglyceride changes the composition and phases of lipids in the intestinal lumen, so that lecithin-cholesterol-bile salt micelles become fatty acid, monoglyceride, lecithin, lysolecithin, diglyceride, and cholesterol bile salt micelles with the appearance of another

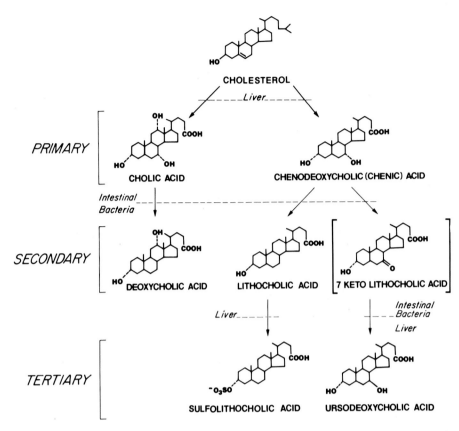

FIG. 2. Major primary, secondary, and tertiary bile salts of man with sites of synthesis and metabolism.

aqueous phase containing the same lipids as liquid crystalline vesicles (29). Both these vehicles apparently shuttle their complement of fat digestive products and other important lipids, such as the lipovitamins and lipophilic drugs, through the unstirred aqueous layers and mucin glycoprotein barriers to enter passively the intestinal absorptive cells. Within these cells, resynthesis of triglycerides and lecithin occurs. Globules of newly formed fat adsorb specific apolipoproteins to form chylomicrons and very low density lipoprotein (VLDL) particles. These are exocytosed into the intestinal lymphatics to transport dietary fat, biliary lecithin, and cholesterol to other organs for metabolic and nutritional purposes (30). Obviously, for a small bile salt pool to transport 25 times its weight of fat from intestinal lumen to lymph each day requires efficient enterohepatic recycling of the transport agents, as shown in Fig. 3.

The ability to form transport vehicles, such as micelles or liposomal vesicles, is totally unrelated to the other functions of bile salts within the enterohepatic circulation. Bile salts are the major osmotic force that promotes water movement from the liver cells into bile (31). In fact, bile flow is inversely related to the micelle-forming abilities of bile salts. Bile salts probably modulate fluid absorption from the small intestine (32), and the dihydroxy species with alpha substituents induce fluid secretion in the large intestine (33,34). Bile

salts have specific effects on a number of digestive enzymes. Human breast milk lipase and the minor lipase of the pancreas (apparently identical enzymes) are dependent on bile salts as cofactors (35). These bile salt-dependent lipases are only activated by primary bile salts (especially the taurine conjugates) and do so at concentrations well below their critical micellar concentrations (35). Moreover, bile salts protect a number of other luminal lipolytic enzymes, such as lingual lipase, pancreatic lipase, and phospholipase A_2, from proteolytic digestion and prevent surface denaturation (28). Because of interfacial competition with bile salts, specific cofactors, such as colipase and Ca^{2+}, are required for physiological activity of these enzymes in the presence of bile salts (36–38). Pancreatic cholesterol esterase, which is secreted as an inactive monomer, requires polymerization in the presence of trihydroxy bile salts for activity (39). Also, intracellular esterification of absorbed cholesterol appears to have a similar requirement (40).

Finally, bile salts returning to the hepatocyte regulate their own synthesis from cholesterol and hence may regulate *de novo* hepatic cholesterol synthesis indirectly (26). The quantity of cholesterol secreted into bile appears to be regulated by a fine balance between the bile salts with 3,7-hydroxyl substituents (chenodeoxycholic and ursodeoxycholic), which decrease its secretion, and bile salts with 3,12-hydroxyl substitu-

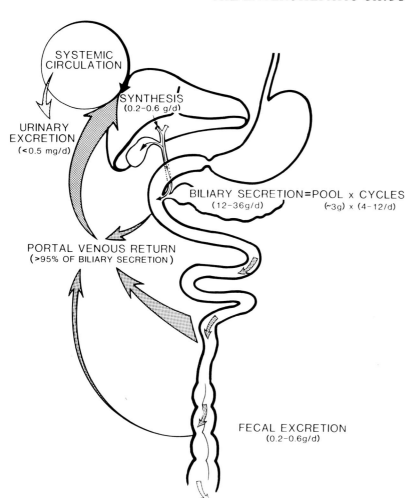

FIG. 3. Enterohepatic circulation of bile salts showing typical kinetic values for healthy man.

ents (deoxycholic and cholic), which increase its secretion (41–49). In addition, the quantity of cholesterol synthesized within the hepatocyte and enterocyte appears to be dependent on the bile salt-mediated cholesterol movement by feedback inhibition. Because bile salts have these multiple functions, they are intimately involved in the pathogenesis of several hepatic, biliary, and intestinal diseases (8).

HISTORY

During the middle ages, it was suspected that bile entering the intestine was absorbed and reutilized. Giovanni Borelli, a 17th century Neopolitan mathematician, was the first to calculate that the total amount of bile entering the duodenum each day was many times the amount of bile present in the biliary tree at any one time (50). He inferred a "particular circulation of the bile through the abdomen, performed by the Venae mesaraicae into the trunk of the Porta, thence to the liver, thence through the bilious vessels into the Duodenum to return again by the Mesaraick veins." Seventy-five years later, an Irish physician, Edward Barry, Professor of Medicine at Dublin University, developed this idea further and made a most

astonishing prediction (51). He asserted in 1759 that bile was a most complicated fluid ("concocted Humour") and that its more acid ("acrid") and active part remained dissolved within the intestines until "after the Chyle had passed the Lacteals." This active part was only then "received into the Meseraic Veins, which soon return again by this short Circulation to the liver; and by this means supply it with active genuine Materials fit for the more easy Preparation and Secretion of new Bile."

This prescient idea concerning the function of bile salts and accurate description of the enterohepatic circulation is astonishing when one realizes that bile salts were first discovered by Berzelius in 1809 (52), and their enterohepatic recycling was not fully confirmed by experiment for another 150 years. In 1937 and 1941, Sobotka (53) and Josephson (54) clearly described the enterohepatic circulation of bile salts in board outline. Their intellectual synthesis was based on the detailed work of many distinguished 19th century chemists and physiologists. Berzelius (52) had known that bile contained an acid fraction, but it was Gmelin in 1826 (55) who identified sodium cholate and taurine in ox bile and Liebig in 1843 (56) who coined the term bile acid (56). In 1855, Lehmann (57) distinguished between glycine and taurine conjugates of cholic acid and realized that these salts were responsible for solubilizing cholesterol in bile. Berzelius, Liebig, and Pettenkofer (53) recognized the paucity of bile products in the stool but considered that it was metabolized and excreted either in the breath (Liebig) or urine (Pettenkofer). In the mid-19th century, Hoffmann (58) and Hoppe-Seyler (59) resurrected Barry's postulate of the continuous circulation of bile salts but were unable to verify it by experiment. In an ingenious series of experiments performed between 1870 and 1892, however, Schiff (53,60) and Weiss (61) independently showed that bile salts were reabsorbed from the intestine to subsequently appear in bile.

In the last 50 years, investigators have fused these concepts and defined the preferred sites and mechanisms of absorption of bile salts (62–65), the frequency of cycling and secretion (9,54,66–69), fecal bile salt loss (9,69–71), and pool size and turnover (72). The importance of maintaining the integrity of the enterohepatic circulation during physiological studies was not appreciated until the studies of Thureborn (73) and Dowling (74,75). In recent years, quantitative measurements of the enterohepatic circulation in man have employed Lindstedt's isotope-dilution technique (76,77) for pool size and synthesis rates and direct multilumen perfusion techniques to estimate bile salt secretion (78,79). Although the existence of a dynamic equilibrium between synthesis and secretion was realized by Berman (80), the details of the homeostatic mechanisms controlling bile salt synthesis, pool size, turnover frequency, bacterial metabolism, fecal loss, and bile salt secretion rates in health and disease are still poorly understood. For further details of the history of the enterohepatic circulation, the authoritative reviews by Hislop (81) and Heaton and Morris (82) should be consulted.

BIOLOGY AND CHEMISTRY OF BILE SALTS

Hepatic Synthesis

In the synthesis of cholate and chenodeoxycholate, the two primary bile salts, from unesterified cholesterol in the liver (12,13), the sequence of intermediate products involved is complex and incompletely defined for man (83,84). The initial biochemical transformation is catalyzed by a mixed function oxidase in the smooth endoplasmic reticulum and involves hydroxylation of the C-7 position on the steroid skeleton to form 7α-hydroxycholesterol. The activity of the 7α-hydroxylase enzyme is rate limiting (85) in bile salt synthesis and is regulated primarily by the magnitude of the bile salt return to the liver in the portal vein (75,86). Subsequent reactions lead to the formation of 7α-hydroxycholest-4-en-3-one, which involves a shift

in the position of the double bond. In the sequence derived for the rat, this is the branch point which leads to cholate or chenodeoxycholate synthesis under the influence of 12α-hydroxylase also localized in the endoplasmic reticulum (87). Once the branch point has been passed, soluble cytosolic enzymes reduce the 3-oxo group of both intermediates to di- and triols. It is only then that mitochondrial (and perhaps microsomal) enzymes cleave the C-27 side chain of the cholestane nucleus, eliminating an isopropyl group to form the C-24 steroids. In man, a second quantitatively important pathway also leads to the synthesis of chenodeoxycholate (84). In this scheme, the side chain is oxidized before the nuclear transformations are completed and proceeds via the 26-hydroxylation of 7α-hydroxycholest-4-en-3-one in the endoplasmic reticulum (84). The final chemical results are more polar molecules than cholesterol with 3α, 7α, or 3α, 7α, 12α-hydroxyl groups, which lie to one side of the fused hydrocarbon ring system, a saturated double bond, a shortened carboxylated side chain, and an A-B ring juncture which is cis or kinked (Figs. 2 and 4).

Prior to secretion into bile, both cholic and chenodeoxycholic acids are conjugated as N-acyl conjugates (peptide linkage) with glycine or taurine (Fig. 4). This chemical modification is essential; in the unconjugated form, both primary bile acids are only sparingly soluble (15) at physiological pH (460 and 256 μM, respec-

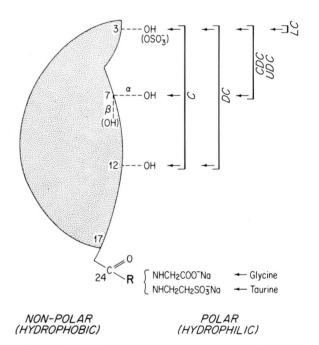

FIG. 4. Amphiphilic structure of the common bile salts of man. In bile and small intestine, the R of the side chain is glycine or taurine. After bacterial deconjugation in the colon, R (conjugate) is replaced by an OH group. C, cholate (3α-, 7α-, 12α-OH); DC, deoxycholate (3α-, 12α-OH); CDC, chenodeoxycholate (3α-, 7α-OH); UDC, ursodeoxycholate (3α-, 7β-OH); LC, lithocholate (3α-OH or 3α-OSO$^-_3$).

tively). Conjugation not only suppresses or abolishes the pH at which bile acids precipitate but allows them to be freely soluble in the aqueous milieu of bile and gut over a wide range of ionic strengths, calcium concentrations, bile salt concentrations, and pH values (24). Taurine conjugates are more water soluble than are glycine conjugates, and trihydroxy bile salts are in general more water soluble than are dihydroxy bile salts. The taurine and glycine conjugates are often called bile salts by virtue of the fact that they are completely ionized at physiological pH, whereas the free bile acids are not. Perhaps the term "bile salt" should be reserved for any bile acid, free or unconjugated, that is ionized and hence very water soluble, and "bile acid" should be reserved for protonated bile salts which are generally only sparingly soluble. Not only do the bile "acids" and bile "salts" differ in aqueous solubility but also in a host of other physicochemical properties (88) and are found in man at distinctly different anatomic locations.

Bacterial Alterations

During passage through the cecum and colon, a percentage of conjugated cholates and chenodeoxycholates is altered biochemically by specific enzymes produced by the indigenous bacterial flora (89,90). The physiologically important bacterial alterations are of three distinct types (17–19,91): (a) deconjugation catalyzed by bacterial cholylamidases liberating unconjugated bile acids; (b) 7α-dehydroxylation, which converts cholate to deoxycholate and chenodeoxycholate to lithocholate; and (c) 7α-dehydrogenation, which converts chenodeoxycholate to 7-oxo-lithocholate which can, in turn, be epimerized by bacterial enzymes to ursodeoxycholate (Fig. 2; Table 1). About 20% of glycine conjugates and 10% of taurine conjugates are deconjugated during an enterohepatic cycle (92–94). The majority of these bile acids are reabsorbed to return to the liver where they are reconjugated with glycine or taurine. Strict anaerobic bacteria (bacteroids, clostridia, and eubacteria) are responsible for the 7α-dehydroxylation of bile salts (95–98); the reaction is induced by bile salts (99,100). The initial reaction step is believed to proceed by a diaxial transelimination of water resulting in the release of the 7α-hydroxy group and the 6β-hydrogen (101,102). The resulting Δ^6-intermediate is subsequently reduced by transhydrogenation at the 6α and 7β positions to yield the secondary bile acid (101,102). The reductive nature of this biotransformation suggests that the anaerobes use this reaction as a mechanism to dispose of electrons generated by fermentative metabolism (103). The 7α-dehydrogenation reaction is currently under intense scrutiny (17–19), and a number of strict intestinal anaerobes have been identified which not only dehydrogenate the 7α-hydroxy group but further reduce and epimerize the 7-oxointermediate to ursodeoxycholic (and ursocholic) acids. Novel epimerization of 7α-hydroxyl groups may also be achieved in the colon by the combined action of bacterial species with 7α- and 7β-dehydrogenating capacities (104). Thus colonic bacteria not only oxidize primary bile acids to secondary 7-oxo bile acids but are capable of further reducing them to tertiary bile acids.

Hepatic Modifications

The fate of the major secondary bile acids differs. About 30 to 50% of the deoxycholic acid formed is absorbed (93) to return to the liver where it is conjugated with glycine and taurine and in man is not rehydroxylated (105). Deoxycholic acid after its absorption resembles a primary bile acid in its subsequent metabolism. The other 50% of deoxycholic acid appears in the stool with and without further bacterial metabolism (106). Only about 20% of the lithocholic acid formed is absorbed from the colon (107) since it is much less soluble than is deoxycholic acid at intestinal pH and body temperature (15,108). Like deoxycholic acid, this fraction is transported to the liver in the portal vein, efficiently extracted, not rehydroxylated (109), and conjugated with glycine or taurine (Fig. 5). Glycine and taurine conjugation, however, does not render lithocholic acid more soluble than its unconjugated form (14). The liver sulfates about 80% of conjugated lithocholates at the 3-position to render it water soluble for secretion into bile (20,110,111). Glycolithocholate is sulfated to a greater extent than taurolithocholate (20,21) but is less soluble than taurolithocholate sulfate (108). The sulfated conjugates are not well absorbed from the gut (112,113) either passively or actively unless desulfation takes place (Fig. 5). Biliary lithocholate levels are generally low because the sulfated species are end products of their metabolism and are lost from the enterohepatic circulation in the feces (107,114). If desulfation occurs, the unsulfated fraction is absorbed with low efficiency to be resulfated by the liver (Fig. 5).

Most of the 7-oxo-lithocholate formed by specific anaerobic bacteria is quantitatively converted to ursodeoxycholate by the same or other bacteria in the colon (104). This tertiary bile acid is absorbed, conjugated in the liver with glycine or taurine, and, in many individuals, is the fourth most common bile acid in bile (Table 1). Small amounts of 7-oxo-lithocholate, however, reach the liver where they are reduced to both ursodeoxycholate and chenodeoxycholate (mainly the latter) (115). These are conjugated and secreted into bile to enter the intestine where they may be again dehydroxylated to lithocholic acid (116) or the 7-oxointermediate. They may again be further metabolized

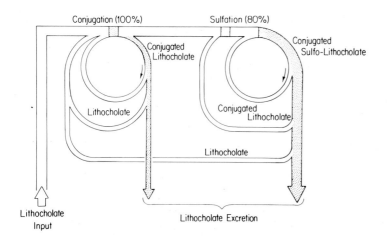

FIG. 5. Enterohepatic circulation of lithocholate formed by intestinal microbial 7-dehydroxylation of chenodeoxycholic or ursodeoxycholic acids. In the liver, conjugation with taurine or glycine is complete, and the efficiency of 3α-sulfation is ≈80%. In contrast to the other common bile salts, the sulfates are poorly conserved by the intestine, so that the enterohepatic circulation of lithocholate sulfates is interrupted after a single pass through the liver. (From refs. 20 and 107).

by bacteria and lost in the feces or absorbed to reach the liver where the metabolic events just outlined are repeated. Thus chenodeoxycholic and ursodeoxycholic acids are precursor and product of each other, and both are precursors of lithocholate.

Bile normally contains traces of other secondary and tertiary bile acids, (Table 1), including 7-oxo-lithocholate (117); but in view of the host of possible bacterial metabolites of bile acids in the colon (106) and urine (118), human bile is remarkably clean (Table 1) since most bacterial metabolities are poorly absorbed and/or poorly cleared by the liver and do not have a continuing biological life within the enterohepatic circulation. In disease, especially cholestasis, a number of additional bile acid-metabolizing functions of the human liver appear. These render even the common bile salts more polar and form less toxic derivatives which have high urinary clearances. These include increases in taurine conjugation, novel 1 and 6-C hydroxylations, sulfation, and glucuronidation of all primary and secondary bile acids (118–126).

PHYSICOCHEMISTRY OF BILE SALTS

General Properties

Conjugated bile salts have powerful detergent-like properties (14,24,25,127,128) which are important in stabilizing the physical state of bile and in promoting fat digestion and absorption (129). The bile salt molecules are rigid planar amphiphiles which possess a hydrophilic side that also has hydrophobic elements and a pure hydrophobic side (Fig. 4). The polar function on the hydrophilic side comes from the hydroxyl (and sulfate) substituents and the charged end group of the side chain. The hydrophobic properties of this side are attributable to the intrinsic hydrocarbon surface which is uncovered with polar substituents together with the aliphatic side chain which subtends the charged end group. The hydrophobic side is formed by the convex convoluted side of the rigid hydrocarbon ring system. It is spiked with three methyl groups at

the C-18,19, and 21 positions. Bile salt molecules aggregate to form polymolecular aggregates called micelles over a narrow concentration range (0.6 to 5 mM); this is called the critical micellar concentration (CMC) (14). The micelles formed just above the CMC are called primary micelles (14); they are globular in shape and contain from two to 15 bile salt molecules that interact hydrophobically via their hydrophobic sides to decrease the hydrocarbon-water contact of the individual monomers (14,127). At higher bile salt concentrations, particularly in high ionic strengths, the primary micelles polymerize via their hydrophilic surfaces to form large, rod-like secondary micelles (14). The driving force for polymerization is also an unfavorable hydrocarbon-water contact on the outside of the primary micelles (127). For these reasons, the distinct aggregation patterns of bile salt molecules have some properties in common with the open-ended self-association of dye and drug molecules (130), particularly in the case of cholates (131,132), and the cooperative micellization of typical detergent molecules (133,134), as occurs with more hydrophobic bile salts (135).

Bile salt micelles can solubilize other important biological amphiphilic molecules that are otherwise water insoluble, such as cholesterol, lipovitamins, lecithin, fatty acid-soaps, and monoglycerides, to form mixed micelles (129). In fact, bile salt micelles also solubilize their own sparingly soluble protonated species as mixed micelles (14,15). It is often considered that cholesterol is poorly solubilized by bile salts in the absence of other solubilized polar lipids, such as lecithins. Examination of the solubility values shows that this is not the case. For example, the solubility of cholesterol monohydrate in water is ≈1 nM (136), but 10 mM can be solubilized by a 200 mM solution of deoxycholate, which is a 10 million-fold increase (137). With the addition of lecithin (138) to deoxycholate, this value is at most tripled. Physiological solutions of all the common bile salts possess the capacity to solubilize cholesterol; the conjugates are less efficient than are the free species, and the taurine conjugates are less efficient than are glycine conjugates (137). Bile salt micelles possess marked capacities to solubilize important polar lipids, which by themselves can form liquid crystalline aggregates (129). These include lecithin, acid soaps, and monoglycerides (insoluble swelling amphiphiles), which can be solubilized by bile salts in ≈2:1 M ratios or greater (14,129,138). The micellar sizes can grow from ≈60 Å to approach the size of microemulsion particles (400 Å) when close to the phase limit (128,139). In such mixed micelles, bile salts and polar lipid molecules are arranged in disk-like bilayers. The bile salts coat the perimeter of the disks and occupy the inside in high concentrations as "reversed micelles" (Fig. 6), i.e., mixed-disk micelles (128).

When mixed micellar systems are bile salt-rich, such

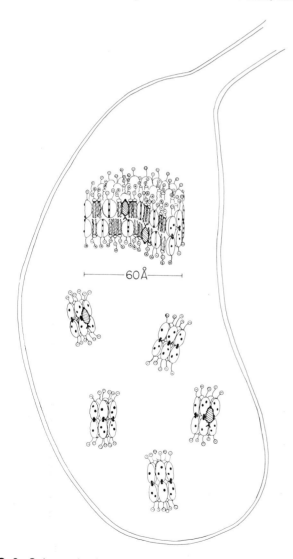

FIG. 6. Schematic view of the physical state of bile in the gall bladder of man. With typical lipid compositions, simple bile salt and mixed bile salt-lecithin micelles coexist. The site of attachment for cholesterol molecules on simple micelles is on the exterior (hydrophilic) surface. In mixed micelles, cholesterol is solubilized within the micelles. (From refs. 25, 128, and 135.)

as in human bile, simple bile salt micelles and mixed-disk micelles coexist (Fig. 6) in varying proportions (128). These mixed bile salt micelles increase the micellar solubility of cholesterol over that of the pure bile salt micelles by about three- to 10-fold. It is now considered that molecules of cholesterol bind to the outside (hydrophilic face) of simple bile salt micelles (135) but are dissolved in the liquid hydrocarbon interior of mixed micelles (25). The incorporation of cholesterol into simple and mixed micelles results in only small perturbations (2 to 3 Å) in micellar size and apparently does not induce or require any appreciable reorganization of the micellar structures (25). When mixed bile salt-lecithin-cholesterol micelles (in bile) or bile salt-acid soap-monoglyceride-cholesterol micelles (in the gut lumen) are induced to grow in size either by dilution (which alters the bile salt-swelling amphiphile ratio in the mixed micelles) or by addition of more swelling amphiphiles, a critical size is reached (≈400 Å) where micelles spontaneously fold into closed, unilamellar vesicles or liposomes (25,128,139,140).

Bile

Native bile of man and animals has been conclusively shown to be a mixed micellar system of bile salt-lecithin-cholesterol coexisting with simple bile salt-cholesterol micelles (Fig. 6) (140). Upon dilution of the total lipid concentration, the size of the micellar particles (≈60 Å) demonstrates all the physical characteristics of model systems, with an abrupt growth in size as the phase limit is approached and subsequent formation of liposomes. Electron microscopy and light-scattering techniques show that about 0.1 to 1% of particles in bile are much larger than micelles (≈1,000 Å). These may be aggregated biliary proteins and/or self-aggregates of bilirubin conjugates (141).

Human bile is generally about 50% saturated with lecithin but saturated or supersaturated with cholesterol; hepatic bile is more supersaturated than is gall bladder bile (138). Available evidence suggests that the excess cholesterol in concentrated gall bladder bile is within the micelles, whereas the excess cholesterol in dilute hepatic bile forms separate 300 to 400 Å amorphous particles containing lecithin and are quite stable (142). It is not known whether these "microemulsion" particles differ in lithogenic versus nonlithogenic supersaturated biles.

Intestinal Lumen

In the small intestine during fat (triglyceride) digestion, the physical state of bile undergoes a number of important changes. During fasting or in the early stages of a meal, the relative lipid composition and chemical components of duodenal bile are the same as in the gall bladder (143) although slightly more dilute (5 to 7 g/dl). As fat digestion progresses, however, bile is diluted further, micelles enlarge (140), and a portion of the bile lipids acting as emulsifiers absorb *en mass* to the triglyceride interface (144,145). Interfacial micellar uptake of lipolytic products saturates the micelles with acid soaps, monoglycerides, lysolecithin, and cholesterol; further dilution induces the large mixed-disk micelles to fold into vesicles. During established fat digestion in man, saturated mixed micelles and vesicles containing the same lipids coexist (Fig. 7) in the aqueous phase of intestinal contents (139). The micelles and vesicles probably enhance transport of lipolytic products from the oil (triglyceride) phase to the surface of the enterocyte for absorption. It is not known whether these large lipid vehicles deliver their digestion products into the enterocyte by bulk fusion or monomer diffusion; evidence for these distinct possibilities is lacking. The presence of bile salt micelles, while not essential for the absorption of triglyceride

lipolytic products, appears to be required for the absorption of cholesterol and lipovitamins (146).

Stomach and Colon

Most bile salts precipitate as bile acids in the stomach and colon because their precipitation pH values are higher than the luminal pH (14,15). When bile refluxes into the stomach, glycine conjugates precipitate, but taurine conjugates do not. If the ambient pH of the duodenum is more acid than normal, such as in certain diseases associated with gastric hypersecretion (147) or pancreatic insufficiency (148), glycine conjugates also precipitate. In the colon, bile salts that escape from the enterohepatic circulation ($\approx$200 to 500 mg/day) and are deconjugated to form free bile acids also precipitate because of their high pKa values and, in the case of lithocholates, because of their high Krafft points (14). If the pH of the colon is slightly alkaline, free bile acids ionize, and a higher proportion will be in solution in the aqueous phase. When the bile salt concentration exceeds 3 to 5 mM, mixed bile salt-bile acid micelles can form. If the colonic pH is more acid, nearly all bile acid molecules precipitate as bile acid crystals (149).

PHYSIOLOGY OF BILE SALTS: DRIVING FORCES OF THE ENTEROHEPATIC CIRCULATION

Overview

The sequential process of bile salt secretion into the intestine, efficient absorption from the intestine, and recapture by the liver is the essence of the enterohepatic circulation (1,2,8,9). Hepatic bile is sequestered in the gallbladder and concentrated interdigestively, then emptied into the intestine in response mainly to cholecystokinin, a duodenal-jejunal hormone released by fatty acids and amino acids entering the duodenum. The majority of bile salts undergo little absorption until the lower third of the small intestine is reached. Here high affinity receptor sites actively absorb bile salts and transfer them to the portal blood where they are carried to the liver in the portal vein bound principally to serum albumin and lipoproteins. In the liver, they again encounter a high affinity binding and uptake site on the sinusoidal membranes of hepatocytes. Thus, they are almost entirely cleared on a single pass through the intrahepatic circulation. The efficiency of the two active transport systems results in little bile salt spillage into feces and extremely low peripheral blood levels (<5 μM). The enterohepatic circulation is powered by the continuous active production of bile into the biliary tree, intermittent contraction of the gallbladder, peristaltic activity of the

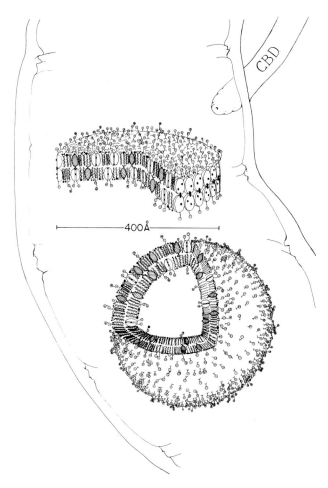

FIG. 7. Schematic view of the physical state of bile in the lumen of the upper small intestine in man. Here the mixed micelles are maximally enlarged with the products of fat digestion and coexist with unilamellar liposomal vesicles composed of the same lipids. (From refs. 29 and 139.)

small bowel, active transport by the ileocytes, and the portal venous flow (2). It is now apparent that, since the bile salts of man vary markedly in polarity, there are three enterohepatic circuits: one fast, one intermediate, and one slow (8). A high proportion of glycine-conjugated dihydroxy bile acids are mainly absorbed passively in the jejunum (150,151); taurine (and glycine) conjugates of the dihydroxy and trihydroxy bile salts are absorbed actively in the distal ileum (152); and unconjugated bile acids are absorbed passively from the colon (153). Conversely, at the sinusoidal membranes, the most polar bile salts are those most efficiently taken up in a single passage (154–156). While the conjugates predominate, peripheral blood is disproportionately enriched in mono- and dihydroxy bile salts rather than trihydroxy bile salts (8). A brief review of the mechanism of the various driving forces in the enterohepatic circulation follows.

Bile Secretion

The active secretion of bile salts from liver cells across the canalicular membranes into bile is the primary metabolic pump of the enterohepatic circulation. This is the rate-limiting step in the overall transport of a bile salt from blood or from *de novo* hepatic synthesis to bile (157). Most of canalicular water flow is a passive process that occurs in response to the transport of bile salts. A linear relationship is found between bile flow and secretion rates in man and other mammals (31). In man, about 10 μl of bile is formed per micromole bile salt secreted. Of the micelle-forming bile salts, all promote the same volume of bile flow per micromole (158). With an intact enterohepatic circulation in man, about 15 μmoles bile salt encumbers a bile salt-dependent flow of ≈ 0.15 ml/min (8). It is not yet clear whether in man bile salt-independent flow of water and electrolytes occurs at the level of the canaliculus; nor is it known how bile salts, with their complement of lecithin and cholesterol, physically exit from the hepatocytes and gain entrance to the canalicular lumen. Since diluted bile is transformed to a vesicle form, it is likely that mixed vesicles of bile salt-lecithin and cholesterol are formed intracellularly, somehow transported vectorially to fuse with the canalicular membranes, and exocytosed into bile. In fact, morphometric studies in animals suggest an increase in number and density of 1,000 Å vesicles in the pericanalicular cytoplasm during increased bile salt secretion (159). If this is the mechanism, the active concentration of bile lipids along the biliary tree could transform mixed vesicles into mixed micelles. The total metabolic driving forces within the biliary tree result in the continuous production of 800 to 1,000 ml of bile per day in an intact man; flow fluctuates greatly, however, and is reduced at night and accelerates with feeding.

Role of the Gallbladder

The gallbladder concentrates bile about five- to 10-fold by the coupled active absorption of sodium and chloride ions with passive movement of water (160). It is not essential for bile secretion but facilitates its storage in preparation for fat digestion. Interdigestively, it remains relaxed, possibly mediated by the antagonists, vasoactive intestinal polypeptide, somatostatin, and pancreatic polypeptide, and the absence of neurohumoral stimulation (161). Many mammals and birds have no gallbladder; humans after cholecystectomy do not suffer from maldigestion or malabsorption of fat. Recent studies in baboons and man (162,163) demonstrate that about one-half the hepatic bile enters the gallbladder for concentration and storage; the other half bypasses the gallbladder to enter the duodenum and undergoes continuous enterohepatic cycling. In response to cephalic and hormonal influences during eating, possibly via the vagus, cholecystokinin, and motilin (161,164,165), the gallbladder contracts over a 15- to 45-min period (166), during which up to 80% of its contents is discharged into the duodenum. The gallbladder, therefore, participates as a holding tank and mechanical pump in the enterohepatic circulation.

Intestinal Bile Salt Absorption

Bile salts are absorbed passively from all anatomic sites of the gastrointestinal tract (64), including slight absorption from the gallbladder (167). The active transport sites are localized in the ileum and, like the absorption of most other water-soluble materials, are dependent on the presence of sodium ions (168). While bile salts are absorbed passively to some extent all along the intestine, this is the major site of bile salt reabsorption in animals and in man (69,75). Passive absorption across the small intestine and colon may occur by ionic or by nonionic diffusion (64). For practical purposes, however, bile salt absorption by nonionic diffusion (i.e., of bile acids) is about 10 times greater than is diffusion of the ionized species (i.e., bile salts). Hence the relative contribution of each process is dependent on the prevailing intraluminal and membrane pH, the dissociation constant (pKa) of the individual bile salts (Fig. 8), the maximum solubilizing capacity of bile salt micelles for their own protonated bile acids (Fig. 8), and the partition coefficients of the ionic and nonionic species into absorptive membranes. At the normal upper intestinal pH (pH 5.5 to 6.5), about 50% of free (unconjugated) bile salts (pKa 5.0 to 6.5) will be protonated (un-ionized); a minor amount of glycine-conjugated bile salt will be protonated (pKa 3.5 to 5.2); and no taurine-conjugated bile salt (pKa < 1.8) will be protonated (Fig. 8). To be absorbed by passive nonionic diffusion, undissociated bile acids must remain in solution. This is achieved by a sufficient sup-

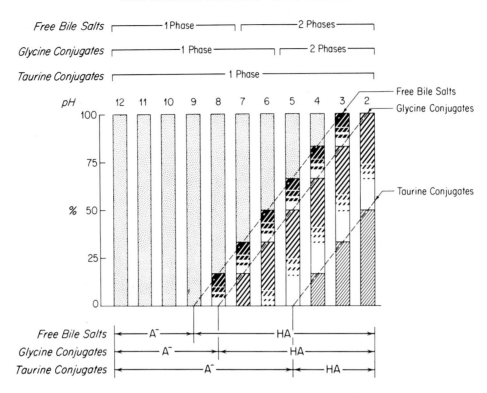

FIG. 8. Percent of bile salts ionized (A⁻) and unionized (HA) and the physical state of unconjugated and glycine- and taurine-conjugated bile salt solutions as functions of pH (14, 15).

ply of the ionized species, which can solubilize the protonated species as mixed micelles. An index of this function is provided by the pKa-pHppt difference of these solutions (Fig. 8). When large, it indicates that the bile salt solubilizes the bile acids poorly; when small, it indicates a high solubilizing efficiency (15). The precipitation pH values are pH 6.4 to 8.1 (free bile

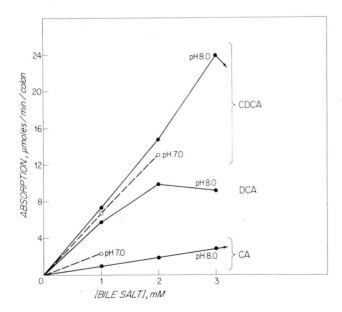

FIG. 9. Rate of colonic absorption of unconjugated bile salts in man as functions of bile salt concentration (abbreviations as in Fig. 4) and solution pH. (From ref. 153).

acids) and 4.3 to 7.4 (glycine conjugates) with ursodeoxycholate > chenodeoxycholate > deoxycholate > cholate. However, the taurine conjugates do not precipitate even at a pH of 1.0. Because the pHppt of chenodeoxycholate and deoxycholate and their glycine conjugates lie within the range of prevailing pH values in the upper small intestine, and because they are also less hydrophilic than are cholate or ursodeoxycholate (169), they are easily absorbed by passive nonionic diffusion. Similarly, free chenodeoxycholate and deoxycholate are absorbed better in the colon than is ursodeoxycholate (which precipitates at pH 8.0) or cholate (which is ionized at pH 6 to 7) (153) (Fig. 9).

The ionized taurine conjugates are almost totally dependent on the active transport sites in the ileum for their absorption (64). A reciprocal relationship exists between active and passive transport rates of bile salts. The most polar bile salts, which are absorbed poorly by passive diffusion in the upper intestine, have the highest maximal transport rates across the ileum. Conversely, the less polar bile salts, which are absorbed well in the upper intestine by passive diffusion, have lower rates of maximal transport in the ileum. As far as is known, bile salts with two or more ionic charges, e.g., sulfated and glucuronidated bile salts, are poorly absorbed from the intestine by active or passive means (113).

The quantitative significance of bile salt absorption at extraileal versus ileal sites is not known in man (8);

estimates based on studies in primates (75) and recently in man (150–153) suggest that as much as 50% of bile salts in the enterohepatic circulation may be absorbed passively at upper small intestinal and colonic sites. This fraction may increase as a compensatory measure in conditions of severe bile salt malabsorption (e.g., ileal disease) (170) when the fraction of the bile salt pool conjugated with glycine may increase up to fivefold owing to the rapid depletion of available taurine pools within the liver (171). It is not known what role intestinal motility plays in distributing bile salts to the various sites of intestinal absorption. Diminished motility may allow for a greater proportion of bile salts to be absorbed at proximal intestinal sites, whereas increased intestinal motility may drive bile salts caudal to the active ileal pump. Since the capacity of the ileal pump is easily saturated (173,174), this could lead to an overflow into the cecum and colon, increased deconjugation and increased absorption of free bile acids at colonic sites, and increased loss of bile acids from the enterohepatic circulation.

Portal Transport

All bile acids and bile salts absorbed from the intestine are transported in portal blood to the liver. Assays for absorbed bile salts in intestinal or thoracic duct lymph show negligible concentrations (176). In one report (175), the total concentration of bile salts in portal venous blood of anesthetized fasting patients undergoing cholecystectomy was $22.2 \pm 5.1 \mu M$. This value is six times greater than the levels in peripheral venous blood ($3.5 \pm 1 \mu M$). In the rat (176,177), values between 50 and 170 μM have been reported for the total portal blood bile salt concentrations; presumably similar values can be reached in portal blood of humans after a meal. Blood flow in the portal vein of man has been reported to be about 500 ml/min (8). Hence, ignoring the contribution from bile salt synthesis, a total portal vein bile salt concentration of 20 μM would give a bile salt inflow to the liver of about 600 μmoles/hr. This figure is in agreement with the calculated nocturnal bile salt secretion rate in man (350 to 900 μmoles/hr) (8,163). Even though the concentration of cholates and chenodeoxycholates in hepatic bile is about equal, portal vein blood is enriched in chenodeoxycholate over cholates (175), consistent with its more rapid absorption, i.e., in the upper small intestine (178), and more efficient conservation compared with the more polar cholates (1,2).

In blood, bile salts are tightly bound to both serum albumin (179) and specific lipoprotein classes, particularly high density lipoproteins (HDL) (180). There is apparently no binding to immunoglobins, fibrogen, or VLDL (180), at least in the fasting state. Both unconjugated and conjugated bile salts bind to serum albumin at pH 7.4, with free bile salts more tightly bound

than conjugated. The extent of binding is greatest with the least polar bile salts (e.g., lithocholates) and decreases with the dihydroxy and trihydroxy species (179). The presence of an oxo-group at either the 3-, 7-, or 12-carbon position of the steroid ring system completely suppresses the affinity for albumin, as does an elevation of pH (179). These studies suggest that a combination of hydrophobic interactions with albumin and an electrostatic bond are the primary forces responsible for binding. Since lowering the pH to 5.9 has no effect on the binding of deoxycholic acids to albumin, hydrophobic interactions are the dominant binding force. While serum lipoproteins were suggested earlier (179) as responsible for binding a considerable proportion (about 25 to 50%) of serum bile salts, the details of this interaction have only recently become available (180). When photoaffinity-labeled taurocholate is added to human peripheral blood in physiological concentrations (2.1 μM), about 30 to 40% of the label binds to HDL and about 15% to low density lipoproteins (LDL) (180). Within the HDL fraction, the bulk of the labeled bile salt associates with the lipids of the lipoprotein, while 10 to 20% binds to the apolipoproteins, predominantly apolipoproteins A-I and A-II (180). More work is needed to define the quantitative significance of each mode of blood transport.

Current evidence suggests that albumin and HDL may share equally the capacity of serum to transport bile salts with the more hydrophobic bile salts (e.g., glycodeoxycholate), being shared more equally than are the more hydrophilic ones (e.g., taurocholate), which are less well bound to lipoproteins (179). Obviously, both transport systems possess great reserve capacities. Portal blood and serum levels of bile salts can rise greatly under physiological and pathological circumstances. Patients with analbuminemia (181 to 185) apparently suffer no hematological or enterohepatic-biliary disorders attributed to overloading of the reserve capacity of the HDL and perhaps LDL to transport bile salts.

Hepatic Uptake

Hepatocellular uptake of bile salts is an extremely efficient process, clearing portal venous blood of more than 80% of bile salts carried to it in a single hepatic passage (1,2,8). Studies in animals (186–188) suggest that bile salt uptake is mediated by a sodium-dependent active transport system which exhibits Michaelis-Menton kinetics, specificity for bile salts, and is competitively inhibited by bile salts. Uptake is probably carrier-mediated since sodium-dependent bile salt receptors have been demonstrated in isolated liver surface membranes (189). Hepatic uptake is apparently related to the polarity of the bile salt and, therefore, is inversely related to the strength of binding to albumin and perhaps lipoproteins (179,180).

Studies on the first-pass hepatic clearance of serum bile salts in animals and man suggest that extraction of cholates is >90% compared with significantly lower extraction efficacies (75 to 80%) for chenodeoxycholates and deoxycholates (1,2,8). The fractional hepatic clearance of bile salts seems to be independent of their perfusate level, suggesting that the capacity of the liver for bile salt uptake exceeds the excretory transport maximum for bile salts into bile (157,190). Under normal physiological conditions, the uptake system of the liver for bile salts functions at concentrations well below its V_{max} for bile salts. That cholates are more rapidly cleared than are chenodeoxycholates suggests that the higher free monomer fraction of the more hydrophilic bile salts in serum may be responsible for their more efficient uptake. This suggestion is not supported by the observation that ursodeoxycholate, the most hydrophilic of all the major bile salts (135,169), gives rise to higher peripheral blood levels when fed to patients than does either cholate or chenodeoxycholate (8,191).

Extraenterohepatic Bile Salts

Feces

Free (unconjugated) bile salts are not found in the small intestine in the healthy subject. Conversely, conjugated bile salts are rarely present (192) in the feces. The conditions necessary for bacterial metabolism of bile salts are the presence of obligate anaerobes in concentrations above $10^4/mm^3$ (193,194). Such conditions occur only in the distal ileum close to the ileocecal sphincter, in the cecum, and in the colon. The possible number of metabolic products produced by anaerobic fecal flora is enormous. They include deconjugation, dehydroxylation, oxidation, desulfation, reduction, epimerization, and even desaturation of the steroid rings (192). Since the most common biotransformations of bile salts are deconjugation and 7α-dehydroxylations, the fecal bile acids in health are composed of deoxycholic and lithocholic acids (70 to 80%) and unmetabolized primary bile salts, cholic and chenodeoxycholic acids (7 to 8%) (106,192). Ursodeoxycholic acid is invariably detected in concentrations of 1 to 2% of the total acidic steroids. About 10% of fecal bile acids are iso-(3β)-lithocholic and iso-deoxycholic acids and a wide variety of oxo-bile acids, particularly 7- and 12-oxo-derivatives; lesser amounts of 3-oxo derivatives have been detected (106,192). The total number of the minor metabolites may extend into the thousands; most have been poorly characterized. Because in man the common hepatic metabolite of lithocholate is sulfolithocholate (Figs. 2 and 5) (20), and because secondary and tertiary bile salts may be involved as cocarcinogens or tumor promoters in colon cancer (195–198), the intestinal bacterial me-

tabolism of this conjugate has been carefully defined (199). The microfloral metabolism of conjugated sulfolithocholate involves deconjugation and desulfation with subsequent transformation of free lithocholate into a number of poorly polar derivatives. These include epimerization of the hydroxyl group at the 3-C position to isolithocholic acid, the formation of 3β-fatty acyl (palmitoyl, palmitoleyl, stearyl, and oleyl) esters of isolithocholic acid, and desaturation of the A ring of the steroid nucleus to yield the Δ^3-cholenoate derivative. That these and other specific intestinal metabolites of the bile acids may be possible biochemical markers of neoplasia is under active investigation in a number of laboratories.

Peripheral Blood

Based on the plasma disappearance of injected labeled bile salts in man and the rapid appearance of labeled bile salts in bile, all bile salts—whether acids or salts, free or conjugated, primary, secondary, or tertiary, sulfated or unsulfated—are rapidly taken up by the liver and excreted into bile (1,2). For this reason, the half-life of any circulating bile salt is probably no longer than a few minutes; yet peripheral blood levels in fasting healthy patients generally fall in the 1 to 5 μM range (8) and show little difference with prolonged fasting (Fig. 10) (200) or between arterial or venous blood (175). Since no appreciable flux of bile salts from hepatocytes into blood occurs in the healthy state and

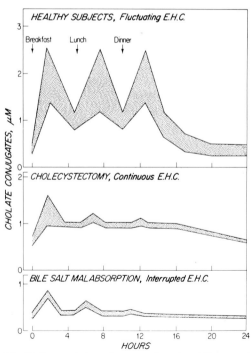

FIG. 10. Daily peripheral serum levels of the conjugates of cholate detected by radioimmunoassay. (Modified from refs. 200 and 201.)

because serum levels decrease with interruption of the enterohepatic circulation (Fig. 10) (8), the maintenance of appreciable peripheral blood levels is a result of continuous intestinal absorption and incomplete plasma clearance during enterohepatic cycling through the liver (1,2,8). This is consistent with the finding that ≈ 50% of secreted hepatic bile bypasses the gall bladder (163) which, therefore, undergoes continuous secretion into and reabsorption from the intestine. It is obvious that in the steady state, differences in the input from the intestinal side and output from the hepatic side result in constant levels during fasting (200). The relative bile salt composition is different between portal venous blood, peripheral venous blood, and hepatic bile. Venous serum contains fewer cholates since not only are they less well conserved by absorption from the intestines but the hepatocellular uptake and clearance are greater than for the dihydroxy species (1,2). The predominant bile salts in fasting peripheral blood, therefore, are chenodeoxycholate conjugates with smaller amounts of deoxycholates and cholates (175,200). The majority of peripheral blood bile salts are conjugated, but unconjugated species can be regularly detected (8), consistent with colonic absorption of the unconjugated species (Fig. 9).

During eating and gallbladder contraction, a striking rise in serum bile salts occurs (Fig. 10). In fact, monitoring of peripheral blood levels by sensitive radioimmunoassay techiques gives an index of the fluctuations of the enterohepatic circulation (200–202). The levels can increase two- to fivefold postprandially (Fig. 10) and are attributed to incomplete hepatic clearance during increased intestinal absorption of bile salts during digestion (1,2). In general, the conjugates of chenodeoxycholate increase more rapidly (peak 60 min) and to a greater extent than do the conjugates of cholate (peak 90 min) (150,200). Between meals, however, the serum values rarely fall as low as the levels detected before the first meal of the day (Fig. 10), consistent with the possibility that gastric emptying and duodenal/jejunal digestion and absorption continue between meals over a 12-hr eating cycle (200). The faster and more abrupt rise in the chenodeoxycholate conjugates compared with cholate conjugates is attributed to the more rapid proximal intestinal absorption of these bile salts together with their less efficient hepatic clearance.

The spikes in serum levels of bile salts persist after cholecystectomy (202) (Fig. 10), indicating that the common bile duct together with a competent sphincter of Oddi takes on a reservoir function. In the cholecystectomized dog, fasting common duct bile can be as concentrated as gallbladder bile (140). In severe bile salt malabsorption, the fasting serum levels of bile salts are low (Fig. 10); usually only a single large spike in peripheral blood levels is observed after breakfast (201,202). These results are consistent with studies of the jejunal concentration of bile salts in such patients in whom intraluminal levels are greatest after the first meal of the day (203). The pattern of rise in free (unconjugated) bile acids is different. When cholic, chenodeoxycholic, or ursodeoxycholic acids are ingested, rapid (30 min) elevations in peripheral bile levels occur. This results from absorption in the upper intestine and is consistent with passive nonionic diffusion of the less polar unconjugated species (191).

Urine

That arterial and venous blood levels of bile salts are not different (175) is in keeping with the belief that renal clearance and urinary excretion (Fig. 3) of the common bile salts are negligible (<10 μmoles/24 hr) in health (2,8). These values can increase dramatically in patients with liver disease, especially cholestasis (119–122,204,205) (>400 μmoles/24hr); the bile salt patterns change dramatically. In one study (126), the conjugates of cholate and chenodeoxycholate predominated (50 to 78%); deoxycholate and other 3,12-disubstituted bile salts constituted between 1.3 and 12%; and monohydroxy bile salts 7 to 15% of urinary bile acids. A high proportion of novel tetrahydroxy bile salts, hydroxylated at C-1 or C-6 positions, constituted 5 and 15% of bile acids, respectively. The glycine-to-taurine ratio is decreased (as occurs in many forms of liver disease) to about 1:1. A high proportion of bile salts is monosulfated in urine, reaching 100% for the monohydroxy, 90% for the dihydroxy, 30% for the trihydroxy, and zero for the tetrahydroxy species. In adults and children with cholestasis (205), significant amounts of the common bile salts are found in bile and urine as glucuronide derivations (sulfate-to-glucuronidate ratio 2:1); conjugates of 3β-hydroxy-delta-5-cholenoate are found in the latter group. Obstruction of the enterohepatic circulation of bile salts leads to increased hydroxylation at unusual positions on the steroid nucleus, increased conjugation with taurine, glucuronidation of hydroxyl functions, and sulfation of one or more hydroxyl functions, all of which lead to the formation of highly polar metabolites. These have weak abilities to solubilize membrane components (169), increased solubility in water, less affinity for albumin and HDL, and a high degree of clearance by the kidney (8). The contributing role of renal metabolism in inducing the formation of some of the metabolites remains to be elucidated.

KINETICS OF THE ENTEROHEPATIC CIRCULATION

In his doctoral thesis, Lindstedt (72) described the kinetics of 24-C¹⁴ cholate in healthy volunteers by a single pool model. With this, he introduced the isotope-dilution technique for the measurement of bile salt kinetics. Subsequent experiments in man have validated Lindstedt's results for cholate and have shown that the metabolism of chenodeoxycholate, deoxycholate, and lithocholate may be similarly described (1).

Definitions and Principles of the Isotope-Dilution Technique

The pool size of a bile salt is that mass of bile salt that dilutes an injected tracer dose of the same bile salt (206,207). Experimentally, a radioactive or stable isotope-labeled bile salt of known specific activity (SA) [distingegrations per minute (DPM) per mass, or atoms % excess in the case of stable isotopes] is injected; small samples of fasting gallbladder bile are obtained daily by aspiration of a well-mixed portion of the pool, i.e., bile-rich duodenal fluid after gall bladder contraction with the use of cholecystokinin or its octapeptide analog. The SA is measured daily for 5 to 7 days from the DPM or atoms excess of a stable isotope and the mass by chromatographic separation. A regression analysis of the natural logarithm of the SA decay is plotted versus time (Fig. 11).

Two reasonable assumptions are necessary: (a) the bile salt pool must behave as a single compartment; and (b) the pool size must be in a steady state, i.e., constant over the 5- to 7-day study period. The conventional exponential decay equation of a one-compartmental system in a steady state then can be used.

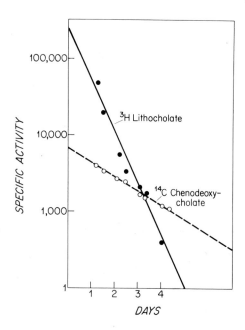

FIG. 11. Specific activity decay versus time (days) curves for a radiolabeled primary (chenodeoxycholate) and secondary (lithocholate) bile salt. (From ref. 1.)

$$SA_{(t)} = SA_{(0)}e^{-kt}$$

$SA_{(t)}$ and $SA_{(0)}$ are the specific activities at time t and time zero, respectively; e is the base of a natural logarithm and k the fractional turnover rate of the pool in dimensions of reciprocal time (time^{-1}). Taking the natural logarithm of both sides, we obtain

$$\ln SA_{(t)} = \ln SA_{(0)} + (-kt)$$

From this equation, it is obvious that the SA will decay with a slope of $-k$ (Fig. 11) and that the intercept at time zero will be ln $SA_{(0)}$. This value gives the SA of the bile salt pool if instantaneous mixing with the labeled bile salt had occurred. From $SA_{(0)}$ and SA of the injected dose, the mass of bile salts in the pool can be calculated:

$$\text{pool size} = \frac{SA \text{ inj}}{SA_{(0)}}$$

The first order decay of the SA decay curve represented by the slope $-k$ represents the fraction of the bile salt pool that is replaced by unlabeled bile salt per unit of time (Fig. 11); it is a function of the synthesis rate of that particular bile salt. Therefore, daily synthesis rate = pool size × fractional turnover rate:

$$\text{daily synthesis} = \frac{SA \text{ inj}}{SA_{(0)}} \times -k$$

Recently, simpler and more rapid variations on the Lindstedt principle have been introduced for the estimation of pool size (208), turnover rate, and synthesis (209). Both these variations employ a single intubation and single sample of duodenal bile. In the first (208), 24 hr after administration of the radiolabel, pool size is estimated, as in the Lindstedt method. In the other (209), ³H and ¹⁴C labeled bile salts are administered intravenously with an interval of 24 hr; the pool is sampled 24 hr later. From the ratio of SA values, the value of k, pool size, and synthesis rates can be estimated (209). Since both these methods have been validated against the classic Lindstedt technique and correlate well (208,209), they are likely to find wide applicability in the clinical as opposed to the experimental situation.

The synthesis rate of primary bile salts, such as chenodeoxycholic acid (Fig. 11), refers to the quantity formed from cholesterol in the liver each day (Table 2). In the case of secondary bile salts, such as lithocholic acid (Fig. 11), synthesis refers to the amount absorbed each day, i.e., total synthesis from the primary bile salt by bacteria minus that lost directly in the feces (Table 2). There is obviously a more rapid turnover rate of secondary bile salts, as shown in Fig. 11. When bile salts are ingested, the Lindstedt synthesis rate overestimates true synthesis since it represents the sum of both endogenous bile salt synthesis and intestinal input from absorption of exogenous bile salt (1,2).

TABLE 2. *Kinetics of individual bile salts in healthy subjects*[a]

Bile salt	Pool size (mg)	Fractional turnover rate (days^{-1})	Daily synthesis (mg)	Daily input (mg)
Cholate	500–1,500	0.20–0.50	180–360	—
Deoxycholate	200–1,000	0.2 – 0.3	—	40–200
Chenodeoxycholate	500–1,400	0.2 – 0.3	100–250	—
Lithocholate	50–100	1.0	—	40–100
Total	1,250–4,000	—	280–610	80–300

[a] Data are rounded off values from many investigations (see refs. 1 and 8).

Direct Measurements of Enterohepatic Circulatory Dynamics

The bile salt pool can be directly measured from the mass of bile salts drained by an acute bile fistula (210). While easy to perform in experimental animals (74,75,211), it is obviously impractical in man. Not only does the mass of bile salts in the area under the "washout" curve (Fig. 12) provide the size of the pool, but basal and derepressed (hepatic compensation) synthesis rates are also obtained (75,211). Despite the suggestion that istotope dilution gives pool sizes that are as much as 50% larger than that by the washout technique (212), there have been no rigorous validation studies in animals or man of the direct versus the indirect measurement by the Lindstedt technique (2,8,9). To achieve this, it would be necessary to measure bile salt synthesis (including input) rates and pool sizes of all the common bile salts by the latter method, since evidence suggests that the rate of enterohepatic cycling of all the primary, secondary, and perhaps ter-

tiary bile salts may be different. Hence, extrapolation based on the findings with one labeled bile salt cannot be related directly to the physiological pool of mixed bile salts whose composition, pool sizes, and synthetic rates may fluctuate continuously.

Synthesis can be measured in man and experimental animals by chemical assay of fecal bile acids utilizing balance techniques (192,213). Provided all acidic steroids are quantitatively assayed, this is probably the most valid method; in the steady state, fecal excretion is equal to synthesis. Synthesis estimated by the Lindstedt method has been claimed to overestimate synthesis by the balance method by up to 30% (212). In individuals with liver disease and biliary obstruction, it is necessary to perform balance measurements on urine, due to the substantial bile salt loss by this route, as well as on feces. The balance method may be the only valid measurement of synthesis rates in patients with severe bile salt malabsorption (1,2,8).

The amount of bile salt that enters the duodenum per unit of time is termed biliary secretion. To approximate hepatic secretion over short time intervals, the gallbladder must be kept in a tonically contracted state. If three meals and a fasting period are simulated, biliary secretion as measured by influx into the duodenum will equal hepatic secretion, provided the study period is sufficiently long (1,2). Only with recent developments in intestinal-perfusion technology has it become possible to measure directly biliary secretion of bile salts in man with intact enterohepatic circulations (78,79). Because the pool was easily measured by the Lindstedt method, it was assumed in the past that one could estimate secretion by assuming a constant recycling frequency and multiplying it by the pool size. With direct measurements of secretion, however, it is apparent that this intuitive concept may be incorrect (206) and that biliary secretion and recycling rate may in fact be inversely proportional to pool size.

Two methods are available for measuring biliary secretion: one may be termed the dynamic method (42,214), and the other the steady state method (78). In the first method, ^{3}H cholesterol, ^{14}C lecithin, and polyethylene glycol, as lipid and aqueous phase recovery markers, respectively, are perfused continuously into the duodenum. Three calorie-balanced liquid meals

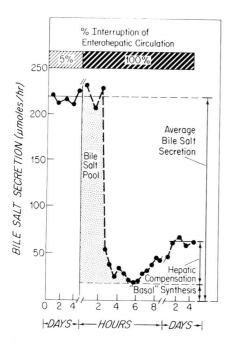

FIG. 12. Direct (washout) measurements of bile salt pool size and basal and compensated bile salt synthesis rates in a 5-kg rhesus monkey. (From ref. 211.)

containing traces of cholesterol and phospholipids, together with a ^{51}Cr meal marker, are infused into the stomach at meal times. Duodenal contents are aspirated continuously in 30-min portions through a tube with a port located at the ligament of Treitz. A fourth tube is utilized for reinfusion of the intestinal contents after *ex vivo* mixing and sampling. Thus the infused sonicated liquid crystalline dispersion of radiolabeled lecithin and cholesterol is used to correct for absorption of secreted biliary lecithin and cholesterol; secreted bile salts are assumed to be unabsorbed in the mixing segment for the 24-hr duration of the perfusion. This method yields dynamic physiological values for daily outputs of bile acids, lecithin, and cholesterol in relation to gastric emptying of meals, gallbladder storage, contraction, and subsequent refilling, as well as during an overnight fast.

In the second method (78,215), the patient is intubated with a three-lumen tube positioned so that two proximal outlets are adjacent to the ampulla of Vater; the third is 10 cm distal just past the ligament of Treitz. Liquid formula containing fat, carbohydrate, and protein calculated to provide the subject's daily caloric requirements and β-sitosterol as a nonabsorbable lipid phase marker are infused through one proximal outlet at a constant rate. Hourly outputs of bile salts and other biliary lipids are determined by marker dilution principles from the samples withdrawn proximally and distally. This method measures biliary lipid secretion under conditions of maximal stimulation and does not estimate the physiological fluctuations in the daily outputs and the markedly diminished output at night. Estimates of the 24-hr outputs of biliary lipids by both techniques actually agree quite well (1,2; Table 3). The hourly secretion rate by the steady (continuous infusion) method $\times$ 24 closely approximates secretion rates for a 24-hr period as measured directly (the dynamic method). More recently, Mok and colleagues (163) demonstrated that the hepatic secretion of endogenous bilirubin is constant and is unrelated to bile salt secretion. Thus bilirubin secretion could be employed as an endogenous marker to determine the rates of biliary lipid secretion and gallbladder storage during fasting.

Derived Measurements of Enterohepatic Circulatory Dynamics

From the direct measurements of 24-hr biliary secretion rates, daily hepatic synthesis by balance or isotope dilution methods and the semidirect measurement of bile salt pool size by Lindstedt's technique (72), two additional parameters of the enterohepatic circulatory dynamics can be derived (215), namely, (a) intestinal absorption efficiency of bile salts and (b) recycling frequency of the bile salt pool. The daily absorption efficiency is derived from the formula

$$\text{absorption efficiency} = \frac{\text{bile salt secretion} - \text{fecal excretion}}{\text{bile salt secretion}}$$

and the daily recycling frequency; the number of times the bile salt pool circulates during a day is derived from the formula

$$\text{recycling frequency} = \frac{\text{bile salt secretion/24 hr}}{\text{bile salt pool size}}$$

Values of Bile Salt Kinetics for Healthy Subjects

In healthy subjects (Table 2), the sizes of the cholate and chenodeoxycholate pools are similar. However, since daily synthesis of chenodeoxycholate is about half that of cholate, the average turnover of chenodeoxycholate is lower (Table 2). As discussed above, this is attributed to the more efficient conservation of chenodeoxycholate conjugates in the upper intestine (150,151) and unconjugated chenodeoxycholate in the colon (153) and is supported by the higher portal blood levels (175). Hence, there is a larger pool size of chenodeoxycholate for a given synthesis rate. The input of deoxycholate from bacterial catabolism of cholate is somewhat less than chenodeoxycholate synthesis (105). Since the fractional turnover rates are similar, the deoxycholate pool is somewhat smaller than the chenodeoxycholate pool (Table 2), and measured levels in bile are invariably less (Table 1). The scanty data available suggest that both input and pool size of lithocholate, the common bacterial catabolite of chenodeoxycholate, is much less than that of the other major bile salts (107). The pool size is kept small ($\approx$4 to 6% of biliary bile acids) (Table 1); when lithocholate passes through the liver, it is not only conjugated with glycine and taurine but also $\approx$80% is sulfated at the 3-OH position (20,21,107). These sulfates are poorly absorbed, either actively or passively (112,113); consequently, intestinal conservation is small (Fig. 5). As a result, its fractional turnover rate is as much as five times larger (1,107) than that of deoxycholate or chenodeoxycholate (Fig. 11).

Using classic or curtailed Lindstedt methods (72, 208,209), the size of the total bile salt pool has been estimated from the ratio of an administered isotopically labeled bile salt to total bile acids (SA) rather than employing individual isotopes for each major bile salt in the pool (8). In fact, measurement of the bile salt pool can be combined with bile salt secretory studies utilizing marker dilution techniques (214,215). These estimates (Table 3) are in fair agreement with the summed data in Table 2 giving total bile salt pools in the range of 1,400 to 4,800 mg. Recent attention has been drawn to the fact that the fasting bile acid pool, as measured in the classic or curtailed Lindstedt method, may not be equal to the circulating pool, as measured

TABLE 3. *Kinetics of the total bile salt pool in healthy 70-kg man*[a]

Method	Pool size (mg)	Synthesis by balance (mg/day)	Secretion		Cycling frequency	Absorption %
			(mg/hr)	(g/day)	(day^{-1})	
Steady state	1,500–4,400	250–500	700–1,700	17–40	6–15	97–99
Dynamic	1,400–4,800	200–800	400–920	11–22	4–10	93–96

[a] Based on data in refs. 213–215.

during marker-dilution secretory studies (216). The fasting pool size may exceed the circulatory pool size by 33 ± 20% when assayed in the same healthy volunteers. Since the differences in the two pool sizes were inversely related to the percentage of the pool emptied during the first perfusion hour, the circulating pool size may be artifactually reduced due to incomplete gall bladder emptying (216).

When bile salt secretion rates are measured by the dynamic or steady-state methods (41–59,214,215), the results are slightly different (Table 3). In general, the dynamic method gives somewhat higher values, suggesting that the higher flux of bile salts returning to the liver may suppress basal bile salt synthesis rates. The potency of the stimulus for gall bladder emptying is of pivotal importance in such investigations and probably accounts for the variations reported between different studies (216) using the steady-state method (215,217). The use of amino acid solutions without fat (217) has been shown (218) to be especially ineffectual in stimulating gallbladder contraction and in stimulating small bowel transit time. As a result, the secretion of biliary lipids into the duodenum is less with amino acids alone, compared with liquid formula infusion (218). The cycling frequency of the pool and the absorption efficiency derived from these data suggest that the pool cycles four to 15 times per day in a healthy subject (Table 3). The recycling frequency depends on the stimulus to the two mechanical pumps that drive the enterohepatic circulation, i.e., gallbladder contraction and intestinal transit time (216), and hence may vary for the same pool size (216). The absorption efficiency in all studies is high (93 to 99%) and varies only slightly with secretion rate (Table 3).

Regulation of the Enterohepatic Circulation in Man

Only in recent years have the various regulatory components of the enterohepatic circulation been investigated in detail in man. Because of the complexity of the methodologies involved, much of our present knowledge has been generated in a small number of specialized laboratories. The best data available have been derived from measurements of bile salt pool size and secretion rates by intestinal perfusion methods incorporating an adequate stimulus for gallbladder con-

traction and where bile salt synthesis was determined by balance techniques or by modified Lindstedt methods (41–47,163,214,215). From these measurements, the recycling frequency of the pool and intestinal absorption efficiency of bile salts were derived. On the assumption that the size of the bile salt pool is the dependent variable, recycling frequency (days^{-1}), total bile salt secretion rate (micromoles per kilogram per hour), total bile salt synthesis (micromoles per kilogram per day), and absorption efficiency (percent) are the factors that should regulate the pool size.

The first and most striking correlation is that there is a significant inverse relationship between recycling frequency and pool size, normalized per kilogram body weight (Fig. 13); that is, the smaller the pool size, the faster the recycling frequency, and the larger the pool size, the slower the recycling frequency. This homeostatic relationship appears to be constant, irrespective of the clinical status of the subject in relation to gallstones, obesity, hyperlipidemia, or bile salt (chenodeoxycholate, cholate, and deoxycholate) ingestion (Fig. 13). The question then arises: Does the recycling frequency control the size of the pool, or does the pool size control the recycling frequency? Inspection of the schematic diagram in Fig. 14 shows that the engineering of the enterohepatic circulation can be considered to be four pumps in series, two metabolic pumps without storage capacity ("scrubbers") and two mechanical pumps with storage capacity ("holding tanks"). In addition, the liver in a "reactor" where *de novo* bile salt synthesis occurs in order to balance fecal bile salt wastage. The synthetic "rheostat" in the liver is under feedback control by the magnitude of the bile salt flux (mass hr^{-1}) returning to the liver in the portal vein. Since leakage and synthesis are balanced in the steady state, the system can be considered a closed loop where the rates of gallbladder contractions and small bowel transit times should govern the bile salt flux to the liver and *de novo* synthesis, which in turn will govern pool size.

A number of critical experiments support this principle. Institution of a 95% carbohydrate diet reduces gall bladder emptying in volunteers and diminishes bile salt pool size (219). The individual pool sizes of both cholic and chenodeoxycholic acids in volunteers significantly correlated with gallbladder emptying rate (220). The larger pool sizes found in subjects with

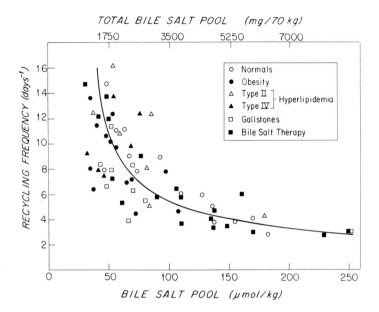

FIG. 13. Relationship of recycling frequency and bile salt pool size. (Data normalized for weight; collated from refs. 41, 42, 47, 163, 215, and 217.)

slower gallbladder emptying rates resulted from reduced fractional turnover rates, whereas synthesis rates of both bile acids were virtually independent of gall bladder emptying rates (220). In contrast, small bowel transit time was a determinant of bile salt pool size, possibly operating via feedback control of bile salt synthesis (220,221). Ingested sorbitol, a nonabsorbable sugar, markedly reduced small bowel transit times (84 → 44 min) in volunteers as determined by the rise in exhaled H_2 and induced a 27% reduction in the size of both total and individual bile salt pools (221). A reduction in bile salt synthesis and an increase in fractional turnover rate of the pool occurred concomitantly. In normal subjects eating three meals per day, larger pool sizes of cholic and chenodeoxycholic acids tend to be associated with slower small bowel transit times (220,221). This relationship is also dependent on synthesis rate of bile salt rather than fractional turnover rate. These relationships suggest that any factor

that increases intestinal motility, such as multiple small meals or ingestion of a high carbohydrate load, will accelerate delivery of the bile salts secreted into the intestine to the sites of absorption and will result in a diminution of the bile salt pool from reduced synthesis. Conversely, when the recycling rate is diminished from impaired gallbladder contractibility or prolongation of intestinal transit time, the bile salt pool will be dramatically expanded as a result of both a reduction in fractional turnover and an increase in synthesis rates. For example, propantheline bromide, an anticholinergic drug, slows gallbladder emptying rates slightly and intestinal transit times markedly (39 → 94 min) and results in a 50% increase in cholic and a 25% increase in chenodeoxycholic acid pools (222). Patients with celiac sprue (223–225) have abnormally slow gall bladder emptying rates as a result of impaired release of cholecystokinin (223) and sluggish transit through the small bowel (225). These abnormalities result in marked expansion of the bile salt pool, decreased cycling frequency, and reduced fractional turnover rates of the bile salts (224,225).

A number of animal experiments corroborate these studies in humans. In the rhesus monkey with an exteriorized enterohepatic circulation, an artificial increase in bile salt cycling frequency results in reduced bile salt synthesis (226); acute administration of atropine to slow intestinal transit times markedly reduces hepatic secretion of bile salts, presumably by slowing enterohepatic circulation of the bile salt pool (227). In addition, expansion of the bile salt pool by feeding one of the common bile salts results in diminished recycling (Fig. 13).

The question as to whether the size of the bile salt pool itself could determine its own recycling frequency remains unanswered. Also unknown is whether the inverse correlation of the recycling rate and total bile salt pool derived from bile salt secretory studies (Fig. 13) is

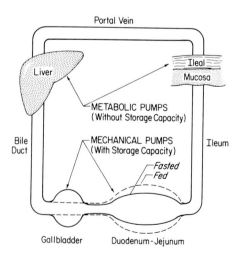

FIG. 14. Schematic engineering of the enterohepatic circulation to show four "pumps" and two "holding tanks" in series.

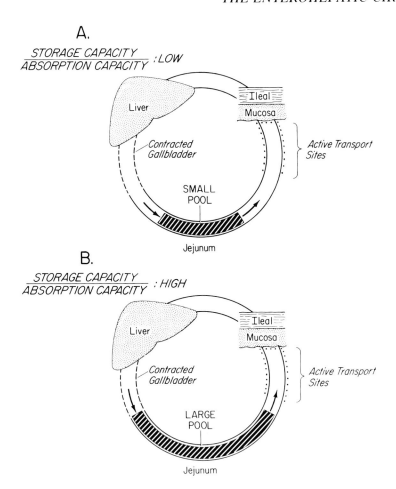

FIG. 15. Bile salt pool size per se may influence its own recycling frequency.

an artifact of the perturbation induced by the invasive nature of the investigation. Since the gallbladder must be kept contracted for steady-state secretory studies, it can be considered for the present discussion that the sequestering function of the contracted gall bladder (Fig. 15) is eliminated from the enterohepatic circulatory schema shown in Fig. 14.

In the case of both a small (Fig. 15A) or large (Fig. 15B) bile salt pool, the storage capacity of the enterohepatic circulation can be considered to reside solely in the upper small intestine. The recycling frequency will then be determined by the balance of the storage capacity versus the absorptive capacity (but not efficiency). In the case of the small pool (Fig. 15A), the storage capacity is high, occupancy is low, and all the pool can move rapidly to the distal ileal transport sites and be absorbed efficiently. In the case of the large pool (Fig. 15B), the storage capacity is higher but occupancy is also high and the ileal absorptive capacity is continually saturated; bile salts must wait their turn to gain attachment to the active transport sites. These considerations are based on the premise that bile salt synthesis is solely under the feedback control of enterohepatically recycling bile salts. A number of poorly understood humoral, circadian, and neural factors may also be involved. In particular, food ingestion is an important stimulus to bile acid synthesis

in man. For example, short-term fasting is associated with a three- to fourfold reduction in bile salt synthesis (228), and high calorie diets and obesity are associated with increased synthesis (229).

As shown in Fig. 16, there is only a weak correlation between secretion rate and pool size when the bile salt pool is small (<65 μmoles/kg) and no correlation between pool size and secretion rates for larger pools (215). For an individual subject, knowledge of the pool size is not an accurate prediction of the bile salt secretion rate. The weak correlation shown for small pool sizes may be important, however, since this is within the range of pool sizes reported to be more common in patients with cholesterol gallstones (76,163,230). Figure 16 also shows a tendency for these with low pools and gallstones (whether or not treated with cholate or chenodeoxycholate) to have an inappropriate lower total bile salt secretion rate for the same pool size when compared with those who do not have gallstones.

In Fig. 17, the total bile salt synthesis rate also bears a weak curvilinear relationship with total bile salt pool size. This is consistent with the previous discussion that as the pool size becomes smaller, recycling frequency is augmented, the flux of bile salts returning to the liver is increased, and bile salt synthesis is diminished. The role of bile salt return to the liver in the

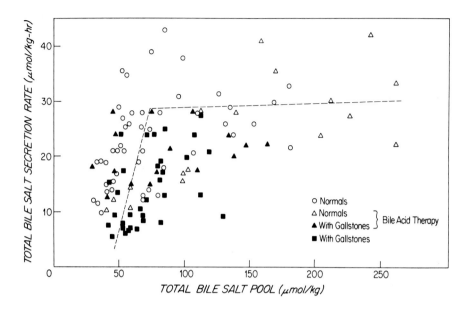

FIG. 16. Relationship of bile salt secretion rates to bile salt pool size. Data normalized for body weight. (From refs. 41, 42, 47, 163, 215, and 217.)

regulation of bile salt synthesis, is incompletely defined for man. The data generated from physiological studies on subhuman primates (74,75,211) allow one to extrapolate to man the important pathophysiological principle illustrated in Fig. 18. Bile salt synthesis from cholesterol in the liver is normally repressed to low levels (Tables 2 and 3) by the high flux of bile salts returning to the liver in the enterohepatic circulation. Synthesis is sensitive to the magnitude of this flux; increased synthesis occurs with decreased return, (Fig. 18), such as with ileal resection or a bile fistula. A maximum synthesis rate is attained and occurs with a reduction to ≈20 g return for man and does not increase with further decreases in bile salt return. In the rhesus monkey, maximum hepatic synthesis is five- to 10-fold the basal level (Fig. 12). Hence, in man with a

total bile fistula, bile salt synthesis can reach levels of ≈5,000 mg/70 kg/day. In contrast, basal synthesis can be decreased further, as with bile salt ingestion (Fig. 18), and reaches a steady but measurable level when the capacity of intestinal absorption is reached.

Finally, as shown in Fig. 19, there is a weak correlation between absorption efficiency and the total bile salt pool size in man (215). If this is real, then a small pool with its high cycling frequency affects not only synthesis but also fecal loss to a slight degree. This mechanism is operative in patients with ileal disease or resection; in patients with normal absorptive mechanisms, however, enhanced recycling of the smaller pools increases the flux of bile salts through the intestine. This in turn promotes a greater fecal loss which, although small, is sufficient to reduce absorption effi-

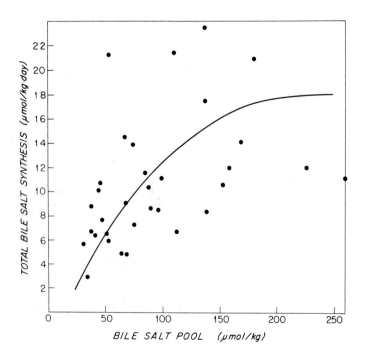

FIG. 17. Relationship between bile salt synthesis rate and pool size. Data normalized for body weight. (From refs. 42, 214, and 215.)

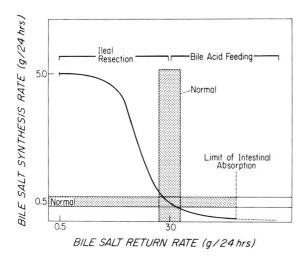

FIG. 18. Bile salt synthesis and secretion rates in man showing the influence of interruption of the enterohepatic circulation and bile salt ingestion.

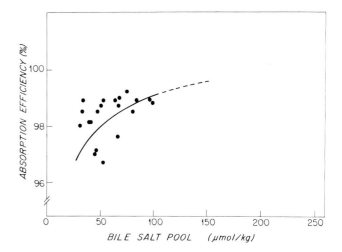

FIG. 19. Dependence of intestinal absorption efficiency on bile salt pool size. Data normalized for body weight. (From ref. 215.)

ciency slightly. This reduced absorption efficiency could also keep the pool small in the face of inappropriate *de novo* synthesis (215). Table 4 gives typical values and deviations for bile salt kinetics in man in relation to increments in pool size. The best correlations of pool size are with cycling frequency and less so with secretion.

In summary, the size of the bile salt pool is related to the balance between input from hepatic synthesis (plus bacterial metabolism) and intestinal loss. Regulatory mechanisms of the bile salt pool that influence these are multifactorial. As discussed, the chief one appears to be the recycling frequency. The information accumulated on the normal physiological control of recycling frequency suggests that it reflects a complex interplay of gallbladder storage and emptying dynamics, intestinal transit time, and efficiency of bile salt absorption. What relationship the fast, intermediate, and slow components of enterohepatic cycling due to bile salts of different polarities and the rates of secondary bile acid formation and absorption in the large intestine may play in controlling bile salt synthesis and recycling rates is unsettled at this time. Furthermore, the role played by cholesterol returning to the liver in lipoproteins as substrates for *de novo* bile salt synthesis is also unclear. In addition, the qualitative difference in the proportion of unconjugated versus conjugated bile salts and primary versus secondary versus tertiary bile

salts returning to the liver needs serious scrutiny since each may exhibit different effects on the feedback control of bile salt synthesis. More attention must be paid to the role of diet and the anaerobic flora of the colon in general regulation of the enterohepatic circulation in man.

PHYSICOCHEMICAL CORRELATES OF THE ENTEROHEPATIC CIRCULATION

Bile Salt Secretion and Cholesterol Saturation of Bile

The major functions of bile salts within the biliary tree are to promote the secretion of endogenous lipids and stabilize the physical state of bile; within the intestine, they aid fat digestion and absorption. The principal malfunctions of bile salts within these organs, i.e., cholesterol gallstones and fat malabsorption, are a result of a relative deficiency of bile salts within the enterohepatic circulation. Cholesterol gallstones have received much attention and have been a stimulus for recent pathophysiological studies on the enterohepatic circulation. Figure 20 shows that in animals and in man, curvilinear relationships exist between cholesterol and lecithin secretion rates as functions of bile salt secretion rate (42,48,214,217,231). Not only is the lecithin secretion rate greater than the cholesterol se-

TABLE 4. *Bile salt kinetics in relation to pool size in man*[a]

Group	Pool size (mg)	Synthesis (mg/day)	Secretion (g/day)	Cycling frequency (day⁻¹)	Absorption efficiency (%)
I (N = 8)	1,649 ± 275	334 ± 98	17.0 ± 5.5	10.3 ± 2.6	97.5 ± 0.6
II (N = 12)	2,464 ± 290	452 ± 262	27.2 ± 7.3	11.0 ± 2.6	98.3 ± 0.8
III (N = 7)	3,436 ± 409	436 ± 50	26.8 ± 7.6	8.4 ± 3.1	98.7 ± 0.2
IV (N = 6)	5,162 ± 1,087	394 ± 111	33.3 ± 6.7	6.7 ± 1.8	98.9 ± 0.1

[a] From ref. 215.

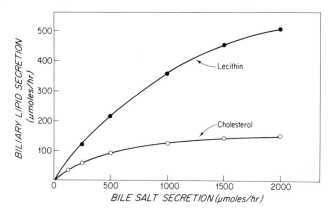

FIG. 20. Influence of bile salt secretion rates on lecithin and cholesterol secretion rates in man. (Means of data from refs. 48, 214, 217, and 231.)

$$X_{Ch} = \frac{\dot{Ch}}{\dot{BS} + \dot{L} + \dot{Ch}}$$

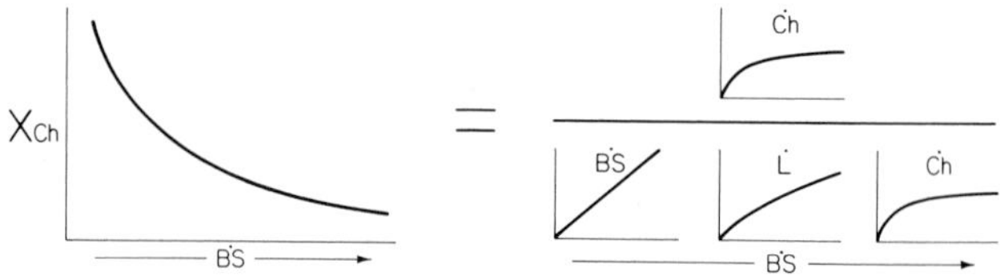

FIG. 21. Simple explanation of curvilinear relationship between cholesterol mole fraction in bile (X_{Ch}) and bile salt secretion rate ($\dot{BS}$). L, lecithin secretion; Ch, cholesterol secretion.

cretion rate, but both outputs asymptotically approach plateau levels at distinctly different secretion rates.

Because bile salt secretion is a linear funtion of itself and because cholesterol and lecithin secretion rates are different (Fig. 21), the cholesterol mole fraction in bile is relatively high at low bile salt secretion rates and decreases in a curvilinear fashion to fairly constant values at high bile salt secretion rates (Fig. 21). In fact, when the secretion rate falls profoundly in the fasting state, the cholesterol/phospholipid molar ratio of bile can increase from a normal of 0.25 to 0.33 at high bile salt outputs to 0.5 to 1.5 at low bile salt outputs (163). When the cholesterol mole fraction as a function of bile salt secretion rate is related to the capacity of human bile to solubilize cholesterol (Fig. 22), even in otherwise healthy subjects, bile becomes supersaturated with cholesterol at bile salt secretion rates of 1,700 μmoles (25 μmoles/kg^{-1}) per hour. Because the meta-

stable solubility of cholesterol in dilute bile is greater than in concentrated bile, bile does not become unstable in the normal individual (Fig. 22) until the bile salt output falls below ($\simeq$6 μmoles/kg^{-1}) per hour.

The Enterohepatic Circulation in Cholesterol Gallstone Disease

There is general agreement that, while normal fasting gallbladder bile is generally saturated with cholesterol, bile from patients destined to form gallstones or who actually harbor gallstones is greatly supersaturated with cholesterol (138) (Fig. 23). In hepatic bile, which is three to five times more dilute than gallbladder bile (138), the equilibrium capacity to solubilize cholesterol is reduced, and both control and gallstone patients demonstrate supersaturated bile. In both cases, the bile of gallstone patients is more supersaturated

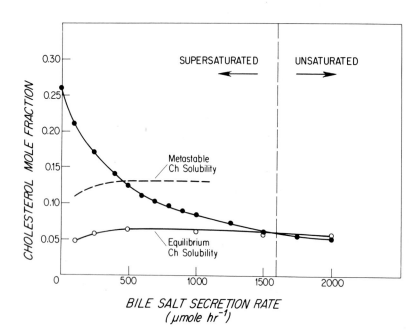

FIG. 22. Biliary cholesterol mole fraction and the physical state of bile (138) as functions of bile salt secretion rates in healthy man (48,214,217,231).

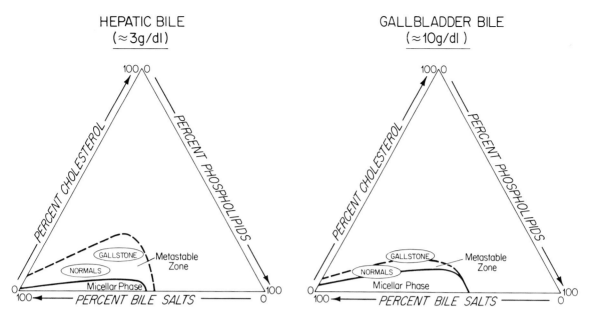

FIG. 23. Relative lipid compositions and micellar and metastable zones of human hepatic and gall bladder biles (138).

with cholesterol; but because of differences in metastability between dilute (≈ 3 g/dl) and concentrated bile (≈ 10 g/dl), only in the gallbladder does supersaturated bile become lithogenic in the gallstone patient.

The bile salt pool of many patients with cholesterol gallstones is smaller than in control subjects (76,232), and it has been suggested that the total pool size is diminished prior to the development of stones (230). Other studies (163) have found that, when compared with the mean total pool sizes of bile acids in control subjects, these differences are not statistically significant. Most studies demonstrating small pools were done on Indian subjects because of their high prevalence of gallstones (230,232). More recent work (233) in Indians and Caucasians confirms that the average bile acid pool in healthy women (who are at higher risk to form gallstones) was significantly smaller than in men (76,230,232,234) but bore no statistically significant relationship to age, race, and body size or to the percent cholesterol saturation of bile.

It was found (233) that the chenodeoxycholic acid pool size showed a significant inverse correlation with biliary cholesterol saturation. Because of the high recycling frequency of small pools, the bile salt secretory rates do not appear to discriminate accurately between gallstone patients and controls (Fig. 16), even though there is a weak correlation of lower secretory rates with small pool sizes. The fasting mean hourly outputs of bile salts estimated by Mok et al. (163) had a wide range [4 to 22 (mean, 11) μmoles/kg/hr] and did not correlate with whether or not the patient had gallstones. The most important pathophysiological relationship is shown in Fig. 24, where the percent cholesterol saturation of control subjects and cholesterol gallstone patients is compared (214) as a function of

bile salt secretion rate. Cholesterol saturation reaches supersaturated levels in gallstone patients at somewhat higher total bile salt outputs than in controls. In addition, owing to the steeper slope in the low range of bile salt outputs in gallstone patients, a transition of metastable to labile supersaturated bile also occurs to higher total bile salt outputs. This implies that (a) more cholesterol is secreted per mole of bile salt in gallstone patients if the bile salt outputs are the same as in controls; and/or (b) their average bile salt secretion is lower than controls and, therefore, their outputs are set on a lower part of the bile salt output axis. Consistent with the former hypothesis, the activity of hepatic HMG-CoA reductase, the rate-limiting enzyme in

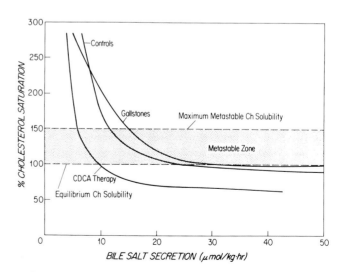

FIG. 24. Dependence of percent cholesterol saturation of bile (controls, gallstone patients, and gallstone patients on therapy with chenodeoxycholate) on bile salt secretion rate. (Means of data in refs. 42 and 214.)

cholesterol synthesis, is increased in cholesterol gall-stone patients and the activity of 7α-hydroxylase, the rate-limiting enzyme in bile salt synthesis, is reduced (235). Consistent with the latter are reports of diminished bile salt pools and low secretory rates (Fig. 16) in gallstone patients.

Recent studies (236) show that postprandial gall-bladder emptying is increased in patients with cholesterol gallstones and remains so after dissolution of the stones. This appears to result from increased gall bladder sensitivity to cholecystokinin (237). Thus altered biliary dynamics may be involved in reducing the bile salt pool. The synthesis and pool size-secretory hypotheses may not be mutually exclusive, but the exact relationships await further elucidation. It is likely that control of synthesis and pool size of endogenous chenodeoxycholic acid may be the major factor. When chenodeoxycholic acid is ingested, the relationship of percent cholesterol saturation to total bile salt secretion rate is dramatically altered (Fig. 24), indicating that, at bile salt outputs greater than ≈10 μmoles/kg/hr, bile is unsaturated with cholesterol.

As shown in recent studies (41–49,238), only chenodeoxycholic and ursodeoxycholic acids, but not cholic or deoxycholic acids, selectively decrease the secretion rates of cholesterol into bile (Fig. 25). Even though this effect is greater with ursodeoxycholic acid, replacement of the total bile salt pool with the conjugates of ursodeoxycholic acid does not desaturate bile at any bile salt output (Fig. 26). Even in the presence of physiological lecithin concentrations, the capacity of this micellar system to solubilize cholesterol is greatly reduced (239). Hence, the cholesterol saturation of bile is probably a delicate balance between the effects of endogenous chenodeoxycholate in depressing cholesterol output and cholate and deoxycholate, which elevate cholesterol output (relative to chenodeoxycholate). Since this pattern is also found acutely (238), it is likely that the decreased secretion of cho-

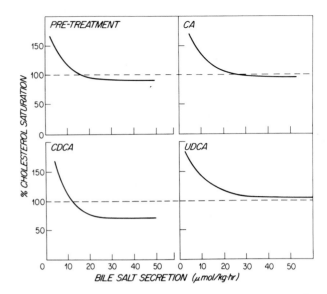

FIG. 26. Influence of bile salt pool replacement on cholesterol saturation of bile. (From refs. 41–48, and 238).

lesterol into bile effected by chenodeoxycholate and ursodeoxycholic acids results neither from their influence on cholesterol absorption nor on hepatic cholesterol synthesis. The most likely reason is altered cholesterol-lecithin-bile salt coupling during intracellular mass-transfer of lipids; the reasons for this are not yet understood.

PATHOPHYSIOLOGY OF BILE SALTS WITHIN THE ENTEROHEPATIC CIRCULATION

This section highlights a number of other derangements of the enterohepatic circulation of bile salts which lead to clinical disease and where, in many cases, the pathophysiology is better delineated than in cholesterol gallstone disease and the methods for characterizing the abnormal bile salt metabolism are better worked out. Because the enterohepatic circulation is interrupted in many of these syndromes, lithogenic bile and gallstones are often associated.

Defective Synthesis

Liver Cirrhosis

In liver cirrhosis, the metabolism of bile salts is markedly disturbed and is multifactorial in origin. The pathogenesis involves parenchymal liver cell diseases, portosystemic shunts, and altered lipoprotein metabolism. Kinetic studies have shown that patients with cirrhosis have a diminished total bile salt pool (240–242), which results from marked reduction in cholate pool size (240–243), reduction or absence of deoxycholate, and relatively normal pool sizes of chenodeoxycholate (240–243). The reduction in cho-

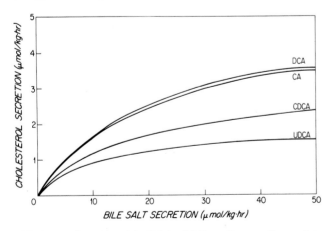

FIG. 25. Influence of individual bile salt secretion rates on cholesterol secretion rates in man. (Adapted from refs. 41–48 and 238.)

late pools appears to be explained by impaired synthetic rates of this primary bile salt, which result from selective reduction of the microsomal 12α-hydroxylation of cholate precursors (244). However, there appear to be multiple defects at different levels of the cholate and chenodeoxycholate pathways (244) in severe cirrhosis.

Based on fecal bile salt analysis (245,246) and *in vitro* cholate metabolism by cultures of fecal bacteria (246), reduction of the deoxycholate pool in cirrhotic patients results from impaired conversion of cholate to deoxycholate by anaerobic bacteria in the cecum. An alternative suggestion (8) is that deoxycholate is formed but is rapidly metabolized further by bacterial enzymes to tertiary bile salts. This mechanism is less likely since the fractional turnover rate of radiolabeled cholate is reduced in cirrhotic patients (240,241). A large fraction of primary bile salts is sulfated in cirrhotic individuals (247): approximately 27% of newly synthesized chenodeoxycholate and 8% of cholate. Similar to sulfated monohydroxy bile salts, these sulfates have a faster turnover rate appearing in both feces and urine (247–250). Hence, in the steady state, the sulfated pool accounts for less than 1% of the total cholate and for ≈5% of the total chenodeoxycholate pool (247). As a consequence of these multifactorial disturbances, the serum concentrations of nonsulfated, sulfated, and unconjugated bile salts are elevated (247,249,250); deoxycholate concentrations are reduced or absent (250–252) and, because of the liver disease, the plasma clearance of infused bile salts is reduced (8,253).

Because biliary secretion rates of cholesterol are apparently suppressed, presumably because of parenchymal liver disease, and/or the absence of deoxycholate, bile is unsaturated with cholesterol in cirrhotic patients (254). Consequently, cholesterol gallstones are rare in this condition, but the prevalence of pigment gallstones is increased (255,256).

Cerebrotendinous Xanthomatosis

Cerebrotendinous xanthomatosis (CTX) is a rare inherited disorder characterized by progressive neurological dysfunction, cataracts, xanthomatosis, premature atherosclerosis, low plasma cholesterol concentrations, and extraordinarily high levels of dihydrocholesterol (cholestanol) in all tissues, including bile and cholesterol/cholestanol gallstones (257). Bile salt production in these patients is diminished by about one-half and is attributed to incomplete oxidation of the cholesterol side chain (257), possibly as a result of inherited 26-hydroxylase deficiency (258). Appreciable levels of many tetrahydroxy and pentahydroxy bile alcohols accumulate in bile (257), and virtually none, or only trace amounts (3 to 5%), of chenodeoxycholate can be detected (257). Curiously, all the bile alcohols in the bile

of CTX patients are conjugated with glucuronic acid (259). Chenodeoxycholate therapy can be helpful in this condition by suppressing the abnormally high rate of cholesterol and cholestanol biosynthesis (257).

Cholesterol 12α-Hydroxylase Deficiency

Cholesterol 12α-hydroxylase deficiency is a rare syndrome (260) associated with lithogenic bile and cholesterol gallstones in the first decade of life, steatorrhea, intractable constipation, and often fecal impaction and low levels of duodenal (1 to 4 mM) and fecal bile salts (37 versus 250 to 500 mg/day in normals).

In the best studied example of this syndrome (260), the liver and intestine were histologically and functionally normal, but the pool of cholate was 153 mg and chenodeoxycholate 215 mg—each ≈ five- to sevenfold smaller than in matched control subjects. Synthetic rates were correspondingly reduced to 33 and 95 mg/day, respectively. Hepatic microsomal cholesterol 12α-hydroxylase activity was markedly diminished, and 7α-hydroxylase levels were in the low normal range. Cholate comprised only 17% of total bile salts, whereas chenodeoxycholate made up 77%. A patient with a similar clinical picture was shown to secrete large amounts of the glucuronide of unconjugated hyodeoxycholate (3α,6α-dihydroxy-5β-cholanoate) in her urine (261). This syndrome may represent a block in the synthesis of both primary bile salts with secondary induction of the primitive 6α-hydroxylase system to convert the high microsomal levels of cholesterol into polar bile salt glucuronides, which are cleared by the kidneys and excreted in the urine.

Types II and IV Hyperlipoproteinemia

Most subjects with types IIa and IIb lipoprotein patterns have subnormal synthetic rates of cholate and a diminished cholate pool size (262,263). In hyperlipoproteinemia type IV, the pattern is different; the total bile salt synthesis is above normal in about 75% of patients, mainly because of an abnormally high production rate of cholate (262,263). Cholestyramine therapy increases cholate synthesis in type II and chenodeoxycholate synthesis in type IV hyperlipoproteinemia (264). Following oral administration of cholate (265), the synthesis rates of both primary bile salts are inhibited. Subjects with type IV lipoprotein patterns appear to lose administered cholate more rapidly from the enterohepatic circulation, implying a reduced absorption efficiency and/or increased turnover of this bile salt. When chenodeoxycholate is administered (266), its pool size increased in both types of hyperlipoproteinemia, and cholic acid synthesis is diminished. However, for comparable biliary cheno-deoxycholate concentrations, feedback control of cholate synthesis was less sensitive in type IV than in type II patients. The metabolic origin of these anomalies of bile salt metabolism are not understood, but they have important clinical relevance since cholesterol gallstones occur with high frequency ($\approx 50\%$) in types IIb and IV hyperlipoproteinemia (267,268).

Defective Secretion

Other than defective bile salt secretion, which may be associated with gallstones and which appears to be secondary to dynamic dysfunction of the enterohepatic circulation, the other common causes of defective bile salt secretion are cholestatic syndromes and bile salt malabsorption, both of which interrupt the enterohepatic circulation (8). To these may be added a third, that of neurohumoral dysfunction or a biliary motor disorder due to defective gallbladder contractility and/or defective relaxation of the sphincter of Oddi (225).

Cholestasis

Any functional or mechanical obstruction from liver cell to duodenum may result in bile secretory failure (cholestasis). The most common causes are gallstones, neoplasms, drugs, and hepatitis. The end results are that the biliary lipids are shunted into the systemic circulation, leading to choluric jaundice and the appearance of abnormal LDL (269), one of which is a unilamellar (liposomal) vesicle (270) containing biliary lecithin and unesterified cholesterol in its lipid bilayer (271). In bile and blood, secondary bile salts disappear, and hepatic enzymes are induced to hydroxylate, sulfate, and glucuronidate, the primary bile salts (118–126,204,205,248–250), thus facilitating their renal clearance and urinary excretion. High blood and skin levels of biliary organic anions (perhaps some less common bile salt anions) may be responsible for the severe pruritus often seen. The decreased output of bile salts into the intestine reduces the duodenal-jejunal levels required for normal fat digestion and absorption (<4 to 8 mM); moderate steatorrhea (<30 g/day) is the result (27). With prolonged obstruction, progressive liver parenchymal cell damage ensues and ultimately leads to biliary cirrhosis.

Neurohumoral Imbalance

Celiac sprue is the best studied example of an intestinal enteropathy associated with an endocrinopathic component which alters the dynamics of the enterohepatic circulation (223–225). Defective release of gut hormones with eating leads to diminished gall

bladder contractibility and failure of the sphincter of Oddi to relax. Studies employing oral and isotopic cholecystography and direct measurements of biliary lipid output after an appropriate stimulus for cholecystokinin release indicate that the gallbladder either fails to contract or contracts late or incompletely in most patients with celiac sprue. Radiokinetic studies (223,224) suggest infrequent cycling of the bile salt pool and stagnation of bile in the biliary tree of celiac sprue patients. The taurocholate pool is increased two- to threefold; the half-life is prolonged; and decreased formation and/or recirculation of deoxycholic acid, the bacterial metabolite of taurocholate, has been demonstrated. Propulsive motility of the gut is also impaired in celiac sprue and contributes to sluggishness of the enterohepatic cycling of bile salts. This low cycling frequency should promote intestinal conservation of bile salts, yet the fecal bile salt output is slightly greater than in controls (272), suggesting impaired bile salt absorption in some patients with severe disease, probably reflecting involvement of ileal active transport sites and passive jejunal absorption sites. It is probable that other enteropathies with diffuse upper intestinal mucosal involvement, such as Whipple disease, tropical sprue, radiation enteritis, and diffuse jejunoileitis, may also be associated with neurohumoral imbalance of the gallbladder-biliary tree axis. A similar defect probably also occurs in the rare somatostatinoma syndrome, where contraction of the gall bladder is inhibited by suppression of the release of cholecystokinin, resulting in fat malabsorption and gallstones (273).

Defective Absorption

Since active transport of bile salts by the distal ileum plays an important role in the integrity of the enterohepatic circulation, any disease of the ileum (e.g., Crohn's, enteritis, resection, or bypass) can give rise to bile salt malabsorption (8,27). Depending on whether derepressed synthesis of new bile salts by the liver can keep pace with the loss, the symptoms of this condition may be bile acid diarrhea with little fat malabsorption (cholerrheic enteropathy) (274) or steatorrhea ± fatty acid diarrhea with little or no bile acid diarrhea (steatogenic enteropathy) (275). The critical length of distal ileal disease or resection which subdivides the two subclasses appears to be ≈ 100 cm as measured from the ileocecal valve (1,274,275).

Cholerrheic Enteropathy (Bile Acid Diarrhea)

In this disorder, increased hepatic bile salt synthesis can maintain the concentration of bile salts in the proximal small intestine within the normal levels required for fat digestion and absorption (27,274). The

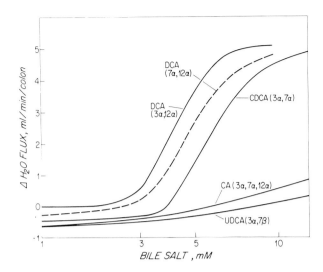

FIG. 27. Influence of bile salt species and concentration on colonic H_2O movement in man. (From refs. 32–34.)

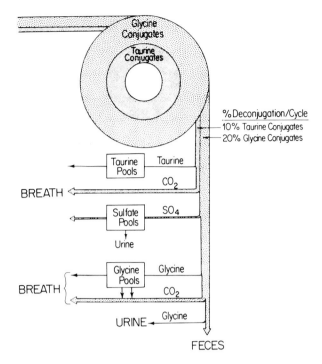

FIG. 28. Metabolism of the amino acid moiety of conjugated bile salts in the colon and in extraintestinal tissues. (Modified from ref. 1.)

patients may have watery diarrhea due to the effects of increased amounts of bile salts reaching the colon. Animal and human studies show that chenodeoxycholate and deoxycholate, but not cholate or ursodeoxycholate, (34,276,277) are responsible for fluid and electrolyte secretion when present in concentrations of >3 mM; the mechanisms have not been elucidated (Fig. 27). Bile salt sequestrants are effective in treating diarrhea in most patients with ileal disease or ileal resection of less than 100 cm (274,278).

Steatogenic (Fatty Acid) Diarrhea

With more extensive ileal disease or resection, i.e., > 100 cm, hepatic bile acid synthesis is inadequate to balance the magnitude of fecal bile loss and keep the bile salt pool intact. This leads to impaired micellar solubilization of dietary lipid in the intestine and steatorrhea (27). Like bile acids, many normal fatty acids stimulate colonic secretion (279); but hydroxylated fatty acids, which result from bacterial enzymatic hydroxylation of the double bonds of oleic and linoleic acids, have even greater secretory effects on the colon (280). The magnitude of the bile salt flux rate into the colon may keep anaerobic counts low. In addition, the colonic pH is more acid as a result of the fermentation action of bacteria and the loss of alkali (149). Because of their high precipitation pH values (15), free deoxycholate and chenodeoxycholate acids are precipitated (149), accounting for the relative unimportance of bile acid diarrhea in the more severe ileal resection syndromes. Increased bacterial metabolism of the amino acid moiety of deconjugated bile salts to mainly CO_2 in the colon (Fig. 28) can be detected with ease by oral administration of ^{14}C glycocholate and measurement of the levels of $^{14}CO_2$ in the exhaled air (1–3,8).

Measurements of the fecal levels of bile salts are necessary to differentiate this cause of an abnormal breath test from small bowel bacterial overgrowth (281). Both syndromes of bile salt malabsorption are associated with lithogenic bile (282) and an increased incidence or cholesterol gallstones (283,284). In addition, bile salts increase absorption of dietary oxalate from the colon with resulting hyperoxaluria (285) and an increased incidence of calcium oxalate kidney stones (286).

Small Bowel Bacterial Overgrowth

Often called the stagnant or blind loop syndrome, small bowel bacterial overgrowth is associated with massive contamination of the small bowel with anaerobic colonic bacteria secondary to stasis and fistulae. The anatomic and motor derangements responsible include surgical blind loops (e.g., Billroth II anastomosis), small bowel diverticulosis, scleroderma, diabetes, and jejunocolic and jejunoileal fistulae (8). In the classic example of this syndrome, the bile salt-metabolizing anaerobic gut flora deconjugate and dehydroxylate bile salts and lead to formation of sparingly soluble unconjugated deoxycholic and lithocholic acids within the small intestine (287–289). Only rarely do these hydrophobic bile acids precipitate intraluminally to form bile acid-fatty acid (choleic acid) stones (enteroliths) (290). More commonly, the bile acids are ab-

TABLE 5. *Methods for characterizing bile acid metabolism in man*[a]

Organ	Function	Test
Hepatic	Uptake	Bile acid clearance
	Synthesis	Bile acid kinetics (isotope dilution)
		Bile acid balance (chemical determination of fecal bile acids)
	Conjugation	Chromatography of biliary bile acids
		Kinetics of amino acid moiety of conjugated bile acids
Intestinal	Absorption	Fecal excretion of labeled bile acids
		Postprandial serum levels
		Bile acid breath test
		Bile acid kinetics (isotope dilution)
Enterohepatic	Secretion	Intestinal perfusion techniques
	Pool size	Isotope dilution
	Absorption and uptake	Fasting state serum levels
		Immunoassay; chemical measurement
Bacterial degradation	Deconjugation	Bile acid breath test
		Kinetics of amino acid moiety of conjugated bile acid
		Aspiration of small intestinal content for chromatographic identification of unconjugated bile acids or isolation of deconjugating bacteria
	Dehydroxylation	Input of secondary bile acids by isotope dilution
		Chromatographic analysis of fecal bile acids

[a] From ref. 2.

sorbed by passive nonionic diffusion to enter portal venous blood and thereby short-circuit the enterohepatic circulation (8). By this means, intraluminal bile salt micelle formation is compromised (27), and unconjugated bile acids together with the bacterial overgrowth injure the small intestinal mucosa (8). This syndrome may lead to severe malabsorption of fat and other nutrients, including vitamin B_{12}, which bacteria absorb and render unavailable for ileal absorption (8). High serum levels of bile salts, particularly the unconjugated variety, are typically observed, but pruritus has not been reported (288). The ^{14}C glycocholate breath test has also been employed to make the diagnosis in clinically significant cases (291). When the fecal output of bile salts is not increased, an abnormal breath test differentiates small bowel bacterial overgrowth from bile salt malabsorption (281).

METHODS FOR CHARACTERIZING BILE SALT METABOLISM IN MAN

With the exception of the bile acid clearance technique, these methods (1,2) are summarized in Table 5 and have been discussed elsewhere in this review. For a discussion of the techniques of clearance tests and their possible usefulness as tests of hepatic function, the reader is recommended to read the excellent review by Matern and Gerok (8).

SUMMARY AND FUTURE PERSPECTIVES

Dramatic progress in understanding the molecular biology, physicochemistry, metabolism, and enterohe-

patic circulation of bile salts has been achieved within the last 25 years. As a result, important advances in our understanding of the pathophysiology of bile salt malfunction in relation to many gastrointestinal diseases have been made. Challenges remain, but we are likely to see much fruit from continued research with these fascinating molecules over the next 25 years.

ACKNOWLEDGMENTS

The author's research is supported by NIH Research Grant AM 18559 and Research Career Development Award AM 00195.

I am extremely grateful to the copyright owners and principal investigators who have allowed me to reproduce directly or in modified form several figures and tables from their original articles or reviews. I also wish to thank a number of authors for furnishing me with preprints of their work. Miss Elizabeth Steeves and Miss Krista Birardi typed the manuscript, and Mrs. Grace Ko helped to compile the bibliography.

REFERENCES

1. Hofmann, A. F. (1976): The enterohepatic circulation of bile acids in man. In: *Advances in Internal Medicine, Vol. 21,* edited by G. H. Stollerman, pp.501–534. Year Book, Chicago.
2. Hofmann, A. F. (1977): The enterohepatic circulation of bile acids in man. In: *Bile Acids. Clinics in Gastroenterology, Vol. 6,* edited by G. Paumgartner, pp. 3–24. Saunders, Philadelphia.
3. Fromm, H., and Hofmann, A. F. (1975): The importance of bile acids in human diseases. In: *Ergenbnisse der Innere Medizin und Kinderheilkunde, Vol. 37,* edited by P. Frick,

G.-A. von Harnack, G. A. Martini, A. Prader, R. Schoen, and H. P. Wolff, pp. 149–192, Springer-Verlag, New York.

4. Greim, H. (1976): Bile acids in hepato-biliary diseases. In: *The Bile Acids, Vol. 3*, edited by P. P. Nair and D. Kritchevsky, pp. 53–80. Plenum, New York.

5. Small, D. M., Dowling, R. H., and Redinger, R. N. (1972): The enterohepatic circulation of bile salts. *Arch. Intern. Med.*, 130:552–573.

6. Dowling, R. H. (1972): The enterohepatic circulation. *Gastroenterology*, 62:122–140.

7. Heaton, K. W. (1972): *Bile Salts in Health and Disease*. Churchill Livingstone, Edinburgh.

8. Matern, S., and Gerok, W. (1979): Pathophysiology of the enterohepatic circulation. *Rev. Physiol. Biochem. Pharmacol.*, 85:126–204.

9. Heaton, K. W. (1969): The importance of keeping bile salts in their place. *Gut*, 10:857–863.

10. Smith, R. L. (1971): Excretion of drugs in bile. In: *Handbook of Experimental Pharmacology, Vol. 28*, edited by B. B. Brodie and J. R. Gillette, pp. 354–389. Springer-Verlag, New York.

11. Smith, R. L. (1973): *The Excretory Function of Bile*. Chapman and Hall, London.

12. Danielsson, H. (1973): Mechanism of bile acid synthesis. In: *The Bile Acids, Vol. 3*, edited by P. P. Nair and D. Kritchevsky, pp. 1–32. Plenum, New York.

13. Danielsson, H. and Sjövall, J. (1975): Bile acid metabolism. *Ann. Rev. Biochem.*, 44:233–253.

14. Small, D. M. (1971): The physical chemistry of cholanic acids. In: *The Bile Acids, Vol. 1*, edited by P. P. Nair and D. Kritchevsky, pp. 249–356. Plenum, New York.

15. Igimi, H. and Carey, M. C. (1980): pH-solubility relations of chenodeoxycholic and ursodeoxycholic acids. Physical-chemical basis for dissimilar solutions and membrane phenomena. *J. Lipid Res.*, 21:72–90.

16. Haslewood, G. A. D., Murphy, G. M., and Richardson, J. (1973): A direct assay for 7-hydroxy bile acids and their conjugates. *Clin. Sci.*, 44:95–98.

17. MacDonald, I. A., Hutchison, D. M., and Forrest, T. P. (1981): Formation of urso- and ursodeoxycholic acids from primary bile acids by *Clostridium absonum*. *J. Lipid Res.*, 22:458–466.

18. Higashi, S., Setoguchi, T., and Katsuki, T. (1979): Conversion of 7-ketolithocholic acid to ursodeoxycholic acid by human intestinal anaerobic microorganism: Interchangeability of chenodeoxycholic acid and ursodeoxycholic acid. *Jpn. J. Gastroenterol.*, 14:417–424.

19. Edenharder, R., and Knaflic, T. (1981): Epimerization of chenodeoxycholic acid to ursodeoxycholic acid by human intestinal lecithinase lipase-negative clostridia. *J. Lipid Res.*, 22:652–658.

20. Cowan, A. E., Korman, M. G., Hofmann, A. F., and Cass, O. W. (1975): Metabolism of lithocholate in healthy man. I. Biotransformation and biliary excretion of intravenously administered lithocholate, lithocholylglycine and their sulfates. *Gastroenterology*, 69:59–66.

21. Allan, R. N., Thistle, J. L., and Hofmann, A. F. (1976): Lithocholate metabolism during chemotherapy for gallstone dissolution. II. Absorption and sulfation. *Gut*, 17:413–419.

22. Fromm, H., Farivar, S., Carlson, G. L., Hofmann, A. F., and Amin, P. (1977): Hepatic formation of ursodeoxycholic acid and chenodeoxycholic acid from 7-ketolithocholic acid in man. *Gastroenterology*, 73:1221 (*Abstr.*).

23. Small, D. M. (1977): Liquid crystals in living and dying systems. *J. Colloid Interface Sci.*, 58:581–602.

24. Carey, M. C., and Small, D. M. (1972): Micelle formation by bile salts: Physical-chemical and thermodynamic considerations. *Arch. Int. Med.*, 130:506–527.

25. Mazer, N. A., Benedek, G. B., and Carey, M. C. (1982): Micellization, solubilization and microemulsions in aqueous biliary lipid systems. In: *Solution Behavior of Surfactants— Theoretical and Applied Aspects*, edited by E. J. Fendler and K. L. Mittal, Plenum, New York.

26. Wilson, J. D. (1972): The role of bile acids in the overall regulation of steroid metabolism. *Arch. Int. Med.*, 130:493–505.

27. Poley, J. R. (1977): Fat digestion and absorption in lipase and bile acid deficiency. In: *Lipid Absorption: Biochemical and Clinical Aspects*, edited by K. Rommel, H. Goebell, and R. Böhmer, pp. 151–202. MTP Press, Lancaster.

28. Carey, M. C. (1980): Lipases, bile salts and fat digestion: New insights. *Ital. J. Gastroenterol.*, 12:140–145.

29. Stafford, R. J., and Carey, M. C. (1981): Physical-chemical nature of the aqueous lipids in intestinal content after a fatty meal: Revision of the Hofmann-Borgström hypothesis. *Clin. Res.*, 29:511A.

30. Ockner, R. K., and Isselbacher, K. J. (1974): Recent concepts of intestinal fat absorption. In: *Rev. Physiol. Biochem. Pharmacol., Vol. 71*, pp. 107–146. Springer-Verlag, New York.

31. Erlinger, S., and Dhumeaux, D. (1974): Mechanisms and control of secretion of bile water and electrolytes. *Gastroenterology*, 66:281–304.

32. Wingate, D. L., Phillips, S. F., and Hofmann, A. F. (1973): The effect of glycine conjugated bile acids with or without lecithin on water and glucose absorption in the perfused human jejunum. *J. Clin. Invest.*, 52:1230–1236.

33. Mekhjian, H. S., Phillips, S. F., and Hofmann, A. F. (1971): Colonic secretion of water and electrolytes induced by bile acids: Perfusion studies in man. *J. Clin. Invest.*, 50:1569–1577.

34. Chadwick, V. S., Gaginella, T. S., Carlson, G. L., Debongnie, J. C., Phillips, S. E., and Hofmann, A. F. (1979): Effect of molecular structure on bile acid-induced alterations in absorptive function, permeability and morphology in the perfused rabbit colon. *J. Lab. Clin. Med.*, 94:661–674.

35. Hernell, O. (1975): Human milk lipases III. Physiological implications of the bile salt-stimulated lipase. *Eur. J. Clin. Invest.*, 5:267–272.

36. Borgström, B., Erlanson-Albertsson, C., and Wieloch, T. (1979): Pancreatic colipase: Chemistry and physiology. *J. Lipid Res.*, 20:805–816.

37. Pieterson, W. A., Volwerk, J. J., and deHaas, G. H. (1974): Interaction of phospholipase A$_2$ and its zymogen with divalent metal ions. *Biochemistry*, 13:1439–1445.

38. Volwerk, J. J., Pieterson, W. A., and deHaas, G. H. (1974): Histidine at the active site of phospholipase A$_2$. *Biochemistry*, 13:1446–1454.

39. Hyun, J., Kothari, H., Herm, E., Mortenson, J., Treadwell, C. R., and Vahouny, G. V. (1969): Purification and properties of pancreatic juice cholesterol esterase. *J. Biol. Chem.*, 244:1937–1945.

40. Borja, C. R., Vahouny, G. V., and Treadwell, C. R. (1964): Role of bile and pancreatic juice in cholesterol absorption and esterification. *Am. J. Physiol.*, 206:223–228.

41. LaRusso, N. F., Hoffman, N. E., Hofmann, A. F., Northfield, T. C., and Thistle, J. L. (1965): Effect of primary bile acid ingestion on bile acid metabolism and biliary lipid secretion in gallstone patients. *Gastroenterology*, 69:1301–1314.

42. Northfield, T. C., LaRusso, N. F., and Hofmann, A. F. (1975): Biliary lipid output during three meals and an overnight fast. II. Effect of chenodeoxycholic acid treatment in gallstone subjects. *Gut*, 16:12–17.

43. Adler, R. D., Bennion, L. J., Duane, W. C., and Grundy, S. M. (1975): Effects of low doses of chenodeoxycholic acid feeding on biliary lipid metabolism. *Gastroenterology*, 68:326–334.

44. Einarsson, K., and Grundy, S. M. (1980): Effects of feeding cholic acid and chenodeoxycholic acid on cholesterol absorption and hepatic secretion of biliary lipids in man. *J. Lipid Res.*, 21:23–34.

45. von Bergmann, K., Gutsfeld, M., Schulze-Hagen, K., and von Unruh, G. (1979): Effects of ursodeoxycholic acid on biliary lipid secretion in patients with radiolucent gallstones. In: *Biological Effects of Bile Acids*, edited by G. Paumgartner, A. Stiehl, and W. Gerok, pp. 61–66. MTP Press, Lancaster.

46. Roda, E., Mazzella, G., Roda, A., Gerinau, S., Festi, D., Aldini, R., and Barbara, L. (1981): Effect of chenodeoxycholic acid and ursodeoxycholic acid administration on biliary lipid secretion in normal weight and obese gallstone patients. In: *Bile Acids and Lipids*, edited by G. Paumgartner, A. Stiehl, and W. Gerok, pp. 189–193. MTP Press, Lancaster.

47. LaRusso, N. F., Szezepanik, P. A., and Hofmann, A. F. (1977): The effect of deoxycholic acid ingestion on bile acid metabolism and biliary lipid secretion in normal subjects. *Gastroenterology*, 72:132−140.

48. Lindblad, L., Lundholm, K., and Schersten, T. (1977): Influence of cholic and chenodeoxycholic acid on biliary cholesterol secretion in man. *Eur. J. Clin. Invest.*, 7:383−388.

49. Schersten, T., and Lindblad, J. (1979): Biliary cholesterol output during ursodeoxycholic acid secretion in man. In: *Biological Effects of Bile Acids*, edited by G. Paumgartner, A. Stiehl, and W. Gerok, pp. 53−60. MTP Press, Lancaster.

50. Gibson, T. (1684): *The Anatomy of Humane Bodies*, 2nd edition. Thomas Fisher, London.

51. Barry, E. (1759): *A Treatise on the Three Different Digestions and Discharges From the Human Body*. A. Miller, London.

52. Berzelius (1809): Cited by Sobotka, H. (1938): *The Chemistry of Steroids*. Bailliére, Tindall and Cox, London.

53. Sobotka, H. (1937): *Physiological Chemistry of the Bile*. Bailliére, Tindall and Cox, London.

54. Josephson, B. (1941): The circulation of the bile acids in connection with their production, conjugation and excretion. *Physiol. Rev.*, 21:463−486.

55. Gmelin, L. Cited by Strecker, A. (1848): Untersuchung der Ochsengalle. *Justus Liebigs Annln. Chem.*, 65:1−37.

56. Liebig, J. (1843): *Animal Chemistry, or Chemistry in its Applications to Physiology and Pathology*, 2nd edition. Taylor and Watton, London.

57. Lehmann, C. G. (1855): *Physiological Chemistry*, 2nd edition. Blanchard and Lee, Philadelphia.

58. Hoffmann, H. (1844): Zur Verdauungslehre. *Arch. Ges. Med.*, 6:157−188.

59. Hoppe-Seyler, F. (1863): Ueber die Schicksale der Galle in Darmkanale. *Virchows Arch. Path. Anat. Physiol.*, 26:519-537.

60. Schiff, M. (1870): Bericht über einige Versuchsreichen I. Gallenbildung, alhängig der Aufsaugung der Gallstoffe. *Pflugers Arch. Ges. Physiol.*, 3:598−613.

61. Weiss, A. (1884): Ce que devient la bile dans le canal digestif. *Bull. Soc. Imp. Nat. Moscou*, 59:22−32.

62. Tappeiner, H. (1878): Über die Aufsaugung der gallensäuren Alkalien im Dünndarme. *Sber. Akad. Wissen. Wien. Abt. III.*, 77:281−304.

63. Lack, L., and Weiner, I. M. (1961): In vitro absorption of bile salts by small intestine of rats and guinea pigs. *Am. J. Physiol.*, 200:313−317.

64. Dietschy, J. M. (1968): Mechanisms for the intestinal absorption of bile acids. *J. Lipid Res.*, 9:297−309.

65. Borgström, B., Lundt, G., and Hofmann, A. F. (1963): The site of absorption of conjugated bile salts in man. *Gastroenterology*, 45:229−238.

66. Whipple, G. H., and Smith, H. P. (1928): Bile salt metabolism IV. How much bile salt circulates in the body? *J. Biol. Chem.*, 80:697−707.

67. Borgström, B., Dahlquist, A., Lundh, G., and Sjövall, J. (1957): Studies of intestinal digestion and absorption in the human. *J. Clin. Invest.*, 36:1521−1536.

68. Hofmann, A. F. (1965): Clinical implications of physiochemical studies on bile salts. *Gastroenterology*, 48:484−494.

69. Hofmann, A. F. (1967): The syndrome of ileal disease and the broken enterohepatic circulation. *Gastroenterology*, 52:752−757.

70. Schmidt, C. R., Beazell, J. M., Berman, A. L., Ivy, A. C., and Atkinson, A. J. (1939): Studies on the secretion of bile. *Am. J. Physiol.*, 126:120−135.

71. Irvin, J. L., Johnston, C. G., and Sharp, E. A. (1946): The enterohepatic circulation of foreign bile acids: The circulation of cholates in hogs with biliary fistulae. *Am. J. Physiol.*, 146:293−306.

72. Lindstedt, S. (1957): The turnover of cholic acid in man. *Acta Physiol. Scand.*, 40:1−9.

73. Thureborn, E. (1962): Human hepatic bile: Composition changes due to altered enterohepatic circulation. *Acta Chir. Scand.* [*Suppl.*], 303:5−63.

74. Dowling, R. H., Mack, E., Picott, J., Berger, J., and Small, D. M. (1968): Experimental model for the study of the en-

terohepatic circulation in Rhesus monkeys. *J. Lab. Clin. Med.*, 72:169−176.

75. Dowling, R. H., Mack, E., Small, D. M., and Picott, J. (1970): Effects of controlled interruption of the enterohepatic circulation of bile salts by biliary diversion and by ileal resection on bile salt secretion, synthesis and pool size in the Rhesus monkey. *J. Clin. Invest.*, 49:232−242.

76. Vlahcevic, Z. R., Bell, C. C., Buhac, I., Farrar, J. T., and Swell, L. (1970): Diminished bile acid pool size in patients with gallstones. *Gastroenterology*, 59:165−173.

77. Vlahcevic, Z. R., Miller, J. R., Farrar, J. T., and Swell, L. (1971): Kinetics and pool size of primary bile acids in man. *Gastroenterology*, 61:85−90.

78. Grundy, S. M., and Metzger, A. L. (1972): A physiological method for estimation of hepatic secretion of biliary lipids in man. *Gastroenterology*, 62:1200−1217.

79. Brunner, H., Northfield, T. C., Hofmann, A. F., Go, V. L. W., and Summerskill, W. H. J. (1974): Gastric emptying and secretion of bile acids, cholesterol and pancreatic enzymes during digestion: Duodenal perfusion studies in healthy subjects. *Mayo Clin. Proc.* 49:851−860.

80. Berman, A. L., Snapp, E., Ivy, A. C., and Atkinson, A. J. (1941): On the regulation or homeostasis of the cholic acid output in biliary-duodenal fistula dogs. *Am. J. Physiol.*, 131: 776−782.

81. Hislop, I. G. (1970): The absorption and entero-hepatic circulation of bile salts: An historical review. *Med. J. Aust.*, 1:1223−1226.

82. Heaton, K. W., and Morris, J. S. (1971): Bitter humour. The development of ideas about bile salts. *J. R. Coll. Physicians Lond.*, 6:83−97.

83. Vlahcevic, Z. R., Schwartz, C. C., Gustafsson, J., Halloran, L. G., Danielsson, H., and Swell, L. (1980): Biosynthesis of bile acids in man. Multiple pathways to cholic and chenodeoxycholic acid. *J. Biol. Chem.*, 255:2925−2933.

84. Swell, L., Gustaffson, J., Schwartz, C. C., Halloran, L. G., Danielsson, H., and Vlahcevic, Z. R. (1980): An *in vivo* evaluation of the quantitative significance of several potential pathways to cholic and chenodeoxycholic acids from cholesterol in man. *J. Lipid Res.*, 21:455−466.

85. Shefer, S., Hauser, S., Berkersky, I., and Mosbach, E. H. (1970): Biochemical site of regulation of bile acid biosynthesis in the rat. *J. Lipid Res.*, 11:404-411.

86. Shefer, S., Hauser, S., Bekersky, I., and Mosbach, E. H. (1969): Feedback regulation of bile acid biosynthesis in the rat. *J. Lipid Res.*, 10:646−655.

87. Björkhem, I. (1975): Microsomal 12α hydroxylation of 7α[12α, 12β-^{2}H$_2$] hydroxy-4-cholesten-3-one. *Eur. J. Biochem.*, 51: 137−143.

88. Carey, M. C., and Igimi, H. (1981): Physical-chemical basis for dissimilar intraluminal solubility and intestinal absorption efficiency of bile salts. In: *Bile Acids and Lipids*, edited by G. Paumgartner, A. Stiehl, and W. Gerok, pp. 123−132. MTP Press, Lancaster.

89. Gustafsson, B. E. and Norman, A. (1962): Comparison of bile acids in intestinal content of germ-free and conventional rats. *Proc. Soc. Exp. Biol.*, 110:387−389.

90. Midtvedt, T., and Norman, A. (1967): Bile acid transformations by microbial strains belonging to genera found in intestinal contents. *Acta Pathol. Microbiol. Scand.*, 71:629−638.

91. Nair, P. P. (1973): Enzymes in bile acid metabolism. In: *The Bile Acids, Vol. 2*, edited by P. P. Nair and D. Kritchevsky, pp. 259−271. Plenum, New York.

92. Hepner, G. W., Hofmann, A. F., and Thomas, P. J. (1972): Metabolism of steroid and amino acid moieties of conjugated bile acids in man. I. Cholylglycine. *J. Clin. Invest.*, 51:1889−1897.

93. Hepner, G. W., Hofmann, A. F., and Thomas, P. J. (1972): Metabolism of steroid and amino acid moieties of conjugated bile acids in man. II. Glycine conjugated dihydroxy bile acids. *J. Clin. Invest.*, 51:1898−1905.

94. Hepner, G. W., Sturmann, J. A., Hofmann, A. F., and Thomas, P. J. (1973): Metabolism of steroid and amino acid moieties of conjugated bile acids in man. III. Cholyltaurine (taurocholic acid). *J. Clin. Invest.*, 52:433−440.

95. Aries, V., and Hill, M. J. (1970): Degradation of steroids by intestinal bacteria. II. Enzymes catalyzing the oxidoreduction of the 3α, 7α, and 12α-hydroxyl groups in cholic acid and the dehydroxylation of the 7α-hydroxyl group. *Biochim. Biophys. Acta*, 202:535–543.

96. Ferrari, A., and Beretta, L. (1977): Activity on bile acids of a *Clostridium bifermentans* cell-free extract. *FEBS Lett.*, 75:163–165.

97. Hylemon, P. B., Cacciapuoti, A. F., White, B. A., Whitehead, T. R., and Fricke, R. J. (1980): 7α-Dehydroxylation of cholic acid by cell extractions of *Eubacterium* species V. P. I. 12708. *Am. J. Clin. Nutr.*, 33:2507–2510.

98. Stellwag, E. J., and Hylemon, P. B. (1979): 7α-Dehydroxylation of cholic acid and chenodeoxycholic acid by *Clostridium leptum*. *J. Lipid Res.*, 20:325–333.

99. White, B. A., Lipsky, R. H., Fricke, R. J., and Hylemon, P. B. (1980): Bile acid induction specificity of 7α-dehydroxylase activity in an intestinal *Eubacterium* species. *Steroids*, 35:103–109.

100. Lipsky, R. H., and Hylemon, P. B. (1980): Characterization of an NADH: Falvin oxidoreductase induced by cholic acid in a 7α-dehydroxylating intestinal *Eubacterium* species. *Biochim. Biophys. Acta*, 612:328–336.

101. Samuelsson, B. (1960): Bile acids and steroids. On the mechanism of the biological formation of deoxycholic acid from cholic acid. *J. Biol. Chem.*, 235:361–366.

102. Ferrari, A., Scolastico, C., and Beretta, L. (1977): On the mechanism of cholic acid 7α-dehydroxylation by a *Clostridium bifermentans* cell-free extract. *FEBS Lett.*, 75:166–168.

103. White, B. A., Cacciapuoti, A. F., Fricke, R. J., Whitehead, T. R., Mosbach, E. H., and Hylemon, P. B. (1981): Cofactor requirements for 7α-dehydroxylation of cholic and chenodeoxycholic acid in cell extracts of the intestinal anaerobic bacterium, *Eubacterium* species, V. P. I. 12708. *J. Lipid Res.*, 22:891–898.

104. Hirano, S., and Masuda, N. (1981): Isolation and characterization of a bacterium capable of 7β-dehydrogenating bile acids and epimerization of the 7-hydroxyl group by combined action of this bacterium with 7α-dehydrogenating bacteria. *J. Lipid Res.*, 22:1060–1068.

105. Einarsson, K., and Hellström, K. (1974): The formation of deoxycholic acid and chenodeoxycholic acid in man. *Clin. Sci. Mol. Med.*, 46:183–190.

106. Eneroth, P., Gordon, B., Ryhage, R., and Sjövall, J. (1966): Identification of mono- and dihydroxy bile acids in human feces by gas-liquid chromatography and mass spectrometry. *J. Lipid Res.*, 7:511–523.

107. Cowan, A. E., Korman, M. G., Hofmann, A. F., Cass, O. W., and Coffin, S. B. (1975): Metabolism of lithocholate in healthy man. II. Enterohepatic circulation. *Gastroenterology*, 69:67–76.

108. Carey, M. C., Wu, S.-F., and Watkins, J. B. (1979): Solution properties of sulfated monohydroxy bile salts. Relative insolubility of the disodium salt of glycolithocholate sulfate. *Biochim. Biophys. Acta*, 575:16–26.

109. Norman, A., and Palmer, R. H. (1964): Metabolism of lithocholic acid-24-^{14}C in human bile and feces. *J. Lab. Clin. Med.*, 63:986–1001.

110. Palmer, R. H. (1967): The formation of bile acid sulfates. A new pathway of bile acid metabolism in humans. *Proc. Natl. Acad. Sci. USA*, 58:1047–1050.

111. Palmer, R. H., and Bolt, M. G. (1971): Bile acid sulfates. I. Synthesis of lithocholic acid sulfates and their identification in human bile. *J. Lipid Res.*, 12:671–679.

112. Low-Beer, T. S., Tyor, M. P., and Lack, L. (1969): Effects of sulfation of taurolithocholic and glycolithocholic acids on their intestinal transport. *Gastroenterology*, 56:721–726.

113. DeWitt, E. H., and Lack, L. (1980): Effects of sulfation patterns on intestinal transport of bile salt sulfate esters. *Am. J. Physiol*, 238:G34–G39.

114. Palmer, R. H. (1971): Bile acid sulfates. II. Formation, metabolism and excretion of lithocholic acid sulfates in the rat. *J. Lipid Res.*, 12:680–687.

115. Fromm, H., Carlson, G. L., Hofmann, A. F., Farivar, S., and Amin, P. (1980): Metabolism in man of 7-ketolithocholic acid.

Precursor of cheno- and ursodeoxycholic acids. *Am. J. Physiol.*, 239:G161–G166.

116. Bazzoli, F., Sarva, R. P., Fromm, H., Ceryak, S., and Sembrat, R. F. (1981): Lithocholic acid is formed from chenodeoxycholic and ursodeoxycholic acids at a similar rate. *Gastroenterology*, 80:1107 (*Abstr.*).

117. Hofmann, A. F., Thistle, J. L., Klein, P. D., Szczepanik, P. A., and Yu, P. Y. S. (1978): Chenotherapy for gallstone dissolution. II. Induced change in bile composition and gallstone response. *JAMA*, 239:1138–1144.

118. Almé, B., Bremmelgaard, A., Sjövall, J., and Thomassen, P. (1977): Analysis of metabolic profiles of bile acids in urine using a lipophilic anion exchanger and computerized gas-liquid chromatography-mass spectometry. *J. Lipid Res.*, 18:339–362.

119. Makino, I., Shinozaki, K., and Nakagawa, S. (1973): Sulfated bile acid in urine of patients with hepatobiliary diseases. *Lipids*, 8:47–49.

120. Stiehl, A. (1974): Bile salt sulphates in cholestasis. *Eur. J. Clin. Invest.*, 4:59–63.

121. Summerfield, J. A., Billing, B. H., and Shackleton, C. H. L. (1976): Identification of bile acids in the serum and urine in cholestasis. *Biochem. J.*, 154:507–516.

122. Thomassen, P. A. (1979): Urinary bile acids in late pregnancy and in recurrent cholestasis of pregnancy. *Eur. J. Clin. Invest.*, 9:425–432.

123. Back, P., Spaczynski, K., and Gerok, W. (1974): Bile salt glucuronides in urine. *Hoppe-Seylers Z. Physiol. Chem.*, 355:749–752.

124. Back, P. (1975): Evidence for bile salt glucuronides in cholestasis. In: *Advances in Bile Acid Research*, edited by S. Matern, J. Hackenschmidt, P. Back, and W. Gerok, pp. 149–152. Schattauer, New York.

125. Fröhling, W., and Stiehl, A. (1976): Bile salt glucuronides. Identification and quantitative analysis in the urine of patients with cholestasis. *Eur. J. Clin. Invest.*, 6:67–74.

126. Bremmelgaard, A., and Sjövall, J. (1979): Bile acid profiles in urine of patients with liver diseases. *Eur. J. Clin. Invest.*, 9:341–348.

127. Mazer, N. A., Carey, M. C., Kwasnick, R. F., and Benedek, G. B. (1979): Quasielastic light scattering studies of aqueous biliary lipid systems. Size, shape and thermodynamics of bile salt micelles. *Biochemistry*, 18:3064–3075.

128. Mazer, N. A., Benedek, G. B., and Carey, M. C. (1980): Quasielastic light scattering studies of aqueous biliary lipid systems. Mixed micelle formation in bile salt-lecithin solutions. *Biochemistry*, 19:601–615.

129. Carey, M. C., and Small, D. M. (1970): The characteristics of mixed micellar solutions with particular reference to bile. *Am. J. Med.*, 49:590–608.

130. Mukerjee, P. (1974): Micellar properties of drugs. Micellar and non-micellar patterns of self-association of hydrophobic solutes of different molecular structures—monomer fraction, availability and misuses of micelle hypothesis. *J. Pharm. Sci.*, 63:972–981.

131. Mukerjee, P., and Cardinal, J. R. (1976): Solubilization as a method for studying self-association. Solubility of naphthalene in the bile salt, sodium cholate and the complex pattern of its aggregation. *J. Pharm. Sci.*, 65:882–886.

132. Djavanbakht, A., Kale, K. M., and Zana, R. (1977): Ultrasonic absorption and density studies of the aggregation in aqueous solutions of bile acid salts. *J. Colloid Interface Sci.*, 59:139–148.

133. Mazer, N. A., Benedek, G. B., and Carey, M. C. (1976): An investigation of the micellar phase of sodium dodecyl sulfate in aqueous sodium chloride solutions using quasielastic light scattering spectroscopy. *J. Phys. Chem.*, 80:1075–1085.

134. Missel, P. J., Mazer, N. A., Benedek, G. B., Young, C. Y., and Carey, M. C. (1980): Thermodynamic analysis of the growth of sodium dodecyl sulfate micelles. *J. Phys. Chem.*, 84:1044–1057.

135. Carey, M. C., Montet, J. C., Phillips, M. C., Armstrong, M. J., and Mazer, N. A. (1981): Thermodynamic and molecular basis for dissimilar cholesterol solubilizing capacities by micellar solutions of bile salts. The cases of sodium

chenodeoxycholate, and sodium ursodeoxycholate and their glycine and taurine conjugates. *Biochemistry*, 20:3637–3648.

136. Saad, H. Y., and Higuchi, W. I. (1965): Water solubility of cholesterol. *J. Pharm. Sci.*, 54:1205–1206.

137. Igimi, H., and Carey, M. C. (1981): Cholesterol gallstone dissolution in bile: Dissolution kinetics of crystalline cholesterol (anhydrate and monohydrate) with chenodeoxycholate, ursodeoxycholate and their glycine and taurine conjugates. *J. Lipid Res.*, 22:254–270.

138. Carey, M. C., and Small, D. M. (1978): Physical-chemistry of cholesterol solubility in bile. Relationship to gallstone formation and dissolution in man. *J. Clin. Invest.*, 61:998–1026.

139. Stafford, R. J., Donovan, J. M., Benedek, G. B., and Carey, M. C. (1981): Physical-chemical characteristics of aqueous duodenal content after a fatty meal. *Gastroenterology*, 80:1291 (*Abstr.*).

140. Mazer, N., Schurtenberger, P., Kanzig, W., Carey, M., and Preisig, R. (1981): Quasielastic light scattering (QLS) studies of native dog bile—comparison with model systems. *Gastroenterology*, 80:1341(*Abstr.*).

141. Carey, M. C. (1980): The physical-chemistry of bile. In: *Drugs Affecting Lipid Metabolism*, edited by R. Fumagalli, D. Kritchevsky, and R. Paoletti, pp. 75–87. Elsevier, New York.

142. Mazer, N. A., and Carey, M. C. (1982): Quasielastic light scattering studies of aqueous biliary lipid systems. Cholesterol solubilization and precipitation in model bile solutions. *Biochemistry* (*in press*).

143. Vlahcevic, Z. R., Bell, C. C., Jr., Juttijudata, P., and Swell, L. (1971): Bile-rich duodenal fluid as an indicator of biliary lipid composition and its applicability to detection of lithogenic bile. *Am. J. Dig. Dis.*, 16:797–802.

144. Lairon, D., Nalbone, G., Lafont, H., Leonardi, J., Domingo, N., Hauton, J. C., and Verger, R. (1978): Possible role of bile lipids and colipase in lipase adsorption. *Biochemistry*, 17:5263–5269.

145. Lairon, D., Nalbone, G., Lafont, H., Leonardi, J., Vigne, J-L., Chabert, C., and Hauton, J. (1980): Effects of bile lipids on the adsorption and activity of pancreatic lipase on triacylglycerol emulsions. *Biochim. Biophys. Acta*, 618:119–128.

146. Hofmann, A. F. (1968): The function of bile in the alimentary canal. In: *Handbook of Physiology, Vol. 5*, edited by C. F. Code, pp. 2507–2533. Am. Physiol. Soc., Washington, D.C.

147. Go, V. L. W., Poley, J. R., Hofmann, A. F., and Summerskill, W. H. J. (1970): The disturbances of fat digestion induced by acid jejunal pH due to gastric hypersecretion in man. *Gastroenterology*, 58:638–646.

148. Regan, P. T., Malagelada, J-R., Dimagno, E. P., and Go, V. L. W. (1979): Reduced intraluminal bile acid concentrations and fat maldigestion in pancreatic insufficiency. Correction by treatment. *Gastroenterology*, 77:285–289.

149. McJunkin, B., Amin, P., and Fromm, H. (1981): The role of fecal pH in the mechanism of diarrhea in bile acid malabsorption. *Gastroenterology*, 80:1454–1464.

150. Angelin, B., and Björkhem, I. (1977): Postprandial serum bile acids in healthy man. Evidence for differences in absorptive pattern between individual bile acids. *Gut*, 18:606–609.

151. Angelin, B., Einarsson, K., and Hellström, K. (1976): Evidence for the absorption of bile acids in the proximal small intestine or normo- and hyperlipidaemic subjects. *Gut*, 17:420–425.

152. Krag, E., and Phillips, S. F. (1974): Active and passive bile acid absorption in man. Perfusion studies of the ileum and jejunum. *J. Clin. Invest.*, 53:1686–1694.

153. Mekhjian, S. H., Phillips, S. F., and Hofmann, A. F. (1979): Colonic absorption of unconjugated bile acids. Perfusion studies in man. *Am. J. Dig. Dis.*, 24:545–550.

154. O'Maille, E. R. L., Richards, T. G., and Short, A. M. (1967): The influence of conjugation of cholic acid on its uptake and secretion. Hepatic extraction of taurocholate and cholate in the dog. *J. Physiol.* (*Lond.*), 188:337–350.

155. O'Maille, E. R. L. (1977): Bile salt secretion. *Ir. J. Med. Sci.*, 146:190–198.

156. Hoffman, N. E., Donald, D. E., and Hofmann, A. F. (1975):

The effect of chenodeoxycholyl taurine or cholyl taurine on bile lipid secretion from the perfused dog liver. *Am. J. Physiol.*, 229:714–720.

157. Poupon, R. E., Poupon, R. Y., Dumont, M., and Erlinger, S. (1976): Hepatic storage and biliary transport maximum of taurocholate and taurochenodeoxycholate in the dog. *Eur. J. Clin. Invest.*, 6:431–437.

158. Lindblad, L., and Scherstén, T. (1976): Influence of cholic and chenodeoxycholic acid on canalicular bile flow in man. *Gastroenterology*, 70:1121–1124.

159. Jones, A. L., Schmucker, D. L., Renston, R. H., and Murakami, T. (1980): The architecture of bile secretion. A morphological perspective of physiology. *Dig. Dis. Sci.*, 25:609–629.

160. Dietschy, J. M. (1966): Recent developments in solute and water transport across the gallbladder epithelium. *Gastroenterology*, 50:692–707.

161. Bloom, S. R., Adrian, T. E., Mitchenere, P., Sagor, C. R., and Christofides, N. D. (1981): Motilin-induced gallbladder contraction—a new mechanism. *Gastroenterology*, 80:1113 (*Abstr.*).

162. O'Brien, J. J., Shaffer, E. A., Williams, L. F., Small, D. M., Lynn, J., and Wittenberg, J. (1964): A physiological model to study gallbladder function in primates. *Gastroenterology*, 67:119–125.

163. Mok, H. Y. I., von Bergman, K., and Grundy, S. M. (1980): Kinetics of the enterohepatic circulation during fasting. Biliary lipid secretion and gallbladder storage. *Gastroenterology*, 78:1023–1033.

164. Rock, E., Malmud, L., and Fisher, R. S. (1981): Gallbladder emptying in response to sham feeding. *Gastroenterology*, 80:1263 (*Abstr.*).

165. Spellman, S. J., Shaffer, E. A., and Rosenthall, L. (1979): Gallbladder emptying in response to cholecystokinin. A cholescintigraphic study. *Gastroenterology*, 77:115–120.

166. Everson, G. T., Braverman, D. Z., Johnson, M. L., and Kern, F., Jr. (1980): A critical evaluation of real-time ultrasonography for the study of gallbladder volume and contraction. *Gastroenterology*, 79:40–46.

167. Ostrow, J. D. (1969): Absorption by the gallbladder of bile salts, sulfobromophthalein, and iodipamide. *J. Lab. Clin. Med.*, 74:482–494.

168. Gallagher, K., Mauskopf, J., Walker, J. T., and Lack, L. (1976): Ionic requirements for the active bile salt transport system. *J. Lipid Res.*, 17:572–577.

169. Armstrong, M. J., and Carey, M. C. (1982): The hydrophobic-hydrophilic balance of bile salts. Inverse correlation between reverse-phase high performance chromatographic mobilities and micellar cholesterol solubilizing capacities. *J. Lipid Res.*, 23:70–80.

170. Hofmann, A. F. (1973): Consequences of bile acid malabsorption. *Mayo Clin. Proc.*, 48:656–659.

171. Sturman, J. A., Hepner, G. W., Hofmann, A. F., and Thomas, P. J. (1976): Taurine pool sizes in man. Studies with ^{35}S taurine. In: *Taurine*, edited by R. Huxtable and A. Barbeau, pp. 21–33. Raven Press, New York.

172. Hofmann, A. F. (1972): Bile acid malabsorption caused by ileal resection. *Arch. Intern. Med.*, 130:597–605.

173. Thistle, J. L., Hofmann, A. F., Ott, B. J., and Stephens, D. H. (1978): Chenotherapy for gallstone dissolution. I. Efficacy and safety. *JAMA*, 239:1041–1046.

174. Sjövall, J., and Akesson, I. (1955): Intestinal absorption of taurocholic acid in the rat. *Acta Physiol. Scand.*, 34:273–278.

175. Ahlberg, J., Angelin, B., Björkhem, I., and Einarsson, K. (1977): Individual bile acids in portal venous and systemic blood serum of fasting man. *Gastroenterology*, 73:1377–1382.

176. Olivecrona, T., and Sjövall, J. (1959): Bile acids in rat portal blood. *Acta Physiol. Scand.*, 46:284–290.

177. Cronholm, T., and Sjövall, J. (1967): Bile acids in portal blood of rats fed different diets and cholestryamine. *Eur. J. Biochem.*, 2:375–383.

178. Einarsson, K., Grundy, S. M., and Hardison, W. G. M. (1979): Enterohepatic circulation rates of cholic acid and chenodeoxycholic acid in man. *Gut*, 20:1078–1082.

179. Rudman, D., and Kendall, F. E. (1957): Bile acid content of human serum. II. The binding of cholanic acids by human plasma protein. *J. Clin. Invest.*, 36:538–542.

180. Kramer, W., Buscher, H-P., Gerok, W., and Kurz, G. (1979): Bile salt binding to serum components. Taurocholate incorporation into high-density lipoproteins revealed by photoaffinity labelling. *Eur. J. Biochem.*, 102:1–9.

181. Benhold, H., Peters, H., and Roth, E. (1954): Uber einem Fall von Kompletter Analbuminaemie ohne wesentliche Klinische Krankheitszeichen. *Verh. Dtsch. Ges. Inn. Med.*, 60:630–634.

182. Keller, H., Morell, A., Noseda, G., and Riva, R. (1972): Analbuminamie Pathophysiologische Untersuchungen an einen Fall. *Schweiz. Med. Wochenschr.*, 102:33–41.

183. Cormode, E. J., Lyster, D. M., and Israels, S. (1975): Analbuminemia in a neonate. *J. Pediatr.*, 86:862–864.

184. Bowman, H., Hermodson, M., Hammond, C. C., and Motulsky, A. G.: Analbuminemia in an American Indian girl. *Clin. Genet.*, 9:513–526.

185. Goule, J. P., Laine, G., Sanger, F., Maitrot, B., Bouillerot, A., Gray, H., Blondet, P., and Dieryck, B. (1976): Etude biochemique de premier ces d'analbuminémie en France. *Ann. Biol. Clin.*, 34:403–409.

186. Reichen, J., and Paumgartner, G. (1975): Kinetics of taurocholate uptake by the perfused rat liver. *Gastroenterology*, 68:132–136.

187. Reichen, J., and Paumgartner, G. (1976): Uptake of bile acids by perfused rat liver. *Am. J. Physiol.*, 321:734–742.

188. Reichen, J., Preisig, R., and Paumgartner, G. (1977): Influence of chemical structure on hepatocellular uptake of bile acids. In: *Bile Acid Metabolism in Health and Disease*, edited by G. Paumgartner and A. Stiehl, pp. 113–123. MTP Press, Lancaster.

189. Accatino, L., and Simon, R. F. (1976): Identification and characterization of a bile acid receptor in isolated liver surface membranes. *J. Clin. Invest.*, 57:496–508.

190. Paumgartner, G., Reichen, J., von Bergmann, K., and Preisig, R. (1975): Elaboration of hepatocytic bile. *Bull. NY Acad. Med.*, 51:455–471.

191. Matern, S., Tietjen, K., Fakler, O., Hinger, K., Herz, R., and Gerok, W. (1978): Bioavailability of ursodeoxycholic acid in man; studies with a radioimmunoassay for ursodeoxycholic acid. In: *Biological Effects of Bile Acids*, edited by W. Gerok, G. Paumgartner, and A. Stiehl, pp. 109–118, MTP Press, Lancaster.

192. Grundy, S. M., Ahrens, E. H., Jr., and Miettinen, T. A. (1965): Quantitative isolation and gas-liquid chromatographic analysis of total fecal bile acids. *J. Lipid Res.*, 6:397–410.

193. Draser, B. S., and Shiner, M. (1969): Studies on the intestinal flora. Part II. Bacterial flora of the small intestine in patients with gastrointestinal disorders. *Gut*, 10:812–819.

194. Gorbach, S. L., and Tabaqchali, S. (1969): Bacteria, bile and the small bowel. *Gut*, 10:963–972.

195. Reddy, B. S., Weisburger, H. J., and Wynder, E. L. (1978): Colon cancer: Bile salts as tumor promoters. In: *Carcinogenesis, Vol. 2. Mechanisms of Tumor Promotion and Cocarcinogenesis*, edited by T. J. Slaga, A. Sivak, and R. K. Boutwell, pp. 453–464. Raven Press, New York.

196. Silverman, S. J., and Andrews, A. W. (1977): Bile acids. Comutagenic activity in the Salmonella/mammalian-microsome mutagenicity test. *J. Natl. Cancer Inst.*, 59:1557–1559.

197. Kawalek, J. C., and Andrews, A. W. (1977): The effect of bile acids on the metabolism of benzo(a)pyrene and 2-aminoanthracene to mutagenic products. *Fed. Proc.*, 36:844–848.

198. Narisawa, T., Magnadia, N. E., Weisburger, J. H., and Wynder, E. L. (1974): Promoting effect of bile acids on colon carcinogenesis after intrarectal instillation of N-methyl-N'-nitro-N-nitrosoguanidine in rats. *J. Natl. Cancer Inst.*, 53:1093–1097.

199. Kelsey, M. I., Molina, J. E., Huang, S-K. S., and Hwang, K-K. (1980): The identification of microbial metabolites of sulfolithocholic acid. *J. Lipid Res.*, 21:751–759.

200. Ponz de Leon, M., Murphy, G. M., and Dowling, R. H. (1978): Physiological factors influencing serum bile acid levels. *Gut*, 19:32–39.

201. LaRusso, N. F., Korman, M. G., Hoffman, N. E., and Hofmann, A. F. (1974): Dynamics of the enterohepatic circulation of bile acids. *N. Engl. J. Med.*, 291:689–692.

202. Hofmann, A. F., Simmonds, W. J., Korman, M. G., LaRusso, N. R., and Hofmann, N. E. (1975): Radioimmunoassay of bile acids. In: *Advances in Bile Acid Research*, edited by S. Matern, J. Hackenschmidt, P. Back, and W. Gerok, pp. 95–98. Schattauer, New York.

203. Van Deest, B. W., Fordtran, J. S., Morawski, S. G., and Wilson, J. D. (1968): Bile salt and micellar fat concentrations in proximal small bowel contents of ileectomy patients. *J. Clin. Invest.*, 47:1314–1324.

204. Thomassen, P. A. (1979): Urinary bile acids during development of recurrent cholestasis of pregnancy. *Eur. J. Clin. Invest.*, 9:417–423.

205. Stiehl, A., Becker, M., Czygan, P., Fröhling, W., Kommerell, B., and Rothauwe, H. W. (1980): Bile acids and their sulfated and glucuronidated derivatives in bile, plasma and urine of children with intrahepatic cholestasis: Effect of phenobarbitol treatment. *Eur. J. Clin. Invest.*, 10:307–310.

206. Hofmann, A. F., and Hoffman, N. E. (1974): Measurements of bile acid kinetics by isotope dilution in man. *Gastroenterology*, 67:314–323.

207. Hofmann, A. F., Schoenfield, L. J., Kottke, B. A., and Poley, J. R. (1970): Methods for the description of bile acid kinetics in man. *Methods Med. Res.*, 12:149–180.

208. Duane, W. C., Adler, R. D., Bennion, L. J., and Ginsberg, R. L. (1975): Determination of bile acid pool size in man. A simplified method with advantages of increased precision, shortened analysis time and decreased isotope exposure. *J. Lipid Res.*, 16:155–158.

209. Vantrappen, G., Rutgeerts, P., and Ghoos, Y. (1981): A new method for the measurement of bile acid turnover and pool size by a double label, single intubation technique. *J. Lipid Res.*, 22:528–531.

210. Eriksson, S. (1957): Biliary excretion of bile acids and cholesterol in bile fistula rats. *Proc. Soc. Exp. Biol.*, 94:578–582.

211. Campbell, C. B., Burgess, P., Roberts, S. A., Dowling, R. H., and White, J. (1971): The use of Rhesus monkeys to study biliary secretion with an intact enterohepatic circulation. *Aust. NZ J. Med.*, 1:49–56.

212. Mok, H. Y. I., and Dowling, R. H. (1975): How well can we measure bile acid pool size. In: *Advances in Bile Acid Research*, edited by J. Hackenschmidt, P. Back, and W. Gerok, pp. 315–323. Schattauer, New York.

213. Grundy, S. M., and Ahrens, E. H., Jr. (1966): An evaluation of the relative merits of two methods for measuring the balance of sterols in man. Isotopic balance versus chromatographic analysis. *J. Clin. Invest.*, 45:1503–1515.

214. Northfield, T. C., and Hofmann, A. F. (1975): Biliary lipid output during three meals and an overnight fast. I. Relationship to bile acid pool size and cholesterol saturation of bile in gallstone and control subjects. *Gut*, 16:1–11.

215. Mok, H. Y. I., von Bergmann, K., and Grundy, S. M. (1977): Regulation of pool size of bile acids in man. *Gastroenterology*, 73:684–690.

216. Rutgeerts, P., Ghoos, Y., Vantrappen, G., and Hellemans, J. (1981): The fasting bile acid pool size is not equal to the circulating pool size. *Gastroenterology*, 80:1266 (*Abstr.*).

217. Shaffer, E. A., and Small, D. M. (1977): Biliary lipid secretion in cholesterol gallstone disease. The effect of cholecystectomy and obesity. *J. Clin. Invest.*, 59:828–840.

218. Everson, G., Lawson, M., McKinley, C., Showalter, R., and Kern, F., Jr. (1981): Differential effects of liquid formula and amino acid solutions on gallbladder emptying, small bowel transit and biliary lipid secretion. *Gastroenterology*, 80:1145 (*Abstr.*).

219. Hepner, G. W. (1975): Effects of decreased gallbladder stimulation on enterohepatic cycling and kinetics of bile acids. *Gastroenterology*, 68:1574–1581.

220. Duane, W. C., and Hanson, K. C. (1978): Role of gallbladder emptying and small bowel transit in regulation of bile acid pool size in man. *J. Lab. Clin. Med.*, 92:859–872.

221. Duane, W. C. (1978): Simulation of the defect of bile acid me-

tabolism associated with cholesterol cholelithiasis by sorbitol ingestion in man. *J. Lab. Clin. Med.*, 91:969–978.

222. Duane, W. C., and Bond, J. H., Jr. (1980): Prolongation of intestinal transit and expansion of bile acid pools by propantheline bromide. *Gastroenterology*, 78:226–230.

223. Low-Beer, T. S., Harvey, R. F., Davis, E. R., and Reed, A. E. (1975): Abnormalities of serum cholecystokinin and gallbladder emptying in celiac disease. *N. Engl. J. Med.*, 292:961–963.

224. Low-Beer, T. S., Heaton, K. W., Pomare, E. W., and Reed, A. E. (1973): The effect of celiac disease upon bile salts. *Gut*, 14:204–208.

225. Trier, J. S., Falchuck, Z. M., Carey, M. C., and Schreiber, D. S. (1978): Celiac sprue and refractory sprue. *Gastroenterology*, 75:307–316.

226. Motson, R., Hammerman, K., Admirand, W., and Way, L. (1973): Effects of altered bile salt enterohepatic cycling upon bile salt kinetics and biliary lipid composition. *Gastroenterology*, 72:A–150/1173.

227. Hardison, W. G. M., Tomaszewski, N., and Grundy, S. M. (1979): Effects of acute alterations in small bowel transit time upon biliary excretion rate of bile acids. *Gastroenterology*, 76:568–574.

228. Duane, W. C., Ginsberg, R. L., and Bennion, L. J. (1976): Effects of fasting on bile acid metabolism and biliary lipid composition in man. *J. Lipid Res.*, 17:211–219.

229. Bennion, L. J., and Grundy, S. M. (1975): Effects of obesity and caloric intake on biliary lipid metabolism in man. *J. Clin. Invest.*, 56:996–1011.

230. Bell, C. C., Vlahcevic, Z. R., Prazich, J., and Swell, L. (1973): Evidence that a diminished bile acid pool precedes the formation of cholesterol gallstones in man. *Surg. Gynecol. Obstet.*, 136:961–965.

231. Wagner, C. I., Trotman, B. W., and Soloway, R. D. (1976): Kinetic analysis of biliary lipid excretion in man and dog. *J. Clin. Invest.*, 57:473–477.

232. Vlachevic, Z. R., Bell, C. C., and Gregory, D. H. (1972): Relationship of bile acid pool size to the formation of lithogenic bile in female Indians of the Southwest. *Gastroenterology*, 62:73–83.

233. Bennion, L. J., Drobny, E., Knowler, W. C., Ginsberg, R. L., Garnick, M. B., Adler, R. D., and Duane, W. C. (1978): Sex differences in the size of bile acid pools. *Metabolism*, 27:961–969.

234. Danziger, R. F., Hofmann, A. F., Thistle, J. L., and Schoenfield, L. J. (1973): Effect of oral chenodeoxycholic acid on bile acid kinetics and biliary lipid composition in women with cholelithiasis. *J. Clin. Invest.*, 52:2809–2821.

235. Marks, J. W., Bonorris, G. G., and Schoenfield, L. J. (1976): Pathophysiology and dissolution of cholesterol gallstones. In: *The Bile Acids, Vol. 3*, edited by P. P. Nair and D. Kritchevsky, pp. 81–113. Plenum, New York.

236. Maudgal, D. P., Kupfer, R. M., Zentler-Munro, P. L., and Northfield, T. C. (1980): Postprandial gallbladder emptying in patients with gallstones. *Br. Med. J.*, 280:141–143.

237. Northfield, T. C., Kupfer, R. M., Maudgal, D. P., Zentler-Munro, P. L., Meller, S. T., Garvie, N. W., and McCready, R. (1980): Gallbladder sensitivity to cholecystokinin in patients with gallstones. *Br. Med. J.*, 280:143–145.

238. Sama, C., LaRusso, N. F., Lopez del Piño, V., and Thistle, J. L. (1982): Effects of acute bile acid administration on biliary lipid secretion in healthy volunteers. *Gastroenterology*, 82:515–525.

239. Carey, M. C. (1978): Critical tables for calculating the cholesterol saturation of native bile. *J. Lipid Res.*, 19:945–955.

240. Vlahcevic, Z. R., Buhac, I., Farrar, J. T., Bell, C. C., Jr., and Swell, L. (1971): Bile acid metabolism in patients with cirrhosis. I. Kinetics aspects of cholic acid metabolism. *Gastroenterology*, 60:491–498.

241. Vlahcevic, Z. R., Juttijudata, P., Bell, C. C., Jr., and Swell, L. (1972): Bile acid metabolism in patients with cirrhosis. II. Cholic and chenodeoxycholic acid metabolism. *Gastroenterology*, 62:1174–1181.

242. McCormick, W. C., Bell, C. C., Jr., Swell, L., and Vlahcevic, Z. R. (1973): Cholic acid synthesis as an index of the severity of liver disease in man. *Gut*, 14:895–902.

243. Einarrson, K., Hellström, K., and Schersten, T. (1975): The formation of bile acids in patients with portal liver cirrhosis. *Scand. J. Gastroenterol.*, 10:299–304.

244. Patterson, T. E., Vlahcevic, Z. R., Schwartz, C. C., Gustafsson, J., Danielsson, H., and Swell, L. (1980): Bile acid metabolism in cirrhosis. VI. Sites of blockage in the bile acid-pathways to primary bile acids. *Gastroenterology*, 79:620–628.

245. Vlahcevic, Z. R., Gregory, D. H., and Swell, L. (1975): Characterization of factors responsible for abnormal metabolism of deoxycholic acid in patients with alcoholic cirrhosis. In: *Advances in Bile Acid Research*, edited by S. Matern, J. Hackenschmidt, P. Back, and W. Gerok, pp. 382–389. Schattauer, New York.

246. Knodell, R. G., Kinsey, M. D., Boedeker, E. C., and Collin, D. P. (1976): Deoxycholate metabolism in alcoholic cirrhosis. *Gastroenterology*, 71:196–201.

247. Stiehl, A., Ast, E., Czygan, P., Fröhling, W., Raedsch, R., and Kommerell, B. (1978): Pool size, synthesis, and turnover of sulfated and nonsulfated cholic acid and chenodeoxycholic acid in patients with cirrhosis of the liver. *Gastroenterology*, 74:572–577.

248. Makino, I., Hashimoto, H., Shinozaki, K., Yoshino, K., and Nakagawa, S. (1975): Sulfated and nonsulfated bile acids in urine, serum and bile of patients with hepatobiliary diseases. *Gastroenterology*, 68:545–553.

249. Back, P., and Gerok, W. (1977): Differences in renal excretion between glycotauroconjugates, sulfoconjugates and glucuronoconjugates of bile acids in cholestasis. In: *Bile Acid Metabolism in Health and Disease*, edited by G. Paumgartner and A. Stiehl, pp. 93–100. MTP Press, Lancaster.

250. Berge-Henegouwen, G. P. van, Brant, K. H., Eyssen, H., and Parmentier, G. (1976): Sulphated and unsulphated bile acids in serum, bile and urine of patients with cholestasis. *Gut*, 17:861–869.

251. Matern, S., Krieger, R., Hans, C., and Gerok, W. (1977): Radioimmunoassay of serum conjugated deoxycholic acid. *Scand. J. Gastroenterol.*, 12:641–647.

252. Struthers, J. E., Jr., Mehta, S. J., Kaye, M. D., and Naylor, J. L. (1977): Relative concentration of individual nonsulfated bile acids in serum and bile of patients with cirrhosis. *Am. J. Dig. Dis.*, 22:861–865.

253. Kaye, M. D., Struthers, J. E., Jr., Tidball, J. S., DeNiro, E., and Kern, F., Jr. (1973): Factors affecting plasma clearance of ^{14}C cholic acid in patients with cirrhosis. *Clin. Sci. Mol. Med.*, 45:147–161.

254. Angelin, B., Einarsson, K., Ewerth, S., and Leijd, B. (1980): Biliary lipid composition in patients with portal cirrhosis of the liver. *Scand. J. Gastroenterol.*, 15:849–852.

255. Bouchier, I. A. D. (1969): Post-mortem study of the frequency of gallstones in patients with cirrhosis of the liver. *Gut*, 10:705–710.

256. Nicholas, P., Rinaudo, P. A., and Conn, H. O. (1972): Increased incidence of cholelithiasis in Laennec's cirrhosis. *Gastroenterology*, 63:112–121.

257. Salen, G., and Mosbach, E. H. (1976): The metabolism of sterols and bile acids in cerebrotendinous xanthomatosis. In: *The Bile Acids, Vol. 3*, edited by P. P. Nair and D. Kritchevsky, pp. 115–153. Plenum, New York.

258. Oftebro, H., Björkhem, I., Stormer, F. C., and Pederson, J. I. (1981): Cerebrotendinous xanthomatosis. Defective liver mitochondrial hydroxylation of chenodeoxycholic acid precursors. *J. Lipid Res.*, 22:632–640.

259. Hosita, T., Yasuhara, M., Une, M., Kibe, A., Itoga, E., Kito, S., and Kuramoto, T. (1980): Occurrence of bile alcohol glucuronides in bile of a patient with cerebrotendinous xanthomatosis. *J. Lipid Res.*, 21:1015–1021.

260. Iser, J. H., Dowling, R. H., Murphy, G. M., Ponz de Leon, M., and Mitroupoulos, K. A. (1977): Congenital bile salt deficiency associated with 28 years of intractible constipation. In: *Bile Acid Metabolism in Health and Disease*, edited by G. Paumgartner and A. Stiehl, pp. 231–234. MTP Press, Lancaster.

261. Almé, B., Norden, A., and Sjövall, J. (1978): Glucuronides of unconjugated 6-hydroxylated bile acids in urine of a patient with malabsorption. *Clin. Chim. Acta*, 86:251–259.

262. Einarsson, K., Hellström, K., and Kallner, M. (1974): Bile acid kinetics in relation to sex, serum lipids, body weights and gallbladder disease in patients with various types of hyperlipoproteinemia. *J. Clin. Invest.*, 54:1301–1311.

263. Einarsson, K., and Hellström, K. (1972): The formation of bile acids in patients with three types of hyperlipoproteinemia. *Eur. J. Clin. Invest.*, 2:225–230.

264. Einarsson, K., Hellström, K., and Kallner, M. (1974): The effect of cholestyramine on the elimination of cholesterol as bile acids in patients with hyperlipoproteinemia Types II and IV. *Eur. J. Clin. Invest.*, 4:405–410.

265. Einarsson, K., Hellström, K., and Kallner, M. (1974): Effect of cholic acid feeding on bile acid kinetics and neutral fecal steroid excretion in hyperlipoproteinemia (Types II and IV). *Metabolism*, 23:863–873.

266. Kallner, M. (1975): The effect of chenodeoxycholic acid feeding on bile acid kinetics and fecal netural steroid excretion in patients with hyperlipoproteinemia Types II and IV. *J. Lab. Clin. Med.*, 86:595–604.

267. Singh, A. (1975): Familial hyperlipoproteinemia and gallstones. *Can. Med. Assoc. J.*, 113:733–735.

268. Ahlberg, J., Angelin, B., Einarsson, K., Hellström, K., and Leijd, B. (1979): Prevalence of gallbladder disease in hyperlipoproteinemia. *Am. J. Dig. Dis.*, 24:459–464.

269. Kostner, G. M., Laggner, P., Prexl, H. J., Holasek, A., Ingolic, E., and Geymayer, W. (1976): Investigation of the abnormal low density lipoproteins occurring in patients with obstructive jaundice. *Biochem. J.*, 157:401–407.

270. Laggner, P., Glatter, O., Muller, K., Kratky, O., Kostner, G., and Holasek, A. (1977): The lipid bilayer structure of the abnormal human plasma lipoprotein X: An x-ray small angle-scattering study. *Eur. J. Biochem.*, 77:165–171.

271. Picard, J., Veissiere, D., Voyer, F., and Bereziat, G. (1972): Composition en acides gras des phospholipides dans les lipoproteins serique abnormales de la cholestase. *Clin. Chim. Acta*, 36:247–250.

272. Weber, A. M., Roy, C. C., Morin, C. L., and Lasalle, R. (1973): Malabsorption of bile acids in children with cystic fibrosis. *N. Engl. J. Med.*, 289:1001–1005.

273. Krejs, G. J., Orci, L., Conlon, J. M., Ravazzola, M., Davis, G. R., Raskin, P., Collins, S. M., McCarthy, D. M., Baetens, D., Rubenstein, A., Aldor, T. A. M., and Unger, R. H. (1979): Somatostatinoma syndrome. Biochemical, morphologic and clinical features. *N. Engl. J. Med.*, 301:285–292.

274. Hofmann, A. F., and Poley, J. R. (1972): Role of bile acid malabsorption in pathogenesis of diarrhea and steatorrhea in patients with ileal resection. I. Response to cholestyramine or replacement of dietary long chain triglyceride by medium chain triglyceride. *Gastroenterology*, 62:918–934.

275. Poley, J. R., and Hofmann, A. F. (1976): Role of fat maldigestion in pathogenesis of steatorrhea in ileal resection. Fat digestion after two sequential test meals with and without cholestryamine. *Gastroenterology*, 71:38–44.

276. Mekhijian, M. S., and Phillips, S. F. (1970): Perfusion of the canine colon with unconjugated bile acids. Effect on water and electrolyte transport, morphology and bile acid absorption. *Gastroenterology*, 59:120–131.

277. Mekhijian, M. S., Phillips, S. F., and Hofmann, A. F. (1971): Colonic secretion of water and electrolytes induced by bile acids. Perfusion studies in man. *J. Clin. Invest.*, 50:1569–1577.

278. Hofmann, A. F., and Poley, J. R. (1969): Cholestyramine treatment of diarrhea associated with ileal resection. Factors influencing response. *N. Engl. J. Med.*, 281:397–402.

279. Ammon, H. V., and Phillips, S. F. (1973): Inhibition of colonic water and electrolyte absorption by fatty acids in man. *Gastroenterology*, 65:744–749.

280. Bright-Astare, P., and Binder, H. J. (1973): Stimulation of colonic secretion of water and electrolytes by hydroxy fatty acid. *Gastroenterology*, 64:81–88.

281. Thayssen, E. H. (1977): Diagnostic value of the ^{14}C-cholylglycine breath test. In: *Clinic in Gastroenterology, Vol. 6*, edited by G. Paumgartner, pp. 227–245. Saunders, Philadelphia.

282. Dowling, R. H., Bell, G. D., and White, J. (1972): Lithogenic bile in patients with ileal dysfunction *Gut*, 13:415–420.

283. Cohen, S., Kaplan, M., Gottlieb, L, and Patterson, J. (1971): Liver disease and gallstones in regional enteritis. *Gastroenterology*, 60:237–245.

284. Heaton, K. W., and Read, A. E. (1969): Gallstones in patients with disorders of the terminal ileum and disturbed bile salt metabolism. *Br. Med. J.*, 3:494–496.

285. Chadwick, V. S., Modha, K., and Dowling, R. H. (1973): Mechanism for hyperoxaluria in patients with ileal dysfunction. *N. Engl. J. Med.*, 289:172–176.

286. Dowling, R. H., Rose, G. A., and Sutor, D. J. (1971): Hyperoxaluria and renal calculi in ileal disease. *Lancet*, 1:1103–1106.

287. Northfield, T. C., Drasar, B. S., and Wright, J. T. (1973): Value of small intestinal bile acid analysis in the diagnosis of the stagnant loop syndrome. *Gut*, 14:341–347.

288. Tabaqchali, S., and Booth, C. C. (1970): Bacteria and the small intestine. In: *Modern Trends in Gastroenterology, Vol. 4*, edited by W. I. Card and G. Creamer, pp. 143–179. Butterworths, London.

289. Tabaqchali, S., Harzioannou, J., and Booth, C. C. (1968): Bile salt deconjugation and steatorrhea in patients with the stagnant loop syndrome. *Lancet*, II:12–16.

290. Fowweather, F. S. (1949): Bile acid enteroliths. With an account of a recent case. *Biochem. J.*, 44:607–610.

291. Fromm, H., and Hofmann, A. F. (1971): Breath test for altered bile-acid metabolism. *Lancet*, II:621–265.

The Liver: Biology and Pathobiology, edited by
I. Arias, H. Popper, D. Schachter, and D. A. Shafritz.
Raven Press, New York © 1982.

Chapter 28

Cholesterol Metabolism and Excretion

Stephen D. Turley and John M. Dietschy

Cholesterol,[1] an essential constituent of living tissues, plays critical roles as a structural component of most biologic membranes and as the immediate precursor for a number of essential vitamins, steroid hormones, and bile acids. It is of critical importance, therefore, that the cells of the major tissues of the body be assured a continuous supply of this compound. To meet this need, a complex series of transport, biosynthetic, and regulatory mechanisms has evolved. Generally, cholesterol can be acquired from the environment through the absorption of dietary cholesterol or synthesized *de novo* from acetyl CoA within the body. More cholesterol usually enters the body through these two mechanisms than is used during normal metabolic turnover, so that the excess must be metabolized and/or excreted to prevent a potentially hazardous accumulation of sterol. Unfortunately, mammalian tissues do not possess enzymes capable of extensive degradation of the sterol nucleus. The best that can be done is to modify certain of the substituent groups on the hydrocarbon tail or on the ring structure of the sterol molecule. Hence, cholesterol is excreted from the body either as the unaltered molecule or after biochemical modification to other sterol products, such as bile acids and steroid hormones.

The availability of cholesterol in the diets of different animal species varies enormously and even in the same species, including man, may change markedly from day to day. Thus it is apparent that regulatory mechanisms must be operative that adjust the rate of cholesterol synthesis within the body and/or the rate of cholesterol excretion from the body to accommodate the varying amounts of sterol that are being absorbed from moment to moment from the diet. Generally these regulatory mechanisms function well, so that there is little net accumulation of cholesterol during the lifetime of many animals, yet sufficient sterol is always available to meet the metabolic needs of the various tissues. In a few species, and in particular in man, subtle imbalances do develop that can lead to elevation in circulating levels of plasma cholesterol or to excessive secretion of cholesterol into bile. In the first instance, this metabolic abnormality may lead to cholesteryl ester accumulation in cells within the walls of arteries and produce clinically apparent atherosclerotic disease. In the second instance, the bile may become supersaturated with sterol, leading to the pre-

---

[1] Sterols other than cholesterol are absorbed from the diet and synthesized within the cells of the various organs of the body. Generally, these sterols are not quantitatively important. In most organs, such as the liver, cholesterol makes up the majority of the newly synthesized sterols. Thus in this chapter, we use the terms "cholesterol" and "sterol" interchangeably and make no attempt to deal with the metabolism of noncholesterol sterol molecules.

cipitation of cholesterol and, ultimately, to clinically apparent cholelithiasis.

This chapter reviews the quantitative differences that exist in various animal species with respect to rates of cholesterol absorption and synthesis. Insofar as data are available, the mechanisms that control these two processes are discussed. Finally, the determinants of the rate of biliary cholesterol secretion are examined in detail. In each of these areas, data derived from different animal species and from man are reviewed and contrasted. Such a comparison is necessary not only because fundamental information on many of these processes is often not available in man, but, more importantly, by understanding the differences that exist in the various aspects of cholesterol metabolism among the different animal species, one may better understand the normal physiology of cholesterol metabolism in man and the ways in which this physiology may go awry, permitting cholesterol gallstone formation to take place.

GENERAL FEATURES OF CHOLESTEROL BALANCE IN MAN AND VARIOUS EXPERIMENTAL ANIMALS

The general features of cholesterol balance that must be taken into consideration in man and in various experimental animals are shown in Fig. 1 (1). The body pool of cholesterol in the adult remains essentially constant. The content of sterols in various tissues varies markedly, from about 0.5 g/kg muscle to 15 g/kg brain but averages approximately 1.4 g/kg tissue for the body as a whole. Thus a 70-kg man contains about 100 g cholesterol, while a 0.2-kg rat has only 0.3 g total sterol (2–4). Not all compartments of this body pool are equally accessible to metabolic interactions or to exchange with cholesterol carried in the blood. Based on an analysis of die-away curves, for example, the body pool of cholesterol has been divided into three functionally distinct areas (5–8). These include a rapidly miscible pool (pool A), a more slowly exchangeable pool (pool B), and a pool of cholesterol that is either only very slowly miscible or nonexchangeable (pool C). In the baboon, the size of pool A equals about 0.3 g/kg body weight and includes nearly all the sterol present in such tissues as blood, small intestine, lung, liver, and spleen, and a lesser proportion of the cholesterol in a variety of other organs, including skeletal muscle. Pool B is larger, equaling about 0.6 g/kg body weight, and includes a portion of the cholesterol present principally in tissues, such as adipose tissue, skeletal muscle, and skin. Pool C, the nonexchangeable cholesterol pool, contains about 0.5 g sterol/kg body weight and is made up largely of cholesterol present in brain, bone, skin, skeletal muscle, and adipose tissue (7,9,10).

New cholesterol can be added to the body pool from only two sources. Either preformed sterol is absorbed from dietary sources across the gastrointestinal mucosa or, alternatively, the cholesterol molecule is synthesized *de novo* from acetyl CoA in a variety of different tissues within the body. The sum of these two processes constitutes the total input of cholesterol into the body pool each day. Similarly, there are only two major pathways for the removal of cholesterol from the body. The unmodified cholesterol molecule may be lost directly from the body pool. This takes place through the sloughing of oily secretions and cells from the skin, through the desquamation of cells from the stomach, small intestine, and colon, and through the movement of cholesterol into pancreatic, gastric, intestinal, and canalicular secretions. Of these various routes, secretion of cholesterol through the canalicular membrane of the hepatocyte is usually of greatest quantitative importance. Alternatively, the cholesterol molecule may first be metabolized to another product, such as bile acids, adrenocorticosteroids, or testosterone, which in turn is excreted from the body through the urine or gastrointestinal tract.

In the growing animal, there is necessarily a greater input than output of cholesterol into the body; on the average, there is a net accumulation of about 1.4 g sterol for each kilogram body weight gained. Once adulthood is reached and body weight becomes con-

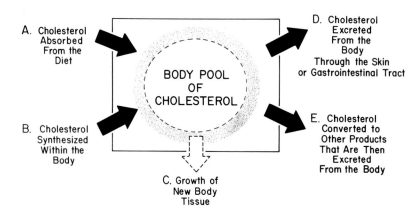

FIG. 1. General schema for the balance of cholesterol across the body. There are only two sources for cholesterol in the body: absorption of sterol from the diet, and synthesis of cholesterol in the various organ systems. Similarly, cholesterol can be excreted intact from the body through the skin or gastrointestinal tract or after conversion to various products, such as bile acids or steroid hormones. In the steady state, total input of cholesterol into the body must equal total output, so that the body pool of cholesterol remains essentially constant.

stant, however, the input of cholesterol into the system must equal output. Thus, even though there may be net accumulation of a small quantity of cholesterol in critical locations, e.g., in the walls of the coronary arteries, the content of cholesterol in the blood and in the other organs remains essentially constant over many years (3).

CHOLESTEROL ABSORPTION RATES IN DIFFERENT SPECIES

The first of the two major sources for sterol in the body pool is dietary cholesterol absorbed through the gastrointestinal tract. Apparently, every animal is capable of absorbing dietary cholesterol to at least some degree, although there are remarkable differences among the various species in the rate of such intestinal transport. Most data indicate that cholesterol movement into the intestinal epithelial cell is a passive process that does not depend on the expenditure of metabolic energy or on the intervention of membrane receptors (11–15). Thus the magnitude of the unidirectional flux of cholesterol across the brush border is a linear function of the concentration of this molecule in the luminal fluid, is independent of the presence of structurally related sterol molecules, and manifests a relatively low temperature dependency and, hence, a low activation energy. It has been shown that it is not the rate of membrane translocation that limits the overall velocity of cholesterol uptake into the intestinal epithelial cell but, rather, the rate at which the cholesterol molecule can diffuse from the bulk phase of the intestinal contents through the unstirred water layers overlying the intestinal microvilli (16–18). Thus, as with most nonpolar, poorly soluble substances, the rate of intestinal uptake of cholesterol is limited by the rate of diffusion up to the brush border and not by the rate at which this solute penetrates this limiting membrane. It is at the level of these unstirred water layers that bile acid micelles appear to exert their critical function in facilitating cholesterol absorption (17,19). Mixed micelles, composed of bile acids and the products of lipolysis of dietary lipids, such as fatty acids and β-monoglycerides, solubilize dietary cholesterol. These micellar structures can carry large amounts of sterol up to the aqueous-microvillar interface overcoming, in effect, the resistance engendered by the unstirred water layers to cholesterol absorption and greatly increasing the velocity of sterol uptake per unit length of intestine. In the intact animal or in man, adequate concentrations of bile acids must be present in the intestinal contents to have relatively rapid sterol absorption. In the absence of such surface active agents, the rate of cholesterol absorption is markedly reduced (17,20,21).

The overall process of net cholesterol absorption from the intestinal lumen to the blood is still more complex than these considerations of brush border translocation might imply. A number of enzymatic reactions in the intestinal contents and within the intestinal epithelial cell could influence the rate of net uptake. Following ingestion, for example, complex foods must be digested by the peptidases and lipases secreted into the intestinal lumen by the pancreas in order to release the largely unesterified dietary sterols. The small amount of dietary cholesteryl esters is hydrolyzed by another pancreatic enzyme, cholesteryl esterase (21–23). This unesterified cholesterol from the diet, along with the unesterified cholesterol reaching the intestinal lumen from the bile, is then solubilized in the complex structure of the mixed micelle (11,24). Following the movement of this carrier up to the brush border, the dietary sterol diffuses into the cytosolic compartment of the intestinal absorptive cell, where it presumably mixes with a pool of newly synthesized cholesterol (25). A large proportion of this intracellular cholesterol pool is esterified to long chain fatty acids and incorporated into the structure of the nascent chylomicron (26). This lipoprotein particle is then secreted from the epithelial cell by an exocytotic process, enters the intestinal lymphatic system, and eventually reaches the circulating blood (27,28). It is apparent that under different physiologic circumstances or in different animal species, significant variation in the velocity of any one of these steps might ultimately limit the rate of net cholesterol uptake into the body pool from the diet.

While few data are available delineating the velocity of each of these steps in different animals, measurements have been made of the overall rates at which dietary cholesterol is absorbed in several species. The methods used to make these measurements are relatively insensitive and are the subject of continuing discussion and controversy (29–31). Nevertheless, as summarized in Table 1, these data do suggest that there are remarkable differences in the amounts of cholesterol that can be absorbed by man and by different experimental animals. A 70-kg man, for example, can absorb several hundred milligrams cholesterol per day. A much smaller animal, such as a 0.2-kg rat or a 1.5-kg rabbit, may absorb, in absolute terms, nearly as much. These differences are made more apparent when the rate of net cholesterol absorption is expressed per kilogram body weight. On a relatively high cholesterol intake, man absorbs only about 2 to 4 mg cholesterol/day/kg body weight. In contrast, other species, such as the rat, rabbit, and dog, can absorb from 35 to 50 times this amount. On the basis of such findings, it has been postulated that this limited capacity to absorb cholesterol may be one of the major mechanisms that protects man against the detrimental effects of excessive dietary cholesterol intake (1).

TABLE 1. *Comparison of rates of cholesterol absorption in four different animal species*[a]

Species	Representative body weight (kg)	Dietary cholesterol intake (mg/day)	Cholesterol absorption rate	
			Per animal[b] (mg/day)	Per kg body weight[c] (mg/day/kg body weight)
Rat	0.2	50–300	44–102	220–510
Rabbit	1.5	465–500	450	300
Dog	10.0	1,100–1,600	70–1,000	70–100
Man	70.0	300–2,950	140–280	2–4

[a] Representative values are shown for the amount of cholesterol absorbed from the diet in four different species. Data are presented in terms of the absolute milligram cholesterol absorbed per day in an animal of average weight[b] and expressed as the milligram sterol absorbed per kilogram body weight[c].
These data were adapted from a variety of studies (32–40).

CHOLESTEROL SYNTHESIS RATES IN THE WHOLE ANIMAL

The second of the major sources for cholesterol in the body pool is *de novo* synthesis of sterol by the major organ systems. The rate at which cholesterol is synthesized within the body of man or the experimental animal has been measured by two different types of procedures. One method involves measuring sterol balance across the body. With this technique, the amount of cholesterol excreted from the body in the feces as neutral (cholesterol and its bacterial degradation products) and acidic (bile acids) sterols is quantitated in the steady state. After taking into account the amounts of cholesterol that are eaten in the diet and lost from the skin or converted to steroid hormones, and after correcting for any sterol that may be completely degraded by intestinal bacteria, it is possible to calculate the rate of total cholesterol synthesis per day in the experimental subject.

The rate of whole body sterol synthesis has been determined more directly by measuring the rate at which an animal incorporates [^{3}H]water into sterols under *in vivo* conditions. By assuming that 1.45 μg atoms of carbon are incorporated into cholesterol for every microgram atom of ^{3}H, it is possible to calculate the absolute amount of cholesterol that is synthesized under a given circumstance from the amount of ^{3}H that appears in the body sterol pool over a relatively short period of time (41). While this carbon/^{3}H incorporation ratio has been shown to be correct in the liver and several other major tissues of different animals, it has not yet been shown to be applicable to all other tissues in the body. Furthermore, these two methods have not yet been rigorously compared in the same experimental setting. Despite these shortcomings, however, the external sterol balance technique and the [^{3}H]water incorporation procedure yield comparable results. For example, the rate of sterol synthesis in the squirrel monkey equals about 30 to 34 mg cholesterol/day/kg body weight whether measured by sterol balance or by

isotope incorporation (41,42). Similarly, about 20 to 24 mg cholesterol are synthesized each day in a 0.2-kg rat when quantitated by either technique (41,43).

Using such methods, rates of whole body cholesterol synthesis have been measured in man and in a variety of animals under conditions where dietary cholesterol intake was low. These values are summarized in Table 2. As is apparent, the absolute amount of cholesterol synthesized varies markedly from animal to animal and even differs between animals of similar weight, e.g., rat and hamster or guinea pig and squirrel monkey. As was the case with species differences in cholesterol absorption, these variations in rates of sterol synthesis are emphasized by expressing the data as the amount of cholesterol synthesized per kilogram body weight. Thus man can synthesize about 9 mg cholesterol/day/kg body weight, while the rat is capable of making over 13 times more sterol, or about 118 mg/day/kg body weight. In general, there is an inverse although imperfect relationship between the rate of whole animal sterol synthesis and body weight. The larger animals and man generally synthesize much less sterol per unit weight than the small animals, particularly the rat.

From these data on the rates of cholesterol absorption (Table 1) and rates of cholesterol synthesis (Table 2), it is possible to begin to appreciate the quantitative importance of each of these input processes as sources for the body pool of cholesterol. Obviously, when man or an experimental animal is maintained on a cholesterol-free diet, 100% of the sterol in the body pool, circulating in the plasma, and secreted into the bile must ultimately be derived from cholesterol synthesized endogenously. As the content of cholesterol in the diet is increased, the extent to which the body pool is derived from this exogenous source will vary and, in a given species, will be largely determined by the amount of cholesterol that can be absorbed from the gastrointestinal tract relative to the amount that can be synthesized under a particular experimental

TABLE 2. *Comparison of rates of whole animal cholesterol synthesis in eight different animal species*[a]

Species	Representative body weight (kg)	Rates of cholesterol synthesis	
		Per animal[b] (mg/day)	Per kg body weight[c] (mg/day/kg body weight)
Rat	0.2	23.6	118
Hamster	0.15	5.8	39
Squirrel monkey	0.6	20.6	34
Rabbit	1.5	46.1	31
Guinea pig	0.5	11.2	22
Baboon	25.0	525.0	21
Dog	10.0	120.0	12
Man	70.0	630.0	9

[a] Representative values are shown for the amount of cholesterol synthesized in the whole body of eight different species. Data are presented in terms of the absolute amount of cholesterol synthesized per day in an animal of average weight[b] and expressed as the milligram cholesterol synthesized per day per kilogram body weight[c].

This table was compiled from data determined either by external balance techniques and reported from a number of different laboratories or by determining the rate of incorporation of [³H]water into cholesterol *in vivo* and then calculating the absolute rate of cholesterol synthesis (41–50).

circumstance. In man, for example, the low rate of cholesterol absorption (2 to 4 mg/day/kg body weight) relative to the capacity for endogenous sterol synthesis (9 mg/day/kg body weight) would suggest that even on a fairly high cholesterol intake, most of the body pool would still be derived from endogenous synthesis. This conclusion is supported by experiments in which human subjects were fed a diet high in radiolabeled cholesterol until an isotopic steady state was achieved. It could then be calculated directly that approximately 60% of the plasma cholesterol pool was still derived from endogenous synthesis, despite the intake of a relatively large amount of dietary cholesterol. In contrast, when the rat is placed on a high cholesterol diet, it absorbs much more dietary cholesterol (220 to 510 mg/day/kg body weight) relative to the rate of endogenous synthesis (<118 mg/day/kg body weight), so that less than 10% of the plasma cholesterol is derived from newly synthesized sterols (32,51).

TECHNICAL PROBLEMS ASSOCIATED WITH DETERMINING THE RATE OF CHOLESTEROL SYNTHESIS IN THE LIVER AND IN OTHER TISSUES

The question of the extent to which the synthesis of endogenous cholesterol takes place in the liver as opposed to the extrahepatic tissues is particularly relevant to the problem of cholesterol gallstone formation in man. It has been postulated that a causal relationship may exist between the rate of cholesterol synthesis in the whole body and, more particularly in the liver, and the amount of cholesterol secreted into bile. Despite the importance of this problem, quantitation of the contribution of hepatic sterol synthesis to whole body cholesterol synthesis has proved to be a difficult and perplexing problem.

Two general approaches have been made to this problem. The first takes advantage of the technique of external sterol balance. Since it is known that cholesterol feeding suppresses sterol synthesis in the liver, it is possible to estimate indirectly the contribution of the liver to total body synthesis by measuring the rate of endogenous cholesterol production in man or an experimental animal on a low and high dietary cholesterol intake. The difference between these two values has been taken as a measure of the rate of hepatic cholesterol synthesis. Such a method is critically dependent on the following assumptions: (a) cholesterol feeding suppresses sterol synthesis only in the liver; and (b) the suppression of hepatic synthesis is essentially complete. In reality, neither of these assumptions is entirely true. In man in particular, cholesterol feeding results in only partial suppression of sterol synthesis in the liver (52,53).

The alternative approach to this problem has been to measure the rates of sterol synthesis in the liver and other tissues in the body under *in vitro* conditions using radiolabeled substrates, such as [¹⁴C]acetate. The amount of sterol synthesis found in the liver can then be expressed as a percentage of the synthetic activity found in all the tissues combined. Such an approach has been used in many species, including man, and has led to the commonly held belief that the liver is the major source for cholesterol in the body. In both the rat and squirrel monkey, for example, more than 80% of the incorporation of [¹⁴C]acetate into cholesterol that can be detected *in vitro* in the different organs of the body takes place in the liver (1,54,55).

More recent data suggest that this conclusion is in error, and that the importance of the liver to whole body sterol synthesis has been grossly overestimated. The reason for this error concerns certain technical problems that are associated with the use of radiolabeled compounds to estimate rates of sterol synthesis. The sources of these problems are shown diagrammatically in Fig. 2. If a preparation of liver cells (or other tissues) is incubated *in vitro* with a precursor compound, such as [14C]acetate (pathway A), the radiolabeled acetate is activated to [14C]acetyl CoA in the cytosolic compartment, which in turn is utilized for the synthesis of cholesterol. The rate of cholesterol synthesis is calculated by dividing the total radioactivity appearing in the sterols by the specific activity (SA) of the [14C]acetate added to the incubation flask. The SA of the cytosolic acetyl CoA pool, however, has been diluted by the generation of unlabled acetyl CoA in the mitochondrial compartment from unlabeled substrates, such as fatty acids. Hence the rate of cholesterol synthesis is underestimated to the degree that such dilution occurs.

To calculate the true rate of cholesterol synthesis, it would be necessary to divide the amount of radioactivity in the cholesterol by the SA of the cytosolic [14C]acetyl CoA and not by the SA of the [14C]acetate added to the incubation mixture. Similar effects are encountered with almost any other 14C-labeled substrate that can be used. For example, the SA of the [14C]acetyl CoA generated from [14C]glucose is massively diluted, both because of unlabeled glucose generated within the cytosolic compartment and because of the production of unlabeled acetyl CoA in the mitochondrial compartment (pathway B). Even the SA of [14C]acetyl CoA generated directly within the mito-

chondria from the oxidation of [14C]octanoate will be diluted to the extent that oxidation of other unlabeled fatty acids is also taking place (pathway C) (56–58).

The magnitude of these errors is illustrated in Fig. 3, where apparent rates of cholesterol synthesis, expressed as the nanomole of acetyl CoA incorporated into sterols, were determined in the same group of liver slices using these three different [14C]substrates. In this tissue, the absolute rate of acetyl CoA incorporation equaled 755 nmoles/hr/g. The rate determined with [14C]glucose was only about 2% of the actual rate and equaled 17 nmoles/hr/g, while the rates determined with [14C]acetate and [14C]octanoate equaled 45 and 76%, respectively, of the absolute value (58). These marked differences reflect the varying degrees of dilution that take place in the liver cell under the conditions of this experiment. Thus the SA of the [14C]acetyl CoA generated from [14C]glucose (pathway B, Fig. 2), [14C]acetate (pathway A), and [14C]octanoate (pathway C) was diluted by 98, 55, and 24%, respectively. Obviously, the apparent rate of sterol synthesis thus determined in the liver depends more on the [14C]substrate used to make the measurement than on the actual rate of synthesis that is occurring within the tissue. Furthermore, there may be serious problems, even when the same [14C]substrate is used to compare rates of synthesis in the liver with those obtained in other tissues; the degree of dilution of the SA of the [14C]acetyl CoA may vary in different types of cells (58).

Because of these problems, investigators have turned

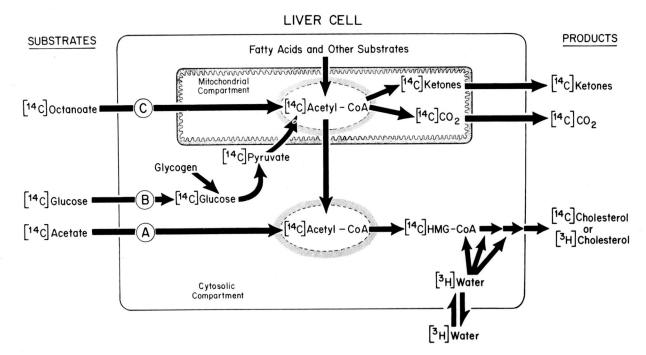

FIG. 2. Illustration of the technical problems associated with the determination of rates of cholesterol synthesis using various radioactive substrates. In this diagram, the liver cell is divided into mitochondrial and cytosolic compartments. The general pathways that must be followed in order to incorporate radioactivity from the various 14C– or 3H-labeled substrates into cholesterol are shown. (Adapted from data largely presented in refs. 56–58.)

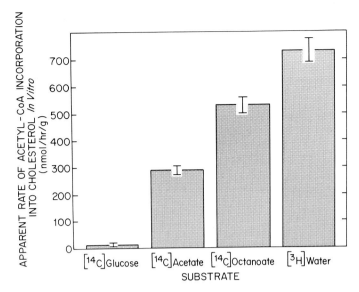

FIG. 3. Rates of cholesterol synthesis in the liver of the rat determined *in vitro* with various radiolabeled substrates. *Vertical axis,* apparent rate of acetyl-CoA incorporation into cholesterol in tissue slices obtained from the same livers using four different radiolabeled substrates. Marked differences in the apparent rates of sterol synthesis are due to variable dilution of the specific activity of the various precursors or their intermediate products. Mean values ± 1 SEM. (Based on data presented in ref. 58.)

labeled water are generated metabolically during the course of the experiment. Thus, in contrast to the situation encountered when [^{14}C]substrates are used, there is essentially no detectable dilution of the SA of the [^{3}H]water. The SA of the water in the incubation media can be taken as a direct measure of the SA of the intracellular water being incorporated into the cholesterol molecule. Second, assuming that the C/^{3}H incorporation ratio is accurately known, then rates of [^{3}H]water incorporation into cholesterol can be converted directly into the mass of cholesterol synthesized. The incorporation of 500 μmoles [^{3}H]water into sterols, for example, would correspond to the synthesis of 15.6 mg cholesterol (41,58).

By simultaneously measuring rates of cholesterol synthesis *in vitro* with a [^{14}C]substrate and with [^{3}H]water, it is possible to determine directly the magnitude of the errors that have been introduced into the determination of the relative importance of various organs in whole body sterol synthesis utilizing such [^{14}C]substrates. As illustrated in Fig. 4, for example, the rate of cholesterol synthesis determined with [^{14}C]acetate is about 45% of the rate found with [^{3}H]water in the liver, small bowel, and spleen. The percentages are even lower in other organs; and in the skin and muscle, two tissues that account for a large proportion of body weight, the rates of [^{14}C]acetate incorporation into sterols are less than 10% of the true rates. Findings such as these strongly imply that rates of sterol synthesis have been disproportionately underestimated in many extrahepatic tissues utilizing [^{14}C]-substrates which, if true, would suggest that the synthesis of cholesterol by the liver is quantitatively far less important than has heretofore been considered to be the case.

to the use of [^{3}H]water as a more appropriate substrate for measuring rates of synthesis in such *in vitro* experiments. As shown in Fig. 2, ^{3}H atoms may be incorporated into the cholesterol molecule either directly from tritiated water or during certain reductive steps involving reduced diphosphopyridine nucleotide (NADPH). The degree to which NADPH becomes labeled with ^{3}H in the presence of [^{3}H]water in turn depends to some extent on the source of the reduced diphosphopyridine nucleotide (58,59). During the biosynthesis of cholesterol, 18 μmoles acetyl CoA give rise to 1 μmole cholesterol containing 27 μg atoms of C and 46 μg atoms of H, 15 of which are derived from NADPH, while seven come directly from water in the medium. Thus the number of microgram atoms of ^{3}H incorporated into cholesterol will depend on the degree of equilibration of the H of NADPH with the ^{3}H of [^{3}H]water (59). Most available evidence suggests that equilibration between the reductive H of NADPH and the ^{3}H of [^{3}H]water is complete (58,60–63). Therefore, about 22 μg atoms of ^{3}H should be incorporated into each micromole newly synthesized cholesterol. Stated differently, 1.45 μmole acetyl CoA should be incorporated into cholesterol for every 1.0 μmole [^{3}H]water; i.e., the C/^{3}H incorporation ratio equals about 1.45.

Two points warrant emphasis concerning the use of [^{3}H]water to quantitate rates of sterol synthesis *in vitro*. First, only infinitesimally small amounts of un-

RATES OF HEPATIC CHOLESTEROL SYNTHESIS *IN VITRO* AND *IN VIVO*

[^{3}H]Water should be the ideal substrate with which to quantitate rates of cholesterol synthesis in the liver, since this method is not subject to the serious errors inherent in the use of various [^{14}C]substrates. Furthermore, recent experimental work has demonstrated that the C/^{3}H incorporation ratio is approximately the same in liver tissue derived from a variety of animal species (41). Hence, the rates of [^{3}H]water incorporation into cholesterol should provide an accurate appraisal of both the relative and absolute rates of hepatic sterol synthesis as measured under *in vitro* conditions.

Rates of cholesterol synthesis have been measured in liver specimens obtained from a variety of animal species that had been maintained on a low intake of dietary cholesterol. As summarized in Fig. 5, large variations are seen among the different species when

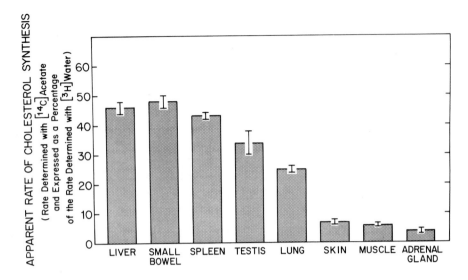

FIG. 4. Rates of cholesterol synthesis in different tissues of the rat measured *in vitro* using [¹⁴C]acetate and [³H]water. In these studies, rates of incorporation of both [¹⁴C]acetate and [³H]water into cholesterol were measured in tissue slices from various organs. *Vertical axis,* apparent rate of sterol synthesis determined with [¹⁴C]acetate expressed as a percentage of the true rate of cholesterol synthesis as determined with [³H]water. Mean values ± 1 SEM. (Adapted from data presented in ref. 58.)

these rates of synthesis are expressed per gram liver tissue. The rat again manifests an extremely high rate of cholesterol synthesis, reflecting the high rate of whole body sterol synthesis found in the same species (Table 2). Rates of sterol synthesis are all much lower in other species, including man. Another point to be emphasized is that there is no general correlation between the rates of hepatic cholesterol synthesis and the relative amounts of cholesterol secreted into the bile of each of these species or of their respective propensities to develop cholesterol gallstones.

These comparisons, although interesting do not answer the fundamentally important question about the quantitative importance of the liver to whole body sterol synthesis in each of these species, particularly under *in vivo* conditions. Fortunately, [³H]water also can be utilized to make such measurements. When administered intravenously, this substrate rapidly equilibrates with the total pool of body water. Hence, the SA of the intracellular water that is being incorpo-

rated into cholesterol presumably equals the SA of water in the circulating plasma; this can be easily sampled. Furthermore, provided that the experimental subject is not given any exogenous water, the SA of the body pool remains essentially constant for long periods of time. Rates of incorporation of [³H]water into cholesterol under these conditions also provide an accurate measure of rates of sterol synthesis *in vivo* (64).

Figure 6 shows the amount of newly synthesized sterol that is found in 1 g of the major organs of the rat (panel A) and squirrel monkey (panel B) 1 hr after the intravenous administration of [³H]water. The highest content of [³H]cholesterol is found in the liver, endocrine glands, and various parts of the gastrointestinal tract. All other tissues contain some newly synthesized sterol, but the amounts are low when expressed per gram tissue (41,65).

To relate these values to whole body synthesis rates, the weight of each organ must be taken into considera-

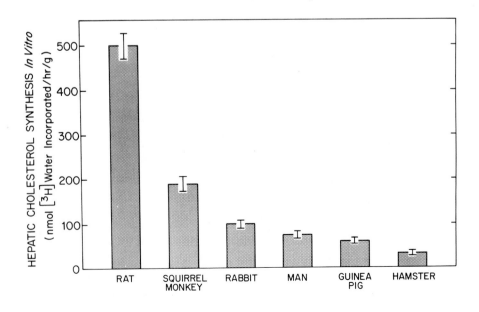

FIG. 5. Rates of cholesterol synthesis in the livers of different species determined *in vitro* using [³H]water, showing rates at which liver slices incorporate [³H]water into cholesterol. In all cases, hepatic tissue was obtained from donors that had been maintained on a low cholesterol intake for several weeks before the studies were carried out. Mean values ± 1 SEM. (Based on unpublished observations in this laboratory as well as on data presented in ref. 41.)

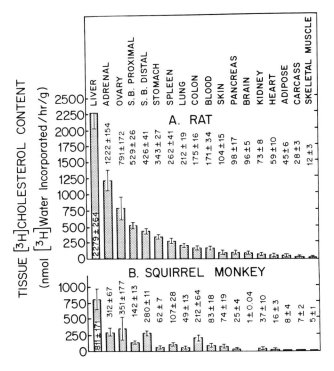

FIG. 6. Content of newly synthesized cholesterol in various organs of the rat and squirrel monkey determined *in vivo*. In these experiments, [³H]water was administered intravenously into the animals, which were killed 1 hr later. The amount of newly synthesized cholesterol present in each tissue is expressed as nanomole [³H]water incorporated into the sterols contained in 1 g of each tissue at 1 hr. Mean values ± 1 SEM. S.B., small bowel. (These data are reported in detail in refs. 41 and 65.)

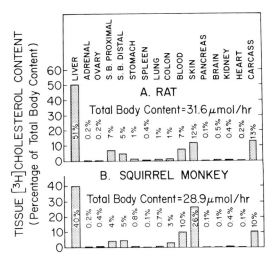

FIG. 7. Importance of the major organ systems as sites for cholesterol synthesis *in vivo* in the rat and squirrel monkey. As described in the legend to Fig. 6, the animals were administered [³H]water intravenously and killed 1 hr later. The content of newly synthesized cholesterol in each major tissue was then determined and is expressed as a percentage of the rate of synthesis found in the whole animal. Rates of cholesterol synthesis in the whole animal are also shown and are expressed as micromoles [³H]water incorporated into sterols by the whole animal per hour. (Data derived from experiments detailed in refs. 41 and 65.)

tion (Fig. 7). The whole rat incorporates 31.6 μmoles/hr [³H]water into sterol; in the squirrel monkey, this value equals 28.9 μmoles/hr. These incorporation rates correspond to the synthesis of 24 and 22 mg/day cholesterol in these two species, respectively. In the rat, 51% of the newly synthesized sterol is found in the liver, 12% in the small intestine, 12% in the skin, and 13% in the carcass (mainly muscle and bone). This same group of organs also contains the majority of the newly synthesized sterol found in the monkey. Thus, while the rates of synthesis per gram skin and muscle are very low, these two organs make up such a large fraction of the body weight of the animals that they also are major sites for the synthesis of sterols.

Under these *in vivo* conditions there have been small shifts of newly synthesized cholesterol from the sites of origin to other organs. Quantitatively, the most important shifts occur out of the liver and small intestine (65). In the rat, for example, nearly half the cholesterol that has been synthesized in the intestine is transferred to the liver within 1 hr, and approximately 30% of that synthesized in the liver has moved out into the plasma and extrahepatic tissues. Taking these shifts into consideration, it has been reported in this species that only about 50% of total body sterol synthesis occurs in the

liver, 24% in the small intestine, 8% in the skin, and 18% in the remaining tissues in the body.

Based on this type of analysis, the quantitative importance of the liver to total body sterol synthesis in different animal species under the condition of low dietary cholesterol intake has been measured in a number of different species, as shown in Fig. 8. In the rat and squirrel monkey, approximately half of whole body sterol synthesis takes place in the liver. In the other species in which such measurements have been made, however, hepatic cholesterol synthesis contributes less than one-third of the sterol synthesized in the body each day. These results confirm that previous work utilizing a variety of [¹⁴C]substrates to quantitate the importance of the major organ systems for endogenous sterol synthesis has grossly underestimated the role of extrahepatic tissues. In a number of species the contribution of gastrointestinal tract, muscle, and skin equals or exceeds that of the liver.

Unfortunately, as also indicated in Fig. 8, such measurements have not been made in man, and only tentative conclusions can be drawn concerning the importance of the liver in this species. Rates of hepatic cholesterol synthesis measured *in vitro* in biopsy specimens are low when compared to similar measurements made in other species, such as the monkey and rat, and are comparable to those obtained in the rabbit and guinea pig (Fig. 5), two animals in which the liver accounts for only about 20% of endogenous cholesterol

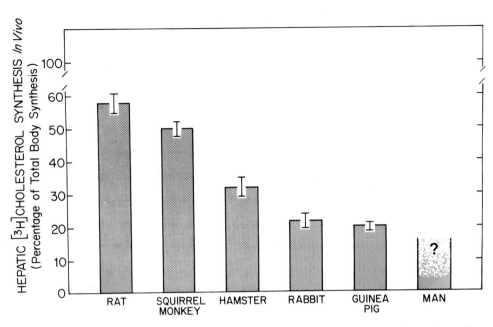

FIG. 8. Importance of the liver as a site for cholesterol synthesis in different species. Data show the amount of sterol synthesized in the liver *in vivo* and are expressed as a percentage of the total rate of cholesterol synthesis found in the whole animal. As discussed in the text, no data of this type are available for man, and the value can be only roughly estimated. In all cases, data refer to the situation where the animals had been maintained on a low cholesterol intake, so that the rates of sterol synthesis in the liver are essentially maximal. To the extent that cholesterol is added to the diet, these values would be proportionately lower.

synthesis (Fig. 8). Such *in vitro* measurements, however, have necessarily been made in tissue obtained from patients who were fasted overnight and who had some degree of liver dysfunction; hence, the validity of this extrapolation is uncertain.

In external balance studies performed in normal man, cholesterol feeding has been reported to have an inconstant effect on total body synthesis. Several investigators have reported studies in which cholesterol feeding had either no effect or only a modest effect on endogenous cholesterol synthesis rates (32,46,47,66). Such a result might imply that the liver of man is not subject to feedback suppression of cholesterol synthesis by dietary cholesterol. Several studies have shown that this is not the case, and that sterol synthesis is at least partially suppressed by cholesterol feeding (52, 53). The alternative explanation is that in man, as in other species that have been investigated, the liver makes only a modest contribution to total body sterol synthesis. Whether or not this conclusion is correct requires further investigations.

CHOLESTEROL TRANSPORT THROUGH THE PLASMA

The liver remains the key organ for the regulation of cholesterol balance within the intact animal. It (a) largely compensates for changes in cholesterol input into the body from the diet, (b) synthesizes various lipoprotein particles which deliver sterol to certain peripheral tissues, (c) takes up other lipoprotein particles carrying cholesterol from the extrahepatic tissues back to the liver, and (d) secretes cholesterol and bile acids from the body. The movement of cholesterol through plasma and its targeted uptake by specific tissues is articulated by special classes of lipoproteins interacting with specific cell surface receptors present on the parenchymal cells of many organs. The major pathways for the transport of cholesterol among the various tissue compartments of the body are outlined in Fig. 9. The amounts of cholesterol shown entering and leaving the body pool through the various input and output pathways are representative for normal man.

Dietary cholesterol, along with endogenous cholesterol that has been secreted into the intestinal lumen in bile and other secretions, is taken up by absorptive cells located predominantly in the proximal portion of the small intestine. There is mixes with an additional pool of cholesterol that has been synthesized locally and, after being largely esterified, is incorporated into the nascent chylomicron (CM) particle. Thus, while most exogenous or dietary cholesterol enters the body carried in the CM, a significant proportion of the cholesterol present in this particle may be of endogenous origin, since the amount of biliary cholesterol entering the bowel lumen or synthesized within the intestinal wall may be large compared to the amount of cholesterol available for absorption from the diet.

The nascent particle contains predominantly apo-

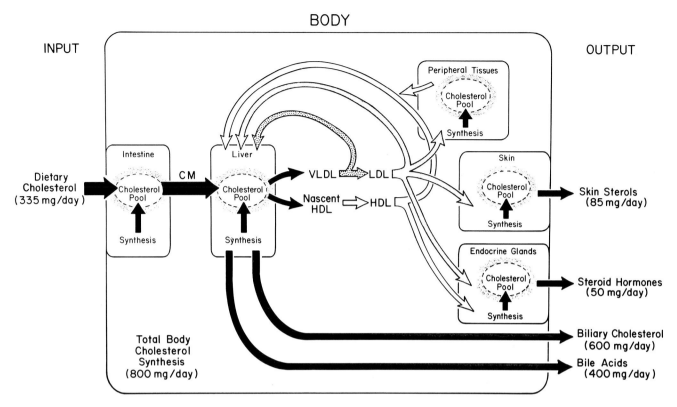

FIG. 9. Major steps in the transport of cholesterol between the different tissue compartments of the body. Many additional details concerning each of these steps are described in the text. Amounts of cholesterol shown as being absorbed, synthesized, and excreted are representative values for normal man.

proteins A-I (apoA-I) and B (apoB). Once it enters the lymph, however, the CM acquires apoproteins E (apoE) and C (apoC) through interaction with other lipoproteins, such as high density lipoproteins (HDL) (67–69). This family of C apoproteins serves two important functions. First, the presence of large amounts of apoC, relative to apoE, appears to prevent uptake of the particle by the liver. Second, one component of this family, apoC-II, activates the enzyme lipoprotein lipase (LPL). This enzyme is situated on the luminal surface of capillaries found predominantly in muscle and adipose tissue and rapidly hydrolyzes much of the triglyceride present in the core of the CM. This liberates large amounts of free fatty acid that are then taken up and stored or metabolized in adjacent tissues. As the triglyceride in the core of the CM is removed, the particle becomes smaller in size and loses some of its surface components, including unesterified cholesterol, phospholipid, and apoproteins A-I and C (70). Presumably because of the decrease in the ratio of apoC to apoE, the partially metabolized CM, or CM remnant, is recognized by the hepatocyte and is rapidly and essentially quantitatively cleared by the liver (69,71–73). This uptake occurs by way of a high velocity, saturable transport system that probably depends on the presence of receptors on the liver parenchymal cells that interact with the apoE of the remnant

(74–78). Since the effective K_m for this transport process is so low, the plasma is cleared essentially completely of the particle within minutes (75). Much of the cholesterol from the diet or bile that is absorbed across the intestine or synthesized within the bowel wall is delivered directly to the liver by this mechanism.

As the CM serves to transport triglyceride and cholesterol out of the intestine, the very low density lipoproteins (VLDL) serve a similar function in transporting triglyceride and cholesterol out of the liver. These particles also contain apoB (although of higher molecular weight than the apoB of the CM), apoC, and apoE (79–81). The triglyceride carried in VLDL is largely disposed of in peripheral tissues as this nonpolar lipid in the core of the lipoprotein is hydrolyzed by LPL and a remnant particle is formed. This remnant, like that formed by the action of LPL on the CM, is rapidly and quantitatively taken up by the liver (82).

An alternative pathway exists for VLDL in that this particle may be metabolized through an intermediate density lipoprotein fraction to low density lipoproteins (LDL), which contain essentially only the B apoprotein. It is unclear where this transformation takes place, although the liver may be involved. In some species, such as the rat, the majority of VLDL produced by the liver is metabolized through the remnant pathway; in man, a much larger proportion of the

VLDL is metabolized to LDL (83,84). Hence, depending on the species, a variable proportion of the cholesterol derived from the hepatic sterol pool and incorporated into VLDL ends up circulating in the plasma LDL fraction.

Many tissues of the body, including the liver, possess specific cell surface receptors that recognize and bind lipoproteins containing the B and/or E apoproteins. These binding sites are referred to as LDL receptors (85–93). Tissues that contain these receptor sites bind and internalize the LDL particle and so acquire cholesterol to partially meet their metabolic needs. Although there is still uncertainty as to the quantitative importance of different organ systems in the uptake and catabolism of LDL, several lines of evidence suggest that approximately 35 to 50% of the LDL cleared from the plasma each day may be taken up by the liver (94,95). Other tissues also depend on LDL as a major source for tissue cholesterol, including the endocrine glands, skin, lung, kidney, intestine, spleen, and several other peripheral tissues (65,96–98).

The liver is one of the sites for the synthesis of nascent HDL, which consist of discoid particles containing predominantly unesterified cholesterol, phospholipid, and the apoproteins A-I and E (99, 100). Similar structures can also be synthesized in the intestine or can be derived from the loss of excess surface material during the metabolism of CM by LPL (100–102). The apoA-I present in these discoid structures acts as a cofactor for the plasma enzyme lecithin-cholesterol acyltransferase (LCAT) that promotes the formation of cholesteryl esters. This nonpolar lipid then moves to the center of the discs, forming spherical, mature HDL particles (99,100,103). Additionally, free cholesterol may move to the HDL particles from other lipoprotein fractions or from the cell membranes of various tissues. There the free sterol is esterified through the action of LCAT and enters the pool of cholesteryl esters carried in the plasma HDL (104).

The mechanisms responsible for the removal of HDL, or of the cholesterol carried in HDL, from the plasma are complex and poorly understood. On one hand, the entire HDL particle may be removed from the plasma and catabolized. This might occur, for example, in those species where the HDL contains significant amounts of apoE that will allow the particles to bind to the LDL receptors in the liver and other tissues (87,88,95,105–107). It has also been suggested that the adrenal gland, ovary, and testes of some species have a second type of transport mechanism that specifically takes up HDL so that the cholesterol may be utilized as a substrate for steroid hormone production (108–115). Although the quantitative importance of such processes are poorly documented, the limited experimental data available suggest that in some species at least, HDL is primarily metabolized in

extrahepatic tissues (95,104,115,116). On the other hand, the cholesteryl esters may be dissociated from the remainder of the HDL structure and transferred to other lipoproteins, such as LDL or the remnants of CM and VLDL (104,117,118). If such transfers are quantitatively important, then considerable amounts of cholesterol may be shuttled to the liver and to the other tissues responsible for the uptake and degradation of these respective lipoprotein fractions.

COMPARTMENTALIZATION AND REGULATION OF CHOLESTEROL BALANCE WITHIN THE LIVER

From these various considerations, the major pathways for the movement of cholesterol into and out of the liver cell can be summarized as shown in Fig. 10. There can be net input of sterol into the metabolically active hepatic cholesterol pool from at least three sources: (a) dietary cholesterol or cholesterol synthesized in the intestine that reaches the liver in CM, (b) cholesterol synthesized in other extrahepatic tissues that reaches the liver carried in HDL, LDL, or remnants of VLDL, and (c) synthesis of cholesterol within the liver itself. Similarly, net loss of sterol from the liver can take place through (a) synthesis and secretion of lipoproteins, (b) secretion of cholesterol into bile, and (c) synthesis of bile acids from cholesterol and their subsequent secretion into bile. Generally, these processes are so well balanced that little or no net accumulation of cholesterol takes place in the hepatocyte.

In theory, at least, it is possible that there is preferential channeling of cholesterol from one input process to a specific excretory pathway. It has been postulated, for example, that a portion of the sterol in bile may be derived directly from cholesterol that is carried to the liver in the form of HDL (119,120). Still other experimental work has suggested that the rate of biliary cholesterol secretion is primarily determined by the amount of cholesterol reaching the liver in CM or, alternatively, by the amount of cholesterol that is newly synthesized within the liver (121–124). Finally, several lines of evidence indicate that newly synthesized cholesterol may be preferentially utilized for the synthesis of bile acids (125,126).

Despite these various observations, however, there are actually few unequivocal data supporting the contention that cholesterol from one source is preferentially utilized for export in one particular pathway. Thus under basal conditions, a portion of cholesterol used for bile acid synthesis or for secretion in bile may be synthesized *de novo* in the liver (127,128). If the input of dietary cholesterol into the body is increased, the fraction of newly synthesized cholesterol used for

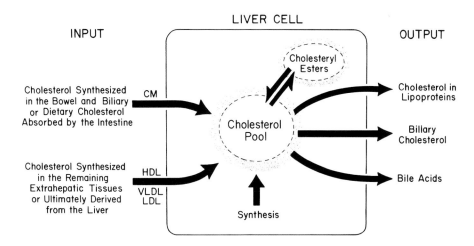

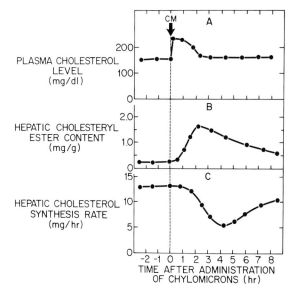

FIG. 10. Cholesterol balance across the liver. Major sources for cholesterol entering the hepatocyte and the major pathways for the disposition of the sterol from the liver are summarized. The intracellular, metabolically active pool of unesterified cholesterol is shown as a single compartment although, as discussed in the text, this pool may be compartmentalized into several functionally distinct subpools.

bile acid synthesis or secreted into bile markedly decreases, and the sterol absorbed from the diet is readily used in its place for these two metabolic processes (127–129). Although it is still possible that some degree of compartmentalization exists within the liver, it is more reasonable to assume that the hepatocyte contains a single functional pool of metabolically active cholesterol. This pool is maintained by the input of cholesterol from the three sources shown diagrammatically in Fig. 10 and can be utilized for lipoprotein and biliary cholesterol and for bile acid synthesis.

Mechanisms must exist, however, to keep this pool relatively constant in the face of the marked changes that may occur in either the input or output of sterol from the liver cell. As the amount of cholesterol in the diet varies from day to day, the amount of cholesterol entering the liver in CM will also vary. The regulatory events that occur in the liver in this situation are shown in Fig. 11. When a large amount of cholesterol carried in CM is introduced into the plasma through the absorption of dietary cholesterol (130) or, experimentally, through the intravenous administration of CM, the lipoprotein particles are rapidly metabolized to remnants that disappear from the plasma and are taken up by the liver (72,73). This causes an increase in the concentration of cholesteryl esters in the liver and a reciprocal suppression of the rate of hepatic sterol synthesis. If no additional CM cholesterol enters the plasma, then the cholesteryl ester pool is slowly utilized, and the rate of cholesterol synthesis slowly increases to its original rate. Thus total input of cholesterol into the metabolically active pool from all sources remains essentially constant and equals output.

Similar adaptations take place when there is excessive loss of cholesterol from the liver, as may occur with interruption of the enterohepatic circulation of bile acids. In this situation, there is an increased rate of bile acid production from cholesterol, coupled with an increased rate of cholesterol synthesis in the liver

(64,131–135). The increment in cholesterol synthesis may balance the increment in bile acid synthesis, so that sterol balance across the liver cells is maintained (95). If not, the liver may pull in additional amounts of cholesterol from the plasma by increasing the number of functional LDL receptors on the sinusoidal membrane (136,137). This lowers the circulating levels of plasma cholesterol and presumably results in the delivery of additional amounts of sterol from the peripheral tissues to the liver. Once again, these adaptive responses are aimed at maintaining a balance between the total input of cholesterol into the liver and the total output.

Even though these adaptive responses generally function well, there is increasing evidence that subtle

FIG. 11. Regulation of hepatic cholesterol synthesis by CM. This diagram illustrates what happens to levels of esterified cholesterol in the liver and to the rates of hepatic cholesterol synthesis when cholesterol carried in CM is introduced into the bloodstream. See text for details. (Based on data largely presented in refs. 72 and 73.)

imbalances in hepatic cholesterol metabolism may occur under certain physiologic conditions or in association with specific disease states. Such imbalances may lead to excessive cholesterol secretion in the bile and set the stage for cholesterol gallstone formation. The remainder of this chapter deals specifically with the process of cholesterol secretion from the liver cell into the bile and examines in detail the factors that appear to regulate this secretory process in man and other species.

COUPLING OF BILIARY CHOLESTEROL SECRETION TO BILE ACID AND PHOSPHOLIPID SECRETION

Under normal conditions, the secretion of cholesterol into bile is closely linked to the secretion of bile acid and phospholipid. This coupling is brought about by the capacity of bile acids to form micelles. These structures incorporate relatively large amounts of phospholipid to form mixed micelles, which normally facilitate the complete solubilization of all cholesterol that enters the bile. For reasons that are as yet poorly understood, this coupling reaction can become disrupted, so that more cholesterol enters the bile than can be solubilized by the bile acid and phospholipid present. The production of such lithogenic bile is the initiating event in the pathogenesis of cholesterol gallstone disease and can involve a variety of secretory defects ranging from excessive cholesterol secretion without any change in bile acid and phospholipid secretion rates to decreased bile acid and phospholipid secretion without any change in cholesterol output (138,139).

The precise manner in which cholesterol and phospholipid output is normally coupled to bile acid secretion is not known. One possibility is that complete micelle formation occurs within the canaliculus, where bile acids that have been actively transported across the canalicular membrane trap cholesterol and phospholipid that have passively entered the lumen. An alternative mechanism is that the assembly of the micelle is already complete as it enters the lumen, the bile acids having entrained cholesterol and phospholipid during their transport across the canalicular membrane (140,141).

Although the mechanism of biliary lipid transport remains unclear, the general features of the kinetics of biliary lipid secretion have been well characterized in several species, including the rat, dog, rhesus monkey, and man (140,142–148). It has generally been found that cholesterol and phospholipid secretion vary as a curvilinear function of bile acid output. The rates of bile acid secretion at which maximal rates of cholesterol and phospholipid output are attained, however, are lower in man than in other species. Figure 12 shows the relationship between biliary cholesterol and bile acid secretion in the rat and man. Data for the rat were obtained by subjecting animals to various experimental manipulations, including chronic biliary diversion, infusion or feeding of bile acids, fasting, and cholesterol and cholestyramine feeding (148). Cholesterol output increases in direct proportion to bile acid output until the latter reaches about 240 μmoles/hr/kg. The output of cholesterol then begins to plateau, reaching a maximum rate of about 4 to 5 μmoles/hr/kg. Data for man were derived from studies with patients undergoing chronic biliary diversion (146,147). Maximal cholesterol output is similar to that in the rat but is attained at a bile acid secretion rate of only about 40 μmoles/hr/kg.

The data shown in Fig. 13 describe the relationship between phospholipid and bile acid output under the same experimental conditions as in Fig. 12. In the rat, phospholipid secretion varies with bile acid output in an almost identical manner to that of cholesterol, with a maximal rate of phospholipid output of about 30 μmoles/hr/kg being attained once bile acid secretion reaches 240 μmoles/hr/kg. In contrast to the similar kinetics of cholesterol and phospholipid secretion in the rat, phospholipid secretion in man approaches its maximal rate at a bile acid output well above that at which cholesterol secretion reaches a plateau (146–148).

The relationships among cholesterol, phospholipid, and bile acid output in the dog are similar to those described for the rat (140,144,145). Thus in these particular species, the relative cholesterol content of bile is lower and tends to remain constant over a broader range of bile acid secretion rates than in man. Once bile acid output attains a sufficiently high rate, however, the relative cholesterol content falls, as it does in man.

The tight coupling that exists between cholesterol and phospholipid secretion while the enterohepatic circulation is intact is disrupted when hepatic bile acid output falls to low levels. Under these conditions, small amounts of cholesterol continue to enter the bile in the near absence of phospholipid (140,146,148). Thus, as illustrated in Fig. 14, there is a dramatic rise in the cholesterol:phospholipid ratio; consequently, the level of saturation increases significantly.

The dissociation of cholesterol and phospholipid secretion at low rates of bile acid output is thought to be an important factor in the pathogenesis of cholesterol gallstone disease in man. Detailed studies of biliary lipid secretion in man throughout the normal daily feeding and fasting cycle have shown that during the fasting phase, there is a physiologic interruption to the enterohepatic circulation; about half the bile acid pool is sequestered in the gall bladder, and there is a marked fall in hepatic bile acid output. Phospholipid secretion falls in parallel with that of bile acid, but

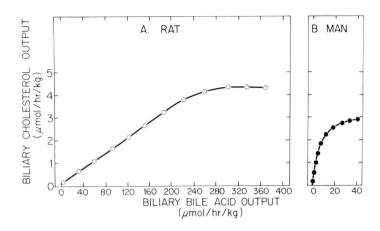

FIG. 12. Relationship between biliary secretion rates of cholesterol and bile acid in the rat and man. Relationship for the rat is based on data adapted from ref. 148. In those studies, the rate of bile acid output was varied by subjecting rats to various experimental manipulations, including chronic biliary diversion, infusion or feeding of bile acids, fasting, and feeding cholesterol or cholestyramine. Relationship for man is based on data adapted from refs. 146 and 147. These studies were carried out in patients undergoing chronic biliary diversion.

there is only a slight fall in cholesterol output. Consequently, the level of cholesterol saturation rises markedly (149,150). The production of such lithogenic bile during the fasting phase might contribute to gallstone formation if this bile did not mix completely with the contents of the gall bladder, thereby allowing localized cholesterol precipitation (149,150).

SPECIES DIFFERENCES IN BILIARY CHOLESTEROL SECRETION

The cholesterol content of bile is usually defined as a molar percentage, which is the ratio of the concentration of cholesterol to the total concentration of bile acid, phospholipid, and cholesterol multiplied by 100. This ratio is simply a measure of the total amount of cholesterol secreted relative to total lipid output and does not necessarily indicate the actual degree of cholesterol saturation and hence the potential for precipitation to occur, because the level of saturation is also determined by other factors, including the concentration of total lipid in bile (151). Thus bile samples with widely different total lipid concentrations may have the same relative cholesterol content, but the actual degree of saturation will be different, the more concentrated sample being less saturated.

An as yet unexplained phenomenon is that the molar percentage of cholesterol in bile varies greatly between different species. This is evident in the data given in Table 3, which shows the molar percentage of cholesterol in hepatic bile for 10 species, including man. In contrast to most other mammalian species, man and the baboon produce bile with relatively much more cholesterol that often reaches complete saturation (152,153,159). These are the only species in which spontaneous cholesterol gallstone formation is known to occur. Although as a group the primate species produce bile that is relatively more cholesterol rich, there is wide variability among these species, as evidenced by the values shown for the baboon and squirrel monkey (153,157). The more commonly utilized laboratory animals, such as the rat, hamster, and rabbit, secrete bile that is relatively poor in cholesterol (148,155,156, 158). The wide range of values reported for the hamster may reflect the use of different animal strains or, more likely, differences in the basal cholesterol content of stock diets used in different laboratories.

The wide variability among species in the relative cholesterol content of bile principally reflects differences in the absolute level of cholesterol. For example, the absolute concentration of cholesterol in baboon bile is several times higher than that in the rat and hamster. The bile of these species in turn contains

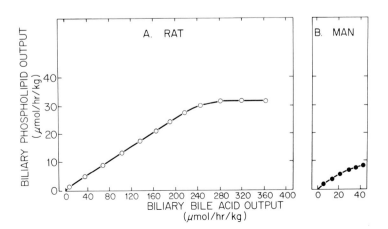

FIG. 13. Relationship between biliary secretion rates of phospholipid and bile acid in the rat and man. (Based on data adapted from refs. 146–148.)

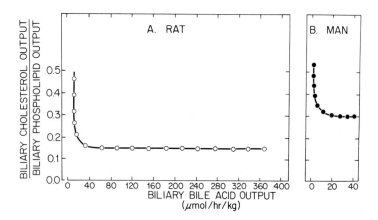

FIG. 14. Ratio of cholesterol to phospholipid output in the bile as a function of bile acid output in the rat and man. (Based on data adapted from refs. 146–148.)

much more cholesterol than the bile of the guinea pig, in which there are only trace amounts of sterol. The absolute concentrations of bile acid and phospholipid also vary from species to species, but the differences are less than those for cholesterol.

Although data are limited, there is no obvious correlation among the various species between biliary cholesterol secretion and other variables, such as plasma cholesterol levels, efficiency of cholesterol absorption (Table 1), rate of cholesterol synthesis in the liver (Fig. 8) or in the body as a whole (Table 2), or composition of the bile acid pool. The major regulatory step that determines biliary cholesterol output must occur at either the level of the coupling reaction involved in micelle formation or at events within the hepatocyte related to the synthesis of cholesterol and the uptake of lipoproteins from the plasma. Whether the pronounced differences in biliary cholesterol secretion among the various species is a manifestation of fundamentally different mechanisms of control remains to be determined.

FACTORS AFFECTING BILIARY CHOLESTEROL SECRETION

As illustrated in Fig. 10, biliary cholesterol must be derived ultimately either from cholesterol that is synthesized in the liver cell and then secreted directly across the canalicular membrane or from preformed cholesterol, which includes not only CM cholesterol (composed of cholesterol synthesized in the bowel as well as biliary or dietary cholesterol absorbed by the intestine), but also newly synthesized cholesterol of both hepatic and extrahepatic origin that was initially utilized for the production of various lipoproteins (HDL, VLDL, LDL) that are eventually catabolized in the liver.

Recent research on the control of biliary cholesterol secretion focuses on quantitating the proportion of biliary cholesterol normally derived from each of these sources and, more particularly, on determining whether

or not the availability of such newly synthesized or preformed cholesterol plays any role in determining the overall rate of transport of cholesterol into bile. In addition to these types of studies, an extensive literature has accumulated on nutritional and environmental factors that can alter biliary cholesterol output.

Rate of Cholesterol Synthesis in the Liver and Other Tissues

On the basis of several lines of evidence obtained from studies in man, it has been hypothesized that the rate of biliary cholesterol output is determined by the rate of cholesterol synthesis in the tissues. One such line of evidence is that cholesterol gallstone patients show higher than normal levels of β-hydroxy-β-methylglutaryl CoA reductase (HMG CoA reductase) activity in the liver (122,123); but this has not always been a consistent finding (160).

A second line of evidence derives from studies involving the administration of chenodeoxycholic acid to cholesterol gallstone patients. Under these conditions,

TABLE 3. *Species differences in the relative cholesterol content of hepatic bile*

Species	Molar percentage of cholesterol
Baboon	14.5
Man	5.0, 8.1
Rhesus monkey	6.0
Squirrel monkey	2.8
Prairie dog	2.4, 4.7
Hamster	1.6, 2.1, 3.6
Rat	1.8
Dog	0.9
Rabbit	0.5
Guinea pig	0.2

Values represent those commonly reported for normal man and animals.

All values were obtained from references 124,140,142, 148, and 152–159, except those for the rabbit and guinea pig, which were derived from unpublished studies in this laboratory.

the rate of biliary cholesterol secretion is reduced, and there is a corresponding fall in the activity of HMG CoA reductase in the liver (123,161,162). The obvious inference that derives from this observation has been undermined considerably by the more recent finding that ursodeoxycholic acid, which is equally or more effective in reducing biliary cholesterol secretion, either has little effect or may actually enhance the rate of hepatic cholesterol synthesis (162–166). Added to this is the recent report that deoxycholic acid, while markedly inhibiting hepatic HMG CoA reductase, has no effect on biliary lipid composition (167,168). Perhaps the strongest evidence for a direct link between biliary cholesterol output and cholesterol synthesis comes from studies in obese subjects. Under such conditions, there is a strong positive correlation between biliary cholesterol secretion and total body cholesterol synthesis, as measured by the sterol balance technique (50). It is unclear whether the liver or some extrahepatic tissue is the source of the additional newly synthesized cholesterol and, if it is of extrahepatic origin, how such cholesterol is delivered to the liver and utilized for biliary secretion.

The rate of sterol synthesis may be a determinant of biliary cholesterol secretion in obesity. In general, however, there is no correlation between the rates of hepatic or whole body cholesterol synthesis and biliary cholesterol output among the various mammalian species. For example, rates of hepatic and whole body cholesterol synthesis in the rat are much higher than in the hamster (Table 2; Fig. 5), but biliary cholesterol output is similar in both species.

The relationship between the rate of cholesterol synthesis in the liver and biliary cholesterol output has been extensively studied in the rat. It was found that when the rate of hepatic sterol synthesis was varied over a wide range by subjecting rats to various experimental manipulations, the rate of biliary cholesterol secretion remained essentially constant (148). In addition, it was shown that biliary cholesterol output could be driven to a similar degree by bile acid infusion in rats with widely different rates of hepatic cholesterol synthesis (148). Although such findings make it apparent that the rate of hepatic cholesterol synthesis does not ultimately determine the rate of biliary cholesterol secretion, some of the cholesterol secreted in bile is derived directly from newly synthesized sterol. This can be demonstrated using [³H]mevalonate or [¹⁴C]acetate (169,170). Such data cannot be used to accurately quantitate the proportion of biliary cholesterol that is newly synthesized, however, because these precursors undergo an unknown degree of intracellular dilution; hence the SA of the precursor within the hepatocyte is unknown (Fig. 2). Consequently, any such measurements based on the use of these precursors necessarily underestimate the actual contribution of newly synthesized sterol to biliary cholesterol.

Such problems can be avoided by using [³H]water, which rapidly equilibrates with total body water, thereby resulting in a SA that is both uniform and measurable (64,128). Since the relative rates of incorporation of ³H and C into the cholesterol molecule have been determined for liver in the rat and several other species, the quantity of newly synthesized cholesterol that is secreted directly into the bile can be determined (128). Using this technique, it has been found that in normal rats, only about 18% of biliary cholesterol is newly synthesized. When the rate of hepatic cholesterol synthesis is enhanced by cholestyramine feeding, 34% of biliary cholesterol is newly synthesized, but when liver cholesterol synthesis is inhibited by either cholesterol feeding or by fasting, the contribution of newly synthesized sterol to biliary cholesterol is reduced to less than 4% (128). Despite the variable proportion of biliary cholesterol that is newly synthesized, total biliary cholesterol output is not significantly changed. Similar conclusions have been drawn by quantitating the output of desmosterol in the bile during treatment with triparanol. These studies showed that approximately 28% of biliary cholesterol was derived directly from newly synthesized sterol (127).

The technique using [³H]water has also been applied to hamsters in which cholesterol gallstone formation has been induced by feeding a fat-free diet. Under such conditions, both liver cholesterol synthesis and total biliary cholesterol output are increased many fold. In parallel with the enhanced rate of hepatic cholesterol synthesis, the amount of labeled sterol secreted in the bile is also greatly elevated. Nevertheless, the fraction of biliary cholesterol derived directly from newly synthesized sterol remains small (171). Thus, at least in this model of experimentally induced cholelithiasis, most of the excess cholesterol secreted in the bile appears to be derived from some preformed source. Although the mechanism involved in the formation of saturated bile under these conditions has not been elucidated, it cannot be attributed to the excessive secretion of newly synthesized sterol across the canalicular membrane.

The contribution of newly synthesized sterol to biliary cholesterol in man has not been directly quantitated. Some indirect evidence has been obtained from studies involving the combined use of isotopic methods and mathematical modeling. This suggests that only 20% of biliary cholesterol in man is newly synthesized (119).

Dietary Cholesterol Intake

As shown in Fig. 10, dietary cholesterol carried from the intestine to the liver in CM represents one of the potential sources of cholesterol for biliary secretion. Although the influence of dietary cholesterol intake on biliary cholesterol output has been studied in several animal models (and in man to a limited extent), there is no conclusive evidence that the amount of cholesterol secreted in bile is directly regulated by dietary cholesterol intake.

In several species, including the squirrel monkey, prairie dog, and hamster, the feeding of a high cholesterol diet results in the production of saturated bile and gallstone formation (124,154,172,173). In most cases, these findings are difficult to interpret because the cholesterol content of the diets greatly exceeded normal levels. This often led to the production of varying degrees of hypercholesterolemia and ultrastructural changes in the liver.

The response of the rat to increased dietary cholesterol intake differs from that found in other animals. Under conditions of a modest increase in dietary cholesterol, rats show no change in biliary cholesterol levels; but when the cholesterol content of the diet is raised to 1 to 2%, biliary cholesterol secretion actually declines (148,174). Similar results are obtained if rats are acutely administered CM cholesterol (148).

In one study with human subjects maintained on a formula diet, it was found that the consumption of 750 mg/day cholesterol led to a significant increase in biliary cholesterol saturation (121). Plasma cholesterol levels also increased significantly, indicating that some other aspect of cholesterol metabolism had been altered. In another study in which a more standard type of diet was used, the intake of large amounts of cholesterol did not increase biliary cholesterol levels (175).

If the liver compensated for an increased dietary cholesterol intake by directly secreting more CM cholesterol in the bile, then the administration of agents that block cholesterol absorption might be expected to have the reverse effect on biliary cholesterol output. Several studies in the rat and man have shown that such agents either have no effect or may actually enhance biliary cholesterol secretion (174,176,177).

There are two main mechanisms by which the liver compensates for an increased dietary cholesterol intake. The first is suppression of its own rate of cholesterol synthesis in direct proportion to the amount of CM cholesterol taken up. The second is induction of bile acid synthesis. Although this has been demonstrated to occur in the rat, dog, guinea pig, and in some but not all squirrel monkeys, the mechanism appears to be absent in the rabbit and hamster (42–44,49,129, 178,179). Similarly, it has been found in most but not all studies that man is not able to produce more bile acids when dietary cholesterol increases (44,47,66). Since cholesterol absorption is relatively inefficient in man, the apparent inability to induce bile acid synthesis may be attributable to the absorption of an insufficient quantity of cholesterol.

Unless excessive amounts of cholesterol are fed, by suppressing synthesis and enhancing catabolism, the liver can fully compensate for the increased uptake of CM cholesterol following a meal. Although some of this CM cholesterol is probably utilized as a source of biliary cholesterol, it is doubtful that its availability has any direct influence on determining the overall rate of biliary cholesterol output.

Hepatic Lipoprotein Uptake

In addition to the cholesterol obtained from *de novo* synthesis and the uptake of CM, the liver also derives cholesterol from the uptake of various plasma lipoproteins (Fig. 10). Although the proportion of biliary cholesterol normally obtained from this source is unknown, it is apparent from studies with the fasted rat that cholesterol carried in plasma lipoproteins can become a major supplier of biliary cholesterol. This is suggested by the finding that biliary cholesterol output remains normal during fasting, even though the supply of newly synthesized cholesterol from within the liver and of CM cholesterol is markedly reduced. Plasma cholesterol levels fall significantly, suggesting the utilization of lipoprotein cholesterol for biliary secretion in this circumstance (148).

The more critical question that remains to be resolved is whether cholesterol carried in any particular lipoprotein particle can be preferentially utilized for biliary secretion. The relative contribution of LDL and HDL cholesterol to biliary secretion has been studied in man and the squirrel monkey using an isotope kinetic method (120,180). It was found that following the administration of LDL and HDL in which the cholesterol had been labeled with different isotopes, the labeled cholesterol originally present in HDL appeared in the bile at a faster rate than the labeled cholesterol from LDL. Although this implies a preferential utilization of HDL free cholesterol as a source of biliary cholesterol, the full extent to which the different rates of secretion of the two isotopic labels into bile may have reflected a difference in the rate at which the labeled cholesterol in the LDL or HDL exchanged with unlabeled cholesterol from other sources is uncertain.

If such selective utilization of free cholesterol from HDL or any other lipoprotein source does occur, the extent to which this may directly influence the overall rate of biliary cholesterol secretion would depend on the mechansim by which such sterol entered the bile. If, for example, it first mixed with cholesterol from other sources in a common pool and was then transported into bile by coupling to the transport of bile acid and phospholipid, total biliary cholesterol output would remain independent of the amount of cholesterol entering the liver cell from any particular lipoprotein particle. Alternatively, if such sterol was delivered directly into the canalicular lumen by some vesicular transport mechanism, then the preferential utilization of cholesterol from any lipoprotein could be an important determinant of the final rate of biliary cholesterol secretion.

Clearly, further studies are needed to resolve whether the preferential utilization of cholesterol from any lipoprotein does actually occur and, if so, whether it has any role in the formation of supersaturated bile in man.

Bile Acid Pool Size and Composition

The size of the bile acid pool and the frequency with which it recycles exert a major regulatory effect on biliary cholesterol secretion. It is now recognized that diminished bile acid pool size is one of the causes of cholelithiasis in man (139,181). The size of the bile acid pool can be reduced to less than normal by various defects, including gross malabsorption of bile acids from the intestine as occurs in patients with ileal disease, an inability to synthesize bile acids at a normal rate, and excessive feedback suppression of bile acid synthesis as a result of an accelerated rate of recycling of bile acids. These defects are discussed in more detail in a recent review (139).

The composition of the bile acid pool is a key factor in determining biliary cholesterol output. This provides the basis for the use of chenic and ursodeoxycholic acid in treating cholesterol gallstone disease. These dihydroxy bile acids, when administered chronically to patients with cholesterol gallstones, effect a significant reduction in the degree of biliary cholesterol saturation by decreasing the absolute rate of cholesterol secretion (161–163,182). This generally results in gallstone dissolution. In contrast to this effect, treatment with deoxycholic acid, also a dihydroxy bile acid, and cholic acid, a trihydroxy bile acid, does not change biliary cholesterol saturation (167, 168,182). The desaturating effect of chenic and ursodeoxycholic acid in man has also been demonstrated acutely. Thus when gallstone patients that had undergone cholecystectomy were subjected to depletion of the bile acid pool followed by repletion with either cholic, chenic, or ursodeoxycholic acid, less cholesterol was secreted in the bile during the infusion of chenic and ursodeoxycholic acid than during the infusion of cholic acid (147,183).

The discovery of the desaturating effect of chenic acid in man has led to the study of the effects of several bile acids on biliary cholesterol secretion in various species, including dog, cat, hamster, and rat. The results of these studies are summarized in Table 4. It is evident that the response of these species is different to that of man. The only exception appears to be the

TABLE 4. *Effect of various bile acids on the relative cholesterol content of bile in different species*

Species	Chronic administration				Acute administration			
	CDC	UDC	DC	C	CDC	UDC	DC	C
Man	↓	↓	⇌	⇌	↓	↓	ND	⇌
Hamster	↓	↓	ND	ND	↑	ND	ND	⇌
Rat	⇌	⇌	ND	⇌	↓	ND	ND	↓
Dog	ND	ND	ND	ND	↑	ND	ND	⇌
Cat	ND	ND	ND	ND	↑	ND	↑	⇌

Studies described in this table are detailed in references 144,145,147,161–163,167,168,173, and 183–186, except those involving the chronic administration of bile acids to rats, which are unpublished observations from this laboratory.

CDC, chenodeoxycholic acid; UDC, ursodeoxycholic acid; DC, deoxycholic acid; C, cholic acid; ND, not determined.

hamster fed a diet containing an elevated content of cholesterol and ethinyl estradiol, as well as either chenic or ursodeoxycholic acid. In contrast to the animals given the diet containing cholesterol and ethinyl estradiol only, those receiving supplementation with either of these bile acids produced bile with an almost normal degree of cholesterol saturation; none developed cholesterol gallstones (173). While this response clearly mimics the effects observed with chenic and ursodeoxycholic acid therapy in patients with cholesterol gallstones, it is opposite the effect found when these bile acids are given acutely. The bile produced in hamsters during intravenous infusion of chenic acid had a significantly higher relative cholesterol content than when cholic acid was given (184). The same response has been demonstrated in the dog and cat (144,145,186). In contrast to these effects, when rats were subjected to depletion of the bile acid pool followed by repletion with either cholic or chenic acid, biliary cholesterol secretion decreased to a similar extent with both bile acids (185).

The mechanism(s) by which changes in the composition of the bile acid pool modify biliary cholesterol saturation is not understood. The highly variable effect on cholesterol saturation that each of the major bile acids has been found to produce *in vivo* clearly indicates that other factors, in addition to the solubilizing capacity of each of the bile acids present within the pool, must be involved in determining the final rate of biliary cholesterol secretion.

Drug Treatments

Although few drug treatments, apart from bile acid therapy, have been developed for specifically desaturating bile, many have been found to influence biliary cholesterol secretion. As is evident from the information given in Table 5, there is no consistent

TABLE 5. *Effect of various drugs on the relative cholesterol content of bile in different species*

Drug treatment	Species		
	Man	Rat	Hamster
Clofibrate	↑	⇌	ND
Cholestyramine	⇌ or ↑	⇌	↑
Colestipol	⇌	ND	ND
β-Sitosterol	⇌	↑	ND
Probucol	ND	⇌	ND
Zanchol	↓	⇌	ND
Pregnenolone-16α-carbonitrile	ND	↑	ND
Spironolactone	ND	↑	ND
Phenobarbital	↓	↓	↑
Ethinyl estradiol or other Estrogens	↑	⇌	↑

Data taken from studies reported in references 123, 173,176,177,187–189, and 191–198.
ND, not determined.

pattern in the effect of any of the drugs between different species. Furthermore, of those treatments that do influence biliary cholesterol secretion, in no case is there a clear explanation for the effect. This is perhaps best exemplified by the studies with clofibrate.

It is now well established that clofibrate therapy in man leads to an increase in biliary cholesterol output and to an increased incidence of cholesterol gallstone formation (187,188). In contrast, clofibrate has no effect on biliary cholesterol secretion in the rat, even though it reduces plasma cholesterol levels in this species as it does in man (189). The source of the additional biliary cholesterol that is secreted during clofibrate therapy has not been established. It almost certainly does not represent newly synthesized cholesterol, since it has been shown to either inhibit or have no effect on the rate of cholesterol synthesis in the liver and several other tissues (189,190). It is more generally accepted that the extra biliary cholesterol derives from the increased mobilization of cholesterol in the tissues, although there is no explanation for the mechanism by which such cholesterol is delivered to the liver and utilized for biliary secretion (187). At least in the rat and man, clofibrate has been shown to inhibit bile acid synthesis; whether this effect has any role in the formation of more saturated bile in man is unclear (187,190).

The various data on drug-induced changes in cholesterol metabolism and biliary lipid secretion demonstrate that there is no simple relationship between biliary cholesterol output and the absorption, transport, synthesis, and degradation of cholesterol. For example, β-sitosterol decreases cholesterol absorption but either has no effect or increases the cholesterol content of bile in man and the rat (176,177). Similarly, under conditions where the rate of conversion of cho-

lesterol to bile acids is enhanced, such as occurs during treatment with cholestyramine or colestipol, the degree of biliary cholesterol saturation is unchanged, at least in man and the rat (189,192,197). In baboons, however, treatment with cholestyramine raises the level of saturation (199). The dissociation of drug-induced changes in biliary cholesterol secretion from cholesterol synthesis is seen by the studies with phenobarbital. These show that despite its effect in enhancing the rate of hepatic cholesterol synthesis, phenobarbital desaturates bile in man, rhesus monkey, and rat but not in the hamster (123,193,195,200).

The lack of a readily available animal model in which saturated bile and cholesterol gallstones form spontaneously has created the need for drug treatments that are effective in producing such conditions in some of the more commonly utilized laboratory animals. In this regard, the hamster treated with ethinyl estradiol is potentially useful because saturated bile and gallstone formation can be induced readily at very low doses of the drug (173). Although rats lack a gallbladder and therefore cannot develop gallstones, the formation of near-saturated bile can be induced by the administration of either pregnenolone-16α-carbonitrile or spironolactone (195). It is not known whether these drugs have a similar effect in other species.

The potential value of some drugs, such as diosgenin, for these types of studies is probably limited; although they may markedly alter the absolute concentration of cholesterol in bile, this may not necessarily involve a change in the relative cholesterol content. If the metabolites of such drugs are secreted in the bile, as they are in the case of diosgenin, they may exert a bile acid- or phospholipid-like effect in solubilizing cholesterol; thus overall, there may be very little change in the actual degree of cholesterol saturation (201).

SUMMARY

All mammalian species continually add cholesterol to the body pool of sterol either by absorbing it from the diet or by synthesizing it *de novo*. The rates of these two processes, however, vary markedly among the different species. In general, small animals have very high rates of cholesterol synthesis within the body and have high capacities to absorb dietary sterol. Larger animals, and particularly man, have much lower rates of whole body synthesis and even lower capacities to absorb cholesterol from the diet. Hence, even in the face of a modestly high dietary cholesterol intake, the majority of the cholesterol present in the body pool of man is derived from synthesis in the major organ systems. Virtually every tissue in the body can synthesize cholesterol to some extent, although the liver, gastrointestinal tract, skin, and muscle are the sites of greatest quantitative importance in most species. Here again, however, marked differences in synthetic capacity exist in different animals. On one hand, the liver accounts for approximately 50% of whole body synthesis in the rat but is quantitatively less important in other species that have been studied.

Nevertheless, in all species, the liver plays a central role in the regulation of cholesterol balance in the body in general, and as the immediate source for biliary cholesterol in particular. Newly synthesized and dietary cholesterol are delivered to the liver in CM where they mix with a pool of sterol newly synthesized within the hepatocytes. A portion of this sterol is exported from the liver in VLDL or nascent HDL or after being utilized for the synthesis of bile acids. The majority of the cholesterol that is synthesized in extrahepatic tissues, along with much of that that had been exported from the liver, ultimately returns to the liver carried in a variety of lipoprotein particles. There is little evidence to support the hypothesis that biliary cholesterol might predominantly come from sterol reaching the liver in a particular fraction, such as CM, LDL, or HDL, or from the pool of newly synthesized cholesterol in the liver. Rather, biliary cholesterol likely is derived from an intrahepatic pool of sterol that has many different sources, the quantitative importance of which will depend on many factors, including the amount of sterol in the diet, the degree of obesity, the metabolic state of the animal, and even the intake of certain drugs. Hence the rate of sterol secretion into the bile probably depends less on the ultimate source of the cholesterol than on the process actually responsible for sterol translocation across the canalicular membrane. Furthermore, the rate of biliary cholesterol secretion cannot be explained simply in physicochemical terms. While the composition and size of the bile acid pool does have a significant influence on biliary cholesterol output, the qualitative nature of such effects varies markedly among different species.

The movement of cholesterol from the liver cell into bile is tightly coupled to the simultaneous secretion of phospholipid and bile acid. For reasons that are not well understood, this coupling process can become disrupted, so that more cholesterol enters the bile than can be solubilized by the bile acid and phospholipid present. The production of such abnormal bile is the initiating event in the pathogenesis of cholesterol gallstone disease. In man, there is a direct correlation among the degree of obesity, the rate of cholesterol synthesis in the whole body, and the secretion of abnormally large amounts of cholesterol in the bile. However, while there is a positive correlation between biliary cholesterol output and whole body sterol synthesis in such subjects, it is not clear whether the liver or some extrahepatic tissue is the source of the addi-

tional newly synthesized cholesterol and, if it is of extrahepatic origin, how such cholesterol is delivered to the liver and utilized for biliary secretion.

Although during the last decade there have been major advances both in identifying the risk factors for cholelithiasis and in the treatment of the disease by bile acid therapy, the fundamental cause(s) of the disease remains to be determined. Since the types of experiments that can be done in man are limited, further study of the regulation of biliary cholesterol secretion will depend on the use of animal models. None of the commonly utilized laboratory animals spontaneously develops cholesterol gallstones; nevertheless, there are marked differences among these various species in the relative cholesterol content of bile. The elucidation of the basic mechanism(s) responsible for these wide species differences may have some significance in further understanding the etiology of cholesterol gallstone disease in man.

ACKNOWLEDGMENTS

This work, as well as some of the original research reported in this chapter, were supported in part by U.S. Public Health Service research grants HL 09610 and AM 19329.

REFERENCES

1. Dietschy, J. M., and Wilson, J. D. (1970): Regulation of cholesterol metabolism. *N. Engl. J. Med.*, 282:1128–1138, 1179–1183, 1241–1249.
2. Cook, R. P. (1958): Distribution of sterols in organisms and in tissues. In: *Cholesterol. Chemistry, Biochemistry, and Pathology*, edited by R. P. Cook, pp. 145–180. Academic Press, New York.
3. Crouse, J. R., Grundy, S. M., and Ahrens, E. H., Jr. (1972): Cholesterol distribution in the bulk tissues of man: variation with age. *J. Clin. Invest.*, 51:1292–1296.
4. Williams, H. H., Galbraith, H., Kaucher, M., and Macy I. G. (1945): The influence of age and diet on the lipid composition of the rat. *J. Biol. Chem.*, 161:463–474.
5. Goodman, D. S., and Noble, R. P. (1968): Turnover of plasma cholesterol in man. *J. Clin. Invest.*, 47:231–241.
6. Manning, P. J., Clarkson, T. B., and Lofland, H. B. (1971): Cholesterol absorption, turnover, and excretion rates in hypercholesterolemic rhesus monkeys. *Exp. Mol. Pathol.*, 14:75–89.
7. Wilson, J. D. (1970): The measurement of the exchangeable pools of cholesterol in the baboon. *J. Clin. Invest.*, 49:655–665.
8. Goodman, D. S., Smith, F. R., Seplowitz, A. H., Ramakrishnan, R., and Dell, R. B. (1980): Prediction of the parameters of whole body cholesterol metabolism in humans. *J. Lipid Res.*, 21:699–713.
9. Chobanian, A. V., and Hollander, W. (1962): Body cholesterol metabolism in man. I. The equilibration of serum and tissue cholesterol. *J. Clin. Invest.*, 41:1732–1737.
10. Chobanian, A. V., Burrows, B. A., and Hollander, W. (1962): Body cholesterol metabolism in man. II. Measurement of the body cholesterol miscible pool and turnover rate. *J. Clin. Invest.*, 41:1738–1744.
11. Hofmann, A. F., and Borgström, B. (1964): The intraluminal phase of fat digestion in man: The lipid content of the micellar

and oil phases of intestinal content obtained during fat digestion and absorption. *J. Clin. Invest.*, 43:247–257.

12. Simmonds, W. J., Hofmann, A. F., and Theodor, E. (1967): Absorption of cholesterol from a micellar solution: Intestinal perfusion studies in man. *J. Clin. Invest.*, 46:874–890.

13. Sylvén, C., and Borgström, B. (1968): Absorption and lymphatic transport of cholesterol in the rat. *J. Lipid Res.*, 9:596–601.

14. Watt, S. M., and Simmonds, W. J. (1971): Uptake and efflux by everted intestinal sacs of micellar cholesterol in bile salts and in non-ionic detergent. *Biochim. Biophys. Acta*, 225:347–355.

15. Dietschy, J. M. (1978): General principles governing movement of lipids across biological membranes. In: *Disturbances in Lipid and Lipoprotein Metabolism*, edited by J. M. Dietschy, A. M. Gotto, Jr., and J. A. Ontko, pp. 1–28. American Physiological Society, Bethesda.

16. Westergaard, H., and Dietschy, J. M. (1974): Delineation of the dimensions and permeability characteristics of the two major diffusion barriers to passive mucosal uptake in the rabbit intestine. *J. Clin. Invest.*, 54:718–732.

17. Westergaard, H., and Dietschy, J. M. (1974): Normal mechanisms of fat absorption and derangements induced by various gastrointestinal diseases. *Med. Clin. North Am.*, 58:1413–1427.

18. Dietschy, J. M. (1978): The uptake of lipids into the intestinal mucosa. In: *Physiology of Membrane Disorders*, edited by T. E. Andreoli, J. F. Hoffman, and D. D. Fanestil, pp. 577–592. Plenum, New York.

19. Westergaard, H., and Dietschy, J. M. (1976): The mechanism whereby bile acid micelles increase the rate of fatty acid and cholesterol uptake into the intestinal mucosal cell. *J. Clin. Invest.*, 58:97–108.

20. Siperstein, M. D., Chaikoff, I. L., and Reinhardt, W. O. (1952): ^{14}C-Cholesterol. V. Obligatory function of bile in intestinal absorption of cholesterol. *J. Biol. Chem.*, 198:111–114.

21. Treadwell, C. R., and Vahouny, G. V. (1968): Cholesterol absorption. In: *Handbook of Physiology, Section 6. Alimentary Canal, Vol. III*, edited by C. F. Code, pp. 1407–1438, American Physiological Society, Washington, D.C.

22. Gallo, L. L., and Treadwell, C. R. (1963): Localization of cholesterol esterase and cholesterol in mucosal fractions of rat small intestine. *Proc. Soc. Exp. Biol. Med.*, 114:69–72.

23. Borja, C. R., Vahouny, G. V., and Treadwell, C. R. (1964): Role of bile and pancreatic juice in cholesterol absorption and esterification. *Am. J. Physiol.*, 206:223–228.

24. Hofmann, A. F., and Small, D. M. (1967): Detergent properties of bile salts: Correlation with physiological function. *Annu. Rev. Med.*, 18:333–376.

25. Dietschy, J. M., and Gamel, W. G. (1971): Cholesterol synthesis in the intestine of man: Regional differences and control mechanisms. *J. Clin. Invest.*, 50:872–880.

26. Johnston, J. M. (1978): Esterification reactions in the intestinal mucosa and lipid absorption. In: *Disturbances in Lipid and Lipoprotein Metabolism*, edited by J. M. Dietschy, A. M. Gotto, Jr., and J. A. Ontko, pp. 57–68. American Physiological Society, Bethesda.

27. Zilversmit, D. B. (1969): Chylomicrons. In: *Structural and Functional Aspects of Lipoproteins in Living Systems*, edited by E. Tria and A. M. Scanu, pp. 329–368. Academic Press, London.

28. Zilversmit, D. B. (1978): Assembly of chylomicrons in the intestinal cell. In: *Disturbances in Lipid and Lipoprotein Metabolism*, edited by J. M. Dietschy, A. M. Gotto, Jr., and J. A. Ontko, pp. 69–81. American Physiological Society, Bethesda.

29. Borgström, B. (1960): Studies on intestinal cholesterol absorption in the human. *J. Clin. Invest.*, 39:809–815.

30. Quintão, E., Grundy, S. M., and Ahrens, E. H., Jr. (1971): An evaluation of four methods for measuring cholesterol absorption by the intestine in man. *J. Lipid Res.*, 12:221–232.

31. Zilversmit, D. B., and Hughes, L. B. (1974): Validation of a dual-isotope plasma ratio method for measurement of cholesterol absorption in rats. *J. Lipid Res.*, 15:465–473.

32. Wilson, J. D., and Lindsey, C. A., Jr. (1965): Studies on the influence of dietary cholesterol on cholesterol metabolism in

the isotopic steady state in man. *J. Clin. Invest.*, 44:1805–1814.

33. Grundy, S. M., Ahrens, E. H., Jr., and Miettinen, T. A. (1965): Quantitative isolation and gas-liquid chromatographic analysis of total fecal bile acids. *J. Lipid Res.*, 6:397–410.

34. Grundy, S. M., and Ahrens, E. H., Jr. (1966): An evaluation of the relative merits of two methods for measuring the balance of sterols in man: Isotopic balance versus chromatographic analysis. *J. Clin. Invest.*, 45:1503–1515.

35. Abell, L. L., Mosbach, E. H., and Kendall, F. E. (1956): Cholesterol metabolism in the dog. *J. Biol. Chem.*, 220:527–536.

36. Wojciech, R., Janecek, H. M., and Ivay, A. C. (1961): Endogenous excretion and intestinal capacity for absorption of cholesterol in the dog. *Am. J. Physiol.*, 201:190–193.

37. Favarger, P., and Metzger, E. F. (1952): La résorption intestinale du deutério-cholestérol et sa répartition dans l'organisme animal sous forme libre et estérifiée. *Helv. Chim. Acta*, 35:1811–1819.

38. Cook, R. P., and Thomson, R. O. (1951): The absorption of fat and of cholesterol in the rat, guinea pig and rabbit. *Q. J. Exp. Physiol.*, 36:61–74.

39. Cook, R. P., Kliman, A., and Fieser, L. F. (1954): The absorption and metabolism of cholesterol and its main companions in the rabbit—with observations on the atherogenic nature of the sterols. *Arch. Biochem.*, 52:439–450.

40. Kaplan, J. A., Cox, G. E., and Taylor, C. B. (1963): Cholesterol metabolism in man: Studies on absorption. *Arch. Pathol.*, 76:359–368.

41. Spady, D. K., and Dietschy, J. M. (1982): Comparison of rates of sterol synthesis in the liver and extrahepatic tissues in five species. *J. Lipid Res.* (*in press.*)

42. Lofland, H. B., Jr., Clarkson, T. B., St. Clair, R. W., and Lehner, N. D. M. (1972): Studies on the regulation of plasma cholesterol levels in squirrel monkeys of two genotypes. *J. Lipid Res.*, 13:39–47.

43. Raicht, R. F., Cohen, B. I., Shefer, S., and Mosbach, E. H. (1975): Sterol balance studies in the rat. Effects of dietary cholesterol and β-sitosterol on sterol balance and rate-limiting enzymes of sterol metabolism. *Biochem. Biophys. Acta*, 388:374–384.

44. Hellström, K. (1965): On the bile acid and neutral fecal steroid excretion in man and rabbits following cholesterol feeding. Bile acids and steroids 150. *Acta Physiol. Scand.*, 63:21–35.

45. Grundy, S. M., and Ahrens, E. H., Jr. (1969): Measurements of cholesterol turnover, synthesis, and absorption in man, carried out by isotope kinetic and sterol balance methods. *J. Lipid Res.*, 10:91–107.

46. Grundy, S. M., Ahrens, E. H., Jr., and Davignon, J. (1969): The interaction of cholesterol absorption and cholesterol synthesis in man. *J. Lipid Res.*, 10:304–315.

47. Quintão, E., Grundy, S. M., and Ahrens, E. H., Jr. (1971): Effects of dietary cholesterol on the regulation of total body cholesterol in man. *J. Lipid Res.*, 12:233–247.

48. Wilson, J. D. (1972): The relation between cholesterol absorption and cholesterol synthesis in the baboon. *J. Clin. Invest.*, 51:1450–1458.

49. Pertsemlidis, D., Kirchman, E. H., and Ahrens, E. H., Jr. (1973): Regulation of cholesterol metabolism in the dog. I. Effects of complete bile diversion and of cholesterol feeding on absorption, synthesis, accumulation, and excretion rates measured during life. *J. Clin. Invest.*, 52:2353–2367.

50. Grundy, S. M., Mok, H. Y. I., and von Bergmann, K. (1976): Regulation of biliary cholesterol secretion in man. In: *The Liver. Quantitative Aspects of Structure and Function*, edited by R. Preisig, J. Bircher, and G. Paumgartner, pp. 393–403. Editio Cantor, Aulendorf.

51. Wilson, J. D., Lindsey, C. A., and Dietschy, J. M. (1968): Influence of dietary cholesterol on cholesterol metabolism. *Ann. N.Y. Acad. Sci.*, 149:808–821.

52. Taylor, C. B., Cox, G. E., Nelson, L. G., Davis, C. B., Jr., and Hass, G. M. (1955): In vitro studies on human hepatic cholesterol synthesis. *Circulation*, 12:489.

53. Bhattathiry, E. P. M., and Siperstein, M. D. (1963): Feedback

control of cholesterol synthesis in man. *J. Clin. Invest.,* 42:1613–1618.

54. Dietschy, J. M., and Siperstein, M. D. (1967): Effect of cholesterol feeding and fasting on sterol synthesis in seventeen tissues of the rat. *J. Lipid Res.,* 8:97–104.
55. Dietschy, J. M., and Wilson, J. D. (1968): Cholesterol synthesis in the squirrel monkey: Relative rates of synthesis in various tissues and mechanisms of control. *J. Clin. Invest.,* 47:166–174.
56. Dietschy, J. M., and McGarry, J. D. (1974): Limitations of acetate as a substrate for measuring cholesterol synthesis in liver. *J. Biol. Chem.,* 249:52–58.
57. Dietschy, J. M., and Brown, M. S. (1974): Effect of alterations of the specific activity of the intracellular acetyl CoA pool on apparent rates of hepatic cholesterogenesis. *J. Lipid Res.,* 15:508–516.
58. Andersen, J. M., and Dietschy, J. M. (1979): Absolute rates of cholesterol synthesis in extrahepatic tissues measured with ³H-labeled water and ¹⁴C-labeled substrates. *J. Lipid Res.,* 20:740–752.
59. Lakshmanan, M. R., and Veech, R. L. (1977): Measurement of rate of rat liver sterol synthesis in vivo using tritiated water. *J. Biol. Chem.,* 252:4667–4673.
60. Alfin-Slater, R. B., Deuel, H. J., Jr., Schotz, M. C., and Shomoda, F. K. (1950): *University of Southern California, Consolidated Engineering Corp., Group Report No. N.3.*
61. Loud, A. V., and Bucher, N. L. R. (1958): The turnover of squalene in relation to the biosynthesis of cholesterol. *J. Biol. Chem.,* 233:37–41.
62. Foster, D. W., and Bloom, B. (1963): The synthesis of fatty acids by rat liver slices in tritiated water. *J. Biol. Chem.,* 238:888–892.
63. Brunengraber, H., Sabine, J. R., Boutry, M., and Lowenstein, J. M. (1972): 3-β-Hydroxysterol synthesis by the liver. *Arch. Biochem. Biophys.,* 150:392–396.
64. Jeske, D. J., and Dietschy, J. M. (1980): Regulation of rates of cholesterol synthesis in vivo in the liver and carcass of the rat measured using [³H]water. *J. Lipid Res.,* 21:364–376.
65. Turley, S. D., Andersen, J. M., and Dietschy, J. M. (1981): Rates of sterol synthesis and uptake in the major organs of the rat in vivo. *J. Lipid Res.,* 22:551–569.
66. Connor, W. E. (1970): The effects of dietary lipid and sterols on the sterol balance. In: *Atherosclerosis. Proceedings of the Second International Symposium,* edited by R. J. Jones, pp. 253–261. Springer-Verlag, New York.
67. Imaizumi, K., Fainaru, M., and Havel, R. J. (1978): Composition of proteins of mesenteric lymph chylomicrons in the rat and alterations produced upon exposure of chylomicrons to blood serum and serum proteins. *J. Lipid Res.,* 19:712–722.
68. Imaizumi, K., Havel, R. J., Fainaru, M., and Vigne, J-L. (1978): Origin and transport of the A-1 and arginine-rich apolipoproteins in mesenteric lymph of rats. *J. Lipid Res.,* 19:1038–1046.
69. Havel, R. J. (1980): Lipoprotein biosynthesis and metabolism. *Ann. N.Y. Acad. Sci.,* 348:16–29.
70. Fielding, C. J. (1978): Origin and properties of remnant lipoproteins. In: *Disturbances in Lipid and Lipoprotein Metabolism,* edited by J. M. Dietschy, A. M. Gotto, Jr., and J. A. Ontko, pp. 83–98. American Physiological Society, Bethesda.
71. Redgrave, T. G. (1970): Formation of cholesteryl ester-rich particulate lipid during metabolism of chylomicrons. *J. Clin. Invest.,* 49:465–471.
72. Nervi, F. O., and Dietschy, J. M. (1975): Ability of six different lipoprotein fractions to regulate the rate of hepatic cholesterogenesis in vivo. *J. Biol. Chem.,* 250:8704–8711.
73. Nervi, F. O., Weis, H. J., and Dietschy, J. M. (1975): The kinetic characteristics of inhibition of hepatic cholesterogenesis by lipoproteins of intestinal origin. *J. Biol. Chem.,* 250:4145–4151.
74. Cooper, A. D. (1977): The metabolism of chylomicron remnants by isolated perfused rat liver. *Biochim. Biophys. Acta,* 488:464–474.
75. Sherrill, B. C., and Dietschy, J. M. (1978): Characterization of the sinusoidal transport process responsible for uptake of chylomicrons by the liver. *J. Biol. Chem.,* 253:1859–1867.
76. Carrella, M., and Cooper, A. D. (1979): High affinity binding of chylomicron remnants to rat liver plasma membranes. *Proc. Natl. Acad. Sci. USA,* 76:338–342.
77. Sherrill, B. C., Innerarity, T. L., and Mahley, R. W. (1980): Rapid hepatic clearance of the canine lipoproteins containing only the E apoprotein by a high affinity receptor. Identity with the chylomicron remnant transport process. *J. Biol. Chem.,* 255:1804–1807.
78. Hui, D. Y., Innerarity, T. L., and Mahley, R. W. (1981): Lipoprotein binding to canine hepatic membranes. Metabolically distinct Apo-E and Apo B,E receptors. *J. Biol. Chem.,* 256:5646–5655.
79. Kane, J. P., Hardman, D. A., and Paulus, H. E. (1980): Heterogeneity of apolipoprotein B: Isolation of a new species from human chylomicrons. *Proc. Natl. Acad. Sci. USA,* 77:2465–2469.
80. Krishnaiah, K. V., Walker, L. F., Borensztajn, J., Schonfeld, G., and Getz, G. S. (1980): Apolipoprotein B variant derived from rat intestine. *Proc. Natl. Acad. Sci. USA,* 77:3806–3810.
81. Elovson, J., Huang, Y. O., Baker, N., and Kannan, R. (1981): Apolipoprotein B is structurally and metabolically heterogeneous in the rat. *Proc. Natl. Acad. Sci. USA,* 78:157–161.
82. Faergeman, O., and Havel, R. J. (1975): Metabolism of cholesteryl esters of rat very low density lipoproteins. *J. Clin. Invest.,* 55:1210–1218.
83. Bilheimer, D. W., Eisenberg, S., and Levy, R. I. (1972): The metabolism of very low density lipoprotein proteins. I. Preliminary in vitro and in vivo observations. *Biochim. Biophys. Acta,* 260:212–221.
84. Shaefer, E. J., Eisenberg, S., and Levy, R. I. (1978): Lipoprotein apoprotein metabolism. *J. Lipid Res.,* 19:667–687.
85. Goldstein, J. L., and Brown, M. S. (1977): Atherosclerosis: The low-density lipoprotein receptor hypothesis. *Metabolism,* 26:1257–1275.
86. Basu, S. K., Goldstein, J. L., and Brown, M. S. (1978): Characterization of the low density lipoprotein receptor in membranes prepared from human fibroblasts. *J. Biol. Chem.,* 253:3852–3856.
87. Brown, M. S., and Goldstein, J. L. (1976): Interaction of swine lipoproteins with low density lipoprotein receptor in human fibroblasts. *J. Biol. Chem.,* 251:2395–2398.
88. Innerarity, T. L., Pitas, R. E., and Mahley, R. W. (1979): Binding of arginine-rich (E) apoprotein after recombination with phospholipid vesicles to the low density lipoprotein receptors of fibroblasts. *J. Biol. Chem.,* 254:4186–4190.
89. Brown, M. S., and Goldstein, J. L. (1979): Receptor-mediated endocytosis: Insights from the lipoprotein receptor system. *Proc. Natl. Acad. Sci. USA,* 76:3330–3337.
90. Schneider, W. J., Goldstein, J. L., and Brown, M. S. (1980): Partial purification and characterization of the low density lipoprotein receptor from bovine adrenal cortex. *J. Biol. Chem.,* 255:11442–11447.
91. Beisiegel, U., Kita, T., Anderson, R. G. W., Schneider, W. J., Brown, M. S., and Goldstein, J. L. (1981): Immunologic cross-reactivity of the low density lipoprotein receptor from bovine adrenal cortex, human fibroblasts, canine liver and adrenal gland, and rat liver. *J. Biol. Chem.,* 256:4071–4078.
92. Windler, E. E. T., Kovanen, P. T., Chao, Y-S., Brown, M. S., Havel, R. J., and Goldstein, J. L. (1980): The estradiol-stimulated lipoprotein receptor of rat liver. A binding site that mediates the uptake of rat lipoproteins containing apoproteins B and E. *J. Biol. Chem.,* 255:10464–10471.
93. Pangburn, S. H., Newton, R. S., Chang, C-M., Weinstein, D. B., and Steinberg, D. (1981): Receptor-mediated catabolism of homologous low density lipoproteins in cultured pig hepatocytes. *J. Biol. Chem.,* 256:3340–3347.
94. Pittman, R. C., Attie, A. D., Carew, T. E., and Steinberg, D. (1979): Tissue sites of degradation of low density lipoprotein: Application of a method for determining the fate of plasma proteins. *Proc. Natl. Acad. Sci. USA,* 76:5345–5349.
95. Koelz, H. R., Sherrill, B. C., Turley, S. D., and Dietschy, J. M. (1982): Correlation of low density lipoprotein binding in vivo with rates of lipoprotein degradation in the rat. A comparison of lipoproteins of rat and human origin. *J. Biol. Chem.* (*in press.*)

96. Andersen, J. M., and Dietschy, J. M. (1977): Regulation of sterol synthesis in 16 tissues of rat. I. Effect of diurnal light cycling, fasting, stress, manipulation of enterohepatic circulation, and administration of chylomicrons and triton. *J. Biol. Chem.*, 252:3646–3651.

97. Andersen, J. M., and Dietschy, J. M. (1977): Regulation of sterol synthesis in 15 tissues of rat. II. Role of rat and human high and low density plasma lipoproteins and of rat chylomicron remnants. *J. Biol. Chem.*, 252:3652–3659.

98. Kovanen, P. T., Basu, S. K., Goldstein, J. L., and Brown, M. S. (1979): Low density lipoprotein receptors in bovine adrenal cortex. II. Low density lipoprotein binding to membranes prepared from fresh tissue. *Endocrinology*, 104:610–616.

99. Hamilton, R. L. (1978): Hepatic secretion and metabolism of high-density lipoproteins. In: *Disturbances of Lipid and Lipoprotein Metabolism*, edited by J. M. Dietschy, A. M. Gotto, Jr., and J. A. Ontko, pp. 155–171. American Physiological Society, Bethesda.

100. Tall, A. R., and Small, D. M. (1978): Plasma high-density lipoproteins. *N. Engl. J. Med.*, 299:1232–1236.

101. Glickman, R. M., and Green, P. H. R. (1977): The intestine as a source of apolipoprotein A-I. *Proc. Natl. Acad. Sci. USA*, 74:2569–2573.

102. Green, P. H. R., Tall, A. R., and Glickman, R. M. (1978): Rat intestine secretes discoid high density lipoprotein. *J. Clin. Invest.*, 61:528–534.

103. Glomset, J. A. (1968): The plasma lecithin:cholesterol acyltransferase reaction. *J. Lipid Res.*, 9:155–167.

104. Sigurdsson, G., Noel, S-P, and Havel, R. J. (1979): Quantification of the hepatic contribution to the catabolism of high density lipoproteins in rats. *J. Lipid Res.*, 20:316–324.

105. Mahley, R. W., and Innerarity, T. L. (1977): Interaction of canine and swine lipoproteins with the low density lipoprotein receptor of fibroblasts as correlated with heparin/manganese precipitability. *J. Biol. Chem.*, 252:3980–3986.

106. Innerarity, T. L., Pitas, R. E., and Mahley, R. W. (1980): Disparities in the interaction of rat and human lipoproteins with cultured rat fibroblasts and smooth muscle cells. Requirements for homology for receptor binding activity. *J. Biol. Chem.*, 255:11163–11172.

107. Dietschy, J. M., Munford, R. S., and Andersen, J. M. (1981): Sites of tissue binding and uptake of high density lipoproteins (HDL) and of the lipopolysaccharide-HDL complex in the rat and squirrel monkey. *J. Clin. Invest.*, 68:1503–1513.

108. Gwynne, J. T., and Hess, B. (1978): Binding and degradation of human ¹²⁵I-HDL by rat adrenocortical cells. *Metabolism*, 27:1593–1600.

109. Andersen, J. M., and Dietschy, J. M. (1978): Relative importance of high and low density lipoproteins in the regulation of cholesterol synthesis in the adrenal gland, ovary, and testis of the rat. *J. Biol. Chem.*, 253:9024–9032.

110. Kovanen, P. T., Schneider, W. J., Hillman, G. M., Goldstein, J. L., and Brown, M. S. (1979): Separate mechanisms for the uptake of high and low density lipoproteins by mouse adrenal gland in vivo. *J. Biol. Chem.*, 254:5498–5505.

111. Chen, Y-D. I., Kraemer, F. B., and Reaven, G. M. (1980): Identification of specific high density lipoprotein-binding sites in rat testis and regulation of binding by human chorionic gonadotropin. *J. Biol. Chem.*, 255:9162–9167.

112. Gwynne, J. T., and Hess, B. (1980): The role of high density lipoproteins in rat adrenal cholesterol metabolism and steroidogenesis. *J. Biol. Chem.*, 255:10875–10883.

113. Kita, T., Beisiegel, U., Goldstein, J. L., Schneider, W. J., and Brown, M. S. (1981): Antibody against low density lipoprotein receptor blocks uptake of low density lipoprotein (but not high density lipoprotein) by the adrenal gland of the mouse in vivo. *J. Biol. Chem.*, 256:4701–4703.

114. Schuler, L. A. Langenberg, K. K., Gwynne, J. T., and Strauss, J. F., III. (1981): High density lipoprotein utilization by dispersed rat luteal cells. *Biochim. Biophys. Acta*, 664:583–601.

115. Andersen, J. M., and Dietschy, J. M. (1981): Kinetic parameters of the lipoprotein transport systems in the adrenal gland of the rat determined in vivo. Comparison of low and high density lipoproteins of human and rat origin. *J. Biol. Chem.*, 256:7362–7370.

116. Van Tol, A., Van Gent, T., Van 'T Hooft, F. M., and Vlaspolder, F. (1978): High density lipoprotein catabolism before and after partial hepatectomy. *Atherosclerosis*, 29:439–448.

117. Chajek, T., and Fielding, C. J. (1978): Isolation and characterization of a human serum cholesteryl ester transfer protein. *Proc. Natl. Acad. Sci. USA*, 75:3445–3449.

118. Nestel, P. J., Reardon, M., and Billington, T. (1979): In vivo transfer of cholesteryl esters from high density lipoproteins to very low density lipoproteins in man. *Biochim. Biophys. Acta*, 573:403–407.

119. Schwartz, C. C., Berman, M., Vlahcevic, Z. R., Halloran, L. G., Gregory, D. H., and Swell, L. (1978): Multicompartmental analysis of cholesterol metabolism in man. Characterization of the hepatic bile acid and biliary cholesterol precursor sites. *J. Clin. Invest.*, 61:408–423.

120. Schwartz, C. C., Halloran, L. G., Vlahcevic, Z. R., Gregory, D. H., and Swell, L. (1978): Preferential utilization of free cholesterol from high-density lipoproteins for biliary cholesterol secretion in man. *Science*, 200:62–64.

121. DenBesten, L., Connor, W. E., and Bell, S. (1973): The effect of dietary cholesterol on the composition of human bile. *Surgery*, 73:266–273.

122. Salen, G., Nicolau, G., Shefer, S., and Mosbach, E. H. (1975): Hepatic cholesterol metabolism in patients with gallstones. *Gastroenterology*, 69:676–684.

123. Coyne, M. J., Bonorris, G. G., Goldstein, L. I., and Schoenfield, L. J. (1976): Effect of chenodeoxycholic acid and phenobarbital on the rate-limiting enzymes of hepatic cholesterol and bile acid synthesis in patients with gallstones. *J. Lab. Clin. Med.*, 87:281–291.

124. Ho, K-J. (1976): Comparative studies on the effect of cholesterol feeding on biliary composition. *Am. J. Clin. Nutr.*, 29:698–704.

125. Mitropoulos, K. A., Myant, N. B., Gibbons, G. F., Balasubramaniam, S., and Reeves, B. E. A. (1974): Cholesterol precursor pools for the synthesis of cholic and chenodeoxycholic acids in rats. *J. Biol. Chem.*, 249:6052–6056.

126. Björkhem, I., and Danielsson, H. (1975): 7α-Hydroxylation of exogenous and endogenous cholesterol in rat-liver microsomes. *Eur. J. Biochem.*, 53:63–70.

127. Long, T. T., III, Jakoi, L., Stevens, R., and Quarfordt, S. (1978): The sources of rat biliary cholesterol and bile acid. *J. Lipid Res.*, 19:872–878.

128. Turley, S. D., and Dietschy, J. M. (1981): The contribution of newly synthesized cholesterol to biliary cholesterol in the rat. *J. Biol. Chem.*, 256:2438–2446.

129. Wilson, J. D. (1964): The quantification of cholesterol excretion and degradation in the isotopic steady state in the rat: the influence of dietary cholesterol. *J. Lipid Res.*, 5:409–417.

130. Weis, H. J., and Dietschy, J. M. (1975): The interaction of various control mechanisms in determining the rate of hepatic cholesterogenesis in the rat. *Biochim. Biophys. Acta*, 398:315–324.

131. Danielsson, H., Einarsson, K., and Johansson, G. (1967): Effect of biliary drainage on individual reactions in the conversion of cholesterol to taurocholic acid. *Eur. J. Biochem.*, 2:44–49.

132. Weis, H. J., and Dietschy, J. M. (1969): Failure of bile acids to control hepatic cholesterogenesis: Evidence for endogenous cholesterol feedback. *J. Clin. Invest.*, 48:2398–2408.

133. Percy-Robb, I. W., and Boyd, G. S. (1970): The synthesis of bile acids in perfused rat liver subjected to chronic biliary drainage. *Biochem. J.*, 118:519–530.

134. Grundy, S. M., Ahrens, E. H., Jr., and Salen, G. (1971): Interruption of the enterohepatic circulation of bile acids in man: Comparative effects of cholestyramine and ileal exclusion on cholesterol metabolism. *J. Lab. Clin. Med.*, 78:94–121.

135. Weis, H. J., and Dietschy, J. M. (1974): Adaptive responses in hepatic and intestinal cholesterogenesis following ileal resection in the rat. *Eur. J. Clin. Invest.*, 4:33–41.

136. Slater, H. R., Packard, C. J., Bicker, S., and Shepherd, J.

(1980): Effects of cholestyramine on receptor-mediated plasma clearance and tissue uptake of human low density lipoproteins in the rabbit. *J. Biol. Chem.*, 255:10210–10213.

137. Kovanen, P. T., Bilheimer, D. W., Goldstein, J. L., Jaramillo, J. J., and Brown, M. S. (1981): Regulatory role for hepatic low density lipoprotein receptors in vivo in the dog. *Proc. Natl. Acad. Sci. USA*, 78:1194–1198.

138. Shaffer, E. A., and Small, D. M. (1977): Biliary lipid secretion in cholesterol gallstone disease. The effect of cholecystectomy and obesity. *J. Clin. Invest.*, 59:828–840.

139. Bennion, L. J., and Grundy, S. M. (1978): Risk factors for the development of cholelithiasis in man. *N. Engl. J. Med.*, 299:1161–1167, 1221–1227.

140. Wheeler, H. O., and King, K. K. (1972): Biliary excretion of lecithin and cholesterol in the dog. *J. Clin. Invest.*, 51:1337–1350.

141. Forker, E. L. (1977): Mechanisms of hepatic bile formation. *Annu. Rev. Physiol.*, 39:323–347.

142. Dowling, R. H., Mack, E., and Small, D. M. (1971): Biliary lipid secretion and bile composition after acute and chronic interruption of the enterohepatic circulation in the rhesus monkey. IV. Primate biliary physiology. *J. Clin. Invest.*, 50:1917–1926.

143. Hardison, W. G. M., and Apter, J. T. (1972): Micellar theory of biliary cholesterol excretion. *Am. J. Physiol.*, 222:61–67.

144. Hoffman, N. E., Donald, D. E., and Hofmann, A. F. (1975): Effect of primary bile acids on bile lipid secretion from perfused dog liver. *Am. J. Physiol.*, 229:714–720.

145. Poupon, R., Poupon, R., Grosdemouge, M. L., Dumont, M., and Erlinger, S. (1976): Influence of bile acids upon biliary cholesterol and phospholipid secretion in the dog. *Eur. J. Clin. Invest.*, 6:279–284.

146. Wagner, C. I., Trotman, B. W., and Soloway, R. D. (1976): Kinetic analysis of biliary lipid excretion in man and dog. *J. Clin. Invest.*, 57:473–477.

147. Lindblad, L., Lundholm, K., and Scherstén, T. (1977): Influence of cholic and chenodeoxycholic acid on biliary cholesterol secretion in man. *Eur. J. Clin. Invest.*, 7:383–388.

148. Turley, S. D., and Dietschy, J. M. (1979): Regulation of biliary cholesterol output in the rat: Dissociation from the rate of hepatic cholesterol synthesis, the size of the hepatic cholesteryl ester pool, and the hepatic uptake of chylomicron cholesterol. *J. Lipid Res.*, 20:923–934.

149. Metzger, A. L., Adler, R., Heymsfield, S., and Grundy, S. M. (1973): Diurnal variation in biliary lipid composition. Possible role in cholesterol gallstone formation. *N. Engl. J. Med.*, 288:333–336.

150. Mok, H. Y. I., Von Bergmann, K., and Grundy, S. M. (1980): Kinetics of the enterohepatic circulation during fasting: biliary lipid secretion and gallbladder storage. *Gastroenterology*, 78:1023–1033.

151. Carey, M. C., and Small, D. M. (1978): The physical chemistry of cholesterol solubility in bile. Relationship to gallstone formation and dissolution in man. *J. Clin. Invest.*, 61:998–1026.

152. Admirand, W. H., and Small, D. M. (1978): The physicochemical basis of cholesterol gallstone formation in man. *J. Clin. Invest.*, 47:1043–1052.

153. McSherry, C. K., Javitt, N. B., De Carvalho, J. M., and Glenn, F. (1971): Cholesterol gallstones and the chemical composition of bile in baboons. *Ann. Surg.*, 173:569–577.

154. Brenneman, D. E., Connor, W. E., Forker, E. L., and Den-Besten, L. (1972): The formation of abnormal bile and cholesterol gallstones from dietary cholesterol in the prairie dog. *J. Clin. Invest.*, 51:1495–1503.

155. Wheeler, H. O. (1973): Biliary excretion of bile acids, lecithin, and cholesterol in hamsters with gallstones. *Gastroenterology*, 65:92–103.

156. Robins, S. J., and Fasulo, J. (1973): Mechanism of lithogenic bile production: Studies in the hamster fed an essential fatty acid-deficient diet. *Gastroenterology*, 65:104–114.

157. Osuga, T., Portman, O. W., Tanaka, N., Alexander, M., and Ochsner, J., III. (1976): The effect of diet on hepatic bile formation and bile acid metabolism in squirrel monkeys with and

without cholesterol gallstones. *J. Lab. Clin. Med.*, 88:649–661.

158. Kajiyama, G., Kubota, S., Sasaki, H., Kawamoto, T., and Miyoshi, A. (1980): Lipid metabolism in the development of cholesterol gallstones in hamsters. I. Study on the relationship between serum and biliary lipids. *Hiroshima J. Med. Sci.*, 29:133–141.

159. Ahlberg, J., Angelin, B., and Einarsson, K. (1981): Hepatic 3-hydroxy-3-methylglutaryl coenzyme A reductase activity and biliary lipid composition in man: relation to cholesterol gallstone disease and effects of cholic acid and chenodeoxycholic acid treatment. *J. Lipid Res.*, 22:410–422.

160. Nervi, F. O., Covarrubias, C. F., Valdivieso, V. D., Ronco, B. O., Solari, A., and Tocornal, J. (1981): Hepatic cholesterogenesis in Chileans with cholesterol gallstone disease. Evidence for sex differences in the regulation of hepatic cholesterol metabolism. *Gastroenterology*, 80:539–545.

161. Adler, R. D., Bennion, L. J., Duane, W. C., and Grundy, S. M. (1975): Effects of low dose chenodeoxycholic acid feeding on biliary lipid metabolism. *Gastroenterology*, 68:326–334.

162. Maton, P. N., Murphy, G. M., and Dowling, R. H. (1977): Ursodeoxycholic acid treatment of gallstones. Dose-response study and possible mechanism of action. *Lancet*, ii:1297–1301.

163. Makino, I., and Nakagawa, S. (1978): Changes in biliary lipid and biliary bile acid composition in patients after administration of ursodeoxycholic acid. *J. Lipid Res.*, 19:723–728.

164. Raicht, R. F., Cohen, B. I., Sarwal, A., and Takahashi, M. (1978): Ursodeoxycholic acid. Effects on sterol metabolism in rats. *Biochim. Biophys. Acta*, 531:1–8.

165. Stiehl, A., Czygan, P., Kommerell, B., Weis, H. J., and Holtermüller, K. H. (1978): Ursodeoxycholic acid versus chenodeoxycholic acid. Comparison of their effects on bile acid and bile lipid composition in patients with cholesterol gallstones. *Gastroenterology*, 75:1016–1020.

166. Carulli, N., Ponz De Leon, M., Zironi, F., Pinetti, A., Smerieri, A., Iori, R., and Loria, P. (1980): Hepatic cholesterol and bile acid metabolism in subjects with gallstones: comparative effects of short term feeding of chenodeoxycholic and ursodeoxycholic acid. *J. Lipid Res.*, 21:35–43.

167. LaRusso, N. F., Szczepanik, P. A., and Hofmann, A. F. (1977): Effect of deoxycholic acid ingestion on bile acid metabolism and biliary lipid secretion in normal subjects. *Gastroenterology*, 72:132–140.

168. Carulli, N., Ponz De Leon, M., Zironi, F., Iori, R., and Loria, P. (1980): Bile acid feeding and hepatic sterol metabolism: effect of deoxycholic acid. *Gastroenterology*, 79:637–641.

169. Schwartz, C. C., Vlahcevic, Z. R., Halloran, L. G., Gregory, D. H., Meek, J. B., and Swell, L. (1975): Evidence for the existence of definitive hepatic cholesterol precursor compartments for bile acids and biliary cholesterol in man. *Gastroenterology*, 69:1379–1382.

170. Normann, P. T., and Norum, K. R. (1976): Newly synthesized hepatic cholesterol as precursor for cholesterol and bile acids in rat bile. *Scand. J. Gastroenterol.*, 11:427–432.

171. Turley, S. D., Spady, D. K., and Dietschy, J. M. (1982): Effect of feeding a fat-free diet on biliary lipid secretion and other aspects of cholesterol metabolism in the hamster and rat. *Gastroenterology.* (*in press.*)

172. Osuga, T., and Portman, O. W. (1972): Relationship between bile composition and gallstone formation in squirrel monkeys. *Gastroenterology*, 63:122–133.

173. Pearlman, B. J., Bonorris, G. G., Phillips, M. J., Chung, A., Vimadalal, S., Marks, J. W., and Schoenfield, L. J. (1979): Cholesterol gallstone formation and prevention by chenodeoxycholic and ursodeoxycholic acids. A new hamster model. *Gastroenterology*, 77:634–641.

174. Cayen, M. N., and Dvornik, D., (1979): Effect of diosgenin on lipid metabolism in rats. *J. Lipid Res.*, 20:162–174.

175. Dam, H., Prange, I., Jensen, M. K., Kallehauge, H. E., and Fenger, H. J. (1971): Studies on human bile IV. Influence of

ingestion of cholesterol in the form of eggs on the composition of bile in healthy subjects. *Z. Ernaehrungswiss.*, 10:178–187.

176. Cohen, B. I., Raicht, R. F., and Mosbach, E. H. (1977): Sterol metabolism studies in the rat. Effects of dietary plant sterols and bile acids on sterol metabolism. *Biochim. Biophys. Acta,* 487:287–296.

177. Tangedahl, T. N., Thistle, J. L., Hofmann, A. F., and Matseshe, J. W. (1979): Effect of β-sitosterol alone or in combination with chenic acid on cholesterol saturation of bile and cholesterol absorption in gallstone patients. *Gastroenterology,* 76:1341–1346.

178. Beher, W. T., Casazza, K. K., Filus, A. M., Beher, M. E., and Bertasius, J. (1970): Effects of accumulated tissue cholesterol on bile acid metabolism in hypophysectomized rats and hamsters. *Atherosclerosis,* 12:383–392.

179. Hansma, H., and Ostwald, R. (1974): Effects of dietary cholesterol upon bile acid metabolism in guinea pig. *Lipids,* 9:731–737.

180. Portman, O. W., Alexander, M., and O'Malley, J. P. (1980): Metabolism of free and esterified cholesterol and apolipoproteins of plasma low and high density lipoproteins. *Biochim. Biophys. Acta,* 619:545–558.

181. Swell, L., Bell, C. C., and Vlahcevic, Z. R. (1971): Relationship of bile acid pool size to biliary lipid excretion and the formation of lithogenic bile in man. *Gastroenterology,* 61:716–722.

182. Thistle, J. L., and Hofmann, A. F. (1973): Efficacy and specificity of chenodeoxycholic acid therapy for dissolving gallstones. *N. Engl. J. Med.,* 289:655–659.

183. Scherstén, T., and Lindblad, L. (1979): Biliary cholesterol output during ursodeoxycholic acid secretion in man. In: *Biological Effects of Bile Acids,* edited by G. Paumgartner, A. Stiehl, and W. Gerok, pp. 53–60. University Park Press, Baltimore.

184. Sarfeh, I. J., Beeler, D. A., Treble, D. H., and Balint, J. A. (1974): Studies of the hepatic excretory defects in essential fatty acid deficiency. Their possible relationship to the genesis of cholesterol gallstones. *J. Clin. Invest.,* 53:423–430.

185. Eaton, D. L., and Klaassen, C. D. (1976): Effects of acute administration of taurocholic and taurochenodeoxycholic acid on biliary lipid excretion in the rat. *Proc. Soc. Exp. Biol. Med.,* 151:198–202.

186. Smallwood, R. A., and Hoffman, N. E. (1976): Bile acid structure and biliary secretion of cholesterol and phospholipid in the cat. *Gastroenterology,* 71:1064–1066.

187. Grundy, S. M., Ahrens, E. H., Jr., Salen, G., Schreibman, P. H., and Nestel, P. J. (1972): Mechanisms of action of clofibrate on cholesterol metabolism in patients with hyperlipidemia. *J. Lipid Res.,* 13:531–551.

188. Bateson, M. C., Maclean, D., Ross, P. E., and Bouchier, I. A. D. (1978): Clofibrate therapy and gallstone induction. *Dig. Dis.,* 23:623–628.

189. Turley, S. D., and Dietschy, J. M. (1980): Effects of clofibrate, cholestyramine, zanchol, probucol, and AOMA feeding on hepatic and intestinal cholesterol metabolism and on biliary lipid secretion in the rat. *J. Cardiovasc. Pharmacol.,* 2:281–297.

190. Cohen, B. I., Raicht, R. F., Shefer, S., and Mosbach, E. H. (1974): Effects of clofibrate on sterol metabolism in the rat. *Biochim. Biophys. Acta,* 369:79–85.

191. Dam, H., Prange, I., Jensen, M. K., Kallehauge, H. E., and Fenger, H. J. (1971): Studies on human bile. V. Influence of cholestyramine treatment on the composition of bile in healthy subjects. *Z. Ernaehrungswiss.,* 10:188–197.

192. Wood, P. D., Shioda, R., Estrich, D. L., and Splitter, S. D. (1972): Effect of cholestyramine on composition of duodenal bile in obese human subjects. *Metabolism,* 21:107–116.

193. Lagarriga, J., and Bouchier, I. A. D. (1973): The effect of phenobarbital on cholesterol gallstones in hamsters. *Gut,* 14:956–961.

194. Pertsemlidis, D., Panveliwalla, D., and Ahrens, E. H., Jr. (1974): Effects of clofibrate and of an estrogen-progestin combination on fasting biliary lipids and cholic acid kinetics in man. *Gastroenterology,* 66:565–573.

195. von Bergmann, K., Schwarz, H. P., and Paumgartner, G. (1975): Effect of phenobarbital, spironolactone and pregnenolone-16α-carbonitrile on bile formation in the rat. *Naunyn Schmiedebergs Arch. Pharmacol.,* 287:33–45.

196. Zimmon, D. S., Kerner, M. B., Aaron, B. M., Raicht, R. F., Mosbach, E. H., and Kessler, R. E. (1976): The effect of a hydrocholeretic agent (zanchol) on biliary lipids in post cholecystectomy patients. *Gastroenterology,* 70:640–643.

197. Grundy, S. M., and Mok, H. Y. I. (1977): Colestipol, clofibrate, and phytosterols in combined therapy of hyperlipidemia. *J. Lab. Clin. Med.,* 89:354–366.

198. Kern, F., Jr., Eriksson, H., Curstedt, T., and Sjovall, J. (1977): Effect of ethynylestradiol on biliary excretion of bile acids, phosphatidylcholines, and cholesterol in the bile fistula rat. *J. Lipid Res.,* 18:623–634.

199. Redinger, R. N., and Grace, D. M. (1978): Cholesterol gallstones and biliary lipid metabolism in the primate. *Gastroenterology,* 74:201–204.

200. Redinger, R. N., and Small, D. M. (1973): Primate biliary physiology VIII. The effect of phenobarbital upon bile salt synthesis and pool size, biliary lipid secretion, and bile composition. *J. Clin. Invest.,* 52:161–172.

201. Cayen, M. N., Ferdinandi, E. S., Greselin, E., and Dvornik, D. (1979): Studies on the disposition of diosgenin in rats, dogs, monkeys and man. *Atherosclerosis,* 33:71–87.

Section II

The Cells

C. Sinusoidal Cells

The barrier between the sinusoidal and perisinusoidal spaces consists of capillary endothelial cells, which comprise the major structural elements of the barrier itself, and other cells which are mainly perisinusoidal. Together, the group of sinusoidal cells constitutes a coordinated defense system in which the parenchymal macrophages, the Kupffer cells, are most potent. They are either perisinusoidal or float in the sinusoidal lumen. The star-shaped extensions of Kupffer cells and fat-storing cells may also play a role in regulation of sinusoidal blood flow. In addition, by formation of ectoskeletal matrix substances and probably collagenous reticulin, they participate in organization of the structure of the liver. Sinusoidal cells have a considerably shorter lifespan than do hepatocytes.

In morphometric measurements of rat liver, 44% of sinusoidal cell volume is endothelial cells, 33% is Kupffer cells, and 22% is fat-storing cells (1). Since endothelial cells are smaller than Kupffer cells, their number is even greater than volumetric figures indicate. In addition, a small number of pit cells may have neuroendocrine function. In embryonal life, the liver is an important hematopoietic organ; even in adults, however, occasional perisinusoidal lymphoid cells are present.

The nucleus of sinusoidal cells accounts for 16 to 20% of cell volume, and mitochondria compromise 4.5%. The main difference between the various cells is in the volume of lysosomes, which occupies about 14% in Kupffer cells, 7% in endothelial cells, and hardly any space in fat-storing cells, in which vitamin A fluorescent lipid droplets fill one-fourth of cell volume. In contrast, pinocytotic vesicles provide almost 6% of endothelial and less than 2% of Kupffer cell volume. Kupffer cells account morphometrically for 17% of the lysosomal volume of the liver.

These morphometric data are related to the functional characteristics of sinusoidal cells, which are discussed in this section. The data support the large phagocytotic potential of Kupffer cells, the endocytotic capacities of endothelial cells, and a different function for the fat-storing cells. All sinusoidal cells are characterized by abundant cytoplasmic extensions; more than one-fourth the plasma membrane in the entire liver is derived from sinusoidal cells, particularly endothelial and fat-storing cells rather than Kupffer cells.

Whether or not hepatic endothelial or Kupffer cells have specific functions in relation to comparable cells in other organs is unknown. They constitute a coordinated defense system which protects hepatocytes against injury. For example, the toxin of frog hepatitis virus renders the hepatocytes vulnerable only after destruction of Kupffer cells and endothelial cells; normal liver is unaffected by frog virus. These cells protect the liver from the effects of lipopolysaccharides of endotoxin nature. Specifics of the defense action of the sinusoidal system are discussed in the following chapters, which emphasize immunologic activities, specific receptors, and secretory products. Understanding the role of the sinusoidal defense system in human disease is an exciting and timely challenge.

REFERENCES

1. Blouin, A. (1977): Morphometry of liver sinusoidal cells. In: *Kupffer Cells and Other Liver Sinusoidal Cells,* edited by E. Wisse and K. L. Knook, pp. 61–71. Elsevier, New York.
2. Wisse, E., and Knook, D. L. (editors) (1977): *Kupffer Cells and Other Liver Sinusoidal Cells.* Elsevier, Amsterdam.
3. Liehr, H., and Grün, M. (editors) (1982): *The Reticuloendothelial System and the Pathogenesis of Liver Disease.* Elsevier, Amsterdam (*in press*).

The Liver: Biology and Pathobiology, edited by
I. Arias, H. Popper, D. Schachter, and D. A. Shafritz.
Raven Press, New York © 1982.

Chapter 29

Sinusoidal Endothelial Cells and Perisinusoidal Fat-Storing Cells: Structure and Function*

H. Dariush Fahimi

It has been more than 100 years since the existence of phagocytic mesenchymal cells in the lining of hepatic sinuoids was recognized (for a review, see ref. 1). Because of their general property to take up vital dyes, the sinusoidal cells of the liver, together with reticular cells of spleen and lymph nodes, as well as histiocytes and monocytes, were grouped together and designated as the reticuloendothelial system (RES). Until recently, the concept of RES influenced our thinking about the sinusoidal lining cells of the liver. It was believed that since all hepatic sinusoidal cells are capable of a certain degree of endocytosis, they must be functional variants of the same single cell type, generally referred to as the Kupffer cell. By electron microscopy the wall-forming endothelial cells (EC) were differentiated from the more phagocytic Kupffer cells; but the existence of intermediate forms, particularly after the stimulation of phagocytosis, was also recognized.

The introduction of perfusion fixation (2), the use of peroxidase as a cytochemical marker for mononuclear phagocytes (3), and the recent application of scanning electron microscopy have furthered our understanding of the morphological and functional relationship of hepatic sinusoidal cells. There is now general agreement that the hepatic sinusoids contain two distinct cell types: (a) the wall-forming endothelial cells, with typical fenestrations, and (b) the phagocytic Kupffer cells, which often protrude into the sinusoidal lumen (Figs. 1–3). The Kupffer cells are distinguished from the endothelial cells by their ability to phagocytize large (0.8 to 1 μm) latex particles and in rat liver by the positive peroxidase reaction in their endoplasmic reticulum and nuclear envelope (Fig. 2). By scanning electron microscopy, the fenestrations of endothelial cells form sieve plates along the sinusoidal lining, and Kupffer cells exhibit typical lamellopodia and microvilli-like structures on their surface (Fig. 3). In addition, the perisinusoidal space contains stellate-shaped cells containing prominent lipid vacuoles, the so-called fat-storing cells (FSC) first described by Ito and associates (for a review, see ref. 4). Several designations have been used for these cells, including lipocytes, perisinusoidal cells, adventitial connective tissue cells, vitamin A-storing cells, and stellate cells. In keeping with the original suggestion of Ito, we refer to them as FSC or Ito cells.

In this chapter, the morphological and functional characteristics of EC and FSC are reviewed; some of the alterations of these cells under experimental conditions and in human disease are discussed. The sinusoidal cells of the liver were the subject of a major symposium held in 1977 (5), and an extensive review of the literature on Ito cells has been published recently (6).

---

* This chapter is dedicated to two well-known hepatologists and close friends who died unexpectedly within a short time: Pierre Drochmans and Jean Claude Wanson.

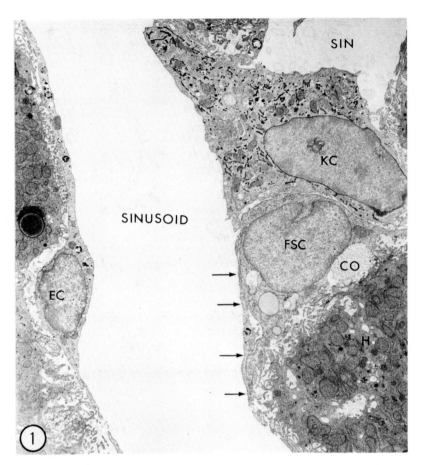

FIG. 1. Rat liver fixed by perfusion. Note the patent sinusoids (SIN) which are free of blood cells. The three cell types encountered are: the wall-forming endothelial cell (EC), the large phagocytic Kupffer cell (KC), and the perisinusoidal fat-storing cell (FSC). The Kupffer cell shows positive reaction for peroxidase in the nuclear envelope and RER. The FSC is closely associated with bundles of collagen (CO) and is separated from the sinusoidal lumen through the extension of an EC (*arrows*). H, hepatocyte. (From ref. 24, with permission.) ×4,680.

ENDOTHELIAL CELLS

Morphologic Characteristics

In livers fixed by perfusion, the sinusoids are patent and free of circulating blood cells. The endothelial cells (EC) have an elongated shape with a small perikaryon, which may either bulge into the lumen or be hidden in a recess. Numerous cytoplasmic processes radiate from the perikaryon with a thin layer of fenestrated cytoplasm stretched between them, lining the sinusoidal wall (Fig. 4). The fenestrations are distributed in clusters of 10 to 50 pores, referred to as sieve plates (7). They are dynamic structures with a mean diameter of 100 nm under physiological conditions (portal vein pressure, 8 mm Hg in rat) which coalesce to form larger holes when the perfusion pressure is increased. Thus the increase of portal pressure to 34 mm

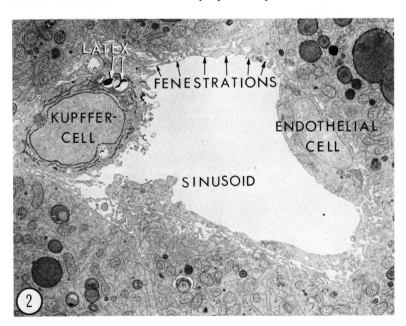

FIG. 2. Distinction between EC and Kupffer cell in rat liver. The EC forms fenestrations along the sinusoidal wall, is peroxidase negative, and does not take up latex particles. The Kupffer cell is peroxidase positive, shows numerous microvilli-like structures on its surface, and takes up injected latex particles. (From ref. 19, with permission of *Am. J. Pathol.*) ×4,950.

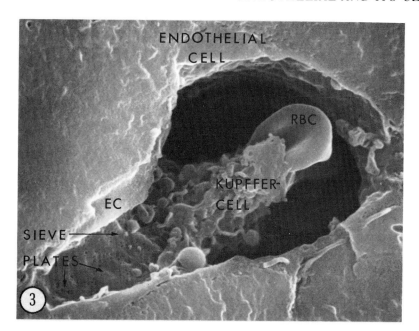

FIG. 3. Scanning electron micrograph of rat liver showing a phagocytic Kupffer cell with typical lamellopodia taking up a red blood cell in contrast to an EC, which stretches along the wall of the sinusoid, forming sieve plates. (Micrograph courtesy of Dr. W. Deimann, Heidelberg.) ×9,000.

Hg in rats causes the formation of holes with a diameter of 240 nm (8). Larger holes (up to several microns) are found by arterial perfusion with pressures above 70 to 90 mm Hg (Fig. 5) (9), as well as by obstruction of the hepatic venous outflow (10). Sieve plates with similar dimensions have also been described in human liver (11).

The neighboring EC touch each other at their periphery, forming poorly defined cell contacts which have been best studied in regenerating liver (12). In freeze-etch preparations, these cell contacts consist of arrays of membrane particles, which remain separated from each other by particle-free intervals. This appearance probably represents an abortive form of tight junction formation, which provides mechanical adhesion without forming a permeability barrier between adjacent EC. It should be emphasized that there are no larger gaps between EC, and the only communication between the space of Disse and sinusoids is through the sieve plates of EC. The Kupffer cells, which usually lie over the endothelium, are attached to the latter with cytoplasmic processes that pass through the fenestrations or penetrate the cytoplasm of EC, extending into the space of Disse. Furthermore, cyto-

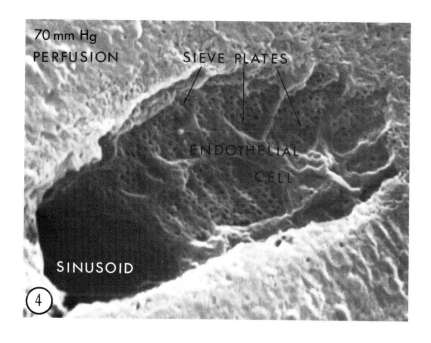

FIG. 4. Perfusion fixation under physiologic conditions (70 mm Hg). An EC with cytoplasmic extensions radiating from its perikaryon is shown. A thin sheet of cytoplasm containing the fenestrations (sieve plates) is stretched between these extensions. (Micrograph courtesy of G. Stöhr, Heidelberg.) ×20,000.

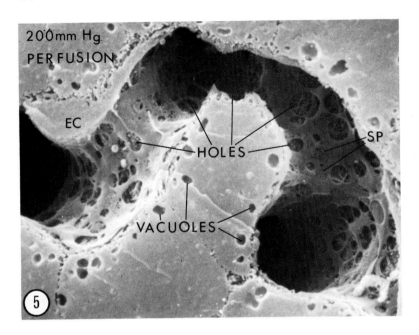

FIG. 5. Perfusion fixation through the abdominal aorta at 200 mm Hg. In addition to sieve plates, there are large holes (up to several microns) in the sinusoidal lining through which the microvilli in the space of Disse are visible. Note also the vacuoles in the cytoplasm of hepatocytes just beneath the endothelial lining. (Micrograph courtesy of Dr. E. Weihe, Heidelberg.) ×2,250.

plasmic processes of perisinusoidal FSC extend into the space of Disse behind the EC, thus providing focally a double lining for the sinusoids (7, 11). Hepatic EC in most mammalian species lack a distinct basement membrane, although abortive structures in the space of Disse have been observed (7). A prominent basement membrane has been described in ruminants (13).

The perikaryon and the cytoplasmic processes of EC contain the usual cell organelles, such as mitochondria, endoplasmic reticulum, microtubules, microfilaments, and a few peroxisomes (14). The lysosomal system is well developed, and large numbers of coated pits and vesicles are seen facing mostly the sinusoidal lumen. Figure 6 shows the uptake of serum

albumin labeled with horseradish peroxidase by an EC in rat liver (Yokota and Fahimi, *in preparation*). The protein binds to specific regions of the plasma membrane, where coated pits are formed. By pinching off, these give rise to coated vesicles with an approximate size of 150 to 200 nm (Fig. 7). The labeled protein is transported to larger vacuoles measuring 700 to 1000 nm in diameter; these are called macropinocytosis vesicles (15). In addition, tubular structures, known as "transfer tubules," are involved in transporting ingested material to phagosomes (Fig. 7).

Treatment of glutaraldehyde-fixed sections with detergents reveals the cytoskeletal proteins, mainly the 10 nm prekaratin filaments in parenchymal cells (16). In this material, the coated vesicles in EC are also

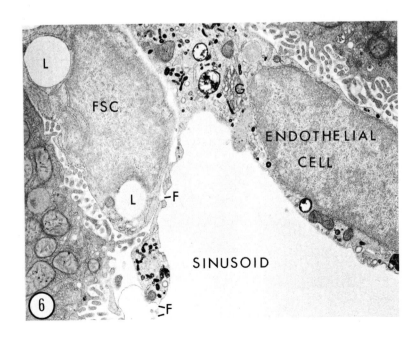

FIG. 6. Rat liver 3 min after the injection of serum albumin labeled with horseradish peroxidase. The labeled protein, which is stained black with the cytochemical method for peroxidase, is localized in small vesicles, in tubules, and in larger phagosomes (macropinocytosis) all in the EC. The FSC does not show any evidence of endocytic activity. F, fenestrations; G, Golgi apparatus; L, lipid droplets. (Micrograph courtesy of Dr. S. Yokota, Heidelberg.) ×6,750.

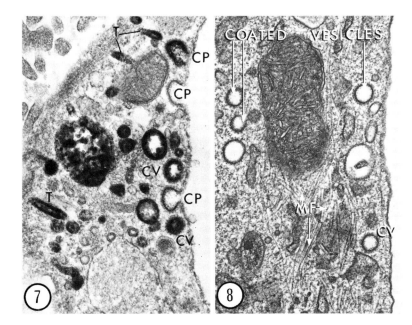

FIG. 7. Higher power view showing the binding of peroxidase-labeled serum albumin to the surface of an EC with the formation of coated pits (CP) and coated vesicles (CV). These seem to lose their bristle coat before discharging their content in the larger phagosome. In addition, there are transfer tubules (T) containing the labeled protein. (Micrograph courtesy of Dr. S. Yokota, Heidelberg.) ×23,400.

FIG. 8. Cytoplasm of an EC containing numerous coated vesicles (CV) and bundles of microfilaments (MF). Tissue treated after glutaraldehyde fixation with detergent to reveal cytoskeletal proteins (16). (Micrograph courtesy of Dr. S. Yokota, Heidelberg.) ×18,000.

distinctly visualized; in addition, bundles of microfilaments are seen in the cytoplasm (Fig. 8). The entire vacuolar apparatus of EC, consisting of coated pits and vesicles, transfer tubules, and the larger phagosomes, as well as the mature (*cis*) cisternae of the Golgi complex, stain strongly with the phosphotungstic acid (17). This suggests a functional relationship between these heterogeneous structures. The Golgi apparatus consists of several stacks and small vesicles; occasionally, small coated vesicles (approximately 100 nm) are found in continuity with its cisternae (15). The nuclei of EC are relatively small, containing aggregates of heterochromatin, a prominent nucleolus, and, in rare instances, a nuclear body or spheridium (15).

After stimulation of the RES with estrogens (18) or zymosan (15) and after partial hepatectomy (19), no evidence of transformation of EC to Kupffer cells is seen. In these conditions, however, many EC in mitosis are observed (Fig. 9), demonstrating the ability of these cells for self-replication. In fetal liver, the EC and Kupffer cells form two separate populations with distinct properties, as in adult animals: EC form fenestrations and sieve plates, and Kupffer cells, identified by the positive peroxidase reaction, exhibit erythrophagocytosis (20). Whereas EC probably arise from the fetal hepatic mesenchyme, Kupffer cells are derived from macrophages of the yolk sack (20). Attention is drawn to the fact that peroxidase reaction for

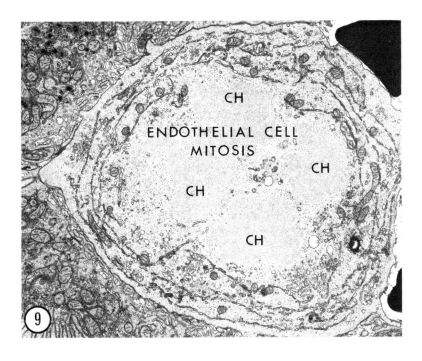

FIG. 9. EC in mitosis from rat liver after partial hepatectomy. Note the clumps of chromatin (CH), small mitochondria, and the few dilated cisternae of the endoplasmic reticulum. (Micrograph from ref. 19 with permission of *Am. J. Pathol.*) ×13,500.

distinction between Kupffer cells and EC is useful only in rat liver; in mouse liver, more than half the EC also exhibit a positive reaction in their nuclear envelope and endoplasmic reticulum (21).

Functional Characteristics

Filtering Function of Sieve Plates

The endothelial lining of hepatic sinusoids provides a continuous filtration barrier with a pore size of approximately 100 nm, shielding the space of Disse from larger particles in circulating blood. The size-dependent selectivity of this sieving system has been demonstrated *in vivo* for chylomicrons (8,22). Isotopically labeled chylomicrons of different sizes were injected into the portal vein, and only small chylomicrons were trapped in the liver. When the perfusion pressure in the portal vein was increased, large chylomicrons were also trapped in the liver. By scanning electron microscopy, it was shown in the latter condition that the size of fenestrations increased significantly (8). Similarly, in neonatal liver, chylomicrons larger than 250 nm were shielded from the space of Disse, but smaller chylomicrons were readily taken up by parenchymal cells (22). The damaging effect of portal venous congestion, hypoxia, and endotoxin on endothelial fenestrations has been demonstrated (9). It has been suggested that the loss of filtration function may be important in the pathogenesis of fatty change seen in chronic venous congestion (8) or in the development of anoxic vacuoles in parenchymal cells (10).

An intact endothelial lining also prevents the entry of viral particles into the space of Disse and may play an important role in the pathogenesis of viral infections of the liver. For example, normal mice are resistant to infection with the vaccinia virus and develop fatal hepatitis if inocculated 4 to 8 hr before with FV_3 virus, which destroys the endothelial lining of liver sinusoids (23). Figures 12 and 13 are from mice infected 5 hr prior to perfusion fixation with the FV_3 virus and show the destruction of sieve plates and the exposure of microvilli in the space of Disse.

Endocytic Function

The sinusoidal lining cells actively participate in clearing the blood of foreign material, such as senescent erythrocytes, microorganisms, and macromolecules. Whereas Kupffer cells are highly efficient in phagocytosis of large particles, EC have a limited capacity for endocytosis of particulate matter (24). The large number of coated endocytic vesicles on their luminal surface indicates that EC are involved in uptake of macromolecules from blood. The involvement of clathrin-coated vesicles in the selective, receptor-mediated endocytosis of several proteins, such as insulin, epidermal growth factor, and α_2 macroglobulin, has been shown in fibroblasts. It has been suggested that all peptide hormones and proteins for which a receptor exists enter the cell through coated pits and vesicles (25). The EC of rat liver are two to six times more efficient than Kupffer cells in binding ligands whose oligosaccharide chains terminate in N-acetylglucosamine or mannose, a finding consistent with the presence of specific receptors on their surface (26). The ligands enter the cell via coated vesicles, which rapidly fuse with existing macropinocytosis vesicles

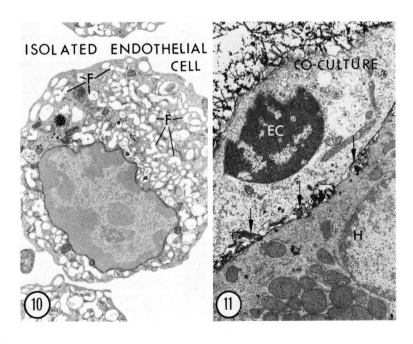

FIG. 10. Isolated EC from rat liver. Note the meandering vacuolar system in the cytoplasm, which corresponds to the fenestrations (F) after detachment from the sinusoidal wall. (Micrograph courtesy of Dr. J. C. Wanson.) ×8,550.

FIG. 11. EC in symbiotic coculture with a parenchymal cell (H). The survival of EC is improved in cocultures, and they form loose contacts with hepatocytes reconstituting a space similar to the space of Disse containing microvilli (*arrows*) and collagen fibers. (Micrograph courtesy of Dr. J. C. Wanson, and with permission of the MTP Press.) ×6,300.

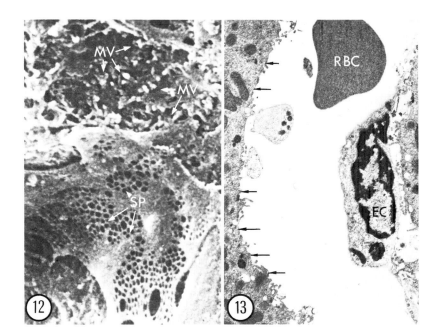

FIGS. 12 and 13. Scanning and transmission electron micrographs of mouse liver 5 min after infection with FV_3 virus. Note the destruction of the endothelial lining with loss of sieve plates. The microvilli (MV) in the space of Disse are directly exposed to the circulating blood in sinusoids. Note also the blunting of such microvilli in Fig. 13 (*arrows*). Some EC seem to survive the infection. RBC, red blood cell. (Micrographs courtesy of Dr. Gendrault and Dr. Kirn, Strassbourg). Fig. 12, ×6,030; Fig. 13, ×9,450.

(at 1 to 15 min) before their ultimate residence in dense bodies (15 min and later intervals) (27). In fibroblasts, the contents of coated pits are internalized into uncoated vesicles, termed "receptosomes" (28), which, at the early interval after endocytosis, selectively fail to fuse with lysosomes and accumulate in the Golgi region. Subsequently (15 to 30 min), the ligand in the receptosomes is delivered to lysosomes, and the receptor molecules are recycled back to the cell surface without destruction (28).

Sinusoidal lining cells have been implicated in the uptake and clearance of lipoproteins, glycoproteins, lipopolysaccharides, and mucopolysaccharides (for a review, see ref. 29), but it is not exactly known which macromolecule is selectively taken up by which cell type. The recent localization of heparin-releasable hepatic lipase on the surface of EC (30) suggests a preferential degradation of lipoproteins in EC. Furthermore, the high concentration of arylsulfatase B in EC (31) is consistent with their involvement in degradation of mucopolysaccharides. The volume density of the plasma membrane of EC is several times larger than that of Kupffer cells, and EC contain substantially more coated vesicles (32). These findings suggest that receptor-mediated selective uptake of macromolecules may be more pronounced in EC than in Kupffer cells, which exhibit a more avid endocytic activity.

Isolation and Cultivation of Sinusoidal Cells

In the last few years, marked improvements have been made in isolation of nonparenchymal cells of liver (5,29). The use of countercurrent centrifugation in an elutriator rotor has resulted in satisfactory separation of nonparenchymal cells into two fractions containing EC and Kupffer cells without disturbing cellular morphology. The EC in such preparations have a spherical shape, with a size of 6 to 9 μm and, in sections, show a meandering cytoplasmic vacuolar system (Fig. 10) which corresponds to the sieve plates after retraction from the lining of sinusoids. Separation of EC from Kupffer cells has provided the basis for study of biochemical differences between these two major sinusoidal lining cells (31).

The sinusoidal lining cells have also been grown successfully in culture, although EC do not survive long in the culture medium (33), perhaps because they do not attach to the culture dish and are lost on changing of medium, or because they require specific growth factors. In symbiotic cocultures with parenchymal cells, the survival of EC is improved, and they form loose contacts with hepatocytes reconstituting a space similar to the space of Disse, which contains microvilli and collagen fibers (Fig. 11) (34).

Involvement in Various Pathologic Conditions

Because of the difficulty in distinguishing the various sinusoidal cells in routine histologic preparations, there have been only few reports of specific lesions of EC in liver disease. A selective involvement of EC containing large foamy vacuoles was described in a case of Morquio disease (35). Neoplastic lesions of EC, angiosarcomas, have been noted in human liver and in experimental animals. Several toxic environmental agents, such as vinyl chloride, arsenic, and thorotrast, have been implicated in the pathogenesis of these lesions (36). The derivation of angiosarcoma cells from the endothelium has been based on the limited phagocytic activity of tumor cells and on electron microscopy. Marked sinusoidal dilatation was noted in most cases of hemangiosarcoma without evidence of passive congestion. Similar forms of sinusoidal dilatations have been described in a variety of unrelated conditions (e.g., Crohn disease, women taking oral contraceptives, hepatic granulomas, and patients receiving anabolic steroids). A basic pathobiologic lesion of the EC may be the common denominator in these conditions.

FAT-STORING CELLS

Morphologic Characteristics

The fat-storing cells (FSC) are difficult to recognize in paraffin-embedded, hematoxylin eosin stained sections; however, they can be selectively stained with the gold impregnation technique (37). Wake (6,37) has noted that the "stellate cells," described originally by von Kupffer in 1876, are not hepatic sinusoidal macrophages but are FSC. This staining is attributable to the reduction of gold chloride by vitamin A, which is present in FSC (37). Vitamin A is also responsible for the quick-fading green fluorescence of FSC seen in frozen sections of formaldehyde-fixed liver. The Ito cells are easily identified in semithin (1 to 2 μm) sections of osmium-fixed and Epon-embedded tissue (38). Because of the capriciousness of gold impregnation techniques and the rapid fading of fluorescence of vitamin A, the latter method is best suited for routine application.

In rat liver, the FSC constitute 13% of the nonparenchymal cells (EC, 48%; Kupffer cells, 39%) (24).

In human liver, there is approximately 1 FSC for every 20 parenchymal cells (38). The Ito cells are located in the perisinusoidal space and contain numerous lipid droplets, which are more prominent in the periportal areas than in the center of hepatic lobules. The size and number of lipid droplets vary with the nutritional status (especially of vitamin A); in addition, species-specific differences exist. For example, man and rodents have numerous small (1 to 3 μm in diameter) droplets, and goats and pigs show a single large droplet (4,39). The FSC have a small perikaryon with a prominent round to ovoid nucleus, which is occasionally indented by the cytoplasmic lipid droplets. The perisinusoidal location with the typical lipid droplets and the absence of phagocytic vacuoles permit easy differentiation of FSC from EC and Kupffer cells by light microscopy.

On electron microscopy, the most prominent ultrastructural feature of FSC is their well-developed rough endoplasmic reticulum (RER). The cisternae of RER are focally dilated (Fig. 14) and often contain finely flocculent material. In addition, a prominent Golgi apparatus with several stacks and few vesicles, features reminiscent of active synthesis and secretion of proteins, are present in the cytoplasm. A few bristle-coated vesicles found below the plasma membrane are probably involved in the secretory process, since FSC do not exhibit endocytic activity (24,39) (Fig. 6). There are also a few multivesicular bodies in FSC, which have been implicated in the esterification of retinol (6). The characteristic lipid droplets usually lack a distinct limiting membrane (38,49), although Wake (6) demonstrated that some are surrounded by a distinct unit membrane. The FSC contain a few small mitochondria, rare peroxisomes (14), and a distinct

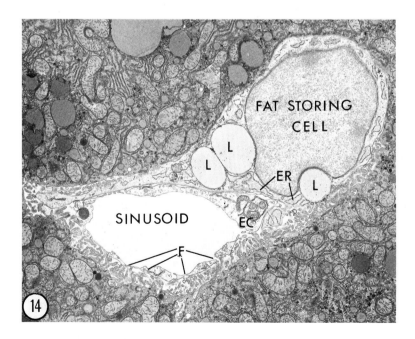

FIG. 14. Perisinusoidal FSC from mouse liver. Note the typical lipid droplets in the cytoplasm, which are lighter than lipid droplets in parenchymal cells. The prominent RER is focally dilated. Note the cytoplasmic extension of the FSC behind the fenestrated (F) endothelium forming focally a double lining for the sinusoid. (Micrograph courtesy of G. Stöhr, Heidelberg.) ×6,300.

centriole. Occasionally, a single cilium projecting into the perisinusoidal space has been observed (40). The cytoplasmic matrix contains bundles of microfilaments and microtubules, which are also seen in extensions of FSC in the space of Disse, the so-called "endothelial processes" (7,40). These processes extend between the EC and the microvilli of parenchymal cells, focally forming a double lining of sinusoids. Functionally, the cytoskeletal proteins in these extensions may reinforce the sinusoidal wall. Distinct cytoplasmic invaginations of FSC surround bundles of collagen, which separate the FSC and parenchymal cells (Fig. 1). There is general agreement that FSC are not engulfed by a basement membrane and, in this respect, differ from the usual pericytes in blood capillaries (4,6,7,40).

Functional Characteristics

Hepatic Fibrogenesis

The involvement of FSC in hepatic lobular fibrogenesis was postulated because of their close association with collagen bundles and their similarity to fibroblasts (41,42). This concept was supported by demonstration of increased uptake of proline by centrilobular perisinusoidal cells in acute hepatic injury with CCl$_4$ (43). Since the centrilobular perisinusoidal cells usually have only a few or no lipid droplets, their exact relationship to FSC remained to be established. Kent et al. (44) demonstrated transition forms with morphologic characteristics of FSC and fibroblasts, and showed association of these cells with type III collagen. Furthermore, they noted evidence of mitosis of FSC, which together with the demonstration of uptake of thymidine (43) indicates that Ito cells are derived locally by self-replication and not from extrahepatic sites.

Marked enlargement of FSC exhibiting only a few lipid droplets but prominent cell organelles has been reported in patients with progressive alcoholic liver disease (45). Myofibroblasts, which are cells with features of smooth muscle cells and fibroblasts, have been reported in liver cirrhosis. It has been suggested that these contractile cells are derived from FSC (46).

Tanaka et al. (47) noted that FSC stain prominently with the cytochemical method for γ-glutamyl transpeptidase, an enzyme possibly involved in the synthesis of fibrous proteins. This staining may provide an excellent marker for FSC, especially in the absence of lipid droplets.

We have recently found that granulomas induced by glucan in rat liver are located in the perisinusoidal space. Hypertrophic FSC with few lipid droplets and a prominent RER occur around these granulomas (Fig. 15). Soluble products, such as lymphokines and monokines from granuloma cells, stimulate fibroblast proliferation and collagen synthesis (48). Spatial proximity in the perisinusoidal space facilitates interaction between granuloma cells and FSC.

Storage of Vitamin A

The presence of vitamin A in hepatic mesenchymal cells was shown by Popper in 1941 (42), who characterized these cells: "vitamin A fluorescence was noted as droplets which filled the cytoplasm thus imparting an outline of the characteristic stellate form of the Kupffer cell." These cells, which have typical lipid droplets and a stellate form, were later identified by Nakane (49) as FSC. The administration of vitamin A

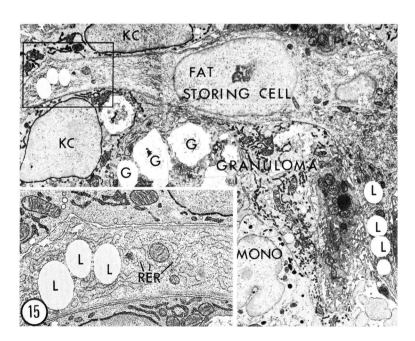

FIG. 15. Large FSC at the periphery of a granuloma induced by the injection of glucan. Note the prominent RER and a few lipid droplets in the cytoplasm of FSC, which is shown at higher magnification in the inset. In the granuloma, Kupffer cells (KC) containing glucan particles (G) and monocytes (MONO) are readily identified by the characteristic peroxidase patterns. (Micrograph courtesy of Dr. W. Deimann, Heidelberg.) ×4,500; inset, ×9,900.

increases lipid droplets in FSC, which exhibit stronger green fluorescence and higher affinity for gold chloride (37). Tritium-labeled vitamin A has been localized by autoradiography over the lipid droplets as early as 10 min after injection (50).

Excessive amounts of vitamin A in rats give rise to massive enlargement of FSC with an increase in their volume density up to ninefold, narrowing of sinusoids, and elevation of portal venous pressure (51). There is, however, no evidence of increased hydroxyproline and fibrosis in the liver of these animals. Russel et al. (52) reported two patients with hypervitaminosis A who presented with ascites and clinical signs of cirrhosis. Liver biopsy revealed many Ito cells with prominent lipid droplets associated with perisinusoidal fibrosis and central vein sclerosis. One of these patients, who continued to take large doses of vitamin A, subsequently developed cirrhosis, as shown by liver biopsy (53). Although Russel et al. (52) suggested that hypervitaminosis A may induce fibrogenesis by FSC, the experimental work in rats does not support a direct relationship (51).

In the cytoplasm of FSC, multivesicular bodies and peroxisomes may be involved in the metabolism of vitamin A. Thus Wake (6) suggested that lipid droplets in FSC are derived from multivesicular bodies, which may be the site of esterification of retinol. The involvement of peroxisomes in the metabolism of vitamin A was suggested by Robison and Kuwabara (54), who noted that injection of vitamin A causes a massive increase of peroxisomes in the pigment epithelium. Fahimi et al. (14) demonstrated the association of peroxisomes with lipid droplets in FSC. Further studies of peroxisomes in FSC in hypervitaminosis A should be helpful in elucidating the role of peroxisomes in this cell.

Involvement in Various Pathologic Conditions

Except for hypervitaminosis A and fibrotic conditions of the liver, there have been only a few reports on the involvement of FSC in systemic diseases. These include patients with mucopolysaccharoidosis and psoriatics receiving methotrexate therapy. The Ito cells appear enlarged and contain numerous vacuoles with a granular content in cases of type I (Hurler) and type II (Hunter) and in chondroitin-4-sulfate mucopolysaccharoidosis (55,56). The finding in FSC is closely related to the generalized storage disease in these patients. A specific lesion of FSC in rat liver induced by the carcinogen N-nitrosomorpholine was noted by Bannasch et al. (57). These cystic lesions, called "spongiosis hepatis," consist of hypertrophic FSC containing large vacuoles with a granular proteinaceous material. A direct effect of the carcinogen

on Ito cells is postulated. A significant increase in number and size of FSC has been reported in patients with psoriasis receiving methotrexate therapy (58). Hepatic fibrosis develops in some of these patients and cirrhosis may be caused by the activation of FSC by methotrexate. Proliferation and enlargement of FSC have also been observed in patients receiving corticosteroids and chlorpromazine (38). Whether these substances affect the growth and function of FSC directly or indirectly through mediators remains conjectural. The recent isolation and cultivation of sinusoidal cells may be useful in studies of the effect of these divergent substances on the growth of Ito cells *in vitro*.

ACKNOWLEDGMENTS

The original experimental work presented in this chapter was supported by grants from the National Institutes of Health, and from Deutsche Forschungsgemeinschaft, Bad Godesberg, FRG.

The author is indebted to the following scientists for supplying micrographs and/or information of their work prior to publication: Dr. P. Bannasch (Heidelberg), Dr. A. Kirn (Strassbourg), Dr. J. C. Wanson (Brussels), and Dr. E. Weihe (Heidelberg). Special thanks are due to my past and present associates who have supplied many of the original micrographs for this review: Dr. W. Deimann, Dr. G. Stöhr, Dr. S. Yokota, and Dr. J. J. Widmann. The technical assistance of Inge Frommer and U. Graber and the secretarial help of Christine Göppel are gratefully acknowledged.

REFERENCES

1. Aterman, K. (1963): The structure of the liver sinusoids and the sinusoidal cells. In: *The Liver. Morphology, Biochemistry, Physiology,* edited by Ch. Rouiller, pp 61–136. Academic Press, New York.
2. Fahimi, H. D. (1967): Perfusion and immersion fixation of rat liver with glutaraldehyde. *Lab. Invest.,* 16:736–750.
3. Fahimi, H. D. (1970): The fine structural localization of endogenous and exogenous peroxidase activity in Kupffer cells of rat liver. *J. Cell Biol.,* 47:247–262.
4. Ito, T. (1973): Recent advances in the study of the fine structure of the hepatic sinusoidal wall: A review. *Gunma Rep. Med. Sci.,* 6:119–163.
5. Wisse, E., and Knook, D. L. (editors) (1977): *Kupffer Cells and Other Liver Sinusoidal Cells.* Biomedical Press, Amsterdam.
6. Wake, K. (1980): Perisinusoidal stellate cells (fat-storing cells, interstitial cells, lipocytes), their related structure in and around the liver sinusoids, and vitamin A-storing cells in extrahepatic organs. *Int. Rev. Cytol.,* 66:303–353.
7. Wisse, E. (1970): An electron microscopic study of the fenestrated endothelial lining of rat liver sinusoids. *J. Ultrastruct. Res.,* 31:125–150.
8. Fraser, R., Bowler, L. M., Day, W. A., Dobbs, B., Johnson, H. D., and Lee, D. (1980): High perfusion pressure damages the sieving ability of sinusoidal endothelium in rat livers. *Br. J. Exp. Pathol.,* 61:222–228.
9. Frenzel, H., Kremer, B., and Hücker, H. (1977): The liver sinusoids under various pathological conditions. A TEM and

SEM study of rat liver after respiratory hypoxia, telecobalt-irradiation and endotoxin application. In: *Kupffer Cells and Other Liver Sinusoidal Cells*, edited by E. Wisse and D. L. Knook, pp 213–223. Elsevier, Amsterdam.

10. Nopanitaya, W., Lamb, J. C., Grisham, J. W., and Carson, J. L. (1976): Effect of hepatic venous outflow obstruction on pores and fenestrations in sinusoidal endothelium. *Br. J. Exp. Pathol.*, 57:604–609.

11. Muto, M., Nishi, M., and Fujita, T. (1977): Scanning electron microscopy of human liver sinusoids. *Arch. Histol. Jpn.*, 40:137–151.

12. Yee, A. G., and Revel, J. P. (1975): Endothelial cell junctions. *J. Cell Biol.*, 66:200–204.

13. Wood, R. L. (1963): Evidence of species differences in the ultrastructure of the hepatic sinusoid. *Z. Zellforsch.*, 58:679–692.

14. Fahimi, H. D., Gray, B. A., and Herzog, V. K. (1976): Cytochemical localization of catalase and peroxidase in sinusoidal cells of rat liver. *Lab. Invest.*, 34:192–201.

15. Wisse, E. (1972): An ultrastructural characterization of the endothelial cell in the rat liver sinusoid under normal and various experimental conditions, as a contribution to the distinction between endothelial and Kupffer cells. *J. Ultrastruct. Res.*, 38:528–562.

16. Yokota, S., and Fahimi, H. D. (1979): Filament bundles of prekeratin type in hepatocytes: Revealed by detergent extraction after glutaraldehyde fixation. *Biol. Cell.*, 34:119–126.

17. de Bruyn, P. P. H., Michelson, S., and Becker, R. P. (1977): Phosphotungstic acid as a marker for the endocytic-lysosomal system (Vacuolar apparatus) including transfer tubules of the lining cells of the sinusoids in the bone marrow and liver. *J. Ultrastruct. Res.*, 58:87–95.

18. Widmann, J. J., and Fahimi, H. D. (1976): Proliferation of endothelial cells in estrogen-stimulated rat liver. A light and electron microscopic cytochemical study. *Lab. Invest.*, 34:141–149.

19. Widmann, J. J., and Fahimi, H. D. (1975): Proliferation of mononuclear phagocytes (Kupffer cells) and endothelial cells in regenerating rat liver. *Am. J. Pathol.*, 80:349–366.

20. Deimann, W., and Fahimi, H. D. (1978): Peroxidase cytochemistry and ultrastructure of resident macrophages in fetal rat liver. *Dev. Biol.*, 66:43–56.

21. Stöhr, G., Deimann, W., and Fahimi, H. D. (1978): Peroxidase-positive endothelial cells in sinusoids of the mouse liver. *J. Histochem. Cytochem.*, 26:409–411.

22. Naito, M., and Wisse, E. (1978): Filtration effect of endothelial fenestrations on chylomicron transport in neonatal rat liver sinusoids. *Cell Tissue Res.*, 190:371–382.

23. Steffan, A. M., and Kirn, A. (1979): Multiplication of vaccinia virus in the livers of mice after frog virus 3-induced damage to sinusoidal cells. *J. Reticuloendothel. Soc.*, 26:531–538.

24. Widmann, J. J., Cotran, R. S., and Fahimi, H. D. (1972): Mononuclear phagocytes (Kupffer cells) and endothelial cells. Identification of two functional cell types in rat liver sinusoids by endogenous peroxidase activity. *J. Cell Biol.*, 52:159–170.

25. Willingham, M. C., Maxfield, F. R., and Pastan, I. H. (1979): α_2Macro-globulin binding to the plasma membrane of cultured fibroblasts. Diffuse binding followed by clustering in coated regions. *J. Cell Biol.*, 82:614–625.

26. Hubbard, A. L., Wilson, G., Ashwell, G., and Stukenbrok, H. (1979): An electron microscope autoradiographic study of the carbohydrate recognition systems in rat liver. I. Distribution of ^{125}I-ligands among the liver cell types. *J. Cell Biol.*, 83:47–64.

27. Hubbard, A. L., and Stukenbrok, H. (1979): An electron microscope autoradiographic study of the carbohydrate recognition systems in rat liver. II. Intracellular fates of the ^{125}I-ligands. *J. Cell Biol.*, 83:65–81.

28. Willingham, M. C., Maxfield, F. R., and Pastan, I. (1980): Receptor-mediated endocytosis of alpha$_2$-macroglobulin in cultured fibroblasts. *J. Histochem. Cytochem.*, 28:818–823.

29. van Berkel, T. J. C. (1979): The role of nonparenchymal cells in liver metabolism. *Trends Biomed. Sci.*, 4:202–205.

30. Kuusi, T., Nikkilä, E. A., Virtanen, I., and Kinnunen, K. J. (1979): Localization of the heparin-releasable lipase *in situ* in the rat liver. *Biochem. J.*, 181:245–246.

31. Knook, D. L., and Sleyster, E. Ch. (1980): Isolated paren-

chymal, Kupffer and endothelial rat liver cells characterized by their lysosomal enzyme content. *Biochem. Biophys. Res. Commun.*, 96:250–257.

32. Blouin, A., Bolender, R. P., and Weibel, E. R. (1977): Distribution of organelles and membranes between hepatocytes and nonhepatocytes in the rat liver parenchyma. A stereological study. *J. Cell Biol.*, 72:441–455.

33. Brouwer, A., Wanson, J. C., Mosselmans, R., Knook, D. L., and Drochmans, P. (1980): Morphology and lysosomal enzyme activity of primary cultures of rat liver sinusoidal cells. *Biol. Cell.*, 37:35–44.

34. Wanson, J. C., Mosselmans, R., Brouwer, A., and Knook, D. L. (1979): Interaction of adult rat hepatocytes and sinusoidal cells in co-culture. *Biol. Cell.*, 36:7–16.

35. Wisse, E., Emeis, J. J., and Daems, W. Th. (1974): Some fine structural considerations on the possible involvement of the liver RES in lysosomal storage diseases, with observations in a case of Morquio's disease. In: *Enzyme Therapy in Lysosomal Storage Diseases*, edited by J. M. Tager, G. J. M. Hooghwinkel, and W. Th. Daems, pp. 95–109. North-Holland, Amsterdam.

36. Popper, H., Thomas, L. B., Telles, N. C., Falk, H., and Selikoff, I. J. (1978): Comparison of hepatic angiosarcoma in man induced by vinyl chloride, thorotrast, and arsenic. *Am. J. Pathol.*, 92:349–376.

37. Wake, K. (1971): "Sternzellen" in the liver; perisinusoidal cells with special reference to storage of vitamin A. *Am. J. Anat.*, 132:429–462.

38. Bronfenmajer, S., Schaffner, F., and Popper, H. (1966): Fat-storing cells (lipocytes) in human liver. *Arch. Pathol.*, 82:447–453.

39. Bartók, I., Tóth, J., Remenár, E., and Virágh, Sz. (1979): Ultrastructure of the hepatic perisinusoidal cells in man and other mammalian species. *Anat. Rec.*, 194:571–586.

40. Ito, T., and Shibasaki, S. (1968): Electron microscopic study on the hepatic sinusoidal wall and the fat-storing cells in the normal human liver. *Arch. Histol. Jpn.*, 29:137–192.

41. Schnack, H., Stockinger, L., and Wewalka, F. (1967): Adventitious connective tissue cells in the space of Disse and their relation to fiber formation. *Rev. Int. Hepatol.*, 17:855–860.

42. Popper, H. (1941): Histologic distribution of vitamin A in human organs under normal and under pathologic conditions. *Arch. Pathol.*, 31:766–773.

43. McGee, J. O. D., and Patrick, R. (1972): The role of perisinusoidal cells in hepatic fibrinogenesis: An electron microscopic study of acute carbon tetrachloride liver injury. *Lab. Invest.*, 26:429–440.

44. Kent, G., Gay, S., Inouye, T., Bahu, R., Minick, O. T., and Popper, H. (1976): Vitamin A-containing lipocytes and formation of type III collagen in liver injury. *Proc. Natl. Acad. Sci. USA*, 10:3719–3722.

45. Balázs, M., Várkonyi, S., and Pintér, A. (1977): Electron microscopic study of alcoholic liver disease with special attention to the changes of mesenchymal cells of the liver. *Exp. Pathol.*, 14:340–350.

46. Irle, C., Kocher, O., and Gabbiani, G. (1980): Contractility of myofibroblasts during experimental liver cirrhosis. *J. Submicrosc. Cytol.*, 12:209–217.

47. Tanaka, M., Kosakai, M., Inomata, I., Takaki, K., and Ishikawa, E. (1976): Enzyme histochemical study on fat-storing cells (so-called Ito's cell) of liver. *Acta Pathol. Jpn.*, 26:581–588.

48. Mergenhagen, S. E., Wahl, S. M., and Wahl, L. M. (1980): Regulation of fibroblast function by lymphokines and monokines. In: *The Reticuloendothelial System and the Pathogenesis of Liver Disease*, edited by H. Liehr and M. Grün, pp. 69–78. Elsevier, Amsterdam.

49. Nakane, P. K. (1963): Ito's fat-storing cell of the mouse liver. *Anat. Rec.*, 145:265–266.

50. Hirosawa, K., and Yamada, E. (1973): The localization of the vitamin A in the mouse liver as revealed by electron microscopic radioautography. *J. Electron Microsc. (Tokyo)*, 22:337–346.

51. Ikejeri, N., and Tanikawa, K. (1977): Effects of vitamin A and

estrogen on the sinusoidal cells in the rat liver. In: *Kupffer Cells and Other Liver Sinusoidal Cells,* edited by E. Wisse and D. L. Knook, pp. 83–93. Elsevier, Amsterdam.

52. Russel, R. M., Boyer, J. L., Bagheri, S. A., and Hruban, Z. (1974): Hepatic injury from chronic hypervitaminosis A resulting in portal hypertension and ascites. *N. Engl. J. Med.,* 291:435–440.

53. Jacques, E. A., Buschmann, R. J., and Layden, T. J. (1979): The histopathologic progression of vitamin A-induced hepatic injury. *Gastroenterology,* 76:599–602.

54. Robison, W. G., Jr., and Kuwabara, T. (1977): Vitamin A storage and peroxisomes in retinal pigment epithelium and liver. *Invest. Ophthalmol. Vis. Sci.,* 16:1110–1117.

55. Freitag, F., Küchemann, K., Schuster, W., and Spranger, J. (1971): Hepatic ultrastructure in chondroitin-4-sulfate mucopolysaccharidosis. *Virchows Arch. Abt. B Zellpathol.,* 8:1–15.

56. Lafon, J., Berard-Badier, M., Chamlian, A., Mariani, R., Casanova, P., and Adechy-Benkoel, L. (1972): Etude ultrastructurale des cellules périsinusoidales du foie dans trois cas de mucopolysaccharidoses. *Pathol. Biol.,* 20:15–21.

57. Bannasch, P., Bloch, M., and Zerban, H. (1981): Spongiosis hepatis. Specific changes of the perisinusoidal liver cells induced in rats by N-nitrosomorpholine. *Lab. Invest.* 44:252–264.

58. Hopwood, D., and Nyfors, A. (1976): Effect of methotrexate therapy in psoriatics on the Ito cells in liver biopsies, assessed by point-counting. *J. Clin. Pathol.,* 29:698–703.

The Liver: Biology and Pathobiology, edited by
I. Arias, H. Popper, D. Schachter, and D. A. Shafritz.
Raven Press, New York © 1982.

Chapter 30

Kupffer Cells

E. Anthony Jones and John A. Summerfield

Kupffer cells are one of four cell types that line hepatic sinusoids; the others are endothelial cells, fat-storing (Ito) cells, and pit cells (1). Kupffer cells are distinguished from other sinusoidal lining cells and hepatocytes on the basis of morphologic, cytochemical, biochemical, and functional criteria. Kupffer cells constitute about 80 to 90% of fixed macrophages of the reticuloendothelial system (2). Sinusoidal cells account for about 30% of the total number of cells in the liver, and Kupffer cells for about 10%. Because sinusoidal cells are much smaller than hepatocytes, however, only 2 to 10% of hepatic protein is in the sinusoidal cells (3). It is becoming increasingly clear that nonparenchymal cells in general and Kupffer cells in particular play a critical role in the maintenance of normal liver function. The functions of Kupffer cells include phagocytosis of particulate matter, various immune reactions, the uptake and catabolism of lipids and enzymes, and the secretion of substances, such as iron. In addition, Kupffer cells probably form part of a cooperative system that interacts with endothelial cells and hepatocytes. This chapter concentrates on aspects of the Kupffer cell in which recent research has

suggested new functions or elucidated further the mechanisms of known function.

METHODOLOGIC CONSIDERATIONS

There are several experimental options for the study of Kupffer cells. *In vivo* studies of the clearance of particles and perfusion fixation for microscopic studies are well described (4–6). Kupffer cells can also be isolated from the liver and studied *in vitro*. Most approaches involve collagenase perfusion of the liver to yield a whole liver cell suspension (7). Until recently, most studies were performed on the crude, nonparenchymal cell fraction obtained by differential centrifugation of liver cell suspensions. These preparations often were reported to be predominantly Kupffer cells. However, they also contain numerous endothelial cells and fat-storing cells.

Methods have been improved to isolate Kupffer cells from the nonparenchymal cell fraction. Three approaches have been used. First, since Kupffer cells in culture stick to the culture plates whereas endothelial cells do not, culture of the nonparenchymal fraction results in plates coated predominantly with Kupffer cells (8). Second, although Kupffer and endothelial cells have similar densities, the Kupffer cells may be selectively loaded *in vivo* with iron and then separated magnetically (9), or Kupffer cells may be separated from endothelial cells by centrifugation on gradients of metrizamide after their density has been selectively increased by loading *in vivo* with Triton WR1339 or Jectofer (10). Techniques that involve the loading of Kupffer cells induce functional alterations that cannot readily be reversed (10). Finally, Kupffer cells may be separated gently and obtained in high yield by centrifugal elutriation. This technique exploits the fact that the Kupffer cell has a different cell volume than that of other hepatic cells and generates a Kupffer cell fraction of high purity (3,10–12). Since pronase, which is also used to isolate Kupffer cells, induces marked surface damage (13), cells are best prepared by collagenase perfusion; or, if pronase is used, cells should be cultured for at least 24 hr to allow replacement of cell surface receptors (8).

Since widely different isolation techniques have been used in various studies, it is important in assessing the results to determine whether a mixture of endothelial and Kupffer cells or a purified preparation of Kupffer cells alone was used. In culture, Kupffer cells undergo cell division and tend to form cell clumps and multinucleate giant cells (14). They can be maintained in culture for several weeks (15), but their capacity to mediate endocytosis becomes diminished when they are cultured for prolonged periods (16).

MORPHOLOGY

Kupffer cells line the lumen of the hepatic sinusoids. They are usually stellate in shape and are preferentially distributed in the sinusoids around the portal tract. They are easily distinguished from the flat, fenestrated endothelial cells. The stellate processes of Kupffer cells are attached to endothelial cells, and some appear to penetrate the sieve plates. There are, however, no junctional attachments between Kupffer cells and endothelial cells or hepatocytes (6). Kupffer cells are also distinguished from other sinusoidal cells by histochemical stains: only Kupffer cells stain for endogenous peroxidase (17) and tartrate-resistant acid phosphatase (18). Stereologic analysis of Kupffer cells in perfusion-fixed rat liver tissue show them to have the following volumetric composition: nuclei, 19%; cytoplasm, 61%; mitochondria, 4.5%: lysosomes, 13.5%; and pinocytotic vesicles, 2% (19). On isolation from liver and separation by centrifugal elutriation, both Kupffer and endothelial cells tend to become spherical. The Kupffer cells have a larger modal cell diameter (8.7 to 9.1 μm) and contain about twice as much pro-

tein (78 to 116 μg/10^6 cells) than do endothelial cells, and Kupffer cells are enriched with lysosomal enzymes, especially cathepsin D (3,20). After centrifugal elutriation, the Kupffer cell population may be heterogeneous as judged by cell size and protein and lysosomal enzyme contents (11).

Kupffer cells have morphologic features typical of macrophages. Their cytoplasm is bulky and contains many well-developed lysosomes and pinocytotic vesicles. The abundance of these organelles is related to the ability of these cells to take up, endocytose, and digest large quantities of foreign or effete endogenous material (21). The preferential location of Kupffer cells in periportal regions of the hepatic sinusoid implies that blood entering the hepatic sinusoid is monitored for particulate matter. Under normal physiologic conditions, digested material rarely is seen in lysosomal vacuoles, and the Kupffer cell is considered to be in a resting state (22).

Kupffer cells have a cell coat that consists of two layers: (a) a thin layer close to the plasma membrane, and (b) a 50 to 70 nm thick filamentous or fuzzy outer layer (22,23). It has been suggested that a receptor for the Fc region of IgG is located in the thin inner cell coat and that a receptor for the conversion product of the third component of complement, C3b, is located in the outer filamentous layer (23). The outer layer reacts for protein and probably also for sugars; the inner layer may consist of glycoproteins and glycolipids (21).

Kupffer cells possess three structures that are related to pinocytosis: (a) bristle-coated micropinocytotic vesicles, which have a diameter of about 100 nm, (b) the thick fuzzy coat on the cell surface, and (c) worm-like structures. These three structures are present in Kupffer cells under normal conditions, and their formation is not dependent on particulate material at the cell surface. Both the vesicles and the worm-like structures have the ability to take up particles 3.5 to 7.5 nm in diameter. The worm-like structures appear to be infoldings of the cell membrane in which a dense midline and cross striations indicate preservation of the fuzzy coat; their width is about 140 nm.

During invagination of the cell membrane, end-to-end fusion of fuzzy coat molecules may lead to worm-like structures (1). They may represent reserves of invaginated membrane to be utilized when increased amounts of cell membrane are required during phagocytosis. Worm-like structures may open into the sinusoidal lumen. The opsonin, fibronectin (24), may interact with the fuzzy coat during the formation of worm-like structures. Consistent with this suggestion is the observation that a 15 nm-thick layer directly apposed to the plasma membrane and a dense midline component of the worm-like structures stain for glycoprotein (23). Kupffer cells also possess fuzzy coat vacuoles, which probably form by invagination of the cell membrane, causing closer apposition or compression of the top layer of the fuzzy coat, thereby facilitating side-to-side attachment of end groups of fuzzy coat molecules. These vacuoles are spherical; their diameter is greater than 1 μm (22).

ORIGIN OF KUPFFER CELLS

Ameboid-like cells, presumed to be Kupffer cells, have been observed at large intercellular gaps between endothelial cells lining hepatic sinusoids of the fetal liver. Cells having surface morphologic features similar to those of Kupffer cells are not confined to sinusoids in the developing liver (25). Kupffer cells in the fetal liver appear to be a separate cell line, which is distinct from all other hepatic sinusoidal cells. No transitional forms are seen, as judged by peroxidase activity, uptake of latex particles, and electron microscope appearance (26,27). Furthermore, the pattern of peroxidase staining and the appearance of fetal hepatic macrophages at the same time as immature leukopoietic cells led to the conclusion that Kupffer cells are a separate line, distinct from monocytes and promonocytes (26). Erythropoiesis in the fetal liver is often associated with phagocytosis of erythroid elements by Kupffer cells (25).

The extent to which the Kupffer cell population in adults results from self replication of Kupffer cells in the liver or immigration of cells from a site outside the liver, such as bone marrow, is controversial. The mechanisms in the physiologic state probably differ from those in states of severe damage to or loss of Kupffer cells (28,29). The normal rat liver shows Kupffer cell division; recent evidence suggests that the growth fraction, i.e., the proportion of Kupffer cells in the proliferative cycle at any time, is about 5% (J. A. Summerfield, J. Vergalla, and E. A. Jones, 1982, *unpublished data*). Kinetic studies suggest, however, that even in the normal state, a proportion of Kupffer cells is derived from the circulation (30). Suppression of Kupffer cell function by blockade or X-irradiation appears to stimulate immigration of Kupffer cells from the bone marrow (30,31). Six months after transplantation of a liver from a donor of the opposite sex in man, the transplanted liver became populated with Kupffer cells that had the sex karyotype of the host (32). Furthermore, after transplantation of bone marrow cells from a donor of the opposite sex in man, Kupffer cells in the liver possessed the sex karyotype of the donor cells (33). Thus a bone marrow origin appears to have been established. Probably this source is quantitatively important in pathologic states involving injury or loss of Kupffer cells. Under normal conditions, the Kupffer cells apparently are maintained largely by local proliferation.

FUNCTIONS OF KUPFFER CELLS

Endocytosis

Kupffer cells have the capacity to endocytose large quantities of materials in the circulation. Many endocytosed materials are continuously produced in small quantities under normal conditions (34). Endocytosis is achieved by pinocytosis and phagocytosis; the latter is responsible for internalization of particulate material. Examples of materials endocytosed by Kupffer cells are virus particles, test substances (such as latex particles, Thorotrast, and colloidal gold), enzymes leaked from cells or the gastrointestinal tract (1,34), fibrinogen derivatives (fibrin monomers and small aggregates), fibrin-fibrinogen complexes, fibrin degradation products (35,36), altered and disintegrated platelets, damaged and desialylated erythrocytes, erythrocyte stroma (37–39), multimolecular complexes (e.g., immune complexes and protease-antiprotease complexes) (40), certain tumor cells, bacteria, bacterial toxins (e.g., endotoxin) (41,42), and lysosomal hydrolases (43).

Pinocytosis

The frequency of the diverse structures associated with pinocytosis in Kupffer cells suggests that these cells continuously pinocytose plasma under normal conditions (22). Using ^{125}I-labeled polyvinylpyrrolidone as a marker of fluid-phase pinocytosis, isolated rat Kupffer cells pinocytose at a rate of 15 ml plasma/ g cell protein/day. Corresponding rates for hepatic endothelial cells and hepatocytes were 13 and 0.96 ml/g/day (44). "Constitutive" or fluid-phase continuous pinocytosis is one of three recognized types of pinocytosis. The other two are pinocytosis following secretion, and pinocytosis of ligand bound to cell surface receptors (45). Apart from carbohydrate recognition systems for receptor-mediated pinocytosis (see below), there is a paucity of data on the mechanisms of pinocytosis by Kupffer cells. Fluid-phase pinocytosis does not require contact of particulate material with the cell membrane for initiation (22). Pinocytosis ends with the delivery of the membrane-bound and fluid-phase contents of pinocytotic vesicles into lysosomal vacuoles (46). Lysosomal enzymes (46) and certain gut-derived substances in portal vein plasma, such as endotoxin (47), probably are cleared by the liver by receptor-mediated pinocytosis.

Phagocytosis

General aspects.

Phagocytosis *in vivo* is initiated by the recognition and attachment of particulate material to the cell surface. The particulate material attaches to and reacts with the fuzzy coat of the Kupffer cell, as a consequence of which the fuzzy coat undergoes compression, contraction, and lateral movement. These phenomena are followed by the formation of a fine, filamentous, organelle-free hyaloplasm in the cytoplasm immediately adjacent to the particle. The hyaloplasm undergoes movements and deformities that engulf the particulate material. The deformities may include the generation of sleeve-like processes, or lamellipodia. The completion of engulfment generates a vacuole, known as a phagosome. Phagosomes are transported through the cytoplasm and fuse with one or more lysosomes. It has been suggested that microtubules function as a cytoskeleton and direct the flow and transport of phagosomes. Depending on the composition of the particulate material phagocytosed, it may be degraded by lysosomal enzymes. Products of lysosomal digestion may be reutilized or excreted, while undigestable components may be stored in lysosomes and subsequently extruded from the cell by reverse endocytosis or alternatively distributed to daughter cells (15,22). It is not known whether recognition signals, which are involved in cell surface recognition, also influence intracellular components of phagocytosis.

The phagocytic capacity of Kupffer cells is influenced by the functional status of Kupffer cells and by humoral components involved in phagocytic clearance (48–50), as well as by hepatic blood flow. Adequate perfusion of the sinusoid with portal venous rather than arterial blood is considered to be a prerequisite for efficient phagocytic function (51). Sinusoidal perfusion with portal venous blood is slow and allows adequate time for phagocytosis. The velocity of sinusoidal perfusion and phagocytic function appear to be reciprocally related (48). Under normal conditions, the prevailing rate of Kupffer cell phagocytosis is low in relation to the maximum capacity for phagocytosis. Factors that influence phagocytosis can be separated into those that affect maximum rates and capacities of phagocytosis and those that affect the phagocytic load. When the phagocytic load exceeds the phagocytic capacity of Kupffer cells, a portion of the load is not phagocytosed. With usual loads, however, the non-phagocytosed portion tends to be minimal (34).

Crucial to phagocytosis is the recognition of appropriate material. This involves distinguishing tissue debris and infectious agents from normal endogenous materials. Recognition occurs at two levels. In the circulation, it is mediated by circulating recognition factors, or opsonins; at the cellular level, it is presumed to be mediated by cell surface receptors. Opsonins can be divided into two groups: those which are nonimmunospecific, such as fibronectin, and those which are immunospecific, in particular IgG and IgM antibodies, which recognize specific antigenic material. Three recognition signals at the cellular level are established. These are particles coated with (a) fibronectin, (b) IgG, or (c) IgM and complement, but others probably exist. Fibronectin, IgG, and IgM are glycoproteins; recognition by Kupffer cells of particles coated with these opsonins may be mediated by their carbohydrate moiety.

In contrast to pinocytosis, phagocytosis by Kupffer cells is not dependent on the presence of preexisting structures. Phagocytosis follows the arrival of particulate material at the surface of Kupffer cells. Particles must be of a certain size to induce phagocytosis. For example, small colloidal particles of less than 10 nm in diameter induce phagocytosis only after aggregation by agglutination (22). Agglutination of small particles usually occurs on entry into the circulation (52) but may occur at the Kupffer cell surface.

Patterns of attachment of particles to the Kupffer cell surface differ. For example, fine colloidal gold (3.5 nm in diameter) and erythrocyte ghosts adhere to the top layer of the fuzzy coat, leaving a space of almost 70 nm between the fuzzy coat and the cell membrane. Larger particles, such as bactolatex (0.8 μm in diameter), erythrocytes, and other cells, become attached by close apposition to the cell surface, leaving a space of 15 nm or less between the fuzzy coat and the cell membrane. It is not known whether the fuzzy coat is removed or subjected to active contraction or passive compression by these processes (22).

Nonimmunospecific, opsonin-mediated.

The surface of foreign or effete endogenous particulate material, when exposed to blood, becomes coated with molecules of opsonin, particularly fibronectin (49,50). This leads to aggregates or complexes of particles. This phenomenon is associated with changed physicochemical properties of both the particles and opsonin molecules. Nonimmunospecific opsonins promote phagocytosis of particles by Kupffer cells as a consequence of interaction between altered opsonin with molecules on the surface of the fuzzy coat. This process may be mediated by receptors that recognize opsonin molecules which have been altered as a result of their interaction with particles. The physicochemical basis of such recognition, however, is unknown. Opsonins normally are present in plasma; in the absence of abnormal loads of circulating particulate material in the circulation, opsonin molecules probably are cleared slowly (22). The level of fibronectin in plasma appears to correlate directly with the capacity of Kupffer cells to mediate nonimmuno-specific clearance and phagocytosis of particulate material (49).

The opsonin fibronectin has been isolated and characterized (24,53,54). It opsonizes endogenous materials, especially those related to thrombotic processes, such as fibrin monomers and fibrin micro-aggregates (34). It may recognize membrane alterations on platelets associated with adhesion and aggregation and it binds to platelets after their exposure to collagen, thrombin, and ADP (55,56). It also has an affinity for native and denatured collagen (34). Fibronectin depletion is associated with intravascular coagulation, platelet aggregation, and increased quantities of circulating altered platelets and fibrin (34).

Immunospecific, opsonin-mediated.

Antigenic particulate material in the circulation may be cleared and phagocytosed by Kupffer cells by immunospecific mechanisms if the material becomes coated with antibody molecules of either the IgG or IgM class.

Fc-receptor mediated. Receptors for the Fc region of cell-bound IgG have been identified on Kupffer cells *in vitro* (8,57–59). A large proportion of IgG-coated sheep red blood cells (EA) (about 80%) are ingested by isolated Kupffer cells. Internalization follows initial binding of EA to Fc receptors on the cell surface and reaches a peak after 30 to 60 min of incubation. The capacity of Kupffer cells to mediate Fc receptor-specific phagocytosis is limited; only a proportion of cell-bound EA is internalized. Thus binding to Fc receptors and subsequent phagocytosis are distinct processes. After maximal phagocytosis of EA, the normal capacity to bind and phagocytose EA is restored after about 40 hr (8). The limiting factor in Fc receptor-dependent phagocytosis appears to be the volume of Kupffer cells rather than the availability of cell surface receptors (57).

Internalization of EA starts and is most rapid in the perinuclear region of the Kupffer cell. The process proceeds at a rate of 3 to 4 EA/Kupffer cell/min. It is associated with striking and rapid activity of the surface membrane. Thin projections of the membrane (sleeve-like lamellipodia) project from the cell surface with subsequent tight engulfment and constriction of EA above the plane of the cell surface prior to movement of phagocytosed EA toward the perinuclear area (58). Binding of EA to Kupffer cells is not appreciably reduced by low temperature or preincubation with trypsin or phospholipase A but is increased by neuraminidase. Internalization of EA is reduced by low temperature or preincubation with trypsin, mercaptoethanol, or cytochalasin B; it is not affected by colchicine but is increased by neuraminidase (57,58).

Thus binding of EA is probably not energy dependent, whereas internalization of EA appears to require energy and to involve the microfilament, but not the microtubule, system. Neuraminidase-induced enhancement of EA binding and internalization suggests the exposure of additional cryptic Fc receptors.

C3b-receptor mediated. Receptors for cell-bound C3, the third component of complement, have been identified on Kupffer cells *in vitro* (8,57–59). Based on *in vivo* studies of the fate of IgM-sensitized erythrocytes in man, the receptor for cell-bound C3 on Kupffer cells is considered to be specific for C3b, a conversion product of C3 (60). Sheep red blood cells coated with IgM and exposed to fresh mouse serum as a source of complement (EAC3b) readily bind to the surface of Kupffer cells *in vitro*. Only a small proportion (about 20%) of cell-bound EAC3b, however, is internalized in the absence of serum (57). In contrast, the majority of Kupffer cell-bound EAC3b is internalized in the presence of newborn calf serum, a phenomenon not attributable to trace amounts of immunoglobulins.

The limiting factor in C3b receptor-mediated phagocytosis also appears to be the volume of Kupffer cells rather than the availability of cell-surface receptors (57). Internalization of EAC3b starts and is most rapid in the perinuclear region of the Kupffer cell. The internalization proceeds at a rate of 5 to 6 EAC3b/Kupffer cell/min. It is associated with depressions in the Kupffer cell surface which may contain more than one EAC3b and coarse projections of the cell membrane which fit loosely between EAC3b. The EAC3b appear to sink slowly into the cytoplasm during this process; membrane activity is less marked than with Fc receptor-mediated internalization (58). Since internalization of EAC3b is not affected by cytochalasin B or colchicine, neither the microfilament nor the microtubule systems appears to be involved (57,58).

Other mechanisms of phagocytosis.

Phagocytosis may be initiated by other mechanisms which do not necessarily require fibronectin or Fc or C3b receptors. Tumor cells are phagocytosed by murine Kupffer cells *in vitro* and *in vivo*. This process may hinder the development of liver metastases. However, there are marked unexplained differences in the avidity of Kupffer cells for different mouse tumor cell lines. The process does not seem to depend on immunologic factors but on recognition of some tumor cell surface component (61). Furthermore, phagocytosis of bacteria by Kupffer cells has been demonstrated in rabbit livers perfused with suspensions of nonopsonized bacteria in saline (62).

Kupffer cells in culture bind and internalize colloidal albumin in the absence of serum. This process is inhibited by cytochalasin B (15,16). Because albumin is not a glycoprotein, these observations suggest that receptors exist on the surface of Kupffer cells which are not carbohydrate recognition systems. They also suggest that the microfilament system may be involved in this model of endocytosis. In contrast, the fluid-phase endocytosis of colloid gold *in vitro* is unaffected by cytochalasin B (63); however, the mechanism of uptake of colloidal gold *in vivo* is different as it involves adsorption of the colloid to cell membranes (1).

Blockade.

The term blockade refers to transient depression of phagocytic function of the reticuloendothelial system (RES), which is induced by intravenous administration of colloid or other phagocytosable particulate material. The dose is usually large enough to exceed the maximum phagocytic capacity of the system and hence temporarily saturates phagocytosis by fixed macrophages. The degree of depression of phagocytic function by agents capable of inducing blockade is not uniform for all fixed macrophages of the RES (4). For example, in normal rats, the clearance from blood of intravenously administered ^{51}Cr-labeled sheep erythrocytes is rapid; 90% of the labeled cells accumulate in the liver. After blockade induced by colloidal dextran sulfate, not only is the clearance of labeled cells slower, but they are taken up preferentially by the spleen and bone marrow. Thus blockade with dextran sulfate appears to induce a greater depression of the phagocytic function of Kupffer cells than of fixed macrophages of the spleen and bone marrow (4).

In some experimental models, blockade of the RES is specific in that blockade induced by one particle does not affect the uptake and phagocytosis of another (64). In other models, the rate of clearance of ^{51}Cr-labeled sheep erythrocytes by the RES is decreased by blockade induced by dextran sulfate, silica, or carbon particles (31). The duration of the depression induced by blockade varies with the dose and type of blockading agent. In the rat, blockade induced by dextran sulfate, silica, or carbon particles lasts for about 4 days (31). Following blockade, phagocytic function usually returns to normal but may be transiently supranormal (4).

After injection of a large bolus of particulate material into the circulation, fibronectin is consumed, and the plasma level of fibronectin falls. This plasma protein influences the clearance of particles by Kupffer cells; low levels are associated with reduction in the phagocytic capacity of Kupffer cells, and vice versa. Thus levels of fibronectin may be decreased during depressed phagocytic function induced by blockade. Furthermore, increased levels of fibronectin may be associated with increased phagocytic function following blockade (34,48–50). Studies employing isolated perfused livers suggest that the mechanism of depression of phagocytic function of Kupffer cells associated with low plasma levels of fibronectin is distinct from that caused by blockade (65).

Effects of Metabolic Inhibitors on Endocytosis

Fluoride, an inhibitor of glycolysis, inhibits pinocytosis of colloidal gold more than do inhibitors of oxidative phosphorylation, such as antimycin A and dinitrophenol (63). Furthermore, endocytosis of formaldehyde-treated albumin by cultured Kupffer cells is more sensitive to fluoride than to antimycin A (16). In contrast, the uptake of heat-aggregated albumin is twice as sensitive to antimycin A than to fluoride (21). Binding of EA to Kupffer cells *in vitro* is not affected by metabolic inhibitors. However, iodoacetate, an inhibitor of glycolysis, abolishes internalization of EA, whereas antimycin A and dinitrophenol have a minimal effect on this process (57,66). These observations provide additional evidence that binding of EA to Kupffer cells is not energy dependent, and that internalization of EA by these cells requires energy, which is probably derived from glycolysis.

Other Agents Modulating Function

Factors that stimulate Kupffer cell function, predominantly phagocytic function, include zymosan (67), glucan (67), C. parvum (68), endotoxin (69), bacillus Calmette Guerin (70), estrogen (71), and hepatitis virus (72). Factors that depress Kupffer cell function, predominantly phagocytic function, include alcohol (73,74), methyl palmitate (67), traumatic shock (75), sepsis (76), neoplastic disease (42), X-irradiation (77), and certain experimental liver disorders (78).

Clearance of Formed Elements of the Blood

Neuraminidase, as either a normal constituent of the body or a component of pathogenic organisms, may desialylate glycoproteins on the surface membranes of formed elements of the blood (see, e.g., ref. 79). When such elements as erythrocytes (38,80), lymphocytes (79), and platelets (81) are desialylated, they are rapidly cleared from the circulation. The cell mediating this phenomenon is probably the Kupffer cell.

Two hypotheses of the mechanism of clearance of desialylated cells have been proposed. The first suggests that exposed galactose residues of glycoproteins on the surface of desialylated cells interact with a galactose-specific receptor on Kupffer cells (82). This theory is not supported by studies which failed to detect galactose-specific receptors on Kupffer cells (13,83). The second theory implicates circulating anti-

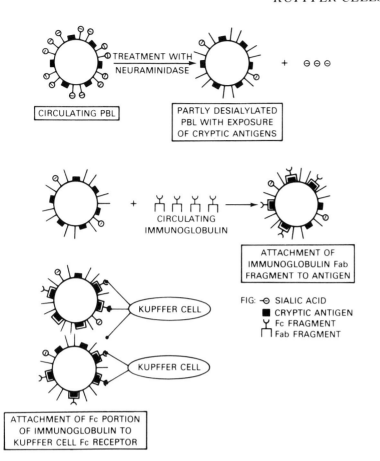

FIG. 1. Schematic representation of a hypothesis for the selective hepatic uptake of desialylated peripheral blood lymphocytes (PBL). Cryptic antigens on the surface of PBL are considered to be exposed by desialylation and are then recognized by naturally occurring, specific IgG antibodies. Exposed Fc regions of cell-bound IgG are recognized by Fc receptors on Kupffer cells. (Reproduced from ref. 79 with permission.)

bodies, which specifically recognize cryptic antigens exposed on the surface of formed elements of the blood by desialylation. Such antibodies for desialylated lymphocytes (see, e.g., ref. 79) and erythrocytes (80) have been detected in the circulation. Circulating desialylated cells may become coated with specific antibody, and their subsequent clearance may be mediated by Fc receptors on Kupffer cells which recognize the Fc region of cell-bound immunoglobulin (79) (Fig. 1). Support for this theory includes the prevention of the selective hepatic uptake of desialylated peripheral blood mononuclear cells by preincubating them with IgG Fab fragments (79) and the demonstration that senescent erythrocytes not only lose sialic acid (38, 80) but also become coated with an IgG autoantibody, which has been implicated in the hepatic sequestration of the senescent cells (80). Kupffer cells play an important role in the clearance of senescent erythrocytes, in the degradation of hemoglobin, and in the storage and release of iron (37).

Antigen Processing

In recent years, the importance of Kupffer cells in immunologic responses has been recognized. Kupffer cells play a central role in mediating immunologic un-

responsiveness to orally administered haptens (the Chase-Sulzberger phenomenon). For example, oral administration of DNCB to dogs suppresses delayed hypersensitivity to this hapten when it is subsequently injected subcutaneously. This effect does not occur in dogs with portacaval shunts (84). The levels of circulating hemagglutinins and hemolysins induced in rats by repeated injections of sheep erythrocytes are less after injection into the portal venous system rather than into the inferior vena cava. Furthermore, cell-mediated immunity, assessed by ear swelling 24 hr after intraauricular injection of antigen, occurred in animals sensitized via the inferior vena cava but not via the portal vein. Organ localization studies using ^{51}Cr-labeled antigen indicated greater hepatic sequestration of antigen when given into the portal vein than into the inferior vena cava (85). These findings suggest that Kupffer cells may influence antibody responses by altering the distribution of antigen.

Kupffer cells may also modulate the immune response by playing a role in the processing of antigen and its presentation to immunocompetent cells. They participate in the induction of antigen-specific immune responses *in vitro*. Isolated murine Kupffer cells can reconstitute antigen-stimulated proliferative responses of antigen-primed, macrophage-depleted lymph node T cells. Murine Kupffer cells also bear the Ia phenotype of accessory cells, which function in antigen presentation (86). These properties of Kupffer cells may modulate the immunologic responses to enterically derived antigens. In addition, antigen-stimulated proliferative responses of antigen-primed macrophage-depleted lymph node T cells are under the control of two immune response genes. The ability of Kupffer cells to select antigenic determinants to induce these immune responses critically depends on their genotype (87).

Carbohydrate Recognition

Recently, several receptor-mediated systems for pinocytosis of glycoproteins in the liver have been described (for review, see ref. 88). Most plasma glycoproteins with a prolonged survival in the circulation bear complex sialic acid-terminated oligosaccharides. Enzymatic removal of the terminal nonreducing sialic acid residues from a glycoprotein usually exposes underlying galactose residues. Galactose-terminated derivatives (i.e., asialoglycoproteins) are rapidly removed from the circulation. Hepatocyte cell surface receptors that specifically bind galactose-terminated glycoproteins mediate this process (89).

Glycoproteins that possess oligosaccharides terminating in N-acetylglucosamine or mannose also disappear rapidly from the plasma and accumulate primarily in the liver. This was first shown for β-glucuronidase and several other glycosidases (43,90–92). The clearance of β-glucuronidase, β-galactosidase, and β-hexosaminidase could be inhibited by agalacto-orosomucoid, a glycoprotein with terminal N-acetylglucosamine residues (93), and by yeast mannan, a mannose polymer, but not by a galactose-terminated glycoprotein (94). These findings are consistent with a receptor in the liver which differs from the galactose recognition system on hepatocytes in that it recognizes different sugar residues, namely, N-acetylglucosamine and/or mannose. Subsequently, this recognition system was demonstrated to be on hepatic sinusoidal cells rather than on hepatocytes (13,95–97).

A similar N-acetylglucosamine/mannose recognition system has been demonstrated on isolated rat alveolar macrophages (98,99). Since the liver is quantitatively the most important site for this recognition system, however, it was pertinent to determine whether the system is present on Kupffer cells and/or endothelial cells. In an electron microscopic autoradiographic study, radiolabeled mannose- and N-acetylglucosamine-terminated glycoproteins accumulated in both Kupffer and endothelial cells but not in hepatocytes. In these studies, however, the uptake and internalization of the radiolabeled ligands by endothelial cells was two to six times greater than that by Kupffer cells (on a cell volume basis) (83,100). Further studies using these

ligands and newer methods to separate Kupffer and endothelial cells should establish whether this recognition system exists primarily on endothelial cells. A single mannose/N-acetylglucosamine receptor may participate in many uptake events, a phenomenon that suggests that these receptors are recycled (46,99). A mannan-binding protein has been isolated recently from rabbit liver (101) and may be the mannose/N-acetylglucosamine receptor.

The function of the mannose/N-acetylglucosamine receptor remains to be defined. Two functions for this receptor have been suggested. First, a variety of intact lysosomal hydrolases are taken up preferentially by hepatic sinusoidal cells by a process mediated by this receptor (see above). Mannose/N-acetylglucosamine-specific receptors may facilitate retrieval of potentially autodestructive lysosomal enzymes which escape into the extracellular space from a variety of tissues as a consequence of normal cellular metabolism or pathologic processes (97). It is not clear whether lysosomal enzymes taken up by Kupffer cells are incorporated into a functional pool. Thus, although one can enzymatically modify the carbohydrate moiety of lysosomal enzymes to favor their selective uptake by hepatic sinusoidal cells (102), it is not known whether such targeting would be beneficial in enzyme replacement therapy for a variety of storage diseases.

Second, clearance of antigen-antibody complexes may be carbohydrate mediated (103,104). Immunoglobulins are also glycoproteins possessing oligosaccharides which do not terminate in sialic acid. In contrast to other glycoproteins, which lack terminal sialic residues, immunoglobulins have a prolonged survival in the circulation. To explain this discrepancy, Baynes and Wold (105) proposed that the oligosaccharide of the normal immunoglobulin molecule in the circulation is sterically protected and that, on interaction with an antigen, a conformational change in the immunoglobulin exposes the carbohydrate residues. Support for this hypothesis came from experiments in rats which demonstrated that IgM-containing immune complexes are cleared rapidly by sinusoidal liver cells; clearance was blocked by mannose- but not galactose-terminated glycoproteins (103). In contrast, IgG-containing immune complexes were rapidly cleared from the circulation by hepatocytes; this process was blocked by galactose- but not mannose-terminated glycoproteins (104). Thus the conformational change induced in IgG by antigen binding to form macromolecular immune complexes exposes galactose residues which mediate the clearance of complexes by the galactose-specific receptor on hepatocytes (89). However, galactose residues exposed on the surface of larger particles, such as cells, may not gain access to the galactose-specific receptors on hepatocytes (79). Clearance of neither enzymes nor immune complexes has been established as the usual or major function of the mannose/N-acetylglucosamine recognition system on liver sinusoidal cells.

Lipoprotein Metabolism

The liver is responsible for key processes in lipoprotein metabolism and is the sole site at which cholesterol and cholesterol esters are removed from the circulation and subsequently secreted in bile as cholesterol or, after biotransformation in the hepatocyte, as bile acids. The role of the sinusoidal liver cells and particularly Kupffer cells in these processes is not yet clear. In early studies (106), Kupffer cells were thought to play a role in the metabolism of chylomicron cholesterol. This role was not confirmed by later studies involving, after injection of labeled cholesterol esters, either isolation of Kupffer cells (107,108) or autoradiography (109,110). Nevertheless, the importance of sinusoidal cells in lipoprotein metabolism has again been stressed. Apoprotein-labeled (111) and cholesterol ester-labeled (112), low density lipoprotein (LDL) and high density lipoprotein (HDL) have been shown to accumulate preferentially in liver sinusoidal cells. The sinusoidal cells contained about four times more radioactivity per milligram cell protein than hepatocytes. This uptake of lipoproteins can be explained by a high concentration of saturable, high affinity binding sites on the surface membrane of sinusoidal cells (113). Unfortunately, it is not possible from these studies to determine whether Kupffer cells and/or endothelial cells are involved in these uptake processes.

Plasma Protein Metabolism

Tracer studies of the turnover of several plasma proteins, including albumin, suggest that they normally undergo catabolism in a compartment closely related to the plasma. It has been suggested but not confirmed that Kupffer cells and other fixed macrophages of the RES may participate in the degradation of plasma proteins (114). A major role for Kupffer cells in the synthesis of plasma proteins has not been established.

KUPFFER CELLS IN DISEASE

The phagocytic function of Kupffer cells may be depressed in disease states as a result of inadequate perfusion of hepatic sinusoids with portal venous blood, hypoxemia, reduced plasma levels of recognition factors, and intrinsic dysfunction of Kupffer cells. In contrast, it may be enhanced in disease states as a result of generation of abnormally large quantities of phagocytosable material over a protracted period of time and increased plasma levels of recognition factors. Even in disease states associated with decreased phagocytic capacity of Kupffer cells, these cells may phagocytose more material than in the normal physiologic state (34).

Liver Disease

In liver diseases associated with necrosis of hepatocytes, histologic study of the liver shows Kupffer cells actively phagocytosing cellular debris (115).

Abnormally high titers of antibodies to E. coli, bacteroides, gluten fraction III, and salmonella, but not to hemophilus influenza B, have been found in the sera of patients with chronic active hepatitis and cirrhosis (116–119). Furthermore, E. coli antibody titers tend to be particularly high in patients with chronic hepatocellular disease who have developed large portal systemic venous shunts or who have a patent portacaval anastomosis (116–117). These findings have been explained by augmented antibody responses to enteric bacterial and dietary antigens if sequestration of antigens by Kupffer cells is diminished due to impaired function secondary to increased portal-systemic shunting of blood (see below). However, the serum titers of antibodies to measles, rubella, and cytomegalovirus are also strikingly increased in patients with chronic active hepatitis (120–122). These viruses may become sequestered in Kupffer cells. Impaired function of these cells in chronic hepatocellular disease may permit the continuous release of viral antigen into the circulation, thereby promoting an augumented antibody response. Enhanced antibody responses to enterobacterial, dietary, and viral antigens may be augmented by tissue breakdown in the liver and absorption of bacterial endotoxin and may contribute to the hypergammaglobulinemia of chronic hepatocellular disease (123,124).

Kupffer cells may play a role in the development of chronic hepatocellular disease. This could occur if they fail to contain a hepatic viral infection because of impaired macrophage function. Possibilities include an intrinsic abnormality of these cells or competitive inhibition of phagocytosis by different antigens, including those released from damaged hepatocytes. Kupffer cells also may contribute to chronic hepatocellular damage because of faulty sequestration of immune complexes and interaction with infiltrating lymphocytes (125).

Experimental evidence indicates that hepatocellular injury may develop secondary to the phagocytic activity of Kupffer cells. This could occur if phagocytosis leads to release of lysosomal enzymes, if toxic material endocytosed by Kupffer cells is subsequently released and taken up by hepatocytes, or, after saturation of phagocytosis, if hepatocytes take up toxic material from the blood (126). Whether such phenomena contribute to hepatocellular injury in man is unknown. Indeed, the importance of the integrity of Kupffer cells in modulating liver diseases in man is uncertain (78).

Endotoxin

Endotoxin derived from enteric bacterial flora is a normal constituent of portal venous blood and appears to be pinocytosed by Kupffer cells and, to a lesser extent, by hepatic endothelial cells (69). Endotoxin is normally not detectable in peripheral blood. In chronic hepatocellular diseases, it is frequently detectable in peripheral blood without gram-negative bacteremia. This finding is attributed to failure of Kupffer cells in chronic hepatocellular disease to clear endotoxin from portal venous blood efficiently. This failure does not necessarily imply impaired Kupffer cell function, but may be due to impaired perfusion with portal venous blood because of intra- and extrahepatic portal-systemic venous shunts (47,69,127–131). It is uncertain whether endotoxin plays a role in the pathogenesis of hepatic injury in man (47,129–131).

Infections

The ability of Kupffer cells to phagocytose bacteria is crucial to the control of many infections (41). Kupffer cells are also responsible for modulating numerous parasitic infections (132). The nature of the interactions between Kupffer cells and viruses varies with different viruses. Some viruses are not taken up by Kupffer cells. In contrast, viruses that are taken up undergo destruction within the Kupffer cell, replication within the Kupffer cell, or passive transfer to hepatocytes. After uptake by a Kupffer cell, a virus may cause injury to the cell, irrespective of whether it replicates in the cell (133). Frog virus III is an example of a virus that causes toxic hepatitis in rodents. It is taken up by Kupffer cells and subsequently mediates the necrosis of these cells with release of lysosomal enzymes (134–136). In a murine model of hepatitis, hepatic sinusoidal cells become infected with virus before hepatocytes (137).

QUANTITATION OF FUNCTION *IN VIVO*

Various approaches for assessment of Kupffer cell function *in vivo* have been proposed and reviewed (138). They can be classified into tests that (a) reflect overall Kupffer cell function and (b) assess individual stages of phagocytosis. Examples of the former include measurements in peripheral blood plasma of endotoxin (127,131), titers of antibodies to enteric bacteria (116–119), and the rate of removal of exogenous test

particles. An example of the latter is measurement of fibronectin in serum (139). The clearance of ^{125}I-polyvinylpyrrolidone from plasma has been studied (140) and may be a quantitative index of fluid-phase pinocytosis by Kupffer cells.

Physiologic Basis of Quantitative Tests of Phagocytic Function

Nonspecific, Opsonin-Mediated Clearance of Colloids

Substances that are cleared from plasma by nonimmunospecific opsonin-mediated uptake and phagocytosis by Kupffer cells, and to a lesser extent by other fixed macrophages, can be used to quantitate nonspecific Kupffer cell phagocytic function *in vivo*. These substances include colloid gold, colloidal lipids, and polystyrene beads (2,141,142). The most widely used test substance is radioiodinated microaggregated (i.e., colloidal) human serum albumin. A tracer dose of this agent (0.025 mg/kg body weight) does not constitute an appreciable phagocytic load to Kupffer cells; its clearance from plasma provides an index of hepatic blood flow (2,141–144). A larger test dose (e.g., 5 mg/kg body weight) is an appreciable phagocytic load; its clearance from plasma is an index of the nonspecific capacity of Kupffer cells to phagocytose circulating colloid particles (2,141,142,144). In practice, after intravenous injection of radioiodinated microaggregated albumin, the initial half-life of radioactivity in plasma is taken as a quantitative index of hepatic blood flow or Kupffer cell phagocytic function. The ratio of the half-life for the test dose to that for the tracer dose (the phagocytic index) is an index of phagocytic function independent of hepatic perfusion (145). Radioiodinated microaggregated albumin, after its uptake by Kupffer cells, undergoes proteolytic degradation in lysosomes with release of free inorganic radioiodine; after a latent interval of about 20 min, there is an appreciable accumulation of nonprotein-bound radioiodine in plasma (145).

Fc Receptor-Mediated Clearance of IgG-Sensitized Particles

When autologous erythrocytes coated with about 2,500 IgG (anti-RhD) molecules per cell and labeled with ^{51}Cr are injected intravenously into normal human subjects, blood radioactivity undergoes a constant monoexponential decline (146,147) (Fig. 2). This is attributable to Fc receptor-mediated clearance and subsequent phagocytosis of labeled cells by fixed macrophages of the RES (148). Although organ localization studies indicate that sequestration of these labeled

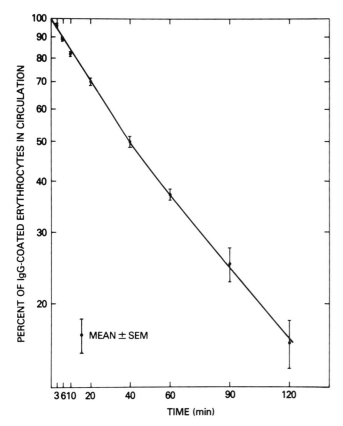

FIG. 2. Fc receptor-mediated clearance in normal human subjects. During the first 2 hr after intravenous administration of IgG-sensitized, ^{51}Cr-labeled autologous erythrocytes, blood radioactivity undergoes a constant monoexponential decline. Clearance is mediated by Fc receptors on fixed macrophages of the RES, including Kupffer cells, but particularly splenic macrophages. Cleared cells are phagocytosed. (Reproduced from ref. 146 with permission.)

cells is primarily in the spleen, Fc receptors on Kupffer cells are presumed to participate in this process (148). The half-life of the labeled cells in the circulation can be taken as a quantitative index of the magnitude of the clearance process.

C3b Receptor-Mediated Clearance of
IgM-Sensitized Particles

C3b receptor-mediated clearance can be studied *in vivo* by defining blood radioactivity curves after intravenous injection of autologous erythrocytes which have been coated with IgM (isoagglutinin or cold agglutinin) molecules and labeled with ^{51}Cr. The IgM-erythrocyte membrane complexes fix C1 of plasma and thereby induce almost instantaneous local activation of the classic complement pathway. This leads to the deposition of opsonically active C3b on the erythrocyte surface (60,149). C3b-coated radiolabeled cells are rapidly cleared from the circulation, predominantly by the liver (60,149,150). This hepatic clearance pro-

cess does not occur if the IgM-sensitized cells do not become coated with C3b. Therefore, it is a C3b-specific process which depends critically on the integrity of the classic complement pathway (60,150,151).

In the rabbit, examination of routine histologic and imprint hepatic preparations by light microscopy after hepatic sequestration of IgM-sensitized erythrocytes showed sinusoidal cells which ingested some erythrocytes and had others adhering to their surface membrane (152). Although the identity of these sinusoidal cells has not been unequivocally determined, it is assumed that they are Kupffer cells. C3b-coated erythrocytes, which are Kupffer cell-bound *in vivo*, are either phagocytosed or the C3b on the surface of the erythrocyte is cleaved by a circulating enzyme (C3b inactivator) into two further fragments: (a) C3d, which remains cell bound, and (b) C3c, which is released into the hepatic sinusoid. As the affinity of the C3d-coated cells for the surface of Kupffer cells is low, C3d-coated radiolabeled erythrocytes are returned to the circulation, producing a secondary rise in blood radioactivity (60,149–151). The degree to which blood radioactivity curves fail to regain their zero time values is an index of the magnitude of phagocytosis of Kupffer cell-bound labeled erythrocytes (147,148) (Fig. 3).

The magnitude of clearance depends on the number of IgM molecules bound per erythrocyte, which in turn determines the number of C1-fixing sites per erythrocyte and hence the amount of C3b deposited on the surface of the sensitized cells. A minimum number of 20 C1-fixing sites per erythrocyte is required to initiate clearance. The nadir value of a clearance curve is an index of the maximal hepatic sequestration of labeled cells and can be used to quantitate the clearance process (60).

Quantitation of Phagocytic Function in Disease States

Nonspecific, Opsonin-Mediated
Clearance of Colloids

Nonspecific phagocytic function of Kupffer cells has been studied using test colloids, particularly radioiodinated microaggregated albumin, in infections, Hodgkin disease, leukemia, reticulum cell sarcoma, rheumatoid arthritis, rheumatic fever, systemic lupus erythematosus (SLE), and acute viral hepatitis; function was either normal or increased (141,142,144,145, 153). This occurred even in diseases in which clearance dysfunction was postulated, such as those with persistence of large amounts of circulating immune complexes (153). An exception to this generalization is the observation of apparently impaired Kupffer cell phagocytic function in a few patients with cholestatic jaundice due to various causes (154). In chronic hepato-

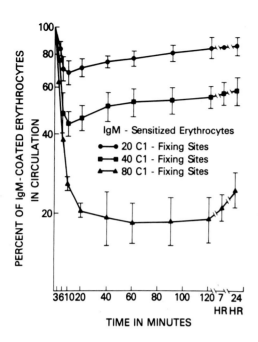

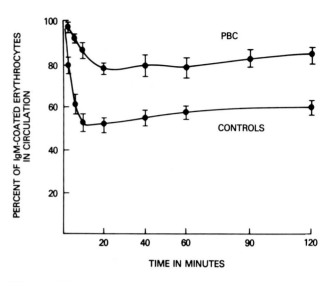

FIG. 3. C3b receptor-mediated clearance in normal human subjects. Blood radioactivity-time curves after intravenous injection of IgM isoagglutinin-sensitized, ^{51}Cr-labeled autologous erythrocytes are shown. The injected cells rapidly become coated with C3b *in vivo*. The three curves depict data obtained employing levels of sensitization of 20 (three individuals), 40 (five individuals), and 80 (three individuals) C1-fixing sites per erythrocyte, respectively. *Vertical lines,* ± 1 SEM. Clearance is mediated by receptors for C3b on Kupffer cells. The nadirs of the curves, which reflect the magnitude of clearance, are lower the larger the number of Cl-fixing sites per erythrocyte. Reaccumulation of blood radioactivity after the nadir reflects the delivery of C3d-coated labeled erythrocytes into the circulation as a consequence of the cleavage by C3b inactivator of C3b on labeled erythrocytes bound to Kupffer cells. The extent to which blood radioactivity curves fail to regain their zero time values is an index of the magnitude of phagocytosis of Kupffer cell-bound labeled erythrocytes. (Reproduced from ref. 60 with permission.)

FIG. 4. C3b receptor-mediated clearance defect in primary biliary cirrhosis (PBC). Data on blood radioactivity after intravenous administration of IgM isoagglutinin-sensitized, ^{51}Cr-labeled autologous erythrocytes in eight normal subjects and four patients with PBC are shown. In each study, the level of sensitization employed was 40 C1-fixing sites per erythrocyte. *Vertical lines,* ± SEM. The initial mean disappearance rate of radioactivity from the circulation is much slower, and the mean nadir of blood radioactivity is much higher ($p < 0.001$) for the group with PBC than for the group of normal subjects. Not included in this figure are corresponding data on two patients with PBC who were studied using an IgM-cold agglutinin, which also indicated defective C3b receptor-mediated clearance. (Reproduced from ref. 146 with permission.)

cellular disease, Kupffer cell phagocytic function is usually well maintained, as judged by an increase in the phagocytic index, but hepatic perfusion is often decreased. In these patients, a close relationship is found between hepatic perfusion and Kupffer cell phagocytic capacity (145). Furthermore, the extent to which Kupffer cells fail to take up radiocolloids used for liver scintiscanning in patients with chronic hepatocellular disease correlates best with indices of the magnitude of portal-systemic shunting of blood (155). The phagocytic capacity of Kupffer cells tends to be decreased in chronic liver diseases because of intra- and extrahepatic portal-systemic shunting of blood rather than because of deficient Kupffer cell function. To date, measurements of the clearance of colloids in many disease states have only rarely demonstrated a defect in nonspecific phagocytosis by Kupffer cells. In general, the clinical usefulness of such measurements is limited.

C3b and Fc Receptor-Mediated Clearance

In patients with primary biliary cirrhosis, an unequivocal defect in C3b receptor-mediated clearance function has been demonstrated (Fig. 4). In contrast, this function is normal in patients with chronic active hepatitis, alcoholic cirrhosis, and large duct biliary obstruction (146,147). Compartmental analysis of blood radioactivity curves indicated that the defect is primarily due to a decreased rate of deposition of C3b-coated cells onto Kupffer cell receptors (147). The defect can not be explained by reduced hepatic blood flow or by a defect in the capacity of Kupffer cells to mediate nonimmunospecific phagocytosis, because the clearance from plasma of tracer and test doses of microaggregated albumin was normal. The defect did not correlate with indices of severity of hepatocellular disease or degree of cholestasis. Furthermore, the defect is not caused by a deficiency of components of the classic complement pathway or by increased activity of C3b inactivator. The specificity of the defect is underscored by the finding that patients with primary biliary cirrhosis exhibit either normal or accelerated Fc receptor-mediated clearance function (146,147).

In contrast to primary biliary cirrhosis, patients with untreated SLE exhibit impaired Fc receptor-mediated clearance function (156). High levels of circulating immune complexes occur in both primary biliary cirrhosis (157–159) and SLE (160). If one assumes that there are fundamental differences in the structure of circulating immune complexes in these two diseases, a potential explanation for the two defects of receptor function is selective partial saturation of C3b receptors by C3b-containing immune complexes in primary biliary cirrhosis and of Fc receptors by IgG-containing immune complexes in SLE. Such saturation of C3b receptors in one disease and of Fc receptors in the other may prolong survival and increase the levels of immune complexes in the circulation. Because immune complexes can cause tissue injury (161), impaired function of C3b and/or Fc receptors on Kupffer cells may play a role in the pathogenesis of tissue injury in certain diseases.

CONCLUDING REMARKS

Recent advances in knowledge of the structure and function of the Kupffer cell emphasize the many roles of this cell in the maintenance of homeostasis under normal conditions and in restoring a normal internal milieu in pathologic states. Elegant ultrastructural studies have shown differences between Kupffer cells and other hepatic sinusoidal cells and provide insights into membrane events and cellular mechanisms involved in pinocytosis and phagocytosis by Kupffer cells. Receptor-mediated pinocytosis may be the mechanism of uptake of many substances by Kupffer cells. In particular, cell surface receptors specific for mannose/N-acetylglucosamine residues appear to mediate the pinocytotic uptake of certain glycoproteins, notably lysosomal hydrolases. These receptors probably also mediate the uptake of IgM-containing immune complexes.

Recognition signals on particulate material which trigger phagocytosis and the roles that cell surface receptors play in phagocytosis are being elucidated. Opsonins, which sensitize particulate material for phagocytosis, may be nonimmunospecific, such as fibronectin, or immunospecific, such as IgG or IgM antibodies against particular antigens. Conformational changes in fibronectin and the Fc region of IgG when these opsonins bind to particulate material may generate signals recognized by specific Kupffer cell receptors. The binding of IgM to particulate antigens creates an antigen-antibody complex that may activate the classic complement pathway and thereby induce deposition of C3b on the surface of the particle. Particle-bound C3b is also a signal which is recognized by a specific Kupffer cell receptor. The precise physicochemical basis of recognition mediated by Kupffer cells has yet to be determined. Kupffer cells may play a critical role in the processing of enterically derived antigens. They appear to present antigen to immunocompetent cells and, in doing so, may modulate immune responses.

In contrast to studies of normal Kupffer cell function, studies of Kupffer cell function in disease states have not been particularly rewarding. An exception is the striking defect in C3b receptor-specific clearance function in primary biliary cirrhosis. This defect may contribute directly to increased levels of circulating immune complexes in this disease and, consequently, may promote tissue deposition of immune complexes and perhaps tissue injury.

Kupffer cells are in intimate contact with endothelial cells and hepatocytes. The ways in which Kupffer cells interact and cooperate with these adjacent cells are only beginning to be explored. Communications between cells probably underlie the observation that when Kupffer and endothelial cells are added to hepatocytes in culture, they reestablish loose intercellular contacts. In addition, hepatocytes form regular liver cell plates and bile canaliculi, and the hepatocytes survive for a longer time (162). The nature of intercellular contacts between Kupffer and endothelial cells and hepatocytes has yet to be clarified. They are not formal structures, such as desmosomes, but they are robust enought to prevent Kupffer cells from being dislodged by the flow of blood in the sinusoid, and they are specific enough to ensure that Kupffer cells are located specifically in the hepatic sinusoid. Future research on the Kupffer cell will clarify the molecular basis of many of the phenomena discussed in this chapter and should provide methods for the manipulation of Kupffer cell functions.

ACKNOWLEDGMENT

John A. Summerfield was the recipient of a United Kingdom Medical Research Council Travelling Fellowship.

REFERENCES

1. Wisse, E., and Knook, D. L. (1979): The investigation of sinusoidal cells: A new approach to the study of liver function. *Prog. Liver Dis.,* 6:153–171.
2. Biozzi, G., and Stiffel, C. (1965): The physiopathology of the reticuloendothelial cells of the liver and spleen. *Prog. Liver Dis.,* 2:166–191.
3. Knook, D. L., and Sleyster, E. Ch. (1976): Separation of

Kupffer and endothelial cells of the rat liver by centrifugal elutriation. *Exp. Cell Res.*, 99:444–449.

4. Bradfield, J. W. B. (1977): Reticuloendothelial blockade: A reassessment. In: *Kupffer Cells and Other Liver Sinusoidal Cells,* edited by E. Wisse and D. L. Knook, pp. 365–372. Elsevier, Amsterdam.

5. Fahimi, H. D. (1967): Perfusion and immersion fixation of rat liver with glutaraldehyde. *Lab. Invest.,* 16:736–750.

6. Wisse, E. (1977): Ultrastructure and function of Kupffer cells and other sinusoidal cells in the liver. In: *Kupffer Cells and Other Liver Sinusoidal Cells,* edited by E. Wisse and D. L. Knook, pp. 33–60. Elsevier, Amsterdam.

7. Berry, M. N., and Friend, D. S. (1969): High yield preparation of isolated rat liver parenchymal cells. Biochemical and fine structural study. *J. Cell. Biol.,* 43:506–520.

8. Munthe-Kaas, A. C., Berg, T., Seglen, P. O., and Seljelid, R. (1975): Mass isolation and culture of rat Kupffer cells. *J. Exp. Med.,* 141:1–10.

9. Rous, P., and Beard, J. W. (1934): Selection with the magnet and cultivation of reticuloendothelial cells (Kupffer cells). *J. Exp. Med.,* 59:577–591.

10. Knook, D. L., and Sleyster, E. Ch. (1977): Preparation and characterization of Kupffer cells from rat and mouse liver. In: *Kupffer Cells and Other Liver Sinusoidal Cells,* edited by E. Wisse and D. L. Knook, pp. 273–288. Elsevier, Amsterdam.

11. Sleyster, E. Ch., Westerhuis, F. G., and Knook, D. L. (1977): The purification of non-parenchymal liver cell classes by centrifugal elutriation. In: *Kupffer Cells and Other Liver Sinusoidal Cells,* edited by E. Wisse and D. L. Knook, pp. 289–298. Elsevier, Amsterdam.

12. Zahlten, R. N., Hagler, H. K., Najtek, M. E., and Day, C. J. (1978): Morphological characterization of Kupffer and endothelial cells of rat liver isolated by counterflow elutriation. *Gastroenterology,* 75:80–87.

13. Steer, C. J., and Clarenburg, R. (1979): Unique distribution of glycoprotein receptors on parenchymal and sinusoidal cells of rat liver. *J. Biol. Chem.,* 254:4457–4461.

14. Pulford, K., and Souhami, R. L. (1980): Cell division and giant cell formation in Kupffer cell cultures. *Clin. Exp. Immunol.,* 42:67–76.

15. Brouwer, A., and Knook, D. L. (1977): Quantitative determination of endocytosis and intracellular digestion by rat liver Kupffer cells in vitro. In: *Kupffer Cells and Other Liver Sinusoidal Cells,* edited by E. Wisse and D. L. Knook, pp. 343–352. Elsevier, Amsterdam.

16. Brouwer, A., Praaning-vanDalen, D. P., and Knook, D. L. (1980): Endocytosis of denatured albumin by rat Kupffer cells in vitro. In: *The Reticuloendothelial System and the Pathogenesis of Liver Disease,* edited by H. Liehr and M. Grun, pp. 107–116. Elsevier, Amsterdam.

17. Wisse, E. (1974): Observations on the fine structure and peroxidase cytochemistry of normal rat liver Kupffer cells. *J. Ultrastruct. Res.,* 46:393–426.

18. McPhie, J. L. (1979): Peroxidase activity in non-parenchymal cells isolated from rat liver: A cytochemical study. *Acta Hepatogastroenterol.,* 26:442–445.

19. Blouin, A., Bolender, R. P., and Weibel, E. R. (1977): Distribution of organelles and membranes between hepatocytes and non-hepatocytes in the rat liver parenchyma. *J. Cell Biol.,* 72:441–455.

20. Knook, D. L. (1974): Distribution of lysosomal enzyme activities between parenchymal and non-parenchymal cells from rat liver. *Hoppe Seyler's Physiol. Chem.,* 255:1217–1219.

21. Knook, D. L., and Brouwer, A. (1980): The biochemistry of Kupffer cells. In: *The Reticuloendothelial System and the Pathogenesis of Liver Disease,* edited by H. Liehr and M. Grun, pp. 17–25. Elsevier, Amsterdam.

22. Wisse, E., and de Zanger, R. B. (1980): On the morphology and other aspects of Kupffer cell function: observations and speculations concerning pinocytosis and phagocytosis. In: *The Reticuloendothelial System and the Pathogenesis of Liver Disease,* edited by H. Liehr and M. Grun, pp. 3–9. Elsevier, Amsterdam.

23. Emeis, J. J. (1976): Morphological and cytochemical heteroge-

neity of the cell coat of rat liver Kupffer cells. *J. Reticuloendothel. Soc.,* 20:31–50.

24. Blumenstock, F., Saba, T. M., Weber, P., and Cho, E. (1976): Purification and biochemical characterization of a macrophage stimulating alpha-2-globulin opsonic protein. *J. Reticuloendothel. Soc.,* 19:157–172.

25. Motta, P. M., and Makabe, S. (1980): Foetal and adult liver sinusoids and Kupffer cells as revealed by scanning electron microscopy. In: *The Reticuloendothelial System and the Pathogenesis of Liver Disease,* edited by H. Liehr and M. Grun, pp. 11–16. Elsevier, Amsterdam.

26. Deimann, W., and Fahumi, H. D. (1977): The ontogeny of mononuclear phagocytes in fetal rat liver using endogenous peroxidase as a marker. In: *Kupffer Cells and Other Liver Sinusoidal Cells,* edited by E. Wisse and D. L. Knook, pp. 487–495. Elsevier, Amsterdam.

27. Naito, M., and Wisse, E. (1977): Observations on the fine structure and cytochemistry of sinusoidal cells in fetal and neonatal rat liver. In: *Kupffer Cells and Other Liver Sinusoidal Cells,* edited by E. Wisse and D. L. Knook, pp. 497–505. Elsevier, Amsterdam.

28. van Furth, R., Crofton, R. W., and Diesselhof-den Dulk, M. M. C. (1977): The bone marrow origin of Kupffer cells. In: *Kupffer Cells and Other Liver Sinusoidal Cells,* edited by E. Wisse and D. L. Knook, pp. 471–480. Elsevier, Amsterdam.

29. Volkman, A. (1977): The unsteady state of the Kupffer cell. In: *Kupffer Cells and Other Liver Sinusoidal Cells,* edited by E. Wisse and D. L. Knook, pp. 459–490. Elsevier, Amsterdam.

30. Crofton, R. W., Diesselhoff-den Dulk, M. M. C., and van Furth, R. (1978): The origin, kinetics and characteristics of the Kupffer cells in the normal steady state. *J. Exp. Med.,* 148:1–17.

31. Souhami, R. L., and Bradfield, J. W. B. (1974): The recovery of hepatic phagocytosis after blockade of Kupffer cells. *J. Reticuloendothel. Soc.,* 16:75–86.

32. Portmann, B., Schindler, A.-M., Murray-Lyon, I. M., Williams, R. (1976): Sarcoma arising after liver transplantation. *Gastroenterology* 70:92–94.

33. Gala, R. P., Sparkes, R. S., and Golde, D. W. (1978): Bone marrow origin of hepatic macrophages (Kupffer cells) in humans. *Science,* 201:937–938.

34. Kaplan, J. E. (1980): Physiological and pathophysiological factors determining phagocytosis. In: *The Reticuloendothelial System and the Pathogenesis of Liver Disease,* edited by H. Liehr and M. Grun, pp. 55–67. Elsevier, Amsterdam.

35. Gans, H., and Lowman, J. (1967): Uptake of fibrin and fibrin degradation products by the isolated perfused rat liver. *Blood,* 29:526–639.

36. Sherman, L. A., Harwig, S., and Lee, J. (1975): In vitro formation and in vivo clearance of fibrinogen-fibrin complexes. *J. Lab. Clin. Med.,* 86:100–111.

37. Fillet, G., Cook, J. D., and Finch, C. A. (1974): Storage iron kinetics. VII. A biological model for reticuloendothelial iron transport. *J. Clin. Invest.,* 53:1527–1533.

38. Landow, S. A., Tenforde, T., and Schooley, J. C. (1977): Decreased surface charge and accelerated senscence of red blood cells following neuraminidase treatment. *J. Lab. Clin. Med.,* 89:581–591.

39. Kaplan, J. E., Saba, T. M. (1978): Platelet removal from the circulation by the liver and spleen. *Amer. J. Physiol.* 235: H314–H320.

40. Haakenstad, A. O., and Mannik, M. (1974): Saturation of the reticuloendothelial system with soluble immune complexes. *J. Immunol.,* 122:1939–1948.

41. Rogers, D. E. (1960): Host mechanisms which act to remove bacteria from the bloodstream. *Bact. Rev.* 24:50–66.

42. Saba, T. M., and Antikatzides, T. G. (1976): Decreased resistance to intravenous tumor cell challenge during periods of reticuloendothelial depression following surgery. *Br. J. Cancer,* 34:381–386.

43. Stahl, P., Rodman, J. S., and Schlesinger, P. (1976): Clearance of lysosomal enzymes following intravenous infusion. Kinetic and competition experiments with β-glucuronidase and N-acetyl-β-D-glucosaminidase. *Arch. Biochem. Biophys.,* 177:594–605.

44. Minniksona, J., Noteborn, M., Kooistra, T., Steinstra, S., Bouna, J. M. W., Gruber, M., Brouwer, A., Praaning-van Dalen, D., and Knook, D. L. (1980): Fluid phase endocytosis by rat liver and spleen. Experiments with ^{125}I-labelled poly(vinylpyrrolidone) in vivo. *Biochem. J.*, 192:613–621.

45. Silverstein, S. C., Steinman, R. M., and Cohn, Z. A. (1977): Endocytosis. *Ann. Rev. Biochem.*, 46:669–722.

46. Stahl, P. D., and Schlesinger, P. H. (1980): Receptor-mediated pinocytosis of mannose/N-acetylglucosamine-terminated glycoproteins and lysosomal enzymes by macrophages. *Trends Biochem. Sci.* 5:194–196.

47. Liehr, H., and Grun, M. (1977): Clinical aspects of Kupffer cell failure in liver diseases. In: *Kupffer Cells and Other Liver Sinusoidal Cells*, edited by E. Wisse and D. L. Knook, pp. 427–436. Elsevier, Amsterdam.

48. Saba, T. M. (1970): Physiology and pathophysiology of the reticuloendothelial system. *Arch. Int. Med.*, 126:1031–1052.

49. Saba, T. M. (1975): Aspecific opsonins. In: *The Immune System in Infections and Diseases*, edited by E. Nater and F. Milgram, pp. 489–504. Karger, Basel.

50. Saba, T. M., Blumenstock, F. A., Weber, P., and Kaplan, J. E. (1978): Physiologic role for cold-insoluble globulin in systemic host defense: Implications of its characterizations as the opsonic α_2-SB-glycoprotein. *Ann. N.Y. Acad. Sci.*, 312:43–55.

51. Grun, M., Brolsch, Ch. E., and Wolter, J. (1980): Influence of portal hepatic blood flow on RES function. In: *The Reticuloendothelial System and the Pathogenesis of Liver Disease*, edited by H. Liehr and M. Grun, pp. 149–158. Elsevier, Amsterdam.

52. Bloch, E. H., and McCuskey, R. S. (1977): Biodynamics of phagocytosis: An analysis of the dynamics of phagocytosis in the liver by in vivo microscopy. In: *Kupffer Cells and Other Liver Sinusoidal Cells*, edited by E. Wisse and D. L. Knook, pp. 21–32. Elsevier, Amsterdam.

53. Blumenstock, F. A., Saba, T. M., Weber, P., and Laffin, R. (1978): Biochemical and immunological characterization of human opsonin α_2SB glycoprotein. Its identity with cold-insoluble globulin. *J. Biol. Chem.*, 253:4287–4291.

54. Blumenstock, F., Weber, P., and Saba, T. M. (1977): Isolation and biochemical characterization of α-2-opsonic glycoprotein from rat serum. *J. Biol. Chem.*, 252:7156–7162.

55. Bennsan, H. B., Koh, T. L., Henry, K. G., Murray, B. A., and Culp, L. A. (1978): Evidence that fibronectin is the collagen receptor on platelet membranes. *Proc. Natl. Acad. Sci. USA*, 75:5804–5868.

56. Plow, E. F., Birdwell, C., and Ginsberg, M. H. (1979): Identification and quantitation of platelet associated fibronectin antigen. *J. Clin. Invest.*, 63:540–543.

57. Munthe-Kaas, A. C. (1976): Phagocytosis in rat Kupffer cells in vitro. *Exp. Cell Res.*, 99:319–327.

58. Munthe-Kaas, A. C., Kaplan, G., and Seljelid, R. (1976): On the mechanism of internalization of opsonized particles by rat Kupffer cells in vitro. *Exp. Cell Res.*, 103:201–212.

59. Steer, C. J., Richman, L. K., Hague, N. E., and Richman, J. A. (1978): Identification of receptors for immunoglobulin and complement on mouse Kupffer cells in vitro. *Gastroenterology*, 75:988 (Abstr.).

60. Atkinson, J. P., and Frank, M. M. (1974): Studies on the in vivo effects of antibody: Interaction of IgM antibody and complement in the immune clearance and destruction of erythrocytes in man. *J. Clin. Invest.*, 54:339–348.

61. Roos, E., and Dingemans, K. P. (1977): Phagocytosis of tumor cells by Kupffer cells in vivo and in the perfused mouse liver. In: *Kupffer Cells and Other Liver Sinusoidal Cells*, edited by E. Wisse and D. L. Knook, pp. 183–190. Elsevier, Amsterdam.

62. Horn, R. G., Koenig, M. G., Goodman, J. S., and Collins, R. D. (1969): Phagocytosis of Staphylococcus aureus by hepatic reticuloendothelial cells, an ultra-structural study. *Lab. Invest.*, 21:406–414.

63. Munthe-Kaas, A. C. (1977): Uptake of macromolecules by rat Kupffer cells in vitro. *Exp. Cell Res.*, 107:55–62.

64. Murray, I. M. (1963): The mechanism of blockade of the reticuloendothelial system. *J. Exp. Med.*, 117:139–147.

65. Jeunet, F. S., Cain, W., and Good, R. A. (1969): Recognition phenomena studied by a liver perfusion system. In: *Cellular Recognition*, edited by R. T. Smith and R. A. Good, pp. 295–304. Appleton-Century-Crofts, New York.

66. van Berkel, T. J. C., and Konter, J. F. (1977): Biochemical characteristics of non-parenchymal liver cells. In: *Kupffer Cells and Other Liver Sinusoidal Cells*, edited by E. Wisse and D. L. Knook, pp. 299–306. Elsevier, Amsterdam.

67. Riggi, S. J., and di Luzio, N. R. (1962): Hepatic function during reticuloendothelial hyperfunction and hyperplasia. *Nature*, 193:1292–1294.

68. Ferluga, J., and Allison, A. C. (1978): Role of mononuclear infiltrating cells in pathogenesis of hepatitis. *Lancet*, 2:610–611.

69. Ruiter, D. J., van der Meulen, J., and Wisse, E. (1980): Some cell histological and pathological aspects of the endotoxin uptake by the liver. In: *The Reticuloendothelial System and the Pathogenesis of Liver Disease*, edited by H. Liehr and M. Grun, pp. 267–277. Elsevier, Amsterdam.

70. Atkinson, J. P., and Frank, M. M. (1974): The effect of bacillus Calmette-Guerin-induced macrophage activation on the in vivo clearance of sensitized erythrocytes. *J. Clin. Invest.*, 53:1742–1749.

71. Ikejiri, N., and Tanikawa, K. (1977): Effects of vitamin A and estrogen on the sinusoidal cells in the rat liver. In: *Kupffer Cells and Other Liver Sinusoidal Cells*, edited by E. Wisse and D. L. Knook, pp. 83–92. Elsevier, Amsterdam.

72. Tanikawa, K., and Ikejiri, N. (1977): Fine structural alterations of the sinusoidal lining cells in various liver diseases. In: *Kupffer Cells and Other Liver Sinusoidal Cells*, edited by E. Wisse and D. L. Knook, pp. 153–162. Elsevier, Amsterdam.

73. Liu, Y. K. (1979): Phagocytic capacity of reticuloendothelial system in alcoholics. *J. Reticuloendothel. Soc.*, 25:605–613.

74. Nola, J. P., Leibowitz, A. I., and Vladntin, A. O. (1980): Influence of alcohol on Kupffer cell function and possible significance in liver injury. In: *The Reticuloendothelial System and the Pathogenesis of Liver Disease*, edited by H. Liehr and M. Grun, pp. 125–136. Elsevier, Amsterdam.

75. Kaplan, J. E., and Saba, T. M. (1976): Humoral deficiency and reticuloendothelial depression after traumatic shock. *Am. J. Physiol.*, 230:7–14.

76. Scovill, W. A., Saba, T. M., Blumenstock, F. A., Bernard, H., and Powers, S. R., Jr. (1978): Opsonic α_2 surface binding glycoprotein therapy during sepsis. *Ann. Surg.*, 188:521–529.

77. Saba, T. M., and di Luzio, N. R. (1969): Effects of X-irradiation on reticuloendothelial phagocytic function and serum opsonic activity. *Am. J. Physiol.*, 216:910–914.

78. Grun, M., and Liehr, H. (1977): Biological significance of altered Kupffer cell function in experimental liver disease. In: *Kupffer Cells and Other Liver Sinusoidal Cells*, edited by E. Wisse and D. L. Knook, pp. 437–446. Elsevier, Amsterdam.

79. Steer, C. J., James, S. P., Vierling, J. M., Hosea, S. W., and Jones, E. A. (1980): The selective hepatic uptake of desialylated peripheral blood mononuclear cells in rabbits. *Gastroenterology*, 79:917–923.

80. Kay, M. M. B. (1978): Role of physiologic autoantibody in the removal of senescent human red cells. *J. Supramol. Struct.*, 9:555–567.

81. Greenberg, J., Packham, M. A., Cazenave, J.-P., Reimers, H.-J., Mustard, J. F. (1975): Effects on platelet function of removal of platelet sialic acid by neuraminidase. *Lab. Invest.* 32:476–484.

82. Kolb, H., Schlepper-Schafer, J., Nagamura, Y., Osburg, M., and Kolb-Bachofen, V. (1980): Analysis of a D-galactose specific lectin on rat Kupffer cells. In: *The Reticuloendothelial System and the Pathogenesis of Liver Disease*, edited by H. Liehr and M. Grun, pp. 117–122. Elsevier, Amsterdam.

83. Hubbard, A. L., Wilson, G., Ashwell, G., and Stukenbrok, H. (1979): An electron microscope autoradiographic study of the carbohydrate recognition systems in rat liver. I. Distribution of ^{125}I-ligands among the liver cell types. *J. Cell Biol.*, 83:47–64.

84. Cantor, H. M., and Dumont, A. E. (1967): Hepatic suppres-

sion of sensitization to antigen absorbed into the portal system. *Nature*, 215:744–745.

85. Triger, D. R., Cynamon, M. H., and Wright, R. (1973): Studies on hepatic uptake of antigen. I. Comparison of inferior vena cava and portal vein routes of immunization. *Immunology*, 25:941–950.

86. Richman, L. R., Klingenstein, R. J., Rochman, J. A., Strober, W., and Berzofsky, J. A. (1979): The murine Kupffer cell. Characterization of the cell serving accessory function in antigen-specific T cell proliferation. *J. Immunol.*, 123:2602–2609.

87. Richman, L. R., Strober, W., and Berzofsky, J. A. (1980): Genetic control of the immune response to myoglobin. III. Determinant-specific, two Ir gene phenotype is regulated by the genotype of reconstituting Kupffer cells. *J. Immunol.*, 124:619–625.

88. Neufeld, E. F., and Ashwell, G. (1980): Carbohydrate recognition systems for receptor mediated pinocytosis. In: *The Biochemistry of Glycoproteins and Proteoglycans*, edited by W. J. Lennarz, pp. 241–266. Plenum Press, New York.

89. Ashwell, G., and Morell, A. G. (1974): The role of surface carbohydrates in the hepatic recognition and transport of circulating glycoproteins. *Adv. Enzymol.*, 41:99–128.

90. Achord, D., Brot, F., Gonzales-Noriega, A., Sly, W., and Stahl, P. (1977): Human β-glucuronidase. II. Fate of infused human placental β-glucuronidase in the rat. *Pediatr. Res.*, 11:816–822.

91. Schlesinger, P., Rodman, J. S., Frey, M., Lang, S., and Stahl, P. (1978): Clearance of lysosomal hydrolases following intravenous infusion. The role of the liver in the clearance of β-glucuronidase and N-acetyl-β-D-glucuronidase. *Arch. Biochem. Biophys.*, 177:606–614.

92. Stahl, P., Six, H., Rodman, J. S., Schlesinger, P., Tulsiani, D. R. P., and Touster, O. (1976): Evidence for specific recognition sites mediating clearance of lysosomal enzymes *in vivo*. *Proc. Natl. Acad. Sci. USA*, 73:4045–4049.

93. Stahl, P., Schlesinger, P. H., Rodman, J. S., and Doebber, T. (1976): Recognition of lysosomal glycosidases *in vivo* inhibited by modified glycoproteins. *Nature*, 264:86–88.

94. Achord, D. T., Brot, F. E., and Sly, W. S. (1977): Inhibition of the rat clearance system for agalactoorosomucoid by yeast mannans and by mannose. *Biochem. Biophys. Res. Commun.*, 77:409–415.

95. Achord, D. T., Brot, F. E., Bell, C. E., and Sly, W. S. (1978): Human β-glucuronidase: In vivo clearance and in vitro uptake by a glycoprotein recognition system on reticuloendothelial cells. *Cell*, 15:269–278.

96. Schlesinger, P. H., Doebber, T. W., Mandell, B. F., White, R., De Schryver, C., Rodman, J. S., Miller, M. J., and Stahl, P. (1978): Plasma clearance of glycoproteins with terminal mannose and N-acetylglucosamine by liver non-parenchymal cells. Studies with N-acetyl-beta-D-glucosaminidase, ribonuclease B and agalacto-orosomucoid. *Biochem. J.*, 176:103–109.

97. Steer, C. J., Kusiak, J. W., Brady, R. O., and Jones, E. A. (1979): Selective hepatic uptake of human β-hexosaminidase A by a specific glycoprotein recognition system on sinusoidal cells. *Proc. Natl. Acad. Sci. USA*, 76:2774–2778.

98. Stahl, P. D., Rodman, J. S., Miller, M. J., and Schlesinger, P. H. (1978): Evidence for receptor-mediated binding of glycoproteins, glycoconjugates and lysosomal glycosidases by alveolar macrophages. *Proc. Natl. Acad. Sci. USA*, 75:1399–1403.

99. Stahl, P., Schlesinger, P. H., Sigardson, E., Rodman, J. S., and Lee, Y. C. (1980): Receptor-mediated pinocytosis of mannose glycoconjugates by macrophages: Characterization and evidence for receptor recycling. *Cell*, 19:207–215.

100. Hubbard, A. L., and Stukenbrok, H. (1979): An electron microscope autoradiographic study of the carbohydrate recognition systems in rat liver. II. Intracellular fates of the ^{125}I-ligands. *J. Cell Biol.*, 83:65–81.

101. Kawasaki, T., Etoh, R., and Yamashina, I. (1978): Isolation and characterization of a mannan-binding protein from rabbit liver. *Biochem. Biophys. Res. Commun.*, 81:1018–1024.

102. Steer, C. J., Furbish, F. S., Barranger, J. A., Brady, R. O., and Jones, E. A. (1978): The uptake of agalacto-glucocerebrosidase by rat hepatocytes and Kupffer cells. *FEBS Lett.*, 91:202–205.

103. Day, J. F., Thornburg, R. W., Thorpe, S. R., and Baynes, J. W. (1980): Carbohydrate-mediated clearance of antibody-antigen complexes from the circulation. The role of high mannose oligosaccharides in the hepatic uptake of IgM-antigen complexes. *J. Biol. Chem.*, 255:2360–2365.

104. Thornburg, R. W., Day, J. F., Baynes, J. W., and Thorpe, S. R. (1980): Carbohydrate-mediated clearance of immune complexes from the circulation. A role for galactose residues in the hepatic uptake of IgG-antigen complexes. *J. Biol. Chem.*, 255:6820–6825.

105. Baynes, J. W., and Wold, F. (1976): Effect of glycosylation on the in vivo circulating half-life of ribonuclease. *J. Biol. Chem.*, 251:6016–6024.

106. Friedman, M., Byers, S. O., and Rosenman, R. H. (1954): Observations concerning the production and excretion of cholesterol in mammals. XII. Demonstration of the essential role of the hepatic reticuloendothelial cell (Kupffer cell) in the normal disposition of exogenously derived cholesterol. *Am. J. Physiol.*, 177:77–83.

107. Nilsson, A., and Zilversmit, D. B. (1971): Distribution of chylomicron cholesteryl ester between parenchymal and Kupffer cells of rat liver. *Biochim. Biophys. Acta*, 248:137–142.

108. Redgrave, T. G. (1970): Formation of cholesteryl ester-rich particulate lipid during metabolism of chylomicrons. *J. Clin. Invest.*, 49:465–471.

109. Shelbourne, F., Hands, J., Meyers, W., and Quartfordt, S. (1980): Effect of apoproteins on hepatic uptake of triglyceride emulsions in the rat. *J. Clin. Invest.*, 65:652–658.

110. Stein, O., Stein, Y., Goodman, D. W., and Fidge, N. H. (1969): The metabolism of chylomicron cholesteryl ester in rat liver. A combined radioautographic-electron microscopic and biochemical study. *J. Cell Biol.*, 43:410–431.

111. van Berkel, T. J. C., and van Tol, A. (1978): In vivo uptake of human and rat low density and high density lipoprotein by parenchymal and nonparenchymal cells from rat liver. *Biochim. Biophys. Acta*, 530:299–304.

112. van Berkel, T. J. C., and van Tol, A. (1979): Role of parenchymal and non-parenchymal rat liver cells in the uptake of cholesterol ester labeled serum lipoproteins. *Biochem. Biophys. Res. Commun.*, 89:1097–1101.

113. van Berkel, T. J. C., Kruijt, J. K., Gent, T. V., and van Tol, A. (1980): Saturable high affinity binding of low density and high density lipoprotein by parenchymal and non-parenchymal cells from rat liver. *Biochem. Biophys. Res. Commun.*, 92:1002–1008.

114. Waldmann, T. A., Strober, W. (1969): Metabolism of immunoglobulins. *Prog. Allergy* 13:1–110.

115. Scheuer, P. J. (1973): *Liver Biopsy Interpretation*, second edition. Williams & Wilkins, Baltimore.

116. Bjorneboe, M., Prytz, H., and Ørskov, F. (1972): Antibodies to intestinal microbes in serum of patients with cirrhosis of the liver. *Lancet*, 1:58–60.

117. Galbraith, R. M., Eddleston, A. L. W. F., Williams, R., Webster, A. D. B., Pattison, J., Doniach, D., Kennedy, L. A., and Batchelor, J. R. (1976): Enhanced antibody responses in active chronic hepatitis: Relation to HLA-B8 and HLA-B12 and porto-systemic shunting. *Lancet*, 1:930–934.

118. Protell, R. L., Soloway, R. D., Martin, W. J., Schoenfield, L. D., and Summerskill, W. H. J. (1971): Anti-salmonella agglutinins in chronic active liver disease. *Lancet*, 2:330–332.

119. Triger, D. R., Alp, M. H., and Wright, R. (1972): Bacterial and dietary antibodies in liver disease. *Lancet*, 1:60–63.

120. Cristie, K. E., and Hankenes, G. (1979): Measles virus specific precipitins in sera from patients with chronic active hepatitis. *Scand. J. Infect. Dis.*, 11:99–106.

121. Laitinen, O., and Vesikari, T. (1972): Chronic hepatitis with very high rubella and measles virus antibody titres. *Lancet*, 2:1141.

122. Triger, D. R., Kurtz, J. B., MacCallum, F. O., and Wright, R.

(1972): Raised antibody titres to measles and rubella viruses in chronic active hepatitis. *Lancet*, 1:665–667.

123. Thomas, H. C., MacSween, R. N. M., and White, R. G. (1973): Role of the liver in controlling the immunogenicity of commensal bacteria in the gut. *Lancet*, 1:1288–1291.

124. Triger, D. R., and Wright, R. (1973): Hyperglobulinaemia in liver disease. *Lancet*, 1:1494–1496.

125. Wright, R. (1973): Hyperglobulinaemia and viral antibodies in liver disease. *Minerva Gastroenterol.*, 22:181–183.

126. Bradfield, J. W. B., and Souhami, R. L. (1980): Hepatocyte damage secondary to Kupffer cell phagocytosis. In: *The Reticuloendothelial System and the Pathogenesis of Liver Disease*, edited by H. Liehr and M. Grun, pp. 165–171. Elsevier, Amsterdam.

127. Jacob, A. I., Goldberg, P. K., Bloom, N., Degenshein, G. A., and Kozinn, P. J. (1977): Endotoxin and bacteria in portal blood. *Gastroenterology*, 72:1268–1270.

128. Liehr, H., and Grun, M. (1979): Endotoxins in liver disease. *Prog. Liver Dis.*, 6:313–326.

129. Mumford, R. S. (1978): Endotoxins and the liver. *Gastroenterology*, 75:532–535.

130. Nolan, J. P. (1975): The role of endotoxin in liver injury. *Gastroenterology*, 69:1346–1356.

131. Prytz, H., Holst-Christensen, J., Korner, B., and Liehr, H. (1976): Portal venous and systemic endotoxaemia in patients without liver disease and systemic endotoxemia in patients with cirrhosis. *Scand. J. Gastroenterol.*, 11:857–863.

132. Soderman, W. A., Rodrick, G. E., and Vincent, A. L. (1980): Parasites, the RES and liver disease. In: *The Reticuloendothelial System and the Pathogenesis of Liver Disease*, edited by H. Liehr and M. Grun, pp. 353–360. Elsevier, Amsterdam.

133. Mims, C. A. (1964): Aspects of the pathogenesis of viral diseases. *Bact. Rev.*, 28:30–71.

134. Gendrault, J.-L., Steffan, A.-M., Bingen, A., and Kirn, A. (1977): Interaction of frog virus 3 (FV3) with sinusoidal cells. In: *Kupffer Cells and Other Liver Sinusoidal Cells*, edited by E. Wisse and D. L. Knook, pp. 223–232. Elsevier, Amsterdam.

135. Gendrault, J.-L., Steffan, A.-M., Bingen, A., and Kirn, A. (1980): Uptake of frog virus 3 by Kupffer cells in vivo and in vitro. In: *The Reticuloendothelial System and the Pathogenesis of Liver Disease*, edited by H. Liehr and M. Grun, pp. 221–228. Elsevier, Amsterdam.

136. Gut, J. P., Steffan, A.-M., and Kirn, A. (1980): Kupffer cell functions and frog virus 3 hepatitis in mice and rats. In: *The Reticuloendothelial System and the Pathogenesis of Liver Disease*, edited by H. Liehr and M. Grun, pp. 211–219. Elsevier, Amsterdam.

137. Reubner, B. H. (1980): The Kupffer cell and viral hepatitis in mice. In: *The Reticuloendothelial System and the Pathogenesis of Liver Disease*, edited by H. Liehr and M. Grun, pp. 229–244. Elsevier, Amsterdam.

138. Bradfield, J. W. B. (1980): Can we measure Kupffer cell function in man? In: *The Reticuloendothelial System and the Pathogenesis of Liver Disease*, edited by H. Liehr and M. Grun, pp. 309–316. Elsevier, Amsterdam.

139. Blumenstock, F. S., Saba, T. M., and Weber, P. (1978): Purification of alpha-2-opsonin protein from human serum and its measurement by immunoassay. *Res. J. Reticuloendothel. Soc.*, 23:119–134.

140. Morgan, A. G., and Soothill, J. F. (1975): Measurement of the clearance function of macrophages with ^{125}I-labelled polyvinylpyrrolidone. *Clin. Exp. Immunol.*, 20:489–497.

141. Biozzi, G., Benacerraf, B., Halpern, B. N., Stiffel, C., and Hillemand, B. (1958): Exploration of the phagocytic function of the reticuloendothelial system with heat denatured human serum albumin labeled with I[131] and application to the measurement of liver blood flow in normal man and in some pathological conditions. *J. Lab. Clin. Med.*, 51:230–239.

142. Sheagren, J. N., Block, J. B., and Wolff, S. M. (1967): Reticuloendothelial system phagocytotic function in patients with Hodgkins's disease. *J. Clin. Invest.*, 46:855–862.

143. Shaldon, S., Chiandussi, L., Guevara, L., Caesar, J., and Sherlock, S. (1961): The estimation of hepatic blood flow and

intrahepatic shunted blood flow by colloidal heat-denatured human serum albumin labeled with I[131]. *J. Clin. Invest.*, 40:1346–1354.

144. Wagner, H. N., Jr., Iio, M., and Hornick, R. B. (1963): Studies of the reticuloendothelial system (RES). II. Changes in the phagocytic capacity of the RES in patients with certain infections. *J. Clin. Invest.*, 42:427–434.

145. Cooksley, W. G. E., Powell, L. W., and Halliday, J. W. (1973): Reticuloendothelial phagocytic function in human liver disease and its relation to haemolysis. *Br. J. Haemotol.*, 25:147–164.

146. Jaffe, C. J., Vierling, J. M., Jones, E. A., Lawley, T. J., and Frank, M. M. (1978): Receptor specific clearance by the reticuloendothelial system in chronic liver diseases. Demonstration of defective C3b-specific clearance in primary biliary cirrhosis. *J. Clin. Invest.*, 62:1069–1077.

147. Jones, E. A., Frank, M. M., Jaffe, C. J., and Vierling, J. M. (1979): Primary biliary cirrhosis and the complement system. *Ann. Intern. Med.*, 90:72–84.

148. Frank, M. M., Schreiber, A. D., Atkinson, J. P., and Jaffe, C. J. (1977): Pathophysiology of immune hemolytic anemia. *Ann. Intern. Med.*, 87:210–222.

149. Jaffe, C. J., Atkinson, J. P., and Frank, M. M. (1976): The role of complement in the clearance of cold agglutinin sensitized erythrocytes in man. *J. Clin. Invest.*, 58:942–949.

150. Schreiber, A. D., and Frank, M. M. (1972): Role of antibody and complement in the immune clearance and destruction of erythrocytes. I. In vitro effects of IgG and IgM complement fixing sites. *J. Clin. Invest.*, 51:575–582.

151. Schreiber, A. D., and Frank, M. M. (1972): Role of antibody and complement in the immune clearance and destruction of erythrocytes. II. Molecular nature of IgG and IgM complement-fixing sites and effects of their interaction with serum. *J. Clin. Invest.*, 51:583–589.

152. Brown, D. L., Lachmann, P. J., and Dacie, J. V. (1970): The in vivo behavior of complement-coated red cells. Studies in C6-deficient, C3-depleted and normal rabbits. *Clin. Exp. Immunol.*, 7:401–421.

153. Salky, N. K., Mills, D., Di Luzio, N. R., and Oppenheim, M. S. (1965): Activity of the reticuloendothelial system in diseases of altered immunity. *J. Lab. Clin. Med.*, 66:952–960.

154. Drivas, G., James, O., and Wardle, N. (1976): Study of reticuloendothelial phagocytic capacity in patients with cholestasis. *Br. Med. J.*, 1:1568–1569.

155. Eddleston, A. L. W. F., Blendis, L. M., Osborn, S. B., and Williams, R. (1969): Significance of increased splenic uptake on liver scintiscanning. *Gut*, 10:711–716.

156. Frank, M. M., Hamburger, M. I., Lawley, T. J., Kimberly, R. P., and Plotz, P. H. (1979): Defective reticuloendothelial system Fc-receptor function in systemic lupus erythrematosus. *N. Engl. J. Med.*, 300:518–523.

157. Gupta, R. C., Dickson, E. R., McDuffie, F. C., and Baggenstoss, A. H. (1978): Circulating IgG complexes in primary biliary cirrhosis. A serial study in forty patients followed for two years. *Clin. Exp. Immunol.*, 34:19–27.

158. Thomas, H. C., de Villiers, D., Potter, B. J., Hodgson, H., Jain, S., Jewell, D. P., and Sherlock, S. (1978): Immune complexes in acute and chronic liver disease. *Clin. Exp. Immunol.*, 31:150–157.

159. Wands, J. R., Dienstag, J. L., Bhan, A. K., Feller, E. R., and Isselbacker, K. J. (1978): Circulating immune complexes and complement activation in primary biliary cirrhosis. *N. Engl. J. Med.*, 298:233–237.

160. Nydegger, U. E., Lambert, P. H., Gerber, H., and Miescher, P. A. (1974): Circulating immune complexes in the serum in systemic lupus erythematosus and in carriers of hepatitis B antigen. Quantitation by binding to radiolabeled C1q. *J. Clin. Invest.*, 54:297–309.

161. Lawley, T. J., James, S. P., and Jones, E. A. (1980): Circulating immune complexes: Their detection and potential significance in some hepatobiliary and intestinal diseases. *Gastroenterology*, 78:626–641.

162. Wanson, J.-C., Mosselmans, R., Brouwer, A., and Knook, D. L. (1979): Interaction of adult rat hepatocytes and sinusoidal cells in co-culture. *Biol. Cell.*, 36:7–16.

The Liver: Biology and Pathobiology, edited by
I. Arias, H. Popper, D. Schachter, and D. A. Shafritz.
Raven Press, New York © 1982.

Chapter 31

Macrophages and the Immune Response

Betty Diamond

Macrophages have long been known to participate in the body's immunologic defenses, but only recently has their range of activity been revealed. This chapter deals with the many facets of macrophage functioning involved in mounting an immune response. Phagocytosis, antigen processing, and secretion of lymphoregulatory molecules are all functions of tissue macrophages in organs throughout the body. In addition, macrophages have a direct microbicidal and tumoricidal capacity. The molecular mechanisms underlying these processes are just beginning to be elucidated. The interaction of macrophages with lymphocytes and the cytocidal potential of the macrophage are discussed herein (Table 1).

ONTOGENY OF THE MACROPHAGE

Mononuclear phagocytes or macrophages are a diverse population of cells. Kupffer cells in the liver, alveolar macrophages in the lung, macrophages in the spleen or lymph nodes, osteoclasts, and microglial cells all derive from a common precursor cell in the bone marrow. The differentiation of a mononuclear phagocyte within the bone marrow occurs in several stages. The stem cell is capable of becoming either a granulocyte or a macrophage (34). If committed to the monocytic line, it becomes a monoblast. The monoblast divides into two promonocytes, and each promonocyte divides into two monocytes (5). The monocyte is released from the bone marrow into the peripheral blood. From the peripheral blood, the monocyte enters the tissue, where it undergoes further differentiation to become a macrophage and perhaps undergoes one further division (6) (Table 2).

Humoral factors control the differentiation of the bone marrow precursor cells to monocytes. Recently, a factor known as colony stimulating factor (CSF) has been identified and purified. It causes the precursor cell to differentiate along the monocytic pathway. It is a sialic acid-containing glycoprotein with a molecular weight of 40,000 to 86,000, depending on the source (7). The precursor cell and cells at all subsequent stages of monocyte development have receptors for CSF. To varying degrees, all cells in the monocytic series can be induced to proliferate in response to CSF *in vitro* (7). The bone marrow cells are most responsive, and the more differentiated cells are less responsive.

In man, CSF is made by macrophages (8). Both tissue macrophages and peripheral blood monocytes have been found to secrete CSF *in vitro*. Endotoxin enhances the secretion of CSF by macrophages; however, the factors that normally regulate CSF production have not yet been defined (9).

A second factor increases monocyte production in the bone marrow. This factor, found in the serum of animals during an inflammatory response (10), has a molecular weight of 30,000 to 40,000. It is derived from serum of an animal in which an inflammatory response has been provoked, and when given to a normal animal, causes an increase in peripheral blood monocytes.

TABLE 1. *Functions of the macrophage in the immune response*

Phagocytosis of immune complexes
Mitogen and antigen presentation
Secretion of lymphoregulatory molecules
Microbicidal and tumoricidal activity

Until recently, the origin of the increased number of tissue macrophages found at sites of inflammation was unclear. It was not known if local proliferation of tissue macrophages or recruitment of peripheral blood monocytes with proliferation in the bone marrow occurred. Recent experiments with radiolabeled bone marrow cells have shown that the major increase in macrophage number is due to recruitment of cells from the bone marrow and not to local proliferation of cells (11). Studies *in vitro* have shown that resting macrophages will not divide, but macrophages exposed to an inflammatory stimulus are capable of dividing when stimulated by CSF (12). Monocyte accumulation, therefore, is primarily a consequence of recruitment from the bone marrow but may also result from local proliferation.

PHARMACOLOGIC AGENTS AFFECTING MONOCYTE NUMBER

Azathioprine in pharmacologic doses decreases peripheral blood monocytes in mice (1). Proliferation of monocytes within the bone marrow is reduced. The kinetics of monocyte maturation and release from the bone marrow are unaffected.

Glucocorticoids also reduce peripheral blood monocytes (1). The proliferation and maturation of cells within the bone marrow appear unaffected, but the cells remain in the bone marrow and are not released into the peripheral blood.

MACROPHAGE ACTIVATION

Monocytes circulate in the peripheral blood for 1 to 4 days before entering the tissues. Once having left the blood and entered tissue, they become macrophages. The macrophage, however, can exist in a number of different morphologic and metabolic states. Resting

TABLE 2. *Ontogeny of the macrophage*

Pluripotential stem cell	Bone marrow
Monoblast	Bone marrow
Promonocyte	Bone marrow
Monocyte	Bone marrow, blood
Macrophage	Tissue

macrophages are adherent. They are capable of phagocytizing antigen-antibody complexes and secrete lysozymes. Activated macrophages morphologically show increased spreading when they attach to a surface. They phagocytize antigen-antibody complexes and antigen-antibody complement complexes through a variety of receptors on their surface. In addition, they secrete several neutral proteases: plasminogen activator, collagenase, and elastase. However, the critical characteristic of an activated macrophage is its ability to engage in tumoricidal and microbicidal activity.

A wide variety of factors activate macrophages. Interferon, immune complexes, and lymphokines transform resting macrophages into activated macrophages (13–15). The complement component C3b also activates macrophages; agents, such as zymosan, dextran sulfate, and endotoxin may activate macrophages through production of C3b in the alternate pathway (16).

Recently, it has become apparent that there is an intermediate state of activation in which macrophages are morphologically activated and show enhanced secretion of proteases; these macrophages have little or no tumoricidal and microbicidal capacity. They are called elicited macrophages to distinguish them from activated macrophages. Such agents as mineral oil, thioglycollate broth, and protease peptone lead to their induction (15).

Resting macrophages are unaffected by treatment with glucocorticoids *in vitro*. Activated and elicited macrophages decrease secretion of proteases *in vitro* in the presence of steroids (17); activated macrophages lose tumoricidal and microbicidal activity when treated with steroids (18).

The behavior of the macrophage in the immune response depends on its state of activation. It is clear that many of the effector functions of macrophages in the immune response are performed by activated macrophages. The interaction of macrophages and lymphocytes involves activation of lymphocytes by macrophages. Macrophages in turn are activated by the products of activated lymphocytes. Both resting and activated macrophages play a role in the immune response.

IDENTIFICATION AND ISOLATION OF MACROPHAGES

Macrophages are versatile cells. They exist in a variety of morphologic states, display different membrane markers, and secrete a large variety of molecules, depending on their state of activation. Until now, there has been no single marker to identify all macrophages. In general, macrophages are identified either by their phagocytic property or their ability to adhere to glass or plastic surfaces. Experiments studying the biologic activity of primary macrophages rely on cell separation techniques that are either not inclusive of the entire macrophage population or contain contaminating nonmacrophage cells, or both. Macrophages purified by virtue of their phagocytic capability are a subpopulation of all macrophages because all macrophages are not phagocytic. Thus the macrophage-depleted population still contains macrophages. Macrophages separated by adherence to a glass or plastic surface are contaminated with other nonmacrophage-adherent cells.

The property that may be most specific and inclusive for identifying macrophages is the presence of receptors for monocytic CSF; however, this property has not been exploited in cell separation techniques. It is also likely that the development of monoclonal antibody will aid in macrophage identification. Antibodies have been described which appear to be specific for macrophages and monocytes (19).

FUNCTIONS OF MACROPHAGES IN THE IMMUNE RESPONSE

The macrophage plays an essential part in the immune response. It has three crucial roles. The first recognized function was the removal and degradation of immune complexes. Second, it processes antigen in such a way that it is recognized by T and B lymphocytes. Third, it secretes a number of molecules that participate in regulating lymphocyte activity.

Removal of Immune Complexes

The macrophage has cell surface receptors that bind immune complexes. There are Fc receptors for IgG molecules and complement receptors for the C3b component of the complement cascade. Fc receptors for immunoglobulin have been studied most extensively in the mouse; three independent Fc receptors capable of binding the Fc portion of an IgG molecule have been identified. One binds specifically IgG2a, one IgG3, and one both IgG1 and IgG2b (20,21). Thus there is an Fc receptor in the mouse for each subclass of IgG. Little is known of the biochemistry of these Fc receptors. It is known, however, that only the receptor for IgG2a is trypsin sensitive (22), and that the receptor for IgG1 and IgG2b contains a glycolipid moiety (23).

Binding of an antigen-antibody complex in the mouse leads to destruction of the complex and activation of the macrophage. Antigen-antibody complexes trigger the macrophage to phagocytize the complexes or to participate in an antibody-dependent, cell-mediated cytotoxicity (ADCC) (24). If the complex is phagocytized, the phagocytic vacuole containing the immune complex fuses with a lysosome, and the com-

plex is degraded within the phagolysosome. If the antibody is bound to a tumor cell, the macrophage is triggered to lyse the cell directly without prior ingestion. ADCC occurs *in vitro*, but it is not known if it is significant *in vivo*.

Human monocytes also have Fc receptors for IgG. Only IgG1 and IgG3 bind to Fc receptors; IgG2 and IgG4 do not (25). It is not known if there is more than one Fc receptor on human monocytes. These cells can be triggered through their Fc receptors to phagocytize or engage in ADCC.

Many factors can increase Fc-mediated phagocytosis. Anything that activates a macrophage (e.g., endotoxin, lymphokines, or interferon) will increase phagocytosis of immune complexes (15). Chemical stimulants to phagocytosis include zymosan, glucan, and glyceryl ester (26).

Other factors decrease phagocytosis. Phagocytosis declines with age and is diminished in protein-deficient conditions (26). *In vitro* experiments have shown that lead acetate, cyclophosphamide, halothane, morphine, and pentobarbital decrease phagocytosis (26). Hydrocortisone and colchicine decrease ADCC but do not affect phagocytosis (26).

Cyclic AMP has been implicated in the regulation of the number of Fc receptors on the macrophage membrane. In human monocytes, increased levels of cyclic AMP appear to reduce the number of Fc receptors on the cell membrane (27). In the mouse system, cyclic AMP appears to increase the number of Fc receptors (28).

In addition to leading to the destruction of antigen-antibody complexes, the binding of immune complex to an Fc receptor on a macrophage activates the cell (15). The cell undergoes morphologic alterations, assumes the configuration of an activated macrophage, and develops nonspecific tumoricidal and microbicidal activity. Binding of immune complexes, therefore, leads to a nonspecific enhancement of macrophage activity.

Macrophages have receptors for the C3b component of complement. Resting macrophages have complement receptors which bind C3b; however, the cell does not ingest the immune complex. Only elicited or activated macrophages are capable of phagocytizing through the complement receptor (29). The complement receptor, like the Fc receptor, provides a mechanism for the removal of immune complexes, but these receptors appear to be under independent regulation.

PRESENTATION OF ANTIGEN

The macrophage plays a role in every stage of lymphocyte activation (30) (Table 3). Interdependency between macrophages and lymphocytes characterizes the immune response. Within this network of cooperation, lymphocytes show specificity for antigen,

TABLE 3. *Activation of lymphocytes by macrophages*

Antibody secretion in response to antigen
Proliferation in response to mitogen
Proliferation of T helper cells in response to antigen
Generation of cytotoxic T cells in response to antigen
Production of lymphokines

whereas macrophages are not antigen specific. A single macrophage is capable of recognizing a multiplicity of antigens.

Although macrophages are not antigen specific, as are lymphocytes, their responsiveness to antigen is genetically determined. The genes that control the ability of the macrophage to respond to protein antigens reside within the major histocompatibility complex; they are called immune response (Ir) genes. Although cell surface antigens encoded by Ir genes are not present on all macrophages, they are critical for recognition of antigen by macrophages and for activation of lymphocytes by macrophages.

Cells bearing Ir gene products are responsible for antigen presentation. It has not been determined absolutely that these cells are derived from the monocyte series. Antigen presentation is performed by an adherent cell population; the cell responsible has been called a macrophage. Recently, the dendritic cell has been described and isolated as a subpopulation of adherent cells (31). These cells arise from bone marrow precursor cells, but their lineage is unknown. They do not possess lymphocyte markers and have neither surface immunoglobulin nor T cell markers. Unlike macrophages, however, they do not have Fc receptors and are not phagocytic. Like macrophages, they are adherent; they have a lower density than macrophages and can be separated from macrophages on the basis of this characteristic. Most important, they have Ia antigens, the products of Ir genes, on their surface. It is this feature that allows them to function as antigen-presenting cells. Dendritic cells are capable of presenting antigen, as can phagocytic, adherent spleen cells (32). The identity of the antigen-presenting cell(s) is not yet fully determined, but it is clear that these cells exist in the spleen, lymph nodes, liver, lungs, and wherever macrophages are present.

Historically, the first observation to suggest a role for macrophages in antigen presentation was the requirement of adherent cells to induce antibody secretion *in vitro* (33). The adherent spleen cell was thought to be a macrophage and appeared to process antigen for the lymphocytes. Adherent cells pulsed with antigen and washed and incubated with lymphocytes could also induce antibody synthesis (34). It has been shown recently that adherent cells from the liver do the same (35) but are less efficient and appear to degrade more antigen and present less in an immunogenic form to lymphocytes. This observation is consistent with experiments *in vivo* which show that antigens that bypass the liver or traverse a nonfunctioning cirrhotic liver provoke an enhanced immune response (36). Liver macrophages degrade antigen more effectively than do spleen macrophages but present antigen to lymphocytes less effectively.

The next observation was that cells that adhered to a glass bead column could enhance the response of lymphocytes to mitogen (37). The processing of mitogen and antigen appeared to be facilitated by adherent cells. Subsequently, an absolute requirement for macrophages in the mitogenic stimulation of lymphocytes was shown; this interaction is mediated by a soluble factor derived from macrophages (38).

Further studies revealed that macrophages *in vivo* appear to stimulate lymphocytes to make specific antibody in response to antigen (34). Peritoneal exudate cells were elicited in mice, which were then immunized with hemocyanin. The macrophages in these experiments retained immunogenicity for as long as 1 month. Thus, while most antigen is quickly degraded by the macrophage, a small portion is retained intact for long periods of time and is immunogenic. In similar experiments, when macrophages are exposed to antigen *in vitro* and then injected into an animal, a greater response occurred than if the antigen were injected in soluble form (39).

As this phenomenon was further dissected, it was demonstrated that the proliferation of T cells in response to antigen is macrophage dependent; furthermore, macrophages and T cells share histocompatibility antigens (40). Antigens encoded by immune response genes must be present on the macrophage for it to stimulate the proliferation of syngeneic antigen-responsive T cells. Treatment of macrophages with antiserum directed against Ia determinants on the cell membrane abrogates this macrophage-dependent proliferative response. T cells that proliferate in response to antigen-pulsed macrophages are capable of providing the helper cell function in B cell synthesis of specific antibody (41). Further studies showed that the antibody response of B cells to T-independent antigens also requires macrophages with the appropriate Ia determinants (42).

Helper T cells are not the only T cell population that displays a requirement for macrophage activation. The generation of cytotoxic T cells is also macrophage dependent (43). To generate a helper T cell population in the murine system, macrophages with appropriate histocompatibility antigens at the Ia region are required; to generate cytotoxic T cells, macrophages syngeneic at the H2d and H2k, which code for the classic transplantation antigens, are needed. Thus for humoral and cell-mediated immunity, macrophages are required to make antigen immunogenic for lymphocytes.

LYMPHOREGULATORY MOLECULES

The third function of macrophages in the immune response is to cooperate with T cells in the production of lymphokines and to secrete lymphoregulatory molecules. Macrophages induce lymphocytes to secrete two lymphokines: macrophage activating factor (MAF) and macrophage inhibition factor (MIF) (44); these factors may be identical.

MAF is assayed by incorporation of radiolabeled glucosamine into macrophage membranes. This correlates with a number of parameters that define an activated macrophage. MAF causes macrophages to adhere more tenaciously, increases adenylate cyclase activity in the macrophage membrane, and increases phagocytic activity with an increased secretion of neutral proteases, such as plasminogen activator, elastase, and collagenase. Macrophages activated by MAF also have enhanced tumoricidal and microbicidal capacities. Most of the alterations in morphology, metabolism, and function occur after 24 to 72 hr of incubation with MAF. MAF, insofar as it has been purified, appears to be a glycoprotein with a molecular weight of 35,000 to 50,000 (45). Antigen-stimulated T cells secrete MAF in the presence of adherent cells but not if macrophages are not present. Curiously, B cells also secrete a factor with MAF-like activity in that it enhances the incorporation of glucosamine into macrophage membranes. B cells secrete this factor when exposed to LPS; crude depletion of macrophages from the B cell population does not alter the ability of B cells to produce this factor.

MIF is also a glycoprotein; on partial purification, it has a molecular weight from 12,000 to 80,000 (46). More recently, using antiserum against guinea pig MIF, lymphokines of molecular weight 15,000, 30,000, 45,000, and 60,000 have been identified and appear to have MIF activity (47). This observation has led to the suggestion that MIF may be oligomers of a covalently linked subunit of molecular weight 15,000. It appears that, in the murine system, MIF is made by both Lyl helper T cell and Ly2,3 suppressor T cell populations (48). MIF is also made by nonlymphoid cells and may represent a heterogeneous group of serologically cross-reacting molecules. MIF inhibits the migration of macrophages or monocytes and is responsible for accumulation of macrophages at sites of inflammation and for participation of macrophages in delayed type hypersensitivity reactions. The mode of action of MIF on macrophages is unknown; it acts directly on the macrophage and not on a serum component which would then inhibit macrophage migration (49). MIF made by lymphocytes in response to antigen is not made in the absence of macrophages, as is MIF made by concanavalin A-stimulated T cells.

Macrophages, therefore, appear to process antigen for lymphocytes before the lymphocyte can produce lymphokines and prior to their participation in cellular immune response or antibody synthesis.

LYMPHOSTIMULATORY MOLECULES

Macrophages secrete lymphostimulatory molecules and induce lymphocytes to secrete MAF and MIF (Table 4). They secrete lymphocyte activating factor (LAF) or mitogenic protein (MP), which has a molecular weight of 15,000 and is trypsin resistant but sensitive to chymotrypsin and papain (50). It causes cell division in thymocytes and, to a lesser degree, in T and B cells and appears to increase helper T cell function. This factor seems to contain Ia antigens. Endotoxin, products of activated lymphocytes, and a phagocytic stimulus increase macrophage secretion of this protein. Interestingly, resting macrophages can be induced to make more of this factor than can activated macrophages.

Macrophages also secrete a factor that acts directly on B cells and causes memory cells to differentiate into immunoglobulin-secreting cells (50). This activity is similar to that of a polyclonal differentiating factor, as no antigen is required. Again, resting macrophages make more of this factor than do activated cells.

TABLE 4. *Lymphoregulatory molecules*

Factor	Molecular weight	Effect
Lymphocyte activating factor LAF Mitogenic protein MP	15,000	Causes proliferation of thymocytes, T, B cells Increases T help
B cell differentiating factor	15,000 140,000	Causes B cells to secrete Ig
Thymic differentiating factor	40,000	Causes maturation of thymocytes
Interferon	15,000–40,000	Modulates T and B cell function
Prostaglandins	300–400	Mediates inflammation Suppresses B cell function

A third factor, thymic differentiating factor, is secreted by macrophages and induces immature thymocytes to become immunocompetent T cells (39). This factor has a molecular weight of 40,000, increases expression of H2 on murine thymocytes, decreases expression of TL antigen, and causes thymocytes to be active in mixed lymphocyte reactions.

Macrophages also produce factors that affect the immune response in a nongenetically restricted fashion. Two of these factors have been important in *in vitro* studies, although it is not clear that they are important *in vivo*. Macrophages secrete thymidine (16), which may have tumoricidal effects *in vivo*. The major consequence of thymidine secretion *in vitro* has been to disrupt proliferation assays in which the incorporation of radiolabeled thymidine is measured as an index of cell division. Thymidine secreted by macrophages competes in these assays with labeled thymidine, and proliferation is underestimated. The other factor is arginase, which is secreted by macrophages and depletes the culture medium of arginine, thereby reducing cell viability and response (51). If supplemental arginine is added to the medium, the response is restored. It is unclear if arginase secretion plays any role *in vivo*.

Macrophages synthesize prostaglandins; they make PGE_2 and α-keto-PGF_{12}, a metabolite of PGI_2 (16). Many inhibitory effects of prostaglandins have been reported. *In vitro*, they depress lymphocyte proliferation in response to mitogen and to antigen. They have been reported to depress antibody synthesis in a sheep RBC response. They reduce secretion of MIF by activated lymphocytes and thereby provide feedback suppression for macrophage activation (16). *In vivo*, they suppress allograft rejection and interfere with induction of adjuvant arthritis in rats. Macrophages from patients with Hodgkins disease suppress a PHA response in lymphocytes; addition of indomethacin to the cultures reverses the defect (52).

Macrophages produce both interferon α (i.e., immune interferon) and interferon γ. The production of interferon by spleen cells in response to antigen requires macrophages (53). Supernatants from activated T cells are capable of inducing interferon production in spleen and bone marrow macrophages (53). Resting macrophages can be induced to make more interferon than do activated macrophages. Both antibody and cell-mediated responses are altered by interferon. Interferon also enhances the activity of cytolytic lymphocytes (54).

In addition, it has been suggested that the cleavage products of complement, specifically C3b, may be an immunosuppressant (16). Macrophages synthesize C3 and can be activated to cleave it to C3a and C3b. While some data suggest that C3a is a cytolytic molecule, the evidence is not conclusive.

Another factor has been identified. It has long been known that patients or animals with myeloma are immunosuppressed and demonstrate a diminished humoral response to antigen. Recent studies show that the plasma cell secretes a factor that causes macrophages to secrete a low molecular weight factor which suppresses antibody production in normal B cells (55). The factor secreted by the macrophages is neither prostaglandin nor interferon; it is as yet unknown if only malignant plasma cells cause macrophages to secrete this factor or if other cells which secrete the same or other factors cause macrophages to secrete this suppression molecule.

CYTOLYTIC CAPACITY

Macrophages function as effector cells in the immune system by destroying microbes and tumor cells. The macrophage recognizes antigen and activates a specific immune response in T and B cells. The immune T cells are capable of activating macrophages by direct contact or through soluble mediators. Activated macrophages appear to be nonspecifically cytocidal.

Resting macrophages show neither microbicidal nor tumoricidal activity. Elicited macrophages, while showing several metabolic changes, reveal little cidal activity. Only macrophages activated by immune T cells or T cell products have a marked capacity to kill tumor cells or intracellular organisms.

Immune T cells at the site of an antigenic challenge secrete chemotactic factors which result in accumulation of macrophages at that site. Although the primary factor is MIF, other chemotactic factors have been identified. The macrophages are recruited from the population of peripheral blood monocytes. There may be some proliferation of macrophages, but the major recruitment is of blood monocytes.

Immune T cells and their products activate the macrophages to be tumoricidal and microbicidal (14). When resting macrophages are incubated with immune T cells and antigen, the macrophages develop cytocidal activity within 24 hr (56). When macrophages are incubated with supernatants from cultures of immune T cells, the process of activation takes 2 to 3 days (56). It is not known if cell-to-cell contact provides another method of activation or if labile soluble mediators of activation are produced.

Although the mediators of activation have not been biochemically analyzed, it is known that an MIF-rich fraction of T cell supernatant possesses these mediators (14). Once activated, macrophages show no specificity in their activity. Macrophages activated by T cells and toxoplasma antigen, for example, acquire resistance to both toxoplasma infection and infection by listeria (39). In addition, macrophages activated by T cells and microbial antigens are capable of killing syngeneic tumor cells.

Macrophages are thought to play a role in tumor rejection. They are found in infiltrating tumors and are present in large numbers at sites of tumor rejection (57). Nonmetastasizing tumors appear more heavily infiltrated than metastasizing tumors. In addition, animals given silica, a treatment that destroys macrophages, show decreased tumor rejection. While *in vitro* experiments show conclusively that macrophages are capable of killing tumor cells, the role of the macrophage *in vivo* in tumor surveillance is still undetermined.

In antimicrobial systems, macrophages accumulate at the site of tuberculosis, brucellosis, listeria, and salmonella infections and possess microbicidal activity.

The mechanism of killing by macrophages is similar to the mechanism used by granulocytes. The cells display an increase in oxidative metabolism through the hexose monophosphate shunt (58), which results in production of superoxide and hydrogen peroxide. The killing capacity of the macrophages correlates with hydrogen peroxide release.

IMMUNITY TO VIRUSES

Macrophages are important in resistance to viruses in two distinct ways: they may (a) resist invasion by viruses and not provide a suitable environment for viral replication, and (b) type virally infected cells.

Resistance to a number of viruses has been studied and correlates with the ability of the macrophage to resist infection by the virus. For example, resistance to arboviruses, mouse hepatitis virus, and myxoviruses are genetically determined traits that correlate *in vitro* with macrophage resistance to infection (59), the mechanism of which is unknown. It has been shown that, in the case of arbovirus, resistant macrophages release more defective interfering virus particles. In the case of myxoviruses, resistance to infection correlates with the ability of the virus to infect macrophages *in vitro* (60). In radiation chimeras where the host is of a resistant mouse strain and the bone marrow cells used to reconstitute the irradiated host are from a susceptible strain, the chimeric animal is resistant. Reconstituting a susceptible animal with bone marrow cells from a resistant animal results in a susceptible animal. Thus the genetic determination of resistance reflects more than the inability of virus to infect macrophages *in vitro*.

The mechanism of macrophage lysis of virally infected cells is thought to be similar to the mechanism of lysis of tumor cells or bacterially infected cells. Immune T cells recruit monocytes and release products that lead to macrophage activation; macrophages then lyse the infected cell.

In addition, macrophages can exacerbate certain viral infections. In dengue fever in man or West Nile virus in mice, macrophages provide an excellent environment for replication of the virus (59). When antibody binds to the virus, the antibody-virus complex is actively phagocytized by macrophages. Virus replicates within the macrophage, leading to increased viremia and more severe infection. Whether or not this mechanism is important in other viral infections is not known.

CONCLUSION

The macrophage is critical in the immune response. It recognizes antigen and, in a genetically restricted manner, presents antigen to lymphocytes. The Ir gene products on the macrophage determine its ability to respond to antigen and to activate syngeneic lymphocytes. Immune lymphocytes transform the macrophage into a potent effector cell. Its functions are genetically unrestricted. It ingests and degrades immune complexes and exhibits both tumoricidal and microbicidal activities. In addition, macrophages secrete a number of molecules that play a role in regulating the immune response and in triggering lymphocyte differentiation.

These functions have been studied extensively in macrophages derived from the spleen or peritoneal exudates. Kupffer cells were found to be capable of performing the same activities. They are clearly phagocytic, and are capable of presenting antigen, although they degrade antigen more readily and thus present less to lymphocytes. Whether or not they are capable of all other macrophage functions remains an area for study.

REFERENCES

1. van Furth, R. (1975): Modulation of monocyte production. In: *Mononuclear Phagocytes*, edited by R. van Furth, pp. 161–172. Blackwell Scientific, Oxford.
2. Oehmichen, M. (1975): Monocytic origin of microglia cells. In: *Mononuclear Phagocytes*, edited by R. van Furth, pp. 223–240. Blackwell Scientific, Oxford.
3. Pike, B. L., and Robinson, W. A. (1970): Human bone marrow colony growth in agar-gel. *J. Cell. Physiol.*, 76:77–84.
4. Metcalf, D. (1971): Transformation of granulocytes to macrophages in bone marrow colonies in vitro. *J. Cell. Physiol.*, 77:277–280.
5. van Furth, R., and Diesselhoff-den Dulk, M. M. C. (1970): The kinetics of promonocytes and monocytes in the bone marrow. *J. Exp. Med.*, 131:813–828.
6. Whitelaw, D. M., and Batho, H. F. (1975): Kinetics of monocytes. In: *Mononuclear Phagocytes*, edited by R. van Furth, pp. 175–187. Blackwell Scientific, Oxford.
7. Stanley, E. R., and Guilbert, L. J. (1980): Regulation of macrophage production by a colony-stimulating factor. In: *Mononuclear Phagocytes*, edited by R. van Furth, pp. 417–434. Martinus Nijhoff, The Hague.
8. Territo, M., and Cline, M. J. (1976): Macrophages and their disorders in man. In: *Immunobiology of the Macrophage*, edited by D. S. Nelson, pp. 593–616. Academic Press, New York.

9. Davies, P., and Allison, A. C. (1976): Secretion of macrophage enzymes in relation to the pathogenesis of chronic inflammation. In: *Immunobiology of the Macrophage*, edited by D. S. Nelson, pp. 427–461. Academic Press, New York.

10. van Waarde, D., Hulsing-Hesselink, E., and van Furth, R. (1971): Humoral regulation of monocytosis during an acute inflammatory reaction. In: *Mononuclear Phagocytes*, edited by R. van Furth, pp. 205–220. Blackwell Scientific, Oxford.

11. van Furth, R., Crofton, R. W., and Diesselhoff-den Dulk, M. M. C. (1977): The bone marrow origin of Kupffer cells. In: *Kupffer Cells and Other Liver Sinusoidal Cells*, edited by E. Wisse and D. L. Knook, pp. 471–480. Elsevier, Amsterdam.

12. van der Zeijst, B. A. M., Stewart, C. C., and Schlesinger, S. (1978): Proliferative capacity of mouse peritoneal macrophages in vitro. *J. Exp. Med.*, 148:1253–1266.

13. Hamburg, S. I., Manejias, R. E., and Rabinovitch, M. C. (1978): Macrophage activation: Increased ingestion of IgG-coated erythrocytes after administration of interferon inducers to mice. *J. Exp. Med.*, 147:593–598.

14. Lazdins, J. K., Kühner, A. L., David, J. R., and Karnovsky, M. L. (1978): Alteration of some functional and metabolic characteristics of resident mouse peritoneal macrophages by lymphocyte mediators. *J. Exp. Med.*, 147:746–758.

15. Ogmundsdottir, H. M., and Weir, D. M. (1980): Mechanisms of macrophage activation. *Clin. Exp. Immunol.*, 40:223–234.

16. Allison, A. C. (1978): Mechanisms by which activated macrophages inhibit lymphocyte responses. *Immunol. Rev.*, 40:3–27.

17. Werb, Z., Foley, R., and Munck, A. (1978): Glucocorticoid receptors and glucocorticoid-sensitive secretion of neutral proteinases in a macrophage line. *J. Immunol.*, 121:115–121.

18. Ralph, P., Ito, M., Broxmyer, H. E., Nakoinz, I. (1978): Corticosteroids block newly induced but not constituitive functions of macrophage cell lines: Myeloid colony-stimulating activity production, latex phagocytosis, and antibody-dependent lysis of RBC and tumor targets. *J. Immunol.*, 121:300–303.

19. Springer, T., Galfré, G., Secher, D. S., and Milstein, C. (1979): Mac-1: A macrophage differentiation antigen identified by monoclonal antibody. *Eur. J. Immunol.*, 9:301–306.

20. Diamond, B., and Scharff, M. D. (1980): IgG1 and IgG2b share the Fc receptor on mouse macrophages. *J. Immunol.*, 125:631–633.

21. Unkeless, J. C. (1979): Characterization of a monoclonal antibody directed against mouse macrophage and lymphocyte Fc receptors. *J. Exp. Med.*, 150:580–596.

22. Unkeless, J. C. (1977): The presence of two Fc receptors on mouse macrophages: Evidence from a variant cell line and differential trypsin sensitivity. *J. Exp. Med.*, 145:931–947.

23. Anderson, C. L. (1980): The murine macrophage Fc receptor for IgG2b is lipid dependent. *J. Immunol.*, 125:538–540.

24. Ralph, P., Nakoinz, I., Diamond, B., and Yelton, D. (1980): All classes of murine IgG antibody mediate macrophage phagocytosis and lysis of erythrocytes. *J. Immunol.*, 125:1885–1888.

25. Huber, H., and Holm, G. (1975): Surface receptors of mononuclear phagocytes: Effect of immune complexes in in vitro function in human monocytes. In: *Mononuclear Phagocytes*, edited by R. van Furth, pp. 291–302. Blackwell Scientific, Oxford.

26. Bjørneboe, M., and Prytz, H. (1976): The mononuclear phagocytic functions of the liver. In: *Immunological Aspects of the Liver and GI Tract*, edited by A. Ferguson and R. N. M. MacSween, pp. 251–290. University Park Press, Baltimore.

27. Ragsdale, C. G., and Arend, W. P. (1980): Loss of Fc receptor activity after culture of human monocytes on surface-bound immune complexes. *J. Exp. Med.*, 151:32–44.

28. Muschel, R. J., Rosen, N., Rosen, O. M., and Bloom, B. R. (1977): Modulation of Fc-mediated phagocytosis by cyclic AMP and insulin in a macrophage-like cell line. *J. Immunol.*, 119:1813–1820.

29. Michl, J., Pieczonka, M. M., Unkeless, J. C., and Silverstein, S. C. (1970): Effects of immobilized immune complexes on Fc- and complement-receptor function in resident and thioglycollate-elicited mouse peritoneal macrophages. *J. Exp. Med.*, 150:607–621.

30. Erb, P., Feldmann, M., Gisler, R., Meier, B., Stern, A., and Vogt, P. (1980): Role of macrophages in the in vitro induction and regulation of antibody responses. In: *Mononuclear Phagocytes*, edited by R. van Furth, pp. 1957–1883. Martinus Nijhoff, The Hague.

31. Steinman, R. M., Kaplan, G., Witmer, M. D., and Cohn, Z. A. (1979): Identification of a novel cell type in peripheral lymphoid organs of mice. V. Purification of spleen dendritic cells, new surface markers, and maintenance in vitro. *J. Exp. Med.*, 149:1–16.

32. Waldron, J. A., Horn, R. G., and Rosenberg, A. S. (1973): Antigen induced proliferation of guinea pig lymphocytes in vitro: Obligatory role of macrophages in the recognition of antigen by immune T lymphocytes. *J. Immunol.*, 122:926–931.

33. Mosier, D. E. (1967): Cell interactions in the primary immune response in vitro. A requirement for specific cell clusters. *J. Exp. Med.*, 129:351–362.

34. Unanue, E. R., and Askonas, B. A. (1968): Persistence of immunogenicity of antigen after uptake by macrophages. *J. Exp. Med.*, 127:915–926.

35. Rogoff, T. M., and Lipsky, P. E. (1980): Antigen presentation by isolated guinea pig Kupffer cells. *J. Immunol.*, 124:1740–1744.

36. Sljivic, V. S., Warr, G. W., and Barrett, J. M. (1977): Stimulation of hepatic phagocytosis and the antibody response. In: *Kupffer Cells and Other Liver Sinusoidal Cells*, edited by E. Wisse and D. L. Knook, pp. 447–456. Elsevier, Amsterdam.

37. Oppenheim, J. J., Leventhal, B. G., and Hirsh, E. M. (1968): The transformation of column-purified lymphocytes with nonspecific and specific antigenic stimuli. *J. Immunol.*, 101:262–270.

38. Rosenstreich, D. L., Farrar, J. J., and Dougherty, S. (1976): Absolute macrophage dependency of T lymphocyte activation by mitogens. *J. Immunol.*, 116:131–139.

39. Unanue, E. R. (1980): Cooperation between mononuclear phagocytes and lymphocytes in immunity. *N. Engl. J. Med.*, 303:977–985.

40. Rosenthal, A. S., and Shevach, E. M. (1973): Function of macrophages in antigen recognition by guinea pig T lymphocytes. I. Requirement for histocompatible macrophages and lymphocytes. *J. Exp. Med.*, 138:1194–1212.

41. Erb, P., and Feldmann, M. (1975): The role of macrophages in the generation of T-helper cells. II. The genetic control of the macrophage-T-cell interaction for helper cell induction with soluble antigens. *J. Exp. Med.*, 142:460–472.

42. Boswell, H. S., Sharrow, S. D., and Singer, A. (1980): Role of accessory cells in B cell activation. I. Macrophage presentation of TNP-Ficoll: Evidence for macrophage-B cell interaction. *J. Immunol.*, 121:989–996.

43. Wagner, H., Feldmann, M., Boyle, W., and Schrader, J. W. (1972): Cell mediated immune response in vitro. II. The requirement for macrophages in cytotoxic reactions against cell-bound and subcellular alloantigens. *J. Exp. Med.*, 136:331–343.

44. Wahl, S. M., Wilton, J. M., Rosenstreich, D. L., and Oppenheim, J. J. (1975): The role of macrophages in the production of lymphokines by T and B lymphocytes. *J. Immunol.*, 114:1296–1301.

45. Nathan, C. F., Karnovsky, M. L., and David, J. R. (1971): Alterations of macrophage functions by mediators from lymphocytes. *J. Exp. Med.*, 133:1356–1376.

46. David, J. R., and Remold, H. G. (1976): Macrophage activation by lymphocyte mediators and studies on the interaction of macrophage inhibitory factor (MIF) with its target cell. In: *Immunobiology of the Macrophage*, edited by D. S. Nelson, pp. 401–426. Academic Press, New York.

47. Sorg, C., and Klinkert, W. (1978): Chemical characterization of products of activated lymphocytes. *Fed. Proc.*, 37:2748–2753.

48. Newman, W., Gordon, S., Hammerling, O., Senik, A., and Bloom, B. R. (1978): Production of migration inhibition factor (MIF) and an inducer of plasminogen activator (IPA) by subsets of T cells in MLC. *J. Immunol.*, 120:927–931.

49. Newman, W., Diamond, B., Flomenberg, P., Scharff, M. D., and Bloom, B. R. (1979): Response of a continuous macrophage-like cell line to MIF. *J. Immunol.*, 123:2292–2297.

50. Unanue, E. R. (1978): The regulation of lymphocyte functions by the macrophage. *Immunol. Rev.*, 40:227–255.

51. Kung, J. T., Brooks, S. B., Jakway, J. P., Leonard, L. L., and Talmage, D. W. (1977): Suppression of in vitro cytotoxic re-

sponse by macrophages due to induced arginase. *J. Exp. Med.,* 146:665–672.

52. Goodwin, J. S., Messner, R. P., Bankhurst, A. D., Peake, G. T., Saiki, J. H., and Williams, R. C. (1977): Prostaglandin-producing suppressor cells in Hodgkin's disease. *N. Engl. J. Med.,* 297:963–967.

53. Stewart, W. E., II (1979): *The Interferon System.* Springer Verlag, Wien.

54. Epstein, L. B. (1976): The ability of macrophages to augment in vitro mitogen and antigen stimulated production of interferon and other mediators of cellular immunity by lymphocytes. In: *Immunobiology of the Macrophage,* edited by D. S. Nelson, pp. 202–234. Academic Press, New York.

55. Kennard, J., and Zolla-Pazner, S. (1980): Origin and function of suppressor macrophages in myeloma. *J. Immunol.,* 124: 268–273.

56. Evans, R., and Alexander, P. (1976): Mechanisms of extracellular killing of nucleated mammalian cells by macrophages. In: *Immunobiology of the Macrophage,* edited by D. S. Nelson, pp. 536–576. Academic Press, New York.

57. Tevethia, S. S., Zarling, J. M., and Flax, M. H. (1976): Macrophages and the destruction of syngeneic virus-induced tumors. In: *Immunobiology of the Macrophage,* edited by D. S. Nelson, pp. 509–533. Academic Press, New York.

58. Nathan, C. F., and Root, R. K. (1977): Hydrogen peroxide release from mouse peritoneal macrophages. *J. Exp. Med.,* 146:1648–1662.

59. Neighbour, P. A., and Bloom, B. R. (1980): Natural resistance to virus infections. *Semin. Infect. Dis.,* III:272–293.

60. Haller, O., Arnheiter, H., and Lindemann, J. (1979): Natural genetically determined resistance toward influenza virus in hemopoietic mouse chimeras. *J. Exp. Med.,* 150:117–126.

Section II

The Cells

D. Extracellular Connective Tissues

The Liver: Biology and Pathobiology, edited by
I. Arias, H. Popper, D. Schachter, and D. A. Shafritz.
Raven Press, New York © 1982.

Chapter 32

The Extracellular Matrix

Marcos Rojkind

Collagen, one of the most abundant proteins in the animal kingdom, is present in small quantities in the liver. However, its distribution is such that small increments are accompanied by dramatic changes in blood flow, structure, and liver function. Collagen in the extracellular matrix is associated with glycoproteins and glycosaminoglycans. These macromolecules interact with each other and with elements of the plasma membrane of different cells. The nature of some of these interactions has been investigated because many normal cells in culture require the extracellular matrix to sustain growth and to maintain specific cellular functions. This chapter reviews the chemical description of the different components of the extracellular matrix, the nature of their interactions, and the possible role of these interactions in cell differentiation (for reviews, see refs. 1–7).

LIVER COMPOSITION

To understand the role of the extracellular matrix in the three-dimensional organization of the liver, it is important to appreciate the compositional relationship between different structural and cellular elements of the liver (8). As shown in Table 1, 84.1% of the total liver volume is occupied by cells and 15.9% by elements of the extracellular space. Of the total cell volume, 92.5% corresponds to hepatocytes and only 7.5% to the sum of endothelial, Kupffer, and fat-storing (Ito) cells. Of the extracellular space, the Disse space and the sinusoidal lumen represent 97.4% of the volume

and are interconnected through fenestrations in the endothelial cells. Accordingly, the contents of the extracellular space are constantly bathing the plasma membrane of cellular elements. It is likely, therefore, that changes in the nature and/or distribution of extracellular components will greatly influence liver function.

EXTRACELLULAR SPACE

The extracellular space of the liver is composed of a large variety of molecules, some of which are "flow-through" elements caught in the two-way traffic between sinusoids and hepatocytes. The other molecules are elements of the connective tissues and constitute the extracellular matrix.

EXTRACELLULAR MATRIX

Three main groups of macromolecules are present in the extracellular matrix: collagens, glycosaminoglycans, and glycoproteins.

Collagen

Collagen is a heterogeneous class of proteins with a unique amino acid composition and structure (9). A collagen molecule is a right-handed coiled-coil structure with a diameter of about 1.4 nm, a length of 300 nm (Fig. 1), and a molecular weight of 300,000. It contains three chains (α-chains), each of which is a left-

TABLE 1. *Liver composition in percent of parenchymal volume*[a]

Location	Actual %	Relative % of cell or space volume
Cells	84.1	
Hepatocytes	77.8	92.5
Nonhepatocytes	6.3	7.5
Endothelial cells	2.8	3.3
Kupffer cells	2.1	2.5
Fat-storing cells	1.4	1.7
Extracellular space	15.9	
Disse space	4.9	30.8
Sinusoidal lumen	10.6	66.6
Biliari canaliculi	0.4	2.7

[a] Modified from ref. 8.

handed helix of 96,000 daltons with approximately 1,050 amino acid residues. About one-third of the total amino acid residues in collagen are glycine residues, and one-fifth is the sum of the imino acids proline and hydroxyproline. Collagen has a highly repetitive sequence of amino acids in which glycine occupies every third position. Its general formula is $(Gly-X-Y)_n$. Proline and hydroxyproline account for one-third of the total X and Y positions of the molecule, and the others are occupied by other amino acid resi-

dues. In interstitial collagens, hydroxyproline occupies the Y position and corresponds to the isomeric form, 4-hydroxyproline. Near the carboxyl-terminal end of the α1 and α2 chains of type I collagen is a 3-hydroxyproline residue (10). In basement membrane collagens, hydroxyproline is present at both X and Y positions of the triplet. In the X position, it is always the 3-hydroxyproline isomer and 4-hydroxyproline in the Y position, as occurs in interstitial collagens (11).

The collagen helix is tight and does not allow accommodation of the side chains of amino acids inside the helix (9). The protein is highly resistant to proteolytic attack (12); in its native state, it is only cleaved by specific proteolytic enzymes named collagenases (13). Nonspecific proteases cleave only the nonhelical extensions, which are present at amino- and carboxyl-terminal ends of the molecule and are remnants of the conversion of procollagen to collagen (14). Type III collagen, however, appears to have some susceptible sites for pepsin and can easily be degraded during extraction procedures (15). In the basement membrane class of proteins, the helix may be discontinuous. These sites are cleaved by pepsin and neutral proteases (16), which probably explains the heterogeneity of peptides obtained during solubilization procedures (17,18).

Specific lysyl and hydroxylysyl residues which are

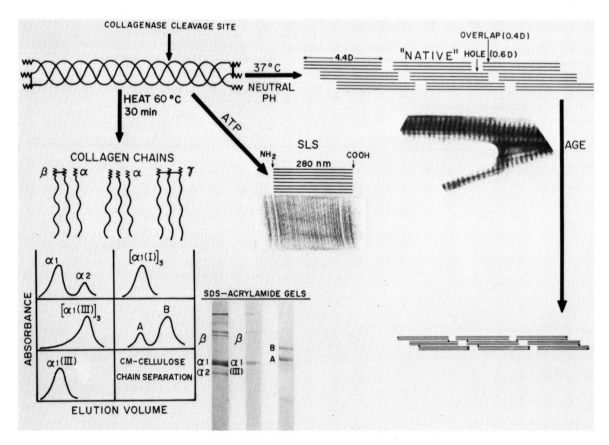

FIG. 1. The extracellular matrix.

located at the amino- and carboxyl-terminal extensions of collagen, are enzymatically oxidized to aldehydes, which are precursors of intra- and intermolecular cross-links in collagen (19). Liver collagen is highly cross-linked and is very insoluble. Only 1 to 2% is solubilized by 1 M NaCl or 0.5 M acetic acid; however, liver collagen can be solubilized at low temperatures following pepsin digestion (20–22).

Collagen α-chains contain glucose and galactose residues, which are attached to the hydroxyl groups of hydroxylysine through a glycosidic linkage (11,12). They exist mainly as disaccharide units (glucosyl-galactosylhydroxylysine), although galactosylhydroxylysine is also present. In general, the degree of glycosylation correlates with the extent of hydroxylation of lysine residues. Collagens with relatively higher hydroxylysine contents are usually more glycosylated (10).

To date, six distinct genetic types of collagen have been characterized on the basis of their individual α-chains (Table 2). Collagens solubilized with pepsin in acetic acid can be precipitated directly with NaCl into discrete fractions, which contain mixtures of collagen, or can be fractionated from Tris-HCl buffer at neutral pH by precipitation with increasing concentrations of NaCl (0.45, 1.7, 2.5, 4.0 M) (Table 2) (21). Individual collagen chains are purified by chromatography on CM-cellulose columns, and identification of the α-chains is monitored by SDS-acrylamide gel electrophoresis (Fig. 1).

Type I Collagen

Type I collagen is present in large concentrations in human liver (20–22). Approximately 33% of total liver collagen is type I and corresponds to the heavy collagen bundles which stain blue with Mallory stains. It is present in portal triads, large vessels, and around terminal venules (23–26). Occasionally, type I collagen fibers are seen within the liver lobule. The amino acid composition of liver type I collagen is shown in Table 3; its general features are described in Table 2.

Trimer of α1 (I)

Although this collagen has not been found in normal human liver (21), it is present in rat liver in 1 to 2% concentration (M. Rojkind and M. A. Giambrone, *unpublished observations*). It is increased in liver disease and in other disease states. It is synthesized by chondrocytes (27–29), fibroblasts (30), and hepatocytes in culture (31). Its distribution in the liver is not known, nor is its role in connective tissue homeostasis. The amino acid composition of [α1(I)]₃ is shown in Table 3.

Type II Collagen

Type II collagen is not present in the liver. It is the cartilage type of collagen and is found in all tissues which contain hyaline cartilage, e.g., notochord, nucleous pulposus, lung, and eye (32–34).

Type III Collagen

Human liver contains approximately 33% of type III collagen (24–26). It corresponds to some but not all reticulin fibers, and stains black with silver stains. It forms fine fibrils because a large proportion is deposited as procollagen (24,26). It is present in portal triads and in terminal venule zones associated with type I collagen. Type III collagen forms the fine framework of the liver and is present in interlobular regions. The amino acid composition of type III collagen is shown in Table 3. Scanning electron microscopy of mouse liver reveals that reticulin fibers are present in the Disse space, and membranous processes of fat-storing cells are associated with reticulin fibers (35). The exact nature of these fibers has to be determined, however, because types III, IV, and V collagens may be present in the same regions.

Type IV Collagen

Type IV collagen may represent up to 10% of total liver collagen (21); because of its heterogeneity after pepsin solubilization (16,36–38) and its fractionation with NaCl into several fractions, however, the actual amount has not been determined. In the portal tract, type IV collagen is present in the basement membrane beneath the endothelial lining of hepatic arteries, portal veins, and lymphatic vessels. It is also present around smooth muscle cells in vessel walls and around bile ducts and ductules and nerve axons (39). In liver parenchyma, type IV collagen is localized along sinusoids between endothelial lining and liver cell plates, and around the central vein. The amino acid composition of two α-size chains (C and D) and a pro-α-size chain (C') derived from basement membrane is shown in Table 3.

Type V or Type AB Collagen

Type V collagen accounts for approximately 7 to 10% of total liver collagen (21). Its exact chain composition is unknown, although from the stoichiometry of the chains isolated on CM-cellulose, liver type V collagen may be αA(αB)₂. In other tissues, the ratios of A/B collagens vary due to the lower denaturation temperature and greater susceptibility of collagen A to proteolysis (40,41). This collagen is present in portal

TABLE 2.

Collagen type	Molecular formula	Tissue distribution	Special features
I	$[\alpha 1(I)]_2 \alpha 2$	All connective tissues: skin, tendon, bone, dentin, liver, lung, heart, fascia.	Lys + hylys = 35 residues, hylys = 7; low glycosylation; heavy collagen bundles of most tissues; solubilized with pepsin and precipitable from neutral pH buffers (Tris-HCl) with 2.5 M NaCl concentrations
I-trimer	$[\alpha 1(I)]_3$	Skin, cartilage, liver, gingiva, chondrocytes.	Present in tissues synthesizing collagen after injury or inflammation; produced by "aged" or dedifferentiated cells; solubilized with pepsin and precipitable from Tris-HCl buffer with 4.0 M NaCl
II	$[\alpha 1(II)]_3$	Hyaline cartilage, nucleus pulposus, notochord, vitreous body.	Lys + hylys = 35, hylys = 13. High glycosylation; forms fine fibers without apparent periodicity; after extraction or removal of glycosaminoglycans, it forms fibers with normal periodicity; solubilized with pepsin and precipitable from Tris-HCl buffer with 4.0 M NaCl
III	$[\alpha 1(III)]_3$	Most connective tissues where type I collagen is present.	Lys + hylys = 35, hylys = 7; low glycosylation; forms disulfide cross-links; corresponds to some but not all the reticulin fibers of the tissues; forms fine fibrils because it is present as procollagen; more abundant in fetal tissues; decreases with age or in fibrotic processes; solubilized with pepsin and precipitable from Tris-HCl buffers with 1.7 M NaCl
IV	$[\alpha 1(IV)]_3$ C and D chains	All basement membranes.	Lys + hylys = 65, hylys = 57; high glycosylation; low alanine content; 3-hydroxyproline present in relatively large concentrations; Heterogeneous; may contain more than a single chain; present as procollagen and shows no periodicity; after solubilization with dilute acid, it forms procollagen-size SLS crystallites; pepsin susceptible site yielding fragments with MW of 55 to 180 K; remains in solution after precipitation of other collagens.
V	$[\alpha A]_3$ $[\alpha B]_3$ $\alpha A[\alpha B]_2$	Present in most tissues in 3–5% concentration; kidney messangium, liver perisinusoidal structures, intestinal basal lamina, lung.	Collagen B: Lys + hylys = 55, hylys = 35; high glycosylation. Collagen A: normal hylys + lys, hylys = 13. Collagen A has a lower melting temperature than collagen B; low alanine content; contains small amounts of 3-hydroxyproline; present in most sites where selectivity of filtration is required, but not defined basement membrane is present; might be associated with the exoskeleton of mesenchymal cells; solubilized with pepsin and precipitable from Tris-HCl buffer with 4.0 M NaCl

triads and central venule areas; however, it is more conspicuous at the sinusoidal site of the hepatocytes. It follows a basket-like pattern and, in some instances, appears to involve the hepatocyte (23). It has been suggested that this collagen may be closely associated with the exoskeleton. Recently, a new chain with amino acid composition similar to collagen B was isolated from placenta (42) and named αC. This chain also occurs in the liver (M. Rojkind, *unpublished observations*). Because of the conflicting lettering of the α-chains in basement membrane and type V collagens, the nomenclature is being reviewed.

Other Collagen-Like Proteins

The sequence Gly-X-Y is not unique to collagen. The Clq subcomponent of complement (43,44) and acetylcholinesterase (45) have collagen-like sequences in short sections of their primary structure. These collagen-like regions may serve as recognition sites for self-aggregation processes or for anchorage in the collagen network of the extracellular matrix (45). Because of the relatively short collagen-like sequences, proteins with this arrangement are not easily detected. Other proteins may have similar features.

TABLE 3. *Amino acid composition of interstitial and basement membrane collagens* [a]

Amino acid	Type I α1(I)[b]	Trimmer {α1(I)}₃[b]	Type III {α1(III)}₃[b]	Type IV			Type V		
				C'[c]	C[c]	D[c]	{A}[d]	{B}[b]	{C}[d]
3-Hydroxyproline	0	0	Trace	1	1	1	1.1	14	0.9
4-Hydroxyproline	102	102	136	118	122	107	107	110	91
Aspartic acid	49	46	56	45	45	50	50	49	42
Threonine	17	15	14	20	19	28	26	24	19
Serine	34	35	35	36	38	30	34	34	34
Glutamic acid	75	80	78	88	78	64	88	85	98
Proline	115	103	96	88	85	73	105	110	99
Glycine	324	340	365	324	334	328	325	332	332
Alanine	120	124	92	30	30	47	57	50	49
½ Cystine	0	0	1–2	2	0	3	0	0	0
Valine	21	21	11	32	33	25	31	29	29
Methionine	6	—	6	14	15	14	10	6	8.1
Isoleucine	12	10	12	32	33	39	18	18	20
Leucine	20	20	18	50	52	56	39	34	56
Tyrosine	1	1	2	8	5	6	2.1	—	2.4
Phenylalanine	12	13	11	28	27	36	11	11	9.2
Hydroxylysine	7	8.6	6	49	50	39	23	31	43
Lysine	30	26	21	7	6	5	13	21	15
Histidine	3.5	2.4	6	6	6	7	9.9	8	14
Arginine	48	48	41	22	22	42	52	40	42

[a] Residues/1,000 amino acid residues.
[b] Human liver collagens (21).
[c] Human placental basement membrane collagens (36).
[d] Human placental type V collagens (42).

Collagen Synthesis

Collagens constantly undergo posttranslational modifications, which begin intracellularly and continue throughout the lifespan of the collagen molecule. The nature of these modifications and the enzymes required have been extensively reviewed (6,7,46–48).

The cell or cells involved in biosynthesis of different types of collagen are not known. It is now acceptable that, at least *in vitro*, every cell can synthesize collagen, including the hepatocyte (31,49).

Proteoglycans

Proteoglycans are high molecular weight aggregates of protein and sugar heteropolymers made of a basic unit named the proteoglycan monomer (5,50). Each monomer is composed of several glycosaminoglycan chains covalently bound to a protein core, which is attached to hyaluronic acid through a link protein. Different connective tissues contain different classes of proteoglycans.

Glycosaminoglycans (Table 4), formerly called

TABLE 4. *Carbohydrate units of glycosaminoglycans* [a]

Glycosaminoglycan	Sugar in repeating disaccharide unit	Average no. of disaccharide units	Position of 0-sulfate groups	Other sugars
Hyaluronic acid	GlcUA; GlcN	500–2,500	—	—
Chondroitin 4- and 6-sulfate	GlcUA; GalN	60–80	GalN-4-S; GalN-6-S	Gal
Heparan and heparan sulfate	GlcN; GlcUA; IdUA	10–20	GlcN-6-S; IdUA-2-S GlcUA-2-S	Gal
Keratan sulfate	GlcN; Gal	10–20	GlcN-6-S; Gal-6-S	NAN = Fuc Man
Dermatan sulfate	GalN; IdUA or GlcUA.	60–80	GalN-4-S	Gal

[a] Modified from ref. 5.

acid mucopolysaccharides, are acidic heteropolymers which consist of a repeating disaccharide unit in which one sugar is an amino sugar (hexosamine) and the other is a uronic acid moiety. The hexosamines are either D-glucosamine or D-galactosamine, and the uronic acid residues are D-glucuronic or L-iduronic acid. There is one exception to this rule; in keratan, galactose units replace uronic acid units.

The polyanionic character of glycosaminoglycans is partly due to the free carboxyl groups of uronic acid residues. In addition, the positive charge of the amino groups is decreased due to substitutions by either N-acetyl groups (N-acetylhexosamines), as occurs in most glycosaminoglycans, or sulfate groups, as occurs in heparin and heparan sulfate. In addition, several glycosaminoglycans have sulfate ester bonds at positions C-4 or C-6 of the hexosamine moiety. In heparin and keratan, the sulfate esters are in the uronic acid and galactose residues, respectively. In heparan, sulfation occurs at position C-2 of uronic acid or glucosamine residues.

The linkage region of the glycosaminoglycans contains two galactose residues; one is bound to the repeating unit (1-3 linkage) and the second is bound to xylose (1-4 linkage). The latter forms a glycosidic linkage with hydroxyl groups of a serine residue in the protein core. In keratans, linkage can occur with hydroxyl groups of serine and threonine or with amide groups of asparagine residues. In this type of glycosaminoglycans, the linking sugar is N-acetylglucosamine or N-acetylgalactosamine rather than xylose.

In cartilage, hyaluronic acid binds to the proteoglycan monomer even in the absence of link protein (51–53). Furthermore, binding is dependent on the availability of free carboxyl groups of uronic acid residues. Chemical modifications of the carboxyl groups (54) or lowering the pH below 5.0 is accompanied by a decrease in proteoglycan binding or by release of proteoglycan previously bound to hyaluronate (50). The link protein stabilizes this binding and prevents release of the proteoglycan monomer at pH 5.0 (50). Hyaluronic acid molecules which contain five or more repeating units suffice to bind the proteoglycan monomer (53).

The organization of the proteoglycan monomer in liver has not been investigated. Although some information exists in relation to liver glycosaminoglycans, the results are conflicting. One group isolated four types of glycosaminoglycans from liver (55). The total amount of glycosaminoglycans reported per liver (10 g) as uronic acid was 318.0 μg glucuronic acid equivalents; approximately 172 μg corresponded to the non-sulfated hyaluronic acid (54% of total glycosaminoglycans) and 146 μg to a mixture of sulfated glycosaminoglycans (30% chondroitin sulfates 4 and 6 and 16% heparin and heparan sulfate). Other investigators (56) used two-dimensional electrophoresis, separated and

quantitated the glycosaminoglycans of normal and lathyritic rat liver, and found that only 10% corresponds to hyaluronic acid, 7% to dermatan sulfate, 7% to chondroitin sulfates, and 75% to heparan sulfate. The very high concentration of heparan sulfate found is not surprising since this is the major glycosaminoglycan of liver plasma membrane (57).

The distribution of each type of glycosaminoglycan in the liver is not known. Similar to other connective tissues, chondroitin sulfates and hyaluronic acid may be in close association with heavy collagen fibers. Heparin and heparan sulfate are associated with plasma membranes and have been isolated from liver as a proteoglycan monomer (57). The core protein of this proteoglycan has a molecular weight ranging from 17,000 to 40,000, depending on the method used for removal of polysaccharide chains. After incubation with alkali, four glycosaminoglycan chains of approximately 14,000 MW are released. The complex proteoglycan monomer has a molecular weight of approximately 75,000.

Heparan proteoglycan monomer, which is bound to the plasma membrane of hepatocytes and other cells (e.g., endothelial cells, fibroblasts) (58–60), may connect cells or maintain continuity of the glycosaminoglycans in the plasma membrane and extracellular matrix. Trypsin treatment removes the proteoglycan monomer from the plasma membrane and inhibits the binding of radioactive heparin and heparan sulfate to the plasma membrane of hepatocytes (61).

It has been suggested that the presence of keratan in the liver does not result from synthesis but reflects hepatic uptake prior to degradation (61).

Glycosaminoglycan biosynthesis is complex, and requires several enzymes. A comprehensive review has been published (5).

It has been shown that hepatocytic cell lines, which maintain the capacity to produce albumin (although not in normal amounts) synthesize glycosaminoglycans. The amount and types synthesized are similar to those found in normal liver (56). These data infer that hepatocytes may produce *in vivo* most if not all liver glycosaminoglycans.

Glycoproteins

The extracellular matrix contains several glycoproteins, two of which have been purified to homogeneity. One, named laminin, is a component of some but not all basement membranes and is present in the liver. The other, fibronectin, is the major membrane component of fibroblasts and is produced by many cell types, including primary cultures of rat hepatocytes.

Laminin is a large molecular weight glycoprotein. It was initially isolated from a murine tumor which produced large amounts of basement membrane collagen (type IV) (62). It contains two subunits of 220,000 and 440,000 daltons which are joined by disulfide cross-links. The protein is enriched in acidic amino acid residues (Table 5) and contains a large number of half cystine residues. Laminin is not related to fibronectin; specific antifibronectin antibodies do not cross-react with laminin, and vice versa (39,62,63). An antilaminin antibody was used recently to determine the distribution of this glycoprotein in the liver. The antibody stained basement membranes beneath the endothelial lining of hepatic arteries, portal veins, and lymphatic vessels. It also showed staining around smooth muscle cells of vessel walls, bile ducts and ductules, and nerve axons. No staining was observed in the sinusoidal lining, however (39). This finding is of interest because types IV and V collagens and fibronectin are present in the sinusoidal lining of the hepatocytes. Depending on their nature and specific function, basement membranes may contain different mixtures of collagen types and glycoproteins.

The physiological role of laminin is unknown. Preliminary studies *in vitro* reveal that, during formation of nephrogenic mesenchyme, laminin appears 24 hr before overt morphogenesis and is present in cells destined to become epithelial cells. Laminin may play an important role in cell-cell aggregation during early morphogenesis (64).

Fibronectin is a large molecular weight glycoprotein made of two subunits of 220,000 daltons joined by a single disulfide bridge near the carboxyl-terminal end (Fig. 2) (3). The protein is highly asymmetric, with a large Stoke's radius (65–69), and contains four carbohydrate side chains clustered in one region of the molecule (68). The sugar chains are linked via asparagine residues (70,71). The structure of the carbohydrate chains has been determined (72).

Fibronectin is present in many tissues in close association with collagen (39,73–76) and is considered as a component of the extracellular matrix. It is also in close association with the cell surface of many cell types, however; in fibroblasts, it is the major cell surface protein (CSP) (77,78). In fibroblasts, the distribution of fibronectin closely resembles that of intracellular actin (79). In transformed fibroblasts, fibronectin is greatly decreased (large external transformation sensitive, LETS) (80).

Cold-insoluble globulin (CIg) is a plasma protein which is slightly larger than fibronectin, but the two are indistinguishable immunologically (81–83) (plasma fibronectin). Its concentration is approximately 30 mg/100 ml (84), and it has a similar subunit composition. Many biochemical and physiological studies have been performed with CIg because it can be obtained in large quantities by simple procedures (85).

Fibronectin binds to native and denatured collagen, fibrin, glycoproteins, glycosaminoglycans, and cells (3). The binding of fibronectin to denatured collagen

TABLE 5. *Amino acid composition of glycoproteins of the basement membrane and extracellular matrix*[a]

Amino acid	Laminin[b]	Biomatrix glycoproteins[c]	Fibronectin[d]	Collagen binding fragment[e]
4-Hydroxyproline	0	0	0	0
Aspartic acid	109	117	100	111
Threonine	58	44	100	87
Serine	77	31	84	52
Glutamic acid	122	117	116	136
Proline	53	57	80	46
Glycine	93	131	88	116
Alanine	76	78	45	32
½ Cystine	30	31	20	78
Valine	48	68	79	51
Methionine	14	7	11	25
Isoleucine	42	57	46	30
Leucine	92	71	57	31
Tyrosine	27	13	48	56
Phenylalanine	31	42	29	30
Hydroxylysine	2	0	0	0
Lysine	52	77	38	36
Histidine	24	21	22	31
Arginine	50	38	62	50

[a] Residues/1,000 amino acid residues.
[b] Laminin from a mouse tumor that produces basement membrane (62).
[c] Noncollagenous glycoproteins of rat liver biomatrix (104).
[d] Human plasma fibronectin (88).
[e] Collagen binding fragment produced after digestion with cathepsin-D and plasmin (91).

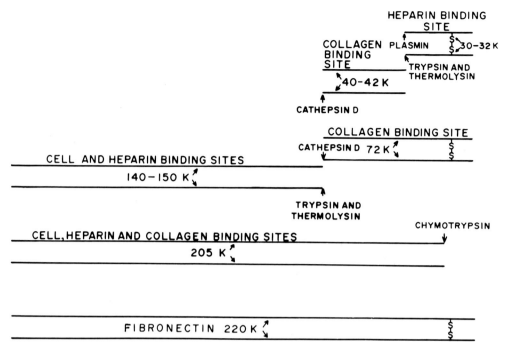

FIG. 2. Fibronectin and fragments obtained after limited cleavage.

is 10 times higher than is its binding to native collagen. Therefore, the physiological role of the process has been questioned (86). In the presence of glycosaminoglycans, binding of fibronectin to native collagen may be stabilized (87).

Fibronectin is an acidic glycoprotein (88) (Table 5) which contains several domains (13). Using limited cleavage with different proteolytic enzymes, it has been possible to map the regions that contain binding sites for collagen, heparin, and cell surface components. A summary of these findings is presented in Fig. 2.

A fragment of 205 K obtained after chymotrypsin treatment is devoid of S-S bonds, including the interchain-disulfide bridge. This fragment promotes cell attachment to collagen and stimulates cell spreading. Two other polypeptides of 40 and 160 K are also produced; the former contains the collagen binding site and the latter the cellular binding site (89). The 205 K fragment does not restore the normal morphology of transformed cells. A peptide of 140 to 150 K, which was obtained after cleavage with trypsin and thermolysin, maintains the binding site for heparin and promotes cell attachment and cell spreading (90). This fragment is derived from the amino-terminal end of the protein and lacks the collagen binding site. A 32 K fragment derived from the C-terminal end of the molecule contains a heparin binding site but does not promote cell attachment and spreading. Finally, a peptide of 42 K located between the pieces of 140–150 and 32 K contains the collagen binding site and was isolated after digestion with cathepsin D and plasmin (91). Although the latter fragment is enriched in

carbohydrate, the role of carbohydrate in collagen binding has been questioned. A nonglycosylated form of fibronectin synthesized in the presence of tunicamycin, which inhibits protein glycosylation through the dolichol pathway, shares the binding properties of fibronectin. The nonglycosylated fibronectin is more sensitive to proteolytic digestion than is glycosylated fibronectin (92). A similar collagen binding fragment of 30 K was obtained after extensive digestion of fibronectin with trypsin (93).

Although the position of the disulfide bond has been firmly established to be at the C-terminal end of fibronectin, recent work suggests that the proteolytic fragments may be derived from the N-terminal end (35,94).

Fibronectin binds to collagen in a region that contains residues 757 to 791. In the $\alpha 1(I)$ chain, it corresponds to a region located in CNBr-derived peptide $\alpha 1(I)CB7$ (95); in the $\alpha 2$ chain, it corresponds to $\alpha 2CB5$ (95). In type II collagen, it is located in peptide $\alpha 1(II)CB10$ (95,96) and in type III collagen, in the peptide $\alpha 1(III)CB5$ (97). Each of these fragments is derived from the same region of the protein and includes the sequence which is cleaved by mammalian collagenases. In fact, cleavage of collagen with mammalian collagenase inhibits binding of fibronectin to collagen (96).

Carbohydrate side chains in fibronectin are not required for cell binding, however, gangliosides (GT_1 and GD_{1a}) inhibit cellular binding of fibronectin. Modifications of the sialic acid residues in gangliosides abolish their inhibitory capacity (98).

Fibronectin can be covalently cross-linked to fibrin and collagen with clothing factor XIIIa (transglutaminase) (99–101). Cellular fibronectin may be cross-linked through either disulfide bridges or cellular transglutaminase; cross-linking may be deficient in transformed cells (102).

The actual amount of fibronectin in liver has not been determined. Primary cultures of hepatocytes synthesize this protein (103). With the use of monospecific immunofluorescent antibodies, the distribution of fibronectin in the liver has been established (39,74). The interstitial matrix of the portal regions is devoid of fibronectin; but fibronectin is in close association with type IV collagen in the perisinusoidal space and in basement membranes beneath the endothelial lining of hepatic arteries, portal veins, and lymphatic vessels, and around bile ducts and ductules and nerve axons (39).

Other Glycoproteins

In addition to fibronectin and laminin, the extracellular matrix of the liver contains several other acidic glycoproteins in concentrations similar to that of collagen (104). Recently, a method was developed for the isolation of "intact" connective tissue elements from the liver (biomatrix) (104). The biomatrix contains all collagens present in the liver (types I, III, IV, and V) and a group of acidic glycoproteins with an amino acid composition similar to that of the acidic structural glycoproteins of the connective tissue (4,105). The nature and function of each individual glycoprotein is not known, but each may be important in cell differentiation and development.

THE ROLE OF THE EXTRACELLULAR MATRIX IN DIFFERENTIATION AND DEVELOPMENT

For many years, the only function assigned to collagen and other components of the extracellular matrix was structural. In the past few years, it has become evident that the extracellular matrix may serve to "connect" and "inform" the cell of events occurring in its surroundings. Changes in the composition of the extracellular matrix may greatly influence cell function (106).

When hepatocytes are removed from their normal habitat after perfusion of the liver with bacterial collagenase and are plated on culture dishes, a small number attach to the dish. These survive for a few days, and most normal hepatocyte functions decline after a few hours in culture (106). It has been suggested that the failure to maintain differentiated epithelial cells in culture is lack of appropriate nutrients in the culture medium and an adequate matrix for the cells to grow upon. The first problem has been solved for a large variety of cells which can grow in small concentrations of serum to which different hormones, cofactors, and vitamins are added (107).

The lack of a matrix for cells has been more difficult because of problems in preparing a matrix that resembles that which is in close contact with the cell membrane of hepatocytes *in vivo*.

Following culture of hepatocytes on dishes precoated with type I collagen (108–110), cell survival has been prolonged for 1 to 2 weeks; hepatocytic functions decline from the first day in culture, however, and all cells die during the first 3 weeks. From the distribution of extracellular matrix components in liver, it is unlikely that hepatocytes are ever in contact with type I collagen and that they are in close proximity with fibronectin, collagens III, IV, and V, and glycosaminoglycans. Accordingly, it was suggested that a reconstituted basement membrane may be the best substratum for hepatocytes (106).

One approach has been to plate hepatocytes on top of a confluent culture of fibroblasts; the latter synthesize components of the extracellular matrix (111). Under this experimental condition, cells were maintained for 1 week and retained phenobarbital-inducible cytochrome P-450. Another approach is to extract the "intact extracellular matrix" from liver and to use it in cell culture (106). Using this technique, hepatocytes have been maintained in a differentiated state for several months (104,112,113). These preliminary results indicate that the extracellular matrix of the liver may serve as a substratum for hepatocytes.

Information obtained from different laboratories using different cells suggests the need for specific cellular factors. Epidermal cells attach preferentially to type IV collagen and appear to synthesize their own specific adhesion factor (114). Chondrocytes in culture require a specific factor (chondronectin) which has been partially characterized (115); it is present in serum and is synthesized by chondrocytes in culture (115). Endothelial cells attach and grow on a matrix produced by a confluent culture of endothelial cells after removal of the cells with dilute detergent (116); the cells grow in either serum or plasma (117). Finally, hepatocytes attach more efficiently to biomatrix from liver than from spleen, lung, kidney, and heart. Hepatocytes maintained on liver biomatrix for at least 4 months synthesize albumin, conjugate bilirubin, contain phenobarbital-activated cytochrome P-450, and bind Azo-carcinogens to ligandin (112,113). These examples indicate the possible specificity of factors required for different cells in culture to attach to a substrate, spread, grow, and maintain specific cellular functions. Since most of these factors facilitate adhesion of cells to collagen, the best source to look for these factors is the connective tissue matrix of particular tissues or cells.

Fibronectin, which is not required for attachment of chondrocytes, epidermal cells (97), and hepatocytes to collagen (108), shows a dedifferentiating effect on chondrocytes and modifies the phenotypic expression of the chondrocytes in culture (119). These results suggest that a balance in different glycoproteins of the extracellular matrix may be required for cells to maintain specific functions. Accordingly, overproduction or decrease in one of the elements may alter the fate of the cell. A possible example of this situation is the decreased production of fibronectin by transformed fibroblasts and metastic tumors (120).

ACKNOWLEDGMENTS

I wish to thank my students for helping me check references and especially Mr. Javier Cordero for proofreading the manuscript. Special thanks to Mrs. Martha Montes and Josefina Quiroga for typing the manuscript. The original work of the author that was summarized in this manuscript was supported in part by Liver Research Center Grant AM 17702, the subcontracts 612-1671 and 612-1749 by the Liver Research Center, Albert Einstein College of Medicine, New York, and Grants 1576 and 790136 from CONACyT-México.

REFERENCES

1. Bornstein, P., and Sage, H. (1980): Structurally distinct collagen types. *Ann. Rev. Biochem.*, 49:957–1003.
2. Eyre, D. R. (1980): Collagen: Molecular diversity in the body's protein Scaffold. *Science*, 207:1315–1322.
3. Pearlstein, E., Gold, L. I., and García-Pardo, A. (1980): Fibronectin: A review of its structure and biological activity. *Mol. Cell. Biochem.*, 29:103–128.
4. Robert, L., Junqua, S., and Moczar, M. (1976): Structural glycoproteins of the intercellular matrix. *Front. Matrix Biol.*, 3:113–142.
5. Roden, L., and Horowitz, M. I. (1978): Structure and biosynthesis of connective tissue proteoglycans. In: *The Glycoconjugates, Vol. II*, edited by M. I. Horowitz and W. Pigman, pp. 3-71. Academic Press, New York.
6. Rojkind, M. (1979): Chemistry and biosynthesis of collagen. *Bull. Rheum. Dis.*, 30:1006–1011.
7. Rojkind, M., and Dunn, M. A. (1979): Hepatic fibrosis. *Gastroenterology, 76:849–863.
8. Blouin, A., Bolender, R. P., and Weibel, E. R. (1977): Distribution of organelles and membranes between hepatocytes and nonhepatocytes in the rat liver parenchyma. *J. Cell. Biol.*, 72:441–455.
9. Bornstein, P., and Traub, W. (1979): The chemistry and biology of collagen. In: *The Proteins, Vol. 4*, edited by H. Neurath and R. L. Hill, pp. 412-605. Academic Press, New York.
10. Piez, K. A. (1976): Primary structure. In: *Biochemistry of Collagen*, edited by G. N. Ramachandran and A. H. Reddi, pp. 1-44. Plenum, New York.
11. Kefalides, N. A. (1977): Basement membranes. In: *Mammalian Cell Membranes, the Diversity of Membranes*, edited by G. A. Jamieson and D. M. Robinson, pp. 298–332. Butterworths, London.
12. Fietzek, P. P., and Kühn, K. (1976): The primary structure of collagen. *Int. Rev. Connect. Tissue Res.*, 7:1–60.

13. Pérez-Tamayo, R. (1978): Pathology of collagen degradation. *Am. J. Pathol.*, 92:507–566.
14. Fessler, J. H., and Fessler, L. I. (1978): Biosynthesis of procollagen. *Ann. Rev. Biochem.*, 47:129–162.
15. Burke, J. M., Balian, G., Ross, R., and Bornstein, P. (1977): Synthesis of Types I and III procollagen and collagen by monkey aortic smooth muscle cells in vitro. *Biochemistry*, 16:3243–3249.
16. Uitto, V. J., Schwartz, D., and Veis, A. (1980): Degradation of basement membrane collagen by neutral proteases from human leukocytes. *Eur. J. Biochem.*, 105:409–417.
17. Hudson, B. G., and Spiro, R. G. (1972): Studies on the native and reduced alkylated renal glomerular basement membrane. *J. Biol. Chem.*, 247:4229–4238.
18. Hudson, B. G., and Spiro, R. G. (1972): Fractionation of glycoprotein components of the reduced alkylated renal glomerular basement membrane. *J. Biol. Chem.* 247:4239–4247.
19. Rojkind, M., Zeichner, M. (1973): Maturation of collagen and elastin. In: *Molecular Pathology of Connective Tissues*, edited by R. Pérez-Tamayo and M. Rojkind, pp. 135–174. Marcel Dekker, New York.
20. Rojkind, M., and Martínez-Palomo, A. (1976): Increase in Type I and Type III collagens in human alcoholic liver cirrhosis. *Proc. Natl. Acad. Sci. USA*, 73:539–543.
21. Rojkind, M., Giambrone, M. A., and Biempica, L. (1979): Collagen types in normal and cirrhotic liver. *Gastroenterology*, 76:710–719.
22. Seyer, J. M., Hutcheson, E. T., and Kang, A. H. (1977): Collagen polymorphism in normal and cirrhotic human liver. *J. Clin. Invest.*, 59:241–248.
23. Biempica, L., Morecki, R., Wu, C. H., Giambrone, M. A., and Rojkind, M. (1980): Immunocytochemical localization of type B collagen. A component of basement membrane in human liver. *Am. J. Pathol.*, 98:591–602.
24. Gay, S., Fietzek, P. P., Remberger, K., Eder, M., and Kühn, K. (1975): Liver cirrhosis: Immunofluorescence and biochemical studies demonstrate two types of collagen. *Klin. Wochenschr.*, 53:205–208.
25. Kent, G., Gay, S., Inouye, T., Bahu, R., Minick, O. T., and Popper, H. (1976): Vitamin A-containing lipocytes and formation of Type III collagen in liver injury. *Proc. Natl. Acad. Sci. USA*, 73:3719–3722.
26. Remberger, K., Gay, S., and Fietzek, P. P. (1975): Immunhistochemische Untersuchungen zur Kollagencharakterisierung im Lebercirrhosen. *Virchows Arch. [Cell Pathol.]*, 367:231–240.
27. Benya, P. D., Padilla, S. R., and Nimni, M. E. (1977): The progeny of rabbit articular chondrocytes synthesize collagen types I and III and type I trimer, but not type II. Verifications by cyanogen bromide peptide analysis. *Biochemistry*, 16:865–872.
28. Mayne, R., Vail, M. S., and Miller, E. J. (1975): Analysis of changes in collagen biosynthesis that occur when chick chondrocytes are grown in 5-bromo-2'-deoxyuridine. *Proc. Natl. Acad. Sci. USA*, 72:4511–4515.
29. Mayne, R., Vail, M. S., Mayne, P. M., and Miller, E. J. (1976): Changes in types of collagen synthesized as clones of chick chondrocytes grow and eventually lose division capacity. *Proc. Natl. Acad. Sci. USA*, 73:1674–1678.
30. Jimenez, S. A., Bashey, R. I., Benditt, M., and Yankowski, R. (1977): Identification of collagen $\alpha 1$(I) trimer in embryonic chick tendons and calvaria. *Biochem. Biophys. Res. Commun.*, 78:1354–1361.
31. Hata, R., Ninomiya, Y., Nagai, Y., and Tsukada, Y. (1980): Biosynthesis of interstitial type of collagen by albumin producing rat liver parenchymal cell (hepatocyte) clones in culture. *Biochemistry*, 19:169–176.
32. Miller, E. J. (1976): Biochemical characteristics and biological significance of the genetically distinct collagens. *Cell Biochem.*, 13:165–192.
33. Reddi, A. H., Gay, R., Gay, S., and Miller, E. J. (1977): Transitions in collagen types during matrix-induced cartilage, bone and bone marrow formation. *Proc. Natl. Acad. Sci. USA*, 74:5589–5592.

34. Von der Mark, K., and Von der Mark, H. (1977): The role of three genetically distinct collagen types in endochondral ossification and calcification of cartilage. *J. Bone Joint Surg.*, 59B:458–464.

35. Oikawa, K. (1979): A scanning electron microscopic study on the liver of mice. *Tohoku J. Exp. Med.*, 129:373–387.

36. Kresina, T. F., and Miller, E. J. (1979): Isolation and characterization of basement membrane collagen from human placental tissue: Evidence for the presence of two genetically distinct collagen chains. *Biochemistry*, 18:3089–3097.

37. Timpl, R., Bruckner, P., and Fietzek, P. (1979): Characterization of pepsin fragments of basement membrane collagen obtained from a mouse tumor. *Eur. J. Biochem.*, 95:255–263.

38. Timpl, R., Martin, G. R., Bruckner, P., Wick, G., and Wiedemann, H. C. (1978): Nature of the collagenous protein in a tumor basement membrane. *Eur. J. Biochem.*, 84:43–52.

39. Hahn, E., Wick, G., Pencev, D., and Timpl, R. (1980): Distribution of basement membrane proteins in normal and fibrotic human liver: Collagen type IV, laminin and fibronectin. *Gut*, 21:63–71.

40. Burgeson, R. E., El Adli, F. A., Kaitila, I. I., and Hollister, D. W. (1976): Fetal membrane collagens. Identification of two new collagen alpha chains. *Proc. Natl. Acad. Sci. USA*, 73:2579–2583.

41. Rhodes, R. K., and Miller, E. J. (1978): Physicochemical characterization and molecular organization of the collagen A and B chains. *Biochemistry*, 17:3442–3448.

42. Sage, H., and Bornstein, P. (1979): Characterization of a novel collagen chain in human placenta and its relation to AB collagen. *Biochemistry*, 18:3815–3822.

43. Porter, R. R. (1977): Structure and activation of early components of complement. *Fed. Proc.*, 36:2191–2196.

44. Porter, R. R., and Reid, K. B. M. (1978): The biochemistry of complement. *Nature*, 275:699–704.

45. Rosenberry, T. L., and Richardson, J. M. (1977): Structure of 18S and 14S acetylcholinesterase. Identification of collagen-like subunits that are linked by disulfide bonds to catalytic subunits. *Biochemistry*, 16:3550–3558.

46. Minor, R. R. (1980): Collagen metabolism: A comparison of diseases of collagen and diseases affecting collagen. *Am. J. Pathol.*, 98:226–280.

47. Prockop, D. J., Kivirikko, K. I., Tuderman, L., and Guzman, N. A. (1979): The biosynthesis of collagen and its disorders. *N. Engl. J. Med.*, 301:13–23.

48. Prockop, D. J., Kivirikko, K. I., Tuderman, L., and Guzman, N. A. (1979): The biosynthesis of collagen and its disorders. *N. Engl. J. Med.*, 301:77–85.

49. Guzelian, P. S., and Diegelmann, R. F. (1979): Localization of collagen prolyl-hydroxylase to the hepatocytes. *Exp. Cell Res.*, 123:269–279.

50. Rosenberg, L., Choi, H., Pal, S., and Tang, L. (1979): Carbohydrate-protein interactions in proteoglycans. In: *Carbohydrate-Protein Interaction*, edited by I. J. Goldstein, pp. 186–216. ACS Symposium Series No. 88.

51. Hardingham, T. E., and Muir, H. (1972): The specific interaction of hyaluronic acid with cartilage proteoglycans. *Biochim. Biophys. Acta*, 279:401–405.

52. Hascall, V. C., and Heinegard, D. (1974): Aggregation of cartilage proteoglycans. I. The role of hyaluronic acid. *J. Biol. Chem.*, 249:4232–4241.

53. Hascall, V. C., and Heinegard, D. (1974): Aggregation of cartilage proteoglycans. II. Oligosaccharide competitors of the proteoglycan-hyaluronic acid interaction. *J. Biol. Chem.*, 249:4242–4249.

54. Christner, J. E., Brown, M. L., and Dziewiatkowski, D. D. (1977): Interaction of cartilage proteoglycans with hyaluronic acid. The role of the hyaluronic acid carboxyl groups. *Biochem. J.*, 167:711–716.

55. Koizumi, T., Nakamura, N., and Abe, H. (1967): Changes in acid mucopolysaccharide in the liver in hepatic fibrosis. *Biochim. Biophys. Acta*, 148:749–756.

56. Ninomiya, Y., Hata, R., and Nagai, Y. (1980): Glycosaminoglycan synthesis by liver parenchymal cell clones in culture and its change with transformation. *Biochim. Biophys. Acta*, 629:349–358.

57. Oldberg, Å., Kjellén, L., and Höök, M. (1979): Cell-surface heparan sulfate. Isolation and characterization of a proteoglycan from rat liver membranes. *J. Biol. Chem.*, 254:8505–8510.

58. Buonassisi, V., and Root, M. (1975): Enzymatic degradation of heparin-related mucopolysaccharides from the surface of endothelial cell cultures. *Biochim. Biophys. Acta*, 385:1–10.

59. Kleinman, H. K., Silbert, J. E., and Silbert, C. K. (1975): Heparan sulfate of skin fibroblasts grown in culture. *Connect. Tissue Res.*, 4:17–23.

60. Kraemer, P. M., and Smith D. A. (1974): High molecular-weight heparan sulfate from the cell surface. *Biochem. Biophys. Res. Commun.*, 56:423–430.

61. Kjellén, L., Oldberg, A., Rubin, K., and Höök, M. (1977): Binding of heparin and heparan sulphate to rat liver cells. *Biochem. Biophys. Res. Commun.*, 74:126–133.

62. Timpl, R., Rohde, H., Gehron-Robey, P., Rennard, S. I., Foidart, J. M., and Martin, G. R. (1979): Laminin—A glycoprotein from basement membranes. *J. Biol. Chem.*, 254:9933–9937.

63. Rennard, S. I., Berg, R., Martin, G. R., Foidart, J. M., and Gehron-Robey, P. (1980): Enzyme-linked immunoassay (ELISA) for connective tissue components. *Anal. Biochem.*, 104:205–214.

64. Ekblom, P., Alitalo, K., Vaheri, A., Timpl, R., and Saxén, L. (1980): Induction of a basement membrane glycoprotein in embryonic kidney. Possible role of laminin in morphogenesis. *Proc. Natl. Acad. Sci. USA*, 77:485–489.

65. Alexander, S. S., Colonna, G., Yamada, K. M., Pastan, I., and Edelhoch, H. (1978): Molecular properties of a major cell-surface protein from chick-embryo fibroblasts. *J. Biol. Chem.*, 253:5820–5824.

66. Hynes, R. O. (1976): Cell surface proteins and malignant transformation. *Biochim. Biophys. Acta*, 458:73–107.

67. Vaheri, A., and Mosher, D. F. (1978): High molecular weight, cell surface-associated glycoprotein (fibronectin) lost in malignant transformation. *Biochim. Biophys. Acta*, 516:1–25.

68. Yamada, K. M., and Olden, K. (1978): Fibonectins-adhesive glycoproteins of cell surface and blood. *Nature*, 275:179–184.

69. Yamada, K. M., Schlesinger, D. H., Kennedy, D. W., and Pastan, I. (1977): Characterization of a major fibroblast cell surface glycoprotein. *Biochemistry*, 16:5552–5559.

70. Carter, W. G., Fukuda, M., Lingwood, C., and Hakomori, S. I. (1978): Chemical composition, gross structure and organization of transformation-sensitive glycoproteins. *Ann. NY Acad. Sci.*, 312:160–177.

71. Yamada, K. M., Olden, K., and Pastan, I. (1978): Transformation-sensitive cell surface protein. Isolation, characterization and role in cellular morphology and adhesion. *Ann. NY Acad. Sci.*, 312:256–277.

72. Takasaki, S., Yamashita, K., Suzuki, K., Iwanaga, S., and Kobata, A. (1979): The sugar chains of cold-insoluble globulin. A protein related to fibronectin. *J. Biol. Chem.*, 254:8548–8553.

73. Hedman, K., Vaheri, A., and Wartiovaara, J. (1978): External fibronectin of cultured human fibroblasts is predominantly a matrix protein. *J. Cell Biol.*, 76:748–760.

74. Linder, E., Stenman, S., Lehto, V. P., and Vaheri, A. (1978): Distribution of fibronectin in human tissues and relationship to other connective tissue components. *Ann. NY Acad Sci.*, 312:151–159.

75. Matzuda, M., Yoshida, N., Aoki, N., and Wakabayashi, K. (1978): Distribution of cold-insoluble globulin in plasma and tissues. *Ann. NY Acad Sci.*, 312:74–92.

76. Stenman, S., and Vaheri, A. (1978): Distribution of a major connective tissue protein fibronectin, in normal human tissues. *J. Exp. Med.*, 147:1054–1064.

77. Yamada, K. M., and Weston, J. A. (1974): Isolation of a major cell surface glycoprotein from fibroblasts. *Proc. Natl. Acad. Sci. USA*, 71:3492–3496.

78. Yamada, K. M., Yamada, S. S., and Pastan, I. (1977): Quantitation of a transformation-sensitive, adhesive cell, surface glycoprotein. *J. Cell Biol.*, 74:649–654.

79. Hynes, R. O., and Destree, A. T. (1978): Relationships between fibronectin (LETS protein) and actin. *Cell*, 15:875–886.

80. Hynes, R. O., and Bye, J. M. (1974): Density and cell cycle

dependence of cell surface proteins in hamster fibroblasts. *Cell,* 3:113–120.

81. Burridge, K. (1976): Changes in cellular glycoproteins after transformation: Identification of specific glycoproteins and antigens in sodium dodecyl sulfate gels. *Proc. Natl. Acad. Sci. USA,* 73:4457–4461.

82. Chen, L. B., Gallimore, P. H., and McDougall, J. K. (1976): Correlation between tumor induction and the large external transformation sensitive protein on the cell surface. *Proc. Natl. Acad. Sci. USA,* 73:3570–3574.

83. Vaheri, A., Ruoslahti, E., Westermark, B., and Pontén, J. (1976): A common cell-type specific surface antigen in cultured human glial cells and fibroblasts: Loss in malignant cells. *J. Exp. Med.,* 143:64–72.

84. Mosesson, M. W., Umfleet, R. A. (1970): The cold-insoluble globulin of human plasma. I. Purification, primary characterization, and relationship to fibrinogen and other cold-insoluble fraction components. *J. Biol. Chem.,* 245:5728–5736.

85. Vuento, M., and Vaheri, A. (1979): Purification of fibronectin from human plasma by affinity chromatography under nondenaturing conditions. *Biochem. J.,* 183:331–337.

86. Engvall, E., Ruoslahti, E., and Miller, E. J. (1978): Affinity of fibronectin to collagens of different genetic types and to fibrinogen. *J. Exp. Med.,* 147:1584–1595.

87. Jilek, F., and Hörmann, H. (1979): Fibronectin (cold-insoluble globulin). VI. Influence of heparin and hyaluronic acid on the binding of native collagen. *Hoppe Seylers Z. Physiol. Chem.,* 360:597–603.

88. Gold, L. I., García-Pardo, A., Frangione, B., Franklin, E. C., and Pearlstein, E. (1979): Subtilisin and cyanogen bromide cleavage products of fibronectin that retain gelatin-binding activity. *Proc. Natl. Acad. Sci. USA,* 76:4803–4807.

89. Hahn, L. E., and Yamada, K. M. (1979): Isolation and biological characterization of active fragments of the adhesive glycoprotein fibronectin. *Cell,* 18:1043–1051.

90. Sekiguchi, K., and Hakomori, S. (1980): Functional domain structure of fibronectin. *Proc. Natl. Acad. Sci. USA,* 77:2661–2665.

91. Balian, G., Click, E. M., Crouch, E., Davidson, J. M., and Bornstein, P. (1979): Isolation of a collagen-binding fragment from fibronectin and cold-insoluble globulin. *J. Biol. Chem.,* 254:1429–1432.

92. Olden, K., Pratt, R. M., and Yamada, K. M. (1979): Role of carbohydrate in biological function of the adhesive glycoprotein fibronectin. *Proc. Natl. Acad. Sci. USA,* 76:3343–3347.

93. Ruoslahti, E., Hayman, E. G., Kuusela, P., Shively, J. E., and Engvall, E. (1979): Isolation of a tryptic fragment containing the collagen-binding site of plasma fibronectin. *J. Biol. Chem.,* 254:6054–6059.

94. Balian, G., Click, E. M., and Bornstein, P. (1980): Location of a collagen-binding domain in fibronectin. *J. Biol. Chem.,* 255:3234–3236.

95. Dessau, W., Adelmann, B. C., Timpl, R., and Martin, G. R. (1978): Identification of the sites in collagen α-chains that bind serum anti-gelatin factor (cold-insoluble globulin). *Biochem. J.,* 169:55–59.

96. Kleinman, H. K., McGoodwin, E. B., Martin, G. R., Klebe, R. J., Fietzek, P. P., and Woolley, D. E. (1978): Localization of binding-site for cell attachment in alpha-1(I) chain of collagen. *J. Biol. Chem.,* 253:5642–5656.

97. Kleinman, H. K., Hewitt, A. T., Murray, J. C., Liotta, L. A., Rennard, S. I., Pennypacker, J. P., McGoodwin, E. B., Martin, G. R., and Fishman, P. H. (1979): Cellular and metabolic specificity in the interaction of adhesion proteins with collagen and with cells. *J. Supramol. Struct.,* 11:69–78.

98. Kleinman, H. K., Martin, G. R., and Fishman, P. H. (1979): Ganglioside inhibition of fibronectin-mediated cell adhesion to collagen. *Proc. Natl. Acad. Sci. USA,* 76:3367–3371.

99. Mosher, D. F. (1975): Cross-linking of cold insoluble globulin by fibrin stabilizing factor. *J. Biol. Chem.,* 250:6614–6621.

100. Mosher, D. F., Schad, P. E., and Kleinman, H. K. (1979):

101. Mosher, D. F., Schad, P. E., and Vann, J. M. (1980): Cross-linking of collagen and fibronectin by factor XIIIa. *J. Biol. Chem.,* 255:1181–1188.

102. Birckbichler, P. J., and Patterson, M. K. (1978): Cellular transglutaminase, growth and transformation. *Ann. NY Acad. Sci.,* 312:354–365.

103. Voss, B., Allam, S., Rauterberg, J., Ullrich, K., Gieselmann, V., and Von Figura, K. (1979): Primary cultures of rat hepatocytes synthesize fibronectin. *Biochem. Biophys. Res. Commun.,* 90:1348–1354.

104. Rojkind, M., Gatmaitan, Z., Mackensen, S., Giambrone, M. A., Ponce, P., and Reid, L. M. (1980): Connective tissue biomatrix: Its isolation and utilization for long-term cultures of normal rat hepatocytes. *J. Cell Biol.,* 87:255–263.

105. Wolff, I., Fuchswans, W., Weiser, M., Furthmayr, H., and Timpl, R. (1971): Acidic structural proteins of connective tissue. Characterization of their heterogeneous nature. *Eur. J. Biochem.,* 20:426–431.

106. Reid, L. M., and Rojkind, M. (1979): New techniques for culturing differentiated cells: Reconstituted basement membrane rafts. *Methods Enzymol.,* 58:263–278.

107. Bottenstein, J., Hayashi, I., Hutchings, S., Masui, H., Mather, J., McClure, D. B., Ohasa, S., Rizzino, A., Sato, G., Serrero, R., Wolfe, R., and Wu, R. (1979): The growth of cells in serum-free hormone-supplemented media. *Methods Enzymol.,* 58:94–109.

108. Rubin, K., Oldberg, Å., Höök, M., and Öbrink, B. (1978): Adhesion of rat hepatocytes to collagen. *Exp. Cell Res.,* 117:165–177.

109. Seglen, P. O., and Fossa, J. (1978): Attachment of rat hepatocytes *in vitro* to substrata of serum protein, collagen, or concanavalin A. *Exp. Cell Res.,* 116:199–206.

110. Sirica, A. E., Richards, W., Tsukada, Y., Sattler, C. A., and Pitot, H. C. (1979): Fetal phenotypic expression by adult rat hepatocytes on collagen gel/nylon meshes. *Proc. Natl. Acad. Sci. USA,* 76:283–287.

111. Michalopoulos, G., Russell, F., and Biles, C. (1979): Primary cultures of hepatocytes on human fibroblasts. *In Vitro,* 15:796–806.

112. Reid, L., Gatmaitan, Z., Arias, I. M., and Rojkind, M. (1979): Prolonged cultures of hepatocytes and other epithelial cells: a progress report. In: *Communications of Liver Cells,* edited by H. Popper, L. Bianchi, F. Gudat, and W. Reutter, pp. 157–166, MTP Press, Lancaster, England.

113. Reid, L. M., Gatmaitan, Z., Arias, I., Ponce, P., and Rojkind, M. (1980): Long-term cultures of normal rat hepatocytes on liver biomatrix. *Ann. NY Acad. Sci.,* 349:70–76.

114. Murray, J. C., Stingl, G., Kleinman, H. K., Martin, G. R., and Katz, S. I. (1979): Epidermal cells adhere preferentially to type IV (basement membrane) collagen. *J. Cell Biol.,* 80:197–202.

115. Hewitt, A. T., Kleinman, H. K., Pennypacker, J. P., and Martin, G. R. (1980): Identification of an adhesion factor for chondrocytes. *Proc. Natl. Acad. Sci. USA,* 77:385–388.

116. Gospodarowicz, D., Delgado, D., and Vlodavsky, I. (1980): Permissive effect of the extracellular matrix on cell proliferation *in vitro. Proc. Natl. Acad. Sci. USA,* 77:4094–4098.

117. Gospodarowicz, D., and Ill, C. R. (1980): Do plasma and serum have different abilities to promote cell growth? *Proc. Natl. Acad. Sci. USA,* 77:2726–2730.

118. Ponce, P., Cordero, J., and Rojkind, M. (1981): A noncollagenous matrix for attachment of rat hepatocytes in culture. *Hepatology,* 1:204–210.

119. West, C. M., Lanza, R., Rosenbloom, J., Lowe, M., Holtzer, H., and Avdalovic, N. (1979): Fibronectin alters the phenotypic properties of cultured chick embryo chondroblasts. *Cell,* 17:491–501.

120. Hynes, R. O., Destree, A. T., Perkins, M. E., and Wagner, D. D. (1979): Cell surface fibronectin and oncogenic transformation. *J. Supramol. Struct.,* 11:95–104.

Cross-linking of fibronectin to collagen by blood coagulation factor XIIIa. *J. Clin. Invest.,* 64:781–787.

SECTION III

Interrelated Cellular Functions

The Liver: Biology and Pathobiology, edited by
I. Arias, H. Popper, D. Schachter, and D. A. Shafritz.
Raven Press, New York © 1982.

Chapter 33

Plasma Membrane Receptors and Function

Pierre De Meyts and Jacques Hanoune

HORMONAL REGULATION OF LIVER METABOLISM

The liver plays a major role in the metabolism of carbohydrates, lipids, and proteins, and its metabolic function is controlled by a network of different hormones. The plasma membrane of the liver cell is a strategic locus for the interaction between intracellular and extracellular factors and, in addition to its various transport functions, constitutes the privileged interface that mediates the coupling between external signals and biological effects (1).

The first step in the action of polypeptide hormones

and catecholamines, as well as other active agents (viruses, drugs, toxins), is their binding to specific molecular structures (often glycoproteins) embedded in the cell membrane, called receptors. The receptor concept, first proposed by J. N. Langley more than a century ago [for historical review, see De Meyts and Rousseau (2)], has undergone an explosive development over the last decade through direct studies with radioactive ligands, and the receptor molecules, some of which are now being isolated and purified, are getting within reach of the sophisticated techniques of molecular biology.

The liver plasma membrane possesses specific receptors for insulin, glucagon, catecholamines, para-thyrin, growth hormone, prolactin, vasopressin, oxytocin, angiotensin, secretin, vasoactive intestinal peptide (VIP), and prostaglandins. Other hormones, such as thyroxine and steroids, act through intracellular receptors in the cytoplasm and nucleus. In this chapter, we will not provide an exhaustive review of the characteristics of all these receptors, but instead focus on those receptors that have been sufficiently studied to provide a meaningful overview of their structure, function, and physiological regulation, as well as of their mode of coupling to intracellular functions (to complement this review, the reader may profitably consult refs. 1, 3, and 4).

Among the many metabolic pathways under hormonal control in the liver, the regulation of glycogen metabolism has been the most comprehensively studied (for review, see ref. 5). The effect of hormones on glycogen metabolism can be classified as "catabolic" (glucagon, adrenergic agonists, vasopressin, angiotensin II, parathyrin, secretin, VIP, oxytocin) and "anticatabolic" (insulin, adrenal steroids). Hormones with catabolic effects, i.e., which stimulate the breakdown of hepatic glycogen, act at least partly by increasing the amount of phosphorylase *a* in the liver. For most hormones, this is done through a mechanism that involves the activation of the adenylate cyclase system and the resultant increase in cyclic AMP (Fig. 1). The catabolic effect of α-adrenergic agonists, vasopressin and angiotensin, however, is under normal circumstances linked to mechanisms which do not involve purine nucleoside cyclic monophosphates, but may involve such intracellular signals as Ca^{2+}, K^+, and phosphatidylinositol breakdown (5).

The mode of action of "anticatabolic" hormones such as insulin, beyond the initial receptor binding step, is still very poorly understood. The membrane receptor for insulin, however, has been one of the most thoroughly investigated hormonal receptors, and its regulation in normal and disease states is now extensively documented.

Understandably, the bulk of this review will focus on insulin receptors, on the one hand, and receptors mediating hormonal responses through the adenylate

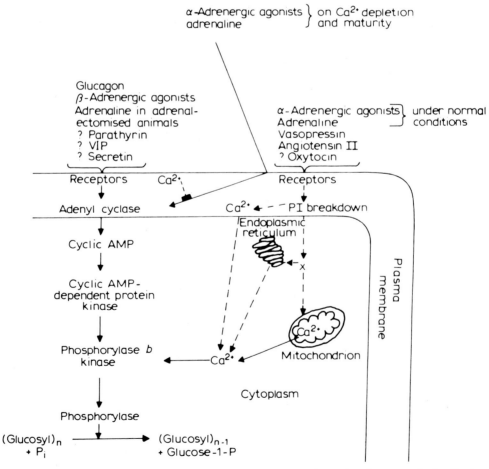

FIG. 1. Possible mechanisms of action of catabolic hormones on rat hepatic glycogenolysis. Dashed lines refer to postulated mechanisms. ■, negative effect. PI, phosphatidyl inositol; VIP, vasoactive intestinal peptide. From ref. 5, with permission.

cyclase system, essentially those for glucagon and catecholamines, on the other.

HISTORICAL ASPECTS OF MEMBRANE RECEPTORS

The localization in the plasma membrane of the receptors for polypeptide hormones has been suspected for a long time; as early as 1949, Levine and co-workers (6) suggested that the primary step in insulin action was at the membrane level, since insulin stimulated the transport of sugar across the plasma membrane. Also in 1949, Stadie et al. (7) found that brief incubation of rat hemidiaphragms with insulin induced a persistent effect on glycogen synthesis.

Seventeen years later, Pastan et al. (8) showed that this persistent effect of insulin was due to the existence of the hormone on the cell surface since washing the tissue with a solution containing anti-insulin antibodies reversed the effect. The same conclusions arose from experiments by Kono (9) who showed that trypsinization of fat cells destroyed their ability to respond to insulin without loss of cellular integrity, without alteration of the glucose transport system, and with an intact response to other hormones. This suggested that a peptide component on the cell surface, presumably the receptor, was necessary for the action of insulin.

This concept was reinforced by another type of indirect experiment done by Schimmer et al. with ACTH (10) and later by Cuatrecasas with insulin (11): hormones linked convalently to beads of large inert polymers such as cellulose or Sepharose were still biologically active, again suggesting that the hormone did not have to enter the cell to be active. Later, however, the beads were shown to leak biologically active hormone, which could account for the observed effect, questioning the validity of the original experiments (12–14).

Direct evidence that hormones bind to surface receptors had to wait until suitable methods for labeling the hormones, while maintaining their biological properties, were devised. As early as 1952, Stadie (15) had attempted to bind labeled insulin to target tissues. However, there were many questions about the biological activity of the labeled insulin and also about the specificity of the small amount of "binding" observed.

In 1969, two groups introduced methods for labeling polypeptide hormones that preserved their biological properties, as well as the use of analogs to define the specificity of the binding (16,17). These methods were the basis for studies of other cell surface receptors, e.g., neurotransmitters, lectins, opiates, LDL, etc. (for general reviews of cell surface receptors, see refs. 18–24).

BASIC TECHNIQUES FOR THE STUDY OF MEMBRANE RECEPTORS

Studying membrane receptors requires ideally:

- a radioactively labeled hormone that is biologically active,
- a suitable target tissue preparation,
- the measurement of a biological response in the tissue studied or, if not possible, evidence that a variety of hormone analogs bind to the tissue studied with a relative potency similar to that observed in a tissue where typical biological effects can be measured.

Radioactive Labeling of the Hormone

Roth (25) has formulated general principles for preparing monoiodo ^{125}I-polypeptide hormones of high specific radioactivity suitable for hormone receptor studies. They are based on the original iodination method of Hunter and Greenwood (26), but with important modifications to avoid the deleterious effects of the excess of chloramine-T or metabisulfite, or of overiodination of the hormone.

One approach is to label a small minority (10% or less) of the molecules with one I atom, followed by chemical separation of the uniodinated molecules from monoidohormone. The final product ("carrier-free" monoiodohormone) has one I atom per molecule but was never exposed to the vigorous conditions of the standard chloramine-T method.

The second approach ("stoichiometric iodination") induces directly, in a carefully controlled stepwise fashion, an average of 0.2 to 0.8 atoms of I per hormone molecule under special conditions, followed by a traditional purification step. A variable percentage of uniodinated hormone subsists in the preparation, but diiodination and loss of activity are minimal. For more specific details, see Roth (25) and Freychet and De Meyts (22).

Radiolabeled catecholamines are not easily prepared by the user and are usually bought from specialized companies. A discussion of the suitable ligands is found below in the section on identification and activation of β-adrenergic receptors.

A Suitable Target Tissue Preparation

Studies of hormone receptors have involved (for review, see refs. 19, 27, and 28):

Whole cells
- freshly isolated from blood, e.g., granulocytes, monocytes, red blood cells
- enzymatically isolated from the intact tissue, e.g., hepatocytes separated by collagenase

Broken cells
- homogenates
- crude plasma membranes
- purified plasma membranes

Soluble receptors
- water-soluble (spontaneously released or removed by trypsin)
- solubilized with a variety of detergents

The Measurement of a Biological Response

This is an ideal requirement to define a hormone-binding protein in a given tissue as the receptor. It is easy to meet for glucagon and hormones which act specifically by stimulating the adenylate cyclase in a restricted number of tissues (see section on the liver adenylate cyclase system, below). It is more complicated for a hormone-like insulin that exerts, besides its role in glucose homeostasis, a large variety of effects on many types of cells in the body. The second messenger for these actions is still unknown. The tissue in which insulin effects are most easy to measure is the adipose tissue, and isolated fat cells provide a sensitive assay system in which several effects of insulin and its analogs can be measured accurately (29). The specificity of insulin binding in a tissue in which no response can be measured must then be established by comparing the relative potencies for binding several insulin analogs in the tissue studied to their relative potencies in eliciting the classical insulin effects in a more respectable target tissue like fat (Fig. 2) (30).

A variety of insulin effects in the liver has been demonstrated (Table 1). However, to date, none of these has been used for detailed structure–activity relationships.

TABLE 1. *Main metabolic effects of insulin in the liver*[a]

Increase	Decrease
Triglyceride synthesis	Fatty acid oxidation to ketone bodies
Triglyceride secretion as VLDL	
Glycolysis	Glucose output
Glycogen synthesis	Glycogenolysis[b]
	Glucagon-stimulated cAMP levels
Amino acid transport (A system)	
Efficiency of ribosomal protein synthesis	
RNA and DNA synthesis	

[a] Compiled by B. Jeanrenaud.
[b] Basal or glucagon and epinephrine stimulated.

INSULIN RECEPTORS

General Properties of Insulin Receptors

Insulin receptors in tissues as different as lymphocytes and placenta, in species as divergent as man and fish, appear strikingly similar in all their properties: specificity, kinetics, pH optimum, regulation of receptor affinity (negative cooperativity). These properties recently have been reviewed extensively by Ginsberg (31).

Since some of the properties of the receptor have been documented in tissues other than liver, but are most likely relevant to liver receptors, given the striking similarity of the receptor in various tissues, we will include in this chapter data collected in nonliver tissue.

Association of ^{125}I-insulin with the receptors is rapid, and reversible upon dilution of the complex or

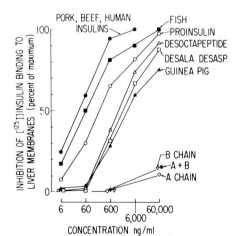

FIG. 2. Effect of insulin and insulin analogs on ^{125}I-insulin binding to liver membranes and on glucose oxidation in fat cells. **Left:** the inhibition of ^{125}I-insulin (porcine) binding to liver membranes expressed as percent of maximum is plotted as a function of the concentration on unlabeled peptide. **Right:** the stimulation of glucose oxidation in isolated fat cells expressed as percent of maximum is plotted as a function of the concentration of unlabeled peptide. From ref. 30, with permission.

addition of an excess of unlabeled insulin. The initial rate of insulin binding increases with temperature (32); as a result, the binding equilibrium shows a complex dependency of temperature suggestive of a reaction driven by hydrophobic forces (33). The pH optimum of binding is sharp with a maximum between 7.8 and 8.0 for most cells and species. In some, but not all, cases other components of the ionic environment also affect the binding (31). The most discriminative characteristic of the insulin receptor is its specificity. Insulins from various animal species, chemically modified insulin analogs, and peptides with insulin-like activity compete with ^{125}I-insulin for binding to the receptors in direct proportion to their biological activity (Fig. 3), in contrast to the type of specificity observed in the anti-insulin antibodies which appears unrelated to the biological potencies. The structure−activity relationships for insulin binding and action are further discussed below in the section on the structure−activity relationship of insulin.

The insulin receptor thus appears remarkably constant in all its properties. However, it should not be conceived as a rigid, fixed structure. In fact, in recent years, two properties of the receptor have been discovered that make the first step in insulin action, its binding to its surface receptor, a highly regulated step: insulin itself regulates the affinity of its receptor (negative cooperativity) (32,34,35) as well as the receptor concentration on the target cells (downregulation) (36,37). These properties have important implications in the pathophysiology of insulin action in man.

Regulation of Insulin Receptor Affinity: Negative Cooperativity

Binding of insulin, like many other polypeptide receptors in cell membranes, does not appear to follow simply the law of mass action (34,35). The Scatchard plot of insulin binding (a linear plot in simple systems)

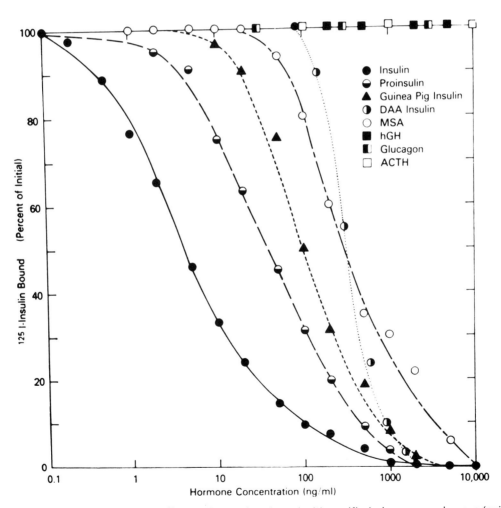

FIG. 3. Specificity of the insulin receptor. ^{125}I-insulin was incubated with purified plasma membranes (avian erythrocyte) in the presence of related and unrelated hormones. Competition for binding sites by each hormone was directly proportional to its biological activity. From ref. 31, with permission.

is curvilinear (Fig. 3). In the case of insulin, this appears to be due not to the presence of distinct classes of receptor sites, but to a regulation of the affinity of the receptors by insulin itself (32,34,35).

The receptor sites appear as a homogeneous class of sites with high affinity at low saturation with insulin, but the affinity of the receptor sites decreases as their occupancy with insulin increases (negative cooperativity) (Fig. 4). This is mediated mostly through a modulation of the dissociation rate of the insulin-receptor complex, which is accelerated when more insulin binds to the receptor sites. This regulation is accomplished by the induction of site–site interactions among the receptors, and not insulin–insulin interactions in the medium or on one receptor site (38,39).

Physiological concentrations of insulin are sufficient to induce a significant loss of affinity in the receptors (33). The precise physical mechanism underlying the negative cooperativity is not known, but has been the object of intense discussions (40–42). What is clear is that the acceleration in the dissociation rate is induced by binding to the receptor of a distinct domain on the surface of the insulin monomer or "cooperative site" (38), see section on structure–activity relationship of insulin, below. Chemical modification of the cooperative site leads to a loss of the negative cooperativity, as in desalanine-desasparagine insulin or desoctapeptide insulin (34,39). Dimerization of insulin, which occurs only at very high insulin concentrations, causes a covering of the cooperative site, and hence the disappear-

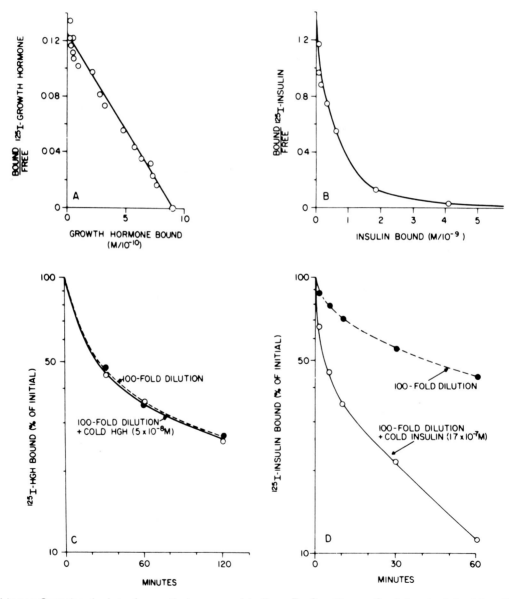

FIG. 4. A: Linear Scatchard plot of growth hormone binding. **B:** Curvilinear Scatchard plot of insulin binding. **C:** Dissociation curve of ^{125}I-growth hormone following a 100-fold dilution in the presence or absence of unlabeled growth hormone. **D:** Dissociation curves of ^{125}I-insulin following a 100-fold dilution in the presence or absence of unlabeled growth hormone. From ref. 34, with permission.

ance of the negative cooperativity at high concentrations of insulin. More recent experiments have used desalanine-desasparagine (DAA) insulin, previously shown to be unable to accelerate the dissociation rate of ^{125}I-insulin. DAA insulin can be labeled like insulin with ^{125}I. ^{125}I-DAA insulin binds to the same number of receptor sites as insulin, with about 10% of the affinity of insulin, but gives linear Scatchard plots.

Also, unlabeled insulin becomes unable to induce the acceleration in the dissociation rate of ^{125}I-insulin if the receptor sites are saturated with unlabeled DAA prior to the addition of the unlabeled insulin (antagonism for the negative cooperativity).

Taken together, these data strongly support the presence of only one class of insulin receptor sites on cells, all with high affinity in the absence of insulin (affinity constant = $\overline{K}_e$), and shifting reversibly to a low affinity state (affinity constant = $\overline{K}_f$) in the presence of increased insulin concentrations because of insulin-induced site–site interactions.

New methods to analyze the data according to this model have been proposed (43,44), which have been applied to various experimental and clinical situations.

Other Regulators of Insulin Receptor Affinity

The affinity of the insulin receptors is affected, not only by insulin, but also by other factors: pH, ions (see above), and probably some metabolic factors still largely unknown. Hence, the affinity of the insulin receptor is enhanced in man after acute fast (in obese patients) or 5 hr after an acute glucose load (45,46). It has also been suggested that ketoacids modulate the affinity of the insulin receptor. The levels of gluco-

corticoids and growth hormone have a marked effect on the affinity of the insulin receptor (47).

Regulation of Insulin Receptor Concentration or "Downregulation"

Insulin receptors, like other membrane proteins, are turning over continuously, and the receptor concentration at any time reflects the net effect of receptor synthesis and receptor degradation. The normal cellular concentration of insulin receptors varies from 27 sites/cell in human erythrocytes to 300,000 sites/cell in human adipocytes. Recent studies both *in vitro* and *in vivo* have shown that the receptor concentration is also subject to regulation and that the major factor regulating the insulin concentration is insulin itself. There is an inverse correlation between the insulin level in the medium and the cellular concentration of receptors; high levels of insulin cause a decrease in the insulin receptor concentration on cells ("downregulation"), and lowered levels of insulin are often followed by a rise in the number of sites per cell.

Studies In Vitro

This downregulation has been shown *in vitro* by Gavin et al. (36). When human lymphocytes were cultured in the presence of concentrations of insulin ranging from 10^{-8} M to 10^{-6} M, there was a time- and concentration-dependent decrease in insulin binding (Fig. 5). Scatchard plots demonstrated that the decreased binding was due solely to a decreased receptor number with no change in affinity for insulin (36) or negative cooperativity (37). The loss of receptors is

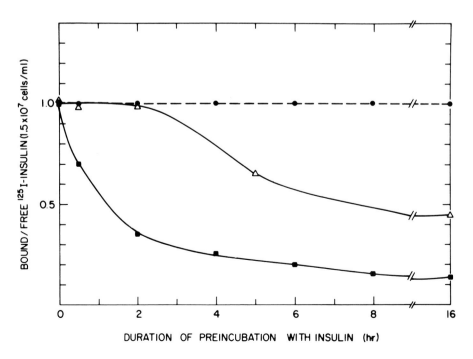

FIG. 5. Down regulation of insulin receptors on cultured human lymphocytes *in vitro* by increased concentrations (10^{-8} M, 10^{-6} M) of ambiant insulin. From ref. 36, with permission.

proportional to the insulin concentration in the medium. The insulin-induced loss of receptors is mediated through binding of insulin to its biologically relevant receptors, since the relative potency analogs in inducing the downregulation is similar to their relative potency in binding to the receptor and inducing the classical biological effects of insulin (48). The exact mechanism of downregulation is unknown but probably involves the now well-documented internalization of the insulin receptor complex (see section on internalization of insulin, below). Receptor occupancy is necessary for downregulation, but is not sufficient. So, the downregulation of insulin receptors is partially blocked by cycloheximide, suggesting that protein synthesis is required (49). Lowering the temperature to 23°C also substantially reduces the downregulation. It is also blocked by energy inhibitors. Removal of insulin from the medium is followed by progressive restoration of the original receptor concentration. This process is also blocked by insulin, at concentration as low as 10^{-9} M. The insulin receptor concentration has also been shown to vary during the growth of cells in culture: cultured mouse fibroblasts bind 5 to 10 times more insulin in the stationary than in the early logarithmic growth phase (50,51). The receptor concentration depends also on the cell cycle: cells arrested in G_0 phase have high levels of insulin binding, drops in levels during the cell cycle, and increases again after mitosis when the cells enter the G_1 phase (51). Fibroblasts transformed by DNA or RNA viruses, X-rays, or chemical carcinogens bind less insulin (50) owing to a reduction in receptor concentration. Glucocorticoids may also have a direct effect on insulin receptor concentration or affinity (47,52,53), as well as direct effects on the glucose oxidation pathway (54,55).

Studies In Vivo

Studies *in vivo* in animals and humans have demonstrated a quasi general relationship between increased insulin levels and decreased insulin receptor concentrations, a direct pathophysiological application of the concept of downregulation.

The best studied animal model of insulin-induced changes in receptor concentration is the genetically obese mouse of the ob/ob strain. These mice have hyperphagia, hyperglycemia, hyperinsulinemia, and marked resistance to endogenous or exogenous insulin (56).

Liver membranes of ob/ob mice bind only 25% of the insulin bound by their thin litter mates; the decreased binding is due purely to a decreased concentration of receptors. The remaining receptors are entirely normal (57–59). The decrease in receptor concentration appears to be generalized and is also found in adipocytes (60), myocardium (61), skeletal muscle

(62), and thymic lymphocytes (63). The decreased receptor concentration was directly related to chronic hyperinsulinemia. Acute injection of insulin prior to killing the mice did not lower the receptor concentration. In contrast, hyperinsulinemia associated with both genetic and acquired obesity led to a loss of receptors (64–66). In gold thioglucose-induced obesity, the loss of receptors was proportional to the body weight and hyperinsulinemia, and after a chronic fast, obese animals returned to normal body weight, normal blood insulin, and normal receptor concentration. Reduction of insulin levels by treatment of ob/ob mice with either streptozotocin or alloxan led to an increased insulin receptor concentration (Freychet P, *personal communication*) and sensitivity to exogenous insulin (67). Fasting of ob/ob mice also led to a decrease in circulating insulin levels and an increase in the concentration of insulin receptors. Thus, reduction in hyperinsulinemia with or without weight loss led to an increased sensitivity to insulin and an increase in insulin receptors.

The inverse relationship between insulin levels and receptor concentration has also been studied extensively in humans, using peripheral mononuclear cells (45,68–70) or adipocytes (71,72). Mononuclear cells from human blood (essentially monocytes) contain insulin receptors that are identical in properties and specificity to receptors in classical target tissues (73) and allow an easy nontraumatic study of insulin receptors in normal and diseased humans. More recently, red blood cells have also been used (74). In human obesity like in animal obesity, increased insulin levels were associated with a proportional reduction in receptor concentration. The results were remarkably similar when studies were done with peripheral blood cells (45) or adipose tissue (72). In contrast, peripheral blood cells from nonobese, nonketotic diabetics bind relatively more insulin than control subjects.

The inverse relationship between insulin levels and receptor concentrations appears to be general, from cultured cells studied *in vitro*, to animal models, to man (Fig. 6).

Structure–Activity Relationship of Insulin

Insulin is synthesized in the β-cell as a single-chain polypeptide, proinsulin (see Chapter by Rubinstein). After folding and correct arrangement of the three disulfide bridges, and removal of the connecting peptide, insulin assumes the now familiar three-dimensional structure revealed by X-ray crystallography (Fig. 7) (70). The biological potency of insulin is crucially dependent on the integrity of this three-dimensional structure. Studies of the biological activities, receptor affinities, and sequences of insulin from different animals strongly suggested that a largely invariant re-

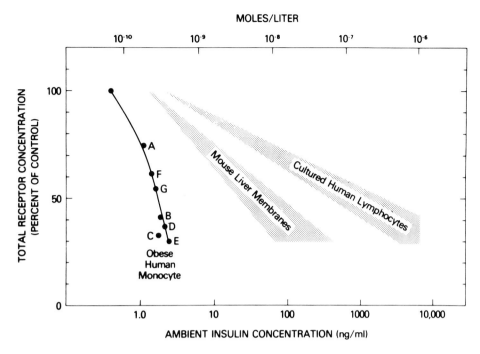

FIG. 6. Insulin receptor concentration as a function of ambiant insulin concentration. Letters A to G refer to individual obese patients. From ref. 45, with permission.

gion of the surface of the insulin monomer may be the receptor-binding region (Fig. 7) (38,75). This region includes both A-chain residues (A_1Gly, A_5Glu, A_{19}Tyr, and A_{21}Asn) and adjacent B-chain residues (B_{24}Phe, B_{25}Phe, B_{26}Tyr, B_{12}Val, and B_{16}Tyr).

More recently, a study of 29 insulin analogs suggested that a discrete invariable region on the surface of the insulin monomer is responsible for inducing the negative cooperativity (38). This domain comprises some of the eight carboxy-terminal residues of the B-chain and the A_{21}-asparagine. Chemical alteration of this "cooperative site" or its burying in the dimer of insulin leads to a loss of negative cooperativity.

Degradation of Insulin at the Cellular Level

Insulin, besides binding to its receptors on the cell surface, is degraded upon exposure to the cells. *In vitro* studies by several laboratories suggested that the majority of insulin degradation occurs at sites other than the receptor site (29,76–80). Indeed, insulin binding and degradation had different pH optima, ionic strength optima, temperature dependence, analog specificity, and ability to be inhibited by antireceptor antibodies. However, in contrast to most previous studies, Terris and Steiner (81,82) suggested that insulin degradation is closely linked to insulin binding. In their hands, the velocity of insulin degradation by isolated hepatocytes showed a first-order dependence on the total concentration of insulin bound at steady state. They also found that various insulin analogs depressed to the same degree the amount of ^{125}I-insulin bound

and the rate of ^{125}I-insulin degradation. Some methodological differences may account for these discrepancies. So Terris and Steiner studied first perfused livers, and then intact hepatocytes, and not purified membranes; bound insulin in their study included nonspecific binding. Further studies are needed to resolve these differences.

The exact enzymatic mechanism by which insulin is normally degraded in cells is not clear, but several enzymes have been described that may be operative, including GSH-insulin transhydrogenase (83,84), a reductase that cleaves S–S bonds, and proteases that act by peptide bond cleavage (85,86) (for review, see ref. 87).

More recent information suggests that, even if the bulk of the insulin degradation is unrelated to receptor binding, the bound insulin itself is nevertheless subject to compartmentalization, processing, and degradation. Kahn and Baird (88) found that insulin bound to adipocytes at 37°C becomes progressively less dissociable with time, suggesting that the bound insulin is rapidly altered or transferred into a "compartment," which is less accessible or less influenced by the effects of dissociating agents in the external milieu. The bound insulin also appeared to be processed to higher and lower molecular weight components, including iodotyrosyl fragments. The observed compartmentalization may be related to internalization of insulin (see the next section on internalization of insulin). Gleimann and Sonne (89), using a different technique, including conditions that minimized insulin degradation in the medium by nonreceptor mechanisms (protease. . .),

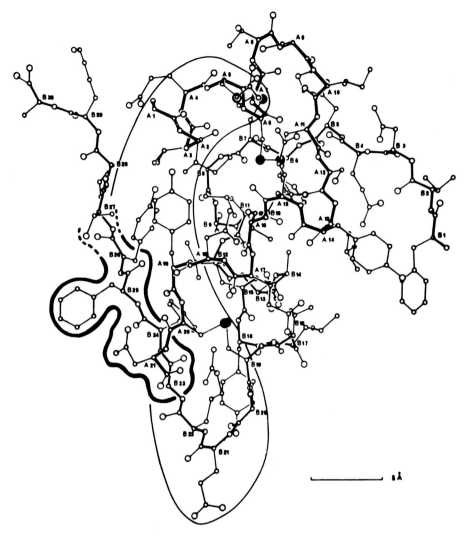

FIG. 7. Structural determinants of insulin receptor binding and negative cooperativity. From ref. 38, with permission.

found that at least 90% of the cell-bound radioactivity was ^{125}I-insulin and less than 5% iodotyrosine. However, about half of the radioactivity dissociated from the cells as iodotyrosine, the other half being iodoinsulin. The same fraction of receptor-bound iodoinsulin was degraded at receptor occupancies ranging from 1 to 90%. They suggested that in the steady state, half of the bound (iodo) insulin molecules are degraded whereas the other half dissociate in intact form. This occurs at any receptor occupancy. Any initially formed labeled peptide is rapidly degraded to iodotyrosine which is immediately released into the medium. Gammeltoft et al. (90), also while minimizing degradation by extracellular proteases, had very similar findings in isolated hepatocytes: the ^{125}I-activity released from the cells was 50% immunoreactive insulin, suggesting that insulin is inactivated in relation to receptor binding. The residual part was released as nonimmunoreactive ^{125}I-activity with a half-life of

about 3 hr, suggesting internalization and degradation of part of the receptor-bound insulin.

The molecular mechanism of receptor-mediated degradation is not known. The receptor and the degrading enzyme may be subunits of the same membrane macromolecule, or the receptor may transfer some insulin molecules to a degrading site in the membrane (89).

A question that remains to be solved is what role compartmentalization and degradation play in the biological action of insulin.

Internalization of Insulin

As we have already noted above, in the section on the general properties of insulin receptors, early studies of insulin effects suggested that the primary action of insulin was at the cell membrane. The direct demonstration that the first interaction is indeed with cell surface receptors led to a strong belief that insulin does not need to enter the cell to act, and that surface binding is both necessary and sufficient. However, there were no objective data showing that the hormone does not penetrate the cell surface after the receptor-binding step, especially after active hormones bound to beads were shown to be leaking.

However, several authors found typical receptors for insulin (20,91–94) and other polypeptides (95,96) on intracellular structures, including the nucleus (92, 93). This was in no way evidence for internalization of the hormone, since these intracellular receptors may be part of the biosynthetic cycle of the receptor, or a consequence of membrane recycling. Yet, evidence has accumulated which suggests that the polypeptide hormones themselves in fact enter the cells, although exactly how they get in is still open to question (97).

Two distinct morphological approaches have been used to demonstrate this internalization.

Autoradiography

Radioactively labeled insulin was allowed to bind to the cells, which were subsequently submitted to light or electron microscopic examination and autoradiography. Using light microscopy and autoradiography, Goldfine et al. (93) saw uptake and subsequent nuclear localization of labeled insulin incubated with human cultured lymphocytes in growth medium at 37°C. They also found some labeled insulin in the nuclei, isolated from other cellular fractions. In contrast, Carpentier et al. (98), using quantitative electron microscopy and autoradiography of cultured human lymphocytes, saw at 37°C only a small but definite translocation of the label, after an initial localization at a line source corresponding to the plasma membrane; this translocation did not extend beyond 10 to 15% of the cell radius. They found no preferential localization to any intracellular organelle. At 15°C, they found no translocation of the label as a function of time. These binding experiments were done in assay buffer and not in growth medium. With isolated hepatocytes, using the same technique, Gorden et al. showed that insulin binding is initially restricted at the plasma membrane, but with increasing time and temperature of incubation, there is a systematic and progressive translocation of autoradiography gains to a highly limited area of the cell periphery representing no more than 15% of the radius of the cell. Gorden and Carpentier showed that after internalization the labeled material becomes associated with lysosomes (99). Gorden et al. found similar data with EGF (epidermal growth factor) (100),

confirming the prediction based on binding studies of Carpenter and Cohen (101).

Video Intensification Microscopy of Fluorescent Hormone Derivatives

Highly fluorescent analogs of insulin and epidermal growth factor were prepared by Schechter et al. (102) by covalent attachment of these peptides to lactalbumin molecules which were highly substituted with rhodamine molecules. These derivatives partially retained their biological activity and ability to bind to the receptors. Using these derivatives, and a sophisticated video intensification microscopic technique, Schlesinger et al. (103) showed that initially, these hormone receptors are distributed diffusely on the cell surface of cultured fibroblasts, that the hormone receptor complexes are initially mobile on the plasma membrane, and that within a few minutes at 37°C the hormone receptor complexes form patches which are immobile. After 30 min at 37°C, the fluorescence could not be removed from the cells by trypsin, suggesting that the hormones had been internalized. Simultaneous and sequential incubations with different fluorescent derivatives of insulin, epidermal growth factor, and α_2 macroglobulin (104) showed that all these ligands concentrate in the same locations on the cell surface and are internalized by a common mechanism in endocytic vesicles, which probably pinch off from specialized (coated) regions of the cell surface. After 24 hr, the fluorescent label is found in phase-dense structures which are probably lysosomal.

In summary, from these studies it seems clear that insulin and other polypeptides, after their initial receptor-binding step, are able to penetrate inside the cell, at least to a limited extent, probably by endocytosis through clathrin-coated pits, and end up in endocytic vesicles possibly associated with lysosomes. Whereas the linkage between this process and receptor-bound degradation of hormone (see section on degradation of insulin at the cellular level, above) is likely, the relationship between internalization and downregulation, on the one hand, and biological effects of the hormone, on the other, remains largely speculative at this point.

Role of the Receptor *In Vivo* as a Reservoir for Plasma Hormones (105)

From measurements *in vivo* of the affinity and the concentration of insulin receptors in various tissues, Zeleznik and Roth estimated that *in vivo* about one-half of the extrapancreatic hormone is actually bound to receptors, and that a receptor compartment should be demonstrable in the whole animal *in vivo*. For this purpose, they injected rabbits intravenously with a labeled insulin that has low affinity for receptors (^{131}I-guinea pig insulin) in combination with a radioiodinated insulin that has high affinity for the receptor (^{125}I-porcine or chicken insulin). Plasma concentrations of the two labeled insulins were measured at selected intervals after injection. Apparent volumes of distribution were calculated by extrapolation of plasma disappearance curves; high affinity insulins consistently distributed into spaces that were two to three times greater than those of the low affinity insulins.

Injections of unlabeled pork insulin before the tracer insulins decreased the distribution space of the high affinity insulin in a dose-dependent manner but with little or no effect on the distribution space of the low affinity labeled insulin. When unlabeled insulin was injected after the tracer insulins, there was an immediate rise in the plasma concentration of the high affinity insulin with only a slight change in the plasma concentration of the low affinity insulin. These results demonstrated that high affinity insulins distributed into a body compartment that has many properties of the insulin receptor previously studied *in vitro*. This receptor compartment recognizes insulins based on their biological potencies, and is saturated by elevated concentrations of insulin. Insulin bound to receptors is in equilibrium with free hormone in the plasma.

Further, the bound:free ratios for hormone, calculated from these data, suggest that *in vivo* 50% of the extrapancreatic insulin is bound to receptors during normal physiological states. This study thus showed another function of the hormone interaction with the receptor, namely, that receptors act as a reservoir or capacitance *in vivo*, rapidly taking up hormone at times when the concentration of hormone in plasma is rising, and releasing hormone back into the plasma at times when the concentration of hormone in plasma is falling.

Evolution of the Insulin Receptor

Muggeo et al. (106) have examined the characteristics of the insulin receptor interaction in different species of vertebrates, including mammals (man, rat, mouse, guinea pig), birds (turkey and chicken), amphibians (frog), bony fish (trout), and a cyclostome (hagfish) (107). That study covers a period of evolution of about 500 million years. The low vertebrates, such as the frog and fish, and even the most primitive one, the hagfish, have insulin receptors that are virtually identical to those of birds and mammals. In particular, we find that the affinity of the insulin receptor for the various insulins and analogs is about the same in all species examined. In all species, chicken insulin bound to the receptor with a higher affinity than pork

insulin, which bound better than fish insulin, guinea pig insulin, hagfish insulin, and the modified insulin derivatives. This difference in affinity reflects the relative biological potency of each insulin in inducing insulin-like effects in mammalian tissues. Thus, the homologous insulin in a given species often bound less well to its own receptor than did insulins of other species.

We also found that in general there was reciprocal correlation between the concentration of the insulin receptor and the biopotency of the homologous insulin: thus, the guinea pig (which has a low affinity insulin) has partially compensated by having the highest concentration of insulin receptor on its cells, while the chicken and turkey (which have superpotent insulins) have the lowest receptor concentration.

In all the species examined, a reduction of receptor affinity, i.e., insulin-induced negatively cooperative site–site interactions among the receptors, was observed.

In addition to very strong functional similarities, insulin receptors from different species are blocked by one very potent serum containing antibodies to the insulin receptor, suggesting some structural similarities as well. However, with other antisera, differences in immunoreactivity were observed, suggesting that the insulin receptor, even if functionally well conserved during the evolution, has undergone some structural changes, probably in regions of the molecule not critical for its insulin-binding properties.

Isolation of the Insulin Receptor

The insulin receptor has been solubilized from a variety of tissues but is still actually far from purification (see refs. 31,108 for review). In work done before 1978, the insulin receptor was shown to be a highly asymmetric protein of molecular weight 300,000. This 300,000 molecular weight receptor may be composed of four subunits, each of about 75,000 daltons (31). Insulin binding seems to promote dissociation of the tetramer into its subunits, possible molecular concomitants of the negative cooperativity which is conserved in the solubilized receptor. In more recent work, two distinct components with distinct physicochemical properties were isolated (109,110). In one of these studies (109), one of the two components had a curvilinear Scatchard plot and the second one a linear plot. There was some interconversion of the two. Another study (110) suggested the interaction of a nonreceptor glycoprotein with another receptor component.

More recently developed affinity-labeling techniques have been used to study the subunit composition and stoichiometry of the insulin receptor. Work from several laboratories (for review, see ref. 108) converges to suggest that the minimum subunit structure consists of two α- and two β-glycoprotein subunits, all disulfide linked in a symmetrical receptor complex reminiscent of the general design of immunoglobulin G molecules (Fig. 8).

Coupling Between Insulin Receptor Binding and Biological Response

In several biological assays *in vitro,* such as those measuring the stimulation by insulin of glucose transport, glucose oxidation, or lipogenesis in isolated rat fat cells, the dose–response curve appears more sensitive by at least an order of magnitude than the concentration dependence of the binding isotherm: maximal biological response is achieved with filling 5 to 10% of the receptor sites. This is referred to as the "spare receptor phenomenon" and implies a rate-limiting step beyond receptor binding (for review, see ref. 111). The precise interpretation of this phenomenon depends on whether a negative cooperative model or a model assuming two classes of sites is considered: with the latter model, the response will be most closely coupled to the class with high affinity. However, sound interpretations of nonlinear coupling within the framework of a negative cooperative model can be proposed, and a detailed discussion of these still highly speculative aspects is beyond the scope of this review.

In isolated rat hepatocytes freshly isolated with collagenase, the degree of nonlinearity of the Scatchard plot at 37°C is minimal and a close coupling between binding to the high affinity sites (the major population) and biological response (transport of α-aminoisobutyric acid) can be demonstrated (112). In these conditions, the kinetic demonstration of negative cooperativity, i.e., the insulin-induced acceleration in the dissociation rate of the insulin receptor complex, is absent. However, after 48 hr of culture in monolayers, the Scatchard plot of binding becomes curvilinear again at 37°C, the kinetic negative cooperativity reap-

pears, and the coupling between binding and response is not close any more : the biological dose–response curve shifts by about an order of magnitude to the left of the binding curve (113). These preliminary data suggest that cooperative interactions may modulate the degree of coupling between binding and response, and that the phenomenon may be blurred by collagenase treatment in hepatocytes.

The nature of the second messenger(s) that mediates the effect of insulin in the target cell is still largely unknown. Several lines of evidence have been recently presented which support the hypothesis that the binding of insulin to adipopocyte plasma membranes activates a membrane protease which results in the production of a soluble factor that stimulates pyruvate dehydrogenase activity when added to mitochondria (114), suggesting that the mediator of insulin effects may be a peptide released by a proteolitic reaction. Such an activity was also observed using skeletal muscle which antagonized cyclic AMP activation of protein kinase and activated glycogen synthase phosphatase (115). The factor isolated from muscle was active in the adipocyte system, suggesting the same mediator was being extracted. These exciting new developments in the study of the mysterious mode of action of insulin are still unraveling as this review is being written.

THE LIVER ADENYLATE CYCLASE SYSTEM

The adenylate cyclase system is a multicomponent enzyme complex which catalyzes the transformation of ATP into cyclic AMP in response to stimulation by a variety of hormones and neuromediators. It is an integral part of the plasma membrane and consists of several distinct subunits. Hormonal receptors are located at the outer surface of the plasma membrane; the catalytic component is located at the inner surface, facing the cytosol. Binding of hormones to their receptors leads to an increase in cyclase activity by a coupling mechanism still largely unknown. Since the early work of Sutherland, numerous studies have been devoted to the hepatic adenylate cyclase system. This is probably due to the development of relatively easy methods to prepare purified plasma membranes and to assay the enzyme. To date, the hepatic adenylate cyclase system is probably one of the best known cyclase systems owing mainly to the activity of the group of Martin Rodbell, who established the kinetic features of the enzyme mechanism and discovered the role of guanosine triphosphate (GTP) in hormone action (116). Several reviews have dealt with adenylate cyclase (117,118); some of them were specifically focused on the hepatic enzyme (119). The human hepatic adenylate cyclase has also been extensively characterized (120).

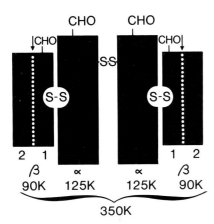

FIG. 8. Minimal subunit structure of the insulin receptor. From ref. 108, with permission.

Hormonal Activation of Liver Adenylate Cyclase

Glucagon activates *in vitro* the adenylate cyclase system in a concentration range from 1 nM to 10 μM. The effect is important (10- to 20-fold increase) and very rapid. Glucagon probably represents the main activator of liver cyclase physiologically: it is generally admitted that all the actions of glucagon upon liver are mediated by an increase in cyclic AMP production, leading to the activation of protein kinase and to the phosphorylation of a number of key enzymes.

The effect of catecholamines upon the cyclase system in liver is less marked and its physiological importance varies from species to species (secondary in rat and man; considerable in dog). It will be described below.

Among the intestinal factors that are endowed with hormonal action, three activate the liver cyclase. Their amino-acid sequence is in part common with that of glucagon: intestinal glucagon has a potency equal to 70% of that of pancreatic glucagon; *VIP* ("vasoactive intestinal peptide") and *secretin* are much less active. These stimulations, of imprecise physiological meaning, occur at two different receptor sites: one common for pancreatic and intestinal glucagon, the other common for secretin and VIP (121,122).

Parathyrin can also activate cyclase in a concentration range from 60 nM to 1 μM and with a potency intermediate between that of glucagon and of epinephrine. The 1-34 moiety of the molecule seems sufficient to activate the enzyme (123).

Prostaglandin PGE_1 also activates cyclase *in vitro* (124) but this might not be of physiological significance since PGE_1 inhibits the action of glucagon in perfused rat liver (125). PGE_1 and PGE_2 bind to a receptor in the plasma membrane which has been characterized and solubilized (126).

Finally, a whole variety of other proteic hormones have no effect upon the hepatic cyclase: gastrin, calcitonin, vasopressin, angiotensin, TSH, ACTH, etc.

Negative Regulation of Liver Adenylate Cyclase

The only compound which consistently inhibits cyclase is *adenosine* (127). The effect can be observed on both basal- and glucagon-stimulated cyclase activities and is highly sensitive to the concentration of bivalent cation in the assay medium. It should be noted that, as discussed by Fain and Shepherd (128), the physiological meaning of this inhibition has yet to be proven, all the more since this nucleotide is known to influence cyclic AMP synthesis in opposite ways depending on the tissue or the type of receptor involved.

An antagonistic action of *insulin* upon glucagon stimulation was shown in mouse liver (129), but was not reproducible in a particulate preparation of rat liver, and was also absent when studied in a purified preparation of plasma membrane from rat liver. Various claims have also been made concerning inhibition of hepatic cyclase activity by somatostatin, acetyl choline, α-adrenergic agonists, etc. The possibility that these inhibitory effects might be mediated by specific inhibitory GTP-binding components, as proposed by Rodbell (130), warrants further and more detailed investigation of these processes.

Role of Guanine Nucleotides

There is now general agreement that GTP plays a pivotal role in both stimulating cyclase activity and in mediating the action of hormones. The latter effect is twofold: GTP is necessary to the action of hormones upon cyclase; at the same time, it increases the dissociation rate of hormones (e.g., glucagon or agonist catecholamines) from their receptors. Reports from several laboratories indicate that GTP acts through one or several proteins, referred to by Rodbell as "nucleotide regulatory protein(s)" (abbreviated as "N", or N_1 and N_2 for the proteins linked to the receptor and the catalytic unit, respectively). There is also, in the cytosol of rat liver, a soluble activator of adenylate cyclase which, in many aspects, appears similar to GTP or to a GTP-protein complex (131) and which might be also involved in the receptor–cyclase coupling (132).

The Coupling Mechanism

The following features of the coupling process are now generally admitted: the nucleotide binding sites are supposed to be located at the inner surface of the plasma membrane, in order to be accessible to intracellular GTP (the concentration of total hepatic GTP is of the order of 0.4 mM, versus ten times as much for ATP). Binding of GTP to N(s) would bring about the functional linkage between receptor and cyclase. In the absence of GTP binding to N_1, the receptor would bind glucagon by a slow process leading to an essentially irreversible binding state of the hormone receptor complex, which cannot bind to the catalytic subunit. In the presence of GTP, the $R-N_1$ complex is able to link to the $E-N_2$ complex. On the other hand, the binding of GTP to N_2 transforms E into a high activity state (high Vmax). In this state, GTP is transformed into inert products GDP and Pi, and the nucleotide regulatory component uncouples, causing the system to revert to the original state.

This model accounts for the rapid on–off characteristics of all cyclase systems in response to hormones and GTP. It also accounts for the fact that analogs of GTP, such as Gpp (NH)p, that are not hydrolyzed at the terminal phosphate, lead to a persistent, high activity state of the enzyme, irrespective of the presence of hormone (133). GTPase activity is involved in degrading GTP at the N_2 site. Cassel and Selinger (134) have recently described a specific, catecholamine sensitive, GTPase in turkey erythrocytes that might be responsible for the turn-off of adenylate cyclase. Maybe as a result of the high level of nonspecific nucleotidase activity (135), a similar enzyme has not been conclusively demonstrated in rat liver plasma membranes. Yet its presence in all cyclase systems is an attractive possibility. Indeed, a confirmation of the possible regulatory role of GTPase has been brought about by the recent progress in the mechanism of action of choleratoxin. This toxin, injected *in vivo* or added *in vitro* to plasma membranes (in the presence of DTT, NAD, and a cytosolic factor), brings about an irreversible high activity state of the enzyme. In turkey erythrocytes, Cassel and Selinger have shown that this was correlated with an inhibition of the GTPase activity (136); the effect of GTP upon the toxin-treated liver membranes becomes similar to that of Gpp (NH)p (137). The mechanism of the action of cholera toxin is now being actively investigated. Several observations suggest that the toxin acts by catalyzing ADP-ribosylation of a membrane protein, which might be the GTP binding protein on the basis of structural (138) and genetic (139) criteria.

Conclusion

The ultimate aim of all investigators in the field is to solubilize the specific components of the adenylate cyclase system (catalytic moiety; regulatory entities; hormonal receptors) in order to reconstitute a complete, physiological system within a simpler environment.

Although the catalytic subunit, the N component, and some of the hormonal receptors have been solubilized and partially purified, this still appears a formidable task, all the more as the number of regulatory components of possible physiological importance keeps steadily increasing. For example, separate N subunits seem to mediate stimulating and inhibitory influences upon adenylate cyclase (130) and milk proteolysis irreversibly activates the hepatic enzyme by a mechanism independent of GTP and of N (140–142). The schematic representation, in Fig. 9, of current opinion regarding the molecular anatomy of the adenylate cyclase system, is an illustration of the complexity of the problem.

GLUCAGON RECEPTORS

Direct Studies with ^{125}I-Glucagon

Although the mode of action of glucagon which acts through the stimulation of adenylate cyclase and pro-

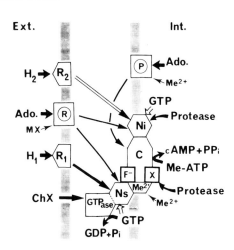

FIG. 9. The adenylate cyclase system. This scheme includes many of the various regulatory components which are thought to alter the activity of the catalytic subunit (C). This subunit, located at the inner surface of the plasma membrane, is under the direct stimulatory control of sites sensitive to fluoride ion (F^-) and divalent cations (Me^{2+}). It can also be directly inhibited by adenosine (Ado) via a specific receptor (P) also located at the inner surface of the membrane and in a manner highly dependent on divalent cation concentration. Stimulating hormones (H_1), after binding to receptors (R_1) at the outer surface of the membrane, activate C via a GTP-binding protein Ns itself endowed with, or connected to, a GTPase activity. Cholera toxin (ChX) inhibits this GTPase by an ADP-ribosylation process, and thereby activates cyclase. Inhibitory hormones (H_2), after binding to specific receptors (R_2), decrease cyclase activity via another GTP binding protein Ni. In some systems, adenosine, after binding to a specific receptor R, located at the outer surface of the membrane and different from the receptor P, can exert either positive or negative regulation on cyclase via Ns or Ni. Finally, the cyclase activity can be enhanced after proteolysis by an action upon Ni, or, more likely in liver, upon another regulatory site (X) and in a manner independent of GTP.

duction of cyclic AMP (143) is far better understood than the mode of action of insulin, studies of the receptor-binding step are much more scarce than those for insulin, and its regulation much less well known. One major problem is that ^{125}I-glucagon appears to be a less reliable tracer than ^{125}I-insulin. Whereas Rodbell and co-workers (144,145) found that iodoglucagon had the same potency as native glucagon in the adenylate cyclase system of liver membranes, Bromer et al. (146) found monoiodoglucagon about five times more potent than the native glucagon. Desbuquois (147) also found an increased receptor affinity and biological activity of iodoglucagon. However, the difference in affinity between glucagon and iodoglucagon is markedly pH dependent and some of the discrepancies between iodoglucagon and glucagon can be accounted for by partial ionization of the hydroxyl group of the iodinated tyrosyl residue due to an alteration of the pK of this group upon iodination (148). Another problem is the ease with which ^{125}I-glucagon is degraded during incubation with cells or cell preparations. This degradation could be reduced, even with whole cells, at 37°C by using bacitracin, low cell concentrations, and relatively short (60 to 90 min) incubation times. Despite these problems, some binding properties of glucagon have been studied in liver (whole cells, membranes, and in solubilized form), adipocytes, and β-cell membranes and are reviewed below.

General Properties of Glucagon Receptors

Few studies have been done with intact cells. In isolated hepatocytes at 37°C, Scatchard plots of glucagon binding were curvilinear (149). Since in these conditions, kinetic experiments did not demonstrate any acceleration of bound ^{125}I-glucagon by unlabeled glucagon, Sonne et al. concluded there was an absence of negative cooperativity, and explained the data by the presence of two classes of saturable binding sites: 2×10^4 sites/cell with a dissociation constant (K_d) of approximately 0.7 nM and approximately 2×10^5 sites with a K_d of approximately 13 nM. In isolated rat fat cells, a single class of sites was found with a dissociation constant of 1.5 nM (150).

Most studies of glucagon binding have been carried out with membrane preparations. Shlatz and Marinetti (151) described two classes of sites in rat liver plasma membranes with very low K_d's (1×10^{-7} M and 3×10^{-5} M) but used only high concentrations of glucagon (10^{-8} to 10^{-5} M). Giorgio et al. (152), using a purified LUBROL-extract of liver plasma membranes, found a K_d for the high affinity binding sites of 0.1 nM but could not determine the K_d for the low affinity receptor. In liver plasma membranes, the affinity of the glucagon receptor has been shown to be dependent on guanyl nucleotides (see below). Desbuquois and Laudat (153) found one dissociation constant of 0.24 nM in adipocyte membranes. Glucagon receptors were also studied in membranes prepared by Goldfine et al. (154) from β-cell tumors which secreted insulin in response to glucagon *in vitro*. The authors did not report the K_d values, but the spread of the competition curve over 4 log units suggests that binding is not accounted for by simple binding to a single class of sites. The binding of glucagon to the receptor depends on the temperature. Sonne reports higher binding at 20°C than at 37°C in whole hepatocytes due to a decrease in the dissociation rate constant (149) whereas Freychet et al. did not find that binding at 20°C was higher, but that a longer time was necessary to reach a plateau at the lower temperature (156) on liver membranes. Rodbell et al. (144) found lower binding at lower temperatures.

The pH dependency of binding is difficult to interpret since pH affects the affinity of iodoglucagon differently than the affinity of glucagon. As in the case for insulin, not all receptors need to be occupied by glucagon to generate a maximal biological response ("spare receptors"). Sonne et al. (149) found in whole hepatocytes a discrepancy between the degree of cyclic AMP accumulation and the occupancy of glucagon binding sites after brief incubation times, indicating a nonlinear relationship between the binding of glucagon and the adenylate cyclase. The accumulation of cyclic AMP was proportional to neither the receptor occupancy nor to the rate of association, as also had been demonstrated by Birnbaumer et al. (155). Rosselin et al. (157) similarly reported a nonlinear relationship between binding and cyclic AMP production, with half-maximal effect when 8% of the receptors only were occupied. Birnbaumer and Pohl (158) also concluded that 80% to 90% of the binding sites need not be occupied for maximal activity. In contrast, Rodbell et al. (159) described in liver membranes a hyperbolic relationship between occupancy and adenylate cyclase activity in the presence of GTP, but complete activation of the enzyme required full occupancy.

Regulation of Glucagon Receptor Affinity: Role of Guanyl Nucleotides

Nobody has yet described any regulation of the affinity of glucagon receptors by glucagon itself (homotropic cooperativity). The kinetic test for negative cooperativity was done by Sonne et al. in isolated fat cells and hepatocytes and found negative (149). However, the dissociation rate of ^{125}I-glucagon was found much faster in the presence of glucagon than de-His-glucagon by Birnbaumer et al. (155), a fact that cannot be explained by noncooperative binding and might suggest site–site interactions (155). In contrast, guanyl nucleotides exert a remarkable effect on the affinity of glucagon receptors and markedly accelerate the dissociation rate of ^{125}I-glucagon, nearly irreversibly bound in their absence (153,160–162). Several models have been advanced by Rodbell's group to explain this effect, from relatively simple two-state models (161) to multitransition states (162) which we will not develop here.

Regulation of Glucagon Receptor Concentrations

There have been relatively few studies on the regulation of glucagon receptors *in vivo* up to now. Freeman et al. (163) reported that hyperglucagonemia reduced both glucagon receptor concentration and basal cAMP production in rat liver membranes, but that stimulation of cAMP production by glucagon was not reduced because of an enhanced adenylate cyclase response to membrane-bound glucagon. The decrease in glucagon binding was due entirely to a decrease in receptor concentration. The same inverse relationship between hyperglucagonemia and decreased glucagon binding was found in starved rats by Fouchereau-Peron et al. (164).

Aging also was reported to have some effect on glucagon binding. Fat cell and fat cell membranes isolated from adult rats bind 40% less glucagon than preparations obtained from young animals (165), and glucagon-stimulated lipolytic activity is reduced. In contrast, aging did not appear to affect glucagon binding to purified liver membranes (166).

Structure–Activity Relationship of Glucagon

In contrast with insulin, which has a well-defined and relatively inflexible globular structure, glucagon is a flexible molecule which easily attains a helical structure in a hydrophobic environment. As underlined by Blundell's group (167), an understanding of the nature of the glucagon receptor interaction depends critically on a proper description of the conformation of the hormone when bound to the receptor. Solution studies show that glucagon exists as an equilibrium population of conformers in dilute aqueous solution, but the structure becomes more ordered on self-association and in the presence of detergents or lipid micelles. X-ray analysis showed (168) that in crystals the polypeptide adopts a mainly helical conformation which is stabilized by hydrophobic interactions between molecules related by threefold symmetry in trimers (Fig. 10). Sasaki et al. (167) presented a plausible model in which the helical conforma-

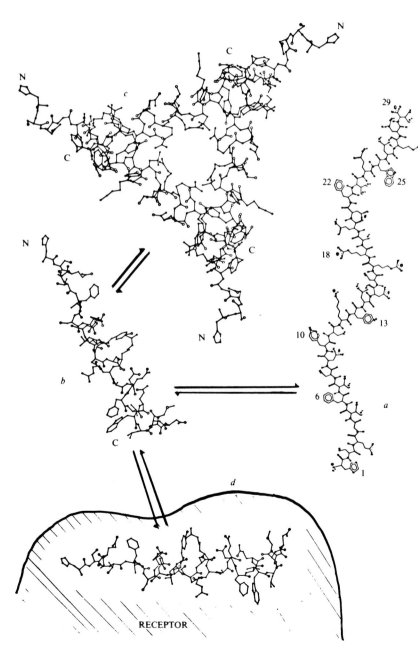

FIG. 10. Schematic representation of the equilibrium among conformers of glucagon **(a)**. Hypothetical random coil structure in equilibrium with a helical form **(b)**. The helical form is stabilized either as trimers **(c)** or by association with a receptor **(d)** by hydrophobic interactions. From ref. 167, with permission.

tion is stabilized by hydrophobic interactions upon receptor binding as it is in the crystalline trimer (Fig. 10c). In contrast with insulin, discrete regions of the glucagon molecule may be involved in receptor binding and biological activity. Rodbell et al. (168) reported that des-His[1]-glucagon (lacking the amino-terminal histidine residue) had no effect on the adenylate cyclase (no efficacy) of rat liver membranes whereas it retained about 16% of the binding affinity of glucagon, suggesting that the presence of the histidine was obligatory for cyclase activation. With β-cell membranes, Goldfine et al. (154) found that des-His[1]-glucagon was one-third less potent as glucagon in inhibiting ^{125}I-glucagon binding but had no effect on adenylate cyclase activity. Des-His[1]-glucagon also antagonized the stimulation of adenylate cyclase by glucagon. But preliminary data from Sonne et al. (169) showed in contrast that both affinity and potency of des-His[1]-glucagon were similarly reduced to a few percent of that of glucagon. Later, Rodbell's group (145) reinvestigated this question with a new batch of highly purified des-His[1]-glucagon and found an efficacy (maximal effect achieved) of 70% of that of glucagon, a biological potency of 2%, and a relative binding affinity of about 7%. Then, Sonne and Gliemann found (150) that des-His[1]-glucagon has an efficacy of about 40% of that of glucagon, and a relative potency and binding affinity which are both reduced to a few percent of that of glucagon. As Sonne and Gliemann concluded (150), the combined evidence therefore shows that the histidine residue is necessary for expression of maximal effects of glucagon even though some effect is still obtained after its removal; in addition, des-His[1]-glucagon shows markedly reduced potency and binding affinity and therefore acts as a weak partial agonist and a weak competitive antagonist.

CATECHOLAMINE RECEPTORS

Classification of α- and β-Adrenergic Effects

Epinephrine acts upon its target organs in varied and often opposite manners. Considerable clarification has resulted from the proposal made by Ahlquist in 1948 that the effects of catecholamines could be classified as α or β, depending on the relative efficiency of five natural and artificial adrenergic agonists. For the α-sites, epinephrine was more active than isoproterenol, while the reverse was found for the β-sites. Later, the availability of adrenergic blockers directed against either the α-sites or the β-sites constituted an elegant confirmation of the proposed classification. Specific antagonists have now been widely used in order to characterize adrenergic receptors in a variety of organs. Further pharmacological subdivisions of both types of receptors into α_1 and α_2 and β_1 and β_2 has been made possible by the use of a large number of specific agonists and antagonists. Some of the pharmacological features of α- and β-adrenergic receptor activation are summarized in Table 2.

Physiological Actions of Catecholamines in Liver

Epinephrine administration to humans or experimental animals is known to elevate blood glucose concentration. The mechanism of this hyperglycemia probably entails several organs. Among them, liver plays a major role: It is now undisputable that epinephrine accelerates both the gluconeogenesis and the glycogenolysis pathways in a variety of species, thus leading to an increase in glucose release from the liver (for review, see ref. 170). Since cyclic AMP was considered to play a role in the effect of epinephrine on hepatic glycogenolysis (171) and since activation of adenylate cyclase is, with few exceptions, mediated by β- rather than by α-receptors, it was natural to suppose that β-receptors mediated the effects of catecholamines in liver.

In the classical work of Sutherland's group (172), the relative potency of several catecholamines in stimulating cyclic AMP formation by dog liver particles, was typically a β-type order. However, Kennedy and Ellis in 1969 (173) showed that the α-adrenergic blocker dihydroergotamine inhibited the epinephrine-induced hyperglycemia and liver glycogen depletion in intact rats, but did not inhibit the muscle or heart glycogenolysis. Furthermore, later experiments using isolated perfused rat liver demonstrated an α-adrenergic mediated glycogenolytic response (174–176).

Recently, additional evidence for the role of α-

TABLE 2. *Pharmacological classification of α- and β-adrenergic drugs*

	α	α_1	α_2	β	β_1	β_2
Selective agonists	Phenylephrine	Methoxamine	Tramazoline Clonidine[a]	Isoproterenol	—[b]	Isoetharine Salbutamol
Selective antagonists[c]	Phenoxybenzamine Phentolamine	Prazosin	Yohimbine	Propranolol	Practolol	Butoxamine

[a] Clonidine behaves mainly as an antagonist upon the α_1-adrenergic receptor in liver (80).
[b] No pure β_1-agonist is actually available.
[c] Labetalol has mixed α- and β-adrenergic effects.

adrenergic mediation of glycogenolysis has been obtained from studies using isolated hepatocytes. An enormous impetus to such work has come from the development of techniques for the preparation of large quantities of isolated hepatocytes. Using these techniques, Tolbert et al. (178) showed that catecholamines could promote gluconeogenesis in rat liver cells by an α-adrenergic activation not related to cyclic AMP variations and insensitive to propranolol; this phenomenon was blocked by the α-adrenergic phentolamine.

It has been demonstrated in the same system that catecholamines could increase glycogenolysis via a mechanism insensitive to β-adrenergic blockade and independent of both cyclic AMP concentration (175, 179,180) and protein kinase activation (180).

Identification and Activation of β-Adrenergic Receptors

Activation of Adenylate Cyclase

Sutherland and Rall first demonstrated that cyclic AMP was produced from ATP by the activation of a membrane-bound enzyme, the adenylate cyclase. Cyclic AMP has since been considered to mediate all the β-adrenergic effects (181). Epinephrine and other catecholamines activate the adenylate cyclase of rat liver plasma membrane (182) via a β_2-type adrenergic receptor (183) (Fig. 11). They lead to the accumulation of cyclic AMP, and in some species and under some conditions, to the classical cascade process of glycogenolysis.

β-Adrenoreceptors in Liver

In order to confirm the hypothesis that the effect of catecholamines in liver is mediated by either α- or β-adrenergic receptors, it is essential to demonstrate the existence of such receptors. A general review on the characterization of α- and β-adrenergic receptors by ligand binding studies can be found in ref. 184.

Early studies using radiolabeled catecholamines to identify β-adrenergic receptors in rat liver plasma membranes as well as in other tissue met with only limited success. This was primarily due to the presence of a high number of nonspecific binding sites, which could be decreased by addition of EDTA (185) or catechol. Recently it has become possible to study β-adrenergic receptors by direct ligand binding techniques, using low concentrations of specific high affinity antagonists and noncatechol ligands, labeled to a high specific radioactivity (see ref. 197). Interestingly, hydroxybenzylisoproterenol, a new potent catecholamine agonist, has been shown to bind to the β-adrenergic receptors of frog erythrocyte membranes with specificity and stereoselectivity, albeit with poor reversibility (186).

β-Adrenergic receptors have been characterized in rat liver, using purified plasma membranes and the specific antagonist dihydroalprenolol. Maximal binding of tritiated dihydroalprenolol takes place rapidly (5 min at 30°C) and reversibly ($t_{1/2} = 5$ min at 3°C), with a high degree of stereospecificity for (−) isomers (187). Displacement of tritiated dihydroalprenolol and iodinated-hydroxybenzylpindolol by agonists (188,189) gave the following order of potency: (−)isoproterenol (0.015 to 0.024 μM) > (−)epinephrine (0.12 to 0.15 μM) > (−)norepinephrine (0.27 to 2 μM) which is in agreement with an interaction with β-adrenergic receptors. Binding data (190) as well as data obtained from cyclase activation (183) revealed that the β-receptor in rat liver belongs to the β_2-subtype. Scatchard plot analysis showed that one class of binding sites was measured in rat liver plasma membranes provided phentolamine, an α-adrenergic blocker, was

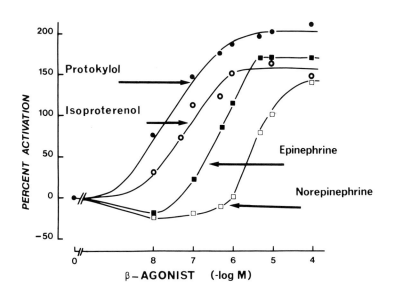

FIG. 11. Effect of various catecholamine agonists on cyclase activity. Normal rat liver plasma membranes were incubated in the presence of increasing concentrations of protokylol ($\bigcirc$), (−)-isoproterenol ($\bullet$); (−)epinephrine ($\triangle$), (−)norepinephrine ($\blacktriangle$). The apparent K_A values for the various agonists determined from this experiment gave an order of potency: (−)isoproterenol (0.2 μM) > (−)epinephrine (0.9 μM) > (−)norepinephrine (4.3 μM), which is typical of β-adrenoreceptors. The very high affinity of protokylol ($K_A = 0.02 \mu$M) suggested that catecholamines activate the hepatic adenylate cyclase via a β_2-type adrenergic receptor. (From ref. 183, with permission).

present in the incubation medium (187,188). Using two different radioligands, Munnich et al. (188) and Wolfe et al. (189) found 75 and 200 fmoles of antagonist bound per mg protein, respectively. The dissociation constant (K_d), calculated from equilibrium studies, was in good agreement with the value obtained from kinetics analysis (1 to 5 nM).

The use of antagonists, instead of agonists, as markers of the β-adrenergic binding sites may be criticized from a physiological standpoint. Nevertheless, a good correlation has been obtained (Fig. 12) between competitive binding studies using labeled antagonists and adenylate cyclase activation in liver. Such a correlation could add further weight to the hypothesis that binding of tritiated antagonists could be physiologically relevant to the β-adrenergic receptor sites (188).

IDENTIFICATION AND ACTIVATION OF α-ADRENERGIC RECEPTORS

α-Adrenergic Receptors in Liver

Only recently, α-adrenergic receptors have been identified and characterized in rat liver plasma membranes by the use of a potent α-adrenergic antagonist, tritiated dihydroergocryptine (187). Binding is rapid (5 min at 37°C), reversible ($t_{1/2} = 1$ min at 37°C), stereospecific, and saturable with a maximal number of binding sites of about 1,400 fmoles/mg membrane protein. Scatchard analysis reveals a single class of noncooperative binding sites with an apparent dissociation constant (K_d) of 1 to 4 nM which is in good agreement with the K_d values calculated from kinetic experiments. From competition dose-response curves, the following order of potency was found for agonists: (−)epinephrine (2.4 μM) > (−)norepinephrine (2.4 μM) > phenylephrine (4.1 μM) > (−)isoproterenol (184 μM) which defines an α-adrenergic receptor (Fig. 13).

Very recent studies have demonstrated that α-adrenergic receptors of rat liver plasma membranes could be solubilized by Lubrol PW and partially purified (191) using a specific irreversible α-adrenergic antagonist, tritiated-phenoxybenzamine (192), as marker. Table 3 summarized the hydrodynamic parameters of the detergent solubilized hepatic adenylate cyclase (193) and α-adrenergic receptor (192), as compared to the β-adrenergic receptor of S49 lymphoma cells (194).

Whether or not this α-adrenergic receptor defined by the binding of either dihydroergocryptine or phenoxybenzamine, and which seems to have similar properties to α-adrenergic receptors of other organs (for details, see Williams and Lefkowitz in ref. 184), represents the physiologic receptor is still open to discussion. A good correlation has been found between competitive binding dose-response curves for tritiated-dihydroergocryptine binding in purified plasma membranes and phosphorylase activity dose-response curves measured in isolated hepatocytes (195). This finding validates the use of tritiated-dihydroergocryptine as a marker of the physiological α-adrenergic receptor in rat liver (Fig. 14). However, El Refai et al. (196), by measuring (−)tritiated-norepinephrine and (±)tritiated-epinephrine binding to rat liver plasma membranes, found two classes of agonist binding sites with high and low affinities for both hormones. Binding to the high affinity sites of the natural agonists was a saturable process within a maximum number of binding sites of about 120 to 160 fmoles/mg protein (as compared with 1,200 fmoles tritiated-dihydroergocryptine bound/mg protein in this system) and a K_d value of 50 nM for both ligands. The limited number of sites of high affinity was believed to represent the physiological α-adrenergic receptor since binding properties correlated well with the effects of catecholamines on phosphorylase activation and calcium efflux in isolated rat hepato-

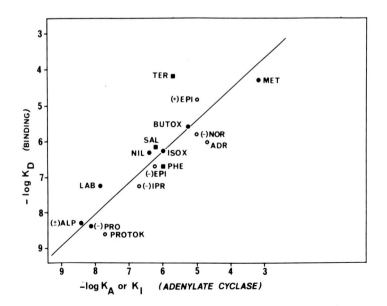

FIG. 12. Correlation between stimulation or inhibition of adenylate cyclase and tritiated dihydroalprenolol displacement from rat liver plasma membranes by adrenergic drugs. This curve represents in ordinate the logarithm of K_D values of adrenergic drugs for the β-adrenoreceptor and in abscissa the logarithm of K_I or K_A values of the same drugs for the adenylate cyclase. The correlation coefficient ($r = 0.95$, $P < 0.001$) and the equation of the straight line were calculated by linear regression. PROTOK: protokylol; (−)PRO: (−)propranolol; (±)ALP: (±)alprenolol; LAB: labetalol; (−)IPR: (−)isoproterenol; PHE: phenylephrine; (−)EPI: (−)epinephrine: NIL: nylidrin; ISOX: isoxsuprine; SAL: salbutamol; ADR: adrenalone; (−)NOR: (−)norepinephrine; BUTOX: butoxamine; (+)EPI: (+)epinephrine; TER: terbutaline; MET: metaraminol. From ref. 188, with permission.

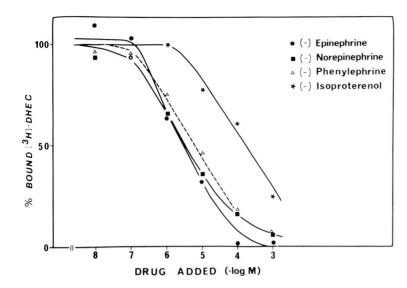

FIG. 13. Displacement curves of tritiated dihydroergocryptine binding by adrenergic drugs. Rat liver plasma membranes were incubated with tritiated dihydroergocryptine (5 nM) and with increasing concentrations of (−)epinephrine (■), (−)norepinephrine (○), (−)phenylephrine (▲), (+)epinephrine (□), and (−)isoproterenol (×). The order of potency of the drugs in competing with the dihydroergocryptine sites is typical of an α-adrenergic receptor. From ref. 187, with permission.

cytes (196). The marked discrepancies between tritiated-catecholamines and tritiated-dihydroergocryptine binding data led to the hypothesis that α-adrenergic agonists and antagonists could bind preferentially but not exclusively to different binding sites or to two different forms of the same receptor in the liver.

The problem has been made more complex by the recent subdivision of the α-adrenergic receptors in two classes. An anatomical distinction was first made between pre- and postsynaptic α-receptors. It was further proposed that postsynaptic α-receptors be named α_1 and presynaptic α_2, and that both types of receptors could be distinguished by pharmacological studies. Subsequently, this concept has been generalized to include the possibility that α_2-receptors also exist in other than presynaptic sites. If it is assumed that adrenergic nerves (containing presynaptic receptors) are connected to the liver, the study of isolated systems (isolated cells, denervated livers), would permit a clearer demonstration of the nature of the α-receptors. Using isolated liver cells, it has been shown

(197) that phosphorylase activation was preferentially inhibited by prazosin while yohimbine was much less effective. Prazosin was also much more effective than yohimbine in displacing tritiated dihydroergocryptine from its binding sites in isolated rat liver membranes (Fig. 15). From these data, it appears that the α-adrenergic receptor in rat liver is of the α_1-subtype.

Mechanisms of α-Adrenergic Action

As has been discussed above, the activation of glycogenolysis in rat liver can be mediated by α-adrenergic receptor activation of phosphorylase via a cyclic AMP-independent, and still unknown, mechanism.

Robison and Sutherland first proposed that a decrease in the cyclic AMP concentration could be provoked by α-adrenergic agonists. This phenomenon has been shown to occur in only a few systems (198). Very recently, Chan and Exton (199) demonstrated that cal-

TABLE 3. *Comparison of the hydrodynamic parameters of rat liver adenylate cyclase and α-adrenergic receptor with the β-adrenergic receptor from S49 lymphoma cells*

	α-Adrenergic receptor[a]	β-Adrenergic receptor[b]	Adenylate cyclase[c]
Stokes radius (nm)	5.7 ± 0.1	6.4 ± 0.03	7.0 ± 0.1
Partial specific volume, v̄ (ml/g)	0.79 ± 0.01	0.83 ± 0.01	0.82 ± 0.01
Sedimentation coefficient ($S_{20,w}$)	4.2 ± 0.1	3.1 ± 0.3	6.8 ± 0.1
Molecular weight (M_r)	128,000	130,000	303,000
Frictional ratio (f/fo)	1.7	1.8	1.5
Lubrol PX bound:			
(mg/mg)	0.3	0.8	0.66
(mol/mol)	60	100	120
Molecular weight of protein	96,000	75,000	183,000

[a] Rat liver, from ref. 191.
[b] S49 lymphoma cells, from ref. 194.
[c] Rat liver, from ref. 193.

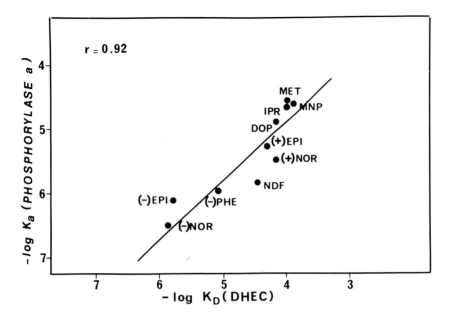

FIG. 14. Correlation between the activation of the glycogen phosphorylase in rat hepatocytes and the displacement of tritiated dihydroergocryptine binding to rat liver plasma membranes by adrenergic agonists. This curve represents K_A for phosphorylase a versus K_D for α-sites. The correlation coefficient ($r = 0.92$, $P < 0.01$) and the equation of the straight line were calculated by linear regression. (−)NOR: (−)norepinephrine; (−)EPI: (−)epinephrine; (−)PHE: (−)-phenylephrine; NDF: nordefrin; (+)-NOR: (+)norepinephrine; (+)EPI: (+)-epinephrine; DOP: dopamine; IPR: isoproterenol; MNP: metanephrine; MET: metaraminol. From ref. 195, with permission.

cium depletion promoted cyclic AMP accumulation in response to the occupancy of α-adrenergic receptors in hepatocytes, and proposed that Ca^{2+} could exert an inhibitory action on the linkage between α-adrenergic receptors and the adenylate cyclase. The physiological implications of these observations are still unclear.

It has been suggested that α-effects of catecholamines were secondary to the elevation of cyclic GMP. However, in rat liver, the increase in cyclic GMP level does not seem to be specific. Thus, insulin, which causes inhibition of glycogenolysis, and carbachol, which has no effect on glycogenolysis, are both able to increase the cyclic GMP level in rat liver isolated cells (200). Thus the role of the cyclic GMP in catecholamine-induced glycogenolysis in liver has to be regarded as uncertain.

The role of calcium as the intracellular messenger in a whole series of cellular events has been extensively

FIG. 15. Inhibition of tritiated-dihydroergocryptine binding to rat liver plasma membranes and inhibition of the (−)epinephrine-stimulated glycogen phosphorylase activity of rat hepatocytes by α-adrenergic antagonists. Prazosin (■, □) and yohimbine (●, ○), two α-adrenergic antagonists known to bind preferentially to α_1- and α_2-receptors, respectively (88), were tested as competitors with dihydroergocryptine for its binding sites. Prazosin ($K_D = 470$ pM) appeared to be 700-fold more potent than yohimbine ($K_D = 0.33$ μM) in displacing tritiated-dihydroergocryptine from the α-adrenoreceptor in purified plasma membranes. Both drugs displaced the tritiated ligand in a monophasic manner. These results showed that there was one class of sites, α_1-receptors, in rat liver plasma membranes, or at least that α_1-sites are much more numerous than α_2-sites. The relative potencies of both prazosin and yohimbine in inhibiting the glycogen phosphorylase stimulated by (−)-epinephrine in isolated rat hepatocytes are also shown. The same order of potencies was found for the inhibition of the enzyme, as for the competition experiments, prazosin ($K_I = 0.85$ nM) being 1300-fold more efficient than yohimbine ($K_I = 11$ μM). From ref. 197, with permission.

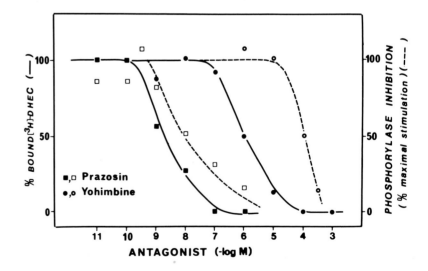

documented, and at the present time the only convincing hypothesis concerning the mechanism of action of the α-adrenergic mediation is a change in the intracellular concentration of calcium [for reviews, see Jones and Michell (201) and Exton (202)]. It has been proposed by Cherrington et al. (180) that Ca^{2+} could also be the second messenger for α-adrenergic-induced activation of glycogenolysis in liver. This hypothesis received further weight from the demonstration of a Ca^{2+} dependence of the hepatic glycogenolytic response to vasopressin, angiotensin II, and oxytocin which do not act via cyclic AMP (203).

Direct measurements have shown an increase in $^{45}Ca^{2+}$ uptake in liver cells in response to α-adrenergic agonists (177), an inhibition of this effect by phenoxybenzamine (204), and a stimulation of the Ca^{2+} efflux from preloaded hepatocytes (204). In rabbit and guinea pig liver slices, Haylett (205) also reported a striking effect of α-agonists on Ca^{2+} efflux which mirrors the action of α-agonists on ^{42}K loss. Thus α-adrenergic activation could lead to change in Ca^{2+} fluxes in parenchymal liver cells.

The activation of glucose release and the stimulation of phosphorylase by the α-adrenergic agonist phenylephrine was impaired in cells in which Ca^{2+} was depleted by EGTA treatment, and restored in these cells by Ca^{2+} addition (204) whereas the effects of a physiological concentration of glucagon were unaffected by these processes (204). Furthermore, experiments with Ca^{2+}-free media have also indicated a Ca^{2+} requirement for the activation by epinephrine of gluconeogenesis in rat hepatocytes (178).

In rat hepatocytes, Assimacopoulos et al. (204) showed that the calcium ionophore A23187 rapidly increased the phosphorylase a activity and the glucose output without altering the cyclic AMP level and the protein kinase activation ratio, provided Ca^{2+} was present in the incubation medium. However, brief exposure of hepatocytes to EGTA still permitted phenylephrine and A23187 activation of phosphorylase, indicating that influx of extracellular Ca^{2+} is not the sole factor involved in the activation of the enzyme (206). Blackmore et al. (206) have provided arguments for an intracellular mobilization of Ca^{2+} and concluded that α-adrenergic agonists, as well as vasopressin and low concentrations of ionophore, activated the phosphorylase in liver cells by mobilizing intracellular calcium and not by promoting Ca^{2+} influx. Thus, calcium which could be released from internal stores (206), presumably mitochondria (207), enters the cytoplasm and thereby activates phosphorylase b kinase, which is a Ca^{2+}-dependent enzyme.

It has been suggested that turnover of phosphatidylinositol plays a role in the coupling between the α-adrenergic receptor activation and the enhanced membrane permeability to Ca^{2+} in smooth muscle. In many tissues, epinephrine stimulates the turnover of phospholipids, in particular phosphatidylinositol [for details, see a review by Michell (208)], and dihydroergocryptine abolishes this effect. It remains to be shown whether the increased phosphatidylinositol metabolism in rat isolated hepatocytes, resulting from α-adrenergic as well as vasopressin-receptor occupancies (209), is responsible for calcium mobilization, or whether it is a separate hormonal effect.

Anatomical Separation of α- and β-Receptors

It has been conclusively demonstrated that the β-adrenergic receptor and adenylate cyclase are distinct molecular entities (194,210–212). While physiological and pharmacological evidence concerning the molecular relationship between α- and β-adrenergic receptors have been inconclusive, biochemical studies have led to the solubilization and further purification of the adrenergic receptors. After solubilization in digitonin, hepatic α- and β-adrenergic receptors have been separated by selective adsorption of the β-receptors to an alprenolol-substituted agarose gel (213). These findings show that the active α- and β-adrenergic binding sites do not simultaneously reside on the same macromolecule and are in agreement with data indicating that these two types of receptors exhibit different sensitivity for SH-group or S–S-bound reagents (214).

Regulation of Adrenergic Receptors

The availability of techniques that permit reliable and simple identification of receptors by direct binding studies has led to rapid and new developments in the understanding of the mechanism involved in regulation of receptor function. Obviously, the receptor, being the first link in the chain of hormone responses, is in a unique position to control tissue sensitivity to hormonal stimulation.

In liver, the activation of phosphorylase and the accumulation of cyclic AMP due to β-adrenergic receptor activation are enhanced when hepatocytes are isolated from hypothyroid rats (215); thyroid hormones have the opposite effect on the hepatic β-adrenergic glycogenolytic response as compared to the response obtained in heart and adipose tissue. Selective changes in the glycogenolytic response of the hepatocytes to various adrenergic agonists have been shown to occur during maturation of rat liver (216) : maturation of the rat appears to be accompanied by a loss of functional β-receptors with epinephrine acting primarily through the α-adrenergic receptor system.

The most studied pathological condition in the liver has been the lack of glucocorticoids: in normal rats, there are relatively few β-adrenergic binding sites (188,189), the response of adenylate cyclase to epinephrine is weak (217), and epinephrine-sensitive glycogenolysis seems to be mediated by α-adrenergic receptors (see above). In adrenalectomized rats, the number of β-adrenergic binding sites is enhanced two- to fourfold, when measured with labeled antagonists (188,189), with no change in the affinity or specificity of the binding of these antagonists; adenylate cyclase activity becomes more sensitive to epinephrine in particulate fractions as well as in purified membrane preparations (217). Under the same conditions, α-adrenergic binding site number remains unchanged (187). Furthermore, glycogenolysis becomes essentially a β-adrenergic receptor mediated effect, whereas the α-adrenergic mediated response is decreased (218). Although the enhanced β-adrenergic response produced by adrenalectomy can be explained by an increased β-adrenergic receptor number, the decreased α-adrenergic response is not due to a change in the α-adrenergic receptor density (187). These data do not explain the well established permissive effect of glucocorticoids on glucagon- and catecholamine-dependent pathways.

The β-adrenergic receptor-coupled adenylate cyclase system in liver has been shown to be modified under several other conditions. Thus, the hormonally induced adenylate cyclase activity is influenced in rat liver during development (219) and aging (220). The catecholamine-sensitive adenylate cyclase is also modified qualitatively in carcinogenesis (221), and quantitatively in cholestasis (222). In the latter case, the increased response of the enzyme to β-adrenergic agonists is linked to a fourfold increase in the β-adrenergic binding site density (222).

While no convincing demonstration of change in adrenergic receptors in human liver has been reported, the adenylate cyclase activity has been studied and shown to be sensitive to adrenergic agonists, with an order typical of a β_2-type receptor (120). Moreover, the level of hormonal activation of the enzyme was higher in fetal liver (epinephrine) and lower in cirrhotic liver (glucagon) than in normal liver (120).

Conclusion

In the mechanism of action of catecholamines in liver, a problem remains as yet unsolved. At what point do the pathways of the α- and β-adrenergic receptor mediated effects on glycogenolysis converge? In both instances, phosphorylase activity is increased, glycogen synthase and pyruvate kinase are inhibited, and the same set of 10 to 12 cytosolic proteins is phosphorylated (223). Yet, the mediation of the β response is cyclic AMP-dependent while that of the α response is due to calcium transfer.

From a physiological viewpoint it is surprising that the same final effect, due to the same hormonal fac-

tors, is mediated by two different intermediary mechanisms depending on the physiological state or on the species (dog versus rat). One possible reason could be that insufficient selection pressure was exerted during the phylogeny, or conversely that no pathway (α- or β-) offered sufficient advantage over the other to be specifically retained. Another possibility, more worrying, albeit less likely, would be that the so-called α- and β-adrenergic phenomena are part of more complex processes and have been dissociated mainly for the sake of convenience.

OTHER RECEPTORS

Vasopressin and Angiotensin II

Vasopressin (224) and angiotensin II (225), in amounts likely to be produced during hemorrhagic shock, cause glycogenolysis in the liver owing to a prompt activation of liver glycogen phosphorylase. In the perfused liver of fed rats vasopressin and angiotensin II were shown to cause glucose release at concentration of about 0.3 nM (170). The effect of vasopressin is mimicked by oxytocin, although with a 1,000-fold lower potency (206). That of angiotensin II is inhibited by the known inhibitor of angiotensin II action, the 1−Sar−8−Ile derivative (225). Vasopressin and angiotensin II cause the phosphorylation of the set of cytosolic proteins, which are also phosphorylated after treatment with an α-adrenergic agonist (223).

It now has been demonstrated clearly that the effect of vasopressin and angiotensin II involves a calcium transfer and it is likely that the actual mechanism of action will appear exactly similar to that of α-adrenergic drugs (177). The nature of the receptor involved in the vasopressin-induced liver glycogenolysis was approached by the use of a variety of derivatives of different potency. It appears that the hepatic receptors for vasopressin share characteristics with, and are related to, those responsible for the suppressive activity of the drug *in vivo*, but are different from those responsible for the antidiuretic activity, namely, the renal receptors (226).

The hepatic receptor of angiotensin has been recently characterized by direct binding studies (227).

Growth Hormone and Prolactin Receptors

In contrast with the insulin receptor, which appears to have been remarkably conserved during the evolution of vertebrates, the receptor for growth hormone (GH) demonstrates marked differences in specificity in various animal tissues. The receptor for human growth hormone (hGH) has been most extensively characterized in human cultured lymphocytes (228,229). It is present as a single class of sites (linear Scatchard plot), and binding is independent of pH over a broad range (6.4 to 8.0). Bovine, porcine, and ovine growth hormones do not compete with human growth hormone binding to this receptor. Human placental lactogen has less than 1% of the potency of human growth hormone in the competition.

The specificity of the "growth hormone" receptors in liver of subprimates is a more complex issue. Tsushima and Friesen (230) described GH receptors in subcellular fractions of liver membranes from pregnant rabbits. The binding specificity correlated with predictions based on the biological specificity of GH in a subprimate: human, monkey, bovine and ovine GH all compete strongly with ^{125}I-hGH for binding whereas turtle and duck GH are much less reactive, and unrelated hormones do not react.

In contrast with the pregnant rabbit liver receptor, identical preparations from pregnant rats have a different specificity more characteristic of a lactogenic receptor (231) (whereas hGH and bovine GH both reacted strongly in the rabbit preparation, the nonlactogenic bovine GH does not react in the rat preparation) (232).

Given the fact that human growth hormone has both somatogenic and lactogenic activities, studies using only ^{125}I-hGH do not clearly differentiate between growth hormone and prolactin receptors; using ovine prolactin as a tracer, sites for this hormone have also been described in addition to the above-mentioned somatogenic receptors (232,233).

It is not clear whether these receptors have any physiological role in the liver, and no correlation between the hormone binding to these sites and any biological effect *in vitro* has been established so far. Since the nature of intracellular events following binding (including a possible second messenger) still entirely escapes our understanding, we will not develop this topic further here and refer the reader to a more detailed discussion in a recent article by Cadman and Wallis (234).

Thyroid Hormones

Triiodothyronine (235) and thyroxine (236) have been reported to bind, with a reasonable degree of specificity, to two apparently different sets of sites located in the plasma membrane of rat liver. The biological role of these binding sites is unknown. It has been proposed that these sites could be involved in the transport of thyroid hormones themselves within the hepatocyte, although this possibility has not been tested. It should be noted that one of the major events in the cellular action of thyroid hormones upon liver is an increase in the number of (Na^+, K^+)ATPase units in the plasma membrane estimated from the concentration of (^{3}H) ouabain binding sites (237). This effect is thought to result from an induction process involving an increased synthesis of the enzyme protein. It is not due to a direct effect on the membrane via the binding sites described above.

Others

The presence of receptors for intestinal glucagon, VIP, secretin, parathyrin, and prostaglandins has been briefly evoked above in the section on the liver adenylate cyclase system. Our lack of understanding of their exact physiological role in the liver does not warrant further development here.

ACKNOWLEDGMENTS

We gratefully acknowledge the expert secretarial assistance of Françoise Lardinois and Thérèse Lambert.

REFERENCES

1. Evans, W. H. (1980): Hepatic plasma-membrane modifications in disease. *Clin. Sci.,* 58:439–444.
2. De Meyts, P., and Rousseau, G. G. (1980): Receptor concepts. A century of evolution. *Circ. Res., (Suppl. 1),* 46:3–9.
3. Baxter, J. D., and Funder, J. W. (1979): Medical progress—hormone receptors. *N. Engl. J. Med.,* 301:1149–1161.
4. Jones, G. A., Vierling, J. M., Steer, C. J., and Reichen, J. (1979): In: *Progress in Liver Disease, Vol. 6,* edited by H. Popper, and F. Schaffner, p. 43. Grune and Stratton, New York.
5. Hue, L., and van den Werve, G. (editors) (1981): *Short-term regulation of liver metabolism.* Elsevier/North Holland Biomedical Press, Amsterdam, New York, Oxford.
6. Levine, R., Goldstein, M. S., Huddlestun, B., and Klein, S. (1950): Action of insulin on the 'permeability' of cells to free hexoses as studied by its effect on the distribution of galactase. *Am. J. Physiol.,* 163:70–76.
7. Stadie, W. C., Haugaard, N., Marsh, J. B., and Itilles, A. G. (1949): The chemical combination of insulin with muscle (diaphragm) of normal rat. *Am. J. Med. Sci.,* 218:265–274.
8. Pastan, I., Roth, J., and Macchia, V. (1966): Binding of hormone to tissue: The first step in polypeptide hormone action. *Proc. Natl. Acad. Sci. (USA),* 56:1802–1809.
9. Kono, T. (1969): Destruction of insulin effector system of adipose tissue cells by proteolytic enzymes. *J. Biol. Chem.,* 244:1772–1778.
10. Schimmer, B. P., Veda, K., and Sato, G. H. (1968): Site of action of adrenocorticotrophic hormone (ACTH) in adrenal cell cultures. *Biochem. Biophys. Res. Commun.,* 32:806–810.
11. Cuatrecasas, P. (1969): Interaction of insulin with the cell membrane: The primary action of insulin. *Proc. Natl. Acad. Sci. (USA),* 63:450–457.
12. Kolb, H. J., Renner, R., Hepp, K. D., Weiss, L., and Wieland, O. H. (1975): Re-evaluation of sepharose insulin as a tool for the study of insulin action. *Proc. Natl. Acad. Sci. (l* 72:248–252.
13. Katzen, H. M., and Vlahakes, G. J. (1973): Biological activity of insulin sepharose. *Science,* 179:1142–1144.
14. Butcher, R. W., Crofford, O. B., Gammeltoft, S., Gliemann, J., Gavin, R. J. III., Goldfine, I. D., Kahn, C. R., Rodbell, M., and Roth, J. (1973): Insulin activity—the solid matrix. *Science,* 182:396–397.
15. Stadie, W. C., Haugaard, N., and Vaughan, M. (1953): The quantitative relation between insulin and its biological activity. *J. Biol. Chem.,* 200:745–751.
16. Lefkowitz, R. J., Roth, J., Pricer, W., and Pastan, I. (1970):

ACTH receptors in the adrenal: Specific binding of ACTH-^{125}I and its relation to adenyl cyclase. *Proc. Natl. Acad. Sci. (USA)*, 65:745–752.

17. Lin, S., Ellis, B., Weisblum, B., and Goodfriend, T. L. (1970): Preparation and properties of iodinated angiotensins. *Biochem. Pharmacol.*, 19:651–662.

18. Roth, J. (1973): Peptide hormone binding to receptors: A review of direct studies in vitro. *Metabolism*, 22:1059–1073.

19. Kahn, C. R. (1975): Membrane receptors for polypeptide hormones. In: *Methods in Membrane Biology. Vol. 3*, edited by E. D. Korn, pp. 81–146. Plenum Press, New York.

20. Kahn, C. R. (1976): Membrane receptors for hormones and neurotransmitters. *J. Cell Biol.*, 70:261–286.

21. Cuatrecasas, P. (1974): Membrane receptors. *Ann. Rev. Biochem.*, 43:169–214.

22. Blecher, M. (1976): Insulin receptors. In: *Methods in Receptor Research. Vol. 2*, edited by M. Blecher. Marcel Dekker, New York.

23. Levey, G. S. (Editor) (1976): *Hormone-Receptor Interaction Molecular Aspects*. Marcel Dekker, New York.

24. Bradshaw, R. A., et al. (Editors) (1976): *Surface Membrane Receptors: Interface Between Cells and Environment*. Plenum Press, New York.

25. Roth, J. (1975): In: *Methods in Enzymology*, edited by S. P. Colowick and N. O. Kaplan, Vol. 37: Peptide Hormones edited by B. W. O'Malley, and J. G. Hardmann, p. 223. Academic Press, New York.

26. Hunter, W. M., and Greenwood, F. C. (1962): Preparation of iodine-131 labelled human growth hormone of high specific activity. *Nature*, 194:495–496.

27. Neville, D. M., Jr. (1975): Isolation of Cell Surface Membrane Fractions from Mammalian Cells and Organs. In: *Methods in Membrane Biology. Vol. 3*, edited by E. D. Korn, pp. 1–49. Plenum Press, New York.

28. Rith, J. (1975): In: *Methods in Enzymology*, edited by S. P. Colowick and N. O. Kaplan. Vol. 37: Peptide Hormones, edited by B. W. O'Malley and J. G. Hardmann, p. 66. Academic Press, New York.

29. Gammeltoft, S., and Gliemann, J. (1979): A procedure for measurement of distribution spaces in isolated fat cells. *Biochem. Biophys. Acta*, 286:1–9.

30. Freychet, P., Roth, J., and Neville, D. M., Jr. (1971): Insulin receptors in the liver: Specific binding of ^{125}I insulin to the plasma membrane and its relation to insulin bioactivity. *Proc. Natl. Acad. Sci. (USA)*, 68:1833–1837

31. Ginsberg, B. H. (1977): In: *Biochemical Action of Hormones, Vol. IV*, edited by G. Litwack, p. 313.

32. De Meyts, P., Bianco, A. R., and Roth, J. (1976): Site-site interactions among insulin receptors. *J. Biol. Chem.*, 251:1877–1888.

33. Waelbroeck, M., and De Meyts, P. (1978): *The Endocrine Society, 60th Annual Meeting*. (Abstr.), 702:428.

34. De Meyts, P., Roth, J., Neville, D. M., Jr., Gavin, J. R., III, and Lesniak, M. A. (1973): Insulin interactions with its receptors: Experimental evidence for negative cooperativity. *Biochem. Biophys. Res. Commun.*, 55:154–161.

35. De Meyts, P. (1976): Cooperative properties of hormone receptors in cell membranes. *J. Supramol. Struct.*, 4:241–258.

36. Gavin, J. R., III, Roth, J., Neville, D. M., Jr., De Meyts, P., and Buell, O. N. (1974): *Proc. Natl. Acad. Sci. (USA)*, 71:84–88.

37. Kosmakos, F., and Roth, J. (1976): *The Endocrine Society, 58th Annual Meeting*. (Abstr.), 69.

38. De Meyts, P., Van Obberghen, E., Roth, J., Brandenburg, D., and Wollmer, A. (1978): Mapping of the residues responsible for the negative cooperativity of the receptor-binding region of insulin. *Nature*, 273:504–509.

39. De Meyts, P., and Michiels-Place, M. (1978): *Diabetologia*, 15:78.

40. Cuatrecasas, P., and Hollenberg, M. D. (1975): Binding of insulin and other hormones to non-receptor materials: Saturability, specificity and apparent "negative cooperativity." *Biochem. Biophys. Res. Commun.*, 62:31–41.

41. Boeynaems, J. M., and Dumont, J. E. (1975): Quantitative analysis of the binding of ligands to their receptor. *J. Cyclic Nucleotide Res.*, 1:123–142.

42. Pollet, R. J., Standaert, M. C., and Haase, B. R. (1977): Insulin binding to the human lymphocyte receptor. *J. Biol. Chem.*, 252:5828–5834.

43. De Meyts, P., and Roth, J. (1975): Cooperativity in ligandin binding: A new graphic analysis. *Biochem. Biophys. Res. Commun.*, 66:1118–1126.

44. Kahn, C. R., Baird, K., Flier, J. S., and Jarrett, D. B. (1977): Effects of autoantibodies to the insulin receptor on isolated adipocytes. *J. Clin. Invest.*, 60:1094–1106.

45. Bar, R. S., Gorden, P., Kahn, C. R., Roth, J., and De Meyts, P. (1976): Fluctuations in the affinity and concentration of insulin receptors on circulating monocytes of obese patients. *J. Clin. Invest.*, 58:1123–1135.

46. Muggeo, M., Bar, R. S., and Roth, J. (1977): Change in affinity of insulin receptors following oral glucose in normal adults. *J. Clin. Endocrinol. Metab.*, 44:1206–1209.

47. Kahn, C. R., Goldfine, I. D., Neville, D. M., Jr., and De Meyts, P. (1978): Alterations in insulin binding induced by changes in vivo in the levels of glucocorticoids and growth hormone. *Endocrinology*, 103:1054–1066.

48. Kosmakos, F., and Roth, J. (1980): Insulin-induced loss of the insulin receptor in IM-9 lymphocytes. *J. Biol. Chem.*, 255:9860–9869.

49. Lesniak, M. A., Gorden, P., Roth, J., and Gavin, J. R., III. (1974): Binding of ^{125}I-human growth hormone to specific receptors in human cultural lymphocytes. *J. Biol. Chem.*, 249:1661–1667.

50. Thomopoulos, P., Roth, J., Lovelace, E., and Pastan, I. (1976): Insulin receptors in normal and transformed fibroblasts: Relationship to growth and transformation. *Cell*, 8:417–423.

51. Thomopoulos, P., Kosmakos, F., Roth, J., and Pastan, I. (1977): Cyclic AMP increases the concentration of insulin receptors in cultured fibroblasts and lymphocytes. *Biochem. Biophys. Res. Commun.*, 75:246.

52. Kahn, C. R., Goldfine, I. D., Neville, D. M., Jr., Roth, J., Garrisson, M., and Bates, R. W. (1973): Decreased binding of insulin to its receptors in rats with hormone induced insulin resistance. *Biochem. Biophys. Res. Commun.*, 53:852–857.

53. Dahms, W. T. (1975): Effect of insulin and cortisol on rat adipose tissue insulin receptors. *Diabetes*, (Suppl. 2), 24:394.

54. Olefsky, J. M., Johnson, J., Lui, F., Jen, P., and Reaven, G. M. (1975): The effects of acute and chronic dexamethasone administration on insulin binding to isolated rat hepatocyte and adepocytes. *Metabolism*, 24:517–527.

55. Livingston, J. N., and Lockwood, D. H. (1975): Effect of glucocorticoids on the glucose transport system of isolated fat cells. *J. Biol. Chem.*, 250:8353–8360.

56. Staufacher, W., Orci, L., Cameron, D. P., Burr, I. M., and Renold, A. E. (1971): Spontaneous hyperglycemia and/or obesity in laboratory rodents: An example of the possible usefulness of animal disease models with both genetic and environmental components. *Recent Progr. Horm. Res.*, 27:41–95.

57. Kahn, C. R., Neville, D. M., Jr., Gorden, P., Freychet, P., and Roth, I. (1972): Insulin receptor defect in insulin resistance: Studies in the obese-hyperglycemic mouse. *Biochem. Biophys. Res. Commun.*, 48:135–142.

58. Kahn, C. R., Neville, D. M., Jr., and Roth, J. (1973): Insulin-receptor interaction in the obese-hyperglycemic mouse. *J. Biol. Chem.*, 248:244–250.

59. Soll, A. H., Kahn, C. R., Neville, D. M., Jr. (1975): Insulin binding to liver plasma membranes in the obese hyperglycemic (ob/ob) mouse. Demonstration of a decreased number of functionally normal receptors. *J. Biol. Chem.*, 250:4702–4707.

60. Freychet, P., Laudat, M. H., Laudat, P., Rosselin, G., Kahn, C. R., Gorden, P., and Roth, J. (1972): Impairment of insulin binding to the fat cell plasma membrane in the obese hyperglycemic mouse. *FEBS Lett.*, 25:339–345.

61. Freychet, P., and Forgue, E. (1974): Insulin receptors in the heart muscle: Impairment of insulin binding to the plasma membrane in the obese hyperglycemic mouse. *Diabetes*, (Suppl. 1), 23:354.

62. Freychet, P., Brandenburg, D., and Wollmer, A. (1974): Receptor-binding assay of chemically modified insulins. *Diabetologia*, 10:1—5.

63. Soll, A. H., Goldfine, I. D., Roth, J., Kahn, C. R., and Neville, D. M., Jr. (1974): Thymic lymphocytes in obese (ob/ob) mice. *J. Biol. Chem.*, 249:4127—4131.

64. Soll, A. H., Kahn, C. R., Neville, D. M., Jr., and Roth, J. (1975): Insulin receptor deficiency in genetic and acquired obesity. *J. Clin. Invest.*, 56:769—780.

65. Baxter, D., Gates, R. J., and Lazarus, N. R. (1973): *Int. Diabetes Fed. 8th Congress. Excerpta Medica Found.*, 280:74.

66. Keven, P., Picard, J., Caron, M., and Veissiere, D. (1975): Decreased binding of insulin to liver plasma membrane receptors in hereditary diabetic mice. *Biochim. Biophys. Acta*, 389:281—289.

67. Mahler, R. J., and Szabo, O. (1971): Amelioration of insulin resistance in obese mice. *Am. J. Physiol.*, 221:980—983.

68. Archer, J. A., Gorden, P., and Roth, J. (1975): Defect in insulin binding to receptors in obese man. *J. Clin. Invest.*, 55:166—174.

69. Olefsky, J. M., and Reaven, G. M. (1974): Decreased insulin binding to lymphocytes from diabetic subjects. *J. Clin. Invest.*, 54:1323—1328.

70. Beck-Nielsen, H., Pedersen, O., Kragballe, K., and Sorensen, N. S. (1977): The monocyte as a model for the study of insulin receptors in man. *Diabetologia*, 13:563—569.

71. Marinetti, G. V., Schlatz, L., and Reilly, K. (1972): In: *Insulin Action*, edited by I. B. Fritz, p. 207. Academic Press, New York.

72. Harrison, L. C., Martin, F. I. R., and Melick, R. A. (1976): Correlation between insulin receptor binding in isolated fat cells and insulin sensitivity in obese human subjects. *J. Clin. Invest.*, 58:1435—1441.

73. Schwartz, R. H., Bianco, A. R., Kahn, R. C., and Handwerger, B. S. (1975): Demonstration that monocytes rather than lymphocytes are the insulin-binding cells in preparations of human peripheral blood mononuclear leukocytes: Implications for studies of insulin-resistant states in man. *Proc. Natl. Acad. Sci. (USA)*, 72:474—478.

74. Archer, J. A. (1978): Characteristics of human erythrocyte insulin receptors. *Diabetes*, 27:701—708.

75. Blundell, T. L., Dodson, G. G., Hodgkin, D. C., and Mercola, D. A. (1972): Insulin: The structure in the crystal and its reflection in chemistry and biology. *Adv. Prot. Chem.*, 26:279—394.

76. Freychet, P., Kahn, C. R., Roth, J., and Neville, D. M., Jr. (1972): Insulin interactions with liver plasma membranes. *J. Biol. Chem.*, 247:3953—3961.

77. Olefsky, J. M., Jen, P., and Reaven, G. M. (1974): Insulin binding to isolated human adipocytes. *Diabetes*, 23:565—571.

78. Hammond, J. M., and Jarrett, L. (1975): Insulin degradation by isolated fat cells and their subcellular fractions. *Diabetes*, 24:1011—1019.

79. Le Cam, A., Freychet, P., and Lenoir, P. (1975): Degradation of insulin by isolated rat liver cells. *Diabetes*, 24:566—573.

80. Flier, J. S., Maratos-Flier, E., Baird, K. L., and Kahn, C. R. (1977): Antibodies to the insulin receptor that block insulin binding fail to inhibit insulin degradation. *Diabetes (Suppl. I)*, 26:354.

81. Terris, S., and Steiner, D. F. (1975): Binding and degradation of ^{125}I-insulin by rat hepatocytes. *J. Biol. Chem.*, 250:8389—8398.

82. Terris, S., and Steiner, D. F. (1975): Retention and degradation of ^{125}I-insulin by perfused livers from diabetic rats. *J. Clin. Invest.*, 57:885—896.

83. Tomizawa, H. H. (1962): Properties of glutathione insulin transhydrogenase from beef liver. *J. Biol. Chem.*, 237:3393—3394.

84. Chandler, M. L., and Varandani, P. I. (1975): Kinetic analysis of the mechanism of insulin degradation by glutathione-insulin transhydrogenase (thiol:protein-disulfide oxidoreductase). *Biochemistry*, 14:2107—2115.

85. Brush, J. S. (1971): Plasma and pancreatic insulin concentra-

86. Duckworth, W. C., Heinemann, M. A., and Kitabchi, A. E. (1972): Purification of insulin-specific protease by affinity chromatography. *Proc. Natl. Acad. Sci. (USA)*, 69:3698—3702. 69:3698—3702.

87. Steiner, D. F. (1977): Insulin today (the Banting memorial lecture, 1976). *Diabetes*, 26:322—340.

88. Kahn, C. R., and Baird, K. L. (1978): Dehydroqunate synthase in bacillus subtilis. *J. Biol. Chem.*, 253:4900—4906.

89. Gliemann, J., and Sonne, I. (1978): Binding and receptor-mediated degradation of insulin in adipocytes. *J. Biol. Chem.*, 253:7857—7863.

90. Gammeltoft, S., Kristensen, L. O., and Sestoft, L. (1978): Insulin receptors in isolated rat hepatocytes. *J. Biol. Chem.*, 253:8406—8413.

91. Bergeron, J. J. M., Evans, W. H., and Geschwind, I. I. (1973): Insulin binding to rat liver golgi fractions. *J. Cell Biol.*, 59:771—776.

92. Horvat, A., Li, T., and Katsoyannis, P. G. (1975): Cellular binding sites for insulin in rat liver. *Biochim. Biophys. Acta*, 382:609—620.

93. Goldfine, I. D., and Smith, G. J. (1976): Binding of insulin to isolated nucleic. *Proc. Natl. Acad. Sci. (USA)*, 73:1427—1431.

94. Posner, B. I., Josefsberg, Z., and Bergeron, J. J. M. (1978): Intracellular polypeptide hormone receptors. *J. Biol. Chem.*, 253:4067—4073.

95. Varga, J. M., Moellmann, G., Fribch, P., Godariska, E., and Lerner, A. B. (1976): Association of cell surface receptors for melanotropin with the melanoma cells. *Proc. Natl. Acad. Sci. (USA)*, 73:559—562.

96. Bergeron, J. J. M., Posner, B. I., Josefsberg, Z., and Sikotrom, R. (1978): Intracellular polypeptide hormone receptors. *J. Biol. Chem.*, 253:4058—4066.

97. Kolata, G. B. (1978): Polypeptide hormones: What are they doing in cells? *Science*, 201:895—897.

98. Carpentier, J. L., Gorden, P., Amherst, M., Van Obberghen, E., Kahn, C. R., and Orci, L. (1978): ^{125}I-insulin binding to cultured human lymphocytes. *J. Clin. Invest.*, 61:1057—1070.

99. Gorden, P., Carpentier, J. L., Freychet, P., Le Cam, A., and Orci, L. (1978): ^{125}I-insulin: Direct demonstration of binding internalization and lysosomal association in isolated rat hepatocytes. *Diabetes (Suppl. 2)*, 27:450.

100. Gorden, P., Carpentier, J. L., Cohen, S., and Orci, L. (1978): Epidermal growth factor: Morphological demonstration of binding internalization and lysosomal association in human fibroblasts. *Proc. Natl. Acad. Sci. (USA)*, 75:5025—5029.

101. Carpentier, G., and Cohen, S. (1976): ^{125}I-labeled human epidermal growth factor. *J. Cell Biol.*, 71:159—171.

102. Schechter, Y., Schlesinger, J., Jacobs, S., Chang, K. J, and Cuatrecasas, P. (1978): Fluorescent labeling of hormone receptors in middle cells. Preparation and properties of highly fluorescent derivatives of epidermal growth factor and insulin. *Proc. Natl. Acad. Sci. (USA)*, 75:2135—2139.

103. Schlesinger, J., Schechter, Y., Willingham, M. C., and Pastan, I. (1978): Direct visualization of binding, aggregation, and internalization of insulin and epidermal growth factor on living fibroblastic cells. *Proc. Natl. Acad. Sci. (USA)*, 75:2659—2663.

104. Maxfield, F. R., Schlesinger, J., Schechter, Y., Pastan, I., and Willingham, M. C. (1978): Direct visualization of binding, aggregation, and internalization of insulin and epidermal growth factor on living fibroblastic cells. *Proc. Natl. Acad. Sci. (USA)*, 75:2659—2663.

105. Zeleznik, A. J., and Roth, J. (1978): Demonstration of the insulin receptor in vivo in rabbits and its possible role as a reservoir for the plasma hormone. *J. Clin. Invest.*, 59:1363.

106. Muggeo, M., Ginsberg, B. H., Roth, J., Kahn, C. R., De Meyts, P., and Neville, D. M., Jr. (1979): The insulin receptor in vertebrates is functionally more conserved during evolution than insulin itself. *Endocrinology*, 104:1393—1402.

107. Muggeo, M., Van Obberghen, E., Kahn, C. R., Roth, J., Ginsberg, B. H., De Meyts, P., Emdin, S. O., and Falkmer, S. (1979): The insulin receptor and insulin of the Atlantic bagfish. Extraordinary conservation of binding specificity and negative

tions in adult squirrel and rhesus monkey. *Diabetes*, 20:151—155.

cooperativity in the most primitive vertebrate. *Diabetes,* 28:175–181.

108. Czech, M. P., Massague, J., and Pilch, P. F. (1981): The insulin receptor: structural features. *Trends in Biochemical Sciences,* 6:222–227.

109. Krupp, M. N., and Livingston, J. N. (1978): Insulin binding to solubilized material from fat cell membranes: Evidence for two binding species. *Proc. Natl. Acad. Sci. (USA),* 75:2593–2597.

110. Maturo, J. M., and Hollenberg, M. D. (1978): Insulin receptor: Interaction with nonreceptor glycoprotein from liver cell membranes. *Proc. Natl. Acad. Sci. (USA),* 75:3070–3074.

111. Kahn, C. R. (1978): Insulin resistance, insulin insensitivity and insulin unresponsiveness: A necessary distinction. *Metabolism (Suppl. 2),* 27:1893–1902.

112. Fehlmann, M. (1981): Insulin and glucagon receptors of isolated rat hepatocytes: Comparison between hormone binding and amino acid transport stimulation. *Endocrinology,* 109:253–261.

113. De Meyts, P., and Fehlmann, M. (1981): Amino acid transport in isolated hepatocytes from streptozotocin-diabetic rats. *Diabetes,* 12:996–1000.

114. Seals, J. R., and Czech, M. P. (1980): Evidence that insulin activates an intrinsic plasma membrane protease in generating a secondary chemical mediator. *J. Biol. Chem.,* 255:6529–6531.

115. Larner, J., Galaski, G., Cheng, K., De Paoli-Roach, A. A., Huang, L., Daggy, P., and Kellog, J. (1979): Generation by insulin of a chemical mediator that controls protein phosphorylation and dephosphorylation. *Science,* 206:1408–1410.

116. Rodbell, M., Birnbaumer, L., Pohl, S. L., and Krans, H. M. J. (1971): The glucagon-sensitive adenyl cyclase system in plasma membranes of rat liver. *J. Biol. Chem.,* 246:1877–1882. 246:1877–1882.

117. Perkins, J. P. (1973): In: *Advances in Cyclic Nucleotide Research, Vol. 3,* edited by P. Greengard and G. A. Robison, p. 1. Raven Press, New York.

118. Birnbaumer, L. (1973): Hormone-sensitive adenylyl cyclases useful models for studying hormone receptor functions in cell-free systems. *Biochim. Biophys. Acta,* 300:129–158.

119. Hanoune, J. (1976): *Biol. Gastroenterol.,* 9:33.

120. Pecker, F., Duvaldestn, P., Berthelot, P., and Hanoune, J. (1979): The adenylate cyclase system in human liver: characterization, subcellular distributions and hormonal sensitivity in normal or cirrhotic adult and in foetal liver. *Clin. Sci.,* 57:313–325.

121. Bataille, D., Freychet, P., and Rosselin, G. (1974): Interactions of glucagon, gut glucagon, vasoactive intestinal polypeptide and secretin with liver and fat cell plasma membranes: Binding to specific sites and stimulation of adenylate cyclase. *Endocrinology,* 95:713–721.

122. Desbuquois, B. (1974): The interaction of vasoactive intestinal polypeptide and secretin with liver cell membranes. *Eur. J. Biochem.,* 46:439–450.

123. Canterbury, J. M., Levey, G., Ruiz, E., and Reiss, E. (1974): Parathyroid hormone activation of adenylate cyclase in liver. *Proc. Soc. Exp. Biol. Med.,* 147:366–370.

124. Sweat, F. W., and Wincek, T. J. (1973): The stimulation of hepatic adenylate cyclase by prostaglandins. *Biochem. Biophys. Res. Commun.,* 55:522–529.

125. De Rubertis, F. R., Zenser, T. V., and Curnow, R. T. (1974): Inhibition of glucagon-mediated increases in hepatic cyclic adenosine 3'-5'-monophosphate by prostaglandin E1 and E2. *Endocrinology,* 94:93.

126. Smigel, M, and Fleischer, S. (1977): Characterization of Triton X-100 solubilized prostaglandin E binding protein of rat liver plasma membranes. *J. Biol. Chem.,* 252:3689–3696.

127. Londos, C., and Preston, M. S. (1977): Regulation by glucagon and divalent cations of inhibition of hepatic adenylate cyclase by adenosine. *J. Biol. Chem.,* 252:5951–5956.

128. Fain, J. F., and Shepherd, R. E. (1977): Adenosine, cyclic AMP metabolism, and glycogenolysis in rat liver cells. *J. Biol. Chem.,* 252:8066–8070.

129. Hepp, K. D. (1971): Inhibition of glucagon-stimulated adenyl cyclase by insulin. *FEBS Lett.,* 12:263–266.

130. Rodbell, M. (1980): The role of hormone receptors and GTP-regulatory proteins in membrane transduction. *Nature,* 284:17.

131. Pecker, F., and Hanoune, J. (1977): Activation of epinephrine-sensitive adenylate cyclase in rat liver by cytosolic protein. Nucleotide complex. *J. Biol. Chem.,* 252:2784–2786.

132. Pecker, F., and Hanoune, J. (1977): Uncoupled B-adrenergic receptors and adenylate cyclase can be recoupled by a GTP-dependent cytosolic factor. *FEBS Lett.,* 83:93.

133. Londos, C., Salomon, Y., Lin, M. C., Hardwood, J. F., Schramm, M., Wolff, J., and Rodbell, M. (1974): 5'-guanylylimidodysphosphate, a potent activator of adenylate cyclase-systems in eukaryotic cells. *Proc. Natl. Acad. Sci. (USA),* 71:3087–3090.

134. Cassel, D., and Selinger, Z. (1976): Catecholamine-stimulated GTPase activity in turkey erythrocyte membranes. *Biochim. Biophys. Acta.,* 452:538–551.

135. Chambaut, A. M., Leray-Pecker, F., Feldmann, G., and Hanoune, J. (1974): Calcium-binding properties and ATPase activities of rat liver plasma membranes. *J. Gen. Physiol.,* 64:104–126.

136. Cassel, D., and Snlinger, Z. (1977): Mechanisms of adenylate cyclase activation by cholera toxin: Inhibition of GTP hydrolysis at the regulatory site. *Proc. Natl. Acad. Sci. (USA),* 74:3307–3311.

137. Lin, M. C., Welton, A. F., and Berman, M. F. (1978): Essential role of GTP in the expression of adenylate cyclase activity after cholera toxin treatment. *J. Cyclic Nucleotide Res.,* 4:159–168.

138. Cassel, D., and Pfeuffer, T. (1978): Mechanism of cholera toxin action: Covalent modification of the guanyl nucleotide-binding protein of the adenylate cyclase system. *Proc. Natl. Acad. Sci. (USA),* 75:2669–2673.

139. Johnson, G. L., Kaslow, H. R., and Bourne, H. R. (1978): Genetic evidence that cholera toxin substrates are regulatory components of adenylate cyclase. *J. Biol. Chem.,* 253:7120–7123.

140. Hanoune, J., Stengel, D., Lacombe, M. L., Feldmann, G., and Coudrier, E. (1977): Proteolytic activation of rat liver adenylate cyclase by a contaminant of crude collagenase from clostridium histolyticum. *J. Biol. Chem.,* 252:2039–2045.

141. Lacombe, M. L., Stengel, D., and Hanoune, J. (1977): Proteolytic activation of adenylate cyclase from rat-liver plasma membranes. *FEBS Lett.,* 77:159–163.

142. Stengel, D., Lad, P. M., Nielsen, T. B., Rodbell, M., and Hanoune, J. (1980): Proteolysis activates adenylate cyclase in rat liver Ac⁻ lymphoma cell independently of the guanine nucleotide regulatory site. *FEBS Lett.,* 115:260.

143. Rodbell, M., Lin, M. C., Salomon, Y., Londos, C., Harwood, J. P., Marin, B. R., Rendell, M., and Berman, M. (1975): Role of adenine and guanine nucleotides in the activity and response of adenylate cyclase systems to hormones: Evidence for multisite transition states. *Adv. Cyclic Nucleotide Res.,* 5:3–29.

144. Rodbell, M., Krans, H. M. J., Pohl, S. L., and Birnbaumer, L. (1971): The glucagon-sensitive adenyl cyclase system in plasma membranes of rat liver. *J. Biol. Chem.,* 246:1861–1871.

145. Lin, M. C., Wright, D. E., Hruby, V. J., and Rodbell, M. (1975): Structure-function relationships in glucagon: Properties of highly purified Des-His'-monoido-, and (Des-Asn²⁸, Thr²⁹) (homoserine lactone²⁷) glucagon. *Biochemistry,* 14:1559–1563.

146. Bromer, W. W., Boucher, M. E., and Patterson, J. M. (1973): Glucagon structure and function, II increased activity of iodoglucagon. *Biochem. Biophys. Res. Commun.,* 53:134–139.

147. Desbuquois, B. (1975): Iodoglucagon-preparation and characterization. *Eur. J. Biochem.,* 53:569–580.

148. Lin, M. C., Nicosia, S., Lad, P. M., and Rodbell, M. (1977): Effect of GTP on binding of [³H]glucagon to receptors in rat hepatic plasma membranes. *J. Biol. Chem.,* 252:2790–2792.

149. Sonne, O., Berg, T., and Christoffersen, T. (1978): Binding of ¹²⁵I-labelled glucagon and glucagon-stimulated accumulation of adenosine 3':5'-monophosphate in isolated intact rat hepatocytes. *J. Biol. Chem.,* 253:3203–3210.

150. Sonne, O., and Gliemann, J. (1977): Receptor binding of glucagon and adenosine 3',5'-monospecific accumulation in isolated rat fat cells. *Biochem. Biophys. Acta.,* 499:259–272.

151. Shlatz, L., and Marinetti, G. V. (1972): Hormone-calcium in-

teractions with the plasma membrane of rat liver cells. *Science*, 176:175.

152. Giorgio, N. A., Johnson, C. B., and Blecker, M. (1974): Hormone receptors. *J. Biol. Chem.*, 249:428–437.

153. Desbuquois, B., and Laudat, M. H. (1974): Glucagon-receptor interactions in fat cell membranes. *Mol. Cell. Endocrinol.*, 1:355–370.

154. Goldfine, I. D., Roth, J., and Birnbaumer, L. (1972): Glucagon receptors in β-cells. *J. Biol. Chem.*, 247:1211–1218.

155. Birnbaumer, L., Pohl, S. L., Rodbell, M., and Sunby, F. (1972): The glucagon-sensitive adenylate cyclase system in plasma membranes of rat liver. *J. Biol. Chem.*, 247:2038–2043.

156. Freychet, P., Rosselin, G., Rancon, F., Fouchereau, M., and Broer, Y. (1974): Interactions of insulin and glucagon with isolated rat liver cells II—dynamic changes in the cyclic AMP induced by hormones. *Horm. Metab. Res. (Suppl. 5)*, 5:78–86.

157. Rosselin, G., Freychet, P., Fouchereau, M., Rancon, F., and Broer, Y. (1974): Interactions of insulin and glucagon with isolated rat liver cells II—dynamic changes in the cyclic AMP induced by hormones. *Horm. Metab. Res. (Suppl. 5)*, 5:78.

158. Birnbaumer, L., and Pohl, S. L. (1973): Relation of glucagon-specific binding sites to glucagon dependent stimulation of adenylyl cyclase activity in plasma membranes of rat liver. *J. Biol. Chem.*, 248:2056–2061.

159. Rodbell, M., Lin, M. C., and Salomon, Y. (1974): Evidence for interdependent action of glucagon and nucleotides on the hepatic adenylate cyclase system. *J. Biol. Chem.*, 249:59–65.

160. Rodbell, M., Krans, H. M. J., Pohl, S. L., and Birnbaumer, L. (1971): The glucagon-sensitive adenyl cyclase system in plasma membranes of rat liver. *J. Biol. Chem.*, 246:1872–1876.

161. Hammes, G. G., and Rodbell, M. (1976): Simple model for hormone-activated adenylate cyclase systems. *Proc. Natl. Acad. Sci. (USA)*, 73:1189–1192.

162. Welton, A. F., Lad, P. M., Newby, A. C., Yamamura, H., Nicosia, S., and Rodbell, M. (1977): Solubilization and separation of the glucagon receptor and adenylate cyclase in guanine nucleotide-sensitive states. *J. Biol. Chem.*, 252:5947–5950.

163. Freeman, D., McCorkle, K., and Srikant, C. B. (1977): Effect of hyperglucagonemia on glucagon binding and biologic activity. *Diabetes (Suppl. 1)*, 26:366.

164. Fouchereau-Peron, M., Rancon, F., Freychet, P., and Rosselin, G. (1976): Effect of feeding and fasting on the early steps and glucagon action in isolated rat liver cells. *Endocrinology*, 98:755–760.

165. Livingston, J. N., Cuatrecasas, P., and Lockwood, D. H. (1974): Studies of glucagon resistance in large rat adipocytes: ^{125}I-labelled glucagon binding and lipolytic capacity. *J. Lipid Res.*, 15:26–32.

166. Lockwood, D. H., and East, L. E. (1978): [^{125}I]glucagon binding by liver membranes from young and adult rats. *Diabetes*, 27:589–591.

167. Sasaki, K., Dockerville, S., Adamiak, D. A., Tickle, I. J., and Blundell, T. (1975): X-ray analysis of glucagon and its relationship to receptor binding. *Nature*, 257:751–757.

168. Rodbell, M., Birnbaumer, L., Pohl, S. L., and Sunby, F. (1971): The reaction of glucagon with its receptor: Evidence for discrete regions of activity and binding in the glucagon molecule. *Proc. Natl. Acad. Sci. (USA)*, 68:909–913.

169. Sonne, O., Gliemann, J., and Gammeltoft, S. (1974): Binding and stimulation of the adenylyl cyclase in isolated rat fat cells by glucagon on Des-His'-glucagon. *Acta Physiol. Scand.*, 91:32A–33A.

170. Hems, D. A. (1977): Short-term hormonal control of hepatic carbohydrate and lipid catabolism. *FEBS Lett.*, 80:237.

171. Exton, J. H., Robison, G. A., Sutherland, E. W., and Park, C. R. (1971): Studies on the role of adenosine 3',5'-monophosphate in the hepatic actions of glucagon and catecholamines. *J. Biol. Chem.*, 246:6166–6177.

172. Murad, F., Chi, Y. M., Rall, T. W., and Sutherland, E. W. (1962): Adenyl cyclase. *J. Biol. Chem.*, 237:1233–1238.

173. Kennedy, B. L., and Ellis, S. (1969): Interactions of catecholamines and adrenergic blocking agents at receptor sites

174. Sherline, P., Lynch, A., and Glinsmann, W. H. (1972): Cyclic AMP and adrenergic receptor control of rat liver glycogen metabolism. *Endocrinology*, 91:680–690.

175. Exton, J. H., and Harper, S. C. (1975): In: *Advances in Cyclic Nucleotide Research*, edited by G. I. Drummond, P. Greengard, and G. A. Robison, p. 519. Raven Press, New York.

176. Saitoh, Y., and Ui, M. (1976): Stimulation of glycogenolysis and gluconeogenesis by epinephrine independent of its beta-adrenergic function in perfused rat liver. *Biochem. Pharmacol.*, 25:841–845.

177. Keppens, S., Vandenheed, J. R., and DeWulf, H. (1977): On the role of calcium as second messenger in liver for the hormonally induced activation of glycogen phosphorylase. *Biochim. Biophys. Acta*, 496:448–457.

178. Tolbert, M. E. M., and Fain, J. N. (1974): Studies on the regulation of gluconeogenesis in isolated rat liver cells by epinephrine and glucagon. *J. Biol. Chem.*, 249:1162–1166.

179. Hutson, N. J., Brumley, F. T., Assimacopoulos, F. D., Harper, S. C., and Exton, J. H. (1976): Studies on the alpha-adrenergic activation of hepatic glucose output. *J. Biol. Chem.*, 251:5200–5208.

180. Cherrington, A. D., Assimacopoulos, F. D., Harper, S. C., Corbin, J. D., Park, C. R., and Exton, J. H. (1976): Studies on the alpha-adrenergic activation of hepatic glucose output. *J. Biol. Chem.*, 251:5209–5218.

181. Robison, A., Butcher, R. W., and Sutherland, E. W. (1971): In: *Cyclic AMP*. Raven Press, New York.

182. Leray, F., Chambaut, A. M., and Hanoune, J. (1972): The glucose effect and cortisone action upon rat liver metabolism. *Biochem. Biophys. Res. Commun.*, 48:1385.

183. Lacombe, M. L., Rene, E., Guellaen, G., and Hanoune, J. (1976): Transformation of the B$_2$ adrenoceptor in normal rat liver into a B$_1$ type in zajdela hepatoma. *Nature*, 262:70–72.

184. Williams, L. T., and Lefkowitz, R. J. (1978): In: *Receptor Binding Studies in Adrenergic Pharmacology*. Raven Press, New York.

185. Lacombe, M. L., and Hanoune, J. (1974): Enhanced specificity of epinephrine binding of rat liver plasma membranes in the presence of EDTA. *Biochem. Biophys. Res. Commun.*, 58:667–673.

186. Lefkowitz, R. J., and Williams, L. T. (1977): Catecholamine binding to the β-adrenergic receptor. *Proc. Natl. Acad. Sci. (USA)*, 74:515–519.

187. Guellaen, G., Yates-Aggerbeck, M., Vauquelin, G., Strosberg, D., and Hanoune, J. (1978): Characterization with [^{3}H]dihydroergocryptine of the alpha-adrenergic receptor of the hepatic plasma membrane. *J. Biol. Chem.*, 253:1114–1120.

188. Munnich, A., Geynet, P., Schmelck, P. H., and Hanoune, J. (1980): The effect of common bile duct ligation upon the rat liver beta-adrenergic receptor-adenylate cyclase system. *FEBS Lett.*, 107:259–263.

189. Wolfe, B. B., Harden, T. K., and Molinoff, P. B. (1976): B-adrenergic receptors in rat liver: Effects of adrenalectomy. *Proc. Natl. Acad. Sci. (USA)*, 73:1343–1347.

190. Yates-Aggerbeck, M., Guellaen, G., and Hanoune, J. (1978): Biochemical evidence for the dual action of labetalol on alpha and beta adrenoceptors. *Brit. J. Pharm.*, 62:543–548.

191. Guellaen, J., Aggerbeck, M., and Hanoune, J. (1979): Characterization and solubilization of the alpha-adrenoreceptor of rat liver plasma membranes labelled with (^{3}H) phenoxybenzamine. *J. Biol. Chem.*, 254:10761–10768.

192. Guellaen, G., and Hanoune, J. (1979): Hepatic alpha-adrenoreceptor: Specific and irreversible labeling of (^{3}H)-phenorybenzamine. *Biochem. Biophys. Res. Commun.*, 89:1178–1185.

193. Stengel, D., and Hanoune, J. (1979): Solubilization and physical characterization of the adenylate cyclase from rat liver plasma membrane. *Eur. J. Biochem.*, 102:21–34.

194. Haga, T., Haga, K., and Gilman, A. G. (1977): Hydrodynamic properties of the beta-adrenergic receptor and adenylate cyclase from wild type and variant S49 lymphoma cells. *J. Biol. Chem.*, 252:5776–5782.

195. Aggerbeck, M., Guellaen, G., and Hanoune, J. (1980): The

alpha-adrenergic mediated effect in rat liver. *Biochem. Pharmacol.*, 29:1653–1662.

196. El-Refai, M., Blackmore, P. F., and Exton, J. H. (1979): Evidence for two alpha-adrenergic binding sites in liver plasma membranes. *J. Biol. Chem.*, 254:4375–4386.

197. Aggerbeck, M., Guellaen, G., and Hanoune, J. (1980): The alpha adrenergic mediated effect in rat liver. *Biochem. Pharmacol.*, 29:143.

198. Jakobs, K. H. (1979): Inhibition of adenylate cyclase by hormones and neurotransmitters. *Mol. Cell. Endocrinol.*, 16:147–156.

199. Chan, T. M., and Exton, J. H. (1977): Alpha-adrenergic-mediated accumulation of adenosine 3':5'-monophosphate in calcium-depleted hepatocytes. *J. Biol. Chem.*, 252:8645–8651.

200. Pointer, R. H., Butcher, F. R., and Fain, J. N. (1976): Studies on the role of cyclic guanosine 3':5'-monophosphate and extracellular Ca^{2+} in the regulation of glycogenolysis in rat liver cells. *J. Biol. Chem.*, 251:2987–2992.

201. Jones, L. M., and Mitchell, R. H. (1978): Stimulus-response coupling at alpha-adrenergic receptors. *Biochem. Soc. Trans.*, 6:673–688.

202. Exton, J. H. (1979): Mechanisms involved in alpha-adrenergic effects of catecholamines on liver metabolism. *J. Cyclic Nucleot. Res.*, 5:277–287.

203. Hems, D. A., Rodrigues, L. M., and Whitton, P. D. (1978): Rapid stimulation by vasopressin, oxytocin and angiotensin II of glycogen degradation in hepatocyte suspensions. *Biochem. J.*, 172:311–317.

204. Assimacopoulos-Jeannet, F. D., Blackmore, P. F., and Exton, J. H. (1977): Studies on alpha-adrenergic activation of hepatic glucose output. *J. Biol. Chem.*, 252:2662–2669.

205. Heylett, D. G. (1976): Effects of sympathomimetic amines on ^{45}Ca efflux from liver slices. *Br. J. Pharmacol.*, 57:158.

206. Blackmore, P. F., Brumley, F. T., Marks, J. L., and Exton, J. H. (1978): Studies on alpha-adrenergic activation of hepatic glucose output. *J. Biol. Chem.*, 253:4851–4858.

207. Blackmore, P. F., Dehaye, J. P., and Exton, J. H. (1979): Studies on alpha-adrenergic activation of hepatic glucose output. *J. Biol. Chem.*, 254:6945–6950.

208. Michell, R. H. (1975): Inositol phospholipids and cell surface receptor function. *Biochim. Biophys. Acta*, 415:81–147.

209. Kirk, C. J., Verrinder, T. R., and Hems, D. A. (1977): Rapid stimulation by vasopressin and adrenaline, of inorganic phosphate incorporation into phosphatidyl inositol in isolated hepatocytes. *FEBS Lett.*, 83:267.

210. Orly, J., and Schramm, M. (1976): Coupling of catecholamine receptor from one cell with adenylate cyclase from another cell by cell fusion. *Proc. Natl. Acad. Sci. (USA)*, 73:4410–4414.

211. Limbird, L. E., and Lefkowitz, R. J. (1977): Resolution of beta-adrenergic receptor binding and adenylate cyclase activity by gel exclusion chromatography. *J. Biol. Chem.*, 252:799–802.

212. Vauquelin, G., Geynet, P., Hanoune, J., and Strosberg, D. (1977): Isolation of adenylate cyclase-free beta adrenergic receptor from turkey erythrocyte membranes by affinity chromatography. *Proc. Natl. Acad. Sci. (USA)*, 74:3710–3714.

213. Wood, C. L., Caron, M. G., and Lefkowitz, R. J. (1979): Separation of solubilized alpha and beta adrenergic receptors by affinity chromatography. *Biochem. Biophys. Res. Commun.*, 88:1–8.

214. Guellaen, G., and Hanoune, J. (1979): Thiol reactivity and the molecular individuality of alpha and beta adrenoreceptors in rat liver plasma membranes. *Biochim. Biophys. Acta*, 587:618–627.

215. Malbon, C. C., Li, S. Y., and Fain, J. N. (1978): Hormonal activation of glycogen phosphorylase in hepatocytes from hypothyroid rats. *J. Biol. Chem.*, 253:8820–8825.

216. Blair, J. B., James, M. E., and Foster, J. L. (1979): Adrenergic control of glucose output and adenosine 3':5'-monophosphate levels in hepatocytes from juvenile and adult rats. *J. Biol. Chem.*, 254:7579–7584.

217. Leray, F., Chambaut, A. M., Perrenoud, M. L., and Hanoune, J. (1973): Adenylate-cyclase activity of rat liver plasma membranes. *Eur. J. Biochem.*, 38:185–200.

218. Chan, T. M., Blackmore, P. F., Steiner, K. E., and Exton, J. H. (1979): Effects of adrenalectomy on hormone action on hepatic glucose metabolism. *J. Biol. Chem.*, 254:2428–2433.

219. Christoffersen, R., Mørland, J., Osnes, J. B., and Øye, I. (1978): Changes in alpha and beta adrenergic activation. *Biochem. Biophys. Acta*, 587:338–344.

220. Kalish, M. I., Katz, M. S., Pineyro, M. A., and Gregerman, R. I. (1977): Epinephrine- and glucagon-sensitive adenylate cyclases of rat liver during aging. *Biochim. Biophys. Acta*, 483:452–466.

221. Boyd, H., and Martin, T. J. (1976): Changes in catecholamine and glucagon responsive adenylate cyclase activity in preneoplastic rat liver. *Mol. Pharmacol.*, 12:195–202.

222. Schmelck, P. H., Billon, M. C., Munnich, A., Getnet, P., Houssin, D., and Hanoune, J. (1979): The effects of common bile duct ligation upon the rat liver beta-adrenergic receptor-adenylate cyclase system. *FEBS Lett.*, 107:259–263.

223. Garrison, J. C., Borland, M. K., Florio, V. A., and Twible, D. A. (1979): The role of calcium ion as a mediator of the effects of angiotensin II, catecholamines, and vasopressin on the phosphorylation and activity of enzymes in isolated hepatocytes. *J. Biol. Chem.*, 254:7147–7156.

224. Keppens, S., and De Wulf, H. (1975): The activation of liver glycogen phosphorylase by vasopressin. *FEBS Lett.*, 51:29–32.

225. Keppens, S., and De Wulf, H. (1976): The activation of liver glycogen phosphorylase by angiotensin II. *FEBS Lett.*, 68:279–282.

226. Keppens, S., and De Wulf, H. (1979): The nature of the hepatic receptors involved in vasopressin-induced glycogenolysis. *Biochim. Biophys. Acta*, 588:63–69.

227. Lafontaine, J. J., Nivez, M. P., and Ardaillou, R. (1979): Hepatic binding sites for angiotensin II in the rat. *Clin. Sci.*, 56:333–337.

228. Lesniak, M. A., and Gorden, P. (1976): In: *Hormone-Receptor Interaction: Molecular Aspects*, edited by G. S. Levy, pp. 201–217. Marcel Dekker, New York.

229. De Meyts, P. (1976): In: *Methods in Receptor Research*, edited by M. Blecher, p. 301. Marcel Dekker, New York.

230. Tsushima, T., and Friesen, H. G. (1973): Radioreceptor assay for growth hormone. *J. Clin. Endocrinol. Metab.*, 37:334–337.

231. Posner, B. I., Kelly, P. A., Shiu, R. P. C., and Friesen, H. G. (1979): Studies of insulin, growth hormone and prolactin binding: Tissue distribution, species variation and characterization. *Endocrinology*, 95:521–531.

232. Kelly, P. A., Posner, B. I., Tsushima, T., Shui, R. P. C., and Friesen, H. G. (1974): In: *Advances in Human Growth Hormone Research*, edited by S. Raiti, p. 567. DHEW, Publication No. NIH-74-612, Washington, D.C.

233. Parke, L., and Forsyth, I. A. (1975): Assay of lactogenic hormones using receptors isolated from rabbit liver. *Endocrine Res. Commun.*, 2:137–149.

234. Cadman, H. F., and Wallis, M. (1981): An investigation of sites that bind human somatotropin (growth hormone) in the liver of the pregnant rabbit. *Biochem. J.*, 198:605–614.

235. Pliam, N. B., and Goldfine, I. D. (1977): High affinity thyroid hormone binding sites on purified rat liver plasma membranes. *Biochem. Biophys. Res. Commun.*, 79:166–172.

236. Gharbi, J., and Torresani, J. (1979): High affinity thyroxine binding to purified rat liver plasma membranes. *Biochem. Biophys. Res. Commun.*, 88:170–177.

237. Lin, M. C., and Akera, T. (1978): Increased (Na^+, K^+)-ATPase concentrations in various tissues of rats caused by thyroid hormone treatment. *J. Biol. Chem.*, 253:723–726.

The Liver: Biology and Pathobiology, edited by
I. Arias, H. Popper, D. Schachter, and D. A. Shafritz.
Raven Press, New York © 1982.

Chapter 34

Cell Membrane Transport Processes: Their Role in Hepatic Uptake

Carl A. Goresky

The effect of the cell membrane on the entry of materials into liver cells varies with the nature of the substance. For labeled water, the permeability is so large that it does not limit the entry of tracer water over the time of exposure encountered during a single sinusoidal transit time (1). Similar characteristics have been found for small, highly soluble lipid materials. For larger, biologically important materials, uptake is characterized by phenomena which, from the general biological point of view, conform to those that are generically categorized as characteristic of "membrane carrier transport." To approach the examination of the uptake of larger materials by the intact perfused liver *in vivo*, one must become familiar with and be able to utilize the major principles and methodology developed for the study of membrane carrier transport processes (chiefly in isolated cell suspensions) and adapt these in such a fashion that they can be utilized in the *in situ* blood-perfused organ and, finally, in man in the study of disease. To perform these studies, methods must be used which were developed to characterize capillary and parenchymal cell permeability in intact perfused organs. They should be modified to take into account the unique characteristics of the liver.

MEMBRANE CARRIER TRANSPORT

In 1961, Wilbrandt and Rosenberg (2) introduced their classic review of the concept of carrier transport and its corollaries as follows:

The cell membrane was once considered a static structure, protecting the cell against the loss of essential constituents by diffusion and allowing molecules and ions to exchange according to their lipid solubility, molecular size, and electric charge. In the past decades, it has proved necessary to revise this view. It has been found that the cell membrane is an active part of the cell machinery that, in many cases, the transfer of substances into and out of cells is due to pump-like devices in the membrane, and that such pumps can be utilized by the cells for different specific cell functions.

Information indicated that, for many substances, especially those which are neither very small nor highly lipid soluble, passage across the membrane could not be explained by simple diffusion through aqueous channels or through continuous lipid layers but rather by their association with some component of the membrane, which was not rigidly fixed but could move across the membrane; hence the introduction of the term "carrier." The development of this mechanism allows for high specificity, high efficacy, and the possibilities of both regulation and modification.

The biological importance of the mechanism is in its operation across the single cell membrane. Where transfer across a whole cell layer is being considered, particularly if there is a polarity to the structure (for example, in the transfer of a substance from liver sinusoidal plasma to canalicular bile), so that two differing sequential membranes are encountered (in this case, the liver sinusoidal membrane and the canalicular membrane), the characterization of the net transfer will reflect not a single barrier but the sequential activity of the two serial barriers. The operating characteristics of each must be determined.

The criteria necessary for establishing the presence of a carrier-mediated mechanism are operational in character and include the following: (a) Demonstration of saturation kinetics: If these are present, initial rates of uptake of material do not increase proportionately but saturate; a maximal rate of uptake is achieved at high external concentration. To explain this, uptake is conceived as occurring as a function of binding to an element in the membrane (the carrier); the limiting maximal rate of transfer occurs because of a finite total to the amount of carrier in the membrane. Initial uptake rates are usually determined, in the case of isolated cells, by placing them in a large volume medium in which a preexisting concentration of substrate has been established. The cells can then be made virtually empty of the substrate whose uptake is being explored. The effect of increasing the concentration on the uptake of substrate by the empty cells is then studied. The analysis of the data involves determination of the initial rate of uptake of substrate (by extrapolation to zero, in the time course of uptake) as a function of external substrate concentration, and the subsequent derivation of a maximal rate of uptake, or V_{max}, and of the concentration at which uptake is half maximal, the K_m, an analog Michaelis constant.

(b) Demonstration of competitive inhibition: The binding of a transported substrate to a specific site carries with it the possibility of competition and competitive inhibition. To the extent that a particular transport process is accumulative or concentrative, rather than nonconcentrative or equilibrative, the probability for inhibition exists at two sites: at the level of the supply of energy and, more directly, at the level of the mechanism itself. In interacting with the carrier mechanism, the competitive substrate may also be transported, or it may fix the carrier at the interface. The interacting penetrating inhibitor will be the type most commonly utilized *in vivo*. The architecture of the particular transport site is important in delineating the structure range of potential inhibitors. Its stereospecificity is particularly important and can be defined easily.

(c) Induction of countertransport: Countertransport is usually defined as an uphill transport, independent of metabolic energy. The necessary energy is derived from the downhill movement of a second substrate using the same carrier. Suppose that a first substrate is equilibrated on the two sides of a cell membrane, and a second substrate is added to the external medium and combines with free carrier. An inwardly directed gradient for the new combination is set up across the cell

membrane. The first substrate meets unequal concentrations of free carrier on the two sides of the cell membrane, so that more of its carrier substrate complex is formed on the inside than on the outside, and a net outward movement of the initial substrate occurs, i.e., an uphill transport. If, on the other hand, one examines a system in which there is an initial equilibration of tracer, and if the phenomenon of countertransport is provoked by addition of unlabeled parent material, one will perceive in the external medium a rise in the activity of tracer, a flush of the tracer material from the cell into the medium. Rosenberg and Wilbrandt (3) showed that the countertransport phenomenon is not to be expected when the competition between substrates concerns fixed sites on the membrane; it occurs only when there is a mobile carrier.

These are the positive three criteria for a carrier mechanism. Saturation kinetics and competition indicate binding, but not necessarily a movable site. The demonstration of countertransport or of isotope countertransport renders the evidence conclusive. On the other hand, it cannot be proved that a specific transfer cannot be mediated by carrier transport. Under low saturation conditions, the kinetics of transfer are indistinguishable from those of simple diffusion, and competition and countertransport are not demonstrable. The only suggestive evidence that might be adduced, if higher concentrations cannot be explored, is the finding of an unexpectedly high structural specificity and stereospecificity.

Substances whose uptake has been explored *in vitro* are usually osmotically free in the medium and in the cells. For nonprotein-bound materials, two differing patterns of behavior are found (4). In steady state, the material taken up either reaches the same concentration within the cell as in the medium (to undergo nonconcentrative or equilibrative uptake) or is concentrated within the cell despite being osmotically free (to undergo accumulative or concentrative transport). In the latter set of circumstances, a net concentration gradient is established and is maintained across the membrane. For substrates concentrated within the cells, the ratio of (intracellular/extracellular) concentrations is high at low external concentrations and decreases toward unity as the external concentration is increased (see Fig. 1). The decrease in concentration ratio with the rise in external concentration may also be expected if an intracellular binding protein were present; this characteristic is not unique to, although it is characteristic of, an intrinsically concentrative transport system.

One other characteristic of concentrative transport may be important *in vivo*; initial concentrations cannot be concisely controlled as with isolated cells. Changes in the internal concentration of osmotically free sub-

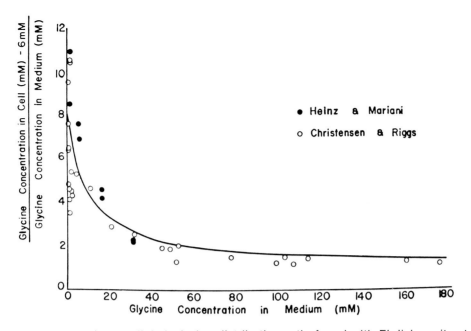

FIG. 1. Steady-state (intracellular/extracellular) glycine distribution ratio found with Ehrlich ascites tumor cells, as a function of external glycine concentration. Complete intracellular binding of glycine up to a concentration of 6 mM was assumed, since accompanying water uptake by these cells occurs only when the gradient across the membrane is greater than 6 mM. (Reproduced from ref. 4, with permission.) The data of Heinz and Mariani (5) (*filled circles*) were obtained from 15-min incubations and those of Christensen and Riggs (6) (*open circles*) from 1-hr incubations. The data from the former group tend to be somewhat higher than those of the latter, perhaps because of a lower proportion of dying cells.

strate affect the initial rate of uptake of labeled substrate from the external medium. As the internal concentration is raised, the initial rate of uptake of labeled substrate increases. This increase in the initial unidirectional uptake flux, which may be termed a preloading effect, is illustrated in Fig. 2. The preloading effect is a variant of the countertransport phenomenon. The efflux of unlabeled amino acids drives the

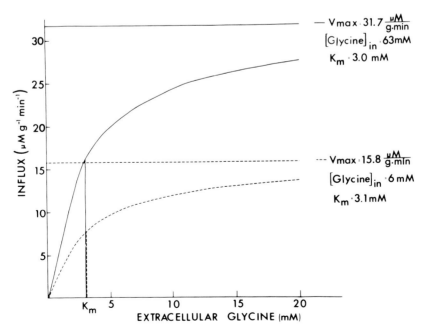

FIG. 2. Effect of preloading (preequilibration with unlabeled glycine) on the initial rate of uptake of labeled glycine by Ehrlich ascites tumor cells. (From ref. 8.)

uptake of labeled amino acid. In this instance, the data from the study of Heinz (7) on the initial rate of uptake of labeled glycine by Ehrlich ascites cells were used as the basis for the figure. When the initial intracellular concentration of glycine was 6 mM, the initial uptake of labeled glycine was characterized by a K_m of 3.1 mM and a V_{max} of 15.8 μmoles g^{-1} min^{-1}. When the initial intracellular concentration was 63 mM, the value for the K_m characterizing the process remained at 3.1 mM but the value for the V_{max} approximately doubled, reaching 31.7 μmoles g^{-1} min^{-1}. Preloading increased the V_{max} dramatically. Where the preloading effect is present, transport should be explored over a wide range of external concentrations with the initial internal concentration fixed. *In vivo*, these conditions are essentially impossible to meet. Instead, it is usually more appropriate to perform a classic tracer experiment and examine the uptake of tracer when varying amounts of substrate are present in the system, being sure that, in each experiment, the system is in a steady state. In experiments of this type, if the transport system being examined is concentrative in nature, the potential for a preloading effect must be kept in mind.

In vivo experiments tend to be more complex than are those *in vitro*. Blood flow will carry substrates to the tissue, and interactions occur from one end of the vasculature to the other; events downstream are modified by those upstream. In addition, other phenomena may be important. For instance, for many substances of interest, protein binding both in the plasma and within hepatocytes is significant.

PERMEABILITY CHARACTERISTICS OF LIVER SINUSOIDS

Hepatocytes subserve the major metabolic functions of the liver. Ultimately, it is the entry of materials into hepatocytes that we examine. Prior to traversing the surfaces of these cells, substrate must first be delivered in some fashion.

The liver sinusoids form channels from terminal portal venule to terminal hepatic vein, lying on each side of single cell-thick sheets of hepatocytes. These channels, which may be regarded as the end organs of the circulation, have a unique structure. They are lined by flattened endothelial cells containing fenestrae of various sizes. Beneath lies the space of Disse, the functional extracellular space of the liver. The fenestrae in the endothelial cells are so large and frequent that they provide continuity between vascular space and the space of Disse. No continuous anatomic barrier exists between the plasma and the Disse space, and hence dissolved substances have free access to the underlying surface of the liver cells. Hepatocytes are attached at mid-depth to their neighbors by tight junctions, which apparently seal the margins of each biliary canaliculus. Each approximately hexagonal cell is thus surrounded by an element in a continuously anastomosing canalicular network. A lateral intercellular cleft penetrates to the tight junction, and communication between plasma and bile is possible for substances that can traverse the tight junctions. The opposing surfaces of hepatocytes bordering the sinusoids are, in contrast, expanded by innumerable microvilli. The plasma membrane of these surfaces is specialized in such a manner as to maximize their area and increase the potential for contact between hepatocyte and blood.

Apart from the ultrastructural examination of the liver sinusoids, the most appropriate way to examine the distribution of materials to the surfaces of hepatocytes is to perform tracer experiments *in vivo*. Goresky (1) adapted the multiple indicator dilution technique (9) for use in the liver. The approach consists of rapid injection of a reference substance and a study substance into the blood flowing into the organ. The reference substance is assumed not to leave the vascular space, to behave similarly to the study substance in the absence of passage out of the circulation. Venous effluent is sampled in a fractionated fashion, and the concentrations of test materials in the blood are measured. To normalize the outflow curves, the concentration of each substance is expressed as a fractional proportion of the material injected per milliliter blood. Displacements of the normalized dilution pattern of the study substance from that of the reference material are assumed to result from passage across the microvasculature.

Rapid, single injection, multiple indicator dilution experiments in the liver were first performed in anesthetized dogs. An injection catheter was placed in the portal vein just above the junction of superior mesenteric and splenic veins, and a venous collection catheter was placed in the left main hepatic vein (1). The substances first examined were those expected to be distributed passively. The substances injected included (a) labeled red cells, which are confined to the vascular space, (b) labeled albumin, which is predominantly confined to the vascular space in organs with a continuous capillary lining, (c) labeled inulin, sucrose, and sodium, which have been viewed as classic extracellular space labels in the liver, and (d) labeled water, which is expected to penetrate cells.

A typical set of normalized hepatic venous dilution curves, resulting from the simultaneous introduction of labeled red cells, albumin, sucrose, sodium, and water into the portal vein, is displayed in the upper and middle panels of Fig. 3. The labeled red cells emerge first. Their outflow fraction per milliliter reaches the highest and earliest peak and decays rapidly until recirculation occurs. The other substances, which were dissolved in the plasma phase, show a systematically

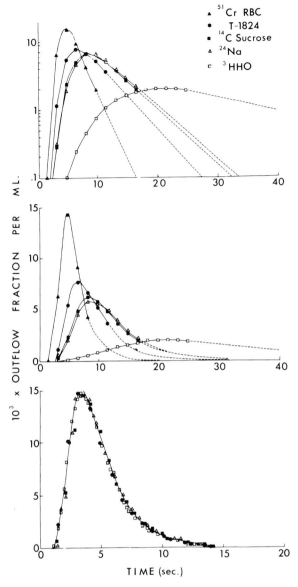

FIG. 3. Normalized hepatic venous outflow curves. T-1824 refers to albumin labeled with Evans blue dye. The ordinate scale is logarithmic in the upper panel and linear in the middle and lower panels. The curves have been corrected for recirculation by linear extrapolation on the semilogarithmic plot. The superimposition of the adjusted diffusible label curves on the labeled red cell curve is illustrated in the bottom panel. (From ref. 9.)

changing behavior. There is a progressive delay in outflow appearance, diminution and delay in reaching their peak, and a progressively retarded downslope decay from labeled albumin to labeled water. Labeled water shows a behavior that extends the continuum exhibited by the extracellular space labels. The delay in outflow appearance, in relation to labeled red cells, is well defined in these experiments.

Bolus flow is expected within the sinusoids (10). The red cells fill the sinusoidal lumina and are deformed by these channels. A mixing motion occurs in the seg-

ments of plasma between them. Both this and the dimensions of the sinusoid [an average diameter of 7.3 μm (11)] assure cross-sectional equilibration within the sinusoid. Beyond the vascular lumen, the small dimensions of the extracellular space are such that virtually immediate lateral diffusional equilibration is expected within the space. [Numerical analysis performed by Bassingthwaighte et al. (12) with realistic dimensions and diffusion coefficients shows that, even with rapid flow, in the absence of a barrier between the vascular space and the Disse space, the concentration profile is so flat that lateral diffusional equilibration can be considered to be established at each point along the length.] Flow-limited distribution of label into the extravascular space will result.

This situation can be modeled. Suppose that an amount of label, q_o, is suddenly introduced as an input at the origin of a sinusoid, and that this is then carried along by the sinusoidal flow, F_s, with the velocity, W. If we solve the partial differential equation describing this, we find that $u(x,t)_{ref}$, the vascular concentration of the reference substance at the position, x, as a function of time, t, can be described by the expression

$$u(x,t)_{ref} = \frac{q_o}{F_s} \delta\left(t - \frac{x}{W}\right) \qquad [1]$$

where the Greek letter stands for the Dirac impulse function. The formalities of the expression are such that the function exists only where $t = x/W$. A single labeled red cell (which is an ideal impulse input) is described as being carried along the sinusoid with the velocity, W, as expected. In mathematical terms, we would say that the impulse function propagates along the sinusoid as a traveling wave. If the sinusoid is of length, L, the red cell will arrive at the outflow at the time, $t = L/W$; that is

$$u(L,t)_{ref} = \frac{q_o}{F_s} \delta\left(t - \frac{L}{W}\right) \qquad [1A]$$

Assume that there are no axial dispersing effects in the capillary, that a bolus of dissolved tracer introduced at the same time as the red cell emerges at the same time as the red cell if none of the dissolved tracer traversed the sinusoidal wall. The structure of the sinusoid, however, will impose a different behavior. As indicated above, we expect flow-limited distribution of tracer into its extravascular space of distribution. If γ is the ratio of the extravascular space of distribution to the vascular space of distribution, its outflow profile is

$$u(L,t)_{diff} = \frac{q_o}{F_s} \delta\left[t - (1 + \gamma)\frac{L}{W}\right] \qquad [2]$$

The impulse function for the diffusible substance travels along the sinusoid as if it were flowing in a larger space, $(1 + \gamma)$ times as large as that for the reference substance. This is best described as delayed wave flow-limited distribution. The behavior is illustrated in Fig. 4. In this extreme, there is no axial dispersion of the tracer. The dissolved tracer input flows along with the velocity, $W/(1 + \gamma)$, slower than that of the vascular reference, and consequently emerges at the delayed outflow.

The relationships between the outflow curves from the whole liver for labeled red cells and that for each of the diffusible substances depends on the relationship between the transit times of the large vessels and those of the sinusoids. Two asymptotic extremes exist in the relationships among these distributions: that in which sinusoidal transit times are uniform, and that in which the large vessel transit times are uniform (13). The forms of the curves in Fig. 3 indicate that the latter probably describes the situation in the liver. If so, after a common large vessel transit time, each point along the diffusible curve will have its transit time increased by the factor $(1 + \gamma)$; since the areas under the normalized curves are the same, its magnitude will be decreased by the factor $1/(1 + \gamma)$. When the diffusible reference curve is transformed in such a manner as to reverse these effects, it should superimpose upon the labeled red cell curve. In the bottom panel of Fig. 3, the diffusible label curves have been appropriately transformed, using a common large vessel transit time. Superimposition occurs for all the labeled diffusible substances in a virtually ideal fashion. Using this superimposition as a criterion, we can infer that there is flow-limited distribution of these substances in the liver, a large heterogeneity of sinusoidal transit times,

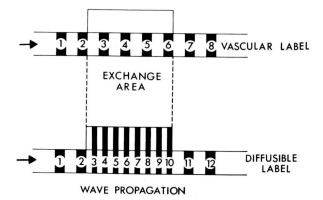

FIG. 4. Principle underlying delayed wave flow-limited distribution. *Upper panel,* vascular label as an idealized impulse at successive intervals of time, traveling with the velocity of flow. *Lower panel,* diffusible label as an impulse function spreading into a space twice as large as that accessible to the vascular label, at the same time intervals. Since the diffusible label effectively flows in a space twice as large, its transit time through the sinusoid is twice as long. (From ref. 9.)

and a common large vessel transit time. Since the liver sinusoids have a relatively common length, there is an underlying heterogeneity of perfusion (probably at a lobular level).

The lack of break in the continuum of behavior from the extracellular space labels to labeled water indicates that, in the liver, where the surfaces of the cells have been increased by formation of microvilli and vascular transit times are relatively long, the retarding effect of the cell membrane on labeled water exchange is not perceptible during a single passage time. Labeled water is distributed into hepatocytes and the extracellular space in a flow-limited fashion.

The volume of distribution of each of the tracers can be calculated as the product of flow and mean transit time. From this point of view, the magnitude of the relative transit times is important. In the dog, the portal vein-hepatic vein mean transit time for labeled red cells is of the order of 8.4 sec; for albumin, 12.4 sec; for sodium and sucrose, 14.7 sec; for inulin, between that for albumin and that for sucrose; and for labeled water of the order of 38 sec. If the flow utilized in the calculation of the volume of distribution for labeled water is that of blood water (calculated from the water content of blood), the amount of water in the liver and its contained blood is estimated. Excellent agreement is found when this is compared to the water content of the organ (1). The dilution probe provides a valid estimate of liver size. The labeled red cell space, calculated from blood flow and the red cell transit time, is found to average 12.8% of the liver weight (1,14). Labeled albumin and the group of extracellular substances are confined to the plasma phase in blood. It is appropriate, therefore, to calculate their spaces of distribution as the product of the plasma flow and their transit time. If we assume that the transit times of these substances are identical to that of the labeled red cells if these did not leave the vascular lumen, the space of distribution available to them, over and above the blood space, can be calculated as the product of the plasma flow and the difference between the transit times of these labels and that for labeled red cells. The result is expressed in terms of equivalent milliliters plasma. Average values, reexpressed as a proportion of liver weight, are presented in Table 1. The proportion of the liver estimated to be occupied by sinusoidal and Disse space corresponds to that estimated from morphometric analysis (11); and the extra space available to albumin corresponds almost exactly to that determined by steady-state tissue analysis (15). This technique provides a valid reflection of the functional composition of the normal liver.

The question remains: How unique is red cell-plasma albumin label separation in the liver? In most other organs, outflow curves for labeled red cells and

TABLE 1. *Relative volumes accessible in the extracellular space of the liver*

Substance	Percent liver weight	Accessible proportion of sodium space
Sodium	8.9	1.00
Sucrose	8.8	0.99
Inulin	7.7	0.87
Albumin	5.7	0.64

labeled albumin are similar. Little outflow displacement of the labeled albumin curve is found. For example, in the pulmonary circulation at low flows, when the labeled red cell mean transit time is of the order of that found in the liver, the ratio of the labeled albumin/red cell mean transit time is 1.04 (16). The value is close to unity and is remarkably different from the value of 1.48, the average found for the liver. In the pulmonary circulation, as in other circulations in which the capillary endothelium is continuous and relatively impermeable, the displacement between the labeled red cell and albumin tracers is minor. The comparatively major difference between the two values, together with the contrasting structure of capillaries and sinusoids, indicates that direct access of dissolved tracer to the Disse or extracellular space (and hence to the surface of the liver cells) sets the microvasculature of the liver apart from that of other organs. This design is optimal for an organ that serves as a chemical factory, which obtains its substrates directly from and discharges its products directly into the bloodstream.

The implicit assumption of our earlier formulations is that albumin and all the extracellular probes enter the Disse space, the extracellular space of the liver. Yet the data in Table 1 indicate that the extracellular space available to these, calculated in terms of plasma equivalents, varies. The accessible space decreases as the size of the probing molecule increases. An apparent exclusion phenomenon increases with the molecular weight. An analogous exclusion phenomenon has been demonstrated *in vitro* for both hyaluronic acid gels (17) and collagen (18); it is evident that similar properties of the ground substance and collagen in the Disse space, which is directly accessible to the soluble probes, are being brought to light by these experiments.

The free accessibility of the Disse space and the exclusion phenomenon imply that, in the use of indicator dilution experiments to study uptake, one must use, in addition to labeled red cells, that specific type of second extracellular space reference that describes the behavior the uptake substance would have if it did not enter the liver cells. For nonprotein-bound, low molecular weight substances, sucrose or sodium are

the most appropriate second references; for albumin-bound substances, labeled albumin is more appropriate.

QUALITATIVE DATA DEMONSTRATING CARRIER TRANSPORT

Those organic anions taken up by the liver and secreted in bile in high concentration (bilirubin, sulfobromophthalein, indocyanine green, and Rose bengal) have been the object of much attention. Bilirubin in particular, because of its high lipid solubility, had been thought likely to enter liver cells passively. Since all these compounds are tightly bound to albumin, if the other compounds also entered the liver in this way, the dominating and virtually exclusively regulating feature for the entry of all would necessarily be the affinity and concentration of hepatic intracellular binding sites and particularly of cytoplasmic binding proteins. It was important, therefore, to determine whether entry through the cell membrane is passive and linear or whether a carrier transport process mediated the entry, with all the potential for specificity and regulation that this mechanism implies.

The problem has been approached in a less detailed fashion by examining the disappearance from plasma of various doses of these organic anions. In each case, it has been clear that the compound is removed from the plasma preferentially by the liver, and that hepatic handling consists of uptake, processing within the cell to form conjugates of bilirubin and sulfobromophthalein, transfer to the excretory system, and biliary excretion. The canalicular excretory step has been examined for bilirubin and sulfobromophthalein and found to be limited; its capacity is the major limiting step in removal under load. The events that occur following injection of a dose of the organic anions into plasma are of interest because, although they do not provide the detail that examination at the level of the liver provides, they illustrate several general phenomena. Ordinarily, following an intravenous dose of these substances, one would expect, if they were being removed by a mechanism functioning as an infinite sink, single exponential disappearance curves (the rates of disappearance would remain proportional to the concentrations). As the materials enter liver cells and their intracellular concentrations increase, it would be reasonable to expect a back flux to plasma, so that the plasma disappearance would become less rapid. A pseudoequilibrium will be established between plasma and liver cells, and the plasma concentrations will be expected to fall more slowly, chiefly as a result of the biliary removal of materials. Exchange across capillaries at the level of other organs has been thought to be minimized by albumin binding; and its contribution to disappearance curves has been neglected. The relative plasma level at which pseudoequilibrium occurs for each dose will be dominated by the intrinsic character of the process underlying transfer across the cell membrane (concentrative or nonconcentrative) and the relative capacity and affinity of binding sites in the plasma and in the cytosol of hepatocytes. With a concentrative process, the plasma concentration at pseudoequilibrium will be much lower. In the case of sulfobromophthalein, for instance, *in vitro* studies of uptake by isolated liver cells suggest that the cellular uptake mechanism is highly concentrative (19); and the *in vivo* steady infusion studies of Wheeler et al. (20) indicate that the space of distribution available to sulfobromophthalein in the liver is larger than the plasma space. Steady state liver intracellular concentrations are higher than those in plasma.

Plasma disappearance curves have been used qualitatively to ascertain whether the three essential operational criteria expected of carrier-mediated transport (saturation of initial uptake, competitive inhibition, and countertransport) are exhibited by the liver uptake process for organic anions (21–24). The slopes of initial disappearance curves on logarithm concentration-linear time plots do not remain constant but decrease as the dose of material is increased. The initial rate of uptake increases with the dose (that is, with the plasma concentration) but not in a linear fashion. It increases in such a way that, at very high concentrations, the initial rate of uptake approaches a maximal value. A saturation phenomenon is present. Initial tracer bilirubin disappearance rates from plasma have also been studied against a background of varied steady-state bilirubin concentrations. Net uptake rates, derived from the rate of disappearance of tracer and the total plasma pool (expressed as a dose), failed to show degrees of saturation comparable to those found in single dose studies.

Scharschmidt et al. (24) interpreted the divergence of the uptake rates for bilirubin in the two instances to provide evidence for a preloading effect on tracer uptake at higher steady-state concentrations. The problem presented by these data exemplifies the difficulties encountered when endeavoring to perform experiments *in vivo* to derive information analogous to that obtained with isolated cells *in vitro*. Second, when any

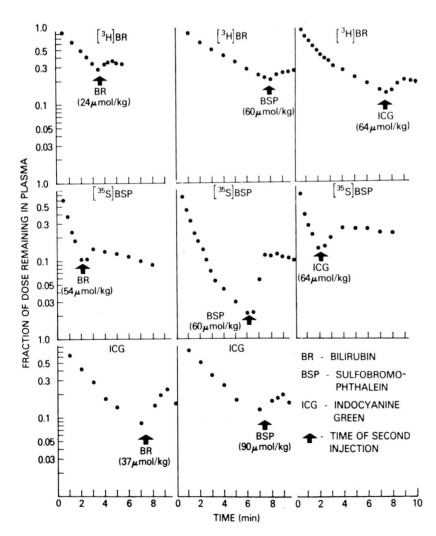

FIG. 5. ^{3}H-Labeled bilirubin, ^{35}S-labeled sulfobromophthalein, and indocyanine green countertransport. A tracer dose of ^{3}H-labeled bilirubin or ^{35}S-labeled sulfobromophthalein or a 0.5 mg/kg dose of indocyanine green was injected intravenously and followed 2 to 7 min later (*arrow*) by a bolus of unlabeled bilirubin, sulfobromophthalein, or indocyanine green. Each of these three organic anions showed reflux from liver to plasma after the second injection. (From ref. 24.)

organic anion is mixed with another, the rate of uptake of each becomes less than if either were presented alone. Competitive inhibition is present. Finally, the phenomena of countertransport can be elicited, both as same-species labeled moiety countertransport and as cross-species countertransport. As a pseudoequilibrium begins to be established, a large dose of counterflush material is added to the plasma. The counterflush material occupies all the available sites on the plasma face of the liver cells but does not acutely inhibit transfer of the material, which has already been equilibrated from cell to plasma, since the intracellular concentrations of the counterflush material will not immediately have been increased. A classic set of findings from a group of countertransport experiments is illustrated in Fig. 5. The phenomena indicate that there is a mobile carrier mechanism in the membrane common to this group of substances and subserving their transport across the sinusoidal face of the parenchymal liver cells.

The canalicular surface of the liver cells is not as easily accessible as is the sinusoidal face of the cells. Knowledge of intracellular concentrations of materials and concentrations and properties of binding proteins will be necessary before transport processes at this level can be analyzed in detail. Nevertheless, the presence of a transport maximum for the biliary excretion of each of these compounds suggests that a second set of carrier processes is present in the canalicular membranes, and that experiments designed from this point of view might provide new knowledge.

INDICATOR DILUTION STUDIES OF HEPATIC UPTAKE

The indicator dilution method permits closer examination of events at the hepatic cell surface and has been used in two major ways: the substance whose uptake is being studied has been supplied as a varying mass bolus (analogous to the intravenous disappearance studies outlined above) or as a tracer bolus, which is superimposed on the steady state. The concentration within the bolus in the former case is unknown (it is mixed with blood during the injection), and parameters characterizing a saturable transport mechanism cannot be accurately determined. The approach is only useful for qualitatively demonstrating that uptake is saturable. In the latter approach (the tracer experiment), in the presence of a steady state with respect to the tracer substrate, the concentrations of substrate across the hepatic sinusoid can be readily defined. If there is no net loss or addition of substrate across the system, input and output cellular concentrations will be the same, and vascular and cellular concentrations will be uniform from input to output. Substrate concentrations can be varied over a wide range of concentrations. If there is net removal of substrate across the system, however, uptake will create two characteristic effects at the lobular level: a steadily falling concentration from input to output, and an abrupt fall in concentration across the hepatocyte plasma membrane if the membrane is a barrier to passage of the material being sequestered in the liver cells.

The two major mechanisms of sequestration within the liver are either conversion to another metabolic product or excretion into bile. Either process produces these effects. The sequestration process also usually exhibits saturation kinetics: if the uptake mechanism is enzymic, Michaelis-Menten kinetics are evident. Biliary secretory mechanisms also exhibit transport maxima, presumably because of a carrier-mediated membrane transport mechanism. Both these processes are nonlinear, but tracer handling is linear. The most economical way to describe the process is to relate the transfer coefficient to space average bulk concentrations in sinusoidal plasma and cellular spaces. The former (the plasma concentration) is easily found, but the cellular concentration becomes available only if one analyzes data to establish the average relationship between cellular and plasma concentrations. The calculated concentrations at the sequestration site then can be related to operation of a specific mechanism. Steady-state falling lobular concentration profiles have been documented autoradiographically for labeled galactose (25) and cholylglycylhistamine (26), a bile acid derivative excreted in bile. The interrelationships among vascular and cellular profiles for substances removed in net fashion across the system are of particular interest when the sequestration mechanism saturates at lower concentrations than does the membrane carrier uptake mechanism (i.e., when the Michaelis constant of the enzymic process is lower than the analog constant for the carrier process). When the concentration of substrate is very low, proportional extraction of substrate will be large (the proportional drop in concentration along the sinusoid will be large), the profiles in vascular and cellular space will be exponential, and the proportional drop in concentration across the liver cell membrane is greatest. As the substrate concentration increases, the proportional drop in concentration from input to output decreases, the longitudinal profile becomes linear, and the proportional drop in concentration across the liver cell membrane becomes very small. Divergence between the average sinusoidal vascular and cellular concentrations is greatest at the lowest concentrations.

Tracer Uptake in the Steady State

The indicator dilution approach, which shows that extracellular space references penetrate to the liver cell membrane in a flow-limited fashion, provides an

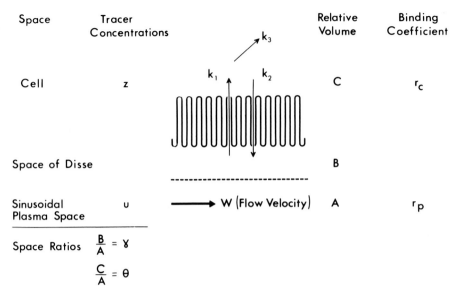

FIG. 6. Kinetic model utilized to derive fitted parameters from experimental indicator dilution curves. (From ref. 27.)

appropriate background for design of experiments to elucidate the steady-state kinetics of tracer transfer across the liver cell membrane. To study cellular uptake, the injection mixture must contain not only labeled red cells and the tracer whose behavior is to be documented, but an appropriate extracellular space reference as well. The labeled substrate would be expected to emerge at the outflow with a profile identical to the appropriate second or extracellular space reference if uptake did not occur, i.e., if the liver cell membranes were impermeable to the tracer. With uptake, the outflow profile will consist of two parts: a throughput component (i.e., that part of the tracer that reaches the outflow without entering the liver cells), and a returning component, which represents the tracer that entered the liver cells and returned to the vascular space to be added to the outflow. If there is no sequestration of tracer, and if outflow mass conservation is present, the total area under the tracer substrate curve will match that under either the red cell curve or that of the second reference. If there is sequestration of tracer, the area under the returning component will be reduced by the uptake process, and the accumulated area under the tracer outflow response will be correspondingly reduced. The phenomena being considered are distributed in time and space. The expressions describing them are simple in terms of understanding the components, as outlined above, but are complicated in terms of detail.

In terms of modeling, we can superimpose uptake at the liver cell surface (Fig. 6). Consider that flow subserves longitudinal transport in the hepatic sinusoid and that solutes in plasma immediately equilibrate within the extracellular space in the liver. In the case of substances which are tightly bound to albumin,

steric exclusion of carrier molecule, i.e., albumin, in the Disse space has an appreciable effect on the immediately accessible extracellular space. If γ is the ratio of the volume of the Disse space to that of plasma, and p is the proportion of that space accessible to the tracer, $p\gamma$ represents the ratio of the apparent volume accessible in Disse space to the sinusoidal plasma volume. With this background, set the rate of change of labeled material in the hepatic parenchymal cells at any point, x, along the length of the sinusoid at the time, t, equal to the difference between rates of influx and loss (the latter occurring either by efflux to plasma or by sequestration, by removal from the intracellular pool) (25,28). In describing the uptake process, we must also take into account the relative binding of protein-bound substrates to albumin in the sinusoid and extracellular space and to binding proteins within cell cytosol (the phase in intimate approximation to the inner surface of the liver cell sinusoidal membranes). To account for this, define a set of binding coefficients, r_p and r_c, which detail the effect in plasma and cell space, respectively. If free concentrations mediate the process, r_p and r_c will be the ratio of total to free concentrations in the respective phases. Each coefficient will increase as the concentration of the binding protein increases and will decrease whenever competitors decrease the average affinity of the protein for the substrate. When there is no binding, r_p and r_c will be unity. With the definitions given in Fig. 6, we arrive at the equation

$$\frac{\partial z(x,t)}{\partial t} = \frac{k_1}{r_p} u(x,t) - \frac{k_2}{r_c} z(x,t) - \frac{k_3}{r_c} z(x,t) \qquad [3]$$

The implication is that in the steady state, if the sequestration process is inoperative,

$$z = \left(\frac{k_1}{k_2}\right)\left(\frac{r_c}{r_p}\right)u \qquad [4]$$

The ratio of cellular to plasma concentrations will reflect not only the membrane activity ratio k_1/k_2 (this will be unity when a nonconcentrative process is considered and will be larger than unity when the process at the membrane is concentrative) but also the binding coefficient ratio r_c/r_p. For protein-bound materials, the ratio r_c/r_p will be controlled not only by the relative concentrations of the proteins but by the numbers and affinities of their unoccupied and occupied binding sites. Increase in the concentration of intracellular binding proteins will be reflected primarily in an increase in the ratio r_c/r_p.

After an impulse response at the origin, the plasma response of the sinusoid will be

$$u(x,t) = \frac{q_o}{F_s} e^{-\frac{k_1\theta}{r_p}\frac{x}{W}} \delta\left[t - (1 + p\gamma)\frac{x}{W}\right]$$
$$+ \frac{q_o}{F_s} e^{-\left(\left[\frac{k_2}{r_c} + \frac{k_3}{r_c}\right]\left[t - (1 + p\gamma)\frac{x}{W}\right]\right)} e^{-\frac{k_1\theta}{r_p}\frac{x}{W}}$$
$$\times \sum_{n=1}^{\infty} \frac{\left(\frac{k_1\theta}{r_p}\frac{k_2}{r_c}\frac{x}{W}\right)^n \left(t - (1 + p\gamma)\frac{x}{W}\right)^{n-1}}{n!\ (n-1)!} S\left[t - (1 + p\gamma)\frac{x}{W}\right]$$

$$[5]$$

where $S[t-(1 + p\gamma)x/W]$ is a step function at the time $(1 + p\gamma)x/W$. The description of the outflow response (the response at $x = L$) is made up of the expected two parts: a first term, the throughput material, the part of the original impulse which survives and reaches the outflow without entering the liver cells, and a second term, the returning material, which enters the liver cells and escapes sequestration to later exit at the vascular outflow. When $k_3 = 0$, all the tracer will emerge at the outflow, and outflow conservation will be complete. When $k_3 = 0$, the transit time for the outflow response will be $[1 + p\gamma + (k_1/k_2) (r_c/r_p)\theta] (L/W)$. The outflow transit time will be expected to increase as (k_1/k_2) increases (that is, as the membrane process becomes more concentrative) and as (r_c/r_p) increases (that is, as the relative concentration of binding sites in the cell is increased).

The approach used above may be termed parametric. The modeling can also be approached from a more physical point of view, in which analog permeabilities P'_{in} and P'_{out}, corresponding to the transport rate constants, the surface area S of the cells, the expanded plasma space $(1 + p\gamma)V_{pl}$, and the cell volume, V_c, are considered. Use of equation [5] over the set of transit times corresponding to the second reference will then enable one to optimize estimates of the lumped coeffi-

cients listed in Table 2. Estimates for influx, efflux, and sequestration coefficients can then be derived from appropriate sets of indicator dilution curves for each compound whose behavior is explored.

Uptake of Tracer Bilirubin, a Substance Bound Bound to Proteins in Either Plasma or Intracellular Spaces

The uptake of glucose by the liver is nonconcentrative. The intracellular concentration of free glucose in the liver is equal to the concomitant plasma concentration, as long as it is not substantially below the normal range (29). The process at the liver cell membrane will be expected to be carrier mediated, if we reason by analogy with the entry processes for glucose in

other cells. The indicator dilution method provides a way to characterize this transport process *in vivo*. The experiments must be performed with tracer glucose when the underlying bulk concentration has been set beforehand and when the system is in a steady state. The outflow profiles from a dilution experiment will be expected to vary somewhat, depending on the intrinsic character of the entry process. When the membrane process is highly concentrative, the returning component will be protracted in time and low in magnitude; hence any substantial throughput component will be

TABLE 2. *Equivalent forms of influx, efflux, and sequestration coefficients*

Coefficient	Parametric modeling	Physical modeling
Influx	$\dfrac{k_1\theta}{r_p(1 + p\gamma)}$	$\dfrac{P'_{in} S}{r_p(1 + p\gamma)V_p}$
Efflux	$\dfrac{k_2}{r_c}$	$\dfrac{P'_{out} S}{r_c}$
Sequestration	$\dfrac{k_3}{r_c}$	$\dfrac{k_3'}{r_c V_c}$

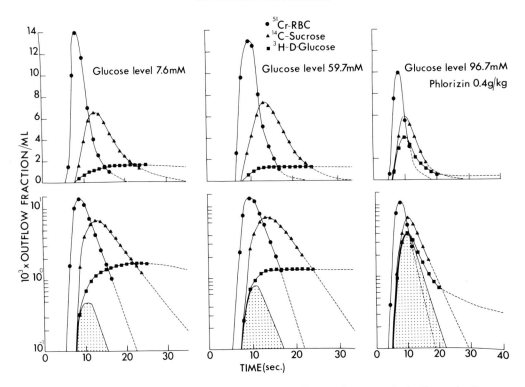

FIG. 7. Labeled glucose multiple indicator dilution experiments. The ordinate scale is linear in the upper panels and logarithmic in the lower. *Left-hand panels,* glucose level is normal for a fasting animal; *middle panels,* quite high; *right-hand panels,* glucose levels have been raised to very high levels, and a phlorhizin infusion (0.4 g/kg) has been carried out for the 20 min prior to and during an experimental run. Computed throughput components are shaded in the lower panels. (From ref. 31.)

laid bare. The influx coefficient can then be estimated simply from the relationship between the second reference and tracer substrate curves (28). This is not so in a nonconcentrative case. Both throughput and returning components are expected to be substantially intermixed; the task of separating throughput and returning components, while optimizing estimates of influx and efflux coefficients, becomes substantial and can be performed only with a digital computer (30). The addition of a sequestration process adds to this complexity. In the asymptotic extreme, when the uptake process is massive, the returning component will be so reduced in magnitude that the throughput component will once again be laid bare. It will be difficult to determine efflux and sequestration coefficients as separable entities and to distinguish between massive net uptake and a highly concentrative entry process from outflow curves.

Multiple indicator dilution studies performed in dogs to characterize tracer glucose uptake are illustrated in Fig. 7. Labeled red cells are used as the vascular reference, and labeled sucrose as the second or extracellular reference. [In nonprimate mammalian species, the time for equilibration of glucose in red cell water is prolonged; in the dog, it is of the order of one day (32).] The glucose label is added to plasma from the animal to make up the injection mixture just before the ex-

periment and can be considered to be confined to the plasma phase of the blood, as is the labeled sucrose; the experiment is a tracer experiment in a steady state (plasma glucose levels are set by a preceding infusion of glucose). In all three panels of Fig. 7, the labeled sucrose curve is related to the labeled red cell curve in the manner expected for flow-limited distribution: the outflow appearance is delayed, the curve rises to a later and lower peak, and its downslope decays more slowly. The areas under the two curves are identical. The relative shapes of the glucose curves change as the conditions of the experiment are changed. In the left-hand panels, where the glucose level was normal, the labeled glucose curve begins to rise at the same time as that of the labeled sucrose but increases slowly to a peak which is later and substantially lower than that for sucrose; it then begins slowly to drop. When the model analysis was fitted to the data, a small throughput component was resolved. As the glucose level was raised, the relative shapes of the labeled glucose curves slowly changed. In the middle panel, where the glucose levels are high, the labeled glucose curve assumes a more squared-off initial shape on the semilogarithmic plot, rising relatively quickly to a prolonged low and flattened peak with an ultimate slow decay. In both these experiments, as expected, a substantial proportion of the returning component emerges at the outflow early in time (the throughput components are shaded in the lower panels). It would have been impossible to resolve the throughput and returning components from the curves without the use of a digital computer. In these experiments, tracer glucose was not consumed metabolically in any important quantitative sense, and the sequestration constant was zero.

The data show an overall trend. As the plasma glucose level is increased, the throughput component increases in magnitude (the proportion of the tracer entering the liver cells decreases). The calculated parameters corresponding to uptake and return, the influx and efflux coefficients, decrease. The unidirectional fluxes of material, the products of the flux coefficients and the concentrations on each side of the membrane, increase with increase in concentration but not in a linear fashion. Instead, they show saturation. Analysis of the data (30) indicates that the K_m for influx and efflux is the same, 122 mM, a high value. The degree of saturation that occurs across the physiological range of concentrations, therefore, is small. The maximal transport rate is 0.028 ml sec^{-1}/ml liver intracellular space. This value is of the order of three times the transport maximum for D-glucose in human erythrocytes (2), in which glucose transport is rapid, in contrast to dog red cells. The average value for the ratio (influx coefficient/efflux coefficient) is of interest; from Table 2, it corresponds to $V_c/[(1 + p\gamma)V_p]$, the ratio of the cellular volume to the expanded plasma sinusoidal volume (in a nonconcentrative system $P'_{in}/P'_{out} = 1$; in the absence of protein binding, r_p and $r_c = 1$). The average value for the ratio was 2.3.

Intuitively, one would trust the model analysis to a greater degree if, at the experimental level, the conditions could be altered in such a way as to make the throughput component emerge from the labeled glucose curve as a separately recognizable component. To this end, in animals with high glucose levels, a competitive glycone, phlorizin, was infused into the portal vein before and during an experimental run. A dramatic effect is illustrated in the right-hand panels of Fig. 7. An early peak has emerged from the D-glucose curve, related to and contained within the overlying sucrose reference curve. On the downslope, the glucose curve approaches and crosses over the sucrose curve. The analysis illustrated in the lower panel demonstrates that the preponderant part of this early peak is a throughput component. The influx and efflux coefficients for tracer D-glucose are reduced to about 40% of the values otherwise expected at the underlying glucose level. Galactose loading produces similar effects. Competitive inhibition is produced at the transport site by either of these maneuvers.

The specificity of the receptor in the transport site can also be made evident by challenging with a related molecule, one with an altered structure but without major change in its chemical properties or molecular weight. The mirror image isomer, L-glucose, is found to enter liver cells very slowly (30), tracer equilibration occurring during 40 min (33); β-methyl D-glucoside enters liver cells at a low rate (30). Countertransport of D-glucose tracer has also been demonstrated *in vivo* (30). Counterflush of D-glucose label occurs after previous equilibration of tracer in the liver cells.

These *in vivo* studies show that the uptake of D-glucose by hepatocytes exhibits the major operational characteristics of a membrane carrier transport system: (a) saturation of rates of initial uptake of tracer at higher underlying glucose concentrations, (b) competitive inhibition, (c) stereospecificity, and (d) isotope countertransport.

D-Galactose, in contrast to D-glucose, is removed in substantial net fashion by the liver by means of an intracellular enzymic sequestration mechanism. Exploration of the disposal of tracer galactose illustrates that the same principles operate at the level of the cell membrane entry mechanism with addition of a saturable intracellular disposal mechanism (25). Rather than reviewing these findings, we examine uptake of a protein-bound material, bilirubin, to show that more detailed knowledge concerning uptake and disposal mechanisms can be found by designing experiments that focus on the accessory effects expected from protein binding.

Uptake of Tracer Bilirubin, a Substance Bound to Both Albumin in the Plasma Space and to Intracellular Binding Proteins

Bilirubin is tightly bound to albumin in plasma. During hepatic uptake, flow carries this pigment protein complex through the hepatic sinusoid, where it will traverse the space of Disse in a flow-limited manner to reach the plasma membranes of the hepatocytes. A proportion of the bilirubin but not albumin (34) is transferred across the cell membrane into the hepatocyte, where it is bound to soluble proteins. Intracellularly, bilirubin binds primarily to ligandin (glutathione S-transferase B) and, to a lesser extent, to other glutathione S-transferases and Z protein (35). Bilirubin within the cell is normally either conjugated and excreted in bile or returned to the plasma without conjugation.

The qualitative intravenous disappearance data presented earlier indicate that bilirubin entry into the liver occurs by a mechanism that fulfills the broad criteria for carrier-mediated membrane transport. Both Goresky (34) and Paumgartner and Reichen (36) have performed indicator dilution load experiments and found substantial evidence of saturation of the entry mechanism. Even under no load conditions,

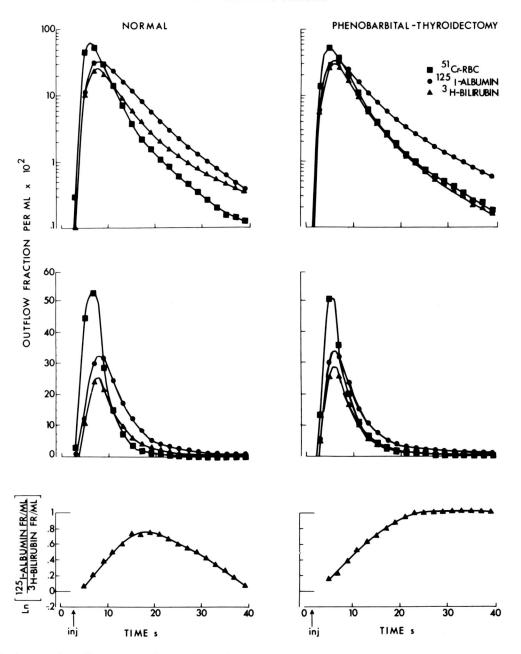

FIG. 8. Typical sets of outflow curves from labeled bilirubin multiple indicator dilution experiments. *Upper panels,* curves plotted in a semilogarithmic fashion; *middle panels,* curves plotted on rectilinear coordinates; *lower panels,* natural logarithm of the ratio of albumin/bilirubin outflow fractions per milliliter are plotted against time. The signal on the time scale represents the transport lag in the input and collection systems. (From ref. 27.)

however, a substantial proportion of the tracer comes through to the outflow in the throughput component. A major proportion of the total has not entered the liver cells (34). With this background information, Wolkoff et al. (27) asked the question: What is the role of the intracellular binding proteins and particularly of ligandin in the uptake of bilirubin, and how do these proteins function, from the kinetic point of view? The authors carried out nonrecirculating multiple indicator dilution tracer studies in the isolated perfused rat liver.

They utilized livers from normal animals and animals in which the ligandin levels were increased by phenobarbital pretreatment or thyroidectomy and performed the experiments in the absence of load, so that the returning components would make up a larger proportion of the outflow curves.

Outflow patterns from a typical set of labeled bilirubin multiple indicator dilution experiments are illustrated in Fig. 8. In each instance, the labeled albumin second reference is displaced from the labeled red cell

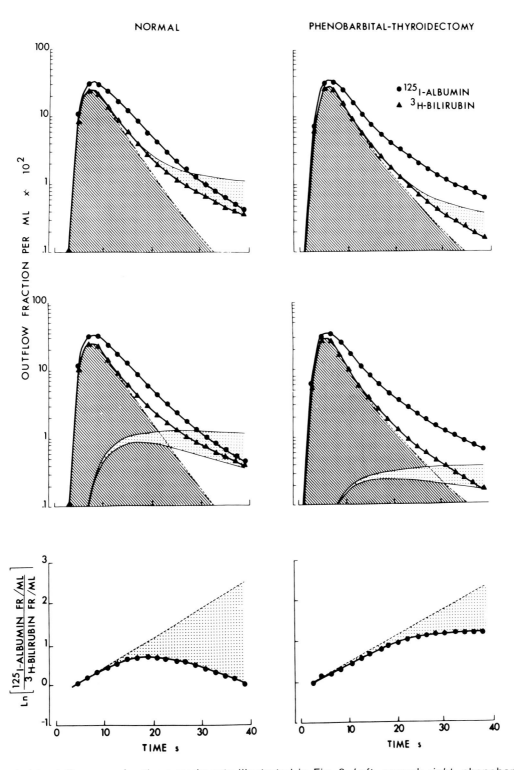

FIG. 9. Computed best fit curves for the experiments illustrated in Fig. 8. *Left,* normal; *right,* phenobarbital-treated thyroidectomized case. Throughput components in upper and middle panels have been emphasized by hatched shading; in the upper two panels, the differences between the returning components and the profiles expected if there had been no sequestration are emphasized by dotted shading. Natural logarithm ratio curves are plotted in the lower panels. (From ref. 27.)

curve in the fashion characteristic of flow-limited distribution. The labeled bilirubin curve is related to that of its carrier molecule, albumin. In the normal animals (left panels), the bilirubin curve progressively diverges from the albumin curve on the semilogarithmic plot until the mid-downslope and then begins to approach the labeled albumin curve. If collections had been continued for a longer period, the bilirubin curve would have crossed the albumin curve. Model analysis indicates that when the throughput component is the bulk of the early part of the curve, the natural logarithm of the ratio of the outflow fractions per milliliter for albumin/bilirubin versus time plot will be expected to have an initial slope corresponding to the influx coefficient and then to deviate progressively from this line as the returning component contributes increasingly to the outflow profile (28). The ratio rises until the sense of the relationship between the curves changes and falls thereafter. The data acquired from the liver of a thyroidectomized animal treated with phenobarbital (right panels) are characteristically different. The late approach to the albumin curve is not evident on the semilogarithmic plot; on the ratio plot, the curve merely levels off, late in time, rather than falling.

The fitted components of the bilirubin outflow dilution curves are illustrated in Fig. 9. The throughput components are similar in the two instances when compared to their respective albumin reference curves. The returning components are different. In the normal instance, the returning component is large enough that the downslope of the labeled bilirubin curve obviously approaches that for albumin; in the middle panel, where this component is plotted separately, it is seen to quantitatively dominate the downslope, late in time. The form of the complete profile and of the returning component, if no sequestration had occurred, is illustrated in the upper and middle

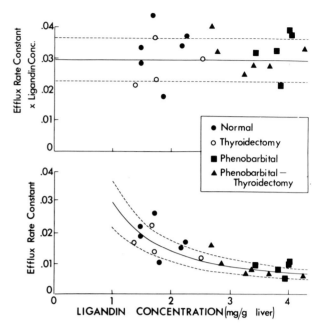

FIG. 10. *Lower panel,* relationship between efflux coefficient and ligandin concentration; *upper panel,* that between the product (efflux rate constant times ligandin concentration) and ligandin concentration. *Solid line,* regression line through the data; *dashed lines,* SE of the fit. Corresponding loci are plotted in the lower panel. (From ref. 27.)

panels, respectively. The difference between these and the observed outflow profiles has been emphasized by hatched shading in both instances. This difference represents the net effect of the sequestration flux and increases with time. In the phenobarbital-treated rat, the second component is grossly reduced in magnitude. The quantitative contribution of the returning component to the outflow profile is small and late in time. Even the second component predicted in the absence of sequestration is de-

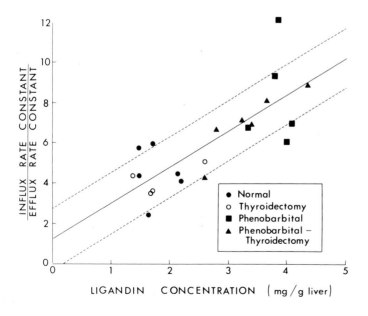

FIG. 11. Relationship between the ratio (influx coefficient/efflux coefficient) and ligandin concentration. *Solid line,* linear regression through the data; *dashed lines,* SE of the fit. (From ref. 27.)

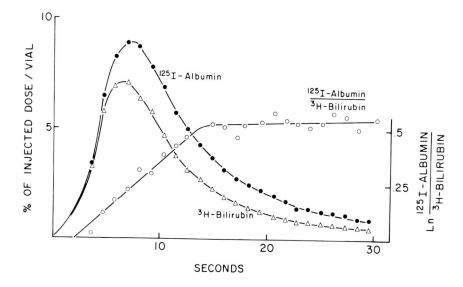

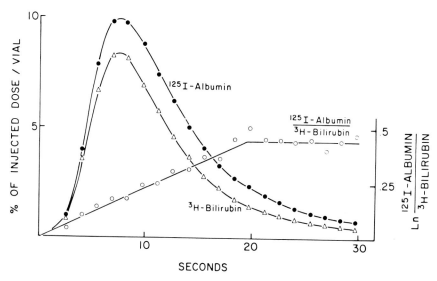

FIG. 12. Indicator dilution outflow curves for ^{125}I-albumin (*closed circles*) and ^{3}H-bilirubin (*open triangles*) in sham-operated liver (*upper panel*) and regenerating liver 48 hrs after two-thirds hepatectomy (*lower panel*). Initially the ^{3}H-bilirubin curve diverges from its ^{125}I-albumin reference. The rate of divergence, as measured by the initial slope of the log(^{125}I-albumin/^{3}H-bilirubin) curve is proportional to the bilirubin influx coefficient. As determined thus, the influx coefficient is independent of liver mass. Cellular proliferation is maximal 48 hr after two-thirds hepatectomy. In the experiment, the initial slope on the log plot is substantially decreased. The influx coefficient of ^{3}H-bilirubin has been reduced by approximately 50%. (The illustration was supplied by Dr. Allan Wolkoff, to whom appreciation is expressed.)

creased in magnitude. The lines corresponding to the throughput components have been placed on the bottom panels (their slopes and hence influx coefficients are almost identical). The deviation from this line late in time is obviously much decreased in phenobarbital-treated rats, where the returning component is reduced in magnitude.

Influx coefficients did not vary significantly between the groups. Efflux coefficients, illustrated in Fig. 10, varied inversely with the ligandin concentrations (the product of the efflux coefficient and the ligandin concentration was essentially constant). Sequestration coefficients did not change in significant fashion.

The ratio (influx coefficient/efflux coefficient) is of interest. The influx coefficient is the ratio $\{P'_{in}S/[r_p(1 + p\gamma)V_p]\}$. This has the form of a PS product divided by the product of r_p and the relative volume $(1 + p\gamma)V_p$ of the compartment which is the origin of the flux. The efflux coefficient is $(P'_{out}S/r_c V_c)$ and again has the form of a PS product divided by the product of

r_c and the relative volume V_c, which is the origin of the flux. The ratio

$$\frac{\text{influx coefficient}}{\text{efflux coefficient}} = \frac{P'_{in}}{P'_{out}} \cdot \frac{V_c}{(1 + p\gamma)V_p} \cdot \frac{r_c}{r_p}.$$

In these experiments, the volume ratio $V_c/(1 + p\gamma)V_p]$ will not have changed, and there is no reason to suspect a change in the permeability parameters. The ratio r_c/r_p, however, would be expected to increase directly with r_c, with increase in the ligandin concentration. The expected pattern of change is illustrated in Fig. 11. In our control experiments, the average value for this ratio is 4.11. The space ratio predicted on the basis of the glucose experiment is 2.30. Hence the value for the product $(P'_{in}/P'_{out})(r_c/r_p)$ is 1.64 in this case. The concentration of albumin in plasma is approximately 0.60 mM and that of ligandin inside the liver cells 0.04 mM. The ratio of cell to plasma concentrations for the two proteins is 0.067. If the affinity of albumin for bilirubin is higher than that of ligandin for bilirubin, as other data suggest, the ratio r_c/r_p will be less. This implies that the ratio (P'_{in}/P'_{out}) must be substantially above 1, that the membrane is acting in a concentrative fashion. Steady-state observations in the Gunn rat (in which conjugation of bilirubin and excretion of conjugates into bile do not occur) support this conclusion. The average ratio of bilirubin concentrations in liver/plasma is 0.40 in the steady state (37), substantially above the ratio of concentrations of ligandin/albumin.

These studies demonstrate a decrease in the efflux of labeled bilirubin from the liver cell as the ligandin concentration is increased. This occurs because of a decrease in the efflux coefficient with increase in ligandin concentration and an increase in the volume of distribution available to labeled bilirubin in the tissue, as perceived from the plasma space, with increased concentrations of ligandin. The multiple indicator dilution approach has allowed a more precise analysis of the process than would otherwise have been possible.

The data on the cell entry of bilirubin validate the idea that entry of this pigment across the liver cell membranes occurs via a carrier-mediated process (despite the lipid solubility of bilirubin). The presence of such a process in the membrane introduces the possibility of variation in its activity. Gartner et al. (38) have specifically sought such evidence in the regenerating rat liver. They have shown that 48 hr after a two-thirds hepatectomy, the influx coefficient for bilirubin is reduced by approximately 50% (an example of such an experiment is presented in Fig. 12). The findings suggest that similar changes should be sought in the immature neonate. The major importance of the findings is that it reemphasizes the individuality of the transfer step in the membrane.

SUMMARY

The principles underlying the entry of various substrates into the liver parenchymal cells have been explored. Carrier-mediated membrane transport is the usual process underlying this entry process, and uptake can usually be shown to exhibit the three operational features characteristic of this process: (a) saturation of initial rates of uptake, (b) competitive inhibition, and (c) countertransport. These phenomena, first documented for monosaccharides, are also characteristic of the process underlying the uptake of organic anions.

ACKNOWLEDGMENTS

The author wishes to express his appreciation to the Medical Research Council of Canada and the Québec Heart Foundation for their support, and to Margaret Mulherin for typing this manuscript.

REFERENCES

1. Goresky, C. A. (1963): A linear method for determining liver sinusoidal and extravascular volumes. *Am. J. Physiol.*, 204:626–640.
2. Wilbrandt, W., and Rosenberg, Th. (1961): The concept of carrier transport and its corollaries in pharmacology. *Pharmacol. Rev.*, 13:109–184.
3. Rosenberg, Th., and Wilbrandt, W. (1957): Uphill transport induced by counterflow. *J. Gen. Physiol.*, 41:289–296.
4. Silverman, M., and Goresky, C. A. (1965): A unified kinetic hypothesis of carrier mediated transport: its applications. *Biophys. J.*, 5:487–509.
5. Heinz, E., and Mariani, H. A. (1957): Concentration work and energy dissipation in active transport of glycine into carcinoma cells. *J. Biol. Chem.*, 228:97–111.
6. Christensen, H. N., and Riggs, T. R. (1952): Concentrative uptake of amino acids by Ehrlich mouse ascites carcinoma cell. *J. Biol. Chem.*, 194:57–68.
7. Heinz, E. (1962): Some remarks on active transport and exchange diffusion of amino acids in Ehrlich cells. In: *Amino Acid Pools: Distribution, Formation, and Function of Free Amino Acids*, edited by J. T. Holden, pp. 539–544. Elsevier, New York.
8. Goresky, C. A. (1976): The design and analysis of uptake experiments. In: *The Liver—Quantitative Aspects of Structure and Function, Vol. II*, edited by R. Preisig, J. Bircher, and G. Paumgartner, pp. 106–125. Editio Cantor, Aulendorf, Switzerland.
9. Goresky, C. A., and Rose, C. P. (1977): Blood-tissue exchange in liver and heart: The influence of heterogeneity of capillary transit times. *Fed. Proc.*, 36:2629–2634.
10. Prothero, J., and Burton, A. C. (1961): The physics of flow in capillaries. I. The nature of the motion. *Biophys. J.*, 1:565–579.
11. Hess, F. A., Weibel, E. R., and Preisig, R. (1973): Morphometry of dog liver: Normal and baseline data. *Virchows Archiv. B. [Cell Pathol.]*, 12:303–317.
12. Bassingthwaighte, J. B., Knopp, T. J., and Hazelrig, J. B. (1970): A concurrent flow model for capillary-tissue exchanges. In: *Capillary Permeability*, edited by C. Crone and N. A. Lassen, pp. 60–80. Munksgaard, Copenhagen.
13. Goresky, C. A., Ziegler, W. H., and Bach, G. G. (1970): Capillary exchange modeling: Barrier-limited and flow-limited distribution. *Circ. Res.*, 27:739–764.
14. Goresky, C. A., and Silverman, M. (1964): Effect of correction of catheter distortion on calculated liver sinusoidal blood volumes. *Am. J. Physiol.*, 207:883–892.
15. Allen, T. H., and Reeve, E. B. (1953): Distribution of "extra plasma" in the blood of some tissues in the dog measured with P^{32} and T-1824. *Am. J. Physiol.*, 175:218–223.
16. Goresky, C. A., Warnica, J. W., Burgess, J. H., and Cronin, R. F. P. (1978): Measurement of the extravascular water space in the lungs: Its dependence on alveolar blood flow. *Microvasc. Res.*, 15:149–167.
17. Ogston, A. G., and Phelps, C. F. (1961): The partition of solutes between buffer solutions and solutions containing hyaluronic acid. *Biochem. J.*, 78:827–833.
18. Wiederhielm, C. A., and Black, L. L. (1976): Osmotic interaction of plasma proteins with interstitial macromolecules. *Am. J. Physiol.*, 231:638–641.
19. Van Bezooijen, C. F. A., Grell, T., and Knook, D. L. (1976): Bromsulfophthalein uptake by isolated liver parenchymal cells. *Biochem. Biophys. Res. Commun.*, 69:354–361.
20. Wheeler, H. O., Epstein, R. M., Robinson, R. R., and Snell, E. S. (1960): Hepatic storage and excretion of sulfobromophthalein sodium in the dog. *J. Clin. Invest.*, 39:236–247.
21. Hunton, D. B., Bollman, J. L., and Hoffman, H. N. (1961): The plasma removal of indocyanine green and sulfobromophthalein: effect of dosage and blocking agents. *J. Clin. Invest.*, 40:1648–1655.

22. Paumgartner, G., Probst, P., Kraines, R, and Leevy, C. M. (1970): Kinetics of indocyanine green removal from the blood. *Ann. NY Acad. Sci.,* 170:134–147.

23. Goresky, C. A. (1965): The hepatic uptake of sulfobromophthalein and bilirubin. *Can. Med. Assoc. J.,* 92:851–857.

24. Scharschmidt, B. F., Waggoner, J., and Berk, P. D. (1975): Hepatic organic anion uptake in the rat. *J. Clin. Invest.,* 56:1280–1292.

25. Goresky, C. A., Bach, G. G., and Nadeau, B. E. (1973): On the uptake of materials by the intact liver: The transport and net removal of galactose. *J. Clin. Invest.,* 52:991–1009.

26. Jones, A. L., Hradek, G. T., Renston, R. H., Wong, K. Y., Karlaganis, G., and Paumgartner, G. (1980): Autoradiographic evidence for hepatic lobular gradient of bile acid derivative. *Am. J. Physiol.,* 238:G233–G237.

27. Wolkoff, A. W., Goresky, C. A., Sellin, J., Gatmaitan, Z., and Arias, I. M. (1979): Role of ligandin in transfer of bilirubin from plasma into liver. *Am. J. Physiol.,* 236:E638–E648.

28. Goresky, C. A., Bach, G. G., and Nadeau, B. E. (1973): On the uptake of materials by the intact liver: The concentrative transport of rubidium-86. *J. Clin. Invest.,* 52:975–990.

29. Cahill, G. F., Jr., Ashmore, J., Earle, A. S., and Zottu, S. (1958): Glucose penetration into the liver. *Am. J. Physiol.,* 192:491–496.

30. Goresky, C. A., and Nadeau, B. E. (1974): Uptake of materials by the intact liver: The exchange of glucose across the cell membranes. *J. Clin. Invest.,* 53:634–646.

31. Goresky, C. A., Huet, P.-M., and Villeneuve, J. P. (1982): Blood-tissue exchange and blood flow in the liver. In: *Textbook of Hepatology,* edited by D. Zakim and T. D. Boyer. Saunders, Philadelphia (*in press*).

32. Laris, P. C. (1958): Permeability and utilization of glucose in mammalian erythrocytes. *J. Cell. Comp. Physiol.,* 51:273–307.

33. Williams, T. F., Exton, J. H., Park, C. R., and Regen, D. M. (1968): Stereospecific transport of glucose in the perfused rat liver. *Am. J. Physiol.,* 215:1200–1209.

34. Goresky, C. A. (1974): The hepatic uptake process: Its implications for bilirubin transport. In: *Jaundice,* edited by C. A. Goresky and M. M. Fisher, pp. 159–174. Plenum, New York.

35. Arias, I. M., Fleischner, G., Kirsch, R., Mishkin, S., and Gatmaitan, Z. (1976): On the structure, regulation, and function of ligandin. In: *Glutathione: Metabolism and Function,* edited by I. M. Arias and W. B. Jakoby, pp. 175–188. Raven Press, New York.

36. Paumgartner, G., and Reichen, J. (1976): Kinetics of hepatic uptake of unconjugated bilirubin. *Clin. Sci. Mol. Med.,* 51:169–176.

37. Hammaker, M. S., and Schmid, R. (1967): Interference with bile pigment uptake in the liver by flavaspidic acid. *Gastroenterology,* 53:31–37.

38. Gartner, U., Stockert, R. J., and Wolkoff, A. W. (1981): Modulation of the transport of bilirubin and asialoorosomucoid during liver regeneration. *Hepatology,* 1:99–106.

The Liver: Biology and Pathobiology, edited by
I. Arias, H. Popper, D. Schachter, and D. A. Shafritz.
Raven Press, New York © 1982.

Chapter 35

Hepatocyte Regeneration, Replication, and Differentiation

H. L. Leffert, K. S. Koch, P. J. Lad, H. Skelly, and B. deHemptinne

CONCEPTS AND QUESTIONS

Proliferation and differentiation are the essential manifestations of living organisms. Mammalian cells generally express these exquisitely controlled properties reciprocally. Mature tissues in higher animals, for example, contain cell populations whose specialized functions are expressed optimally during proliferative quiescence. Without these conditions, neither phenotypic stability nor life as we know it could exist. Consequently, the quiescent state is a critical one.

With respect to hepatocyte growth as studied in the rat, quiescence does not imply a zero proliferation rate. Instead, it reflects a spontaneous rate of about 0.05 and 0.005% for adult rat hepatocytes in regard to S-phase tritiated thymidine nuclear labeling indices ([³H]dT LI) and labeled mitotic indices (LMI), respectively. These are standard proliferation parameters measured *in vivo* and *in vitro* (see refs. 1–3 for reviews). Therefore, the quiescent state (termed G_0) is characterized by low frequencies of differentiated hepatocyte "entry" into the cell "cycle" that are balanced by equivalently low rates of hepatocyte aging and death.

The cell cycle concept is useful to quantitate kinetic changes as cells multiply. When adult rats are subjected to hepatoproliferogenic stimuli (e.g., 70% hepatectomy), hepatocyte LI and LMI frequencies increase 600-fold, but not immediately. First, G_0-exit into the "prereplicative" phase occurs. This period, the "onset time" (S_t) (3,4), lasts between 12 and 16 hr. When it ends, hepatocytes synthesize nuclear DNA

semiconservatively (S-phase). As measured by slopes of LI curves after 12 to 18 hr (S_Δ) (3,4), S-phase entry rates often vary, depending on the animals' age and the type of growth stimulus and its "dose" (2). This variance reflects asynchronous S-phase entry times among the hepatocyte population. By contrast, temporal durations of nuclear DNA replication per cell are rather constant (approximately 8 hr) and independent of the stimulus and its dose (5,6). When S-phase ends, 4 to 6 hr of further preparation for cell division are needed (G_2 phase). Ultimately, the mitotic process begins, and within 30 to 60 min, two hepatocytes are formed from one (M-phase). In the regenerating rat liver, most hepatocytes proliferate at least once within 24 to 36 hr after a suitable growth stimulus. Nonparenchymal cells also proliferate but later in time (7). If hepatocytes proliferate continuously, progeny cells enter another temporal "gap" (G_1) between M-phase and the ensuing S-phase. During regeneration, some hepatocytes undergo second and third "rounds" of proliferation. Under these conditions, hepatocyte G_1 durations last between 6 and 8 hr, noticeably less than the duration of S_t (8). Therefore, liver proliferative responses are neither specific nor synchronous (3,7); nonetheless, they are elegantly controlled.

When chronic proliferation occurs, specialized hepatocyte function is reduced. As proliferation normally ceases, diminished functions are restored, some rapidly, others more gradually. This usually happens within 7 to 28 days after birth or 70% hepatectomy in the rat. If abnormal proliferation occurs, however, differentiated function may be permanently reduced or even extinguished. These phenomena have been described in detail in many liver developmental, regeneration, and carcinogenesis studies (9–11).

Given these fundamental concepts, three major questions emerge: (a) What factors control hepatocyte proliferation? (b) How do these factors work? (c) What are the molecular and cellular linkages between proliferative and differentiated states?

This chapter describes current progress toward solutions to these questions. Despite progress, definitive answers are not yet known. In certain areas, we try to clarify what additional knowledge is needed. It is assumed that information from animal cell studies will be relevant to human liver cells. At this time, however, defined growth control studies with human hepatocytes have not been reported. Only during the last decade have advances in rat hepatocyte culture, biochemistry, and molecular biology provided experimental methods to study these complex problems using defined conditions and powerful analytical tools. The groundwork is just beginning.

PROLIFEROGENIC GROWTH FACTORS

Biologic or xenobiotic substances that alter hepatocyte LI and LMI values positively or negatively are growth factors if, and only if, they act directly upon the liver. To prove that such factors are physiologically relevant requires additional criteria (3).

One might expect *a priori* that three growth factor classes exist: (a) stimulatory, (b) inhibitory, and (c) a class with both properties determined by its ambient concentration (for example, stimulating at low or inhibiting at high extracellular concentrations). The existence and identity of natural blood-borne stimulatory and/or inhibitory hepatotrophic factors was controversial for many years (12). Recent work mitigated this controversy somewhat, at least with respect to stimulatory factors (1). It now appears that certain peptides and a variety of amino acids (nutrients) are hepatocyte proliferogens (13–16). A list of the peptides and some of their chemical properties is given in Table 1.

How is it known that these peptides are proliferogens? First, all stimulate adult or neonatal rat hepatocyte DNA synthesis or [^{3}H]dT incorporation into DNA directly *in vitro* under appropriate conditions (4,13,14,17–20; H. Leffert, K. S. Koch, H. Skelly, *unpublished results*). Figures 1, 2A–D, G, and H show photomicrographs of representative primary "monolayer" adult hepatocyte cultures used in these studies (4,17,21). The cultures are made, following liver perfusion with collagenase buffers, from single cell adult hepatocyte suspensions (that immunofluorescently

TABLE 1. *Blood-borne peptides that stimulate adult rat hepatocyte DNA synthesis* in vitro

Peptide[a]	Abbreviation	Molecular weight	Isoelectric point	Biologic properties	"Cell-cycle" action
Epidermal growth factor	EGF	6,100	4.6	Synergisms with G and NSILAs	$G_{0,1}$ (early)
Glucagon	G	3,600	7.5–8.5	Synergisms with EGF and NSILAs	Late G_1
Insulin	I	6,000	5.35	Synergisms with EGF, G; additive or competitive with NSILAs	Late G_1
Insulin-like growth factor[b]	IGF$_1$[c]	7,649	acidic	Synergisms with EGF, G; additive or competitive with other NSILAs	? Late G_1
Insulin-like growth factor[b]	IGF$_2$	7,471	acidic	Synergisms with EGF, G; additive or competitive with other NSILAs	? Late G_1
Somatomedin-C[b]	SC	7,500	8.0–8.7	Synergisms with EGF, G; additive or competitive with other NSILAs	? Late G_1

[a] See text for references related to these peptides and their biologic effects on cultured hepatocytes.

[b] These factors are collectively termed a family of nonsuppressible (by insulin antiserum) insulin-like activities or NSILAs.

[c] IFG$_1$ and SC are similar, and possibly identical, peptides (see text for details).

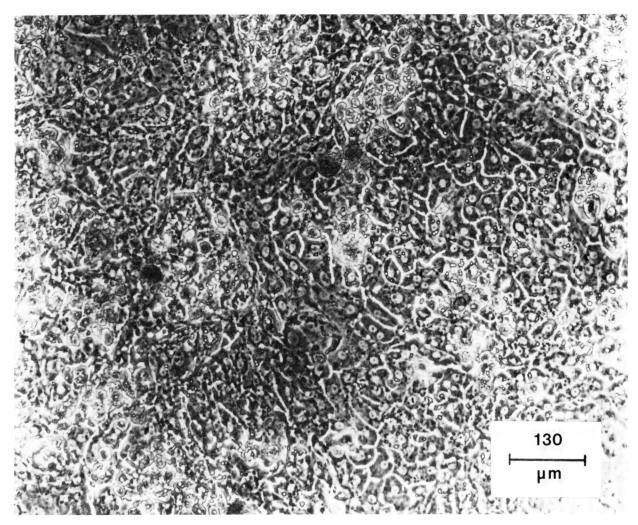

FIG. 1. Hepatocytes in culture. Photomicrograph of 30-day-old living adult rat hepatocytes in primary "monolayer" culture. Cells were cultured as described elsewhere (4). *Inset bar,* relative dimensions in microns.

stain for albumin, as shown in Fig. 2A). The cells are seeded into small tissue culture dishes (Fig. 2D) along with supplemented nutrient media (22–24).

Cultured hepatocytes initially express many growth state-dependent differentiated functions (Fig. 3) (23). When asynchronous proliferation starts between 2 and 10 days after plating, differentiated functions decline. The cultures reach a stationary phase 10 to 14 days postplating, at which time they substantially regain many of their specialized adult functions, including total albumin synthesis (see Figs. 2B and 2C) and other enzymatic capabilities (Fig. 3) (21–23). At this point, hepatocyte LI values fall to <5%, visualized autoradiographically in Fig. 2G; few mitoses are seen. Such cultures contain quiescent hepatocytes that, under chemically defined conditions, synthesize DNA and divide again in response to various exogenous peptides (Fig. 2H) (17).

Second, three peptides that have been studied in detail using adult culture systems [epidermal growth factor (EGF), insulin (I), and glucagon (G)] (see Table 1) act at nanogram levels. The kinetics of hepatocyte S-phase entry and the appearance of [³H]dT-labeled mitotic figures in the responding cultures (Fig. 2G, H, and Fig. 4) closely simulate hepatocyte proliferation kinetics *in vivo* following 70% hepatectomy (17). Further "similarities" *in vitro* to the *in vivo* state are seen. For example, a minority population of non-parenchymal cells in the stationary cultures (Figs. 2D-F) also is stimulated to grow but, like the *in vivo* response to 70% hepatectomy, after hepatocyte proliferation has begun (Fig. 4).

Third, several lines of evidence strongly suggest that insulin, glucagon, and EGF are physiologically relevant *in vivo*. Evidence that insulin and glucagon are obligatory for normal rat liver regeneration rests on the following observations: (a) Pancreatic ablation (by gastrointestinal tract evisceration) markedly impairs liver regeneration, whereas insulin and glucagon repletion fully repair the proliferative "lesion," mea-

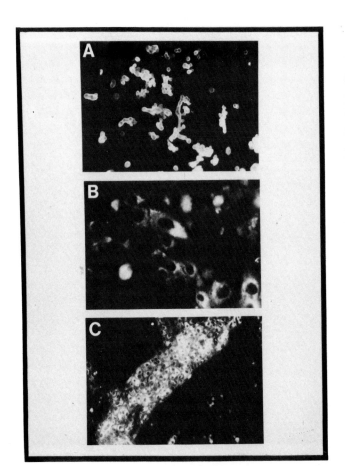

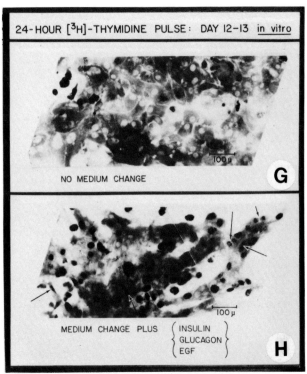

NO MEDIUM CHANGE

G

100μ

MEDIUM CHANGE PLUS { INSULIN GLUCAGON EGF }

H

100μ

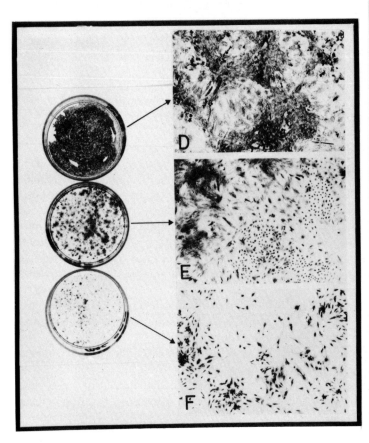

D

E

F

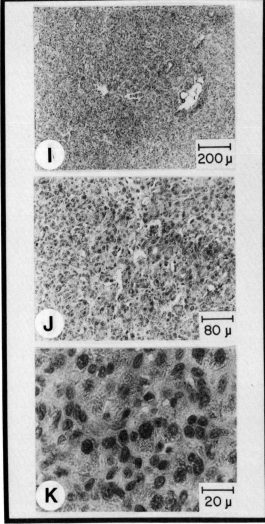

I

200μ

J

80μ

K

20μ

sured by [³H]dT uptake into hepatocyte DNA (25); insulin and glucagon are produced by and secreted from β- and α-cells of the islets of Langerhans, respectively; (b) glucagon infusions stimulate some hepatocyte proliferation in the intact animal (15), whereas antiinsulin antiserum infusions blunt DNA-synthesis induced by 70% hepatectomy (26); (c) proliferative stimuli dose-dependent changes in arterial and portal venous blood insulin and glucagon levels occur prior to proliferative changes (8,27–29); (d) proliferative stimuli dose-dependent changes in glucagon and insulin hormone receptor or receptor-associated components occur prior to proliferative changes (8,27–31); and (e) proliferative stimuli-dependent changes in hepatic insulin and glucagon uptake and/or turnover precede proliferative changes (1).

For EGF, in addition to cell culture studies, the current evidence is suggestive but not yet conclusive that it too is involved obligatorily *in vivo*: (a) EGF infusions markedly potentiate the effects of [I + G] mixtures in stimulating hepatocyte proliferation (26); and (b) within minutes after 70% hepatectomy, but not after sham operations, exogenously administered radioactive EGF is specifically concentrated by liver remnant (caudate and accessory lobes) (1).

Attempts to block liver regeneration with EGF antisera have not yet been successful. The reasons are unclear. Other endogenous stimulatory factors may be active, or appropriate antisera or conditions to neutralize the biologic effects of EGF or its rapid interactions with liver tissue, have yet to be found. Monoclonal EGF antibodies might help to resolve this problem. Similar reagents directed against glucagon would permit additional studies of proliferative requirements of this peptide, hindered to date because of extraordinary costs of available glucagon antisera needed in growth factor "neutralizing" studies.

Are EGF, insulin, and glucagon unique, natural regulators of hepatocyte proliferation? Although they produce significant responses together *in vitro* and regarding [I + G] are obligatory for proliferation *in vivo*, a number of reasons suggest that additional factors are involved. This view stems not from unsubstantiated claims of "new" factors (32,33), but rather from observations that concern the virtual specificity and, with respect to growth factors, the degenerative nature of the proliferative response. For example, all the peptides listed in Table 1 (with the possible exception of glucagon), stimulate nonliver cell proliferation *in vitro* and possibly *in vivo* (34–38). Does this mean, therefore, that none of these peptides, except for glucagon, is normally hepatoproliferogenic? The answer is unclear.

Glucagon receptors are found only in hepatocytes in the liver; but kidney, fat pad, and cardiac muscle cells also contain glucagon receptors, and their metabolic responses could facilitate regeneration *in vivo* (8). Specificity, if it exists (because of the rapid hepatocyte proliferative response compared to the delayed nonparenchymal response during regeneration) could be determined in various ways without postulating that specific growth factors exist (see also ref. 29). For example, the relative combinations of a set of factors, the cell-surface receptor display to them (see below), and/or the chemical equilibria that exist between hepatocyte populations and growth factor repertoires at any instant in time all might be critical variables through which these factors act (1,3,4,8,14,18,29). Still another consideration is that one peptide, if present in limiting amounts, may obviate the requirement for another. This is best illustrated by recent findings *in vitro* that three nonsuppressible insulin-like peptides (NSILAs) (38,39), including IGF$_1$ (40), IGF$_2$ (41), and somatomedin-C (42) stimulate adult hepatocyte DNA synthesis when EGF and glucagon but not insulin are present (19). The potencies of certain NSILAs *in vitro* appear to be higher than insulin. The role of NSILAs in liver regeneration, first implicated by *in vitro* results in 1974 (14), nonetheless remains unclear.

In summary, several I-like factors are hepatoproliferogenic *in vitro* like insulin *in vivo*. Factors, such as glucagon, seem unique since other peptides have not yet been found to mimic its effects *in vivo*. Additional EGF-like factors probably exist in rat serum; if all six peptides (Table 1) are added in large excess to culture fluids (10 ng/ml), rat serum still causes a marked stimulation of hepatocyte DNA synthesis *in vitro* (19). The observed degenerative nature of the

---

FIG. 2. Normal liver cells in primary culture and liver sections from rats fed a choline-devoid diet containing *N*-acetyl-2-aminofluorene (AAF). **A–H:** Various aspects of adult liver cells in primary culture. **A–C:** Appearance of normal adult rat hepatocytes, immunofluorescently stained for albumin, at 1 to 2 hr, 4 to 5 days, and 11 and 12 days, postplating respectively (relative magnifications: ×100, ×400, and ×100). (Adapted from ref. 21.) **D:** Crystal violet-stained culture fixed with neutral formalin, similar in age to the cells shown in **C**. Nonhepatocytes are interspersed cells with poorly stained cytoplasms. **E** and **F:** Cells obtained from pronase-treated, freshly isolated liver cell suspensions. In order to grow, these cells require arginine **(E)**, and ornithine will not replace it **(F)**, as ornithine normally does for hepatocytes under routine plating conditions **(D)** (4). **G** and **H:** DNA synthesizing hepatocytes before **(G)** and after **(H)** reinitiation of proliferation by a shift into fresh culture medium plus 50 ng I, G, and EGF/ml (crystal violet stained). (Adapted from ref. 17.) **I, J,** and **K:** Hematoxylin- and eosin-stained paraffin-embedded liver sections from rats fed AAF in a choline-devoid diet illustrating oval cell replacement of normal liver parenchyma (S. Sell and H. L. Leffert, *unpublished results;* see text and refs. 92 and 97 for details). *Inset bars,* relative dimensions in microns.

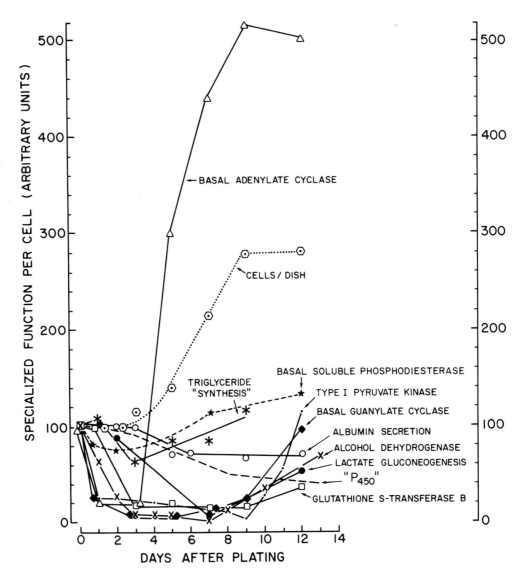

FIG. 3. Relationships between hepatocyte growth state and specialized function in primary culture. Ten functions were measured during the growth cycle (*dotted line*) and changes relative to normal tissue levels given (on the Y-axis) for a 2-week period *in vitro*. Seven of the functions (excluding adenylate cyclase, phosphodiesterase, and guanylate cyclase) are hepatocyte specific. The general trends are reciprocal relationships between growth state and function (i.e., an S-shaped growth curve versus U-shaped function curves). Total albumin synthesis and mRNA$_{ALB}$ sequences/cell (not shown) give U-shaped curves (*unpublished results*). [See refs. 103 (gluconeogenesis) and 4, 21–24, and 104 (alcohol dehydrogenase) for further details.

proliferative response may be fortuitous; it may be important teleologically (18); or there may be as yet unknown explanations at the molecular and cellular levels (see below).

Any serious claim to finding a new hepatocyte proliferogenic factor, unaccompanied by complete chemical identification and purification, must contend with the kinds of biologic interactions mentioned above plus the fact that all of the peptides (Table 1) are found in serum or plasma in high molecular weight form in covalent or noncovalent associations with large carrier proteins, or as cleaved protein fragments (35,43–46). At this time, the proliferogenic activities of the high

molecular weight forms are unknown. NSILAs are produced by hepatocytes and other liver-derived cells (e.g., somatomedin-C [47,48]). Hence new proliferogenic factors isolated from liver or from other sources must be distinguished chemically from these known molecules.

PROLIFEROGENIC MECHANISMS

A major reason for considerable effort identifying blood-borne growth factors is based on the assumption that once they are known, the problem of hepatocyte

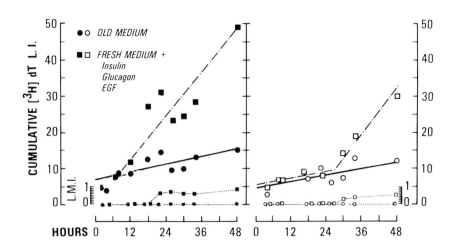

FIG. 4. Proliferation kinetics of liver cells in primary culture. (Data adapted from ref. 4, where full details are given.) Stationary cultures (see Fig. 2G) were stimulated to grow under conditions similar to those shown in Fig. 2H. [³H]dT (1.25 µCi/ml, 3 × 10⁻⁶ M unlabeled TdR) was added at 0 hr and autoradiography performed on groups of cultures at the times indicated on the X-axis. Control cultures (old medium) were similarly perturbed but received old (i.e., unchanged day 12) media. Labeled hepatocyte **(left)** and nonhepatocyte **(right)** nuclei were counted to obtain cumulative LI values (Y-axis). Labeled mitoses also were scored in these populations (see inset LMI curves for each panel).

growth control can be defined in terms of (a) the growth factor mechanisms of action, and (b) how the factors become available in nonrate-limiting sinusoidal or Disse space concentrations to the quiescent hepatocyte.

These simple views are useful as a first approach toward answering mechanistic questions. They are partly inadequate, however, because available information suggests that no single factor is sufficient to fully stimulate or inhibit hepatocyte proliferation. For example, several interactions among the six peptides have been observed that are important in considering how the peptides work.

First, they act synergistically to control hepatocyte DNA synthesis. Stimulatory synergisms occur between [I + G] in the presence of EGF (17,20,49) or between [G + EGF] in the presence of I (or any one of the three NSILAs listed in Table 1); this means that how one peptide works alone is not necessarily how it might work when other peptides are present. It also suggests that more than one rate-limiting event is necessary for proliferation (see below).

Second, hepatocyte responses to peptides depend not only on the ratio [cells]/[peptide] but on relative ambient peptide concentrations as well (8). This means that stimulatory effects of a peptide under one condition might be observed under other conditions either as no effects or as inhibiting effects (8,14,50,51). Regarding the latter possibility, although "pure" hepatocyte proliferogenic inhibitors may exist (1,29); the available evidence has not yet satisfied criteria that prove this definitively (3,52).

Third, to obtain optimal proliferative responses, hepatocytes prefer exposure to EGF (or factors like it) for at least 3 hr, followed by exposure to insulin and glucagon for at least 9 hr in the presence of nutrients (particularly amino acids). In other words, the hepato-

cellular response to proliferogenic factors suggests that they can work sequentially and require unlimiting amounts of simple nutrients. Both *in vitro* and *in vivo* studies of interactions among EGF, insulin, glucagon, and amino acids support this view (15–17,25,49). Figure 5 schematically depicts these relationships. Such conditions might actually prevail upon G_0-hepatocytes *in vivo*, for example, after 70% hepatectomy (4,17).

A simple hypothesis is suggested. Two nutrient-dependent, rate-limiting events must be activated by at least three classes of peptides. The first event is postulated to consist of an EGF (or EGF-like)-activated process that causes the formation inside the cell of

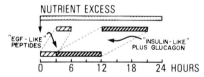

↑SIGNAL ① (ALTERED MONOVALENT CATION FLUXES)
↑MEMBRANE POTENTIAL, INTRACELLULAR pH CHANGES

(DEPOLARIZING PHASE)

↑"A" SYSTEM AMINO ACID TRANSPORT FUNCTION (MET, GLY, GLU-NH₂)

↑ALTERED RNA, PROTEIN, AND LIPID METABOLISM

↑SIGNAL ② (CA⁺⁺ FLUX-Cyclic AMP SURGE)

(HYPERPOLARIZING PHASE)

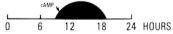

↑DEOXYRIBONUCLEOSIDE TRIPHOSPHATE SYNTHESIS

↑"DELAY" PROTEINS (or, INITIATOR SUBSTANCES) REACH CRITICAL THRESHOLD

↑INCREASED DNA SYSTHESIS INITIATION RATES

↑INCREASED MITOTIC INDEX

FIG. 5. Model of normal hepatocyte proliferation control. (See text and references cited therein for details.)

molecules required to initiate DNA replication (perhaps a so-called complex of "delay proteins"). Such molecules would not act until they reach threshold intracellular concentrations (hence, the prereplicative delay, S_t). Presumably, they build up and decay slowly to subthreshold levels 20 to 22 hr poststimulus (to account for the finding that [G + I] additions in vitro need not be administered immediately after EGF, whose presence is needed for ≥ 3 hours, as shown in Fig. 5 (8,17,18). The second event, an EGF-primed and [G + I]-dependent process, is postulated to occur and decay rapidly (late in the prereplicative or G_1 phase) to account for observations of delayed and rather prolonged exposure time requirements of hepatocytes for [G + I] in vivo and in vitro (after prior EGF additions) (see Fig. 5) (8,17,18,25). To facilitate discussion, we refer to the activation of these virtually distinct events as signal one and signal two, respectively (4,17,53).

In considering signaling mechanisms in general, it is necessary to understand how the cells interact chemically with peptides. The current view is that peptides bind noncovalently and reversibly to specific, saturable, high affinity ($K_{D[apparent]} \sim 10^{-11}$-$10^{-9}$ M) sinusoidal surface membrane protein receptors. Binding (that is, ligand/receptor occupancy and/or interaction time between the ligand and the receptor) but not subsequent cellular uptake (of the peptide, the peptide-receptor complex, or fragments of both) is thought to initiate signaling (54,55). None of the hepatocyte proliferogen receptors has been purified, but it is known that both EGF and glucagon receptors are distinct entities (56,57) that differ from the insulin receptor (58). Recent work suggests that somatomedin-C and IGF_1 share similar if not identical receptors which, in turn, are closely related to insulin receptors (59; J. J. Van Wyk, personal communication). A distinct MSA receptor has been reported; it may be more closely related to the IGF_2 receptor (60). Evidence is needed to prove that all relevant NSILA receptors are present in hepatocyte sinusoidal plasma membranes.

The dual signaling model shown in Fig. 5 must be considered only as a working hypothesis. At least four reasons account for this present situation. First, biochemical, biophysical, and functional characterization of the above-mentioned ligand-receptor interactions are poorly understood, even with respect to the one most widely studied (glucagon activation of adenylate cyclase to produce cAMP). All these interactions involve multiple components [e.g., glucagon signaling requires guanine nucleotides and at least nine proteins (8,61)].

Second, in certain instances, although evidence has been presented for possible rapid biochemical effects of ligand-receptor interactions, there is little evidence available to link such effects to initiating DNA synthesis. For example, the phosphorylation of tyrosine residues in tumor cell membrane proteins after EGF exposure has been reported (62). This finding has not yet been confirmed in hepatocyte systems; pending such results, it remains an observation in search of a specific inhibitor in order to ultimately show that such phosphorylations are necessary to stimulate hepatocyte proliferation. A similar situation prevails for the mechanism of insulin action, recently suggested to proceed through an intracellular peptide activator formed after the ligand/receptor complex activates a plasma membrane protease (63). Whether any of the proliferogenic NSILAs exert similar effects is unknown. However, other effects of [EGF; I + G]-receptor interactions may involve modulation of monovalent cation fluxes across the cell surface and of intracellular cAMP levels. Thse might be causally related to proliferation.

Third, it is not yet clear, in the case of insulin, for example, if the peptide is acting at an NSILA receptor (64). While this might again reflect a relevant biologic degeneracy (even a desirable one with respect to proliferation), it is important to learn whether or not the hepatocyte insulin receptor is designed to modulate metabolic changes exclusively as opposed to mitogenic ones (the latter might be thought of as modulated by NSILA receptors). The distinction is not trivial because some proliferation control models regard mitogenic activation as the consequence of overall metabolic rate increases, whereas other models postulate that mitogenic activation is a highly specific activation process (like a differentiated function). Further work is needed to clarify this potentially important aspect of hepatocyte growth control.

Last, certain peptides may exert as yet undefined mediated effects. For example, glucagon may alter cellular Ca^{2+} depots through a non-cAMP-mediated mechanism (65).

As suggested above, available evidence links signals one and two to the activation of monovalent cation fluxes (Na^+ and K^+) and a transient surge (i.e., a rise and fall) of intrahepatocellular cAMP levels, respectively (Fig. 5). The experimental evidence has been discussed critically (1,4,8,17,18,53). At present, the model rests mainly on pharmacologic studies, for example, findings that specific, nontoxic drugs (that neither inhibit peptide-receptor interactions nor DNA synthesis, once stimulated) block rapid cellular responses to the peptides and the initiation of hepatocyte DNA synthesis and mitosis [observed as increases in S_t and M_t (4,18)].

Thus, EGF (or an EGF-like factor) stimulates a Na^{2+} flux transient in G_0 or early G_1 which in turn slowly depolarizes the cell surface membrane, increases intracellular pH (via a Na^+/H^+ antiport system), and transiently activates the Na^+/K^+-ATPase

(4,17,18,66–68). These early functional membrane changes are postulated, by mechanisms that include the eventual activation of Na^+-dependent amino acid "A-system" transport, to stimulate macromolecular RNA and protein syntheses (or decrease their degradation). Both macromolecular classes must be synthesized for hepatocyte proliferation to occur (17). Late in G_1, macromolecular changes in protein levels may be driven by [G + I] sustained A-system activation in consequence of elevated cAMP levels and chronic electrogenic hyperpolarizing changes across the cell surface, that is, an electrically more negative cellular interior (8,69). As sufficient delay or other rate-limiting DNA replication proteins are formed (70,71), together with DNA substrates, such as deoxyribonucleoside triphosphates whose formation is $Ca^{2+}/cAMP$ dependent (72), DNA replication would start. In terms of the physical meaning of measurements of the rates of initiation of hepatocyte DNA synthesis in a liver cell population (i.e., S_Δ determinations), these rates might reflect the probability that in any single cell, the overall rate constants for two independent events both attain threshold values. In chemical terms, if such rate constants are first order, the cellular concentrations of both reaction products needed to start DNA replication are proportional to these constants. How hepatocytes are driven through G_2 and M is unknown. Presumably, the molecules needed for these transitions are produced also as a consequence of both signals (49,53).

In summary, several peptides appear to activate at least two cellular processes sequentially, via rapid transients in membrane ion fluxes and delayed transients in cAMP production. These early and late prereplicative events are postulated to result in the formation of excess levels of molecules required to start DNA replication and the mitotic process per se. According to this model, a quiescent liver is defined by a low steady-state equilibrium between hepatocyte surface membrane receptors and activating ligands, whereas an actively growing liver is one in which activating ligands have come to occupy more receptors, in the presence of excess nutrients, and thereby shifted the steady state to a high equilibrium value. As more cells grow, receptor-ligand equilibria are restored, and proliferation rates fall to preexisting levels.

The model is speculative but testable. Various kinds of studies are needed to support or to refute it in order to assess its validity. For example, the model need not exclude the concept of endogenous growth inhibitors produced by hepatocytes (1). Signal one and/or two might be associated with deactivation of at least two classes of such putative inhibitors: $G_0 \rightarrow G_1$ and/or $G_1 \rightarrow S$ (1,18,29,52). Still another possibility, not inconsistent with the model, involves signal-dependent formation of endogenous liver growth stimulators. For

example, might EGF and/or glucagon cause liver cells to synthesize NSILAs? This possibility needs scrutiny because liver cells synthesize and secrete NSILAs both constitutively (47) and in response to somatotropin and insulin (48). Consequently, NSILAs might act within producer cells or, after secretion, from without. Cell-cell interactions, facilitated by either signal, might also explain why hepatocytes and nonhepatocytes have unequal onset times (1,2,4,7,14,29) (see Fig. 4).

PROLIFERATION-DIFFERENTIATION LINKAGES

Despite the virtual complexity of normal control of hepatocyte proliferation, recent developments suggest that multifaceted approaches can reveal mechanisms coupling differentiation to proliferation. New developments in molecular biology, biochemistry, cell biology, and carcinogenesis feeding regimens have facilitated progress in this area.

With respect to developmental changes, available evidence suggests that transcriptional alterations largely account for fetal gene expression (when hepatocytes are proliferating rapidly) and for adult gene expression (when the quiescent state is reached). One of the best examples of this regulatory mode comes from studies of hepatocyte alpha-fetoprotein (AFP) and albumin (ALB) gene expression *in vivo* (73–75) and *in vitro* (76). To perform these experiments, ALB and AFP DNA nucleic acid sequences complementary to polysomal mRNA molecules coding for these specialized proteins are constructed (73). The radioactive cDNA-probes are used to quantitate the tissue or cellular homogenate levels of the specific $mRNA_{AFP}$ or $mRNA_{ALB}$ directly by DNA-RNA molecular hybridization R_0t analyses (77). The results show that fetal hepatocytes contain thousands of $mRNA_{AFP}$ sequences per cell, whereas adult hepatocytes contain <5 to 10 of these sequences per cell (74,76). The converse is true for $mRNA_{ALB}$ with respect to adult hepatocytes, which contain 10 to 20 thousand functional sequences per cell.

Notably, [G + I] mixtures stimulate AFP (but not ALB) production synergistically in cultured fetal hepatocytes (78). This observation might illuminate the nature of the [G + I] synergy that stimulates hepatocyte proliferation. The latter observation also provides a conceptual approach to the "linkage" problem. Since proliferation is related to differentiation reciprocally (see Fig. 3), transient overall reductions of specialized function could be related to growth factor mechanisms of action. A corollary of this view, consistent with earlier studies (21,79,80), is that membrane fluxes and cellular cAMP levels control the expression of specialized functions in embryonically committed and adult hepatocytes.

LOSS OF GROWTH CONTROL

Two broad areas are under active investigation. One comprises the possibility that abnormal hepatocytes produce tumor virus-like gene products (81) that exert pleiotropic effects, for example, protein regulators that "shut off" adult gene expression and "turn on" fetal gene expression (and the mitogenic program).

This view should gain (or lose) support in a testable way in lieu of the recent development of temperature-sensitive DNA tumor virus transformed fetal hepatocyte cell lines (82). The SV40-DNA viral gene product [the "T" antigen (83)], a protein that confers malignancy (in fibroblasts transformed with this virus), is temperature sensitive. This gene is retained in the cultured hepatocyte chromosomes. When the cells are cultured at low temperatures, they grow rapidly and produce AFP but not ALB. When cultured at high temperatures, at which the malignant gene product is inactivated, slow growth is observed, AFP production ceases, and ALB production is restored (82). Studies of relationships between proliferation and fetal and adult specialized functions in this system and in normal primary fetal (78,84–86) and adult (23) hepatocyte cultures (Fig. 3) should yield considerable information. If consistent trends are found, mechanisms that regulate growth-dependent linkages will be greatly clarified.

The other area involves recent studies suggesting that subtle changes in hepatocyte gene structure modify the expression of differentiated function. For example, gene rearrangement does not account for the failure of hepatocytes to express salivary gland functions like α-amylase (87). However, hypomethylation of deoxycytidine residues may be a signal for increased transcriptional activity at many genetic loci (for review, see ref. 88). Such molecular mechanisms may be involved in the differentiation changes that accompany normal hepatocyte proliferation during development or during liver regeneration. Alternatively, they may be important in embryonic life, when the commitment to produce a hepatocyte is made. At this time, little along these lines is known. The hypomethylated DNA concept is intriguing; it may have bearing upon some rather unconventional cellular mechanisms that alter hepatic gene expression in the adult rat, following exposure to certain chemical carcinogens.

Most hepatocarcinogenesis models state that hepatomas descend from parenchymal hepatocytes that have interacted with carcinogens during the life of the animal. Specifically, the hepatoma is taken to have descended from a liver nodule or an atypical hepatocyte, both of which originated from parenchymal cells, as shown in Fig. 6 (89,90). Many fast-growing hepatomas eventually produced by these chemical regimens, although poorly differentiated, synthesize and secrete AFP (91). The putative premalignant nodules, however, do not produce AFP (92). By contrast, a number of laboratories, following earlier observations (93–95) have shown that chemical carcinogens fed in choline-deficient diets (96) cause normal rat livers to become inundated with small "oval" cells (see Figs. 2I, J, and K.) This occurs rapidly, within 4 weeks of dietary treatment (97–99). Oval cells contain both AFP and ALB, proliferate explosively, and invade the entire liver lobule (97,98). Oval cells do not metastasize outside the liver. Under appropriate conditions, they are transplantable into choline-deficient recipient rats, whereas liver nodule cells and normal hepatocytes are not (100,101).

It is not known yet if rat oval cells are hepatoma progenitors. Conditions that give rise to their formation *in vivo* and their transplantability might also cause DNA hypomethylation at deoxycytidine residues (102) and generalized methylation defects as a consequence of choline deficiency. All liver cell lineage classes are candidates (92), but in what liver cells do these chemical changes occur, if at all? What may be the proliferative and functional consequences? Do parenchymal cell functions normally suppress oval cell proliferation, and are these functions blocked by carcinogens?

This latter discussion illustrates the complexity of conceptual attempts to relate the results of growth control studies with normal parenchymal hepatocytes (fetal or adult) to current studies of the generation of abnormal hepatocytes. Nonetheless, combined physiologic and molecular biologic studies of the various available *in vitro* and *in vivo* models should lead to simpler views than those currently available. Ten years ago, the field of hepatocyte growth control had not reached the stage where numerous models were testable.

SUMMARY

A current view of hepatocyte growth control is that two liver cell types must be considered in models of "normal" and "abnormal" proliferation and differentiation and of the relationships that reciprocally link these properties.

The first type involves parenchymal cells: the hepatocytes. Available evidence suggests that three kinds of peptide families—EGF-like, insulin-like (insulin and/or the NSILA family), and glucagon—interact synergistically and temporally to alter normal proliferation rates. These interactions usually are perceived as stimulatory and seem to operate in the form of chemical equilibria among these ligands and their plasma membrane receptors. It is proposed that growth stimuli *in vivo,* like partial hepatectomy or liver injury, shift such equilibria toward higher steady

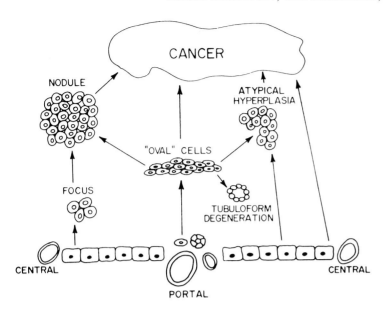

FIG. 6. Cell lineage model for hepatoma formation. (From ref. 90; see text for details.) "Tubuloform degeneration" refers to new ductular structures stained for AFP that arise by cell proliferation in rats fed AAF in a choline-devoid diet. Liver cell "foci" are discussed elsewhere (10,87,88).

states, reversibly. Receptor-mediated events may set into motion a dual signaling mechanism that activates transients of monovalent cation fluxes (first) and cAMP formation (second), leading to intracellular production of molecules required to synthesize DNA and to divide. Cell-cell interactions may participate via endogenous and exogenous liver-derived growth regulators. It is postulated that the suppression of specialized functions (during development or liver regeneration) is regulated by growth factor-related mechanisms that stimulate growth. At the macromolecular level, transcriptional changes have been identified in the growth state-dependent expression of prominent hepatocyte secretory functions, such as AFP and ALB. A delineation of mechanisms by which hepatoproliferogens alter gene expression appears to be a major challenge of future growth control research.

The second cell type involves what may actually be a liver "stem" cell: the oval cell. Its mode of growth control is a complete mystery. Recent models developed to study its proliferation and differentiation dynamics suggest that it should be considered as a serious progenitor candidate of rat hepatocellular carcinoma induced by chemicals. No clear-cut explanations of hepatocarcinogenesis are available; but alterations in liver cell-cell communication, in gene expression, and in modification of gene structure in hepatocytes or their stem cells may be involved.

ACKNOWLEDGMENTS

Work from this laboratory was supported by USPHS grants from the National Institutes of Arthritis, Metabolism and Digestive Disease (AM28215, AM28392) and Alcohol Abuse (AA03504). Purified preparations of somatomedin-C, and of IGF$_1$ and IGF$_2$ were the generous gifts of J. J. Van Wyk and M. E. Svoboda, and R. E. Humbel, respectively. We thank Margie Williams and Sandra Dutky for technical and computerized typographical assistance, respectively.

REFERENCES

1. Leffert, H. L., Koch, K. S., Moran, T., and Rubalcava, B. (1979): Hormonal control of rat liver regeneration. *Gastroenterology*, 76:1470–1482.
2. Bucher, N. L. R., and Malt, R. A. (1971): *Regeneration of Liver and Kidney*. Little, Brown, Boston.
3. Leffert, H. L., Koch, K. S., Lad, P. J., Skelly, H., and de-Hemptinne, B. (1982): Hepatocyte growth factors. In: *Hepatology*, edited by D. Zakim and T. D. Boyer, Saunders, Philadelphia, Toronto (*in press*).
4. Koch, K. S., and Leffert, H. L. (1980): Growth regulation of adult rat hepatocytes in primary culture. In: *Annals of the New York Academy of Sciences, Vol. 349: Differentiation and Carcinogenesis in Liver Cell Cultures*, edited by G. M. Williams and C. Borek, pp. 111–127. New York Academy of Sciences, New York.
5. Fabrikant, J. (1968): The kinetics of cellular proliferation in regenerating liver. *J. Cell Biol.*, 36:551–565.
6. Rabes, H. M. (1978): Kinetics of hepatocellular proliferation as a function of the microvascular structure and functional state of the liver. In: *Hepatotrophic Factors*, edited by R. Porter and J. Whelan, pp. 31–53. CIBA Foundation Symposium no. 55. Elsevier, Amsterdam.
7. Grisham, J. W. (1962): A morphologic study of deoxyribonucleic acid synthesis and cell proliferation in regenerating rat liver; autoradiography with thymidine-H³. *Cancer Res.*, 22:842–849.
8. Leffert, H. L., Koch, K. S., Lad, P. J., de Hemptinne, B., and Skelly, H. (1982): Glucagon and liver regeneration. In: *Handbook of Experimental Pharmacology*, edited by P. Lefebvre. Springer-Verlag, Berlin (*in press*).
9. Weber, G. (1969): Hormonal control of metabolism in normal and cancer cells. In: *Exploitable Molecular Mechanisms and Neoplasia*, pp. 521–560. Williams & Wilkins, Baltimore.
10. Knox, W. E. (1976): *Enzyme Patterns in Fetal, Adult, and Neoplastic Rat Tissue*. Karger, New York.
11. Pitot, H. (1978): *Fundamentals of Oncology*. Marcel Dekker, New York.

12. Starzl, T. E., Porter, K. A., Francavilla, J. A., Benichou, J., and Putnam, C. W. (1978): A hundred years of the hepatotrophic controversy. In: *Hepatotrophic Factors,* edited by R. Porter and J. Whelan, pp. 111–129. CIBA Foundation Symposium no. 55. Elsevier, Amsterdam.

13. Koch, K., and Leffert, H. L. (1974): Growth control of differentiated fetal rat hepatocytes in primary monolayer culture. VI. Studies with conditioned medium and its functional interactions with serum factors. *J. Cell Biol.,* 62:780–791.

14. Leffert, H. L. (1974): Growth control of differentiated fetal rat hepatocytes in primary monolayer culture. VII. Hormonal control of DNA synthesis and its possible significance to the problem of liver regeneration. *J. Cell Biol.,* 62:792–801.

15. Short, J., Brown, R. F., Husakova, A., Gilbertson, J. R., Zemel, R., and Lieberman, I. (1972): Induction of DNA synthesis in the liver of the intact animal. *J. Biol. Chem.,* 247:1757–1766.

16. Short, J., Armstrong, N. B., Zemel, R., and Lieberman, I. (1973): A role for amino acids in the induction of deoxyribonucleic acid synthesis in liver. *Biochem. Biophys. Res. Commun.,* 50:430–437.

17. Koch, K. S., and Leffert, H. L. (1979): Increased sodium ion influx is necessary to initiate rat hepatocyte proliferation. *Cell,* 18:153–163.

18. Leffert, H. L., and Koch, K. S. (1980): Ionic events at the membrane initiate rat liver regeneration. In: *Annals of the New York Academy of Sciences, Vol. 339: Growth Regulation by Ion Fluxes,* edited by H. L. Leffert, pp. 201–215. New York Academy of Sciences, New York.

19. Leffert, H. L., and Koch, K. S. (1982): Hepatocyte growth regulation by hormones in chemically defined medium. A two-signal hypothesis. In: *Conferences on Cell Proliferation, Vol. 9.* Cold Spring Harbor Laboratory, New York (*in press*).

20. Richman, R. A., Claus, T. H., Pilkis, S. J., and Friedman, D. L. (1976): Hormonal stimulation of DNA synthesis in primary cultures of adult rat hepatocytes. *Proc. Natl. Acad. Sci. U.S.A.,* 73:3589–3593.

21. Leffert, H. L., and Koch, K. S. (1979): Regulation of growth of hepatocytes. In: *Progress in Liver Diseases,* edited by H. Popper and F. Schaffner, pp. 123–134. Grune & Stratton, New York.

22. Leffert, H. L., Moran, T., Boorstein, R., and Koch, K. S. (1977): Procarcinogen activation and hormonal control of cell proliferation in differentiated primary adult rat liver cell cultures. *Nature,* 267:58–61.

23. Leffert, H., Moran, T., Sell, S., Skelly, H., Ibsen, K., Mueller, M., and Arias, I. (1978): Growth state dependent phenotypes of adult hepatocytes in primary monolayer culture. *Proc. Natl. Acad. Sci. U.S.A.,* 75:1834–1838.

24. Leffert, H. L., Koch, K. S., Moran, T., and Williams, M. (1979): Liver cells. In: *Methods in Enzymology* Vol. 58, edited by W. B. Jakoby and I. H. Pastan, pp. 536–544. Academic Press, New York.

25. Bucher N. L. R., and Swaffield, M. N. (1975): Regulation of hepatic regeneration by synergistic action of insulin and glucagon. *Proc. Natl. Acad. Sci. U.S.A.,* 72:1157–1160.

26. Bucher, N. L. R., Patel, U., and Cohen, S. (1978): Hormonal factors concerned with liver regeneration. In: *Hepatotrophic Factors,* edited by R. Porter and J. Whelan, pp. 95–107. CIBA Foundation Symposium no. 55. Elsevier, Amsterdam.

27. Leffert, H., Alexander, N. M., Faloona, G., Rubalcava, B., and Unger, R. (1975): Specific endocrine and hormonal receptor changes associated with liver regeneration in adult rats. *Proc. Natl. Acad. Sci. U.S.A.,* 72:4033–4036.

28. Leffert, H. L. (1977): Glucagon, insulin, and their hepatic "receptors": An endocrine pattern characterizing hepatoproliferative transitions in the rat. In: *Glucagon, its Role in Physiology and Clinical Medicine,* edited by P. O. Foá, J. S. Bajaj, and N. L. Foá, pp. 305–319. Springer-Verlag, New York, Berlin.

29. Leffert, H. L., and Koch, K. S. (1978): Proliferation of hepatocytes. In: *Hepatotrophic Factors,* edited by R. Porter and J. Whelan, pp. 61–82. CIBA Foundation Symposium no. 5. Elsevier, Amsterdam.

30. Mourelle, M., and Rubalcava, B. (1979): Changes in the insulin and glucagon receptors in the regenerating liver following intoxication with carbon tetrachloride. *Biochem. Biophys. Res. Commun.,* 88:189–198.

31. Mourelle, M., and Rubalcava, B. (1981): Regeneration of the liver after carbon tetrachloride. *J. Biol. Chem.,* 256:1656–1660.

32. La Brecque, D. R., and Pesch, L. A. (1975): Preparation and partial characterization of hepatic regenerative stimulator substances from rat liver. *J. Physiol.,* 248:273–284.

33. Morley, C. G. D., and Boyer, J. L. (1977): Stimulation of hepatocellular proliferation by a serum factor from thioacetamide-treated rats. *Biochim. Biophys. Acta,* 477:165–176.

34. Hintz, R. L., Clemmons, D. R., Underwood, L. E., and Van Wyk, J. J. (1972): Competitive binding of somatomedin to the insulin receptor of adipocytes, chondrocytes, and liver membranes. *Proc. Natl. Acad. Sci. (USA),* 69:2351–2353.

35. Giordano, G., Van Wyk, J. J., and Minuto, F. (editors) (1979): *Somatomedins and Growth.* Academic Press, London.

36. Salmon, W. D., and Daughaday, W. H. (1957): A hormonally controlled serum factor which stimulates sulfate incorporation by cartilage in vitro. *J. Lab. Clin. Med.,* 49:825–836.

37. Van Wyk, J. J., and Underwood, L. E. (1978): The somatomedins and their actions. In: *Biochemical Actions of Hormones,* edited by G. Litwack, vol. 5, pp. 101–148. Academic Press, New York.

38. Zapf, J., Rinderknecht, E., and Humbel, R. E. (1978): Non-suppressible insulin-like activity (NSILA) from human serum: Recent accomplishments and their physiologic implication. *Metabolism,* 27:1803–1827.

39. Blundell, T. L., Bedarkar, S., Rinderknecht, E., and Humbel, R. E. (1978): Insulin-like growth factor: A model for tertiary structure accounting for immunoreactivity and receptor binding. *Proc. Natl. Acad. Sci. U.S.A.,* 75:180–184.

40. Rinderknecht, E., and Humbel, R. E. (1978): The amino acid sequence of human insulin-like growth factor I and its structural homology with proinsulin. *J. Biol. Chem.,* 253:2769–2776.

41. Rinderknecht, E., and Humbel, R. E. (1978): Primary structure of human insulin-like growth factor II. *FEBS Lett.,* 89:283–286.

42. Svoboda, M. E., Van Wyk, J. J., Klapper, D. G., Fellows, R. E., Grissom, F. E., and Schlueter, R. J. (1980): Purification of somatomedin-C from human plasma: Chemical and biological properties, partial sequence analysis, and relationship to other somatomedins. *Biochemistry,* 19:790–797.

43. Antoniades, H. N., Simon, J. D., and Stathakos, D. (1973): Conversion of exogenous insulin into high molecular weight forms in vivo. *Biochem. Biophys. Res. Commun.,* 53:182–187.

44. Carpenter, G., and Cohen, S. (1979): Epidermal growth factor. *Ann. Rev. Biochem.,* 48:193–216.

45. Lefebvre, P. (1982): Glucagon. In: *Handbook of Experimental Pharmacology,* edited by P. Lefebvre. Springer-Verlag, Berlin (*in press*).

46. Leffert, H. L. (1974): Growth control of differentiated fetal rat hepatocytes in primary monolayer culture. V. Occurrence in dialyzed fetal bovine serum of macromolecules having both positive and negative growth regulatory functions. *J. Cell Biol.,* 62:767–779.

47. Spencer, E. M. (1979): Synthesis by cultured hepatocytes of somatomedin and its binding protein. *FEBS Lett.,* 99:157–161.

48. Shapiro, B., Waligora, K., and Pimstone, B. L. (1978): Generation of somatomedin activity in response to growth hormone and insulin from isolated perfused livers of normal and protein-malnourished rats. *J. Endocrinol.,* 79:369–373.

49. Andreis, P. G., and Armato, V. (1981): Effects of epidermal growth factor/urogastrone and associated pancreatic hormones on mitotic cycle phases and proliferation kinetics of neonatal rat hepatocytes in primary culture. *Endocrinology,* 108:1954–1964.

50. Price, J. B., Takeshige, K., Max, M. H., and Voorhees, A. B. (1972): Glucagon as the portal factor modifying hepatic regeneration. *Surgery,* 72:74–82.

51. Strecker, W., Goldberg, M., Feeny, D. A., and Ruhenstroth-Bauer, G. (1979): The influence of extended glucagon infusion

on liver cell regeneration after partial hepatectomy in the rat. *Acta Hepatogastroenterol.*, 26:439–441.

52. Leffert, H. L., and Weinstein, D. B. (1976): Growth control of differentiated fetal rat hepatocytes in primary monolayer culture. IX. Specific inhibition of DNA synthesis initiation by very low density lipoprotein and possible significance to the problem of liver regeneration. *J. Cell. Biol.*, 70:20–32.

53. Leffert, H. L., and Koch, K. S. (1981): Two ionic signals as prominent regulators of liver regeneration. In: *Frontiers of Science and the Liver*, edited by P. D. Berk, pp. 54–60. Thieme-Straton, New York.

54. Le Cam, A., Maxfield, F., Willingham, M., and Pastan, I. (1979): Insulin stimulation of amino acid transport in isolated rat hepatocytes is independent of hormone internalization. *Biochem. Biophys. Res. Commun.*, 88:873–881.

55. Maxfield, F. R., Davies, P. J. A., Klempner, L., Willingham, M. C., and Pastan, I. (1979): Epidermal growth factor stimulation of DNA synthesis is potentiated by compounds that inhibit its clustering in coated pits. *Proc. Natl. Acad. Sci. U.S.A.*, 76:5731–5735.

56. Das, M., and Fox, C. F. (1978): Molecular mechanism of mitogen action: Processing of receptor induced by epidermal growth factor. *Proc. Natl. Acad. Sci. U.S.A.*, 75:2644–2648.

57. Johnson, G. L., MacAndrew, V. I., and Pilch, P. F. (1981): Identification of the glucagon receptor in rat liver membranes by photoaffinity crosslinking. *Proc. Natl. Acad. Sci. U.S.A.*, 78:875–878.

58. Jacobs, S., Hazum, E., and Cuatrecasas, P. (1980): The subunit structure of the rat liver insulin receptor. *J. Biol. Chem.*, 255:6937–6940.

59. Van Wyk, J. J., Svoboda, M., and Underwood, L. E. (1980): Evidence from radioligand assays that somatomedin-C and insulin-like growth factor-I are similar to each other and different from other somatomedins. *J. Clin. Endocrinol. Metab.*, 50:206–208.

60. Kasuga, M., Obberghen, E. V., Nissley, S. P., and Rechler, M. M. (1981): Demonstration of two subtypes of insulin-like growth factor receptors by affinity cross-linking. *J. Biol. Chem.*, 256:5305–5308.

61. Rodbell, M. (1980): The role of hormone receptors and GTP-regulatory proteins in membrane transduction. *Nature*, 284:17–22.

62. Ushiro, H., and Cohen, S. (1980): Identification of phosphotyrosine as a product of epidermal growth factor-activated protein kinase in A-431 cell membranes. *J. Biol. Chem.*, 255:8363–8365.

63. Seals, J. R., and Czech, M. P. (1980): Evidence that insulin activates an intrinsic plasma membrane protease in generating a secondary chemical mediator. *J. Biol. Chem.*, 255:6529–6531.

64. King, G. L., Kahn, C. R., Rechler, M. M., and Nissley, S. P. (1980): Direct demonstration of separate receptors for growth and metabolic activities of insulin and multiplication-stimulating activity (an insulin-like growth factor) using antibodies to the insulin receptor. *J. Clin. Invest.*, 66:130–140.

65. Kelley, D. S., Evanson, T., and Potter, V. R. (1980): Calcium-dependent hormonal regulation of amino acid transport and cyclic AMP accumulation in rat hepatocyte monolayer cultures. *Proc. Natl. Acad. Sci. U.S.A.*, 77:5953–5957.

66. Fehlmann, M., and Freychet, P. (1981): Insulin and glucagon stimulation of (Na^+-K^+)-ATPase transport activity in isolated rat hepatocytes. *J. Biol. Chem.*, 256:7449–7453.

67. Fehlmann, M., Canivet, B., and Freychet, P. (1981): Epidermal growth factor stimulates monovalent cation transport in isolated rat hepatocytes. *Biochem. Biophys. Res. Commun.*, 100:254–260.

68. Hasegawa, K., Namai, K., and Koga, M. (1980): Induction of DNA synthesis in adult rat hepatocytes cultured in a serum-free medium. *Biophys. Res. Commun.*, 95:243–249.

69. Wondergem, R., and Harder, D. R. (1980): Membrane potential measurements during rat liver regeneration. *J. Cell. Physiol.*, 102:193–197.

70. Chang, L. M. S., and Bollum, F. J. (1972): Variation of deoxy-ribonucleic acid polymerase activities during rat liver regeneration. *J. Biol. Chem.*, 247:7948–7950.

71. Stetler, G. L., King, G. J., and Huang, W. M. (1979): T_4 delay proteins, required for specific DNA replication, form a complex that has ATP-dependent DNA topoisomerase activity. *Proc. Natl. Acad. Sci. U.S.A.*, 76:3737–3741.

72. Whitfield, J. F., Boynton, A. L., MacManus, J. P., Rixon, R. H., Sikorska, M., Tsang, B., and Walker, P. R. (1980): The roles of calcium and cyclic AMP in cell proliferation. In: *Annals of the New York Academy of Sciences, Vol. 339: Growth Regulation by Ion Fluxes*, edited by H. L. Leffert, pp. 216–240. New York Academy of Sciences, New York.

73. Sala-Trepat, J. M., Sargent, T. D., Sell, S., and Bonner, J. (1979): α-Fetoprotein and albumin genes of rats: No evidence for amplification-deletion or rearrangement in rat liver carcinogenesis. *Proc. Natl. Acad. Sci. U.S.A.*, 76:695–699.

74. Sala-Trepat, J. M., Dever, J., Sargent, T. D., Thomas, K., Sell, S., and Bonner, J. (1979): Changes in expression of albumin and alphafetoprotein genes during rat liver development and neoplasia. *Biochemistry*, 18:2167–2178.

75. Sell, S., Thomas, K., Michaelson, M., Scott, J., and Sala-Trepat, J. M. (1979): Alphafetoprotein production by normal and abnormal liver cells. In: *Carcino-Embryonic Proteins. Vol. I*, edited by F. G. Lehmann, pp. 121–128. Elsevier, Amsterdam.

76. Leffert, H., Bonner, J., Brown, J., Moran, T., Sala-Trepat, J., Sell, S., Skelly, H., and Thomas, K. (1979): Molecular studies of retrodifferentiation phenomena in proliferation-competent adult hepatocyte cultures. In: *Gene to Protein*, Vol. 16, p. 606. Academic Press, New York.

77. Galau, G. A., Britten, R. J., and Davidson, E. H. (1974): Measurement of the sequence complexity of polysomal messenger RNA in sea urchin embryos. *Cell*, 2:9–17.

78. Leffert, H. L., Koch, K. S., Rubalcava, B., Sell, S., Moran, T., and Boorstein, R. (1978): Hepatocyte growth control: In vitro approach to problems of liver regeneration and function. *Natl. Cancer Inst. Monogr.*, 48:87–101.

79. Friedmann, N., and Dambach, G. (1973): Effects of glucagon, 3′-5′-AMP and 3′-5′-GMP on ion fluxes and transmembrane potential in perfused livers of normal and adrenalectomized rats. *Biochim. Biophys. Acta*, 307:399–403.

80. Friedmann, N., and Dambach, G. (1980): Antagonistic effect of insulin on glucagon-evoked hyperpolarization. A correlation between changes in membrane potential and gluconeogenesis. *Biochim. Biophys. Acta*, 596:180–185.

81. Spector, D. H., Varmus, H. E., and Bishop, J. M. (1978): Nucleotide sequences related to the transforming gene of avian sarcoma virus are present in DNA of uninfected vertebrates. *Proc. Natl. Acad. Sci. U.S.A.*, 75:4102–4106.

82. Chou, J. Y., and Schlegel-Hauter, S. E. (1981): Study of liver differentiation in vitro. *J. Cell Biol.*, 89:216–222.

83. Tjian, R., and Robbins, A. (1979): Enzymatic activities associated with a purified simian virus 40 T-antigen related protein. *Proc. Nat. Acad. Sci. U.S.A.*, 76:610–614.

84. Leffert, H. L., and Sell, S. (1974): Alpha₁-fetoprotein biosynthesis during the growth cycle of differentiated fetal rat hepatocytes in primary monolayer culture. *J. Cell. Biol.*, 61:823–829.

85. Sell, S., Leffert, H., Mueller-Eberhard, U., Kida, S., and Skelly, H. (1975): Relationship of the biosynthesis of alpha₁-fetoprotein, albumin, hemopexin, and haptoglobin to the growth state of fetal rat hepatocyte cultures. In: *Annals of the New York Academy of Sciences, Vol. 259: Carcinofetal Proteins: Biology and Chemistry*, edited by H. Hirai and E. Alpert, pp. 45–58. New York Academy of Sciences, New York.

86. Watabe, H., Leffert, H., and Sell, S. (1976): Developmental and maturational changes in alpha₁-fetoprotein and albumin production in cultured fetal rat hepatocytes. In: *Oncodevelopmental Gene Expression*, edited by W. Fishman and S. Sell, pp. 123–130. Academic Press, New York.

87. Young, R. A., Hagenbüchle, O., and Schibler, U. (1981): A single mouse α-amylase gene specifies two different tissue-specific mRNAs. *Cell*, 23:451–458.

88. Lindahl, T. (1981): DNA methylation and the control of gene expression. *Nature*, 290:363–365.

89. Farber, E. (1980): The sequential analysis of liver cancer induction. *Biochim. Biophys. Acta,* 605:149–166.

90. Pitot, H. C., and Sirica, A. E. (1980): The stages of initiation and promotion in hepatocarcinogenesis. *Biochim. Biophys. Acta,* 605:191–215.

91. Sell, S., and Morris, H. (1974): Rate α_1-fetoprotein: Relationship to growth rate and chromosomal composition of Morris hepatomas. *Cancer Res.,* 34:1413–1417.

92. Sell, S., and Leffert, H. L. (1982): An evaluation of cellular lineages in the pathogenesis of experimental hepatocellular carcinoma. *Hepatology,* 2:77–86.

93. Dempo, K., Chisaka, N., Yoshida, Y., Kaneko, A., and Onoe, T. (1975): Immunofluorescent study on α-fetoprotein-producing cells in the early stage of 3'-methyl-4-dimethylaminoazobenzene carcinogenesis. *Cancer Res.,* 35:1282–1287.

94. Hering, E. (1871): Kapitel 18. In: *Stricker's Handbuch der Lehre von den Geweben.* Leipzig.

95. Steiner, J. W., and Carruthers, J. S. (1961): Studies of the fine structure of the terminal branches of the biliary tree. I. The morphology of normal bile canaliculi, ile preductules (ducts of Hering) and bile ductules. *Am. J. Pathol.,* 6:639–661.

96. Rogers, A. E. (1975): Variable effects of a lipotrope-deficient diet, high fat on chemical carcinogenesis in rats. *Cancer Res.,* 35:2469–2475.

97. Sell, S., Osborn, K., and Leffert, H. L. (1981): Autoradiography of oval cells appearing rapidly in the livers of rats fed N-2-fluorenylacetamide in a choline-devoid diet. *Carcinogenesis,* 2:7–14.

98. Sell, S., Leffert, H. L., Shinozuka, H., Lombardi B., and N.

Gochman (1981): Rapid development of large numbers of AFP-containing "oval" cells in the liver of rats fed N-2-fluorenylacetamide in a choline-devoid diet. *GANN,* 72: 479–487.

99. Shinozuka, H., Lombardi, B., Sell, S., and Iaminarino, R. M. (1978): Early histological and functional alterations of ethionine liver carcinogenesis in rats fed a choline-deficient diet. *Cancer Res.,* 38:1092–1098.

100. Lombardi, B., Takahashi, S., and Sells, M. A. (1980): On a possible role of "oval" cells in chemical hepatocarcinogenesis. *Proc. Am. Assoc. Cancer Res.,* 21:389.

101. de Hemptinne, B., Skelly, H., Lad, P. J., Leffert, H. L., and Sell, S.: Studies of "oval" cell transplantation in Fisher/344 rats following 70% hepatectomy or dietary feeding of choline-devoid diets. (*In preparation.*)

102. Salas, C. E., Pfohl-Laszkowicz, A., Lang, M. C., and Dirheimer, G. (1979): Effects of modification by N-acetoxy-N-2'-acetylaminofluorene on the levels of DNA methylation. *Nature,* 278:71–72.

103. Brown, J. W., Leffert, H. L., Sell, S., and Ho, R.-J. (1980): Rapid radioisotopic analysis of glucose synthesis from lactate in primary adult rat hepatocyte cultures. *Anal. Biochem.,* 109:284–290.

104. Lad, P. J., Skelly, H., de Hemptinne, B., Koch, K. S., and Leffert, H. L. (1982): Ethanol metabolism, albumin production, and alcohol dehydrogenase activity during the growth cycle of adult rat hepatocytes in primary culture. In: *Ethanol and Protein Synthesis in Cerebral Tissue and Other Organs,* edited by S. Tewari and E. P. Noble (*in press*).

The Liver: Biology and Pathobiology, edited by
I. Arias, H. Popper, D. Schachter, and D. A. Shafritz.
Raven Press, New York © 1982.

Chapter 36

Communication and Gap Junctions

Norton B. Gilula and Elliot L. Hertzberg

A variety of mechanisms can be used for transmitting signals throughout the liver parenchyma. Although much of the signaling occurs via the movement of molecules in the extracellular space, some takes place as a result of cell-to-cell transmission of small molecules. This latter form requires a specialized physical contact or junction between hepatocytes and is referred to as intercellular or cell-to-cell communication. This chapter provides a basic introduction to the property of cell-to-cell communication and a contemporary perspective on the recent progress that has been made in this area of research.

DEFINING CELL-TO-CELL COMMUNICATION

Three basic approaches can be used to study cell-to-cell communication: (a) ionic coupling measurements, (b) determination of the cell-cell transfer of radiolabeled molecules or metabolic coupling, and (c) detection of gap junctional contacts via electron microscopy.

IONIC COUPLING

Communication was first described as an electrical event between excitable cells in the invertebrate nervous system (1) and the mammalian myocardium (2,3). It was also described as an electrical or electrotonic synapse as a result of low-resistance pathways for the transmission of current between adjacent cells. Signals can be transmitted rapidly between cells via such

pathways. In excitable tissues, the electrical synapse provides a useful mechanism for eliciting rapid responses (4) and for synchronizing the activities of cells in a tissue, such as the myocardium (2). In studies on nonexcitable epithelial cells, similar low-resistance pathways were detected (5–8). The communication pathways between nonexcitable cells were defined by their permeability to microinjected low molecular weight dyes (7,9), such as sodium fluorescein (MW 330). At present, low-resistance pathways or ionic coupling have been described in a wide range of animal and plant tissues both *in vivo* and in culture (for reviews, see refs. 4, and 20).

Biophysical observations on ionic coupling can be used to project several properties for the low-resistance pathways or channels: (a) The pathways are specialized regions of the cell surface membranes with resistance properties similar to cytoplasm (10 to 100 Ωcm^2) rather than the nonjunctional cell surface membrane (10^6 to 10^8 Ωcm^2). (b) The current that is passed from cell to cell probably is in the form of inorganic ions, such as Na^+, K^+, or Cl^-. (c) The pathways must have finite dimensions or channels with appropriate polar or hydrophilic properties that would permit the movement of inorganic ions with these hydrated molecular dimensions. Channels of 12 to 15 Å in diameter would be required.

METABOLIC COUPLING

Another approach for demonstrating communication has been to study the contact-dependent transfer of radiolabeled metabolites (10–14). This type of communication can be shown by utilizing one cell type with a known metabolic capacity as a preradiolabeled donor and another cell type without the same metabolic capacity as a recipient. After coculturing the donor and recipient, the communication of this metabolic capacity is revealed in autoradiographs as a contact-dependent transfer of radiolabeled molecules to the recipient. In the initial studies, recipient cells were deficient in inosinic pyrophosphorylase activity (IPP$^-$ or HGPRT$^-$), and the donor cells were prelabled with the exogenous purine ^{3}H-hypoxanthine. Thus the donor cells were able to "rescue" the recipient cells in HAT medium by transferring an important metabolite related to purine metabolism. In subsequent studies, data indicated that a small molecule, presumably a nucleotide, was transferred, and not a large polynucleotide or enzyme-related macromolecule (13,15). An approach has been developed using ^{3}H-uridine nonspecifically to demonstrate contact-dependent nucleotide transfer or exchange between metabolically competent cells (13).

IONIC AND METABOLIC COUPLING

A close relationship between ionic and metabolic coupling has been established in two separate studies (12,16). In coculture combinations of communication-competent and communication-defective cells, both ionic and metabolic coupling were examined. In cocultures comprised of two communication-competent cell types, both ionic and metabolic coupling were present. However, ionic and metabolic coupling were not detected between communication-competent and communication-defective cells. Therefore, it was concluded that both contact-dependent phenomena can occur simultaneously, and both require the presence of a similar pathway. Although likely, it cannot be concluded from those studies that both inorganic ions and metabolites are transmitted through the same pathway. The gap junction was implicated as the structural pathway for communication in the cocultures, since it was not detected between cells that failed to communicate, whereas it was readily detected between cells that were able to communicate (12).

JUNCTIONAL BASIS FOR COMMUNICATION

A specific cell membrane specialization, the gap junction, or nexus, has been strongly implicated as a structural pathway for communication on the basis of several experimental observations: (a) The gap junction is present at the site of electrical synaptic activity between neurons in the nervous system (4,17). (b) It connects adjacent myocardial cells for the electrotonic

propagation of impulses in the myocardium (18,19). This was elegantly demonstrated by utilizing selective cell contact dissociation procedures, such as EDTA treatment or perfusion with hypertonic sucrose; for example, EDTA treatment disrupts myocardial desmosome contacts but not gap junctions (or electrotonic coupling) without affecting desmosomes (19). (c) The gap junction is consistently present *in vivo* and in culture between cells that are communicating (for reviews, see refs. 9,20, and 21). (d) It is not expressed by a mouse cell culture line that is not able to communicate (12,22); this mouse A9 cell line is currently used as the universal communication-defective fibroblast. These observations have provided a substantial basis for gap junctional involvement in communication; however, other junctional structures, such as tight junctions or septate junctions, may also serve as low resistance pathways. It has not yet been possible to resolve this issue, since these junctions invariably coexist with gap junctions.

The gap junction was initially resolved by Revel and Karnovsky in 1967 (23; for review of early history, see ref. 24). It is currently synonymous with the structure that was called the nexus by Dewey and Barr in 1962 (25). In thin-section electron microscopy, the gap junction can be detected as a unique apposition between adjacent cells (Fig. 1). At the site of contact, the junction can be resolved as a seven-layered (septilaminar) structure, the entire width of which is 15 to 19 nm. The septilaminar image represents the parallel apposition of two 7.5 nm unit membranes that are separated by a 2 to 4 nm gap or electron-lucent space. This thin-section appearance led to the use of the term gap junction to describe this structure.

The precise clarification of the gap junctional structure in thin sections relied on the use of electron-opaque materials, or tracer substances, that are able to fill the extracellular space. Currently, colloidal lanthanum hydroxide, pyroantimonate, and ruthenium red can all be utilized for this tracing or staining purpose (23,26,27). The tracer substances are capable of penetrating a central region of the junction that corresponds to the location of the gap. In oblique or *en face* views of tracer-impregnated gap junctions, it is possible to visualize a unique polygonal lattice of 7 to 8 nm subunits. The tracer outlines the subunits, which have a 9 to 10 nm center-to-center spacing, as a result of penetrating the regions of the lattice that are continuous with the extracellular space (23). A 1.5 to 2 nm electron-dense dot is frequently present in the central region of these subunits. A similar lattice was described by Robertson (see discussion in ref. 17) at the site of an electrotonic synapse in a study that preceded the use of the tracer approaches. When gap junctions have been examined in detergent-treated isolated membrane fractions with negative stain procedures, a simi-

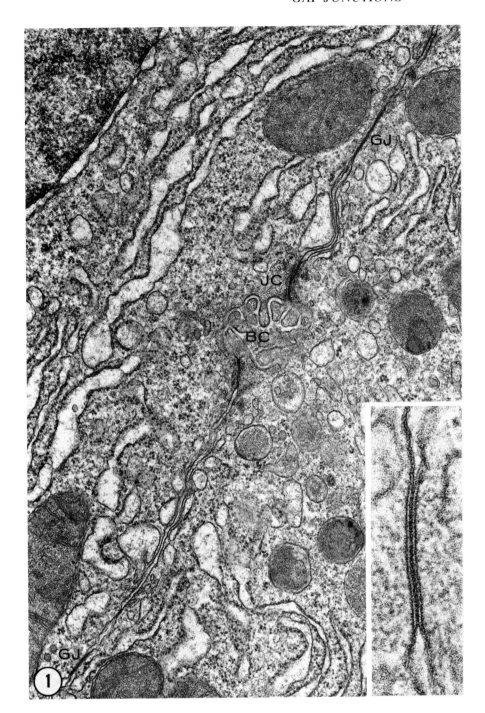

FIG. 1. Thin-section electron micrograph of cell-cell contact region between adjacent rat hepatocytes *in vivo*. A series of cell contacts is present in the region of the junctional complex (JC), which is adjacent to the bile canaliculus (BC). Gap junctional contacts (GJ) of variable size also are present in this region. ×30,000. **Inset:** High magnification, thin-section image of the hepatocyte gap junction. ×150,000.

lar polygonal lattice of subunits has been observed (28–31) (see Fig. 4).

The freeze-fracture technique has been utilized to obtain important complementary information about the gap junctional structure. This procedure provides detailed information about the internal content of the junctional membranes. In general, specialized membranes, such as those present at the sites of cell junctions, have significant internal membrane structural modifications (for review, see refs. 24 and 33). The freeze-fractured gap junctional membranes contain two complementary membrane halves or fracture faces (Fig. 2). The cytoplasmic or inner membrane half contains a polygonal lattice of homogeneous 7 to 8 nm intramembrane particles; the outer membrane half contains a complementary arrangement of pits or depressions. In many instances, a 2 to 2.5 nm dot is detectable in the central region of these junctional particles. These fracture face characteristics and membrane particle dispositions have now been documented as a constant feature of most nonarthropod gap junctions that have been examined (24,27,33). The junctional membrane lattices can exist in a variety of pleiomorphic forms, but the variations surround a

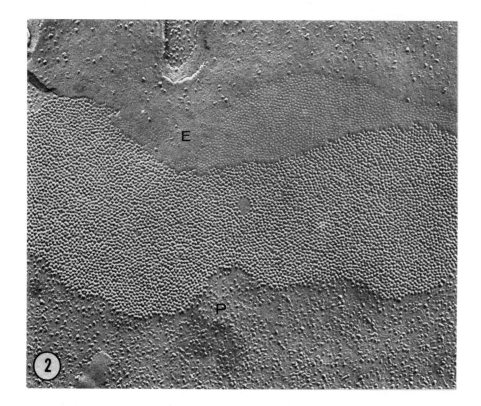

FIG. 2. Freeze-fracture appearance of a gap junctional membrane specialization in rat liver. The inner membrane half (fracture face P) contains a polygonal arrangement of intramembrane particles; a complementary arrangement of depressions or pits is present on the outer membrane half (fracture face E). ×96,000.

single theme: a plaque-like or localized (focal) contact between interacting cells. Gap junctions are usually present as oval or circular plaques; however, various forms, including linear strands (34), have been reported.

Gap junctions are structurally resistant to treatments with proteases and other agents that are used to dissociate cells (2a,35). One satisfactory procedure has been reported for splitting or separating gap junctional membranes in intact tissues. This procedure involves the perfusion of tissues with hypertonic sucrose solutions (18,36). In intact mouse liver, the junctional membranes are separated by this treatment somewhere in the central region of the extracellular gap (36). The separated junctional membranes still contain the characteristic particle lattices in freeze-fractured replicas, and the particles appear to be more tightly packed when the membranes are separated.

Gap junctions have been described in a variety of arthropod tissues with both thin-section and freeze-fracture techniques (for review, see ref. 37). The structural features of the arthropod gap junctions are sufficiently different from nonarthropod gap junctions to be considered a unique structural variation. In thin sections, the arthropod gap junctions are similar to nonarthropod gap junctions, although the intercellular gap is slightly larger (about 3 to 4 nm). In freeze-fracture replicas, the junctional particles are associated with the outer membrane half (fracture face E); the membrane particles are large (11 nm or larger in

diameter) and often heterogeneous in size; they are frequently present as fused aggregates of two or more particles. In addition, the particles are not usually in a highly ordered polygonal array.

STRUCTURE-FUNCTION RELATIONSHIPS IN COMMUNICATION

Several attempts have been made to relate the structure of gap junctions to low-resistance properties (see refs. 4 and 38). In general, it has been impossible to relate specific resistances or permeability measurements to the number of presumptive channels that can be detected ultrastructurally. The difficulties have been related primarily to the problem of finding a well-defined system (preferably a two-cell system) where the coupling and other membrane properties are relatively stable and where the number of gap junctional particles can be reliably quantitated.

Several studies have focused on correlating gap junctional structure with junctional conductance. Uncoupling treatments caused tighter, more regular particle packing within gap junctional plaques when compared to those in control specimens of the crayfish septate lateral giant axon (41). Similar particle rearrangements in response to various uncoupling treatments have also been observed in the myocardium (39), rat liver, and stomach by both conventional (40) and rapid freezing techniques (14). At present, it is not clear whether such structural changes can be observed in the junctions associated with vertebrate lens fibers (41a−43).

In one recent study on myocardial cell aggregates (44), normal junctional conductance was observed under conditions where few, if any, junctional structures were detected. Thus the structure-function relationship may be difficult to study, particularly when channels may exist as isolated rather than aggregated units in the cell surface membrane.

REGULATION OF JUNCTIONAL PERMEABILITY

The permeability properties of low-resistance junctions have been analyzed primarily by utilizing: (a) dye injections (visualization of the cell-to-cell transfer of fluorescence or color) (7,9), (b) injections of radiolabeled molecules (visualization of cell-to-cell transfer in autoradiographs or direct chromatographic analysis in tissue slices) (45,58), (c) transfer of radiolabeled molecules between cells in cocultures (visualization in autoradiographs) (15,46), and (d) injections of synthetic molecules conjugated to fluorescein or rhodamine (visualization of fluorescence movement) (47). On the basis of the information from these approaches, several general statements can be made: (a) Cell-to-cell transfer appears to be a relatively passive process; there has been no conclusive demonstration that energy is directly required for channel function. (b) Cell-to-cell transfer occurs at a slow rate, on the order of passive cytoplasmic diffusion. (c) Junctional permeability appears to be determined primarily on the basis of molecular size and perhaps charge. Molecules of 1,200 daltons and smaller can pass through the junctional channels, whereas larger molecules cannot be transferred from cell to cell (47). In essence, the junctional channels appear to function as a molecular sieve. These data suggest that a large number of cytoplasmic molecules, such as inorganic ions, amino acids, nucleotides, and sugars, can move from cell to cell. Macromolecular species, such as proteins, nucleic acids, and polysaccharides, however, cannot move through these pathways.

Three major physiological parameters have been implicated in regulating junctional permeability: (a) intracellular calcium concentration (48,49), (b) intracellular pH (50), and (c) voltage dependence (51). All three can influence junctional permeability in specific biologic systems, and none except pH has widespread regulatory effects. Both Ca^{2+} and pH can cause a complete loss of permeability, but the Ca^{2+} effect is usually irreversible, whereas the pH effect is readily reversible (48−50). The voltage dependence is characterized by a reversible modulation in the permeability or junctional resistance, without a complete loss in function (51).

BIOCHEMICAL AND BIOPHYSICAL ANALYSIS OF ISOLATED GAP JUNCTIONS

Gap junctions have been successfully isolated from liver plasma membranes of rats (31,52) and mice (30) (Figs. 3 and 4). There is now general agreement that gap junctions from mammalian liver are comprised predominantly of a 27,000 dalton polypeptide (Fig. 5). Lipid analysis indicates a composition similar to that of the plasma membranes from which they are derived (30,31), although an enrichment for cholesterol has been demonstrated (30). Thus far, no glycosylation has been detected on any material in the isolated junction. Junctions similar to those isolated from liver can be obtained from mammalian lens fibers, and such material contains a predominant 25,000 dalton polypeptide (41a,53,54). Although the structures are similar, the two polypeptides (liver and lens) do not appear to be closely related (55). At present, it is not clear what, if any, relationship might exist between the lens fiber junctions and the gap junctions present in other tissues.

Structural analysis of liver gap junctions has been carried out by optical diffraction of images of negatively stained samples and X-ray diffraction of pelleted gap junctions (32,56,57). In one study (32,56), a major variable feature observed was the lattice constant, which varied from 8 to 9 nm. The smaller lattice constant was associated with a partial collapse of the gap between apposing membranes. These observations were included in a model in which tighter particle packing and partial collapse of the gap occur with a narrowing of the gap junctional channel; this would be associated with a loss of channel conductance (32,56).

In another study on isolated gap junctions from mouse liver (57), no significant variation in the lattice constant was detected. However, two forms were observed: one was obtained in the isolated (detergent-treated) junction fraction (type A); the second was induced by prolonged dialysis (type B), presumably by removing traces of residual detergent. The B form is reversibly converted into the A form by addition of small amounts of detergent. These observations indicate that the A form contains an open channel, and that the B form is generated by a radial motion of the subunits at the cytoplasmic surface, resulting in closure of the channel. Although a mechanism dependent on relative motion of protein subunits is attractive, it is difficult to extrapolate from these findings to an *in vivo* regulatory mechanism.

POTENTIAL ROLE OF COMMUNICATION IN HORMONAL STIMULATION

A model coculture system was generated in order to study the potential role of cell communication in the

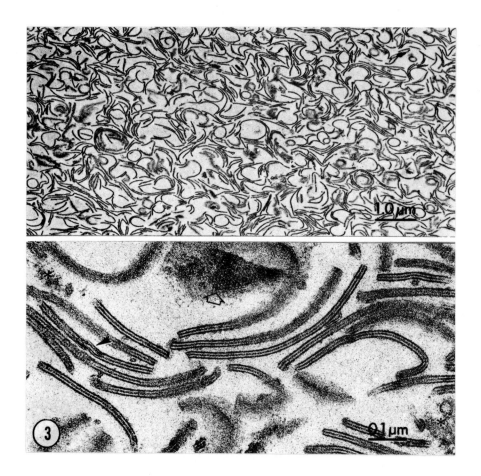

FIG. 3. Appearance of the enriched gap junctional fraction isolated from rat liver. **Upper image:** Low magnification, thin-section sampling of the pellet from the fraction. **Lower image:** Higher magnification view of the same fraction. Note that the fraction contains isolated junctional membranes that still retain their structural characteristics. (From ref. 31.)

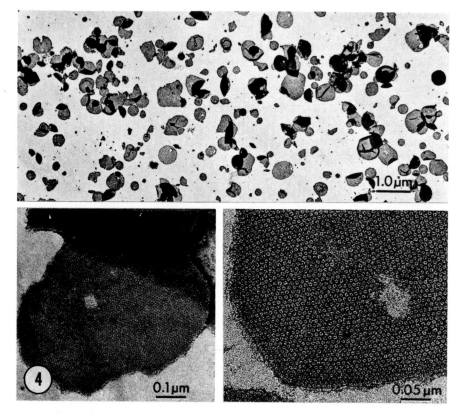

FIG. 4. Negative stain appearance of the isolated gap junctions from rat liver at low **(upper),** intermediate **(lower left),** and high **(lower right)** magnification. Such negative stain preparations of the isolated gap junctions reveal the characteristic polygonal arrangement of particles that are 8 to 9 nm in diameter. (From ref. 31.)

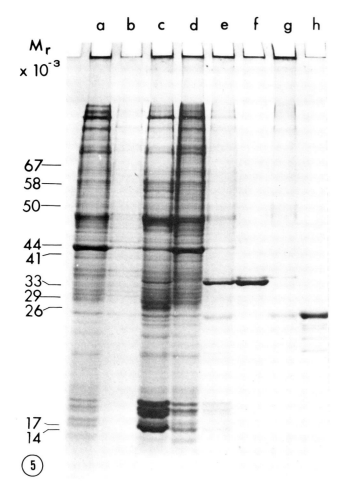

FIG. 5. Electrophoretic gel composite illustrating the polypeptide content of various fractions obtained during the procedure for isolating gap junctions from rat liver. The various fractions were solubilized in the detergent SDS and separated electrophoretically prior to staining with Coomassie blue. Lane (a) contains the polypeptides resolvable in the total plasma membrane fraction, while lane (h) contains a sample from the enriched gap junction fraction. The most prominent polypeptide component in the gap junction fraction has an apparent molecular weight of 27,000 daltons, although it can vary in mobility in different gel systems. (From ref. 59.)

transmission of hormonal stimulation in multicellular systems (58a). Two hormonally responsive cell phenotypes were selected for this purpose: the follicle stimulating hormone (FSH)-responsive rat ovarian granulosa cell, and the catecholamine-responsive mouse neonatal ventricular myocardial cell.

In initial experiments, the two cell types were fully characterized for both hormonal responsiveness and communication competency. The rat ovarian granulosa cells were treated with a saturating dose of FSH, and their response was measured as either the production of a secreted cell product, plasminogen activator, or a morphologic change in cell shape. Both FSH-stimulated responses are preceded by a dose-

dependent increase in intracellular cAMP; this effect is potentiated by cyclic nucleotide phosphodiesterase inhibitors and it is mimicked by dibutyryl cAMP. The mouse ventricular myocardial cells were stimulated with the catecholamine norepinephrine, and the response was measured as either an increase in beat frequency or a change in the action potential properties. The catecholamine stimulation is accompanied by a rapid elevation of intracellular cAMP. This stimulation can be potentiated by cyclic nucleotide phosphodiesterase inhibitors, such as theophylline and methylisobutylxanthine, and can be mimicked by dibutyryl cAMP.

The communication properties of the two cell types were examined in both homologous and heterologous cultures. Both cell types could be characterized as communication competent by ionic coupling, metabolic coupling, and the presence of gap junctional contacts. In fact, communication was as prominent between heterologous cells as it was between homologous cells. The transmission of hormonal communication between heterologous cells was examined initially by treating myocardial cells cultured alone or in contact with granulosa cells with FSH. The myocardial cells cultured alone had no detectable response to FSH, whereas the myocardial cells in contact with the granulosa cells had a marked increase in beat frequency together with the characteristic stimulated action potential properties. In a similar fashion, it was possible to stimulate the production of plasminogen activator by treating granulosa cells in contact with myocardial cells with norepinephrine. In both cases, the transmission of hormonal stimulation was directly dependent on direct contact between the heterologous cell type. The observed effect does not appear to be related to either a hormone-induced change in electrical properties of the cell membrane or to a movement of hormone receptors between the heterologous cells. In this system, both hormonal responses are cAMP dependent; therefore, the cyclic nucleotide is a likely candidate for the mediator of hormonal stimulation.

COMMUNICATION IN THE LIVER

The liver has played a central role in our present understanding of the property of communication between cells. As a cell type in culture, the communication properties of both normal and tumorigenic liver cells have been studied in an attempt to determine if a relationship exists between communication and growth regulation (for an extensive review of this area, see ref. 20). Some but not all tumorigenic cells have communication defects; therefore, it has been difficult to establish such a proposed correlation between the two properties. Nevertheless, a relationship may exist that can be clarified as more sensitive probes for communication are developed.

Liver regeneration has been another unique resource for studies on the modulation and/or formation of cell junctional structures. In an early study, ultrastructural observations indicated that there are substantial rearrangements of the cell junctions between hepatocytes during the regeneration process (60,61). In essence, the particle aggregates ascribed to gap junctional elements undergo either reorganization or disappear, while the tight junctional ridges (occluding zonule elements) are still detectable. This apparent loss of gap junctional particle aggregates occurs around the peak of mitotic activity during regeneration; subsequently, the junctional particle aggregates reappear in close association with the tight junctional ridges. In a recent study on this process using combined electrophysiologic and electron microscopic techniques, junctional conductance was still detectable between the hepatocytes at the time during regeneration when the junctional particle aggregates are not detectable (37a,62). These observations provide a graphic example of the difficulty of correlating structure and function; and perhaps more interestingly, they suggest the possibility of a close relationship between the tight junctional and gap junctional elements. Such a relationship may be established by determining the biochemical and biophysical properties of the tight junctional ridges.

Finally, the liver has been the major source for identifying and characterizing the molecular components of the vertebrate gap junction. This has been a product of three factors: (a) the liver provides a favorable homogeneous tissue for subcellular fractionation; (b) the tissue is readily available in large quantities; and (c) the hepatocytes are joined by a population of large gap junctional structures that are insoluble under most conditions. The subcellular fractions that have been isolated from liver have been extremely useful for both biochemical and structural analysis, as indicated previously. Currently, the predominant liver gap junctional polypeptide is being used in several laboratories to develop appropriate immunological probes that can be used in the future to study the biosynthesis and biologic role of gap junctional communication.

REFERENCES

1. Furshpan, E. J., and Potter, D. D. (1959): Transmission at giant motor synapse of the crayfish. *J. Physiol.,* 143:289–325.
2. Weidmann, S. (1952): The electrical constants of Purkinje fibers. *J. Physiol. (Lond.),* 118:348–360.
2a. Amsterdam, A., and Jamieson, J. D. (1974): Studies on dispersed pancreatic exocrine cells. I. Dissociation technique and morphologic characteristics of separated cells. *J. Cell Biol.,* 63:1037–1056.
3. Woodbury, J. W., and Crill, W. E. (1961): On the problem of impulse conduction in the atrium. In: *Nervous Inhibition,* edited by E. Florey, pp. 124–135. Pergamon, London.
4. Bennett, M. V. L. (1977): Electrical transmission: a functional analysis and comparison with chemical transmission. In: *Cellular Biology of Neurons, Vol. I, Sect. 1. Handbook of Physiology, The Nervous System,* edited by E. Kandel, pp. 357–416. Williams & Wilkins, Baltimore.
5. Furshpan, E. J., and Potter, D. D. (1968): Low-resistance junctions between cells in embryos and tissue culture. *Curr. Top. Dev. Biol.,* 3:95–127.
6. Johnson, R. G., and Sheridan, J. D. (1971): Junctions between cancer cells in culture: Ultrastructure and permeability. *Science,* 174:717–719.
7. Loewenstein, W. R. (1966): Permeability of membrane junctions. *Ann. N.Y. Acad. Sci.,* 137:441–472.
8. Loewenstein, W. R., Socolar, S. J., Higashino, S., Kanno, Y., and Davidson, N. (1965): Intercellular communication: Renal, urinary bladder, sensory, and salivary gland cells. *Science,* 149:295–298.
9. Sheridan, J. D. (1976): Cell coupling and cell communication during embryogenesis. In: *The Cell Surface in Animal Embryogenesis and Development, Cell Surface Reviews, Vol. 1,* edited by G. Poste and G. L. Nicolson, pp. 409–443. North Holland, New York.
10. Cox, R. P., Krauss, M., Balis, M. E., and Dancis, J. (1970): Evidence for transfer of enzyme product as the basis of metabolic cooperation between tissue culture fibroblasts of Lesch-Nyhan and normal cells. *Proc. Natl. Acad. Sci. USA,* 67:1573–1579.
11. Cox, R. P., Krauss, M. R., Balis, M. E., and Dancis, J. (1974): Metabolic cooperation in cell culture: a model for cell-to-cell communication. In: *Cell Communication,* edited by R. P. Cox, pp. 67–96. Wiley, New York.
12. Gilula, N. B., Reeves, O. R., and Steinbach, A. (1972): Metabolic coupling, ionic coupling and cell contacts. *Nature,* 235:262–265.
13. Pitts, J. D., and Simms, J. W. (1977): Permeability of junctions between animal cells: Intercellular transfer of nucleotides but not macromolecules. *Exp. Cell Res.,* 104:153–163.
14. Raviola, E., Goodenough, D. A., and Raviola, G. (1980): Structure of rapidly frozen gap junctions. *J. Cell Biol.,* 87:272–279.
15. Pitts, J. D. (1977): Direct communication between animal cells. In: *International Cell Biology (1976–1977),* edited by B. R. Brinkley and K. R. Porter, pp. 43–49. The Rockefeller University Press, New York.
16. Azarnia, R., Michalke, W., and Loewenstein, W. R. (1972): Intercellular communication and tissue growth. VI. Failure of exchange of endogenous molecules between cancer cells with defective junctions and noncancerous cells. *J. Membr. Biol.,* 10:247–258.
17. Sotelo, C., and Korn, H. (1978): Morphological correlates of electrical and other interactions through low-resistance pathways between neurons of the vertebrate central nervous system. *Int. Rev. Cytol.,* 55:67–107.
18. Barr, L., Berger, W., and Dewey, M. M. (1968): Electrical transmission at the nexus between smooth muscle cells. *J. Gen. Physiol.,* 51:347–368.
19. Dreifuss, J. J., Girardier, L., and Forssman, W. G. (1966): Etude de la propagation de l'excitation dans le ventricule de rat du moyen de solutions hypertoniques. *Pfluegers Arch.,* 292:13–33.
20. Loewenstein, W. R. (1979): Junctional intercellular communication and the control of growth. *Biochim. Biophys. Acta,* 560:1–65.
21. Gilula, N. B. (1977): Gap junctions and cell communication. In: *International Cell Biology (1976–1977),* edited by B. R. Brinkley and K. R. Porter, pp. 61–69. The Rockefeller University Press, New York.
22. Azarnia, R., Larsen, W. J., and Loewenstein, W. R. (1974): The membrane junctions in communicating and non-communicating cells, their hybrids and segregants. *Proc. Natl. Acad. Sci. USA,* 71:880–884.
23. Revel, J. P., and Karnovsky, M. J. (1967): Hexagonal array of subunits in intercellular junctions of the mouse heart and liver. *J. Cell Biol.,* 33:C7–C12.

24. McNutt, N. S., and Weinstein, R. S. (1973): Membrane ultrastructure of mammalian intercellular junctions. *Prog. Biophys. Mol. Biol.*, 26:45–101.

25. Dewey, M. M., and Barr, L. (1962): Intercellular connection between smooth muscle cells: The nexus. *Science*, 137:670–672.

26. Payton, B. W., Bennett, M. V. L., and Pappas, G. D. (1969): Permeability and structure of junctional membranes at an electrotonic synapse. *Science*, 166:1641–1643.

27. Friend, D. S., and Gilula, N. B. (1972): Variations in tight and gap junctions in mammalian tissues. *J. Cell Biol.*, 53:758–776.

28. Benedetti, E. L., and Emmelot, P. (1968): Hexagonal array of subunits in tight junctions separated from isolated rat liver plasma membranes. *J. Cell Biol.*, 38:15–24.

29. Goodenough, D. A., and Stoeckenius, W. (1972): The isolation of mouse hepatocyte gap junctions. Preliminary chemical characterization and X-ray diffraction. *J. Cell Biol.*, 58:646–656.

30. Henderson, D., Eibl, H., and Weber, K. (1979): Structure and biochemistry of mouse hepatic gap junctions. *J. Mol. Biol.*, 132:193–218.

31. Hertzberg, E. L., and Gilula, N. B. (1979): Isolation and characterization of gap junctions from rat liver. *J. Biol. Chem.*, 254:2138–2147.

32. Makowski, L., Caspar, D. L. D., Phillips, W. C., and Goodenough, D. A. (1977): Gap junction structures. II. Analysis of the X-ray diffraction data. *J. Cell Biol.*, 74:629–645.

33. Staehelin, L. A. (1974): Structure and function of intercellular junctions. *Int. Rev. Cytol.*, 39:191–283.

34. Raviola, E., and Gilula, N. B. (1973): Gap junctions between photoreceptor cells in the vertebrate retina. *Proc. Natl. Acad. Sci. USA*, 70:1677–1681.

35. Berry, M. N., and Friend, D. S. (1969): High yield preparation of isolated rat liver parenchymal cells: a biochemical and fine structure study. *J. Cell Biol.*, 43:506–520.

36. Goodenough, D. A., and Gilula, N. B. (1974): The splitting of hepatocyte gap junctions and zonulae occludentes with hypertonic disaccharides. *J. Cell Biol.*, 61:575–590.

37. Lane, N. J., and le B. Skaer, H. (1980): Intercellular junctions in insect tissues. *Adv. Insect Physiol.*, 15:35–213.

37a. Meyer, D. J., Yancey, S. B., and Revel, J. P. (1979): Electronic coupling and dye spread after disappearance of gap junctions. *J. Cell Biol.*, 83:84a.

38. Bennett, M. V. L. (1973): Function of electrotonic junctions in embryonic and adult tissues. *Fed. Proc.*, 32:65–75.

39. Baldwin, K. M. (1979): Cardiac gap junctional configuration after an uncoupling treatment as a function of time. *J. Cell Biol.*, 82:66–75.

40. Peracchia, C. (1977): Gap junctions. Structural changes after uncoupling procedures. *J. Cell Biol.*, 72:628–641.

40a. Peracchia, C. (1980): Structural correlates of gap junction permeation. *Int. Rev. Cytol.*, 66:81–146.

41. Peracchia, C., and Dulhunty, A. F. (1976): Low-resistance junctions in crayfish. Structural changes with functional uncoupling. *J. Cell Biol.*, 70:419–439.

41a. Goodenough, D. A. (1979): Lens gap junctions: A structural hypothesis for non-regulated low-resistance intercellular pathways. *Invest. Ophthalmol. Visual Sci.*, 18:1104–1122.

42. Peracchia, C., and Peracchia, L. L. (1980): Gap junction dynamics: Reversible effects of divalent cations. *J. Cell. Biol.*, 87:708–718.

43. Peracchia, C., and Peracchia, L. L. (1980): Gap junction dynamics: Reversible effects of hydrogen ions. *J. Cell Biol.*, 87:719–727.

44. Williams, E. H., and DeHaan, R. L. (1981): Electrical coupling among heart cells in the absence of ultrastructurally defined gap junctions. *J. Membr. Biol.*, 60:237–248.

45. Rieske, E., Schubert, P., and Kreutzberg, G. W. (1975): Transfer of radioactive material between electrically coupled neurons of the leech central nervous system. *Brain Res.*, 84:365–382.

46. Subak-Sharpe, J. H., Bürk, R. R., and Pitts, J. D. (1969): Metabolic cooperation between biochemically masked mammalian cells in tissue culture. *J. Cell Sci.*, 4:353–367.

47. Simpson, I., Rose, B., and Loewenstein, W. R. (1977): Size limit of molecules permeating the junctional membrane channels. *Science*, 195:294–296.

48. Rose, B., and Loewenstein, W. R. (1975): Permeability of cell junction depends on local cytoplasmic calcium activity. *Nature*, 254:250–252.

49. Rose, B., and Rick, R. (1978): Intracellular pH, intracellular free Ca and junctional cell-cell coupling. *J. Membr. Biol.*, 44:377–415.

50. Turin, L., and Warner, A. (1977): Carbon dioxide reversibly abolishes ionic communication between cells of early amphibian embryo. *Nature*, 270:56–57.

51. Spray, D. C., Harris, A. L., and Bennett, M. V. L. (1979): Voltage dependence of junctional conductance in early amphibian embryos. *Science*, 204:432–434.

52. Finbow, M., Yancey, S. B., Johnson, R., and Revel, J.-P. (1980): Independent lines of evidence suggesting a major gap junctional protein with a molecular weight of 26,000. *Proc. Natl. Acad. Sci. USA*, 77:970–974.

53. Alcala, J., Lieska, N., and Maisel, H. (1975): Protein composition of bovine lens cortical fiber cell membranes. *Exp. Eye Res.*, 21:581–595.

54. Bloemendal, H. (1977): The vertebrate eye lens. *Science*, 197:127–138.

55. Hertzberg, E. L., Anderson, D. J., Friedlander, M., and Gilula, N. B. (1981): Comparative analysis of the major polypeptides from liver gap junctions and lens fiber junctions. *J. Cell Biol.*, 92:53–59.

56. Caspar, D. L. D., Goodenough, D. A., Makowski, L., and Phillips, W. C. (1977): Gap junction structures. I. Correlated electron microscopy and X-ray diffraction. *J. Cell Biol.*, 74:605–628.

57. Unwin, P. N. T., and Zampighi, G. (1980): Structure of the junction between communicating cells. *Nature*, 283:545–549.

58. Tsien, R. W., and Weingart, R. (1976): Inotropic effect of cyclic AMP in calf ventricular muscle studied by a cut-end method. *J. Physiol. (Lond.)*, 260:117–141.

58a. Lawrence, T. S., Beers, W. H., and Gilula, N. B. (1978): Transmission of hormonal stimulation by cell-to-cell communication. *Nature*, 272:501–506.

59. Hertzberg, E. L. (1980): Biochemical and immunological approaches to the study of gap junctional communication. *In Vitro*, 16:1057–1067.

60. Yee, A. G. (1972): Gap junctions between hepatocytes in regenerating liver. *J. Cell Biol.*, 55:294a.

61. Yee, A. G., and Revel, J. P. (1978): Loss and reappearance of gap junctions in regenerating liver. *J. Cell Biol.*, 78:554–564.

62. Yancey, S. B., Easter, E., and Revel, J. P. (1979): Cytological changes in gap junctions during liver regeneration. *J. Ultrastruct. Res.*, 67:229–242.

SECTION IV

The Organ

The Liver: Biology and Pathobiology, edited by
I. Arias, H. Popper, D. Schachter, and D. A. Shafritz.
Raven Press, New York © 1982.

Chapter 37

The Hepatic Circulation

Jose L. Campra and *Telfer B. Reynolds

The hepatic circulation has some unique characteristics. The liver has two afferent blood supplies: one is
the hepatic artery, whose function is primarily nutritional; another, the portal vein, is designed to facilitate
exposure of absorbed nutrients and toxins to hepatocytes and reticuloendothelial cells. Thus toxic materials can be removed, and metabolic conversion of absorbed nutrients can occur. To accomplish the latter
objective, large volume flow is needed together with
close contact between the blood and the microvilli of
the hepatocytes. Since the blood bringing materials
from the digestive tube has already lost much of its
kinetic energy by passing through the capillary system
of the gut, the portal vascular channels in the liver
must offer extremely low resistance to blood flow.
Junction of the high pressure, high resistance hepatic
arterial stream with the low pressure, low resistance
portal stream in the sinusoids requires an ingenious
mechanism for equalization of pressures in order to
avoid turbulent flow.

Department of Internal Medicine, National University of Cordoba, Department of Gastroenterology and Hepatology, Hospital
Privado, Cordoba, Argentina; and *Department of Medicine, University of Southern California, Division of Hepatology, Los Angeles
County-USC Medical Center, Los Angeles, California 90033

MACROCIRCULATION

Portal Vein

The portal vein collects all the blood that leaves the
spleen, stomach, small and large intestine, gall bladder, and pancreas and carries it to the liver. It is most
commonly formed (85 to 93% of cases) (1) by the union
of the superior mesenteric and splenic vein just posterior to the head of the pancreas at the level of the
second lumbar vertebrae (Fig. 1). In about 10% of
cases, it is formed by the confluence of the superior
mesenteric, inferior mesenteric, and splenic veins. It
averages 7 cm in length, with a maximum of 8 and a
minimum of 5.5 cm, and its diameter varies from 1.1 to
3.2 cm, averaging approximately 2 cm (1). Afferent
branches of the portal vein are the superior mesenteric, splenic, inferior mesenteric, pyloric, cystic, and
coronary veins, as well as some irregular pancreatoduodenal vessels. At the porta hepatis, the portal
vein divides into a right and a left branch (74 to 88%
of cases) (2,3), or into three branches, with two going
to the right and one to the left lobe (10% of cases).

Other modes of division are highly unusual. The
major branching usually occurs just outside the liver.

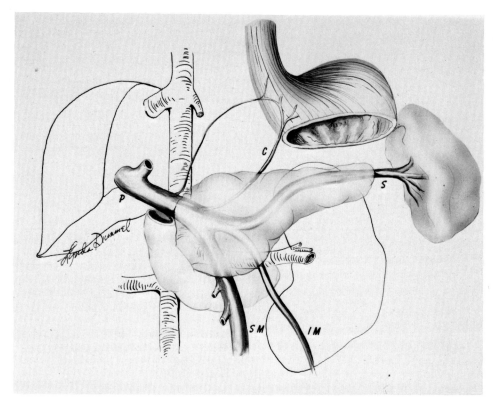

FIG. 1. Extrahepatic portal vein. Its major afferent branches are the splenic (S), inferior mesenteric (IM), superior mesenteric (SM) and coronary (C) veins. (From ref 10.)

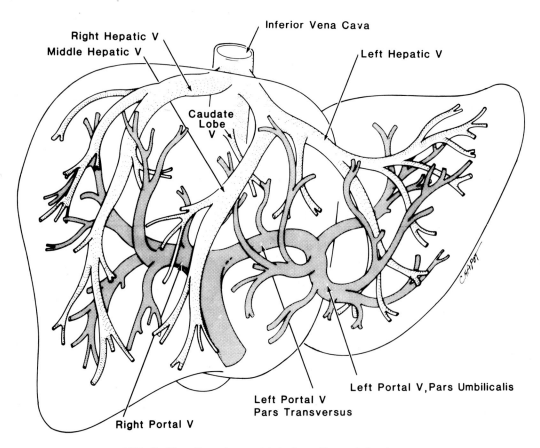

FIG. 2. Hepatic veins and intrahepatic portal vein.

The right branch receives the cystic vein just before entering the liver parenchyma. The left intrahepatic portal trunk consists of two sections, pars transversa and pars umbilicalis (Fig. 2). The latter begins with a sharp angulation or kink caused by the tension from the ligmentum teres, the site of the fetal umbilical vein. Usually, two branches to the lateral segment of the left lobe arise from the pars umbilicalis. Branches to the medial segment of the left lobe also derive from the pars umbilicalis. The short, stout right main branch of the portal vein divides into anterior and posterior segmental veins for the corresponding segments of the right lobe. Each one gives off a superior and an inferior branch. The quadrate lobe receives ascending and descending branches from the right wall of the pars umbilicalis of the left portal vein. The caudate lobe receives most of its portal blood supply from vessels leading from the pars transversa of the left portal vein. The right portion of the caudate lobe is supplied by a branch from the right portal vein or from the main portal vein in about 25% of cases (4). The major intrahepatic branches of the portal vein have a definite spatial arrangement with few anastomoses between them (Fig. 3).

The anatomic features of the portal vein with clinical relevance are as follows: (a) It is valveless, so that elevations of pressure are transmitted to all its branches with ease. (b) Its anatomic location makes access to it for physiologic measurements or surgery relatively difficult. (c) In the hepatoduodenal ligament, it consistently runs behind the bile duct and hepatic artery, which aids in its identification during biliary or portacaval shunt surgery. (d) A segment of portal vein between the highest afferent branch and the porta hepatis, which averages 5 cm and has a minimum

length of 3.5 cm, facilitates dissection and mobilization of the portal trunk without risk of hemorrhage. (e) There are numerous potential anastomoses between the portal venous system and the superior and inferior vena caval systems. These carry no blood and have no functional significance in the normal person. In the presence of portal hypertension, however, they often develop into relatively large channels capable of substantial collateral portal blood flow.

The most important potential anastomoses are the following: (a) At the gastroesophageal junction, blood from the gastric coronary vein or from the short gastric veins may drain toward the superior vena cava, resulting in esophageal and gastric varices. (b) A reopened umbilical vein or newly developed paraumbilical channels may connect the pars umbilicalis of the left intrahepatic portal vein with abdominal wall vessels that lead cephalad to join the superior vena caval system or, less commonly, caudad into branches of the inferior vena cava. This may result in spectacular physical findings, such as a caput medusa and/or a palpable thrill and loud continuous bruit (Cruveilhier-Baumgarten murmur) over tortuous abdominal veins. (c) Anastomoses between distal branches of the inferior mesenteric and rectal veins may create large internal hemorrhoids. (d) Portal blood can reach the inferior vena cava by a variety of retroperitoneal collaterals. Perhaps the most important are large anastomoses that sometimes develop between the splenic vein and the left renal vein, in the area of the adrenal gland. These may achieve such a large size as to result in periodic episodes of otherwise unexplained hepatic encephalopathy, as sometimes seen after surgical portal-systemic shunt (5). (e) Large collateral veins often develop in adhesions that connect the mesentery or intestine to the parietal peritoneum. Usually, these are beneath operative scars, but they may develop between the spleen or liver and the peritoneum, presumably as a consequence of some earlier inflammatory disorder. Collateral veins in adhesions pose a risk of bleeding during paracentesis, laparoscopy, or liver biopsy. Other, less important potential portal collaterals are the diaphragmatic veins of Sappey, which can connect with either superior vena caval branches or pulmonary veins and the ductus venosus, which is rarely partially patent.

Portal collateral flow diverts intestinal blood around the liver, potentially exposing the brain to toxic substances, altering the blood levels of hormones, such as insulin and glucagon, and affecting the metabolism of those ingested drugs that are normally highly extracted during their first passage through the liver.

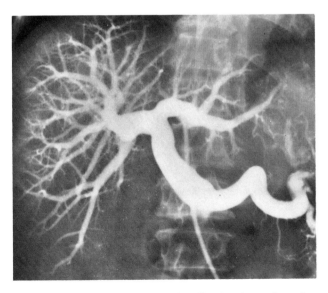

FIG. 3. Intrahepatic portal vein. Contrast medium has been injected through a catheter that has been introduced into the main portal vein via the umbilical vein remnant and the left branch of the portal vein.

Hepatic Artery

Anatomic variations in the hepatic artery are common; the usual pattern is present in only slightly more

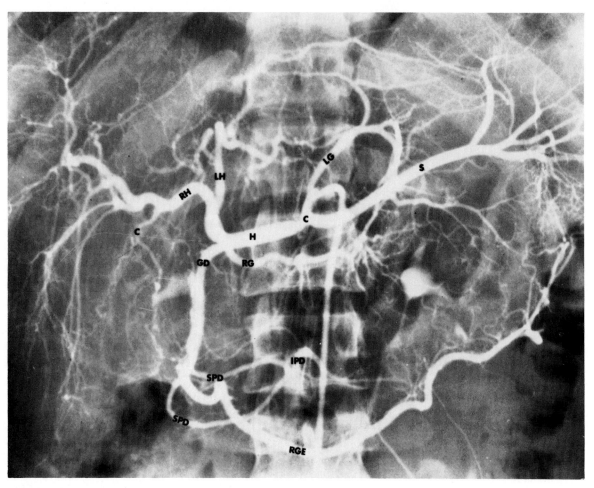

FIG. 4. Celiac axis and the hepatic artery. Contrast medium has been injected through a catheter placed in the celiac axis by way of the femoral artery and aorta. Shown are the celiac trunk (C), and the following arteries: splenic (S), left gastric (LG), hepatic (H), cystic (C), gastroduodenal (GD), right gastric (RG), superior and inferior pancreatoduodenal (SPD and IPD) and right gastroepiploic (RGE).

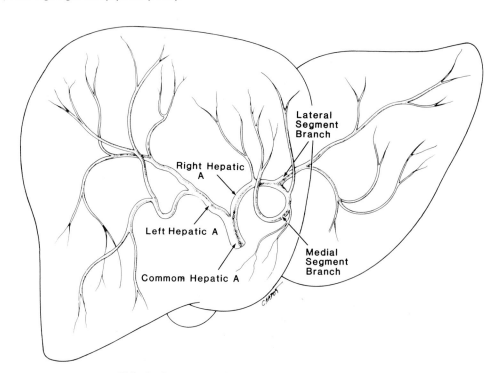

FIG. 5. Branches of the hepatic artery in the liver.

than 50% of individuals (6). In the typical person, the hepatic artery arises from the celiac axis and takes an irregular horizontal trajectory from left to right along the upper border of the head of the pancreas (Fig. 4). Posterior to the duodenum, it gives off the gastroduodenal artery and ascends toward the liver, giving rise to the supraduodenal and right gastric arteries. In the hepatoduodenal ligament, it runs medial to the common bile duct and anterior to the portal vein. From the gastroduodenal artery to the porta hepatis, it is known as the proper hepatic artery. At the porta hepatis, it usually breaks into two branches, right and left, with the left soon dividing into a branch supplying the medial segment of the left lobe (called by some the middle hepatic artery) and a branch to the lateral segment of the left lobe (Fig. 5). Nine additional anatomic variations are described by Michels (6). The most important of these are the right hepatic artery or the entire hepatic artery arising from the superior mesenteric trunk, and the branch to the lateral segment of the left lobe arising from the left gastric artery.

In addition to the parenchymal branches to the liver, the proper hepatic artery also provides vasa vasora, which supply the major vascular structures at the hilum of the liver, and subcapsular branches, which enter into a diffuse subcapsular plexus. This plexus communicates with extrinsic arteries, forming important extrahepatic anastomoses (for example, with the inferior phrenic arteries). The plexus and its extrahepatic anastomoses contribute to the preservation of blood supply to the liver after hepatic artery ligation.

Corrosion casts demonstrate that the arterial vasculature of the liver is arranged in regional units, with few intrahepatic anastomoses (7,8). However, subcapsular anastomoses connect the right and left hepatic arteries. In general, the intrahepatic branches of the hepatic artery follow the corresponding portal and biliary channels, although the major channels often are not precisely parallel.

Anatomic points of clinical interest are as follows: (a) Collateral flow occurs via the gastroduodenal artery, so that ligation of the hepatic artery close to the aorta does not seriously disturb hepatic blood flow. Communication between the subcapsular arterial plexus and extrinsic arteries, such as the inferior phrenic, allows ligation of even the proper hepatic artery with little likelihood of serious consequence. (b) Trauma to the liver resulting in external or biliary tract bleeding may require hepatic arterial ligation. The frequent anatomic variations make preoperative angiography essential. (c) The point of division between the right and left hepatic lobes is at the porta hepatis, where the hepatic artery and portal vein divide, rather than at the indentation formed by the falciform ligament. The latter actually divides the left lobe into medial and lateral portions. Surgical lobectomy proceeds along the line from the porta hepatis (base of the gall bladder) to the

groove of the inferior vena cava on the superior posterior surface of the liver. (d) A replaced right hepatic artery may jeopardize a portacaval shunt because it commonly lies dorsal and lateral to the portal vein. If a portacaval shunt is constructed ventral to the replaced hepatic artery, the portal vein may be angulated and partly obstructed as it courses in a ventral to dorsal direction toward the vena cava (9). (e) The anterior segmental branch of the right hepatic artery often forms a loop close to the gall bladder fossa. This close relationship could lead to inadvertent ligation during cholecystectomy.

Hepatic Veins

Three major hepatic veins (right, middle, and left) empty into the inferior vena cava in the groove on the posterior surface of the liver (Fig. 2); they are enveloped by the coronary ligament. There are numerous anastomoses between the various intrahepatic branches of the hepatic veins (10). The right hepatic vein is actually a bundle of several large veins which converge toward a single (occasionally double) opening in the right anterior wall of the inferior vena cava (11). It is the largest of the three and drains most of the territory to the right of the gall bladder-caval line. It runs along the intersegmental plane between the anterior and posterior segments and drains the entire posterior segment of the right lobe and a variable part of the anterior superior segment. The middle hepatic vein drains the medial segment of the left lobe and a variable portion of the anterior segment of the right lobe. It lies in the lobar fissure and joins the left hepatic vein before emptying into the vena cava in about 80% of dissections (12). The left hepatic vein drains the lateral portion of the left lobe.

In addition to these three major branches, various smaller branches usually are found. These small veins empty into the inferior vena cava below the terminations of the major hepatic veins and drain the posterior superior margins of the right lobe, the caudate lobe, and circumscribed areas around the gall bladder. In about 50% of cadavers, there is a space of at least 1 cm between the vena cava and the first branches of the right hepatic vein (12). This is important in considering venous ligation.

Clinical correlations with hepatic venous anatomy are as follows: (a) The relative inaccessibility of the major hepatic veins makes control of bleeding after trauma difficult. (b) The major hepatic vein trunks must be avoided during hepatic resection in order to prevent major blood loss. (c) The short distance between the vena cava and the first branches of the hepatic veins makes it difficult to clamp and tie the venous trunks during hepatic surgery. (d) If there is thrombosis of the major hepatic venous trunks (Budd-Chiari syndrome), the portions of liver, including caudate lobe and the posterior portions of the right and left lobes, that contain small veins draining directly into the vena cava are not compromised and may undergo hypertrophy.

MICROCIRCULATION OF THE LIVER

The major inflow system, the portal vein, and the outflow system, the hepatic vein, are like large branching trees with their main trunks at a 90° angle (Fig. 2). The fine terminal branches of the two trees do not meet but are regularly interspersed. Each terminal twig is at the greatest possible distance from the twigs of the other tree, and the intervening space is filled with hepatic plates and sinusoids.

Portal Vein

Elias (13) has proposed a distinctive nomenclature for the finer intrahepatic branches of the portal vein. The major trunks ramify progressively to penetrate the liver substance. Veins with a diameter of more than 400 μm are called conducting veins; they are usually interlobular. Smaller veins are called distributing veins, either marginal or axial. Axial distributing veins have a diameter of less than 280 μm and occupy the axis of a portal canal. The distributing portal veins branch repeatedly into smaller terminal divisions that eventually become continuous with sinusoids. Preterminal portal branches lie in small triangular portal spaces and form the axis of complex acini. Terminal portal veins are seen in the smallest round or oval portal spaces and form the vascular axis for the simple acinus (14). The distributing veins connect with the sinusoidal bed by way of short, perpendicular inlet venules, which pierce through the limiting plate. According to Rappaport (15) and Knisely et al. (16), the inlet venules show sphincter-like activity, which regulates the admission of portal blood into the sinusoidal bed.

Hepatic Artery

Hepatic arteries run with the branches of the portal vein in the portal canals. One to five arteries of variable size may be seen within a portal space, anastomosing with one another. Burkel (17) recognizes four types of arteries according to size and wall structure: (a) arterioles, with a caliber of 50 to 100 μm and with two layers of smooth muscle cells; (b) terminal arterioles, 10 to 50 μm in diameter, with the media consisting of a single layer of smooth muscle cells; (c) precapillaries arising from the terminal arterioles in the larger portal spaces, which constitute a transitional vessel surrounded at their origin by cuffs of smooth muscle reportedly with sphincter activity (18); and (d) capillaries, less than 10 μm in diameter, forming a dense network of vessels ramifying throughout the portal space.

Hepatic arterioles and capillaries run along the limiting plate and emit short branches which penetrate it and enter peripheral sinusoids or go deeper into the parenchyma to reach radial sinusoids. The distribution of the terminal branches of the hepatic artery has been divided into (a) general plexus within the portal tract, (b) a special capillary plexus surrounding the bile ducts, and (c) the arterial capillaries emptying directly into the sinusoids (19). The general plexus supplies the structures within the portal tract other than the bile ducts, sending terminal branches into the radial and peripheral sinusoids (20). The peribiliary plexus plays an important role in secretion, absorption, and concentration of bile (21). Terminal branches from this plexus pass into the sinusoidal bed or join the terminal portal venules, forming the so-called "internal roots of the portal vein" (22).

Some authors maintain that terminal hepatic arterioles and capillaries traverse the hepatic parenchyma to join sinusoids in the central lobular area near the terminal hepatic venules (13,23). This concept has been contested by the observations of Rappaport et al. (24), McCuskey (25), Nakata and Kanbe (26), and Reeves, et al. (27), who deny the presence of anastomoses between arterioles and sinusoids in the center of the lobule (zone 3 of the Rappaport acinus). This controversy has not yet been settled. A recent study employing scanning electron microscopy of corrosion casts has shown branches of intralobular arterioles terminating in the vicinity of the central veins, suggesting that there may be anastomoses even in zone 3 of the acinus (28).

Sinusoids

Sinusoids of the liver are specialized capillaries with a remarkably discontinuous basement membrane, lined by Kupffer cells and endothelial cells. The endothelial cells are flat, lobulated, and fenestrated. They overlap loosely without being attached to one another. Their cytoplasm has fenestrae of 0.1 to 0.2 μm disposed in clusters termed sieve plates (Fig. 6). Larger fenestrations up to 2 μm in diameter are found near the portal end of the sinusoids. Because of these openings, sinusoids are fully permeable to substances, even of high molecular weight (up to 250,000). The marked porosity of the sinusoids is of great hemodynamic importance because the low sinusoidal pressure (estimated to be 2 to 3 mm Hg) would not otherwise be appropriate for a rapid perfusion of fluid into the space around the hepatocytes. Sinusoids are 7 to 15 μm wide; this width can increase up to 180 μm when needed. The change in sinusoidal caliber depends on contractile mechanisms not fully understood. According to Rap-

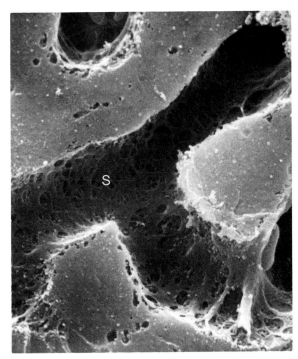 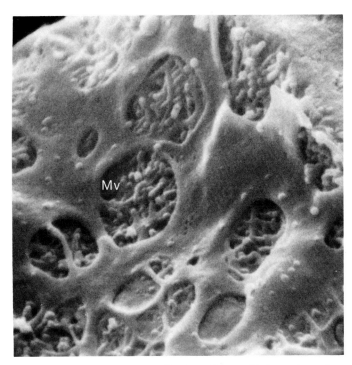

FIG. 6. Hepatic sinusoids. **Left:** These scanning electron micrographs of sinusoids (S) show the multiple and varying sized fenestrations in the endothelial lining cells (×3585). **Right:** Further enlargement (×12,725) shows the microvilli (Mv) of underlying hepatocytes readily exposed to the sinusoidal contents. (From ref. 135.)

paport (29), groups of sinusoids shift their work asynchronously, with the circulatory activity spreading simultaneously to those sectors adjacent to an active axial vessel.

Terminal Hepatic Venules

The majority of the sinusoids empty individually into the terminal hepatic venules (central veins). These venules are lined by a simple endothelium covered by an external adventitia. They have an average diameter of 45 μm. At the periphery of the lobule, the central vein connects at right angles with a sublobular or intercalated vein, which in turn empties through collecting hepatic veins of ever-increasing caliber to become large hepatic veins which drain into the inferior vena cava.

Sphincters: Fact or Fiction?

Hepatic vessels, both afferent and efferent, have a rich innervation, particularly of adrenergic fibers. The complex vascular structure inside the liver provides numerous possible sites for vasomotor mechanisms, which could modulate liver blood flow and its distribution (30,31). Hepatic arterioles may constrict along their entire length. Sphincters have been described at the bifurcation of the arterioles within the portal canals, at the level of the precapillaries, at the entrance of the arterial branches into the sinusoids, and into branches

of the portal vein (25). Sphincters also have been found at the inlet venules. With transillumination technique, using a modified binocular microscope and monochromatic light, McCuskey (25) recognized contractile structures consisting of endothelial cells located at the junction of sinusoids with portal venules (inlet sphincters) and with terminal hepatic veins (outlet sphincters). Finally, outflow sphincters have been reported where central veins join sublobular veins. These observations require further substantiation.

The Microcirculatory Unit

There is total merging of the high pressure hepatic arterial and low pressure portal streams within the sinusoidal bed of the microcirculatory unit. The functional unit of the liver is the simple acinus, consisting of a small parenchymal mass, irregular in size and shape, that is formed about a vascular axis consisting of a terminal portal venule and hepatic arteriole, a bile duct, lymph vessels, and nerves. The microcirculatory unit comprises the terminal portal vein, a glomus of sinusoids branching off it, and arterial capillaries which empty into the terminal portal vein and sinusoids. The glomus of sinusoids is drained by at least two terminal hepatic venules in the periphery of the acinus. Because of the 90° angle between the portal venous and hepatic venous trees, their terminal branches will be in different planes and will not be seen easily in the same microscopic section (Fig. 7). The spatial relationship between the terminal afferent and efferent

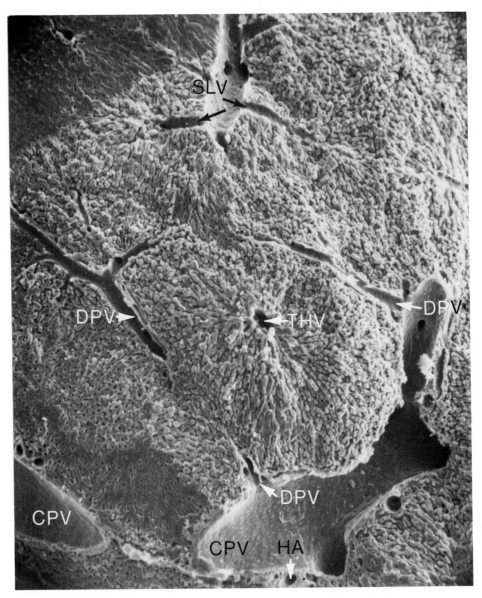

FIG. 7. This scanning electron micrograph (×130) shows the relationship between the terminal branches of the portal vein, distributing portal veins (DPV), and the terminal hepatic venule (THV). Note that they are in different planes. Also shown are conducting portal veins (CPV), hepatic artery branches (HA), and a sublobular hepatic vein (SLV) sectioned to illustrate its continuity (*arrows*) with terminal hepatic veins. (From ref. 135.)

vessels is illustrated in a diagram (Fig. 8) from Rappaport, who pointed out that the smallest hepatic vein branches are at the periphery of the hepatic acinus rather than at the center.

The prime mover and regulator of pressure and flow in these units is the hepatic arteriole (21). The hemodynamics of the hepatic microcirculation depend on the activity of smooth muscle cells around the arterioles and precapillary sphincters. To a lesser degree, the large endothelial cells at the entry and exit of the sinusoids and arterial capillaries, by the activity of the intracellular filaments, may act as the adjusting "microscrews" of the sinusoidal flow (29). Regulation of hepatic microcirculation occurs mainly via the ar-

terioles through nervous stimulation, hormones, metabolites, and bile salts.

PHYSIOLOGY OF THE HEPATIC CIRCULATION

The gastrointestinal and other visceral vascular beds are in a parallel configuration with all the venous blood draining into the portal vein, which provides the liver with 70 to 75% of its blood supply (32,33). The hepatic artery provides the remaining 25 to 30% of the blood supply of the human liver. The portal vein is a low pressure-low resistance circuit while the hepatic ar-

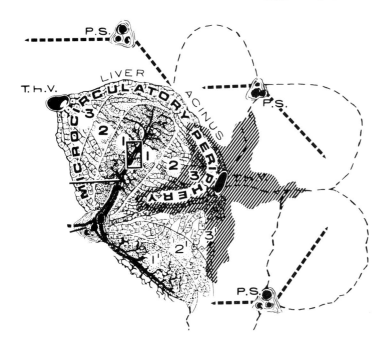

FIG. 8. Hepatic acinus. The terminal afferent vessels, hepatic arterioles, and distributing portal veins leave the larger portal spaces (PS) at right angles and distribute blood to adjacent sinusoids. Zones 1, 2, and 3, respectively, represent areas supplied with blood of first, second, and third quality with regard to oxygen and nutrient contents. Blood from each microcirculatory unit is collected by at least two terminal hepatic venules (ThV). The perivenular area is formed by the most peripheral portions of zone 3 of several adjacent acini. In injury progressing along this zone, the damaged area assumes the shape of a seastar. (From ref. 136).

tery supplies the liver with arterial blood in a high pressure-high resistance system (34).

Hepatic Blood Flow

Under normal resting conditions in man, indirect estimates of total hepatic blood flow showed it to be approximately 25% of cardiac output (35). Using the bromsulphalein (BSP) infusion method, hepatic blood flow ranges between 1,380 and 1,510 ml/min per 1.73 m^2, with a mean figure of 1,497 ml/1.73m^2 (36). When hepatic blood flow is expressed in terms of liver weight, it ranges from 100 to 130 ml/min/100 g liver in different species, such as humans, dogs, and cats (34,37). During daily activity, liver blood flow varies widely in amount. A cyclic pattern is related to respiration. Outflow of blood from the hepatic vein is maximum during expiration and decreases substantially with inspiration (38). This phenomenon has been ascribed to inspiratory increase of pressure on the suspending matrix of the liver vasculature by the diaphragm, causing the vasculature to partially collapse with an impediment to the outflow of splanchnic blood. Hepatic blood flow increases during expiration with relaxation of the diaphragm. The phasic character of hepatic blood flow with respiration is opposite to the phasic flow of blood from the lower portion of the body in the inferior vena cava. The result is a steady inflow of blood to the right atrium from the inferior vena cava. Assumption of the upright posture (35,39) or mild exercise in the decubitus position (39,40) is known to induce splanchnic vasoconstriction with reduction of hepatic blood flow. Food ingestion increases blood flow to the gut and resultant hepatic blood flow (41,42). During vigorous exercise, blood is shunted to the muscles and brain with reduction in hepatic blood flow (43).

Vascular Pressures

The mean pressure in the hepatic artery is similar to that in the aorta, while portal vein pressure ranges between 6 and 10 mm Hg. Both afferent systems merge at the sinusoidal bed, where the pressure is estimated to be from 2 to 4 mm Hg above inferior vena caval pressure. Direct measurement of sinusoidal pressure by the micropuncture technique has not yet been accomplished. Pressures in the major hepatic veins, obtained by retrograde catheterization, are only slightly higher than pressures in the inferior vena cava. Nakata et al. (44) have measured pressures directly in both portal venules and collecting hepatic veins by micropuncture in the transilluminated rat liver. Pressures fell from 130 mm H_2O in the portal vein to 65 mm H_2O in terminal portal venules and to 23 mm H_2O in the collecting tributaries of the hepatic veins. The mean sinusoidal pressure probably is only slightly greater than that in the smallest collecting veins.

Portal pressure depends primarily on the degree of constriction or dilatation of the mesenteric and splanchnic arterioles and on intrahepatic resistance. Normal hepatic arterial pressure is greatly reduced at the point where the arterioles join the sinusoidal bed and has little influence on portal pressures.

Hepatic Blood Volume

Estimations of hepatic blood volume are highly variable. Ordinarily, the liver contains 25 to 30 ml blood/

100 g, accounting for 10 to 15% of the total blood volume (45). It is unclear what proportion of blood is contained within the large versus small blood vessels; a rough estimation suggests that more than 40% of the hepatic blood is held in the large capacitance vessels (portal vein, hepatic veins, and hepatic artery) (34). Increases in central venous pressure are transmitted almost quantitatively back to the sinusoids; for 1 mm Hg rise in hepatic venous pressure, the intrahepatic blood volume may increase by as much as 4 ml/100 g. In cats during blood volume expansion with intravenous fluids, the liver accommodates approximately 20% of the infused volume (46). The compliance of the vascular bed, calculated as the change in blood volume per unit change in venous pressure, was seen to increase with rising distending pressures over the 0 to 9.4 mm Hg range (47). The volume increase is attributed to passive distention of the capacitance vessels with subsequent engorgement of the liver.

Hepatic blood volume may expand considerably in cardiac failure, up to as much as 60 ml/100 g liver (37). The liver also plays an important role as a blood reservoir during bleeding episodes. After a moderate blood loss with a drop in arterial blood pressure to 50 mm Hg, the capacitance vessels of the liver expel enough blood to compensate for 25% of the hemorrhage. The mechanism implicated in this massive response is not well established. Although several factors may be involved, a reflex regulation involving the atrial receptors and the sympathetic innervation of the large capacitance vessels likely is of predominant importance (46).

Hepatic Oxygen Consumption

Oxygen saturation in the hepatic artery is high, as in any other body artery. During the fasting state, portal blood has an oxygen saturation greater than that of systemic veins, ranging up to 85%. Oxygen content falls substantially after food ingestion. Hepatic venous oxygen content (fasting) averages 13 to 14 ml/dl; splanchnic oxygen consumption averages 42 ml/min/m^2 or about 25% of total oxygen consumption (48). In the fasting state, roughly one-half the oxygen supplied to the liver derives from the portal vein and one-half from the hepatic artery.

An interesting feature concerning oxygen delivery and consumption in the liver is the lack of subservience of hepatic blood flow to oxygen requirements of the liver (45). Under conditions of normal blood flow, oxygen extraction by the liver is less than 40% of the amount of oxygen supplied, and oxygen uptake is estimated at 4 to 6 ml/min/100 g liver (48). When liver blood flow or oxygen supply is reduced, hepatic oxygen uptake decreases but to a lesser amount than supply (49). Experimental evidence shows that oxygen extraction by the liver is potentially more efficient than most other tissues (50). In feline liver, oxygen uptake approaches oxygen supply as the latter is reduced either as a result of decreased blood oxygen content or decreased blood flow. The liver oxygen consumption is best described by the following characteristics: (a) The primary mechanism by which a rising oxygen requirement is met by the liver is through increased oxygen extraction. Neither vasodilatation nor increased blood flow is important. (b) Oxygen uptake remains fairly constant for any given oxygen supply, whether the blood flow to the liver arrives by way of the portal vein alone or the hepatic artery alone, or from both afferent vessels at the same time. This suggests that, in the feline liver, all areas have a mixed arterial and portal blood supply.

Autoregulation

Autoregulation is the tendency for local blood flow to remain constant in the face of pressure changes in the arteries perfusing a given organ. This seems to occur in all organs and tissues of the human body. The physiologic mechanism involved in autoregulation probably reflects the sum of effects due to either flow sensitivity or pressure sensitivity at the arteriolar level (51). The purpose of autoregulation is to maintain an adequate nutrient flow to the tissues. In denervated dog liver preparations, Hanson and Johnson (52) showed that a step-wise reduction of hepatic artery pressure from 90 to 30 mm Hg was accompanied by a substantial reduction in hepatic artery resistance. Blood flow was still detectable, in minimal amount, at a hepatic arterial pressure of 10 mm Hg. In another series of experiments in canine livers, Torrance (53), leaving the periarterial nerve plexus intact, studied the effect of gradual reduction of hepatic arterial pressure on hepatic arterial resistance. He found that a 63% pressure reduction was accompanied by a 60% decrease in arterial resistance. This response was abolished by *E. coli* endotoxin and by papaverine infusion, suggesting that the observed events were primarily mediated by a myogenic adaptation of the vasculature to changes in transmural pressure.

Pressure flow studies of the portal venous system do not show evidence of similar autoregulation; in fact, there is evidence for an opposite effect. Hanson and Johnson (52) observed that an 80% reduction of portal inflow in denervated dog liver was accompanied by a portal pressure fall from 6.2 to only 4.5 mm Hg, with a near doubling of intrahepatic portal venous resistance. This suggested that with the reduction of pressure, a partial passive collapse of the portal vascular bed was taking place. Also, a step-wise increase in portal venous pressure was accompanied by a reciprocal decrease in resistance until maximal vessel opening was observed.

Hepatic Artery–Portal Vein Interrelationships

The reciprocal response of the hepatic artery to reduction in portal venous perfusion has been thoroughly studied in man and other species (52,54,55). It has been shown in denervated canine livers that total diversion of portal inflow results in a 31% decrease in hepatic artery resistance and a 22% increase in inflow (54). Other authors have shown that critical reductions of portal inflow by ligation of the superior mesenteric artery or by portacaval shunt resulted in a 50 to 100% increase in hepatic arterial flow (32,56). Despite the significant increase in arterial inflow, total liver blood flow in these studies was always subnormal. As in the case of autoregulation, a myogenic mechanism is thought to be involved. Evidence supporting this theory is that papaverine, a potent vasodilator, obliterates this response to a great extent (55).

Hepatic arterial flow seems to have little influence on portal venous flow. There is no rise in portal inflow on occlusion of the hepatic artery; in fact, there is a tendency for reduction in portal venous flow (57).

Venous–Arteriolar Response

Elevation of venous pressure in some organs, such as the liver, evokes a definite constriction of the arterial bed. Current evidence indicates that this response takes place in the precapillary vessels and is related to intravascular pressure. Both precapillary sphincters and small arterioles constrict when venous pressure is increased (58). In the liver, a rise in hepatic venous pressure elicits hepatic arteriolar constriction. This effect reaches a maximum at venous pressures below 10 mm Hg. Hanson and Johnson (52) proposed a unifying hypothesis that links autoregulation, the hepatic venous arteriolar response, and the effect of portal venous perfusion on hepatic artery resistance. They postulate a common mechanism, the myogenic reaction to a rise in transmural pressure across the arteriolar wall.

METHODOLOGY FOR THE MEASUREMENT OF BLOOD FLOW AND PRESSURES IN THE SPLANCHNIC SYSTEM

Measurement of Hepatic Blood Flow

Bradley (59) has classified all techniques for measurement for hepatic blood flow into three broad categories: (a) techniques relying on hepatic clearance of a substance from the circulation, (b) techniques depending on indicator dilution methodology, and (c) a group of miscellaneous techniques applying a form of physical measurement. Some of these methods are direct, but the majority are indirect. Direct methods are highly accurate but have serious shortcomings because they are invasive procedures introducing extraneous effects on basal circulatory events. Indirect methods also have inherent limitations, such as inability to discriminate between portal vein and hepatic artery flow, and inability to respond to rapid alterations of flow rate.

Methods Relying on Hepatic Clearance

Hepatic clearance basically depends on two physiologic variables: hepatic blood flow and intrinsic efficiency of elimination mechanisms (60,61). Substances with a high intrinsic hepatic clearance, such as propranolol, lidocaine, indocyanine green, and colloidal particles, have a high hepatic extraction ratio; their hepatic clearance is limited by hepatic blood flow (62). Substances well suited for hepatic perfusion measurements should be eliminated by first order kinetics; i.e., the removal rate should be proportional to the blood level, and the fractional clearance (k) should be constant.

Constant infusion method.

The constant infusion method was introduced by Bradley et al. (36) in 1945, who employed BSP as the test substance. It is based on the indirect Fick principle involving the selective removal from blood of the dye by the hepatocytes. It requires hepatic vein catheterization and constant infusion of BSP. Since the uptake of BSP by the liver is not directly measured, this value is indirectly approached by varying the infusion rate to maintain a constant peripheral blood concentration of BSP. If the peripheral blood concentration of BSP is indeed constant, then hepatic uptake of the dye equals the infusion rate. Calculation of the hepatic blood flow is by the following formula:

$$HPF^* = \frac{B}{C_1 - C_0}$$

HPF, hepatic plasma flow/min; B, total amount of BSP removed by the liver/min; C_1, concentration of BSP (mg/dl) in blood plasma entering the liver; C_0, concentration of BSP (mg/dl) in blood plasma leaving the liver; *, convertible to total hepatic blood flow by correction with hematocrit.

This same principle has been applied to the estimation of hepatic blood flow by other materials dependent on hepatic extraction, such as indocyanine green and [131]I Rose Bengal. The validity of this method depends on the following assumptions: (a) the material is removed only by the liver and not by extrahepatic tissues; (b) a blood sample obtained from a single hepatic vein is representative of the total mixed hepatic venous outflow; (c) the concentration of the substance in the portal vein and hepatic artery is the same as in the peripheral circulation; and (d) the efficiency of hepatocyte clearance is not spontaneously variable.

BSP is inexpensive and easily measurable; however, it is partially (5 to 7%) extracted by extrahepatic tissues (63) and is excreted by the kidney in small amounts (64–66). Moreover, there is a certain amount of enterohepatic recirculation of the dye (67). In patients with liver disease, particularly those with jaundice, the hepatic extraction ratio of BSP can fall as low as 5 to 15%, in which case the calculations are unreliable (68).

Indocyanine green seems to be cleared from the plasma only by the liver. Enterohepatic recirculation is negligible, and the extraction ratio may still be adequate in patients with liver disease (69). Indocyanine green is expensive, however, and is quite unstable in aqueous solutions unless albumin is added. Nevertheless, most authorities regard the constant infusion of indocyanine green as the most reliable method available for measurement of hepatic blood flow (70).

Single injection method.

The single injection technique, which can be used with either BSP or indocyanine green, is based on the same concept of clearance and extraction ratio. It is somewhat less reliable than the constant infusion method but offers the advantage of performance in 15 to 20 min and a possibility for a sequential determination. Hepatic vein catheterization is required. The method is based on Lewis' concept of clearance (71,72). The substance used must be removed exponentially from plasma by the liver. The amount of material injected must be measured precisely, preferably by a gravimetric technique. Several pairs (minimum of three) of arterial and hepatic venous plasma samples are obtained during a 15-min period after allowing time for mixing for the injected material. Dye concentrations are plotted on semilogarithmic paper against time, and hepatic blood flow is calculated from the following formula:

$$HBF = \frac{k \times \text{blood volume}}{\text{hepatic extraction ratio}}$$

HBF = hepatic blood flow

$$k = \text{fractional clearance} \left(\frac{0.693}{T\frac{1}{2}} \right)$$

0.693 = log 2 (base n)

T½ = time in minutes for peripheral vein dye concentration to fall 50%

$$\text{plasma volume} = \frac{\text{amount of dye injected}}{\text{extrapolated zero time concentration of dye in peripheral venous plasma}}$$

$$\text{blood volume} = \text{plasma volume} \times \frac{1}{1 - \text{hematocrit}}$$

$$\begin{array}{c}\text{hepatic} \\ \text{extraction ratio}\end{array} = \frac{\text{peripheral vein} - \text{hepatic vein} \atop \text{dye concentration}}{\text{peripheral vein dye concentration}}$$

The single injection method becomes inaccurate when hepatic extraction ratio is small (less than 10%), when there is difficulty in constructing a straight line on semilogarithmic paper for either peripheral venous or hepatic venous dye concentrations, and when these lines are not parallel. This method correlates well with the constant infusion method (69). It has been shown to give falsely low values, in the range of -20 to -30%, following experimental hemorrhage and shock in dogs with intact livers (73,74).

Reticuloendothelial particle clearance.

To avoid dependence on adequate dye extraction by the hepatocytes in liver disease, Dobson and Jones (75) formulated a method of determining total hepatic blood flow using radioactive-tagged colloidal particles, which are removed by the reticuloendothelial cells. Approximately 90% of the reticuloendothelial cells in the body are found in the liver sinusoids. They may continue to function despite hepatocellular insufficiency, resulting in a relatively greater extraction efficiency in patients with liver disease. Several radioactive-tagged colloidal particles have been used, such as P^{32} chromic phosphate (76), heat-denatured I^{131} human serum albumin (77), Fe^{59}-labeled saccharate (78), radioactive gold colloid (79), Cr^{51}-labeled chromic phosphate (80), Tc-99m sulfur colloid (81), and I^{131}-labeled albumin microspheres. Hepatic blood flow is calculated by the same formula used for the single injection dye methods. The accuracy of this form of clearance methodology is dependent on several assumptions: (a) First order kinetics for removal of the colloidal particles must be followed. (b) Either all the marker must be removed on the first pass through the liver, or the extraction efficiency must be assessed by hepatic vein catheterization. (c) The number of particles must be small in relation to the number of binding sites in the liver. (d) The particulate material must be cleared from the blood only by the liver.

The major problem with this method is extrahepatic uptake of colloidal material by the bone marrow, which tends to raise the value for fractional clearance (k). Bone marrow uptake is relatively small in the normal human but increases substantially in chronic liver disease. Splenic uptake of colloid does not affect hepatic blood flow calculation in normal humans since the spleen is in series with the liver. In disease states where blood may be shunted from the splenic vein around the liver, however, the increased splenic uptake of colloid will artificially raise the value for k.

Attempts to simplify the particle clearance method by recording isotope accumulation of the liver externally or by simply recording the rate of decrease in blood isotope concentration without performing hepatic vein catheterization are clearly only approximations that can estimate "minimal hepatic blood flow" but cannot possibly estimate actual hepatic blood flow; hepatic extraction efficiency of the various colloids may decrease markedly in many liver diseases.

Indicator Dilution Methods

In 1958, Reichman et al. (82) first applied the Stewart-Hamilton principle to the volumetric determination of hepatic blood flow. This principle states that the volume of flow in a moving stream can be measured by the dilution of a known quantity of tracer over an accurately measured time period. The tracer is given as a bolus upstream, and its concentration is measured continuously as it passes a point downstream. The objective is a method that is independent of hepatic function, since the extraction techniques fail to give accurate measurement of hepatic blood flow in patients with severe liver disease. The application of dilution techniques rests on several basic assumptions: (a) the marker used is not metabolized by the liver; (b) all the material injected must traverse the liver; i.e., there must be no shunts between the injection site and the sampling site; (c) uniform mixing of the substance in blood at the site of injection is required; (d) the ratio of hepatic arterial to portal venous flow should remain constant in all parts of the liver during the observation period; and (e) the volume of blood contained within the liver should not change while the procedure is being performed.

The test substance can be injected into the spleen (82), the hepatic artery beyond the take-off of the gastroduodenal artery (83), or the splenic or superior mesenteric arteries (84). If the portal vein is catheterized by the transhepatic or umbilical route, then indicator can be injected into the portal vein at the hilum of the liver (85). Continuous sampling of indicator concentration is made from either hepatic vein. Comparison of the hepatic vein dilution curves after injection in various sites has been used to estimate collateral blood flow around the liver from the splenic

and superior mesenteric circulations (84). The markers employed in indicator dilution studies are radioactive substances such as I^{131}-labeled human serum albumin and Cr^{51}-labeled red blood cells. Several factors, such as recirculation, nonuniform mixing, and possibly pooling, make this method of uncertain reliability. Marked discrepancies between actual flow values and those determined by indicator dilution techniques have been noted in controlled model systems (86).

Miscellaneous Techniques

The Kety-Schmidt method has been adapted to the determination of hepatic blood flow (87). Intravenous administration of a rapidly diffusible substance establishes a constant equilibrium between blood and tissue concentration of the marker substance. Examples of marker substances used are the radioactive gases Xe^{133} (88) and Kr^{85} (89). After administration of the isotope ceases, its speed of removal from the liver can be determined by an external probe and is directly proportional to the blood flow. Various routes for administration of these radioactive gases have been used; stomach (90), rectum (91), spleen (92). Administration by the umbilical vein approach can be used for assessment of portal flow. One criticism of these techniques is that they measure flow only through capillary beds and should not detect blood flow through arteriovenous shunts (93).

The electromagnetic flowmeter is a highly accurate method for measuring flow in unopened blood vessels (94). Separate measurements of portal venous and hepatic arterial blood flow can be made. These devices can be employed for measuring blood flow in humans at surgery. The probes can be implanted and left *in situ* to be used later in the unanesthetized animal. The chief problem for human use is the requirement for direct application of the device on a blood vessel, which means anesthesia, surgical trauma, and the possibility of denervation of the perivascular plexus.

Recently, a velocity flowmeter has been incorporated into an angiographic catheter tip. This catheter can be introduced selectively into a blood vessel for the measurement of the velocity of flow (95). To calculate flow rate, the cross-sectional area of the vessel must be obtained from a simultaneous three-dimensional angiogram.

Another method for quantitation of blood flow is by injection of lipiodol droplets into the portal vein via the umbilical vein approach. The cross-sectional area of the portal vein is calculated from biplane fluoroscopy. This is multiplied by the velocity of flow determined by cineradiographic observation of the lipiodol droplets (96).

Approximate hepatic blood flow can be calculated

from pharmacokinetic data after simultaneous oral and intravenous administration of a drug that is completely absorbed and eliminated only by the liver. Propranolol is such a drug and can be given orally as unmodified drug and intravenously as [H³]-propranolol with determination of the "area under the curve (AUC)" for 8 hr subsequently for both propranolol and [H³]propranolol (62,97). The formula used for liver blood flow calculation is:

$$F = \frac{Do \cdot Div}{Do \ AUC_{IV}} - Div \ AUC_o$$

where F, hepatic blood flow; Do, oral dose; Div, IV dose; AUC_{IV}, area under the blood concentration/time curve of [H³]-propranolol; and AUC_o, area under the blood concentration/time curve of propranolol. If liver blood flow is measured directly by another method, such as indocyanine green clearance, then the fraction of liver blood flow that undergoes intrahepatic shunting can be estimated (62).

EFFECTS OF DRUGS AND HORMONES ON THE HEPATIC CIRCULATION

The hepatic circulation is influenced by a host of chemical substances and physical agents capable of exerting significant hemodynamic effects.

Catecholamines

Intravenous epinephrine causes a rapid rise in portal pressure. Typically, the pressure record is biphasic, with an initial rise, paralleled by a similar increase in hepatic arterial pressure, and a second peak occurring while the arterial pressure is falling. The initial pressure rise is ascribed to vasoconstriction of portal and hepatic venules, while the second peak may be attributed to increased flow into the portal vein via the mesenteric arteries (98).

Hepatic arterial and portal resistances show a significant increase after both epinephrine and norepinephrine (99–101). Total hepatic blood flow increases with epinephrine in cats (102), dogs (103), and man (104), with little change in hepatic arterial inflow. The increase in portal flow is caused by intestinal vasodilatation, with this phenomenon known to be blocked by propranolol administration. Epinephrine causes vasodilatation in the intestine, with an increase in portal pO_2, which may be an important mechanism for increasing the portal contribution to the oxygen supply of the liver (105). Phenylepinephrine and methoxamine produce similar effects on portal flow and portal pressure (106). In the isolated, perfused

liver, epinephrine causes a decrease in hepatic volume, whereas it produces an increase in intact dogs. The direct action of epinephrine is constriction of the capacitance vessels; in the intact animal, this effect is masked by a passive dilatation due to increased portal flow (105).

Beta-Adrenergic Agents

Systemic isoproterenol causes an increase in cardiac output and vasodilatation of the hepatic arterial bed which is blocked by propranolol (107,108). Intravenous isoproterenol increases portal flow by intestinal and splenic vasodilatation (109).

Histamine and Cimetidine

Histamine infusion induces vasodilatation of the hepatic arterial bed in dogs and cats (106). In dog liver preparations, it also produces a rise in portal pressure and a decrease in portal flow which is ascribed to a direct effect of the drug on the sphincters of the smaller hepatic veins. Experimental studies in dogs subjected to suprahepatic inferior vena cava constriction have shown that systemic or portal histamine administration increases the rate of ascites formation. These effects were abolished by antihistamine drugs (98). In dogs, Pawlik et al. (110) found mesenteric artery dilatation and increased flow with intravenous histamine; this was reduced by H_1- and H_2-receptor blockers. One report claims cimetidine caused a 30% fall in hepatic blood flow (111) but this conclusion is unwarranted from the data shown.

Serotonin

Serotonin infusion in dogs and man caused a small decrease in total liver blood flow. Both hepatic arterial and portal resistances were increased in isolated, perfused dog liver (112).

Dopamine

Intravenous dopamine induces somewhat different responses in dogs and cats. There is increased hepatic arterial resistance and decreased liver weight in the former (113) and increased mesenteric and decreased hepatic arterial and splenic flow in the latter species (114).

Angiotensin

Chiandussi et al. (115), infused angiotensin at a rate of 0.3 to 0.5 $\mu g/kg/min$ in man and observed a decrease of 17.5% in cardiac output and 26% in hepatic blood flow (measured by constant infusion of indocyanine green). Changes in portal pressure were not significant, while splanchnic resistance was found to increase more than 100%. Infusion of angiotensin in cirrhotic patients has been found to cause substantial increase in portal venous pressure along with reduction in splanchnic blood flow (116). This was ascribed to a direct hepatic venous effect. Both hepatic arterial and portal blood flow fell because of arterial vasoconstriction (117). Williams et al. (118), studied cardiac output and hepatic vein flow during angiotensin infusion in man. They found a rise in mean arterial pressure of about 30% and a fall in cardiac output and hepatic venous flow of about 30 to 35%.

Vasopressin

Vasopressin is the most potent known vasoconstrictor of the mesenteric vasculature. It causes a sustained decrease in portal pressure, portal flow, and total hepatic blood flow by vasoconstriction in the intestinal vascular bed. In dogs, primates, and cirrhotic humans, a fall in portal pressure is accompanied by a similar fall in splanchnic blood flow (119–122). There is usually a decrease in cardiac output during and after vasopressin infusion. It's biologic half-life ranges from approximately 15 min in the experimental animal to 24 min in man (123).

Kerr et al. (124) compared the effects of three routes of administration of vasopressin on blood flow through the hepatic and superior mesenteric artery in dogs. Their experiments confirmed and expanded previous observations, attesting to the following: (a) There was a marked reduction in hepatic arterial flow followed rapidly by autoregulatory escape when infused into either the hepatic artery or the portal vein. Systemic infusions of vasopressin produced no significant change in hepatic arterial blood flow. (b) Regardless of the route of administration, vasopressin caused identical diminution in superior mesenteric arterial blood flow, which did not show autoregulatory escape during infusion. (c) The effect of vasopressin on both arterial and portal venous pressure was similar, whether it was given into the hepatic artery, the portal vein, or a systemic vein.

Other Pharmacologic Agents

Several substances have been found to increase total hepatic blood flow by inducing hepatic arterial dilatation. These include acetylcholine (106), prostaglandin E_1 and E_2 (125), parathyroid hormone, and papaverine (106).

Somatostatin infusion has been shown to cause variable degrees of lowering of portal pressure in man (126,127), probably by reduction of splanchnic inflow. There was little or no effect on systemic hemodynamics.

In a recent study, propranolol lowered portal pressure in humans with portal hypertension, probably by decreasing cardiac output and splanchnic blood flow (128).

Foodstuffs and Gastrointestinal Hormones

A test meal rich in protein has been shown to cause a significant increase in hepatic blood flow and a rise in wedged hepatic vein pressure, in both normal volunteers (41) and cirrhotic patients (129). The increased liver blood flow is largely contributed to by the portal vein and is caused by mesenteric arterial vasodilatation. The mechanism for this response is the interplay of gastrointestinal hormones, digestive by-products, and other chemical substances released into the general circulation. Experimental studies in dogs have shown that systemic infusion of amino acids and fructose induced dilatation of both hepatic arterial and portal vasculature, with an increase in liver blood flow (130,131). Proteins were more effective than carbohydrates; lipid infusions caused minimal hemodynamic changes. Amino acid solutions caused a proportionately greater increase in portal than hepatic arterial blood flow; the dose response curves showed a sigmoid configuration, with a rate change at 0.5 ml/kg/min and a saturation above 1 ml/kg/min.

The enterohepatic circulation of bile salts seems to affect the hepatic circulation, since sodium dehydrocholate is known to cause an increase in portal and hepatic arterial blood flow (132). Some gastrointestinal hormones are known to cause vasodilatation in the mesenteric circulation; pentagastrin, secretin, and cholecystokinin given intravenously in dogs caused mild to moderate increases in portal vein flow (133). Only pentagastrin produced a measurable increase in hepatic artery flow. Vasointestinal peptide caused a substantial increase in both hepatic arterial and portal inflow, but the doses administered in these experiments exceeded the known physiologic ranges. Glucagon (10 mg/kg i.v.) in dogs caused a 90% increase in portal vein flow and a 70% increase in portal pressure (134). Hepatic artery flow increased only transiently. This was followed by a decreased flow, with pressure changing inversely. Insulin, given in sufficient amount to produce hypoglycemia, caused a delayed increase in hepatic blood flow, probably secondary to the release of epinephrine induced by the hypoglycemia.

REFERENCES

1. Gilfillan, R. S. (1950): Anatomic study of the portal vein and its main branches. *Arch. Surg.,* 61:449–461.
2. Gupta, S. C., Gupta, C. D., and Arora, A. K. (1977): Intrahepatic branching patterns of portal vein. A study by corrosion cast. *Gastroenterology,* 72:621–624.
3. Toni, G., Testoni, P. P., Trombetta, N., and Favero, A. (1959): LeZone Epatiche. Instituto di Anatomia Umana Trieste. [Mentioned by Sedgwick, C. E., and Poulantzas, J. K.: *Portal Hypertension.* Little, Brown, Boston.]
4. Healey, J. E., Jr. (1970): Vascular anatomy of the liver. *Ann. N.Y. Acad. Sci.,* 170:8–17.
5. Lam, K. C., Juttner, H. U., and Reynolds, T. B. (1981): Spontaneous portosystemic shunt: Relationship to spontaneous encephalopathy and gastrointestinal hemorrhage. *Dig. Dis. Sci.,* 26:346–352.
6. Michels, N. A. (1966): Newer anatomy of the liver and its variant blood supply and collateral circulation. *Am. J. Surg.,* 112:337–347.
7. Healey, J. E., Jr. (1954): Clinical anatomic aspects of radical hepatic surgery. *J. Intern. Coll. Surgeons,* 22:542–550.
8. Healey, J. E., Jr., Schroy, P. C., and Sorensen, R. J. (1953): The intrahepatic distribution of the hepatic artery in man. *J. Int. Coll. Surgeons,* 20:133–148.
9. Eckhauser, F. E., Strodel, W. E., Thompson, N. W., and Turcotte, J. G. (1980): Technical dilemmas in portacaval shunt operations as a consequence of replaced hepatic artery. *Surg. Gynecol. Obstet.,* 151:533–537.
10. Rappaport, A. M. (1975): Anatomic considerations. In: *Diseases of the Liver,* fourth edition, edited by L. Schiff, pp. 1–50. Lippincott, Philadelphia.
11. Elias, H., and Sherrick, J. C. (1969): *Morphology of the Liver.* Academic Press, New York.
12. Nakamura, S., and Tsuzuki, T. (1981): Surgical anatomy of the hepatic veins and the inferior vena cava. *Surg. Gynecol. Obstet.,* 152:43–50.
13. Elias, H. (1949): A re-examination of the structure of the mammalian liver; the hepatic lobule and its relation to the vascular and biliary systems. *Am. J. Anat.,* 85:379–456.
14. Rappaport, A. M., Borowy, Z. J., Lougheed, W. M., and Lotto, W. N. (1954): Subdivision of hexagonal liver lobules into a structural and functional unit. Role in hepatic physiology and pathology. *Anat. Rec.,* 119:11–33.
15. Rappaport, A. M. (1973): The microcirculatory hepatic unit. *Microvasc. Res.,* 6:212–228.
16. Knisely, M. H., Bloch, E. H., and Warner, L. (1948): Selective phagocytosis 1. Microscopic observations concerning the regulation of blood flow through the liver and other organs and the mechanism and rate of phagocytic removal of particles from the blood. *Det. Kongelige Danske Videnskabernes Selskab. Biol. Skrifter.,* 4:1–93. [Quoted in Bloch, E. H. (1970): The termination of hepatic arterioles and the functional unit of the liver as determined by microscopy of the living organ. *Ann. N.Y. Acad. Sci.,* 170:78–87.]
17. Burkel, W. E. (1970): The fine structure of the terminal branches of the hepatic arterial system of the rat. *Anat. Rec.,* 167:329–349.
18. Rhodin, J. A. (1967): The ultrastructure of mammalian arterioles and precapillary sphincters. *J. Ultrastruct. Res.,* 18:181–223.
19. Hale, A. J. (1951): The minute structure of the liver. A review. *Glasgow Med. J.,* 32:283–301.
20. Olds, J. M., and Stafford, E. S. (1930): On the manner of anastomosis of hepatic and portal circulation. *Bull. Johns Hopkins Hosp.,* 47:176–185.
21. Rappaport, A. M., and Schneiderman, J. H. (1976): The function of the hepatic artery. *Rev. Physiol. Biochem. Pharmacol.,* 76:129–175.
22. Andrews, W. H. H., Maegraith, B. G., and Wenyon, C. E. M. (1949): Studies on the liver circulation. II. The micro-anatomy of the hepatic circulation. *Ann. Trop. Med. Parasitol.,* 43:229–237.
23. Wakim, K. G., and Mann, F. C. (1942): The intrahepatic circulation of blood. *Anat. Rec.,* 82:233–253.
24. Rappaport, A. M., Black, R. G., Lucas, C. C., Ridout, J. H., and Best, C. H. (1966): Normal and pathologic microcirculation of the living mammalian liver. *Rev. Int. Hepat.,* 16:813–828.
25. McCuskey, R. S. (1966): A dynamic and static study of hepatic arterioles and hepatic sphincters. *Am. J. Anat.,* 119:455–478.
26. Nakata, K., and Kanbe, A. (1966): The terminal distribution of the hepatic artery and its relationship to the development of focal liver necrosis following interruption of the portal blood supply. *Acta Pathol. Jpn.,* 16:313–321.
27. Reeves, J. T., Leathers, J. E., and Boatright, C. (1966): I. Microradiography of the rabbit's hepatic microcirculation. The similarity of the hepatic portal and pulmonary arterial circulations. *Anat. Rec.,* 154:103–119.
28. Kardon, R. H., and Kessel, R. G. (1980): Three dimensional organization of the hepatic microcirculation in the rodent as observed by scanning electron microscopy of corrosive casts. *Gastroenterology,* 79:72–81.
29. Rappaport, A. M. (1980): Hepatic blood flow: morphologic aspects and physiologic regulation. *Int. Rev. Physiol.,* 21:1–63.
30. Knisely, M. H., Harding, F., and Debacker, H. (1957): Hepatic sphincters; brief summary of present-day knowledge. *Science,* 125:1023–1026.
31. McCuskey, R. S. (1971): Sphincters in the microvascular system. *Microvasc. Res.,* 3:428–433.
32. Schenk, W. G., Jr., McDonald, J. C., McDonald, K., and Drapanas, T. (1962): Direct measurement of hepatic blood flow in surgical patients: with related observations on hepatic flow dynamics in experimental animals. *Ann. Surg.,* 156:463–471.
33. Chiandussi, L., Greco, F., Sardi, G., Vaccarino, A., Ferraris, C. M., and Curti, B. (1968): Estimation of hepatic arterial and portal venous blood flow by direct catheterization of the vena porta through the umbilical cord in man. Preliminary results. *Acta Hepatosplenol.* (*Stuttg.*), 15:166–171.
34. Greenway, C. V., and Stark, R. D. (1971): Hepatic vascular bed. *Physiol. Rev.,* 51:23–65.
35. Bradley, S. E. (1949): Variations in hepatic blood flow in man during health and disease. *N. Engl. J. Med.,* 240:456–461.
36. Bradley, S. E., Ingelfinger, F. J., Bradley, G. P., and Curry, J. J. (1945): The estimation of hepatic blood flow in man. *J. Clin. Invest.,* 24:890–897.
37. Hanson, K. M. (1978): Liver. In: *Peripheral Circulation,* edited by P. C. Johnson, pp. 285–314. Wiley, New York.
38. Moreno, A. H., Burchell, A. R., Van der Woude, R., and Burke, J. H. (1967): Respiratory regulation of splanchnic and systemic venous return. *Am. J. Physiol.,* 213:455–465.
39. Wade, O. L., and Bishop, J. M. (1962): *Cardiac Output and Regional Blood Flow.* Blackwell, Oxford.
40. Burns, G. P., and Schenk, W. G., Jr. (1969): Effect of digestion and exercise on intestinal blood flow and cardiac output. An experimental study in the conscious dog. *Arch. Surg.,* 98:790–794.
41. Orrego, H., Mena, I., Baraona, E., and Palma, R. (1965): Modifications in hepatic blood flow and portal pressure produced by different diets. *Am. J. Dig. Dis.,* 10:239–248.
42. Shoemaker, W. C., Yanof, H. M., Turk, L. N., III, and Wilson, T. H. (1963): Glucose and fructose absorption in the unanesthetized dog. *Gastroenterology,* 44:654–663.
43. Wade, O. L., Combes, B., Childs, A. W., Wheeler, H. O., Cournand, A., and Bradley, S. E. (1956): The effect of exercise on the splanchnic blood flow and splanchnic blood volume in normal man. *Clin. Sci.,* 15:457–463.
44. Nakata, K., Leong, G. F., and Brauer, R. W. (1960): Direct measurement of blood pressures in minute vessels of the liver. *Am. J. Physiol.,* 199:1181–1188.

45. Lautt, W. W. (1977): Hepatic vasculature: a conceptual review. *Gastroenterology*, 73:1163–1169.
46. Greenway, C. V., and Lister, G. E. (1974): Capacitance effects and blood reservoir function in the splanchnic vascular bed during non-hypotensive haemorrhage and blood volume expansion in anesthetized cats. *J. Physiol. (Lond.)*, 237:279–294.
47. Lautt, W. W., and Greenway, C. V. (1976): Hepatic venous compliance and role of liver as a blood reservoir. *Am. J. Physiol.*, 231:292–295.
48. Myers, J. D. (1947): The hepatic blood flow and splanchnic oxygen consumption of man—their estimation from urea production or bromsulphalein excretion during catheterization of the hepatic veins. *J. Clin. Invest.*, 26:1130–1137.
49. Lutz, J., Henrich, H., and Bauereisene, E. (1975): Oxygen supply and uptake in the liver and the intestine. *Pfluegers Arch.*, 360:7–15.
50. Lutz, J., Decke, B., Bäuml, M., and Schulze, H. G. (1978): High oxygen extraction with extensive oxygen consumption in the rat liver perfused with Fluosal-DA a new perfluoro compound emulsion. *Pflüegers Arch.*, 376:1–6.
51. Johnson, P. C., and Hanson, K. M. (1966): Capillary filtration in the small intestine of the dog. *Circ. Res.*, 19:766–773.
52. Hanson, K. M., and Johnson, P. C. (1966): Local control of hepatic arterial and portal venous flow in the dog. *Am. J. Physiol.*, 211:712–720.
53. Torrance, H. B. (1961): The control of the hepatic arterial circulation. *J. Physiol. (Lond.)*, 158:39–49.
54. Greenway, C. V., and Oshiro, G. (1972): Intrahepatic distribution of portal and hepatic arterial blood flows in anesthetized cats and dogs and the effects of portal occlusion, raised venous pressure and histamine. *J. Physiol. (Lond.)*, 227:473–485.
55. Hanson, K. M. (1973): Dilator responses of the canine hepatic vasculature. *Angiologica*, 10:15–23.
56. Kock, N. G., Hahnloser, P., Roding, B., and Schenk, W. G., Jr. (1972): Interaction between portal venous and hepatic arterial blood flow: an experimental study in the dog. *Surgery*, 72:414–419.
57. Ternberg, J. L., and Butcher, H. R., Jr. (1965): Blood flow relation between hepatic artery and portal vein. *Science*, 150:1030–1031.
58. Baez, S., Laidlaw, Z., and Orkin, L. R. (1974): Localization and measurement of microvascular and microcirculatory responses to venous pressure elevation in the rat. *Blood Vessels*, 11:260–276.
59. Bradley, E. L., III (1974): Measurement of hepatic blood flow in man. *Surgery*, 75:783–789.
60. Perrier, D., and Gibaldi, M. (1974): Clearance and biologic half-life as indices of intrinsic hepatic metabolism. *J. Pharmacol. Exp. Ther.*, 191:17–24.
61. Rowland, M., Benet, L. Z., and Graham, G. G. (1973): Clearance concepts in pharmacokinetics. *J. Pharmacokinet. Biopharm.*, 1:123–136.
62. McLean, A., du Souich, P., and Gibaldi, M. (1979): Noninvasive kinetic approach to the estimation of total hepatic blood flow and shunting in chronic liver disease—a hypothesis. *Clin. Pharmacol. Ther.*, 25:161–166.
63. Bradley, S. E. (1950): Clinical aspects of hepatic vascular physiology. In: *Liver Injury*, edited by F. W. Hoffbauer, pp. 71–81. Josiah Macy Jr. Foundation, New York.
64. Pratt, E. B., Burdick, F. D., and Holmes, J. H. (1952): Measurement of liver blood flow in unanesthetized dog using bromsulfalein dye method. *Am. J. Physiol.*, 171:471–478.
65. Winkler, K. (1961): Urinary elimination of bromsulfalein in man. *Scand. J. Clin. Lab. Invest.*, 13:44–49.
66. Leevy, C. M., Bender, J., Silverberg, M., and Naylor, J. (1963): Physiology of dye extraction by the liver: comparative studies of sulfobromophthalein and indocyanine green. *Ann. N.Y. Acad. Sci.*, III:161–175.
67. Lorber, S. H., Oppenheimer, M. J., Shay, H., Lynch, P., and Siplet, H. (1953): Enterohepatic circulation of bromsulphalein: Intraduodenal, intraportal and intravenous dye administration in dogs. *Am. J. Physiol.*, 173:259–264.
68. Chiandussi, L. (1972): Clinical techniques for the evaluation of changes induced by drugs in hepatic circulation. In: *Liver and Drugs*, edited by F. Orlandi and A. M. Jezequel, pp. 129–144. Academic Press, London.
69. Caesar, J., Shaldon, S., Chiandussi, L., Guevara, L., and Sherlock, S. (1961): The use of indocyanine green in the measurement of hepatic blood flow and as a test of hepatic function. *Clin. Sci.*, 21:43–57.
70. Winkler, K., Larsen, J. A., Munkner, T., and Tygstrup, N. (1965): Determination of the hepatic blood flow in man by simultaneous use of five test substances measured in two parts of the liver. *Scand. J. Clin. Lab. Invest.*, 17:423–432.
71. Lewis, A. E. (1948): The concept of hepatic clearance. *Am. J. Clin. Pathol.*, 18:789–795.
72. Agrest, A., Aramendia, P., and Roncoroni, A. J. (1957): A single injection method for estimation of splanchnic blood-flow with B.S.P. *Acta Physiol. Lat. Am.*, 7:212–218.
73. Teranaka, M., and Schenk, W. G., Jr. (1977): Hepatic blood flow measurement. A comparison of indocyanine green and electromagnetic techniques in normal and abnormal states in the dog. *Ann. Surg.*, 185:58–63.
74. Nxumalo, J. L., Teranaka, M., and Schenk, W. G., Jr. (1978): Total hepatic blood flow measured by ICG clearance and electromagnetic flowmeters in a canine septic shock model. *Ann. Surg.*, 187:299–302.
75. Dobson, E. L., and Jones, H. B. (1952): The behaviour of intravenously injected particulate matter: its rate of disappearance from the blood stream as a measure of liver blood flow. *Acta Med. Scand. [Suppl. 273]*, 144:1–71.
76. Dobson, E. L., Warner, G. F., Finney, C. R., and Johnston, M. E. (1953): The measurement of liver circulation by means of the colloid disappearance rate. I. Liver blood flow in normal young men. *Circulation*, 7:690–695.
77. Shaldon, S., Chiandussi, L., Guevara, L., Caesar, J., and Sherlock, S. (1961): The estimation of hepatic blood flow and intrahepatic shunted blood flow by colloidal heat-denatured human serum albumin labeled with I^{131}. *J. Clin. Invest.*, 40:1346–1354.
78. Fellinger, K., Gisinger, E., and Vetter, H. (1956): Der stoffwechsel Fe 59-markierten kolloidalen eisensaccharates beim menschen. In: *Radioaktive Isotope in Klinik und Forchung, Vol. II*, edited by K. Fellinger and H. Vetter, p. 13. Urban and Schwarzenberg, München. [Quoted in Christie, J. H., and Chaudhuri, T. K. (1972): Measurement of hepatic blood flow. *Semin. Nucl. Med.*, 2:97–107.]
79. Vetter, H., Grabner, G., Hofer, R., Neumayr, A., and Parzer, O. (1956): Comparison of liver blood flow values estimated by the bromsulphalein and by the radiogold method. *J. Clin. Invest.*, 35:825–830.
80. Schapiro, R. L., MacIntyre, W. J., and Schapiro, D. I. (1966): The effect of homologous and heterologous carries on the clearance of colloidal material by the reticuloendothelial system. *J. Lab. Clin. Med.*, 68:286–299.
81. Mundschenk, H., Hromec, A., and Fischer, J. (1971): Phagocytic activity of the liver as a measure of hepatic circulation—A comparative study using ^{198}Au and ^{99m}Tc-sulfur colloid. *J. Nucl. Med.*, 12:711–718.
82. Reichman, S., Davis, W. D., Storaasli, J. P., and Gorlin, R. (1958): Measurement of hepatic blood flow by indicator dilution techniques. *J. Clin. Invest.*, 37:1848–1856.
83. Cohn, J. N., Khatri, I. M., Groszmann, R. J., and Kotelanski, B. (1972): Hepatic blood flow in alcoholic liver disease measured by an indicator dilution technic. *Am. J. Med.*, 53:704–714.
84. Groszmann, R., Kotelanski, B., Cohn, J. N., and Khatri, I. M. (1972): Quantitation of portasystemic shunting from the splenic and mesenteric beds in alcohol liver disease. *Am. J. Med.*, 53:715–722.

85. Huet, P-M, Lavoie, P., and Viallet, A. (1973): Simultaneous estimation of hepatic and portal blood flows by an indicator dilution technique. *J. Lab. Clin. Med.*, 82:836–846.

86. Jacobs, R. R., Schmitz, U., Heyden, W. C., Roding, B., and Schenk, W. G., Jr. (1968): A comparison of the accuracies of the electromagnetic flowmeter and the cardio-green dye dilution blood flow measurement techniques in a model. *Surg. Forum*, 19:113–117.

87. Thompson, A. M., Cavert, H. M., Lifson, N., and Evans, R. L. (1959): Regional tissue uptake of D_2O in perfused organs: Rat liver, dog heart and gastrocnemius. *Am. J. Physiol.*, 197:897–902.

88. Darle, N. (1970): Xenon[133] clearance and liver blood flow. An experimental study in the cat. *Acta Chir. Scand.* [Suppl.], 407:1–64.

89. Leiberman, D. P., Mathie, R. T., Harper, A. M., and Blumgart, L. H. (1978): Measurement of liver blood flow in the dog using Krypton-85 clearance: A comparison with electromagnetic flowmeter measurements. *J. Surg. Res.* 25:147–153. 25:147–153.

90. Stone, R. M., Ten Hove, W., Effros, R., and Leevy, C. M. (1972): Portal venous blood flow: Its estimation and significance. *Gastroenterology*, 62:186 (Abstr.).

91. Castell, D. O., Grace, N. D., Wennar, M. H., Chalmers, T. C., and Moore, E. W. (1969): Evaluation of portal circulation in hepatic cirrhosis: A new method using Xenon. *Gastroenterology*, 57:533–541.

92. Lombardo, C. R., Long, R. T., Braunwald, E., and Morrow, A. G. (1960): The measurement of portal-systemic circulation time: A new method of detecting esophageal varices and determining the patency of a portacaval anastomosis. *Surg. Forum*, 10:275–277.

93. Williams, R., Condon, R. E., Williams, H. S., Blendis, L. M., and Kreel, L. (1968): Splenic blood flow in cirrhosis and portal hypertension. *Clin. Sci.*, 34:441–452.

94. Denison, A. B., Jr., Spencer, M. P., and Green, H. D. (1955): A square wave electromagnetic flowmeter for application to intact blood vessels. *Circ. Res.*, 3:39–46.

95. Kolin, A., Archer, J. D., and Ross, G. (1967): An electromagnetic catheter-flow meter. *Circ. Res.*, 21:889–899.

96. Sovak, M., Soulen, R. L., and Reichle, F. A. (1971): Blood flow in the human portal vein. A cineradiographic method using particulate contrast medium. *Radiology*, 99:531–536.

97. Kornhauser, D. M., Wood, A. J. J., Vestal, R. E., Wilkinson, G. R., Branch, R. A., and Shand, D. G. (1978): Biological determinants of propranolol disposition in man. *Clin. Pharmacol. Ther.*, 23:165–174.

98. Schwartz, S. I. (1970): Influence of vasoactive drugs on portal circulation. *Ann. N.Y. Acad. Sci.*, 170:296–314.

99. Andrews, W. H. H., Hecker, R., and Maegraith, B. G. (1956): The action of adrenaline, noradrenaline, acetylcholine and histamine on the perfused liver by the monkey, cat and rabbit. *J. Physiol. (Lond.)*, 132:509–521.

100. Mahfouz, M., and Geumei, A. (1967): Pharmacodynamic of intrahepatic circulation in shock. *Surgery*, 61:755–762.

101. Shoemaker, W. C., Szanto, P. B., Fitch, L. B., and Brill, N. R. (1964): Hepatic physiologic and morphologic alterations in hemorrhagic shock. *Surg. Gynecol. Obstet.*, 118:828–836.

102. Greenway, C. V., and Lawson, A. E. (1966): The effects of adrenaline and noradrenaline on venous return and regional blood flows on the anesthetized cat with special reference to intestinal blood flow. *J. Physiol. (Lond.)*, 186:579–595.

103. Shoemaker, W. C., Turk, L. N., III, and Moore, F. D. (1961): Hepatic vascular response to epinephrine. *Am. J. Physiol.*, 201:58–62.

104. Bearn, A. G., Billing, B., and Sherlock, S. (1951): The effect of adrenaline and noradrenaline on hepatic blood flow and splanchnic carbohydrate metabolism in man. *J. Physiol. (Lond.)*, 115:430–441.

105. Greenway, C. V., and Stark, D. D. (1970): The vascular responses of the spleen to intravenous infusions of catecholamines, angiotensin and vasopressin in the anesthetized cat. *Br. J. Pharmacol.*, 38:583–592.

106. Greenway, C. V., and Stark, R. D. (1971): Hepatic vascular bed. *Physiol. Rev.*, 51:23–65.

107. Geumei, A., and Mahfouz, M. (1968): The presence of β-adrenergic receptors in the hepatic vasculature. *Br. J. Pharmacol. Chemother.*, 32:466–472.

108. Greenway, C. V., and Lawson, A. E. (1968): Effect of adrenaline and propranolol in the superior mesenteric artery blood flow. *Can. J. Physiol. Pharmacol.*, 46:906–908.

109. Greenway, C. V., and Lawson, A. E. (1969): β-Adrenergic receptors in the hepatic arterial bed of the anesthetized cat. *Can. J. Physiol. Pharmacol.*, 47:415–419.

110. Pawlik, W., Tague, L. L., Tepperman, B. L., Miller, T. A., and Jacobson, E. D. (1977): Histamine H_1- and H_2-receptor vasodilation of canine intestinal circulation. *Am. J. Physiol.*, 233:E219–224.

111. Feely, J., Wilkinson, G. R., and Wood, A. J. J. (1981): Reduction of liver blood flow and propranolol metabolism by cimetidine. *N. Engl. J. Med.*, 304:692–695.

112. Andrews, W. H. H., and Butterworth, K. R. (1958): The vascular action of 5-hydroxytryptamine on the canine liver. *J. Physiol. (Lond.)*, 141:38P.

113. Shanbour, L. L., and Hinshaw, L. B. (1969): Effects of dopamine on the liver before and following administration of endotoxin. *Can. J. Physiol. Pharmacol.*, 47:923–928.

114. Ross, G., and Brown, A. W. (1967): Cardiovascular effects of dopamine in the anesthetized cat. *Am. J. Physiol.*, 212:823–828.

115. Chiandussi, L., Vaccarino, A., Greco, F., Muratori, F., and Cesano, D. I. (1963): Effect of drug infusion on the splanchnic circulation. I. Angiotensin infusion in normal and cirrhotic subjects. *Proc. Soc. Exp. Biol. Med.*, 112:324–326.

116. Segel, N., Bayley, T. J., Paton, A., Dykes, P. W., and Bishop, J. M. (1963): The effects of synthetic vasopressin and angiotensin on the circulation in cirrhosis of the liver. *Clin. Sci.*, 25:43–55.

117. Cohen, M. M., Sitar, D. S., McNeill, J. R., and Greenway, C. V. (1970): Vasopressin and angiotensin on resistance vessels of spleen, intestine and liver. *Am. J. Physiol.*, 218:1704–1706.

118. Williams, S. R., Zimmon, D. S., Thompson, E., and Sherlock, S. (1964): The estimation of segmental hepatic venous flow in man. *Gastroenterology*, 46:525–530.

119. Shaldon, S., Dolle, W., Guevara, L., Iber, F. L., and Sherlock, S. (1961): Effect of pitressin on the splanchnic circulation in man. *Circulation*, 24:797–807.

120. Millette, B., Huet, P-M, Lavoie, P., and Viallet, A. (1975): Portal and systemic effects of selective infusion of vasopressin into the superior mesenteric artery in cirrhotic patients. *Gastroenterology*, 69:6–12.

121. Barr, J. W., Lakin, R. C., and Rösch, J. (1975): Similarity of arterial and intravenous vasopressin on portal and systemic hemodynamics. *Gastroenterology*, 69:13–19.

122. Freedman, A. R., Kerr, J. C., Swan, K. G., and Hobson, R. W., II (1978): Primate mesenteric blood flow: effects of vasopressin and its route of delivery. *Gastroenterology*, 74:875–878.

123. Bauman, G., and Dingman, J. F. (1976): Distribution, blood transport and degradation of antidiuretic hormone in man. *J. Clin. Invest.*, 157:1109–1116.

124. Kerr, J. C., Hobson, R. W., II, Seelig, R. F., and Swan, K. G. (1978): Vasopressin: route of administration and effects on canine hepatic and superior mesenteric arterial blood flow. *Ann. Surg.*, 187:137–142.

125. Hanson, K. M., and Post, J. A. (1976): Splanchnic vascular responses to the infusion of prostaglandins A_1, A_2 and B_1. *Pharmacology*, 14:166–181.

126. Bosch, J., Kravetz, D., and Rodes, J. (1981): Effects of somatostatin on hepatic and systemic hemodynamics in patients with cirrhosis of the liver: Comparison with vasopressin. *Gastroenterology*, 80:518–525.

127. Sonnenberg, G. E., Keller, U., Perruchoud, A., Burckhardt, D., and Gyr, K. (1981): Effect of somatostatin on splanchnic

hemodynamics in patients with cirrhosis of the liver and in normal subjects. *Gastroenterology,* 80:526–532.

128. Lebrec, D., Nouel, O., Corbic, M., and Benhamou, J-P (1980): Propranolol—a medical treatment for portal hypertension? *Lancet,* 2:180–182.

129. Brandt, J. L., Castleman, L., Ruskin, H. D., Greenwald, J., Kelly, J. J., Jr., and Jones, A. (1955): The effect of oral protein and glucose feeding on splanchnic blood flow and oxygen utilization in normal and cirrhotic subjects. *J. Clin. Invest.,* 34:1017–1025.

130. Hallberg, D., and Soda, M. (1974): Hepatic blood flow and portal vein pressure during intravenous infusions of amino acids in dogs. *Acta Chir. Scand.,* 140:232–233.

131. Hallberg, D., and Soda, M. (1974): Effects of various parenteral nutritional solutions on hepatic blood flow in dogs. *Acta Chir. Scand.,* 140:226–231.

132. Mitchell, G. G., and Torrance, H. B. (1966): The effects of a bile-salt sodium dehydrocholate upon liver blood-flow in man. *Br. J. Surg.,* 53:807–808.

133. Post, J. A., and Hanson, K. M. (1975): Hepatic, vascular and biliary responses to infusion of gastrointestinal hormones and bile salts. *Digestion,* 12:65–77.

134. Kock, N. G., Roding, B., Hahnloser, P., Tibbon, S., and Schenk, W. G., Jr. (1970): The effect of glucagon on hepatic blood flow. An experimental study in the dog. *Arch. Surg.,* 100:147–149.

135. Kessel, R., and Hardon, R. H. (1979): *Tissues and Organs: A Text–Atlas of Scanning Electron Microscopy.* W H Freeman and Co.

136. Rappaport, A. M. (1975): Liver architecture and microcirculation. In: *Alcoholic Liver Pathology,* edited by Khanna, Israel, and Kalant. Addiction Research Foundation, Toronto, Ontario.

The Liver: Biology and Pathobiology, edited by
I. Arias, H. Popper, D. Schachter, and D. A. Shafritz.
Raven Press, New York © 1982.

Chapter 38

Liver Cell Heterogeneity

Jorge J. Gumucio and Deborah L. Miller

In 1856, Beale (1), in his lecture entitled *The Minute Anatomy of the Liver*, commented:

> The vertebrate liver may be looked upon as consisting essentially of two distinct systems of channels arranged so as to form networks. . . . In one of these networks lie the secreting cells, often arranged so as to form only a single row. . . . The fluid bile . . . flows towards the surface of the lobule where the ducts lie. In the other network flows the blood but in a precisely opposite direction to that which the bile takes. . . . The cells at the circumference usually contain a much larger quantity of oil than those near the centre, which is just what we should anticipate when we recollect that the portal blood, rich with the freshly absorbed constituents of the food, first reaches these marginal cells. . . . The cells in all parts of the network have no doubt the power of forming bile . . . but in different degrees. . . . The cells near the margins of the lobule take the most active part in the formation of bile.

Almost 70 years later, Noel (2), observing the morphological changes in liver cell mitochondria under various metabolic conditions, proposed the division of the hepatic lobule into three functional zones. Because dietary modifications induced significant changes in mitochondrial shape in hepatocytes near the portal vein, Noel proposed that these changes reflected high metabolic activity in this zone, which he called "zone of permanent function." The appearance of mitochondria in hepatocytes surrounding the central vein, how-

ever, was constant regardless of the metabolic state. Because these hepatocytes were thought to be metabolically inactive, the zone was called the "zone of permanent rest." Finally, Noel recognized an intermediate zone of "variable activity," which would be functionally recruited according to the phase of digestion. These observations remind us that the notions of liver cell heterogeneity, concentration gradients, and zonal and dynamic distribution of labor within the microvascular unit of the liver, the subjects of this chapter, have been discussed for at least 125 years. This chapter summarizes the existing experimental evidence for liver cell heterogeneity and assembles these data within the context of the functional organization of the liver acinus.

MICROVASCULAR UNIT OF THE LIVER: A DETERMINANT OF CELL HETEROGENEITY

Studies of the microcirculation of the liver *in vivo* led Rappaport (3–6) to propose that the simple liver acinus rather than the hepatic lobule represents the microvascular unit of liver parenchyma. As illustrated in Fig. 1, this unit is a microscopic mass of cells, irregular in size and shape, departing from an axis comprised of a terminal portal venule less than 40 μm in diameter, a terminal hepatic arteriole ranging in diam-

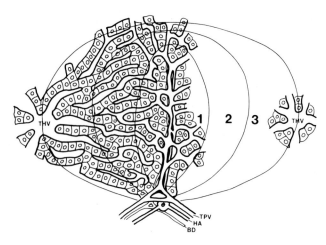

FIG. 1. The microvascular unit of liver parenchyma, the hepatic acinus. The acinar axis is formed by the terminal extensions of the portal venule (TPV), the arteriole (HA), and the bile ductule (BD). Blood empties into acinar sinusoids in this axial area (zone 1) and flows sequentially through zone 2 and into zone 3, where it exits via the terminal hepatic venules (THV). The sinusoids of zone 1 are more highly anastomotic and are characterized by a lower volume fraction and higher surface-to-volume ratio than the sinusoids of zone 3.

eter between 15 and 50 μm, and a bile ductule(s), lymph vessels, and nerves (3). Blood flows from the terminal portal venule into sinusoids, which sequentially distribute this blood to approximately 20 hepatocytes on each side of the axis before emptying into the terminal hepatic venules. The flow of blood from the portal venule to the hepatic venule creates microenvironments around hepatocytes of the simple liver acinus, owing to the transport of the incoming metabolites by the cells closer to the acinar inlet. As solutes are removed by those hepatocytes, the concentration of metabolites in sinusoidal blood decreases toward the acinar outlet. Hepatocytes closer to the terminal portal venule, therefore, are exposed to different concentrations of substrates than those near the terminal hepatic venule. This notion has prompted the arbitrary division of the simple liver acinus into different zones according to their distance from the portal axis. Acinar zone 1 is comprised of the cuff of hepatocytes distributed immediately around the terminal branch of the portal vein. Zone 3 marks the acinar periphery; its landmark is the hepatic venule. The arbitrarily interposed intermediate zone is called acinar zone 2 (3).

It is important to correlate the acinar zones described by Rappaport with the more traditional lobular terms "periportal" and "centrilobular" often used in descriptions of liver pathology. Terminal hepatic venules are commonly called "central veins" in the terminology of the lobular vascular concept developed by Kiernan (7). However, Kiernan's hexagonal lobule does not represent a homogeneous vascular unit as

blood is supplied to lobular hepatocytes by a number of arterioles and portal venules originating from different parent branches (6). Indeed, following the injection of two differently colored gelatin masses into the two main branches of the portal vein of the dog or rabbit, homogeneously colored areas are observed only around terminal portal venules, identifying these areas as the axes of the microvascular units. In contrast, in the area around the terminal hepatic venule (central vein), as well as around the preterminal portal veins, both dyes are seen, showing the heterogeneous blood supply of these areas (3). The hexagonal or lobular vascular pattern is merely the result of the visual effect of the interdigitation of terminal branches originating from three triangular portal spaces surrounding one terminal hepatic venule (5). The acinus represents the smallest structural and functional vascular unit of hepatic parenchyma, since acinar hepatocytes receive blood from a common source (3).

The term centrilobular corresponds to acinar zone 3, since both represent the area surrounding the terminal hepatic venule. The term "periportal," as used in the lobular context, refers most frequently to the area surrounding the preterminal, triangular portal spaces. This area is comprised of hepatocytes of all three acinar zones, as demonstrated by dye-injection studies (3). The terms acinar zone 1 and periportal area are identical only when used to describe the regions surrounding terminal portal venules less than 40 μm in diameter, the acinar landmarks (3); thus it is important to clearly define the landmark used as the reference base when describing experimental observations in liver. To best define the cell population predominantly involved in any metabolic process, it is meaningful to use the simplest structural and functional unit of hepatic parenchyma, the liver acinus, as the basis of description. Many of the studies analyzed in this chapter have used lobular terminology to describe results. In those cases, the term periportal is placed in quotation marks.

SYSTEMS TO STUDY THE FUNCTIONAL ORGANIZATION OF THE LIVER ACINUS

The ample evidence that hepatocytes of the liver acinus represent a heterogeneous cellular group must be organized in a more functional context. It is necessary to determine the relative contribution of the cells of the various acinar zones to the transport and intracellular processing of solutes. It is also important to understand the interrelationships between cellular zones and the modifications of this zonal organization under different metabolic conditions, including damage. The following methods have been used to study liver cell heterogeneity and its functional significance.

In Vivo Approach

Morphology

Light and electron microscopy have been performed to gain, from observations of changes in structure, a better understanding of the functional state of the cell in each zone. Specifically, intracellular changes have been studied following the administration of substances, such as bile salts (8), or after surgical procedures, such as total or selective biliary obstruction (9,10). Similarly, this approach has allowed the definition of cellular zones that represent the targets of drugs, such as phenobarbital (11), and other compounds, such as bromobenzene (12), carbon tetrachloride (13), and allyl alcohol (14). The advent of quantitative morphometric methods has permitted recognition at the zonal level of otherwise subtle qualitative differences between cells (15). Technical refinements, such as the use of a double embedding procedure for electron microscopy, facilitate accurate localization of the acinar landmarks (16).

Autoradiography

Autoradiography has been used successfully to demonstrate cellular gradients for galactose (17) and for a bile acid analog, cholylglycylhistamine (18). The zonal rate of protein synthesis (19−21) and the contribution of each cellular zone to liver regeneration (22, 23) have also been studied using this approach. In these cases, conventional autoradiographic techniques have been used, resulting in extraction of any water-soluble label. The autoradiographic detection of water-soluble compounds presents numerous technical problems, as illustrated by the abundance of methods described in the literature.

Histochemistry

Histochemistry represents one of the first methods used to determine qualitatively the localization of enzymes within the various zones of the hepatic acinus (24,25). Several points should be borne in mind, however, when interpreting any histochemical results. Zonal differences in the apparent concentration of an enzyme might be functionally meaningless unless the enzyme is the rate-limiting step in a metabolic process. The zonal distribution of most enzymes is not static, but varies during the diurnal cycle and with different metabolic states of the liver (26−29). This approach also presents technical problems, such as substrate availability, diffusion or nonspecific deposition of reaction products, and difficulty in quantitation. These techniques have been greatly improved. The use of

immunocytochemistry has permitted detection and localization of proteins within the acinus (30). More recently, a quantitative cytochemical method, involving the reduction of ferricyanide by glutathione and quantitation by microdensitometry, has been used to determine the zonal distribution of glutathione within the rat liver lobule (31).

Microspectrophotometry and Microphotometry

The zonal distribution of cytochrome P-450 has been determined by means of a laser double beam microspectrophotometer (32). This instrument is equipped with a scanning monochromator which allows recording of the difference spectra of reduced and oxidized forms of cytochrome P-450 in various zones of the acinus. In our laboratory, we have determined the zonal distribution of fluorescent compounds by fluorescence microscopy and quantitated the concentration of fluorescent substances in cells of each zone by quantitative fluorescence microphotometry. The fluorescence of an unfixed, unmounted cryostat section is excited by an argon laser. A variable frame diaphragm is used to restrict the detected fluorescence to an area of 6.25 μm^2 and thus to measure fluorescence within the cytoplasm of a single hepatocyte. By scanning the acinus, it is possible to determine the zonal distribution of the fluorescent substance and assess the contribution of each acinar zone to the transport of these substances. Microphotometry of single hepatocytes has also been used to determine the activity of enzymes, such as lactic and succinic dehydrogenases (33).

Zonal Damage

Compounds, such as allyl alcohol (34,35), bromobenzene (34−36), or carbon tetrachloride (35), have been administered *in vivo* to induce selective zonal damage and determine the functional capabilities of the remaining acinar zones. The major problem with this approach is the difficulty in establishing with certainty that morphologically well-preserved zones are also functionally intact.

In Vitro Approach

Microdissection

Most recent data on the zonal localization of carbohydrate metabolism have been obtained by microdissection of acinar zones followed by the enzymatic analysis of the samples (37−40). This tedious approach to the separation of zones requires very sensitive methods of detection. Unfortunately, it cannot be used in studies requiring integrity of the plasma membrane because the cells are not only sliced but subsequently freeze dried. Also, the small areas of parenchyma obtained by microdissection contain hepatocytic and non-hepatocytic cell populations, and the number of cells analyzed represents only a small sample of the total liver cell population.

Isolation of Liver Cell Subpopulations

Subfractionation of isolated hepatocytes has been attempted using density gradient centrifugation in Ficoll or Metrizamide (41–44), velocity sedimentation analysis (45), and partition in phase systems (46). When isolated hepatocytes are centrifuged in Ficoll gradients, two subpopulations can be recognized (41). Light hepatocytes are characterized by a mean diameter of 20.5 μm, a mean volume of 4,800 μm^3, and a density of 1.10; heavy hepatocytes with a mean volume of 3,800 μm^3 and a mean diameter of 19.0 μm equilibrate at a density of 1.14. On the basis of the intracellular distribution of glycogen and smooth endoplasmic reticulum (SER) and the response to phenobarbital administration, it has been proposed that the light cells are enriched in centrilobular hepatocytes; heavy cells consist primarily of "periportal" hepatocytes (41,42). Similar results are obtained when hepatocytes are fractionated in Metrizamide gradients (44). Under these conditions, the administration of phenobarbital for 3 days concomitantly induces the SER of acinar zone 3 cells in tissue and cytochrome P-450 in the light hepatocyte population (44).

When sedimentation velocity analysis is used to separate subpopulations of hepatocytes, volume rather than density is the main determinant of the velocity of sedimentation. This technique resolves the total hepatocytic population into 12 arbitrary fractions with mean volumes ranging from 10,900 to 2,300 μm^3. The analysis of the sedimentation velocity-volume characteristics also suggests the existence of two liver cell populations (45).

Thus subpopulations of hepatocytes may be separated on the basis of differences in cellular density or volume. Also, it has been proposed that the two subpopulations obtained correspond to zone 1 (periportal) and zone 3 (centrilobular) hepatocytes. However, the zonal origin of the fractions requires further study. A reliable marker for hepatocytes of zone 1 or 3 is needed. The *in vivo* administration of the marker ideally should produce a stable, visually detectable concentration gradient predominantly in one zone and should label cells without damaging them or changing their density or volume. This is a major problem when studying the effects of drugs on liver cells, because there is no guarantee that hepatocytes separated at a certain density after drug administration correspond to hepatocytes that separate at the same density from normal liver.

MORPHOLOGICAL CHARACTERISTICS OF THE HEPATOCYTES OF THE ACINAR ZONES

Cell Size

Morphometric determinations in tissue have shown that the average cell diameter of "periportal," midzonal, and centrilobular hepatocytes is 20.8 ± 0.2 (SD), 20.8 ± 0.3, and 21.0 ± 0.3 μm, respectively (15). These results compare well with measurements made on isolated hepatocytes purportedly originating from different cellular zones. While the diameter of the subpopulation enriched in centrilobular cells is 19.0 ± 3.0 μm (SD), that of the subpopulation enriched in "periportal" hepatocytes is 20.5 ± 3.3 μm (41). Cell diameter, therefore, is relatively constant among the various cellular zones. Selective zonal changes in cell diameter, however, can be induced by phenobarbital. After 3 days of phenobarbital administration, the diameter of the subpopulation of light, presumably centrilobular hepatocytes increases from 20 to 23.7 μm, whereas the diameter of the heavier cells is unchanged (42).

Hepatocyte volume has been estimated by morphometric analysis of tissue to be about 5,400 μm^3 and constant across the lobule (15). Differences in cell volume are found after fractionation of isolated hepatocytes by velocity sedimentation. Using this procedure, cellular volumes range between 2,300 and 10,000 μm^3 (45). A different approach—subfractionation of hepatocytes in Ficoll gradients—shows that the mean cell volume of the population enriched in "periportal" hepatocytes is 3,800 μm^3, while that of a band enriched in centrilobular cells is 4,800 μm^3 (41). These volumes increase to 4,100 and 7,300 μm^3, respectively, following phenobarbital administration (42), indicating a selective zonal response to this drug.

Intracellular Characteristics

Glycogen Distribution

Numerous studies have shown that the amount of glycogen in a given acinar zone depends on the metabolic state of the liver (26,47–53). Deane (48), examining the effects of diurnal variation on glycogen contents, found that the storage of glycogen occurs soon after eating. Glycogen is laid down initially in the "peripheral part of the lobule," then more centrally. In contrast, during glycogenolysis, glycogen disappears first from the central region and then from the peripheral region.

Although the total content of glycogen varies among

the cellular zones, electron microscopic studies show that the hepatocytes of each acinar area have a characteristic pattern of intracellular glycogen distribution. Glycogen in cells of acinar zone 1 is seen in large aggregates often gathered into broad areas, while glycogen in hepatocytes of acinar zone 3 is dispersed throughout the cells in small, isolated rosettes, often closely associated with the SER (12,15).

Endoplasmic Reticulum

Quantitative analyses have shown that centrilobular cells contain more SER than do "periportal" hepatocytes (10,15,54). This distribution varies during the day and with age. The amount of SER in centrilobular and midzonal cells is highest at about 10 PM, when the activities of several microsomal enzymes are also highest (27–29,54). No daily variation in SER surface density is found in "periportal" cells (54). In the Fischer rat, the surface density of the SER increases twofold in both zones between the ages of 1 and 10 months, then declines, until at 30 months, the amount is similar to that of 1-month-old rats (55). At all ages, more SER is apparent in centrilobular hepatocytes.

The distribution of rough ER (RER) among hepatocytes of the acinus has not been clearly established. While some studies have shown no differences between zones (9,10,15), others describe a predominant concentration of RER in "periportal" hepatocytes (8,55). Age, however, alters RER distribution in the rat; between 1 and 10 months, the specific surface area of RER in centrilobular hepatocytes increases by 127% (55).

Lysosomes

Histochemical data suggest that the activity of the lysosomal marker acid phosphatase is higher in "periportal" than in centrilobular hepatocytes (24,25,56, 57). Moreover, qualitative and quantitative studies propose that lysosomes are more numerous and larger in "periportal" cells (9,10,24). Other morphometric studies, however, have not confirmed these differences (8,15). Quantitation of lysosomes is difficult because of their small volume fraction in the hepatocytes. Furthermore, lysosomes occur in several forms, including primary and secondary lysosomes and multivesicular and residual bodies. Quantitation of these individual forms of lysosomes across the acinus remains to be performed.

Mitochondria

Quantitative studies by Loud (15) have shown striking differences in mitochondrial characteristics between "periportal" and centrilobular hepatocytes.

"Periportal" cells contain fewer mitochondria and are 2.3 times larger and shorter with a length-to-diameter ratio of 7, as compared with a ratio of 16 found in centrilobular hepatocytes. As a result, periportal mitochondria occupy a greater fraction of the hepatocyte volume than do centrilobular mitochondria. Changes in mitochondrial size and shape during the diurnal cycle (2,48) and after dietary manipulations (2) illustrate the dynamic state of mitochondria.

Golgi, Pericanalicular Ectoplasm, and Secretory Pole

The Golgi apparatus is conspicuously located at the secretory pole of the hepatocyte. As early as 1926, Cramer and Ludford (58) proposed that the Golgi participates in the excretion of bile pigment. More recently (8–10), morphometric studies of the distribution of the Golgi in hepatocytes and particularly in the pericanalicular ectoplasm have been performed. In sham-operated rats, "periportal" hepatocytes contain twice the volume of Golgi-rich area as do centrilobular cells. Following selective biliary obstruction (10), the volume of the Golgi-rich area increases in centrilobular hepatocytes of the unobstructed lobes, suggesting a possible morphological adaptation during enhanced bile secretion by these lobes. Changes in the pericanalicular ectoplasm, the zone of cytoplasm immediately surrounding the bile canaliculus, have been studied following the administration of sodium taurocholate (8). Under these experimental conditions, the size of the bile salt pool increases by a factor of 2, and the transport maximum for taurocholate excretion increases by 50%. While no concomitant changes are observed in the total amount of Golgi-rich area in whole hepatocytes, the volume in the pericanalicular area of centrilobular hepatocytes doubles and that of "periportal" cells triples, suggesting migration of Golgi into the biliary pole. Thus changes in the amount of bile salts to be secreted result in dynamic variations in the volume fraction and intracellular distribution of Golgi within hepatocytes of each cellular zone (8).

Differences in the diameter of the bile canaliculus between "periportal" and centrilobular hepatocytes have also been noted (8–10,59,60). However, reproducible measurements of the volume fraction or diameter of the canaliculi are difficult because of the variability in size and shape of this space. The range of volume fractions reported for centrilobular canaliculi is between 0.004 and 0.009, while measurements between 0.01 and 0.02 have been obtained for "periportal" canaliculi (8,9). Considerable variation has also been noted in the cross-sectional diameter of the bile canaliculus in both the "periportal" and the centrilobular areas (60). Despite this variability, average values indicate that the volume fraction and the cross-sectional diameter of canaliculi are larger in "periportal" than in centrilobular hepatocytes (8,9,60).

Changes in the size and shape of the bile canaliculus after the administration of bile salts have been noted. After a prolonged intraduodenal administration of bile salts (8), an increase in the volume fraction of the canaliculus in both zones is observed, while briefer intravenous infusion of bile salts selectively increases the cross-sectional diameter of centrilobular bile canaliculi (60). These data suggest that bile canalicular structure also varies according to changes in the intracellular concentration of solutes to be transported.

BIOCHEMICAL CHARACTERISTICS OF THE HEPATOCYTES OF ACINAR ZONES

Heterogeneous Enzyme Distribution

Several studies using histochemical techniques or microdissection have found differences in the distribution of enzymes among hepatocytes of the liver acinus. Shank et al. (61) microdissected the liver parenchyma into "periportal," midzonal, and centrilobular areas and determined the activity of several enzymes by quantitative histochemistry. Their findings indicate a gradient of enzyme activities rather than the exclusive localization of enzymes in "periportal" or centrilobular zones. More recently, attempts have been made to organize this incomplete and fragmentary information on the biochemical characteristics of hepatocytes into the more meaningful functional context of zonal metabolism.

Functional Organization of the Hepatic Acinus

Carbohydrate Metabolism

On the basis of histochemical data, Novikoff (24,25) initially suggested that "periportal" hepatocytes, containing long and numerous mitochondria with high levels of cytochrome oxidase and succinic dehydrogenase (62,63), might provide the predominant contribution to oxidative respiration. In addition, Novikoff suggested that the higher levels of glucose-6-phosphatase in "periportal" cells (37,63–65) may be related to the fact that these cells are the first to deposit glycogen, while glycolysis and other oxidative pathways might occur at a relatively high rate in centrilobular cells (24,25). More recently, studies using microdissection of acinar zones followed by enzymatic analysis have shown that phosphoenol-pyruvate carboxykinase, presumably a rate-limiting step in gluconeogenesis (38), and fructose-1,6-diphosphatase (39) are predominantly located in the cells of acinar

zone 1. In contrast, the activity of pyruvic kinase, an enzyme involved in glycolysis, is higher in the hepatocytes of acinar zone 3 (38).

These data support the proposal of zonal heterogeneity for carbohydrate metabolism (26,40,53,66–68). According to this proposal, acinar zone 1 hepatocytes are predominantly engaged in gluconeogenesis, while cells of acinar zone 3 participate predominantly in glycolysis. No sharp border exists between gluconeogenic and glycolytic hepatocytes; enzymes corresponding to each pathway can be detected in both zones. Only the predominance of one or another rate-limiting enzymatic pattern would make the zone either gluconeogenic or glycolytic (38). In addition many other parameters that have not been determined at the zonal level, such as the concentration of substrates, coenzymes, activators, inhibitors, and oxygen in each zone may play important roles in determining these metabolic fluxes at each zone *in vivo* (38).

Protein Metabolism

After the intravenous administration of tritiated leucine, autoradiographic studies show that the majority of the label is localized in acinar zone 1 hepatocytes (19–21). Although interesting, the interpretation of these results is difficult; the label has been incorporated into many proteins. In addition, incorporation of the radioactive tracer into proteins in each cellular zone depends on many factors, including the concentration gradient of the labeled amino acid in sinusoidal blood, the rate of uptake of the tracer, and the rate of excretion of the labeled proteins. A different approach has been used to study the synthesis of specific proteins, such as albumin and fibrinogen. Immunocytochemical techniques have demonstrated that in human liver, between 15 and 35% of hepatocytes contain detectable amounts of albumin under physiological conditions, while about 1% contain fibrinogen (69,70). The albumin- or fibrinogen-containing hepatocytes are apparently randomly distributed throughout the acinus. In nephrotic rats, a situation in which the synthesis of albumin appears to be increased (71,72), all hepatocytes contain albumin and are presumably engaged in albumin synthesis (73). On the basis of these results, it has been suggested that the capacity to synthesize albumin is distributed in all hepatocytes, although for unknown reasons, only some of them (without a specific zonal localization) may engage in albumin synthesis under physiological conditions (69,73).

Lipid Metabolism

Although the amount of visible lipid present in hepatocytes is subject to diurnal and metabolic variation, lipid is more concentrated in the centrilobular zone of recently fed animals (48). Likewise, the activities of the enzymes beta-hydroxybutric dehydrogenase (24,65) and esterase (24,25) are apparently higher in cells of acinar zone 3. Hepatocytes of zone 3 also contain a greater number of microbodies (15). Although the exact function of these catalase-containing organelles in cellular processes is unknown, a possible role in lipid metabolism has been suggested (74–77). Therefore, it has been postulated that these centrilobular hepatocytes are more active in lipid metabolism (5,24,25).

Drug Metabolism

Several lines of evidence suggest that cells closer to the terminal hepatic venule (centrilobular hepatocytes) contribute predominantly to the metabolism of drugs via the cytochrome P-450 mixed function oxidase system. Histochemical studies show that NADPH-dependent hydroxylating systems are predominantly located in hepatocytes in this area. During the first weeks of life, in the rat, the activity of one of these enzymes, NADPH-nitro-BT reductase, increases. This increment is due to increased activity per cell and an increased number of hepatocytes containing the enzyme (78). In female rats, the activity of this enzyme is restricted to cells of acinar zone 3; in males, the gradient of concentration extends into the acinar zone 1 area. This difference between the sexes is seen only after 6 weeks of life (78).

Cytochrome b_5, a component of the microsomal electron transport system, has been localized using immunoperoxidase techniques. The presence of cytochrome b_5 was detected only in centrilobular hepatocytes (79,80).

Spectrophotometric assays of cytochrome P-450, using unfixed cryostat liver sections, show that this cytochrome is also predominantly located in the cells of acinar zone 3 (32). The total cellular content of cytochrome P-450, however, is comprised of a heterogeneous mixture of cytochromes with different substrate specificities (81). A better understanding of the contribution of the different acinar zones to drug metabolism via the cytochrome P-450 system will be achieved only once the zonal localization of each of the various forms of cytochrome P-450 is established. The zonal contribution to the metabolism of drugs which do not primarily interact with the cytochrome P-450 system may depend on the predominant localization of the enzymatic system involved (assuming the enzymatic system is rate-limiting). For example, alcohol dehydrogenase may be located primarily in periportal hepatocytes (82), which may explain lesions induced by toxic doses of allyl alcohol in cells of acinar zone 1 (83).

It is dangerous to derive conclusions as to the zonal contribution to drug metabolism based only on the predominant acinar localization of nonrate-limiting enzymes. The rate of interaction of the drug with its metabolic system determine the contribution of each zone to drug metabolism. This interaction and the rate of drug metabolism in each zone are influenced by the concentration gradient of the drug in sinusoidal blood, the capabilities of cells for intracellular binding, and the cellular concentration gradients of cofactors.

Organization of the Hepatic Acinus for Transport

The hepatic sinusoids

For a solute to interact with the sinusoidal membrane and eventually be taken up by the hepatic cell, it must move out of the sinusoidal space and into the space of Disse. This movement occurs after the solute collides with the endothelial walls of the sinusoid and passes through the sinusoidal fenestrations. One of the elements determining the probability of this collision is the configuration of the sinusoidal space. The cross-sectional area of the sinusoid, its surface-to-volume ratio, and its sinuousity or degree of branching affect the probability of solute-sinusoidal wall interaction.

The configuration of hepatic sinusoids is different in the various acinar zones. Analysis of silicone rubber casts shows that the periportal area is characterized by rich anastomotic channels, whereas those closer to the central vein are more radially arranged (84). Furthermore, the fraction of parenchymal volume occupied by sinusoids is larger in zone 3 than in zone 1. The surface-to-volume ratio, however, is higher in zone 1. These observations suggest a greater probability for solute-sinusoidal wall interaction in the periportal area (85). Other important factors influence the probability of this interaction, such as the velocity of blood flow, in each zone. In this regard, three types of sinusoids—direct, branching, and interconnecting—have been described. The velocity of red blood cell flow is fastest in direct sinusoids, which connect the terminal portal and terminal hepatic venules. Branch sinusoids have intermediate velocity; and the average velocity in the interconnecting sinusoids is slower but fluctuates widely (86). The distribution of these different types of sinusoids and the velocity of blood flow at each acinar zone remains to be determined.

The movement of a solute from the sinusoids into the space of Disse is also affected by the size and distribution of the sinusoidal fenestrations. Initially, it was observed that, in the albino rat, fenestrations were not present in the first 10 to 50 μm of the periportal sinusoids. An intermediate zone, representing about 90% of the total length of the sinusoid, was well fenestrated and devoid of an endothelial basement membrane. In the area immediately surrounding the central vein, the endothelium was again devoid of fenestrations (87). More recent studies by scanning electron microscopy in the Wistar rat show fenestrations that are not only present throughout the length of the sinusoids but also extend into short segments of the terminal portal and hepatic venules (88). Two sizes of fenestrations have been described: large, single ones 1–3 μm in diameter, and smaller, clustered fenestrae measuring 0.04 to about 1 μm. The larger openings are more numerous near the portal venules; closer to the terminal hepatic venules, the fenestrae are smaller and rare. Thus the predominant distribution of large fenestrations in acinar zone 1 may favor the entry of solutes into the space of Disse at the acinar inlet, the periportal area. The size of the fenestrations is subject to change. For example, after obstruction of the hepatic venous outflow, the small fenestrations disappear from the centrilobular area and are replaced by large 2 to 5 μm openings (89). This fusion of small into larger fenestrations has also been observed in freeze fracture studies (90). Further evidence of the dynamic condition of these endothelial openings is provided by the finding that they are surrounded by contractile microfilaments (91).

Concentration Gradients in Sinusoidal Blood

The steepness of the slope describing the zone 1 to zone 3 solute concentration gradient in sinusoidal blood depends on the rate of removal of solutes by the preceding cellular zones. Although it is expected that solutes taken up by hepatocytes by simple diffusion follow the zone 1 to zone 3 concentration gradient, solutes transported into cells by carrier-mediated processes may create different gradients. If carrier sites are equal in number, and the kinetics of transport are similar in hepatocytes of all acinar zones, a zone 1 to zone 3 concentration gradient would be expected, as indicated by kinetic analysis of uptake using either the multiple dilution technique (17,92,100) or other mathematical models (93–95). Kinetic analysis of solute uptake by hepatocytes in each zone has not been performed. In addition, although morphometric studies indicate that the configuration of the sinusoidal space is different in acinar zones 1 and 3, and the probability of solute-sinusoidal wall interaction may differ, the degree to which these findings can affect the results predicted by these models remains to be determined.

One of the most conspicuous solutes considered in explaining the zonal distribution of metabolic processes is oxygen. Even though a zone 1 to zone 3 gradient in oxygen concentration is commonly implied, the concentration of oxygen in sinusoidal blood in each zone has not been measured. Data obtained using surface or needle electrodes suggest that PO_2 decreases along the length of the sinusoids in a nonlinear manner. The range of PO_2 varies between 1 and 65 mm Hg; most of the observed values are 20 to 25 mm Hg (96). The problem of oxygen concentration gradients has been approached indirectly by measuring changes in the activity of two oxygen-dependent enzymes with different affinities for oxygen under conditions of hypoxia (97). On the basis of these studies, a steep zone 1 to zone 3 concentration gradient of oxygen in sinusoidal blood has been proposed (97), suggesting that the concentration of oxygen in zone 3 cells is close to a critical level, as supported also by the centrilobular lesion induced by hypoxia (98).

Recently, three-dimensional recordings of the redox state have been performed in perfused rat liver (99). These results have been interpreted as indicative of a periportal to centrilobular redox gradient. The explanation for this gradient is not clear, as the PO_2 measured in the effluent of the perfused liver is two orders of magnitude higher than the apparent K_m for oxygen in isolated mitochondria. Of interest is the finding that the slope of this redox gradient can be modified by administration of alcohol (99), which provides another example of the dynamic state of the cells of the hepatic acinus.

Cellular Concentration Gradients

Based on indirect measurements of solute concentration in sinusoidal blood, a zone 1 to zone 3 concentration gradient in hepatocytes has been proposed for bilirubin (100), bile salts (35,36,100), and galactose (17). However, such gradients have been directly observed autoradiographically only after administration of labeled galactose (17) and, as seen in Fig. 2, after administration of a lipid-soluble bile acid analog, cholylgylcylhistamine (18). Fluorescent substances have also been used to create visible cellular concentration gradients and thus to study the contribution of hepatocytes to transport (101). Following perfusion of rat liver with low concentrations of rhodamine B (5 $\times$ 10^{-7} M), fluorescence is observed in acinar zone 1 cells (Fig. 3). At concentrations above 5 $\times$ 10^{-6} M, however, progressive recruitment of hepatocytes transporting rhodamine B is observed (Fig. 4). Quantitative measurements by microphotometry indicate that this progressive recruitment for transport is characterized by an increasing concentration of rhodamine B in periportal cells and by enlistment of new hepatocytes for transport. Parameters other than the concentration gradient in sinusoidal blood, such as distribution of transport sites and kinetic characteristics, may influence the direction of cellular gradients, as evidenced

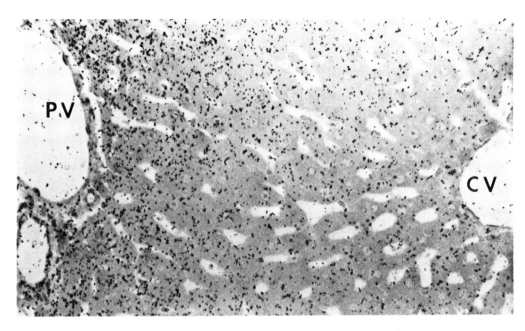

FIG. 2. A "periportal" (PV) to centrilobular (CV) lobular gradient of autoradiographic grains is seen 1 min after the intraportal injection of ¹²⁵I-cholylglycylhistamine. (Photograph reproduced from Jones et al. *Am. J. Physiol.,* 238:G233, 1980, with permission from the authors and publisher.)

by the finding of a cellular concentration gradient in the reverse direction (zone 3 to zone 1) after infusion of high concentrations of fluorescein isothiocyanate (Fig. 5).

Since the intracellular concentration of solutes influences the rate of biliary secretion by the hepatocyte, cellular concentration gradients directly affect the relative contribution of each acinar zone to bile secretion. If, as indicated by the zone 1 to zone 3 concentration gradient created by the bile acid derivative cholylglycylhistamine (Fig. 2), endogenous bile salts are

also transported primarily by acinar zones 1 and 2, these zones should contribute predominantly to the secretion of bile salts. Hepatocytes of acinar zones 1 and 2, therefore, can contribute predominantly to the generation of the bile salt-dependent fraction of canalicular bile (18,34–36). In contrast, it has been proposed that hepatocytes of acinar zone 3 may contribute to the secretion of the bile salt nondependent fraction of canalicular bile (34–36). Additional data are needed to define further the contribution of hepatocytes of each cellular zone to bile secretion.

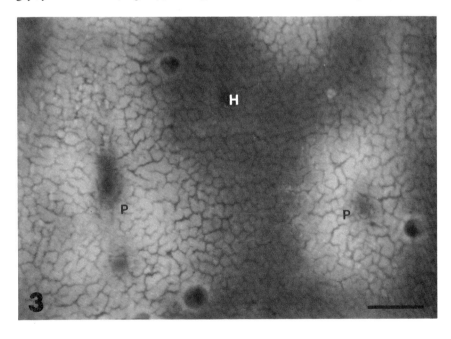

FIG. 3. Fluorescence micrograph of rat liver parenchyma after the perfusion of rhodamine B, 5 × 10⁻⁷ M. Fluorescence is confined to the area surrounding the portal venules (P). H, hepatic venule. *Bar* = 100 μm.

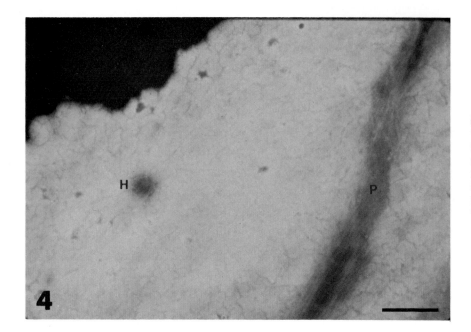

FIG. 4. After the perfusion of 5 × 10⁻⁶ M rhodamine B, all cells contain fluorescent label. Progressive recruitment of hepatocytes for transport of rhodamine B has occurred between 5 × 10⁻⁷ M (Fig. 3) and 5 × 10⁻⁶ M (Fig. 4). H, hepatic venule; P, portal venule. *Bar* = 100 μm.

ZONAL RESPONSES OF ACINAR HEPATOCYTES

Induction of SER and Cytochrome P-450 by Phenobarbital

Following administration of phenobarbital to rats for 5 days, the cellular volume increases. Most of this increment can be accounted for by changes in cytoplasmic volume predominantly due to an increase in SER (102). Thus, after 1 day of phenobarbital administration, there is proliferation of the SER in cells of acinar zone 3 (centrilobular cells). After 2 days, the cytoplasm of acinar zone 3 cells is filled with packed vesicles of SER. Concomitantly, hepatocytes with the ap-

pearance of zone 3 cells (compact cytoplasm with glycogen dispersed within the cytoplasm rather than aggregated into large lakes as in zone 1 cells) extends further into acinar zone 2. After 10 days of phenobarbital administration, most hepatocytes resemble zone 3 cells, and only a few around the terminal portal venule remain unchanged (11). Thus from the morphological standpoint, the initial inductive effect of phenobarbital is reflected by proliferation of SER in acinar zone 3 hepatocytes. As the administration of phenobarbital is prolonged, this inductive effect progresses from cells of zone 3 to include cells closer to the terminal portal venule.

From a functional point of view, it has been shown that phenobarbital induces microsomal cytochrome

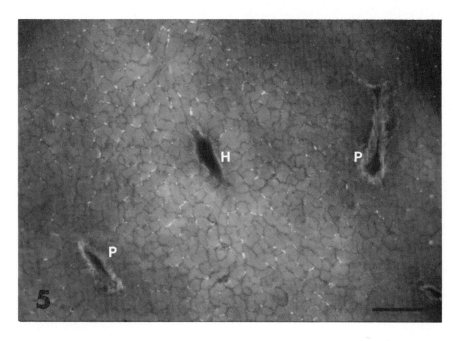

FIG. 5. A reverse gradient is seen after the perfusion of fluorescein isothiocyanate, 8 × 10⁻⁵ M. The perivenular area (H) is fluorescent, while less label is present in periportal cells (P). *Bar* = 100 μm.

P-450, an enzyme that plays a central role in drug metabolism (103). Furthermore, as already described, the total content of cytochrome P-450 corresponds to multiple forms of this cytochrome which have different substrate specificities (81,104). Phenobarbital induces one of these forms with a molecular weight close to 50,000 daltons (104). Spectrophotometric assays indicate that cytochrome P-450 is predominantly located in cells of acinar zone 3 (32). Similarly, studies using subpopulations of isolated hepatocytes (44) and unfixed cryostat liver sections (32) show that phenobarbital induces cytochrome P-450 predominantly in hepatocytes located near the terminal hepatic venule. During short-term administration of phenobarbital, the inductive effects are exerted predominantly in the cells of acinar zone 3. Although the mechanisms responsible for this selective zonal effect of phenobarbital have not been elucidated, several possibilities exist (44): (a) predominant uptake of phenobarbital by hepatocytes of zone 3 (regardless of the postulated zone 1 to zone 3 concentration gradient in sinusoidal blood), (b) predominant interaction due to the presence of phenobarbital binding proteins in cells of zone 3, or (c) the concentration in zone 3 of factors necessary for gene activation by phenobarbital.

Regenerative Responses

Following two-thirds partial hepatectomy, the rat liver rapidly regenerates and regains its original mass (105,106). The mechanism responsible for this restoration is proliferation of hepatocytes in the hepatic remnant. Therefore, regeneration initially involves intact hepatocytes located within intact acini. DNA synthesis and cell proliferation have been studied under these conditions by following the incorporation of ^{3}H-thymidine into DNA (22). Hepatocytes begin synthesizing DNA between 12 and 18 hr after partial hepatectomy. At about 20 hr, 30% of the hepatocytes are involved in DNA synthesis, and this precedes the peak mitotic activity by 6 hr. About 80% of the total DNA synthesized by hepatocytes may be accounted for by labeled cells located in acinar zones 1 and 2 of the liver acinus. This zonal proliferation occurs only when the resected liver mass is at least 20 to 30%; otherwise, all zones of the acinus seem to contribute to the regenerative response. In addition, the fact that all acini are similarly labeled with ^{3}H-thymidine suggests that growth of the residual acini rather than formation of new acini has occurred (22).

In contrast to partial hepatectomy, zonal damage, which results from most forms of liver disease, affects all hepatic acini. Regeneration starts in damaged rather than in intact acini. For example, following selective zone 3 injury by bromobenzene, autoradiographic data

indicate that the contribution of acinar zones 2 and 3 to DNA synthesis is greatest. In contrast, after damage to zone 1 by allyl alcohol, the relative contribution of acinar zone 1 hepatoytes to DNA synthesis is greater (23). Furthermore, after carbon tetrachloride administration (107) in fatty liver (108), and following biliary obstruction, hepatocytes synthesizing DNA are uniformly distributed within the acinus rather than predominantly located in acinar zone 1. These data suggest that regeneration is not an exclusively periportal phenomenon but that the contribution of each acinar zone to cell regeneration depends on the zonal distribution of the damage.

Zonal Liver Damage

One of the most compelling clinical observations leading to the concept of liver cell heterogeneity is the finding that drugs and toxic substances can induce liver damage, which appears to be restricted to a single zone of the liver acinus. Yellow phosphorous (110), allyl formate (83), ngaione at low doses (111), and bile salts (36) damage acinar zone 1 cells. More frequently, however, acinar zone 3 is the target of these toxic effects. Acetaminophen (112–114), bromobenzene (12, 115–117), carbon tetrachloride (118), DDT (119), amanita phalloides (119), halothane (120), herbal remedies (119), and others (119) induce damage which is distributed predominantly in cells of acinar zone 3.

Why is the damage zonal? Is the toxic substance taken up or bound mainly to cells of one zone? Do damaged hepatocytes have a different capacity to metabolize the toxic substance? Is the capacity for repair the determining factor? The question can be restated: Is the geographic location of the cells with respect to incoming metabolites the main determinant of zonal damage, or do intrinsic cellular differences direct selective zonal responses?

Allyl alcohol is metabolized by alcohol dehydrogenase, an enzyme presumably located in hepatocytes of acinar zone 1 (82). The product of this reaction, acrolein, is purportedly the toxic intermediate (14). Thus zonal damage due to allyl alcohol may be the consequence of the predominant location of alcohol dehydrogenase in cells of acinar zone 1.

In contrast, administration of sodium taurocholate in high doses via the portal vein also damages zone 1 cells (36). The zonal damage is secondary, however, most likely to the predominant interaction of bile salts with hepatocytes of acinar zone 1, the zone that seems to transport most of the load of bile acids under physiological conditions (17,18,82,83,86).

Acetaminophen is conjugated mainly with either glucuronic acid or sulfates. A minor metabolic pathway involves interaction with the cytochrome P-450 mixed function oxidase system (121−123). It has been proposed that, after the administration of toxic doses, the glucuronide-sulfate pathways are saturated, and the cytochrome P-450 pathway becomes predominant (121,122). The products of the biotransformation of acetaminophen by the cytochrome P-450 system are reactive, toxic metabolites that can initiate cell damage unless removed by conjugation with glutathione. Depletion of cellular glutathione by a large dose of acetaminophen generates toxic metabolites that can react with nucleophilic cell macromolecules resulting in cell death. Since the cytochrome P-450 system seems to be predominantly located in cells of acinar zone 3 (32), it is conceivable that the concentration of toxic metabolites may be higher in these centrilobular cells. In addition, it has been proposed that the concentration of glutathione is lower in the cells of zone 3 than in hepatocytes closer to the terminal portal venule (31). Both the high concentration of reactive metabolites and the low concentration of glutathione favor zonal damage in the centrilobular area. The concentration of toxic metabolites in each zone, however, also depends on the concentration gradient of acetaminophen in sinusoidal blood. Whether the differences in the relative concentrations of cytochrome P-450 and glutathione are sufficient to upset the presumed higher rate of transport of acetaminophen into cells of acinar zone 1 remains to be determined. The rate at which toxic metabolites are generated by each zone may not significantly differ; other factors, such as the rate of zonal cell repair, the rate of glutathione resynthesis, or the zonal distribution of one of the forms of cytochrome P-450, may play a major role in determining acetaminophen-induced damage of hepatocytes of acinar zone 3. These alternatives have not been tested.

LIVER FUNCTION, A ZONAL EVENT

In 1958, J. W. Wilson (124) wrote:

> In the thinking of biochemists and physiologists, and even sometimes of cytologists, the liver cell has become dangerously near to being The Cell, the typical cell, and with good reason, because it has all the structural characteristics of the typical cell and is amenable to a large number of experimental procedures. . . . The activity of a liver cell at a given moment, is determined by many factors. . . . While all cells presumably are potentially alike, they may not be doing the same things at the same time, and the same cell may not be doing the same things all the time.

This review summarizes the increasing experimental evidence for Wilson's proposal. The liver is comprised of a heterogeneous population of hepatocytes organized within the zones of the microvascular unit. The cells of these zones are constantly adapting to chang-

ing functional demands, a dynamic process that has been recognized morphologically and biochemically. Liver function represents the overall expression of intracellular events occurring at each zone and organized within the framework of the hepatic acinus.

REFERENCES

1. Beale, L. S. (1856): The minute anatomy of the liver. *Med. Times Gazette,* 13:82−85.
2. Noel, R. (1923): Sur la cellule hepatique du mammiferes. *Arch. Anat. Microsc.,* 19:1−158.
3. Rappaport, A. M., Borowy, Z. J., Lougheed, W. M., and Lotto, W. N. (1954): Subdivision of hexagonal liver lobules into a structural and functional unit: Role in hepatic physiology and pathology. *Anat. Rec.,* 119:11−34.
4. Rappaport, A. M. (1958): The structural and functional unit in the human liver (liver acinus). *Anat. Rec.,* 130:673−686.
5. Rappaport, A. M. (1980): Hepatic blood flow. In: *Liver and Biliary Tract Physiology, I,* edited by N. B. Javitt, pp. 1−63. University Park Press, Baltimore.
6. Rappaport, A. M., and Bilbey, D. L. J. (1960): Segmentation of the liver at the microscopic level. *Anat. Rec.,* 136:262−263.
7. Kiernan, F. (1833): The anatomy and physiology of the liver. *Philos. Trans. R. Soc. Lond.,* 123:711−770.
8. Jones, A. L., Schmucker, D. L., Mooney, J. S., Ockner, R. K., and Adler, R. D. (1979): Alterations in hepatic pericanalicular cytoplasm during enhanced bile secretory activity. *Lab. Invest.,* 40:512−517.
9. Jones, A. L., Schmucker, D. L., Mooney, J. S., Adler, R. D., and Ockner, R. K. (1976): Morphometric analysis of rat hepatocytes after total biliary obstruction. *Gastroenterology,* 71:1051−1061.
10. Jones, A. L., Schmucker, D. L., Mooney, J. S., Adler, R., and Ockner, R. K. (1978): A quantitative analysis of hepatic ultrastructure in rats during enhanced bile secretion. *Anat. Rec.,* 192:227−228.
11. Burger, P. C., and Herdson, P. B., (1966): Phenobarbital-induced fine structural changes in rat liver. *Am. J. Pathol.,* 48:793−809.
12. Miller, D. L., Harasin, J. M., and Gumucio, J. J. (1978): Bromobenzene-induced zonal necrosis in the hepatic acinus. *Exp. Mol. Pathol.,* 29:358−370.
13. Jezequel, A. A. (1958): Les effects de l'intoxication aigue au phosphore sur le foie de rat. Etude au Microscopique Electronique. *Aur. Anat. Pathol.* (Paris), 3:512−514.
14. Reid, W. D. (1972): Mechanism of allyl alcohol induced hepatic necrosis. *Experientia,* 28:1058.
15. Loud, A. V. (1968): Quantitative stereological description of the ultrastructure of normal rat liver parenchymal cells. *J. Cell Biol.,* 37:27−46.
16. Miller, D. L., and Gumucio, J. J. (1979): A double embedding technique for the electron microscopic analysis of the acinus. *J. Microsc.,* 115:283−288.
17. Goresky, C. A., Baeh, G. G., and Nadeau, B. E. (1973): On the uptake of materials by the intact liver. The transport and net removal of galactose. *J. Clin. Invest.,* 52:991−1009.
18. Jones, A. L., Hradek, G. T., Renston, R. H., Wong, K. Y., Karlaganis, G., and Paumgartner, G. (1980): Autoradiographic evidence for hepatic lobular concentration gradient of bile acid derivative. *Am. J. Physiol.,* 238:G233−G237.
19. LeBouton, A. V. (1968): Heterogeneity of protein metabolism between liver cells as studied by radioautography. *Curr. Mod. Biol.,* 2:111−114.
20. LeBouton, A. V. (1969): Relations and extent of the zone of intensified protein metabolism in the liver acinus. *Curr. Mod. Biol.,* 3:4−8.
21. LeBouton, A. V. (1971): Protein synthesis in the rat liver acinus after injection of actinomycin D: An autoradiographic study. *Curr. Mod. Biol.,* 3:353−358.

22. Grishaw, J. W. (1962): A morphologic study of deoxyribonucleic acid synthesis and cell proliferation in regenerating rat liver; autoradiography with thymidine-H₃. *Cancer Res.*, 22:842–849.

23. Nostrant, T. T., Miller, D. L., Appelman, H. D., and Gumucio, J. J. (1978): Acinar distribution of liver cell regeneration after selective zonal injury in the rat. *Gastroenterology*, 75:181–186.

24. Novikoff, A. B. (1959): Cell heterogeneity within the hepatic lobule of the rat (staining reactions). *J. Histochem. Cytochem.*, 7:240–244.

25. Novikoff, A. B., and Essner, E. (1960): The liver cell. Some new approaches to its study. *Am. J. Med.*, 29:102–131.

26. Sasse, D. (1975): Dynamics of liver glycogen. *Histochemistry*, 45:237–254.

27. Radzialowski, F. M., and Bousquet, W. F. (1967): Circadian rhythm in hepatic drug metabolizing activity in the rat. *Life Sci.*, 6:2545–2548.

28. Radzialowski, F. M., and Bousquet, W. F. (1968): Daily rhythmic variation in hepatic drug metabolism in the rat and mouse. *J. Pharmacol. Exp. Ther.*, 163:229–238.

29. Jori, A., DiSalle, E., and Santini, V. (1971): Daily rhythmic variation and liver drug metabolism in rats. *Biochem. Pharmacol.*, 20:2965–2969.

30. Feldmann, G., Panaud-Laurewcin, J., Crassous, J., and Benhamou, J. P. (1972): Albumin synthesis by human liver cells: Its morphological demonstration. *Gastroenterology*, 63:1036–1048.

31. Smith, M. T., Loveridge, N., Wills, E. D., and Chayen, J. (1979): The distribution of glutathione in rat liver lobule. *Biochem. J.*, 182:103–108.

32. Gooding, P. E., Chayen, J., Sawyer, B., and Slater, T. F. (1978): Cytochrome P-450 distribution in rat liver and the effect of sodium phenobarbitone administration. *Chem. Biol. Interact.*, 20:299–310.

33. Nolte, J., and Pette, D. (1972): Microphotometric determination of enzyme activity in single cells in cryostat sections. Application of the gel film-technique to microphotometry and studies on the intralobular distribution of succinate dehydrogenase and lactate dehydrogenase activities in rat liver. *J. Histochem. Cytochem.*, 20:567–576.

34. Gumucio, J. J., Balabaud, C. P., Miller, D. L., DeMason, L. J., Appelman, H. D., Stocker, T. J., and Franzblau, D. R. (1978): Bile secretion and liver cell heterogeneity in the rat. *J. Lab. Clin. Med.*, 91:350–362.

35. Gumucio, J. J., Katz, M. E., Miller, D. L., Balabaud, C.P., Greenfield, J. M., and Wagner, R. M. (1979): Bile salt transport after selective damage to acinar zone 3 hepatocytes by bromobenzene in the rat. *Toxicol. Appl. Pharmacol.*, 50:77–85.

36. Gumucio, J. J., and Katz, M. E. (1979): The acinar organization for bile salt transport. In: *The Liver: Quantitative Aspects of Structure and Function*, edited by R. Preisig and J. Bircher, pp. 179–184. Editio Cantor, Aulendorf.

37. Teutsch, H. F. (1978): Quantitative determination of glucose 6 phosphatase activity in histochemically defined zones of the liver acinus. *Histochemistry*, 58:281–288.

38. Guder, W. G., and Schmidt, U. (1976): Liver cell heterogeneity. The distribution of pyruvate kinase and phosphoenol pyruvate carboxykinase (GTP) in the liver lobule of fed and starved rats. *Hoppe Seylers Z. Physiol. Chem.*, 357:1793–1800.

39. Schmidt, U., Schmidt, H., and Guder, W. G. (1978): Liver cell heterogeneity. The distribution of fructose-biphosphatase in fed and fasted rats and in man. *Hoppe Seylers Z. Physiol. Chem.*, 359:193–198.

40. Katz, N., and Jungermann, K. (1975): Autoregulatory switch from glycolysis to gluconeogenesis in rat hepatocyte suspensions. *Hoppe Seylers Z. Physiol. Chem.*, 356:244.

41. Drochmans, P., Wanson, J-C., and Mosselmans, R. (1975): Isolation and subfractionation on Ficoll gradients of adult rat hepatocytes. *J. Cell Biol.*, 66:1–22.

42. Wanson, J-C., Drochmans, P., May, C., Penasse, W., and Popowski, A. (1975): Isolation of centrilobular and perilobular hepatocytes after phenobarbital treatment. *J. Cell Biol.*, 66:23–41.

43. Weigand, K., Otto, I., and Schopf, R. (1974): Ficoll density separation of enzymatically isolated rat liver cells. *Acta Hepatogastroenterol.*, 21:245–253.

44. Gumucio, J. J., DeMason, L., Miller, D. L., Kresoski, S. O., and Keener, M.(1978): Induction of cytochrome P-450 in a selective sub-population of hepatocytes. *Am. J. Physiol.*, 234:C102–C109.

45. Sweeney, G. D., Garfield, R. E., Jones, K. G., and Latham, A. N. (1978): Studies using sedimentation velocity on heterogeneity of size and function of hepatocytes from mature male rats. *J. Lab. Clin. Med.*, 91:432–433.

46. Walter, H., Krob, E. J., Ascher, G. S., and Seaman, G. V. F. (1973): Partition of rat liver cells in aqueous dextran-polyethylene glycol phase systems. *Exp. Cell Res.*, 82:15–26.

47. Forgren, E. (1935): Uber die rhytmik der leverfunktion, des stoffwechsels und des schlafes. *Sven. Lak Sallsk. Handl. Bd.*, 61:S.1–56.

48. Deane, H. W. (1944): A cytological study of the diurnal cycle of the liver of the mouse in relation to storage and secretion. *Anat. Rec.*, 88:39–65.

49. Corrin, B., and Aterman, K. (1968): The pattern of glycogen distribution in the liver. *Am. J. Anat.*, 122:57–72.

50. Welsh, F. A. (1972): Distribution of glycogen within the liver lobule. *J. Histochem. Cytochem.*, 20:112–115.

51. Den Otter, W., and Tuit, G. (1972): Causes of the zonal distribution of glycogen in the liver acinus after a fat-rich diet. *Anat. Rec.*, 173:325–332.

52. Babcock, M. B., and Cardell, R. R. (1974): Hepatic glycogen patterns in fasted and fed rats. *Am. J. Anat.*, 140:229–338.

53. Sasse, D., Katz, N., and Jungermann, K. (1975): Functional heterogeneity of rat liver parenchyma and of isolated hepatocytes. *FEBS Lett.*, 57:83–88.

54. Chedid, A., and Nair, V. (1972): Diurnal rhythm in endoplasmic reticulum of rat liver: Electron microscopy study. *Science*, 175:176–179.

55. Schmucker, D. L., Mooney, J. S., and Jones, A. L. (1977): Age-related changes in the hepatic endoplasmic reticulum: A quantitative analysis. *Science*, 197:1005–1007.

56. Rutenberg, A. M., and Seligman, A. M. (1955): The histochemical demonstration of acid phosphatase by a post-incubation coupling technique. *J. Histochem. Cytochem.*, 3:455–470.

57. Wachstein, M. (1959): Enzymatic histochemistry of the liver. *Gastroenterology*, 37:525–537.

58. Cramer, W., and Ludford, R. J. (1926): On the cellular mechanism of bile secretion and its relation to the Golgi apparatus of the liver cell. *J. Physiol.*, 62:74–80.

59. Biava, C. G. (1964): Studies on cholestasis: A reevaluation of the fine structure of normal bile canaliculi. *Lab. Invest.*, 13:840–864.

60. Layden, T. J., and Boyen, J. L. (1978): Influence of bile acids on bile canalicular membrane morphology and the lobular gradient in canalicular size. *Lab. Invest.*, 39:110–119.

61. Shank, R. E., Morrison, G., Cheng, C. H., Karl, I., and Schwartz, R. (1959): Cell heterogeneity within the hepatic lobule (quantitative histochemistry). *J. Histochem. Cytochem.*, 7:237–239.

62. Seligman, A. M., and Rutenberg, S. H. (1951): The histochemical demonstration of succinic dehydrogenase. *Science*, 113:317–318.

63. Schumacher, H. H. (1957): Histochemical distribution pattern of respiratory enzymes in the liver lobule. *Science*, 125:501–503.

64. Chiquoine, A. D. (1953): The distribution of glucose 6 phosphatase in the liver and kidney of the mouse. *J. Histochem. Cytochem.*, 1:429–435.

65. Wachstein, A., and Meisel, E. (1957): Histochemistry of hepatic phosphatases at a physiologic pH. *Am. J. Clin. Pathol.*, 27:13–23.

66. Katz, N., and Jungermann, K. (1976): Autoregulatory shift from fructolysis to lactate gluconeogenesis in rat hepatocyte

suspensions. The problem of metabolic zonation of liver parenchyma. *Hoppe Seylers Z. Physiol. Chem.*, 357:359–375.

67. Sasse, D., Teutsch, H. F., Katz, N., and Jungermann, K. (1979): The development of functional heterogeneity in the liver parenchyma of the golden hamster. *Anat. Embryol.*, 156:153–163.

68. Brinkmann, A., Katz, N., Sasse, D., and Jungermann, K. (1978): Increase of the gluconeogenic and decrease of the glycolytic capacity of rat liver with a change of the metabolic zonation after partial hepatectomy. *Hoppe Seylers Z. Physiol. Chem.*, 359:1561–1571.

69. Schreiber, G., Lesch, R., Weinssen, U., and Zahringer, J. (1970): The distribution of albumin synthesis throughout the liver lobule. *J. Cell Biol.*, 47:285–289.

70. Hamashima, Y., Harter, J. G., and Coons, A. H. (1964): The localization of albumin and fibrinogin in human liver cells. *J. Cell Biol.*, 20:271–279.

71. Katz, J., Bonoris, G., Okuyama, S., and Sellers, L. (1967): Albumin synthesis of perfused liver of normal and nephrotic rats. *Am. J. Physiol.*, 212:1255–1260.

72. Jensen, H., Rossing, N., Andersen, S. B., and Jarnum, S. (1967): Albumin metabolism in the nephrotic syndrome in adults. *Clin. Sci.*, 33:445–457.

73. Maurice, M., Feldmann, G., Druet, P., Laliberte, F., and Bouige, D. (1979): Immunoperoxidase localization of albumin in hepatocytes of nephrotic rats with special references to changes in the Golgi apparatus. *Lab. Invest.*, 40:39–45.

74. Ahlabo, I., and Bernard, T. (1971): Observations on peroxisomes in brown adipose tissue of the rat. *J. Histochem. Cytochem.*, 19:670–675.

75. Goldficher, S., Rohein, P. S., Edelstein, D., and Essner, E. (1971): Hypolipidemia in a mutant strain of "acatalasemic" mice. *Science.*, 173:65.

76. Inestrosa, N. C., Bronfman, M., and Leighton, F. (1979): Properties of fatty acyl-coenzyme A oxidase from rat liver, a peroxisomal flavoprotein. *Life Sci.*, 25:1127–1136.

77. Inestrosa, N. C., Bronfman, M., and Leighton, F. (1979): Detection of peroxisomal fatty acyl-coenzyme A oxidase activity. *Biochem. J.*, 182:779–788.

78. Koudstaal, J., and Hardonic, M. G. (1970): Histochemical demonstration of enzymes in rat liver during post-natal development. *Histochemistry*, 23:71–81.

79. Muller-Eberhard, U., Yam, L., Tavassolie, M., Cox, K., and Ozols, J. (1974): Immunohistochemical demonstration of cytochrome B₅ and hemopoxin in rat liver parenchymal cells using horseradish peridoxidase. *Biochem. Biophys. Res. Commun.*, 61:983–988.

80. Tavassolie, M., Ozols, J., Suyimoto, G., Cox, K. H., and Muller-Eberhard, U. (1976): Localization of cytochrome B₅ in rat organs and tissues by immunohistochemistry. *Biochem. Biophys. Res. Commun.*, 72:281–287.

81. Haugen, D. A., Van Der Hoeven, T. A., and Coon, M. J. (1975): Purified liver microsomal cytochrome P-450: Separation and characterization of multiple forms. *J. Biol. Chem.*, 250:3567–3570.

82. Greenberger, N. J., Cohen, R. B., and Isselbacher, K. J. (1965): The effect of chronic ethanol administration on liver alcohol dehydrogenase activity in the rat. *Lab. Invest.*, 14:264–271.

83. Rees, R. K., and Tarlow, M. J. (1967): The hepatotoxic action of allyl formate. *Biochem. J.*, 104:757–761.

84. Hase, T., and Brim, J. (1965): Observation of the microcirculatory architecture of the rat liver. *Anat. Rec.*, 156:157–174.

85. Miller, D. L., Zanolli, C. S., and Gumucio, J. J. (1979): Quantitative morphology of the sinusoids of the hepatic acinus. Quantimet analysis of rat liver. *Gastroenterology*, 76:965–969.

86. Koo, A., Liang, I. Y. S., and Cheng, K. K. (1975): The terminal hepatic microcirculation in the rat. *Q. J. Exp. Physiol.*, 60:261–266.

87. Burkel, W. E. and Low, F. (1966). The fine structure of rat liver sinusoids, space of Disse and associated tissue space. *Am. J. Anat.*, 118:769–784.

88. Grisham, J. W., Nopanitaya, W., Compagno, J., and Nagel, A. E. H. (1975): Scanning electron microscopy of normal rat liver; the surface structure of its cells and tissue components. *Am. J. Anat.*, 144:295–322.

89. Nopanitaya, W., Lamb, J. C., Grisham, J. W., and Carson, J. L. (1976): Effect of hepatic venous outflow obstruction on pores and fenestrations in sinusoidal endothelium. *Br. J. Exp. Pathol.* 57:604–609.

90. Montesano, R., and Nicolescu, P., (1978): Fenestrations in endothelium of rat liver sinusoids revisited by freeze-fracture. *Anat. Rec.*, 190:861–870.

91. Wisse, E. (1970): An electron microscopic study of the fenestrated endothelial lining of rat liver sinusoids. *J. Ultrastruct. Res.*, 31:125–150.

92. Goresky, C. A. (1980): Uptake in the liver: The nature of the process. In: *Liver and Biliary Tract Physiology, I,* edited by N. B. Javitt, pp. 65–101. University Park Press, Baltimore.

93. Forker, E. L., and Luxon, B. (1978): Hepatic transport kinetics and plasma disappearance curves: Distributed modeling versus conventional approach. *Am. J. Physiol.*, 235:648–660.

94. Bass, L. (1979): Current models of hepatic elimination. *Gastroenterology*, 76:1504–1505.

95. Bass, L. (1980): On the location of cellular functions in perfused organs. *J. Fluor. Biol.*, 82:347–351.

96. Kessler, M., Gornandt, L., and Lang, H. (1973): Correlation between oxygen tension in tissue and hemoglobin dissociation curve. In: *Oxygen Supply: Theoretical and Practical Aspects of Oxygen Supply and Microcirculation of Tissue,* edited by M. Kessler, pp. 156–159. University Park Press, Baltimore.

97. Sies, H. (1977): Oxygen gradients during hypoxic steady states in liver. Urate oxidase and cytochrome oxidase as intracellular O_2 indicators. *Hoppe Seylers Z. Physiol. Chem.*, 358:1021–1032.

98. Rappaport, A. M., and Hiraki, G. Y. (1958): The anatomical pattern of lesions in the liver. *Acta Anat.*, 32:126–140.

99. Quistorff, B., Chance, B., and Takeda, H. (1978): Two and three dimensional redox heterogeneity of rat liver. Effects of anoxia and alcohol on the lobular redox pattern. In: *Frontiers of Biological Energetics, Vol. 2,* edited by P. L. Dutton, J. S. Leigh, and A. Scarda, pp. 1487–1497. Academic Press, New York.

100. Goresky, C. A. (1975): The hepatic uptake process: Its implications for bilirubin transport. In: *Jaundice,* edited by C. A. Gonesky and M. M. Fisher, pp. 159–174. Plenum, New York.

101. Gumucio, J. J., Miller, D. L., Krauss, M. D., and Cutter-Zanolli, C. (1981): The transport of fluorescent compounds by hepatocytes and the resultant zonal labelling of the hepatic acinus in the rat. *Gastroenterology*, 80:639–646.

102. Staubli, W., Hess, R., and Weibel, E. R. (1969): Correlated morphometric and biochemical studies on the liver cell. II. Effects of phenobarbital on rat hepatocytes. *J. Cell Biol.*, 42:92–112.

103. Orrenius, S., Ericsson, J. L., and Ernster, L. (1965): Phenobarbital-induced synthesis of the microsomal drug-metabolizing enzyme system and its relationship to the proliferation of endoplasmic membranes. *J. Cell Biol.*, 25:627–639.

104. Haugen, D. A., and Coon, M. J. (1976): Induction of multiple forms of mouse liver cytochrome P-450. *J. Biol. Chem.*, 251:1817–1827.

105. Harkness, R. D. (1957): Regeneration of liver. *Br. Med. Bull.*, 13:87–93.

106. Wienbreu, K. (1959): Regeneration of liver. *Gastroenterology*, 37:657–668.

107. Leevy, C. M., Hollister, R. M., Schmid, R., MacDonald, R. A., and Davidson, C. S. (1959): Liver regeneration in experimental carbon tetrachloride intoxication. *Proc. Soc. Exp. Biol. Med.*, 102:672–675.

108. MacDonald, R. A., Schmid, R., and Mallory, G. K. (1960): Regeneration in fatty liver and cirrhosis. Autoradiographic study using titrated thymidine. *Arch. Pathol.*, 69:175–180.

109. MacDonald, R. A., and Pechet, G. (1961): Liver cell regeneration due to biliary obstruction. *Arch. Pathol.*, 72:133–141.

110. LaAne, J. S., Schenken, J. R., and Kuker, L. H. (1944): Phosphorus poisoning: A report of sixteen cases with repeated liver biopsies in a recovered case. *Am. J. Med. Sci.*, 208:223–224.

111. Seawright, A. A., and Hardlicker, J. (1972): The effect of prior

dosing with phenobarbitone and diethylamino ethyl diphenyl-propylacetate (SKF 525-A) on the toxicity and liver lesion caused by ngaione in the mouse. *Br. J. Exp. Pathol.,* 52: 242–252.

112. Davidson, D. G. D., and Eastham, W. N. (1966): Acute liver necrosis following overdose of paracetamol. *Br. Med. J.,* 2:506–507.

113. Rose, P. G. (1969): Paracetamol overdose and liver damage. *Br. Med. J.,* 1:361–362.

114. Clark, R., Thompson, R. P. H., and Borirakchanyavat, V. (1973): Hepatic damage and death from overdose of paracetamol. *Lancet,* 1:66–70.

115. Koch-Weser, D., De la Huerga, J., Yesinick, D., and Popper, H. (1953): Hepatic necrosis due to bromobenzene as an example of conditioned amino acid deficiency. *Metabolism,* 2:248–260.

116. Mitchell, J., Reid, W., Christie, W., Moskowitz, J., Krishna, G., and Brodie, B. (1971): Bromobenzene-induced hepatic necrosis: Species difference and protection by SKF 525-A. *Res. Commun. Chem. Pathol. Pharmacol.,* 2:877–888.

117. Reid, W., Christie, B., Kirshna, G., Mitchell, J., Moscowitz, J., and Brodie, B. (1971): Bromobenzene metabolism and hepatic necrosis. *Pharmacology,* 6:41–55.

118. Oberling, C., and Rouiller, C. (1967): Les effects de l'intoxication aigue au tetrachlorure de carbone sur le foie de rat. Etude au microscope electronique. *Ann. Anat. Pathol.,* 1:401–427.

119. Rouiller, C. H. (1964): Experimental toxic injury of the liver. In: *The Liver, Vol. 2,* edited by C. H. Rouiller, p. 335. Academic Press, New York.

120. Zimmerman, H. (1978): Anesthetic agents. In: *Hepatotoxicity,* edited by H. J. Zimmerman, p. 370. Appleton-Century-Crofts, New York.

121. Mitchell, J. R., Thorgursson, S. S., and Potter, W. Z. (1974): Acetaminophen-induced hepatic injury: Protective role of glutathione in man and rationale of therapy. *Clin. Pharm. Ther.,* 16:676–684.

122. Mitchell, J. R., and Jollow, D. J. (1975): Metabolic activation of drugs to toxic substances. *Gastroenterology,* 68:392–410.

123. Black, M. (1980): Acetaminophen hepatotoxicity. *Gastroenterology,* 78:382–392.

124. Wilson, J. W. (1958): Hepatic structure in relation to function. In: *Liver Function. A Symposium on Approaches to the Quantitative Description of Liver Function,* edited by R. W. Brauer, pp. 175–197. Am. Inst. Biol. Sci., Washington, D.C.

The Liver: Biology and Pathobiology, edited by
I. Arias, H. Popper, D. Schachter, and D. A. Shafritz.
Raven Press, New York © 1982.

Chapter 39

Hepatic Nerve Function

Mark I. Friedman

Given the variety of bodily processes in which the liver plays a part, it is not surprising that the innervation of this organ serves a number of different functions. This chapter reviews the current state of knowledge of these hepatic nerve functions. First, a brief overview of the neuroanatomy of the liver, with special emphasis on its intrinsic innervation, is given. Then, efferent influences on hepatic functions are described, followed by a review of the evidence for various sensory capacities of hepatic nerves. Finally, some general features of hepatic nerve action are discussed.

All the relevant literature is not cited, nor are all aspects of hepatic nerve function covered. Where possible, review articles are cited that deal with various areas of research, and the most recent papers in a series are referenced. Details and a more complete bibliography are presented in two recent reviews covering efferent (1) and afferent (2) functions of the hepatic nerve supply.

ANATOMY

Extrinsic Innervation

Branches of the vagus, splanchnic, and sometimes phrenic nerves enter the liver primarily in association with blood vessels and the bile duct (3). Sympathetic and parasympathetic nerves form two separate but intercommunicating plexuses. The anterior plexus, which surrounds the hepatic artery, is composed of fibers originating from the celiac ganglia and anterior vagus. Ramifications of the right celiac ganglion and posterior vagus form the posterior plexus, which is located behind the hepatic portal vein and bile duct. Several neural inputs to the liver bypass the plexuses, traveling by way of the hepatic vein (4) or originating from the anterior vagus (3) and gall bladder (5). There are a number of species differences in the extrinsic innervation of the liver. The phrenic nerves do not always supply the liver in humans and cats; whereas both vagal trunks send branches to the liver in humans, cats, and dogs, only the anterior vagus provides a projection to the liver in rats.

Intrinsic Innervation

Most intrinsic nerves of the liver also are associated with the vascular system. Numerous fibers ramify with major vessels and form plexuses in the adventitia of arterioles and venules. Branches extending from there to the media terminate on smooth muscle fibers, suggesting that these nerves may modulate vasomotor function (3). Studies with the transmission electron microscope have found nerve fibers associated with endothelial cells at terminal branches of the hepatic artery and with hepatocytes of the portal lamina (6). Along with fibers running through and terminating near the spaces of Disse (7), neurons have been found terminating on Kuppfer cells (7) and the fat-storing cells of Ito (6).

The gall bladder is reported to receive sympathetic and parasympathetic input by nerves associated with the hepatic artery, cystic duct, and cystic artery.

Within the wall of the gall bladder is an extensive network of five interconnecting plexuses (8). Tsai (9), working with human and dog liver, has described club-shaped and splayed, glomerular nerve endings in association with the bile ducts. Innervation of the bile ducts has been described in the rat (10); others (11), however, have found only a sparse innervation that appeared to be associated more closely with blood vessels than with the biliary system.

Despite an early controversy beginning in the late 19th century concerning the existence of an intralobular innervation, recent anatomic studies using more specific and sensitive staining techniques have demonstrated a neural supply to hepatic parenchymal cells. There are a number of descriptions of nerve fibers coursing between, circumscribing, and apparently terminating on hepatocytes (2). On occasion, neurons appear to penetrate the plasma membrane of parenchymal cells. More frequently, nerves are found passing through or terminating within indentations in the parenchymal cells. Such terminals are not encapsulated and, although they contain clear and dense-core vesicles, apposed membrane densifications indicative of neurochemical synapses have not been observed. The intralobular innervation of liver is best described, depending on the species, as sparse to moderate. Tight electrical coupling between hepatocytes, however, may obviate the need for extensive innervation; indeed, in tree shrew livers, the greatest number of nerve fibers are found where gap junctions are rare (7). Similarly, in rat liver which shows relatively few intralobular neurons, gap junctions are numerous (11).

Extent and distribution of intrahepatic adrenergic and cholinergic nerves differ considerably between species. In all species studied, adrenergic nerves, as revealed by fluorescence microscopy, innervate hepatic blood vessels, including the portal vein and branches of hepatic arteries and sinusoids. Primates, including the tree shrew, rhesus monkey, and human, have a rich intralobular catecholaminergic innervation in contrast to rats, in which it appears to be relatively sparse (11). Adrenergic nerves have been found to innervate the spaces of Disse, parenchymal cells, and Kuppfer cells. Evidence for an extensive sympathetic innervation of primate liver is substantial. In the tree shrew, chemical sympathectomy eliminates hepatic nerve fibers shown by fluorescence and electron microscopy; as shown by autoradiography, hepatic nerve fibers take up large amounts of exogenous ^{3}H-norepinephrine (7). Nobin et al. (12) have studied the catecholaminergic innervation of the liver in humans and rhesus monkey. A dense network of monoamine-containing neurons in close contact with blood vessels and hepatocytes was found by Falck-Hillarp fluorescence microscopy. Electron microscopy of tissue incubated with 5-hydroxydopamine to "label" catechol-amine-containing neurons confirmed the presence of sympathetic fibers associated with blood vessels and hepatocytes. Finally, biochemical determinations showed a high concentration of norepinephrine in liver tissue, with that in human liver being the highest found in any species examined thus far.

Evidence for an extensive cholinergic innervation of liver is less clear. Recent studies (7) of primate livers suggest that the intralobular innervation is primarily, if not exclusively, monoaminergic. In an early study, Sutherland (10) found intralobular cholinesterase-positive cells in monkeys; however, treatment of tissue to reduce nonspecific reactions eliminated the structures initially identified as intralobular fibers. Suppression of nonspecific reactions in histochemical studies of the hepatic cholinergic innervation appears necessary since nonspecific butyrylcholinesterase activity is found in a variety of hepatic structures, including membranes of cells forming the bile cannaliculi and lining the sinusoids, as well as in connective tissue. Thus, whereas previous studies (10,13) described an extensive intralobular cholinergic plexus in the rat, Reilly et al. (11) failed to find such innervation when nonspecific activity was suppressed. Consistent with earlier studies, however, Reilly and colleagues (11) found some cholinergic-positive nerve fibers in association with the vessels in the portal space. In addition, they observed fibers that were not contiguous with the vessels which, in some cases, ran to adjacent parenchymal cells where they terminated as end bulbs. So far, of the species studied, only the guinea pig has significant intralobular cholinergic nerves, as demonstrated by histochemical methods in which nonspecific activity was suppressed (14).

Few direct anatomic observations concern relative contributions of efferent and afferent fibers to the hepatic nerve supply. Dense-core vesicles, as well as histofluorescent and histochemical reactions reflecting the presence of catecholamines and acetylcholinesterase activity, indicate effector neurons. However, microvesicles have been found in a number of purely sensory structures, and acetylcholinesterase reactions have been seen in the chemoreceptive glomus cells of the carotid body (2). Morphologic evidence for afferent nerve endings in the liver rests largely on the demonstration of degenerated hepatic neurons following nerve sections that would spare postganglionic efferents (9). Nerve fibrils associated with endothelial cells in the intima of hepatic veins in man and guinea pigs have been thought to be sensory nerve endings by virtue of their location and Tsai (9) has described several types of intralobular nerve endings in man and dog that resemble known sensory processes. One indication that the sensory nerve supply to the liver may be substantial stems from degeneration studies in which it was estimated that up to 90% of fibers in the abdominal vagus and about 50% of sympathetic fibers in the cat splanchnic nerve are afferent processes (2).

Several studies have examined the effects of liver injury on hepatic nerves. Hepatic nerves found in association with the vasculature degenerate in dogs made ascitic by constriction of the thoracic vena cava (4). Deterioration of nerve fibers in the peripheral branches of the portal vein and hepatic artery appeared to follow that in the major vessels. Nerve degeneration in livers from cirrhotic humans has been reported as well; here, nerve fibers showing irregularities were seen in the hepatic vein and near the hilus (4). Ungvary and his colleagues have examined the consequences of partial hepatectomy (15) or bile duct ligation (14) on adrenergic and cholinergic innervation of the liver by histochemical methods. Fluorescence microscopy showed that monoaminergic innervation of portal vein branches in regenerating liver of partially hepatectomized rats can be seen as early as 7 days after hepatectomy, although not until 6 weeks following removal of the major lobes did the regenerated tissue contain a nearly full complement of nerve fibers showing intense fluorescence and distinct varicosities. Ligation of the common bile duct in guinea pigs resulted in a disappearance 4 days later of catecholamine-containing and acetylcholinesterase-positive nerves normally found, respectively, in association with the hepatic vasculature and bile ducts. Two weeks following ligation, livers were fibrotic, and innervation again was demonstrable in the expanded connective tissues.

EFFERENT FUNCTIONS

Hemodynamics

Of the hemodynamic effects of hepatic efferent nerve activity, those on the hepatic resistance vessels are the longest known and best studied. As early as 1910, Burton-Opitz (16) showed that electrical stimulation of the nerve bundle that surrounds the hepatic artery in dogs reduced arterial blood flow conspicuously (17). This decreased conductance is frequently followed, upon termination of stimulation, by a brief period of hyperemia. Stimulation of the hepatic nerves also increased vascular resistance in the portal vein, which is reflected in an increase in portal pressure with no reduction in flow (18). The response of portal resistance vessels to stimulation is less than that seen in the hepatic artery.

These changes in vascular resistance are under α-adrenergic control. Infusions of norepinephrine also decrease hepatic artery conductance (19). Greenway and Stark (26) have shown that the response to nerve stimulation is prevented by α-receptor blockade (17). Although hepatic resistance vessels do not appear to

be under tonic sympathetic tone, as acute nerve section produces no change in blood flow, it is not clear whether some critical hepatic nerves were left intact in denervation studies (1). Inasmuch as stimulation of the vagus did not change hepatic blood flow grossly (20), cholinergic mechanisms do not appear to be involved in the control of hepatic vascular tone. β-Adrenergic nerves, however, may play a part; during α-receptor blockade, nerve stimulation produces a slight dilation in the hepatic artery, which can be prevented in turn by β-blockade (21).

In cats, nerve stimulation produces only a transitory decrease in arterial conductance. During stimulation, blood flow increases and by 4 to 5 min returns to about 80% of normal (18,20). A similar escape effect of smaller magnitude is seen with portal constriction during stimulation. It is not clear how blood flow is restored, despite continuing stimulation, although nerve fatigue, redistribution of blood flow, and accumulation of metabolites appear to have been ruled out (1). Relaxation of smooth muscle due to an accumulation of intracellular sodium has been proposed as an alternative mechanism (1). As Lautt (1) has pointed out, the phenomenon of vascular escape may help to protect the liver from hypoxia when blood flow is restricted because of massive sympathetic activation. Consistent with this hypothesis are the findings that occlusion of the carotid arteries, which would be expected to provoke a dramatic sympathetic response, increases hepatic arterial resistance followed by a partial vascular escape (20). In addition, although blood flow does not recover during nerve stimulation in dogs (16), it is restored following the decline in response to hemorrhage or denervation of the sinoaortic region (22).

Hepatic blood volume decreased markedly (by 50%) in response to hepatic nerve stimulation or infusion of physiologic quantities of catecholamines (18,23). The effect of nerve stimulation on capacitance appears independent of that on vascular resistance since it persists following vascular escape in cats. Approximately 6% of total blood volume in dogs and cats can be mobilized by activation of hepatic nerves; the response is under α-adrenergic control (17).

Changes in hepatic nerve activity appear to have little functional effect on hepatic fluid exchange or diffusion parameters (1). The microcirculation of the liver, however, is not unaffected by changes in nerve activity. Using a transillumination technique and a videomicroscope, Koo and Liang (24) and their associates have obtained substantial evidence that opening and closing of rat liver sinusoids is under neural control. Briefly, they found that stimulation of the vagus increased the caliber of open sinusoids and dilated previously closed ones. Although blood flow velocity increased in individual sinusoids, no change in total flow was seen, a finding consistent with earlier observations (17). Intraportal infusions of acetylcholine or cholinergic agonists also produced dilation of sinusoids, as did the anticholinesterase physostigmine. Conversely, bilateral section of the vagus or injection of the cholinergic blocker atropine constricted sinusoids. These findings indicate that parasympathetic hepatic nerves exert a dilator tone on liver sinusoids. Sympathetic innervation may have the opposite function since intraportal injections of norepinephrine or hemorrhage constrict hepatic sinusoids.

Glucose Metabolism

The neural control of hepatic glucose metabolism is a classic area of investigation that dates back to Claude Bernard, who attributed the hyperglycemia observed after puncture of the fourth ventricle to activity in the splanchnic nerves. Since then, a great deal has been learned about this neural control; most of this knowledge has been obtained from studies in which hepatic nerves were stimulated directly.

It has long been known that splanchnic stimulation produces hyperglycemia (25). Such stimulation, however, may affect the release of glucose through secretion of epinephrine and glucagon as well as by direct actions on hepatocytes. Therefore, only studies in which specific hepatic nerves are stimulated speak directly to the question of the neural influence on hepatic glucose balance. Here, too, care must be taken, since activation of nerve branches from the anterior plexus to the pancreas also contributes to the hyperglycemia produced by periarterial nerve bundle stimulation (26). Nevertheless, there is evidence that activation of the hepatic sympathetic innervation mobilizes glucose from the liver in a variety of species.

Stimulation of the splanchnic nerves in calves, dogs, and cats results in a marked hyperglycemia that is dependent on the integrity of the hepatic innervation (27). In experiments with cats in which activation of pancreatic branches from the anterior plexus was prevented, stimulation of the periarterial hepatic nerve bundle increased hepatic glucose output rapidly. In an experiment that perhaps most clearly rules out any hormonal contribution to neurally mediated hepatic glucose release, Seydoux et al. (28) stimulated the perivascular nerve bundles in mouse liver that was perfused *in situ* with no recirculation of the medium. The authors found a doubling of glucose output within 5 min following stimulation. Finally, in patients operated for gallstones, Nobin et al. (29) observed elevated plasma glucose levels following electrical stimulation of the periarterial hepatic nerve bundle.

In three of the species studied, neural activation of hepatic glucose mobilization appears to be mediated via α-adrenergic receptors. Portal vein infusions of phentolamine, an α-receptor blocker, prevented the release of glucose in cats in response to nerve stimulation (30). In rabbits, α-blockade prevented hyperglycemia following splanchnic nerve stimulation (31). In contrast, β-receptors may mediate hepatic glucose production in the toad (32) and dog (33). In the experiments of Seydoux et al. (42), β-receptor blockade slightly attenuated the increased glucose output in mouse liver during stimulation, whereas the effect of α-blockade was more pronounced. Atropine had no effect, suggesting that parasympathetic nerves play no part in the response. In addition, α-receptor blockade was more effective in preventing increased glucose mobilization seen in response to infusions of norepinephrine or epinephrine.

The increased efflux of glucose from liver in response to nerve stimulation results from glycogenolysis (34); the biochemical basis for the glycogenolytic effect of nerve stimulation in rabbits has been described in a series of studies by Shimazu and Amakawa (35). Briefly, splanchnic nerve stimulation increased the activity of glycogen phosphorylase and glucose-6-phosphatase; adrenalectomy or pancreatectomy did not interfere with these effects. The increase in phosphorylase appeared to occur indirectly as a result of inhibition of phosphorylase phosphatase, which converts phosphorylase to its inactive form; indeed, stimulation increased the amount of the active enzyme from one-fourth to three-fourths of total hepatic phosphorylase. Proost et al. (31), however, failed to observe inhibition of phosphorylase phosphatase in rabbits after splanchnic nerve stimulation, a finding that raised doubts about the mechanism of phosphorylase activation. Nevertheless, in the Shimazu and Amakawa studies, the increase in phosphorylase activity and inactivation of the phosphatase occurred without a rise in cyclic AMP or activation of phosphorylase kinase. The glycogenolytic response to nerve stimulation was thus different from that produced with catecholamine infusions, which produced a rise in cyclic AMP, an activation of the protein kinase, a slower conversion of phosphorylase to its active form, and no change in glucose-6-phosphate.

Hepatic nerves responsible for mobilizing glucose appear to be recruited during physiologic stress. Decreased blood pressure increased firing rates of hepatic nerves in the toad (32). Lautt and Côte (36) showed that selective hepatic sympathectomy produced by infusions of the neurotoxin 6-hydroxydopamine reduced hyperglycemia seen 80 min and longer after laparotomy in anesthetized, fed rats and prevented the early glycemic response to surgery in fasted animals. Adrenalectomy, however, prevented the long-term hyperglycemia in fed animals and had no effect on the response to laparotomy in fasted rats. These findings indicate that stages in the glycemic response to stress may be under differential control by the adrenals and intrahepatic nerves. Injections of 2-deoxyglucose (2-DG), a glucose analog that inhibits glycolysis, produce a counterregulatory sympathetic discharge and hyperglycemia. Browdows et al. (37) have found that this glycemic response, while attenuated compared to normal subjects, is present in adrenalectomized men, suggesting participation of intrahepatic nerves. The failure to observe a statistically significant increase in systemic plasma glucagon levels after 2-DG in the adrenalectomized subjects, despite their marked glycemic response following infusions of glucagon, indicated that glucagon probably was not responsible for the hyperglycemia after 2-DG administration. Subtle changes in portal vein glucagon levels or glucagon/insulin ratios could not be ruled out, however. Thus, while the above studies indicate that changes in hepatic nerve activity may participate in the sympathetic response to stress in man and other species, the extent of this involvement and the role of these nerves under more physiologic conditions remain to be determined.

In contrast to the hepatic sympathetic nerve supply, which appears to function in the mobilization of glucose from the liver, parasympathetic input to the liver appears to promote hepatic glucose uptake. Shimazu (38) and his associates have conducted several studies on the effects of vagus nerve stimulation on hepatic glucose metabolism. Electrical stimulation of the vagus in rabbits increased hepatic glycogen synthetase activity that was nearly maximal by 5 min after the start of stimulation. Vagal stimulation decreased slightly blood glucose levels and substantially the concentration of a previously injected radioactive glucose tracer. Incorporation of radioactive glucose into glycogen increased during vagal stimulation, as did hepatic glycogen levels when glucose was also injected. Vagus nerve stimulation appeared to accelerate glycogen biosynthesis by creating a ''pull'' on glycogen precursors rather than increasing the supply of substrate (38), as evidenced by the decrease observed in liver UDPG and glucose-6-phosphatase. Experiments showing that glycogen synthetase activity increased more slowly following insulin injection than after vagal stimulation and that the effects of stimulation described above occurred in pancreatectomized rabbits indicated that a neurogenic insulin release was not responsible for changes in glucose metabolism induced by nerve stimulation. Comparable findings have been reported by Lautt and Wong (26). Using cats with hepatic chemical sympathectomies, these authors found that stimulation of the periarterial parasympathetic nerves resulted in a pronounced and rapid reduction in hepatic glucose output, even though the branch from the stimulated nerves to the pancreas was ligated.

Shimazu and his associates (48) have also examined the effects of chemical and electrical stimulation of the hypothalamus on hepatic glucose metabolism. Their findings are consistent with a sympathetic control of glucose output and a parasympathetic control of glucose uptake. They note that the effects they describe, however, may have been due to altered adrenal and pancreatic hormone secretion (39). Perhaps the most compelling demonstration of a direct central control over hepatic glucose metabolism stems from the work of Szabo and Szabo (40). Carotid but not jugular injections of 500 μm insulin conspicuously decreased blood glucose levels of normal and diabetic rats. This hypoglycemia occurred even when nondiabetic rats were pancreatectomized and eviscerated and was attenuated when rats were functionally hepatectomized by ligation of the hepatic vasculature, suggesting that a decrease in hepatic glucose output was responsible for the drop in blood sugar following carotid insulin injections. Cervical vagotomy and peripheral injections of atropine attenuated the hypoglycemic effect of insulin, whereas it was abolished by intracarotid injection of atropine. Administration of adrenergic blockers or epinephrine had no effect. The authors concluded that the mechanism responsible for the hypoglycemic effect of carotid insulin is cholinergic (39). This conclusion is consistent with the finding that parasympathetic activation decreases hepatic glucose output (26).

Biliary Function

Little can be said about the direct neural control of the biliary system, since there have been few attempts to specifically stimulate or cut hepatic nerves. Without such specific nerve manipulations, findings are difficult to interpret, since humoral factors or changes in local hydraulic pressure can affect the biliary system. Vagal stimulation, for example, provokes the release of gut and pancreatic hormones as well as gastric acid, which may in turn alter biliary function. Therefore, I touch upon only several reported observations; for more details, the reader is referred to Lautt (1).

Vagus nerve stimulation has been reported to increase bile flow and result in contraction of the gall bladder. Parasympathetic activation also contracted the cholecystocytic and choledochoduodenal sphincters. This latter effect is questionable; when gastric acid is prevented from reaching the duodenum, stimulation of the hepatic and celiac branches of the vagus had no effect (41). Stimulation of the sympathetic nerves, usually the splanchnics, produced a relaxation of the gall bladder and contraction of the sphincters mentioned above. α-Receptors may mediate a weak sympathetic contraction of the gall bladder and biliary sphincters, whereas relaxation of the gall bladder and sphincters may be under β-receptor control.

SENSORY FUNCTIONS

Osmoreceptors

Haberich (52) was the first to suggest that osmoreceptors sensitive to changes in the osmolarity of blood reside in the liver or its portal vessels (42). He and his colleagues showed initially that portal vein infusions of water, which were estimated to reduce plasma osmolarity by 1%, rapidly increased urine flow in conscious rats, and that similar infusions into the vena cava had no significant effect unless a longer infusion period was used (42). In a subsequent experiment (43) to further control the systemic effects of portal vein infusions, they used a double infusion technique in which water was infused into the portal vein while a twice isotonic saline solution was infused simultaneously into the vena cava. Again a diuresis was observed; when the infusates were switched so that saline was infused intraportally, an antidiuresis was seen. Antidiuresis also was observed if mannitol or glucose solutions were infused into the portal vein, suggesting that the alteration in osmolarity, rather than electrolyte concentration, was critical.

Although cross-circulation experiments failed to demonstrate a humoral factor in the diuretic response to hypotonic infusions into the portal vein, transfusion of blood from osmotically stimulated animals caused antidiuresis (44). The suggestion that antidiuretic hormone (ADH) may mediate this antidiuretic response has recently been confirmed by experiments in conscious dogs showing increased plasma ADH levels following intraportal infusions of hypertonic saline that did not raise systemic plasma osmolarity (45). The ADH response occurred within 2 min after the start of infusions; the magnitude was directly related to the concentration of the saline perfusate.

Niijima (46) has provided electrophysiologic evidence for hepatic osmoreceptors; the findings, however, are not unequivocal. In perfused guinea pig livers, the afferent discharge rate of units in nerve filaments dissected from the hepatic vagus showed a direct positive relationship to the concentration of sodium chloride in the perfusate. Addition of hyperosmotic sugars to the perfusate also increased afferent discharge rates and did so to the same degree as sodium chloride added in twice the osmotic concentration. It is not clear, therefore, whether the units that responded were specifically or quantitatively sensitive to osmotic perturbations. In a subsequent study (47), however, units in the hepatic vagus from isolated rat livers were found that responded in a regular fashion to changed concentrations of sodium chloride in the perfusion medium but altered discharge rate only slightly when equiosmotic urea or glucose was added. This relative lack of response was attributed to the diffusibility of urea and glucose, although the findings raise questions of whether the nerve units were responding to sodium ions or to their osmotic properties.

That the hepatic vagus may be involved in transmitting information about changes in osmolarity is further supported by findings showing that section of this nerve abolishes the diuretic and antidiuretic responses in the double infusion paradigm described above (48). Also, in a recent paper, Rogers and his associates (49) reported that right cervical vagotomy eliminated the response of the thalamic and pontine units to portal infusions of hypertonic solutions. Sympathetic nerves may also be involved in the antidiuretic response to portal infusions of hypertonic saline, inasmuch as section of the dorsal roots attenuates the response (50).

The existence of hepatic osmoreceptors in dogs is controversial. Lydtin (51) has found that hypotonic saline given either orally or into the portal vein produces a greater diuresis than peripheral vein infusions, whereas others (52) have been unable to replicate these results. In man, evidence for hepatic osmoreceptors rests on the finding that intragastric infusions of water produce a much greater diuresis (and cutaneous water loss) than does intravenous administration of fluids (42). Others reported similar findings (2). One group compared oral and intravenous routes of administration, and failed to observe any differences in diuresis (53).

Sodium Receptors

Experiments suggest the existence of sodium receptors in the liver or its vasculature which are sensitive to changes in the concentration of the ion independent of its osmotic properties. Portal vein infusions of hypertonic saline (5 to 6%) increased sodium excretion more than comparable femoral vein infusions in anesthetized dogs (54) and cats (55). Because this difference in route of administration was not seen with isosmotic solutions of sucrose or erythritol, the natriuresis following saline appeared to be related specifically to the sodium chloride content rather than to its osmotic properties. In contrast, there are several reported failures to find increased sodium excretion following portal infusions of hypertonic saline (52). Although the use of high infusion rates or a variable end point method of calculating excretion may account for the discrepant findings in two of these experiments (55), it cannot account for the failure to confirm found by Kapteina et al. (56). The basis for these contradictory results has not been established; however, one possibility lies in the fact that anesthetized animals were used in those studies in which evidence for a hepatic sodium receptor was found; conscious dogs were employed in those experiments in which sodium excretion did not increase after portal infusions of hypertonic saline. It is not clear what role hepatic sodium receptors may play under physiologic conditions, inasmuch as their influence is unmasked only in anesthetized animals.

The control of natriuresis by the liver may be mediated by neural or humoral mechanisms. Bilateral cervical vagotomy eliminates increased sodium excretion in cats in response to intraportal infusions of hypertonic saline (55). In dogs, intravenous administration of a globular protein, isolated and partially purified from a concentrated liver perfusate, produces a natriuretic response (54).

Sodium excretion associated with isotonic saline loading also may be mediated in part by a hepatic mechanism. Dogs with portacaval shunts (57) and partially hepatectomized rats (58) show a diminished natriuresis following isotonic saline infusions. Perlmutt et al. (58) have provided more direct evidence for a role of the liver in this response by comparing the effects of portal and caval infusions of isotonic saline. Portal vein infusions produced a greater and specific sodium excretion, which appeared to be independent of any osmotic effects of the infusate since isosmotic glucose had no effect on natriuresis. Unlike the response to hypertonic saline infusions, vagotomy had no effect on the natriuresis following normal saline, a finding that was interpreted to suggest the role of a humoral factor.

Electrophysiologic studies provide the most direct support for hepatic sodium receptors. Andrews and Orbach (76) have found afferent hepatic nerves in rabbits that alter firing rates in response to changes in the sodium chloride concentration of the perfusion medium. The nerves appeared to respond to variations in ion concentrations, rather than osmolarity, because the discharge rate did not change in response to glucose, mannitol, or the varied water content of the perfusate. Schmitt (61), recording from single units in the rat hypothalamus, zona incerta, and ventral thalamus, has found neurons that alter firing rates in response to brief (5 sec) intraportal infusions of hypertonic, but not isotonic, saline. Jugular infusions had no effect, nor did injections of equiosmotic glucose or sucrose, suggesting that the consequences of hepatic infusions were specific to the liver as well as to the alteration in ionic concentration. In addition, sympathetic and parasympathetic involvement in the central effects of portal injections of sodium chloride were suggested by the observations that section of the splanchnic nerves or spinal cord at T5 abolished the response, whereas it was enhanced by vagotomy. More recently, units in the thalamus and pontine parabrachial nucleus have been found that respond to intraportal sodium chloride and choline chloride but not other equiosmotic solutions (49).

Baroreceptors

Alterations in portal venous pressure change urine flow. Ohm and Haberich (62) decreased portal pres-

sure in rats by occluding the mesenteric and celiac arteries and increased it by constricting the portal vein. Raised portal blood pressure caused anuria followed by antidiuresis, whereas a decrease was accompanied by increased urine flow. Liang (63), using dogs, observed an antidiuretic response following only large increases in portal pressure exceeding 15 cm H_2O and an increase in urine output when portal pressure was raised by less than 15 cm H_2O. These responses were abolished by local anesthetics applied to the renal neural plexus or pedicle, suggesting that the efferent limb of the reflex was neural.

Electrophysiologic studies provide more direct evidence for receptors that respond to changes in blood pressure in the hepatic bed. Liver congestion altered afferent discharge rate of hepatic nerves in dogs both *in vivo* and in a perfused liver preparation (64). In addition, Niijima (65) has recorded from nerve filaments in the splanchnic nerve of perfused guinea pig livers and found units that altered firing rates as a function of the perfusion pressure. A stop-flow method showed that the responding nerves were sensitive to changes in pressure and not in volume. Local stimulation of the liver or portal vein also increased firing of afferents; in *in vivo* studies using rabbits, the time course of nerve activity was correlated with changes in portal venous pressure.

Metabolic Receptors

Much of the evidence that hepatic receptors are sensitive to changes in liver metabolism has come from studies on the hepatic control of feeding behavior. Russek (67) was the first to suggest that receptors in the liver monitor changes in metabolism that may signal hunger and satiety. In early studies, the duration and degree of anorexia produced by intraperitoneal or intraportal injections of glucose or various drugs was highly correlated with the uptake of glucose into liver and the hepatic concentration of reducing sugars. In subsequent studies, intraportal infusions of glucose were more effective than jugular infusions in decreasing food intake of previously fasted dogs. Several studies failed to reveal any special effect of portal vein infusions of glucose on food intake (2). Given the many procedural differences between those experiments showing and those not showing the satiating effects of portal glucose infusions, the discrepancies are difficult to resolve; more systematic investigations are needed. To this end, Russek et al. (66) have shown that infusions of sufficiently large amounts of glucose into the portal but not jugular vein produces anorexia in dogs tested using an experimental paradigm in which portal vein infusions of smaller amounts of glucose were previously found to be ineffective (68).

In other behavioral studies, attempts have been made to increase food intake in animals by altering hepatic metabolism. Intraportal injections of 2-DG, which causes hunger in man and animals, were more effective than jugular injections in stimulating eating in rabbits (69) and rats (70), although there is one reported failure to observe this difference in route of administration (71). Several attempts to establish a hepatic site of action of 2-DG (2), however, have not been clear-cut; for example, vagotomy eliminated the special effectiveness of the portal infusions, but no data are presented to show the effects of nerve section on eating following jugular infusions of the analog (69). In addition, because 2-DG disrupts cerebral metabolism, portal injections may be less debilitating than jugular injections, since less of the analog reaches the brain. Thus a greater willingness to eat after portal injections of 2-DG may reflect less malaise.

It is not yet clear which changes in liver metabolism constitute a signal or signals detected by hepatic receptors. Although the effects of drugs or portal infusions of glucose and 2-DG have been interpreted as evidence for hepatic "glucoreceptors" (that is, neural receptors activated by changes in glucose metabolism), the drugs used have a number of actions besides those on glucose metabolism; the metabolic impact of glucose infusions may not be restricted to glycolytic pathways. Studies examining the role of the liver in eating induced by injections of insulin have indicated that other hepatic fuels besides glucose also may be satiating. Here, jugular infusions of fructose, a hexose utilized readily by the liver but not by the brain, inhibited increased food intake during insulin hypoglycemia, whereas infusions of β-hydroxybutyrate, a metabolic fuel oxidized by brain but not by liver, was ineffective or less effective, depending on the concentration used (72,73). In subsequent studies, fructose did not reduce insulin-induced eating in animals with the hepatic branch of the vagus nerve cut, suggesting that the hexose was acting in the liver to decrease eating (74).

Electrophysiologic experiments, which provide the most direct evidence for metabolic receptors, also indicate that the receptors may be sensitive to different metabolic substrates. Niijima (75), using an isolated guinea pig liver preparation, found nerve units in the hepatic vagus that decreased firing rates when glucose, but not other sugars, was added to the perfusion medium. Recordings *in situ* revealed units that responded following intravenous infusions of glucose as well as glucose-6-phosphate, fructose-6-phosphate, and ATP. Schmitt (61) found units also in the hypothalamus of rats that responded following portal injections of glucose but not of an isosmotic solution of sucrose. Andrews and Orbach (76), who failed to find nerve responses from isolated perfused rabbit livers following addition of glucose to the perfusate, have recorded from populations of hepatic nerves that in-

creased firing rates when long-chain fatty acids were added (77).

Experiments on the role of the liver in gastric function provide perhaps the most convincing functional evidence for hepatic affectors responding to changes in metabolism. Portal vein injections of 2-DG in doses that were ineffective when given systemically increased gastric acid secretion in cats with intercollicular brainstem transections (78). Because injections of 2-DG directly into the left vertebral artery provoked a full-blown secretory response, different populations of receptors were suggested. In other studies, infusions of fructose in concentrations that did not raise blood glucose levels, blocked insulin-induced gastric acid secretion and motility, provided the infusions started prior to the onset of gastric activity (59). Portal vein infusions of fructose were more effective than jugular infusions, and section of the hepatic branch of the vagus eliminated the suppressive effects of fructose, but not of glucose, injections. Comparable findings have been reported (79) when the activity of the gastric vagus is monitored during insulin hypoglycemia. Portal vein and carotid artery injections of glucose decreased nerve activity, whereas jugular infusions had no effect. Section of the hepatic vagus eliminated the effects of portal infusions.

GENERAL FEATURES OF HEPATIC NERVE FUNCTION AND CLINICAL IMPLICATIONS

The function of hepatic efferent and afferent nerves, or the processes under their control, appear to be modulated by daily rhythms. Vagal and sympathetic inputs to the liver seem to contribute to the rhythmic activity in hepatic tyrosine activity (80). Similarly, circadian rhythms in the activity of hepatic glycogen synthetase-I (active form), an enzyme that can be affected by vagal nerve activity, may be partly under the control of cholinergic neurons in the hypothalamus (81). With respect to hepatic afferent fibers, Schmitt (82) found that lateral hypothalamic units which fired in response to intraportal injections of saline or glucose showed a circadian rhythmicity in resting discharge rate, and that the response to hepatic stimuli was highly dependent on these diurnal changes in activity. Finally, we have found recently (P. E. Sawchenko, M. I. Friedman, and R. M. Gold, *unpublished observations*) that section of the hepatic branch of the vagus nerve alters the diurnal pattern of eating in rats by attenuating the normal nocturnal bias in food intake. Although it is not clear whether this effect of nerve section is due to interruption of afferent or efferent fibers, this and other findings suggest that studies of hepatic nerve function should include time of day as a variable.

Given the location of the liver, hepatic sensory

nerves are well positioned to detect the postabsorptive consequences of ingestion. These receptors may provide an "early warning" signal of changes in the osmolarity or ion concentration of ingested fluids or foodstuffs so that appropriate renal and pituitary (ADH) responses can be made to accommodate imminent fluctuations in body fluid balance. Similarly, hepatic afferents responding to the metabolic impact of absorbed nutrients appear to recruit responses that contribute to the digestion and assimilation of foodstuffs (74). Findings discussed above suggest that metabolic receptors in the liver provide a feedback signal that may control gastric emptying. Recent experiments by Niijima (83) showing that intraportal but not intrajugular infusions of glucose increase firing rates of the pancreatic branch of the vagus and decrease discharge of neurons in the adrenal nerve indicate that metabolic receptors in the liver also may modulate hormone secretions. Such afferent nerve activity may thus help foster the shift in metabolism from a fasting to a fed state and prepare an organism to incorporate an increased influx of nutrients.

As discussed above, hepatic afferents may contribute to the control of ingestion. How hepatic signals alter food and fluid intake is far from clear; accumulating evidence indicates, however, that a change in taste preference or reactivity may be involved. Infusions of hypertonic saline into the portal vein but not vena cava decrease the preference for isotonic saline in thirsty rats; right cervical vagotomy abolishes this effect (84). Consistent with this finding and with the anatomic overlap of central gustatory and vagal afferent projections (85), neurons in the pontine parabrachial nucleus of rats responded to both application of hypertonic saline to the tongue and infusions of saline into the portal vein (49). With respect to food consumption, Campbell and Davis (86) have shown that intraportal infusions of glucose decrease licking of glucose or sucrose solutions by mildly hungry rats, whereas intrajugular infusions had no effect. In humans, hepatic function also may influence the sense of taste, in that gustatory acuity is depressed in acute or chronic liver diseases (60,87).

Although our understanding of the functions of hepatic nerves is tentative, information currently available may have implications for the diagnosis and treatment of hepatic disease. Anatomic work in animals with experimental liver damage suggests that degeneration of intrinsic hepatic nerves may contribute to problems in human hepatic disease; conversely, regenerative capacity of hepatic nerves may be a factor in the recovery from hepatic damage. Malfunction or deterioration of hepatic osmo-, ion-, or baroreceptors or different efferent inputs may play a role in the disturbances in electrolyte balance in cirrhosis (88,89). Given the probable role of hepatic efferent nerves in

hepatic glucose metabolism and the influence of hepatic afferent signals on gastrointestinal function and endocrine secretions from the adrenals and pancreas, hepatic neuropathy may play a part in metabolic and digestive disease. Also, animal studies suggest that disturbances in hepatic nerve function may be considered in the etiology of eating disorders. Inasmuch as the liver plays an important if not central role in many bodily functions, pathologic states may be associated with malfunctions of hepatic nerves. Since hepatic nerves serve a variety of functions, and the liver is both a neurologically reactive and sensate organ, further clinical investigations into the role of neural impairments in hepatic diseases are warranted.

ACKNOWLEDGMENTS

Preparation of this chapter was supported by NIH grant AM-20022.

The author thanks Karen Gil and Jim Granneman for editorial assistance, and Melanie Bellenoit and Chris Decoteau for typing this manuscript.

REFERENCES

1. Lautt, W. W. (1980): Hepatic nerves: A review of their functions and effects. *Can. J. Physiol. Pharmacol.*, 58:105–123.
2. Sawchenko, P. E., and Friedman, M. I. (1979): Sensory functions of the liver—A review. *Am. J. Physiol.*, 236:R5–R20.
3. Alexander, W. F. (1940): The innervation of the biliary system. *J. Comp. Neurol.*, 72:357–370.
4. Honjo, I., and Hasebe, S. (1965): Studies on the intrahepatic nerves in cirrhotic liver. *Rev. Int. Hepatol.*, 15:595–604.
5. Sutherland, S. D. (1965): The intrinsic innervation of the liver. *Rev. Int. Hepatol.*, 15:569–578.
6. Ito, T., and Shibasaki, S. (1968): Electron microscopic study on the hepatic sinusoidal wall and the fat-storing cells in the normal human liver. *Arch. Histol. Jpn.*, 29:137–192.
7. Forssman, W. G., and Ito, S. (1977): Hepatocyte innervation in primates. *J. Cell. Biol.*, 73:299–313.
8. Nawar, N. N. Y., and Kamel, I. (1975): Intrinsic innervation of the gall bladder in the dog. *Acta Anat.*, 92:411–416.
9. Tsai, T. L. (1958): A histological study of sensory nerves in the liver. *Acta Neuroveg.*, 17:354–385.
10. Sutherland, S. D. (1964): An evaluation of cholinesterase techniques in the study of the intrinsic innervation of the liver. *J. Anat.*, 98:321–326.
11. Reilly, F. D., McCuskey, P. A., and McCuskey, R. S. (1978): Intrahepatic distribution of nerves in the rat. *Anat. Rec.*, 191:55–68.
12. Nobin, A., Baumgarten, H. G., Falck, B., Ingemansson, S., Moghimzadeh, E., and Rosengren, E. (1978): Organization of the sympathetic innervation in liver tissue from monkey and man. *Cell Tissue Res.*, 195:371–380.
13. Skaaring, P., and Bierring, F. (1976): On the intrinsic innervation of normal rat liver. *Cell Tissue Res.*, 171:141–155.
14. Ungvary, Gy., and Donath, T. (1975): Neurohistochemical changes in the liver of guinea pigs following ligation of the common bile duct. *Exp. Mol. Pathol.*, 22:29–34.
15. Ungvary, Gy., Donath, T., and Naszaly, S. A. (1974): Regeneration of the monoaminergic nerves in the liver after partial hepatectomy. *Acta Morphol. Acad. Sci. Hung.*, 22:177–186.
16. Burton-Opitz, R. (1910): The vascularity of the liver: I. The flow of blood in the hepatic artery. *Q. J. Exp. Physiol.*, 3:297–313.
17. Greenway, C. V., and Stark, R. D. (1971): Hepatic vascular bed. *Physiol. Rev.*, 51:23–65.

18. Lautt, W. W. (1977): Effect of stimulation of hepatic nerves on hepatic O$_2$ uptake and blood flow. *Am. J. Physiol.*, 232:H652–H656.

19. Swan, K. G., Kerr, J. C., Wright, C. B., and Reynolds, D. G. (1977): Adrenergic mechanisms in the hepatic arterial circulation of baboons. *Surgery*, 81:326–334.

20. Greenway, C. V., Lawson, A. E., and Mellander, S. (1967): The effects of stimulation of the hepatic nerves, infusions of noradrenaline and occlusion of the carotid arteries on liver blood flow in the anesthetized cat. *J. Physiol. (Lond.)*, 192:21–41.

21. Greenway, C. V., and Lawson, A. E. (1969): β-Adrenergic receptors in the hepatic arterial bed of the anesthetized cat. *Can. J. Physiol. Pharmacol.*, 47:415–419.

22. Mundschau, G. A., Zimmerman, S. W., Gildersleeve, J. W., and Murphy, Q. R. (1966): Hepatic and mesenteric artery resistances after sinoaortic denervation and hemorrhage. *Am. J. Physiol.*, 211:77–82.

23. Greenway, C. V., and Lautt, W. W. (1972): Effects of adrenaline, isoprenaline and histamine on transsinusoidal fluid filtration in the cat liver. *J. Pharmacol.*, 47:415–419.

24. Koo, A., and Liang, I. Y. S. (1979): Stimulation and blockade of cholinergic receptors in terminal liver microcirculation in rats. *Am. J. Physiol.*, 236:E728–E732.

25. Macleod, J. M. (1907): Studies in experimental glycosuria. I. On the resistance of afferent and efferent nerve fibers controlling the amount of sugar in the blood. *Am. J. Physiol.*, 19:388–407.

26. Lautt, W. W., and Wong, C. (1978): Hepatic parasympathetic neural effect on glucose balance in the intact liver. *Can. J. Physiol. Pharmacol.*, 56:679–682.

27. Edwards, A. V. (1972): The hyperglycemic response to stimulation of the hepatic sympathetic innervation in adrenalectomized cats and dogs. *J. Physiol. (Lond.)*, 220:697–710.

28. Seydoux, J., Brunsmann, M. J. A., Jeanrenaud, B., and Girardier, L. (1979): α-Sympathetic control of glucose output of mouse liver perfused *in situ*. *Am. J. Physiol.*, 236:E323–E327.

29. Nobin, A., Falck, B., Ingemansson, S., Jarhult, J., and Rosengren, E. (1977): Organization and function of the sympathetic innervation of human liver. *Acta Physiol. Scand. [Suppl.]*, 452:103–106.

30. Lautt, W. W. (1979): Neural activation of α-adrenoreceptors in glucose mobilization from liver. *Can. J. Physiol. Pharmacol.*, 57:1037–1039.

31. Proost, C., Carton, H., and DeWulf, H. (1979): The α-adrenergic control of rabbit glycogenolysis. *Biochem. Pharmacol.*, 28:2187–2191.

32. Niijima, A., and Fukuda, A. (1973): A reflex effect on glucose release from the liver of the toad. *Jpn. J. Physiol.*, 23:559–567.

33. Hardcastle, J. D., and Ritchie, H. D. (1968): The liver in shock: Comparison of some techniques used currently in therapy. *Br. J. Surg.*, 55:365–368.

34. Shimazu, T., and Fukuda, A. (1965): Increased activities of glycogenolytic enzymes in liver after splanchnic-nerve stimulation. *Science*, 150:1607–1608.

35. Shimazu, T., and Amakawa, A. (1975): Regulation of glycogen metabolism in the liver by the ANS: VI. Possible mechanism of phosphorylase activation by the splanchnic nerve. *Biochim. Biophys. Acta*, 385:242–256.

36. Lautt, W. W., and Côte, M. G. (1977): The effect of 6-hydroxydopamine-induced hepatic sympathectomy on the early hyperglycemic response to surgical trauma under anesthesia. *J. Trauma*, 17:270–274.

37. Browdows, R. G., Pi-Sunyer, F. X., and Campbell, R. G. (1975): Sympathetic control of hepatic glycogenolysis during glucopenia in man. *Metabolism*, 24:617–624.

38. Shimazu, T. (1971): Regulation of glycogen metabolism by the autonomic nervous system. V. Activation of glycogen synthetase by vagal stimulation. *Biochim. Biophys. Acta*, 252:28–38.

39. Matsushita, H., Ishikawa, K., and Shimazu, T. (1979): Chemical coding of the hypothalamic neurones in metabolic control. I. Acetylcholine-sensitive neurones and glycogen synthesis in liver. *Brain Res.*, 163:253–261.

40. Szabo, A. J., and Szabo, O. (1975): Influence of the insulin sensitive central nervous system glucoregulator receptor on hepatic glucose metabolism. *J. Physiol. (Lond.)*, 253:121–133.

41. Hopton, D. S., and White, T. T. (1971): Effect of hepatic and coeliac vagal stimulation on common bile-duct pressure. *Am. J. Dig. Dis.*, 16:1095–1101.

42. Haberich, F. J. (1968): Osmoreception in the portal circulation. *Fed. Proc.*, 27:1137–1141.

43. Haberich, F. J., Aziz, O., Nowacki, P. E., and Ohm, W. (1969): Zur spezifität der Osmoreceptoren in der Leber. *Pfluegers Arch.*, 313:289–299.

44. Aziz, O., and Haberich, F. J. (1967): Versuche zur Humoralen Übertragbarkeit verschiedener Diurese-zustände am gekreuzten Kreislaufprärarat mit wachen Ratten. *Pfluegers Arch.*, 294:R34 (*Abstr.*).

45. Chwalbinska-Moneta, J. (1979): Role of hepatic portal osmoreception in the control of ADH release. *Am. J. Physiol.*, 236:E603–E609.

46. Niijima, A. (1969): Afferent discharges from osmoreceptors in the liver of the guinea pig. *Science*, 166:1519–1520.

47. Adachi, A., Niijima, A., and Jacobs, H. L. (1976): An hepatic osmoreceptor mechanism in the rat: Electrophysiological and behavioral studies. *Am. J. Physiol.*, 231:1043–1049.

48. Dennhardt, R., Ohm, W. W., and Haberich, F. J. (1971): Die Ausschaltung der Leberäste des N. vagus an der wachem Ratte und ihr Einfluss auf die hepatogene Diurese—indirekter Beweis für die afferente Leitung der Leber-Osmoreceptoren uber den N. vagus. *Pfluegers Arch.*, 328:51–56.

49. Rogers, R. C., Novin, D., and Butcher, L. L. (1979): Electrophysiological and neuroanatomical studies of hepatic portal osmo- and sodium-receptive afferent projections within the brain. *J. Autonom. Nerv. Syst.*, 1:183–202.

50. Aisman, R. I., and Finkinshtein, Y. D. (1976): On the liver osmo- and ionic receptors. *Fiziol. Zh. SSSR*, 62:218–236.

51. Lydtin, H. (1969): Untersuchungen über Mechanismen der Osmo- und Volumenregulation. II. Untersuchungen über den einfluss intravenös intraportal und oral zugführter hypotoner Kochsalzlösungen auf die Diurese des Hundes. *Z. Gesamte Exp. Med.*, 149:193–210.

52. Schneider, E. G., Davis, J. O., Robb, C. A., Baumber, J. S., Johnson, J. A., and Wright, F. S. (1970): Lack of evidence for a hepatic osmoreceptor mechanism in conscious dogs. *Am. J. Physiol.*, 218:42–45.

53. Bennett, W. M., Hennes, D., Elliot, D., and Porter, G. A. (1974): In search of a hepatic osmoreceptor in man. *Dig. Dis.*, 19:143–148.

54. Daly, J. J., Roe, J. W., and Horrocks, P. (1967): A comparison of sodium excretion following the infusion of saline into the systemic and portal veins in the dog: Evidence for a hepatic role in the control of sodium excretion. *Clin. Sci.*, 33:481–487.

55. Passo, S. S., Thornborough, J. R., and Rothballer, A. B. (1973): Hepatic receptors in control of sodium excretion in anesthetized cats. *Am. J. Physiol.*, 224:373–375.

56. Kapteina, F. W., Motz, W., Schwartz-Porsche, D., and Gauer, O. H. (1978): Comparison of renal responses to 5% saline infusions into vena portae and vena cava in conscious dogs. *Pfluegers Arch.*, 374:23–29.

57. Wolfmann, E. F., Zuidema, G. D., O'Neal, R. M., Turcotte, J., Kowalczyk, R., and Child III, C. G. (1961): Sodium excretion after intrasplenic and systemic sodium chloride in normal dogs and after portacaval shunt. *Surgery*, 50:231–237.

58. Perlmutt, J. H., Aziz, O., and Haberich, F. J. (1975): A comparison of sodium excretion in response to infusion of isotonic saline into the vena porta and vena cava of conscious rats. *Pfluegers Arch.*, 357:1–14.

59. Granneman, J. and Friedman, M. I. (1980): Hepatic modulation of insulin-induced gastric acid secretion and EMG activity. *Am. J. Physiol.*, 238:R346–R352.

60. Smith, F. R., Henkin, R. I., and Dell, P. B. (1976): Disordered gustatory acuity in liver disease. *Gastroenterology*, 70:568–571.

61. Schmitt, M. (1973): Influences of hepatic portal receptors on hypothalamic feeding and satiety centers. *Am. J. Physiol.*, 225:1089–1095.

62. Ohm, W., and Haberich, F. J. (1969): Über den Einfluss des

Druckes im Portalkreislauf auf die Diurese der wachen Ratte. *Pfluegers Arch.*, 306:227–231.

63. Liang, C. C. (1971): The influence of hepatic portal circulation on urine flow. *J. Physiol. (Lond.)*, 214:571–581.

64. Andrews, W. H. H., and Palmer, J. F. (1967): Afferent nervous discharge from the canine liver. *Q. J. Exp. Physiol.*, 52:269–276.

65. Niijima, A. (1977): Afferent discharges from venous pressoreceptors in liver. *Am. J. Physiol.*, 232:C76–C81.

66. Russek, M. (1971): Heaptic receptors and the neurophysiological mechanisms controlling feeding behavior. In: *Neurosciences Research,* edited by S. E. Ehrenpreis and O. C. Solnitzky, pp. 213–282. Academic Press, New York.

67. Russek, M., Lora-Vilches, M. C., and Islas-Chaires, M. (1980): Food intake inhibition elicited by intraportal glucose and adrenaline in dogs on a 22 hour-fasting/2 hour feeding schedule. *Physiol. Behav.*, 24:157–161.

68. Bellinger, L. L., Trietly, G. J., and Bernardis, L. L. (1976): Failure of portal glucose and adrenaline infusions or liver denervation to affect food intake in dogs. *Physiol. Behav.*, 16:299–304.

69. Novin, D., VanderWeele, D., and Rezek, M. (1973): Infusion of 2-deoxy-D-glucose into the hepatic portal system causes eating: Evidence for peripheral glucoreceptors. *Science*, 181:858–860.

70. Rowland, N., and Nicolaidis, S. (1974): Reponses glycémique et de prise d'aliments à l'injection intraauriculaire et portale de 2-désoxy-D-glucose chez le rat. *C. R. Acad. Sci.*, 279:1093–1096.

71. Russell, P. J. D., and Mogenson, G. J. (1975): Drinking and feeding induced jugular and portal infusions of 2-deoxy-D-glucose. *Am. J. Physiol.*, 229:1014–1018.

72. Friedman, M. I., Rowland, N., Saller, C., and Stricker, E. M. (1976): Different receptors initiate adrenal secretion and hunger during hypoglycemia. *Neurosci. Abstr.*, 2:299.

73. Stricker, E. M., Rowland, N., Saller, C. F., and Friedman, M. I. (1977): Homeostasis during hypoglycemia: Central control of adrenal secretion and peripheral control of feeding. *Science*, 196:79–81.

74. Friedman, M. I. (1980): Hepatic-cerebral interactions in insulin-induced eating and gastric acid secretion. *Brain Res. Bull. [Suppl. 4],* 5:63–68.

75. Niijima, A. (1969): Afferent impulse discharges from glucoreceptors in the liver of the guinea pig. *Ann. N.Y. Acad. Sci.*, 157:690–700.

76. Andrews, W. H. H., and Orbach, J. (1974): Sodium receptors activating some nerves of perfused rabbit livers. *Am. J. Physiol.*, 227:1273–1275.

77. Orbach, J., and Andrews, W. H. H. (1973): Stimulation of afferent nerve terminals in the perfused rabbit liver by sodium salts of some long-chain fatty acids. *Q. J. Exp. Physiol.*, 58:267–274.

78. Kadekaro, M., Timo-Iaria, C., and Vincentini, M. de L. M. (1977): Control of gastric secretion by the central nervous system. In: *Nerves and the Gut,* edited by F. P. Brooks and P. W. Evers, pp. 377–429. Slack, Thorofare, N.J.

79. Sakaguchi, T., and Yamaguchi, K. (1979): Changes in efferent activities of the gastric vagus nerve by administration of glucose in the portal vein. *Experientia*, 35:875–876.

80. Black, I. B., and Reis, D. J. (1971): Central neural regulation by adrenergic nerves of the daily rhythm in hepatic tyrosine transaminase activity. *J. Physiol. (Lond.)*, 219:267–280.

81. Shimazu, T., Ishikawa, K., and Matsushita, H. (1977): Role of hypothalamic cholinergic neurones in generation of the circadian rhythm of liver glycogen synthetase. *Brain Res.*, 138:575–579.

82. Schmitt, M. (1973): Circadian rhythmicity in responses of cells in the lateral hypothalamus. *Am. J. Physiol.*, 225:1096–1101.

83. Niijima, A. (1980): Glucose sensitive afferent nerve fibers in the liver and regulation of blood glucose. *Brain Res. Bull. [Suppl. 4]*, 5:175–179.

84. Blake, W. D., and Lin, K. K. (1978): Hepatic portal vein infusion of glucose and sodium solutions on the control of saline drinking in the rat. *J. Physiol. (Lond.)*, 274:129–139.

85. Norgren, R. (1978): Projection from the nucleus of the solitary tract in rats. *Neuroscience*, 3:207–218.

86. Campbell, C. S., and Davis, J. D. (1974): Licking rate of rats is reduced by intraduodenal and intraportal glucose infusion. *Physiol. Behav.*, 12:357–365.

87. Coltorti, M., Gentile, S., Loguercio, C., and Porcellini, M. (1978): Changes in gustatory acuity in chronic liver disease. *Ital. J. Gast.*, 10:178 (*Abstr.*).

88. Epstein, M. (1979): Deranged sodium homeostasis in cirrhosis. *Gastroenterology*, 76:622–635.

89. Vaamonde, C. A. (1978): Renal water handling in liver disease. In: *The Kidney in Liver Disease,* edited by M. Epstein, pp. 67–89. Elsevier, New York.

90. Smith, F. R., Henkin, R. I., and Dell, P. B. (1976): Disordered gustatory acuity in liver disease. *Gastroenterology*, 70:568–571.

SECTION V

Relation of the Liver to Other Organs

The Liver: Biology and Pathobiology, edited by
I. Arias, H. Popper, D. Schachter, and D. A. Shafritz.
Raven Press, New York © 1982.

Chapter 40

Interaction of Liver and Muscle in the Regulation of Metabolism in Response to Nutritional and Other Factors

Hamish N. Munro

The role of the liver is unique in regulating mammalian metabolism in the body as a whole. Most nutrients absorbed from the intestine encounter the liver before passing to other organs, thus indicating that the liver is likely to exercise some control over their distribution to other organs. This chapter focuses on skeletal muscle as a recipient of nutrients from the liver and assesses the interplay of major metabolites between liver and muscle in both directions as part of the overall economy of metabolism in health and disease.

In this respect, muscle commands attention on the basis of size alone. Table 1 shows that the skeletal musculature of the nonobese young adult human or mature rat represents about 45% of body weight. This proportion is not constant throughout life. At birth, little more than 20% of body weight of both species is muscle, whereas in old age, the human undergoes a considerable reduction in the percentage of body weight accounted for as muscle (Table 1). This is confirmed (1) by studies comparing lean body mass estimated from ^{40}K content of the body with nitrogen content measured by whole body neutron activation analysis. With progressive aging of adults, the body content of ^{40}K, which is more concentrated in skeletal muscle, undergoes a greater decrease than does nitrogen content.

The relative sizes and metabolic roles of liver and muscle are also affected by the species size of mammals (2). In Table 2, selected mammals from the shrew to the horse have been arranged in order of increasing adult body weight. Over this weight range spanning five orders of magnitude, liver weight decreases from 6.1% of the body weight of the shrew to 1.3% of the body weight of the horse, whereas the total skeletal musculature is estimated to remain essentially constant at 45% of body weight. This decrease in the relative size of the liver is undoubtedly related to the diminution in metabolic intensity with increasing species size. For example, basal energy metabolism, expressed in kilocalories per kilogram body weight, is 108 for the mature rat but only 23 for adult man, a fivefold difference; total body protein synthesis in the same two species undergoes a reduction in intensity of equal magnitude. Using total RNA content of liver and skeletal musculature as an index of the intensity of protein synthesis in these tissues, it can be seen (Table 2) that increasing body size of species results in a greater reduction in the total amount of protein made per kilogram body weight in the liver than in the musculature. Since most metabolic data obtained on man must be supplemented by results obtained from small animals, such as the rat, the investigator should bear in

TABLE 1. *Proportion of skeletal muscle in the body of man and the rat at different stages of development*[a]

Stage	Man (%)	Rat (%)
Birth	21	23
Weaning	18	28
Adolescent	36	32
Adult	45	46
Elderly	27	—

[a] From ref. 90.

mind this change in the relative contributions of liver and muscle in species of different body size.

The remainder of this chapter examines the interactions of liver and muscle in the metabolism of protein, carbohydrate, and fat, and how this relationship between the two organs is affected by nutritional status and in various disease states. In some cases, the published evidence includes estimates of the total flux of metabolites across liver and muscle; thus it is possible to provide a quantitative description of changes in their utilization by each of these tissues as they respond to nutritional and other factors. In most cases, the evidence is less complete and we must be content with data that point to the change in metabolite utilization by each organ. The least satisfactory situation is one in which only alterations in the blood levels of lipids, glucose, or amino acids are available, since it is not certain whether an increase in blood concentration is due to increased release of the metabolites from one organ or diminished uptake by another, nor can the magnitude of the flux be obtained.

INTERACTIONS OF LIVER AND MUSCLE IN CARBOHYDRATE AND FAT METABOLISM

Muscle and liver interact in the metabolism of energy-yielding substrates. The following description can be amplified from reviews by Newsholme and Start (3), Robinson and Williamson (4), and McGarry and Foster (5), which should be consulted for details. Figure 1 contrasts the effects of feeding and fasting on the metabolic interchange between liver and muscle. The primary agents causing these changes are insulin and glucagon. In the fed state, the increased level of insulin accelerates the deposition of glycogen in liver and, to a less dramatic extent, in muscle. Carbohydrate becomes the main energy source in both tissues. In the fasting state, not only is the plasma insulin level lower, but the concentration of glucagon rises as fasting progresses.

The reduction in insulin level in fasting affects glycogen deposition adversely in liver and muscle and also causes activation of the lipase in the adipose tissues, so that large amounts of free fatty acids and glycerol are released from the fat depots. The increased level of glucagon has several consequences. It causes loss of liver glycogen (glycogenolysis) and, at the same time, inhibits glycolysis, with the result that the glucose formed from liver glycogen breakdown passes into the bloodstream. Glucagon also determines the partition of the incoming free fatty acids liberated from the adipose tissue. These can either undergo β-oxidation to acetyl-CoA or combine with glycerol to form neutral fats, which are exported by the liver into the plasma as very low density lipoproteins (VLDL). Control over these alternative pathways may be exercised by the concentration in the liver of malonyl-CoA, according to McGarry and Foster (5). After consuming a meal, the high intracellular concentrations of malonyl-CoA inhibit formation of fatty acylcarnitine, an essential step in the transport of fatty acids into the mitochondria for their oxidation, and thus favor release of the fatty acids as neutral fat. Fasting causes a rise in glucagon concentration, which reduces the malonyl-CoA level in the liver; consequently, less

TABLE 2. *Effect of species size on percentage of liver and skeletal muscle in body and on total RNA content of these organs per kilogram body weight*

Species	Mature body weight (kg)	Tissue weight[a]		Total RNA in Tissue[b]		
		Liver	Skeletal muscle	Liver	Skeletal muscle	Ratio muscle/liver
		(% body weight)		(mg RNA/kg body weight)		
Shrew	0.007	6.1	45	—	—	—
Mouse	0.03	5.3	45	455	477	1.0
Rat	0.25	4.2	45	300	396	1.3
Rabbit	2.0	3.0	45	140	288	2.0
Dog	25	2.1	45	96	230	2.4
Man	70	1.9	45	(75)	(210)	(2.8)
Bullock	450	1.4	45	53	212	4.0
Horse	700	1.3	45	40	176	4.4

[a] Data based on best fit to allometric equations (see ref. 2).
[b] Data from ref. 91, with values for human estimated by interpolation.

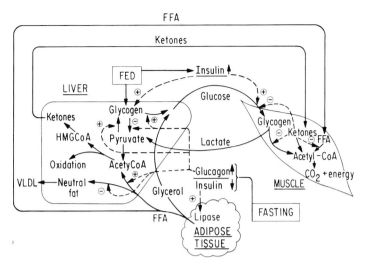

FIG. 1. Role of liver and muscle in the metabolism of carbohydrate and fat in the fed and fasted states.

of the incoming fatty acids are reexported as neutral fats and more are transported by carnitine into mitochondria to undergo β-oxidation. Some of the acetyl-CoA so formed is oxidized to yield energy, while the excess is channeled into formation of hydroxymethylglutaryl-CoA (HMGCoA), the precursor of ketone bodies. The production of ketones thus is determined by free fatty acid excess and glucagon. (Note that HMGCoA is also the precursor of cholesterol, although in a different compartment of the hepatocyte.)

In fasting, metabolic changes occurring in the liver determine that glucose is replaced by free fatty acids and ketone bodies as the major fuel available to muscle (Fig. 1). Accumulation of ketone bodies in muscle inhibits uptake of glucose and also glycolysis, so that blood glucose and muscle glycogen are spared. In addition, the presence of ketone bodies reduces uptake of free fatty acids by muscle; as fasting progresses, ketones become the preferred substrate over free fatty acids. Thus the substrate oxidized in muscle is determined by availability from liver and adipose tissue. In the reverse direction, muscle contributes to liver carbohydrate metabolism in the form of lactate. This is released from muscle fibers under conditions of inadequate oxygenation or on stimulation by epinephrine and is removed by the liver to form pyruvate and thus glucose through gluconeogenesis. The glucose so formed can be released into the blood and used by muscle to form glycogen again (Cori cycle).

INTERACTION OF LIVER AND MUSCLE IN PROTEIN METABOLISM

Amino acids are the currency of protein metabolism and can be considered to have three fates: (a) They are the basic materials for protein synthesis; (b) they provide precursors for the synthesis of nitrogenous small molecules, such as creatine; and (c) amino acids in

excess of requirements for these other two purposes undergo degradation.

Protein Turnover in Muscle and Liver

Figure 2 represents an attempt to quantitate the daily turnover of protein in a 70-kg man. Total body protein turnover has been estimated using stable isotopes (6) to be 250 to 300 g/day. This is 2.5 to three times the daily intake of protein in the Western diet (100 g), indicating that reutilization of amino acids liberated through tissue protein breakdown must be very

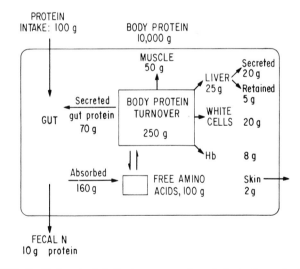

FIG. 2. Estimated daily turnover of protein in the whole body and some organs of a 70-kg man. The basis of the data is provided in an earlier diagram (19), supplemented with a more recent estimate of daily turnover of muscle (11). The total quantity of plasma proteins secreted daily by the liver (20 g) has been estimated from the data of McFarlane (12) for albumin (12 g), gammaglobulins (3 g), and fibrinogen (2.5 g), from Morgan (93) for transferrin (1 g), and from Waldmann et al. (94) for ceruloplasmin (0.2 g), the balance (1.3 g) allowing for the turnover of other plasma proteins.

extensive. About two-thirds of protein synthesis of the body can be identified in Fig. 2 with specific organs. Muscle protein replacement has been estimated (7) from 3-methylhistidine output in the urine. Studies on rat (8) and man (9) show that this amino acid, formed by methylation of specific histidine residues in actin and myosin, is released during myofibrillar breakdown and is quantitatively excreted in the urine. Our data (10) suggest that most of the 3-methylhistidine in urine comes from skeletal muscle. The amount excreted by young adults of 70-kg weight on a flesh-free diet is equivalent to replacement of 50 g muscle protein daily (11).

Proteins formed in the liver consist of retained and secreted (plasma) proteins. The daily turnover of the latter can be estimated reasonably accurately by injecting labeled plasma protein and observing its rate of removal, e.g., 12 g/daily for albumin turnover (12). An approximate value of 20 g protein can be accepted as the amount of plasma proteins made daily by the liver. Since membrane-attached (secreting) ribosomes are four times more numerous than free (retained protein) ribosomes in the liver of the rat (13), we may accept 25 g protein as a rough approximation of the total amount of secreted and retained protein synthesized daily by the liver. This demonstrates that the total amount of protein synthesized in the liver of man is about one-half that made by the total musculature, in agreement with the relative amounts of RNA in these two tissues (Table 2).

Amino Acid Degradative Pathways in Liver and Muscle

The role of the liver and the carcass in amino acid degradation was first investigated systematically by Miller (14), who used perfused rat liver and eviscerated rats without or with the liver. Table 3 shows that the nonessential amino acids were readily oxidized in both liver and carcass. For seven of the essential amino acids (arginine, histidine, lysine, methionine, phenylalanine, tryptophan, and threonine), oxidation was trivial in the eviscerated rat compared with the eviscerated rat with its liver retained or in the perfused rat liver. This indicates that the liver is the major site of oxidation of these essential amino acids. On the other hand, catabolism of the remaining three essential amino acids (leucine, isoleucine, and valine) was low in the perfused liver but brisk in the eviscerated carcass.

It has been shown that degradative enzymes for the three branched-chain amino acids are most active in muscle, kidney, brain, and adipose tissue (15). The first step, catalyzed by the branched-chain amino acid transaminase, yields the corresponding three α-keto acids, which then undergo further degradation through

TABLE 3. *Oxidation of* ^{14}C*-labeled amino acids by the perfused liver and by nonhepatic tissues during 5-hr perfusions*[a]

Amino acid[b]	$^{14}CO_2$ as percent dose		
		Eviscerated rat	
	Liver perfusion	Liver out	Liver in[c]
L-Phenylalanine	25.8	0.13	27.7
DL-Tryptophan-2-^{14}C	16.8	1.6	21.2
L-Arginine·HCl	16.1	3.0	—
L-Threonine	66	1.2	—
DL-Methionine-2-^{14}C	47.7	2.0	22.0
L-Histidine-2-^{14}C HCl	36.7	0.35	—
DL-Lysine-6-^{14}C HCl	25	1.1	—
L-Valine	—	19.3	31
L-Leucine	7.4	13.3	14.3
L-Isoleucine	4.3	27.5	17.7
L-Glutamic acid	47.8	40.2	62.5
L-Glutamine	43.0	20.3	—
Glycine-1-^{14}C	—	8.4	19.0
L-Aspartic acid	—	53	63
L-Proline	—	17.2[d]	—

[a] Adapted from ref. 14.
[b] All amino acids uniformly labeled unless otherwise indicated.
[c] Liver left in supplied with hepatic artery.
[d] Kidneys also removed.

the action of branched-chain keto-acid dehydrogenase, which shortens the chain by removal of the first carbon of the amino acid as CO_2, the remainder becoming the acyl-CoA appropriate for each branched-chain amino acid. Further degradation eventually results in formation of acetyl-CoA from leucine, propionyl-CoA from valine, and a mixture of both from isoleucine.

The extent to which oxidation of branched-chain amino acids is complete in muscle is uncertain. Compared with muscle, the liver has only low transaminase activity for branched-chain amino acids but high activity for dehydrogenation of their keto acids, suggesting that at least part of the branched-chain keto acids are transferred from muscle to liver for oxidation (16). Livesey and Lund (17) have recently shown that the concentrations of branched-chain keto acids in the muscle of fed and 24-hr starved rats are higher than one would expect if they were transient intermediates; even more compelling, in the intact rat, these keto acids are released from muscle and taken up by liver in approximately equal amounts (about 1 mmole/24 hr for a 400-g rat). Although this is much less than the customary intake of branched-chain amino acids by adult rats eating laboratory chow (about 8 mmoles/day), the measurements of Livesey and Lund (17) were made during the day, whereas the rat eats at night, and release of branched-chain keto acids from muscle may have been much greater during the absorptive period.

Accordingly, we can conclude that an unknown proportion of the keto acids derived from branched-chain amino acids is exported from muscle.

Response of Protein Metabolism to a Meal

Before discussing the interchange of amino acids between the viscera and the peripheral tissues, the events occurring after consuming a meal containing protein are summarized (Fig. 3). Although digestion of protein by enzymes secreted into the alimentary tract results in some small peptides and free amino acids being absorbed into the mucosal cells, peptidases in these cells ensure that only free amino acids pass into the portal vein for delivery to the liver (18). In the mucosal cells, some metabolic changes occur involving the absorbed amino acids (19). In particular, glutamine and glutamic acid undergo transamination with pyruvate to form alanine, which passes to the liver and provides carbon for gluconeogensis and nitrogen for urea formation. The same metabolic changes in the mucosa dispose of glutamine coming from the peripheral tissues (Fig. 3).

Most of the absorbed essential amino acids are monitored by the liver according to the needs of the body. For example, in the rat, intake of tryptophan above the requirements needed by the tissues causes induction of tryptophan oxygenase in liver (20). This regulates the amounts of tryptophan passing to the peripheral circulation, including the brain, where it is rate-limiting in the synthesis of the neurotransmitter serotonin (21). On the other hand, the branched-chain amino acids undergo little degradation in the liver but pass to the peripheral tissues, where they can be transaminated, as described earlier. Consequently, the amino acid mixture presented to the peripheral tissues after a meal containing protein is especially rich in branched-chain amino acids. Their entry into muscle and adipose tissue is facilitated by insulin secreted in response to the meal. This can be demonstrated by feeding a meal of carbohydrate, which rapidly causes some reduction in plasma levels of most amino acids, least in the case of tryptophan and most extensively in the case of the branched-chain amino acids (22). The amino acids so removed from the bloodstream contribute to muscle protein synthesis (23). Insulin is also released following a meal of protein (24).

Muscle releases large amounts of alanine and glutamine, the latter being a source of ammonia for the kidney and also of alanine formed in the intestinal mucosa (Fig. 3). Alanine so formed and alanine from muscle then pass to the liver, as described above. This

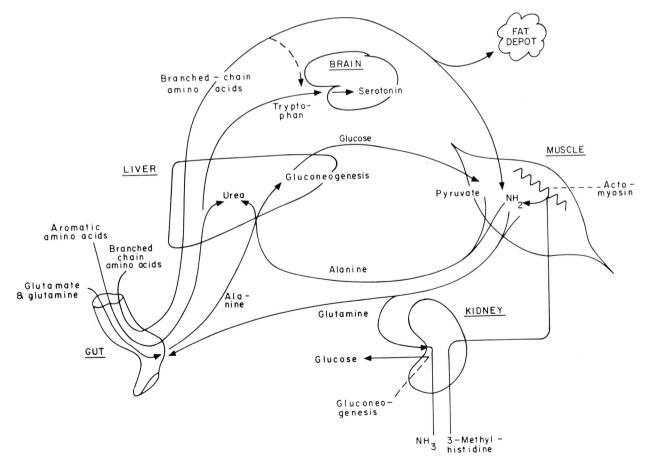

FIG. 3. Interactions of organs in the metabolism of some major amino acids discussed in the text.

gives muscle a dominant role in the metabolism of branched-chain amino acids and of alanine and glutamine. Recently, Goldberg and Tischler (25) have drawn attention to a similar role for adipose tissue. They and their colleagues examined the metabolism of leucine and other branched-chain amino acids by pieces of muscle and adipose tissue taken from fed or fasted rats. Both tissues released $^{14}CO_2$ from 1-^{14}C-leucine, indicating an active branched-chain keto-acid dehydrogenase in both tissues. In comparison with fed animals, fasting of the donor animal increased the *in vitro* rate of catabolism of leucine by muscle but decreased the rate in adipose tissue (26). In agreement with these responses, fasting increased dehydrogenase activity in muscle but decreased its activity in adipose tissue. From a study of the release of $^{14}CO_2$ from 1-^{14}C-leucine and from U-^{14}C-leucine by intact fed or fasted rats, Tischler and Goldberg (26) conclude that food deprivation does not alter the total rate of leucine oxidation but switches it from the fat pads, where it provides carbon for triglyceride formation and thus for fat deposition, to muscle, where it is converted to energy through the tricarboxylic acid cycle. On the other hand, studies of the utilization of leucine *in vitro* by different tissues of the nonfasted rat (27) show that per gram tissue, muscle is twice as active as adipose tissue. Furthermore, adipose tissue (15% of body weight) is one-third as abundant as muscle (45% of body weight) in the young adult. This suggests that body fat can account for only one-sixth as much leucine metabolism as can skeletal muscle.

Amino Acid Exchange Between Muscle and Viscera

Metabolism of substrates by tissues studied *in vitro* should be supplemented by measurements of the uptake and release of amino acids in the intact animal or subject to reflect responses to the complex hormonal and metabolite changes occurring following food intake and other factors. To quantitate such exchanges, the afferent and efferent blood vessels supplying an organ have been catheterized. By measuring differences in amino acid concentration across the organ and rate of blood flow, it is possible to estimate exchange of amino acids and other metabolites by the organ. In the case of muscle, the use of a limb leads to the ambiguity of how much is contributed by adipose tissue. Such measurements of exchange have led to some striking observations, namely (a) the release of large amounts of alanine and glutamine from the peripheral tissues, (b) the metabolism of this alanine and glutamine by the visceral organs, and (c) the transfer of branched-chain amino acids in large amounts from the viscera to the peripheral tissues after the

consumption of protein. Each of these features of the exchange between viscera and muscle is discussed.

Figure 4 illustrates the profiles of amino acids released by the tissues of the legs of human subjects who fasted overnight. Glutamine and alanine each account for about 30 to 40% of the total release of amino acids from the leg in the postabsorptive state. Felig (28) has used the release of lysine (one of the essential amino acids not degraded in muscle) to compute changes in muscle protein turnover in the fasting subject. He demonstrated that only 30% of the alanine released by the arm or leg muscles could be accounted for as coming directly from alanine made available because of reduced protein synthesis or increased breakdown, the remaining 70% being synthesized from other nitrogen sources within muscle. The same applies to the large release of glutamine.

In these experiments on fasting subjects, differences were also measured across the splanchnic viscera (Fig. 4). Exchange of alanine and glutamine represented the predominant change; this time, a reduction in plasma amino acids indicated metabolic removal by the splanchnic viscera. Within the splanchnic area, there is further redistribution. The small intestine consumes glutamine and adds the amino nitrogen as alanine to the portal vein. This alanine is extracted by the liver along with alanine coming directly from muscle and adipose tissue (Fig. 3). Studies on human subjects (29) show that one-half the glutamine taken up by the splanchnic area is accounted for by mucosal metabolism. The extensive studies of Windmueller and Spaeth (30,31) and Hanson and Parsons (32) on rats confirm this picture. The former authors perfused surviving rat intestine and showed that the carbon of glutamine was used as an energy source, while the nitrogen was donated to alanine. Their studies also show that glutamine given by way of the intestinal lumen underwent a similar fate, namely, hydrolysis to glutamate by glutaminase, followed by transamination with pyruvate to yield alanine, and, finally, formation of proline, ornithine, and citrulline, all of which enter the portal vein. With respect to participation of alanine in the exchange between the peripheral and visceral organs, glucose is generated by the liver and becomes available again to the periphery, where it can yield pyruvate for transamination to form alanine. This has been named the glucose-alanine cycle (Fig. 3).

The third feature of amino acid exchange between viscera and peripheral tissues is the response to a meal containing protein. It has been estimated from data such as those shown in Fig. 4, that amino acid output by total musculature of a fasting subject is 0.43 moles/day, equivalent to breakdown of 50 g muscle protein per 24-hr period (33). Clearly, this loss must be compensated by an equivalent replacement of muscle pro-

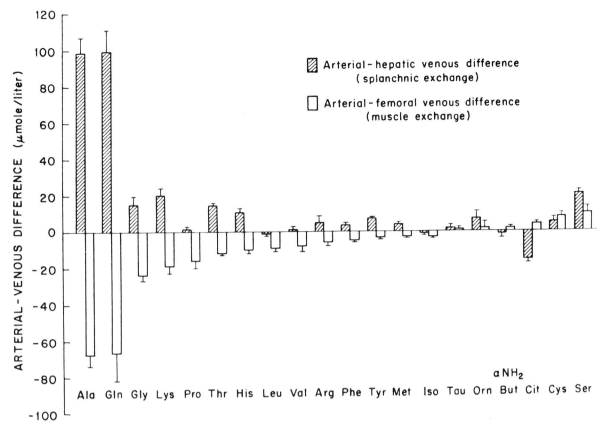

FIG. 4. Splanchnic and leg exchange of amino acids in normal humans after an overnight fast, based on arterial-hepatic and arterial-femoral venous differences (56). Above the line, uptake; below, loss.

tein during the absorptive period after a meal of protein. Table 4 shows relevant data on man, sheep, and dog. In the fasting state, human subjects (24) showed a small release of branched-chain amino acids from the splanchnic area and from the leg. Following a meal of protein, there was a fivefold increase in output of branched-chain amino acids from the hepatic vein (also seen in the protein-fed dogs in Table 4), so that these amino acids constituted more than one-half the amino acids leaving the liver. Since the protein in the meat meal contained only 20% branched-chain amino acids, this confirms other evidence (34) (Table 3) for selective catabolism by the liver of many absorbed essential and nonessential amino acids but not the branched-chain amino acids.

During the absorptive period, the leg changed from losing to gaining branched-chain amino acids. More than one-half the amino acids taken up by the leg at 30 and 60 min after the meal, and essentially all the amino acids taken up at 90, 120, 150, and 180 min, could be accounted for by uptake of branched-chain amino acids. Thus these amino acids are major carriers of amino nitrogen from liver to the peripheral tissues. Since the amino acid mixture taken up by the tissues of the leg during the absorptive period provides branched-chain amino acids out of proportion to the

amount needed for resynthesis of muscle proteins, we conclude that much of the branched-chain amino acids underwent catabolism [a finding confirmed by our studies (35) with ^{13}C-leucine on the fate of excess leucine given as protein to human subjects]. However, the amino nitrogen liberated did not leave the leg, which remained in positive nitrogen balance for at least the first 3 hr after the meal. In particular, output of alanine and glutamine were similar in the postabsorptive and absorptive states. It must be concluded that the amino nitrogen liberated from the branched-chain amino acids remains in the tissue and is used to synthesize nonessential amino acids, which are required for the burst of protein synthesis but are not provided in adequate amounts from the liver.

Since the most striking feature of these studies is the capacity of the limbs to remove large amounts of branched-chain amino acids and to release alanine and glutamine, a relationship between the two events has been sought. Goldberg and Tischler (25) conclude that the glucose-alanine cycle should be renamed the branched-chain-amino acid-alanine cycle. As described above, however, subjects fasted or fed meat show a dissociation between the avid uptake of the branched-chain amino acids during the meal and their release from the legs during fasting, without a correspond-

TABLE 4. *Exchange of amino acids across the splanchnic viscera and the lower limbs of fed and fasting man and animals obtained by measuring amino acid concentrations in blood going to and leaving organs and rate of blood flow*

Species	Status	Organ exchange[a]	Branched-chain amino acids	Alanine	Glutamine
Human[b]	Fed	Splanchnic	−115	+78	+93
		Leg	+42	−24	−37
	Fasting	Splanchnic	−23	+70	+49
		Leg	−12	−24	−30
Sheep[c]	Fed	Portal viscera	−32	−28	+18
		Liver	+14	+38	+25
		Total splanchnic	−18	+10	+43
		Hindquarters	−4	−14	−13
	Fasting	Hindquarters	−18	−25	−21
Dog[d]	Fed	Gut	−260	−230	−50
		Liver	+90	+260	+70
		Total splanchnic	−170	+30	+20
	Fasting	Gut	−25	−55	+30
		Liver	+5	+135	+20
		Total splanchnic	−20	+80	+50

[a] Calculated from published data as total millimoles of amino acid exchanged per 12 hr. +, Uptake by organ; −, output.

[b] Data of Wahren et al. (24) for nondiabetic subjects in the overnight fasting state and at 120 min after a large meal of meat. The entries under glutamine are for glutamine and asparagine combined at 120 min and were obtained by interpolation of data at 90 and 150 min after food consumption.

[c] Data of Bergman and Heitmann (92). Note that the hindquarter output is expressed as micromoles per liter blood, since blood flow was not estimated.

[d] Computed from graphical data of Elwyn (34) for dogs during the first 12 hr after a protein meal (fed) and the second 12 hr (fasting).

ing change in release of alanine and glutamine. Conditions giving rise to increased pyruvate production by muscle favor increased alanine release from muscle. These include exercise (36,37) and a hereditary myopathy causing excessive pyruvate production (38), both of which increase alanine output, and McArdle syndrome, in which reduced alanine output is associated with inhibition of pyruvate production from lack of myophosphorylase (39). Although these observations suggest that glucose may be the main source of pyruvate for transamination, Goldstein and Newsholme (40) provide evidence that the branched-chain amino acids can generate pyruvate in muscle through the action of phosphoenolpyruvate carboxykinase. Such an effect spares glucose during fasting and explains why Sherwin (41) observed an elevation of blood glucose when starving subjects were given leucine. Chang and Goldberg (42) provide additional evidence that leucine can be a significant energy source for muscle in the fasting but not the fed state. Addition of physiologic concentrations of leucine (but not isoleucine or valine) to muscle preparations from fasting rats resulted in reduction of glucose oxidation, indicating that metabolites of leucine were the preferred energy substrates. Ketone bodies have a similar sparing effect on glucose oxidation in muscle (Fig. 1)

but appear to operate by separate mechanisms, since leucine and ketone bodies have additive effects on oxidation of glucose by excised muscle (42). Ketone bodies also reduce the release of amino acids from muscle, both *in vitro* by rat diaphragm (43) and when infused into fasting human subjects (44).

The release of alanine and glutamine from tissues does not always occur in the same proportion. Release of glutamine from the arm is preferentially increased in hepatic cirrhosis as a means of lowering blood ammonia (45) and is also more abundant than alanine when adipose tissue is incubated with leucine (26), whereas muscle preparations made from diabetic or cortisone-treated rats show elevated *in vitro* release of alanine but reduced output of glutamine (46).

Hormones and the Amino Acid Flux Between Muscle and Liver

Several hormones have opposing actions on protein metabolism in liver and muscle, so that one organ loses while the other gains (47). Thus the relative proportions of liver and muscle in the growing rat vary with thyroid status (48). A more striking and better understood example is the action of corticosteroids. Administration of different doses of corticosterone to adrenalectomized rats showed (49) that amounts of the hormone up to 1 mg/100 g body weight daily did not increase plasma corticosterone beyond the diurnal normal range. Doses of 5 and 10 mg, however, raised plasma corticosterone to levels seen only in severe stress and resulted in cessation of growth, increased output of 3-methylhistidine associated with loss of leg muscle weight, and considerable liver enlargement. Thus there is a threshold level above which abnormal metabolic responses occur.

The consequences of corticosteroid administration on amino acid exchange between muscle and liver have been explored by a few investigators. Treatment of rats with corticosteroids increases the concentrations of free amino acids in muscle, especially alanine, glutamic acid, and aspartic acid (52). These also were elevated in the plasma and liver and presumably contributed through gluconeogenesis to the elevated blood sugar levels found in corticosterone-treated rats (49). These observations are generally supported by the *in vitro* studies of Karl et al. (46) on muscles excised from corticosterone-treated rats. Hormone treatment resulted in a higher *in vitro* output of alanine but a diminished output of glutamine. Unfortunately, since their rats were treated chronically with corticosteroid and lost weight, the effects of undernutrition cannot be eliminated.

The participation of muscle and liver has also been explored in the response of tyrosine metabolism to hormone treatment. Release of tyrosine from muscle occurs after administration of corticosteroid (52) or thyroxine (53). In the case of corticosteroid treatment,

the liver enzyme tyrosine transaminase is also induced by the steroid treatment and causes lowering of the level of tyrosine in the plasma (52). In contrast, administration of large amounts of thyroxine also causes release of tyrosine from muscle protein but raises the concentrations of this amino acid in the plasma because there is no corresponding increase in liver tyrosine transaminase activity (54).

In pregnancy, the uterus becomes another sink for alanine and glutamine additional to those shown in Fig. 3. Battaglia and Meschia (55) have shown that a considerable portion of alanine and glutamine released from the muscles of pregnant sheep is needed to meet the requirements of the fetoplacental unit. This presumably accounts for the lower level of plasma alanine in fasting pregnant than in fasting normal women (56) and contributes to the fasting hypoglycemia found in pregnancy.

IMPACT OF NUTRITIONAL AND OTHER FACTORS ON METABOLIC INTERACTIONS BETWEEN LIVER AND MUSCLE

Adaptation to Starvation

During the past 20 years, the use of prolonged starvation for weight reduction has provided an opportunity for studying metabolic adaptation using arteriovenous differences in metabolite concentration across organs. In a recent survey summarizing the main findings, Cahill and Aoki (50) point out that the energy needs of the brain are considerable (about 25%

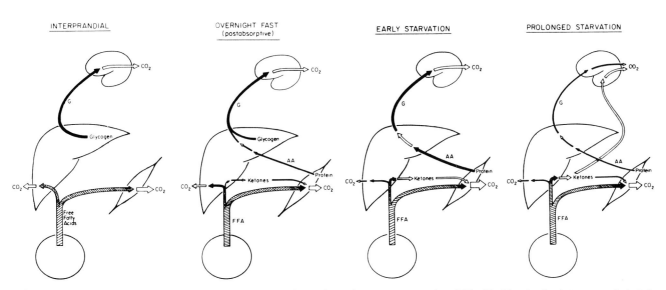

FIG. 5. Sequence of diagrams showing metabolic adaptation of man to starvation (50). (1): Man in the interprandial state with hepatic glycogen providing glucose (G) for brain. (2): Overnight fasting state, with hepatic gluconeogenesis from muscle-derived amino acids (AA) providing glucose (G) for brain. The remainder of the body is using free fatty acids (FFA). (3): Early starvation, with muscle providing the major share of gluconeogenic precursor. (4): Prolonged starvation, with ketoacids being mainly rejected by muscle to elevate blood levels to permit their facilitated diffusion into brain. Thus brain glucose (G) utilization is diminished and, pari passu, muscle proteolysis.

of the total basal metabolism in the adult and about 50% in the child). Because of the blood-brain barrier, these needs must be met by water-soluble energy substrates, namely, glucose in the well-nourished subject and ketones following adaptation to starvation.

Figure 5 illustrates four successive stages between the interprandial state and prolonged starvation. In the interprandial interval, the major source of energy for the brain is glucose released from liver glycogen, while the fuel of muscle is predominantly free fatty acids liberated from the fat stores as a result of reduced plasma insulin levels. Following overnight fasting, glucose is supplied to the brain through gluconeogenesis derived from alanine released by muscle and intestine. Energy also is available to muscle from ketone bodies generated in the liver, which is promoted by the rise in glucagon level. Further starvation results in increased release of alanine from muscle (2 to 3 days); after prolonged starvation (e.g., 3 to 6 weeks), proteolysis of muscle with release of alanine diminishes, less glucose is made in the liver, and ketone bodies take over as the major fuel for the brain (50). It has been suggested (44) that the hyperketonemia of prolonged starvation causes the reduced alanine output, but this relationship has been doubted (51). More likely, the reduced alanine output represents less amino nitrogen available from muscle proteolysis and from reduced uptake of branched-chain amino acids. In prolonged starvation, Sherwin (41) has shown that the capacity of the body to clear leucine from the blood progressively diminishes, possibly because of the lack of insulin needed to transport the branched-chain amino acids into muscle. During the first 2 to 3 days of starvation, this leads to an accumulation of leucine in plasma; with prolonged starvation, leucine release from tissues diminishes, and the plasma leucine level declines.

Exercise

Exercise represents a change in energy metabolism centered on muscle. For more than a century, the effect of muscular exercise on nitrogen balance has been debated, without any definitive evidence of an effect on nitrogen balance in the habitual athlete receiving an adequate energy intake sufficient to compensate for the exercise. This does not imply that metabolic interchange of amino acids between muscle and viscera is unaffected by sudden changes in energy expenditure by muscle. Felig and Wahren (37) have shown that alanine output from an exercising limb increases in proportion to the amount of exertion expended by the fasting subject. The additional alanine added to the effluent blood passes to the liver for gluconeogenesis, but there is no net increase in glucose output because splanchnic uptake of other glucogenic amino acids di-

minishes (37). The nitrogen needed for increased alanine output from the exercising muscle probably comes from catabolism of branched-chain amino acids; it has been observed that exercise of fasting subjects increases the flow of branched-chain amino acids from viscera to muscle (36) and also increases oxidation of leucine (57). Some of the carbon for the extra alanine released may come from breakdown of glucose to pyruvate, since pyruvate is released from muscle in proportion to alanine (37). In experiments performed nearly 50 years ago, we (58) showed that the effect of exercise on nitrogen balance at a constant level of energy intake is more adverse if performed during the absorptive period after a meal than if performed before the meal. This suggests that exercise modifies the patterns of nitrogenous metabolites during the absorptive period.

Diabetes

The patterns of amino acid exchange between liver and muscle of diabetics in the fasting and protein-fed state have been explored by Felig, Wahren, and their colleagues (24,59). In the basal state, splanchnic glucose release from the liver of nonketotic diabetics did not differ from normal values, but alanine uptake was elevated twofold, as was uptake of lactate and pyruvate. This was not matched by a perceptible increase in the release of these glucogenic precursors from the limbs, so that the plasma concentrations were reduced through more vigorous hepatic extraction by diabetic patients. Since glutamine was not measured in these studies, it is possible that, released in larger amounts from muscle, it increases the supply of alanine and other three-carbon compounds by metabolism in the intestinal mucosa (Fig. 3). Although this may seem unlikely since Karl et al. (46) found reduced *in vitro* release of glutamine from muscle taken from diabetic rats along with elevated output of alanine, their animals had lost weight, compared with the nondiabetic controls. Furthermore, output of these amino acids was insensitive to insulin in the medium.

Following a meal of meat (24), the lack of insulin secretion by the human diabetic had predictable consequences. Although splanchnic exchange of amino acids was the same for diabetic as for healthy subjects, the major amino acids released into the peripheral circulation being the branched-chain amino acids, measurement across the leg showed that the increased uptake of branched-chain amino acids after the meal was much less marked for diabetics than for control subjects. This can be related to the lack of insulin secretion following the meal in diabetics. In consequence of this reduced capacity to remove amino acids, the blood levels of the branched-chain amino acids were elevated in the diabetic group. Splanchnic output of glucose was moderately increased during the early part of the absorptive period, in contrast to the control subjects, while uptake of glucogenic precursors (lactate and glycerol) did not decline, as it did in the controls following the meal. In addition, ketone body output was severalfold higher in the diabetics; the meal failed to lower blood levels or splanchnic uptake of free fatty acids, as it did in the controls.

Fever, Sepsis, and Injury

During fever, there is increased production and utilization of energy, along with changes in hormonal and metabolite profiles. Beisel and his colleagues (60) recently summarized the effects of fever and sepsis on intermediary metabolism, including the participation of liver and muscle. Hormonal levels in plasma are mostly increased; elevated insulin and glucagon and raised glucocorticoids (61,62) have predictable effects on metabolism (Figs. 1 and 3). Thus in febrile illnesses, the free fatty acids of plasma decrease (63). Studies on animals with various infections (64) show that the liver increases its conversion of free fatty acids into triglycerides, but the major reason for the reduction in plasma free fatty acids is fever-related elevation of insulin, which inhibits release of free fatty acids from adipose tissue (Fig. 1) and reduces the capacity of the liver to produce ketones. Neufeld and colleagues (64) have shown that febrile illnesses, including those produced by sterile turpentine abscesses, result in diminished production of ketone bodies. When ketonemia was induced in normal animals by starvation, it disappeared when fever was induced, a response coinciding with the secretion of insulin. During a febrile episode, there is also increased uptake of branched-chain amino acids by muscle (65), which is another response compatible with the increased plasma insulin level. Nitrogen made available by this accelerated uptake is reflected in increased release of alanine and glutamine from the muscles of the febrile patient (66), which results in increased gluconeogenesis and glucose turnover, encouraged by the elevated glucagon levels of febrile and septic patients (62). Unlike in normal fasting subjects, gluconeogenesis in septic patients cannot be suppressed by administering infusions of glucose (67). Apart from this observation, the metabolic interaction of liver and muscle in febrile patients is explicable in terms of known hormonal and metabolite regulation (Figs. 1 and 3).

Of importance is the metabolic response of the body to traumatic injury. Although too large a field to summarize here, some relevant observations on the participation of liver and muscle in the metabolic response are discussed. Severe accidental injury, such as femoral fracture, can lead to considerable nitrogen loss over many days. Williamson et al. (68) have shown that an extensive negative nitrogen balance occurs in trauma cases who do not develop ketonemia. In their series, nonketonemic cases had a daily negative balance of 12.4 g nitrogen, whereas those who showed ketonemia had only a small nitrogen loss. 3-Methylhistidine output by the nonketonemic group was elevated by an amount equivalent to loss of 16 g nitrogen daily from muscle protein (similar to the negative nitrogen balance), whereas output of 3-methylhistidine by the ketonemic group was minimally elevated; nitrogen balance of this group was little disturbed. This protective effect of ketonemia on muscle protein breakdown is consistent with the demonstration that infusion of ketone bodies into intact fasting human subjects reduces amino acid output from muscle (44). Although branched-chain amino acid infusion can also reduce nitrogen losses in starvation, Robinson and Williamson (4) point out that branched-chain amino acids nevertheless are elevated in the plasma of patients with extensive negative nitrogen balances following trauma. This suggests some degree of specificity of action of ketone bodies.

Hepatic Cirrhosis

The severe disruption of liver function that occurs in cirrhosis of the liver permits exploration of the metabolic interrelationships between liver and muscle under conditions of hepatic malfunction and allows some speculation on factors involved in hepatic coma. Figure 6 illustrates the extent of these consequences. Ammonia and amines formed by intestinal bacteria are normally removed during passage through the liver; consequently, in severe liver damage, failure to remove them may contribute to hepatic coma (Fig. 6). More recently (69–71), attention has been focused on the distorted free amino acid patterns in the plasma of the cirrhotic patient. The levels of the aromatic amino acids (phenylalanine, tyrosine, and tryptophan) are elevated, while those of the branched-chain amino acids are considerably below normal.

This pattern can be related to impairment of the normal regulatory functions of the liver. Loss of liver function allows the aromatic amino acids to pass unrestricted into the systemic circulation. In addition, half the insulin secreted by the pancreas is normally removed by the liver (72). Consequently, the peripheral plasma of the cirrhotic subject contains excessive levels of insulin, especially after meals (73). This high level of insulin causes excessive uptake of branched-chain amino acids by muscle, so that the levels of these amino acids in the plasma are severely depressed in cases of cirrhosis. Tryptophan competes with the other amino acids, notably, the branched-chain amino

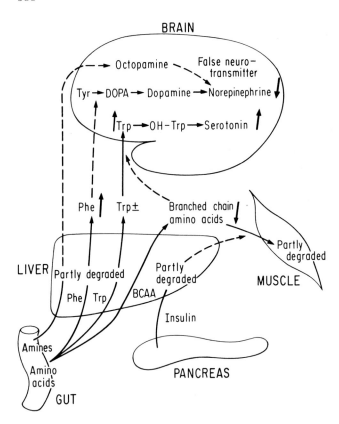

FIG. 6. Diagram illustrating how amino acid imbalance in the plasma of cirrhotic subjects may contribute to the precipitation of hepatic coma (From ref. 95.) Owing to unrestricted passage of insulin into the general circulation, branched-chain amino acids are removed excessively by muscle. In consequence of the lowering of plasma branched-chain amino acids, there is less competition with tryptophan for entry into the brain; thus more serotonin is made.

acids, for entry into the brain. The lowering of plasma levels of branched-chain amino acids and the elevation of tryptophan favors entry of tryptophan into the brain. The higher levels of brain tryptophan result in overproduction of brain serotonin, favoring depressed cerebral function and alertness and contributing to hepatic coma. In confirmation of this action, Hagenfeldt and Wahren (74) have directly demonstrated the effect of branched-chain amino acids on the entry of aromatic amino acids into the brain using measurements of arteriovenous differences between arterial blood and jugular vein blood. The drowsiness of hepatic coma has been reversed by administering branched-chain amino acids in order to reduce the entry of plasma tryptophan into the brain (75).

Muscle also plays a role in disposing of the ammonia bypassing the liver of the cirrhotic patient, in whom Ganda and Ruderman (45) measured the arteriovenous differences in ammonia and amino acids across the forearm. In normal individuals, muscle releases a small amount of ammonia; this release increases on exercise (76). Blood ammonia levels are higher in cir-

rhosis, and the muscles of the cirrhotic take up ammonia, the uptake being less in those with severe muscular wasting (45). Muscle, therefore, may act as a buffer against accumulation of ammonia in cirrhosis. When arteriovenous differences in free amino acid levels were measured on the forearm of fasting cirrhotic subjects, no significant uptake or release of amino acids was observed, except for release of alanine and glutamine. In the case of glutamine, this was three times greater than for alanine, whereas in healthy subjects, alanine is released in amounts similar to (Fig. 4) or greater than glutamine. The authors conclude that the ammonia taken up by muscle generates extra glutamine, which detoxifies ammonia and prepares it for transport to the viscera.

Host Metabolism in Cancer

Cachexia is a feature of advanced malignant disease. The metabolic and hormonal changes associated with cachexia have been studied using a number of animal models; the literature on the interaction between tumor and host has been reviewed by Goodlad (77) and Munro (78). Tumors take up amino acids avidly and release lactate into the circulation for conversion to glucose by the liver. Extensive metabolic changes also occur in the host, which loses protein from muscles but gains liver protein, even when the control and tumor-bearing animals consume the same amount of food (79,80). In muscle, the effect is confined to loss of contractile proteins (81). Adrenocortical enlargement suggests that increased corticosteroid release may contribute to this loss of muscle protein and gain in liver protein. Increased release of corticosteroids could also account for the insulin resistance found in human cancer cases (82). In agreement with the differential effect on liver and muscle protein content, RNA decreases in muscle and increases in the liver, indicating opposite changes in rate of synthesis of protein in the two organs (81).

The effect of a tumor on muscle amino acid metabolism has been examined by Goodlad and Clark (83), who incubated diaphragms from control and tumor-bearing rats with $1\text{-}^{14}\text{C}$-leucine. In the latter, incorporation of leucine into protein was reduced, whereas oxidation was increased, which was confirmed by increased activity of the branched-chain keto-acid dehydrogenase of muscle. The defect in muscle protein synthesis by tumor-bearing rats has been attributed by Clark and Goodlad (84) to a defect in muscle ribosome function. However, the diminished *in vitro* synthesis of protein by isolated muscle can be corrected by adding a complete mixture of amino acids to the medium (85). Subsequent studies by Goodlad et al. (86) on the extensor digitorum longus of the leg confirmed the decrease in protein synthesis and increase in leucine oxidation in the tumor-bearing rat and showed, in addition, that breakdown of protein in this muscle was accelerated. No changes in leucine utilization and protein turnover occurred in the soleus, however, a muscle that does not undergo weight loss in tumor-bearing rats. It might be concluded that, for unknown reasons, some muscles of the tumor-bearing rat oxidize branched-chain amino acids excessively and that administration of branched-chain amino acids may reverse the cachexia. Schaur and colleagues (87) have given branched-chain amino acids to tumor-bearing rats. Survival time was prolonged and loss of carcass protein was reduced, suggesting an increased need for leucine. However, the gastrocnemius muscle of the rats given the branched-chain amino acids lost more weight. This finding is unfortunately confounded by longer survival of branched-chain-treated animals and by their different food intake.

In addition to its capacity for leucine metabolism, muscle in normal subjects releases alanine and glutamine. Output of alanine by the diaphragm of tumor-bearing rats has been studied *in vitro* (83). Despite the increased breakdown of muscle protein evidenced by release of tyrosine, phenylalanine, and methionine into the medium, alanine output was depressed but could be restored by the addition of glucose; at the same time, ammonia output by the piece of muscle was reduced. We can conclude that the alanine added to the medium following glucose addition derived its nitrogen from ammonia or a source generating ammonia, and that glycolysis was the source of the carbon for alanine synthesis. Surprisingly, *in vitro* output of glutamine by the diaphragm of the tumor-bearing host did not differ from nontumor-bearing controls and did not respond to addition of glucose to the medium. This contrasts with the relationship between availability of ammonia and glutamine released by muscle in cases of cirrhosis (45). The reduction in alanine release *in vitro* coincides with low plasma levels of this amino acid observed by Waterhouse and colleagues (88) in cancer patients and the low plasma glucose found in tumor-bearing animals, indicating depressed gluconeogenesis from alanine (89).

REFERENCES

1. Cohn, S. H., Vartsky, D., Yasumura, S., Sawitsky, A., Zanzi, I., Vaswani, A., and Ellis, K. J. (1980): Compartmental body composition based on total-body nitrogen, potassium and calcium. *Am. J. Physiol.*, 239:E524–E530.
2. Munro, H. N. (1969): Evolution of protein metabolism in mammals. In: *Mammalian Protein Metabolism, Vol. III.*, edited by H. N. Munro, pp. 133–182. Academic Press, New York.
3. Newsholme, E. A., and Start, C. (1973): *Regulation in Metabolism*. Wiley, London.
4. Robinson, A. M., and Williamson, D. H. (1980): Physiological roles of ketone bodies as substrates and signals in mammalian tissues. *Physiol. Rev.*, 60:143–187.
5. McGarry, J. D., and Foster, D. W. (1980): Regulation of hepatic fatty acid oxidation and ketone body production. *Ann. Rev. Biochem.*, 49:395–420.
6. Young, V. R., Winterer, J. C., Munro, H. N., and Scrimshaw, N. S. (1976): Muscle and whole body protein metabolism, with special reference to man. In: *Special Review Aging Research*, edited by M. F. Elias, B. E. Eleftherio, and P. K. Elias, pp. 217–252. EAR, Bar Harbor.
7. Young, V. R., and Munro, H. N. (1978): N$^\tau$-methylhistidine (3-methylhistidine) and muscle protein turnover: an overview. *Fed. Proc.*, 37:2291–2300.
8. Young, V. R., Alexis, S. D., Baliga, B. S., Munro, H. N., and Muecke, W. (1972): Metabolism of administered 3-methylhistidine. Lack of muscle transfer ribonucleic acid charging and quantitative excretion as 3-methylhistidine and its N-acetyl derivative. *J. Biol. Chem.*, 247:3592–3600.
9. Long, C. L., Haverberg, L. N., Young, V. R., Kinney, J. M., Munro, H. N., and Geiger, J. W. (1975): Metabolism of 3-methylhistidine in man. *Metabolism*, 24:929–935.
10. Haverberg, L. N., Omstedt, P. T., Munro, H. N., and Young, V. R. (1975): N$^\tau$-methylhistidine content of mixed proteins in various rat tissues. *Biochim. Biophys. Acta*, 405:67–71.
11. Bilmazes, C., Uauy, R., Haverberg, L. N., Munro, H. N., and Young, V. R. (1978): Muscle protein breakdown rates in humans based on N$^\tau$-methylhistidine (3-methylhistidine) content of mixed proteins in skeletal muscle and urinary output of N$^\tau$-methylhistidine. *Metabolism*, 27:525–530.
12. McFarlane, A. S. (1964): Metabolism of plasma proteins. In: *Mammalian Protein Metabolism, Vol. I.*, edited by H. N. Munro, and J. B. Allison, pp. 297–341. Academic Press, New York.
13. Munro, H. N. (1970): A general survey of mechanisms regulating protein metabolism in mammals. In: *Mammalian Protein Metabolism, Vol. IV.*, edited by H. N. Munro, pp. 3–130. Academic Press, New York.
14. Miller, L. L. (1962): The role of the liver and the non-hepatic tissues in the regulation of free amino acid levels in the blood. In: *Amino Acid Pools*, edited by J. T. Holden, pp. 708–721. Elsevier, Amsterdam.
15. Goldberg, A. L., and Chang, T. W. (1978): Regulation and significance of amino acid metabolism in skeletal muscle. *Fed. Proc.*, 37:2301–2307.
16. Krebs, H. A., and Lund, P. (1977): Aspects of the regulation of the metabolism of branched-chain amino acids. *Adv. Enzyme Regul.*, 15:375–394.
17. Livesey, G., and Lund, P. (1980): Enzymic determination of branched-chain amino acids and 2-oxoacids in rat tissues: Transfer of 2-oxoacids from skeletal muscle to liver in vivo. *Biochem. J.*, 188:705–713.
18. Kim, Y. S., and Freeman, H. J. (1977): The digestion and absorption of protein. In: *Clinical Nutrition Update: Amino Acids*, edited by H. L. Greene, M. A. Holliday, and H. N. Munro, pp. 135–141. American Medical Association, Chicago.
19. Munro, H. N. (1977): Parenteral nutrition: Metabolic consequences of bypassing the gut and liver. In: *Clinical Nutrition Update: Amino Acids*, edited by H. L. Greene, M. A. Holliday, and H. N. Munro, pp. 141–146. American Medical Association, Chicago.
20. Young, V. R., and Munro, H. N. (1973): Plasma and tissue tryptophan levels in relation to tryptophan requirements of weanling and adult rats. *J. Nutr.*, 103:1756–1763.
21. Fernstrom, J. D., Madras, B. K., Munro, H. N., and Wurtman, R. J. (1974): Nutritional control of the synthesis of 5-hydroxytryptamine in the brain. In: *Aromatic Amino Acids in the Brain*, pp. 153–166. Assoc. Sci. Publ., Amsterdam.
22. Munro, H. N., and Thomson, W. S. T. (1953): Influence of glucose on amino acid metabolism. *Metabolism* 2:354–358.
23. Munro, H. N., Black, J. G., and Thomson, W. S. T. (1959): The mode of action of dietary carbohydrate on protein metabolism. *Br. J. Nutr.*, 13:475–485.
24. Wahren, J., Felig, P., and Hagenfeldt, J. (1976): Effect of protein ingestion on splanchnic and leg metabolism in normal man and diabetes mellitus. *J. Clin. Invest.*, 57:987–999.
25. Goldberg, A. L., and Tischler, M. E. (1981): Regulatory effects of leucine on carbohydrate and protein metabolism. In: *Metabolism and Clinical Implications of Brain-Chain Amino and*

Keto Acids, edited by M. Walser and J. R. Williamson, pp. 283–288. Elsevier, New York.

26. Tischler, M. E., and Goldberg, A. L. (1980): Leucine degradation and release of glutamine and alanine by adipose tissue. *J. Biol. Chem.,* 255:8074–8081.

27. Rosenthal, J., Angel, A., and Farkas, J. (1974): Metabolic fate of leucine: A significant sterol precursor in adipose tissue and muscle. *Am. J. Physiol.,* 226:411–418.

28. Felig, P. (1981): Inter-organ amino acid exchange. In: *Nitrogen Metabolism In Man,* edited by J. C. Waterlow and J. M. L. Stephen, pp. 45–61. Applied Science, London.

29. Felig, P., Wahren, J., and Rof, L. (1973): Evidence of inter-organ amino acid transport by blood cells in man. *Proc. Natl. Acad. Sci. USA,* 70:1775–1779.

30. Windmueller, H. G., and Spaeth, A. E. (1974): Uptake and metabolism of plasma glutamine by the small intestine. *J. Biol. Chem.,* 249:5070–5079.

31. Windmueller, H. G., and Spaeth, A. E. (1975): Intestinal metabolism of glutamine and glutamate from the lumen as compared to glutamine from blood. *Arch. Biochem. Biophys.,* 171:662–672.

32. Hanson, P. J., and Parsons, D. S. (1977): Metabolism and transport of glutamine and glucose in vascularly perfused small intestine of rat. *Biochem. J.,* 166:509–519.

33. Pozefsky, T., Felig, P., Tobin, J., Soeldner, J. S., and Cahill, G. F. (1969): Amino acid balance across tissues of the forearm in post-absorptive man. Effects of insulin at two dose levels. *J. Clin. Invest.,* 48:2273–2282.

34. Elwyn, D. H. (1970): The role of the liver in regulation of amino acid and protein metabolism. In: *Mammalian Protein Metabolism, Vol. 4,* edited by H. N. Munro, pp. 523–557. Academic Press, New York.

35. Motil, K. J., Matthews, D. E., Bier, D. M., Burke, J. F., Munro, H. N., and Young, V. R. (1981): Whole body leucine and lysine metabolism studied simultaneously with [1-13C]leucine and [α-15N]lysine: Response to altered dietary protein intake in young men. *Am. J. Physiol.,* 240:E712.

36. Ahlborg, G., Felig, P., Hagenfeldt, L., Hendler, R., and Wahren, J. (1974): Substrate turnover during prolonged exercise in man: Splanchnic and leg metabolism of glucose, free fatty acids and amino acids. *J. Clin. Invest.,* 53:1080–1090.

37. Felig, P., and Wahren, J. (1971): Amino acid metabolism in exercising man. *J. Clin. Invest.,* 50:2703–2714.

38. Felig, P., Linderholm, H., and Wahren, J. (1979): Amino acid metabolism in patients with a hereditary myopathy and paroxysmal myoglobinuria. *Acta Med. Scand.,* 206:309–315.

39. Wahren, J., Felig, P., Havel, R. J., Jorfeldt, L., Pernow, B., and Saltin, B. (1973): Amino acid metabolism in McArdle's syndrome. *N. Engl. J. Med.,* 288:774–777.

40. Goldstein, L., and Newsholme, E. A. (1976): The formation of alanine from amino acids in diaphragm muscle of the rat. *Biochem. J.,* 154:555–558.

41. Sherwin, R. S. (1978): Effect of starvation on the turnover and metabolic response to leucine. *J. Clin. Invest.,* 61:1471–1481.

42. Chang, T. W., and Goldberg, A. L. (1978): Leucine inhibits oxidation of glucose and pyruvate in skeletal muscle during fasting. *J. Biol. Chem.,* 253:3696–3701.

43. Palaiologos, G., and Felig, P. (1976): Effects of ketone bodies on amino acid metabolism in isolated rat diaphragm. *Biochem. J.,* 154:709–716.

44. Sherwin, R., Hendler, R., and Felig, P. (1975): Effects of ketone administration on amino acid metabolism in man. *J. Clin. Invest.,* 55:1382–1390.

45. Ganda, O. P., and Ruderman, N. B. (1976): Muscle nitrogen metabolism in chronic hepatic insufficiency. *Metabolism,* 25:427–435.

46. Karl, I. E., Garber, A. J., and Kipnis, D. M. (1976): Alanine and glutamine synthesis and release from skeletal muscle. III. Dietary and hormonal regulation. *J. Biol. Chem.,* 251:844–850.

47. Munro, H. N. (1964): General aspects of the regulation of protein metabolism by diet and hormones. In: *Mammalian Protein Metabolism, Vol. I,* edited by H. N. Munro and J. B. Allison, pp. 381–481. Academic Press, New York.

48. Burini, R., Santidrian, S., Moreyra, M., Brown, P., Munro, H. N., and Young, V. R. (1981): Interaction of thyroid status

and diet on muscle protein breakdown in the rat, as measured by N⁷-methylhistidine excretion. *Metabolism,* 30:679–687.

49. Tomas, F. M., Munro, H. N., and Young, V. R. (1979): Effect of glucocorticoid administration on the rate of muscle protein breakdown in vivo in rats as measured by urinary excretion of Nᵀ-methylhistidine. *Biochem. J.,* 178:139–146.

50. Cahill, G. F., Jr., and Aoki, T. T. (1980): Conditions with abnormal energy balance: Partial and total starvation. In: *Assessment of Energy Metabolism in Health and Disease,* edited by J. M. Kinney and E. Lense, pp. 129–134. Ross Laboratories, Columbus, Ohio.

51. Fery, F., and Balasse, E. O. (1980): Differential effects of sodium acetoacetate and acetoacetic acid infusions on alanine and glutamine metabolism in man. *J. Clin. Invest.,* 66:323–329.

52. Betheil, J. J., Feigelson, M., and Feigelson, P. (1965): The differential effects of glucocorticoid on tissue and plasma amino acid levels. *Biochim. Biophys. Acta,* 104:92–97.

53. Foley, T. H., London, D. R., and Prenton, M. A. (1966): Arterial plasma concentrations and forearm clearances of amino acids in myxedema. *J. Clin. Endocrinol.,* 26:781–785.

54. Rivlin, R. S., and Levine, R. J. (1963): Hepatic tyrosine transaminase activity and plasma tyrosine concentration in rats with altered thyroid function. *Endocrinology,* 73:103–107.

55. Battaglia, F. C., and Meschia, G. (1981): Foetal and placental metabolisms: Their interrelationship and impact upon maternal metabolism. *Proc. Nutr. Soc.,* 40:99–113.

56. Felig, P. (1975): Amino acid metabolism in man. *Annu. Rev. Biochem.,* 44:933–954.

57. Wolfe, R. R., Goodenough, R., Royle, G., Wolfe, M., and Nadel, E. (1981): Leucine oxidation during exercise in humans. *Fed. Proc.,* 40:900.

58. Cuthbertson, D. P., McGirr, J. L., and Munro, H. N. (1937): A study of the effect of over-feeding on the protein metabolism in man. IV. The effect of muscular work at different levels of energy intake, with particular reference to the timing of the work in relation to the taking of food. *Biochem. J.,* 31:2293–2305.

59. Wahren, J., Felig, P., Cerasi, E., and Luft, R. (1972): Splanchnic and peripheral glucose and amino acid metabolism in diabetes mellitus. *J. Clin. Invest.,* 51:1870–1878.

60. Beisel, W. R., Wannemacher, R. W., Jr., and Neufeld, H. A. (1980): Relation of fever to energy expenditure. In: *Assessment of Energy Metabolism in Health and Disease,* edited by J. M. Kinney and E. Lense, pp. 144–150. Ross Laboratories, Columbus, Ohio.

61. Beisel, W. R., and Rapaport, M. I. (1969): Inter-relations between adrenocortical functions and infectious illness. *N. Engl. J. Med.,* 280:541–546; 596–604.

62. Curnow, R. T., Rayfield, E. J., George, D. T., Zenser, T. V., and DeRubertis, F. R. (1976): Altered hepatic glycogen metabolism and glucoregulatory hormones during sepsis. *Am. J. Physiol.,* 230:1296–1301.

63. Beisel, W. R., and Fiser, R. H., Jr. (1970): Lipid metabolism during infectious illness. *Am. J. Clin. Nutr.,* 23:1069–1079.

64. Neufeld, H. A., Pace, J. A., and White, F. E. (1976): The effect of bacterial infections on ketone concentrations in rat liver and blood and on free fatty acid concentrations in rat blood. *Metabolism,* 25:877–884.

65. Imamura, M., Clowes, G. H. A., Jr., Blackburn, G. L., O'Donnell, T. F., Jr., Trerice, M., Bhimjee, Y., and Ryan, N. T. (1975): Liver metabolism and glucogenesis in trauma and sepsis. *Surgery,* 77:868–875.

66. Wannemacher, R. W., Jr. (1977): Key role of various individual amino acids in host response to infection. *Am. J. Clin. Nutr.,* 30:1269–1280.

67. Long, C. L., Kinney, J. M., and Geiger, J. W. (1976): Nonsuppressibility of gluconeogenesis by glucose in septic patients. *Metabolism,* 25:193–201.

68. Williamson, D. H., Farrell, R., Kerr, A., and Smith, R. (1977): Muscle protein catabolism after injury in man, as measured by excretion of 3-methylhistidine. *Clin. Sci. Mol. Med.,* 52:527–533.

69. Fernstrom, J. D., Wurtman, R. J., Hammarstrom-Wiklund, B., Rand, W. M., Munro, H. N., and Davidson, C. S. (1979): Diurnal variations in plasma neutral amino acid concentrations

among patients with cirrhosis: Effect of dietary protein. *Am J. Clin. Nutr.*, 32:1923–1933.

70. Fischer, J. E., Funovics, M., Aguirre, A., James, J. H., Keane, J. M., Wesdorp, R. I. C., Yoshimura, N., and Westman, T. (1975): The role of plasma amino acids in hepatic encephalopathy. *Surgery*, 78:276–280.

71. Munro, H. N., Fernstrom, J. D., and Wurtman, R. J. (1975): Insulin, plasma amino acid imbalance, and hepatic coma. *Lancet*, 1:722–724.

72. Krass, E., Bittner, R., Meves, M., and Beger, H. G. (1974): Insulin-konzentrationen im Pfortaderblut des Menschen nach glucose-infusion. *Klin. Wochenschr.*, 52:404–408.

73. Fernstrom, J. D., Arnold, M. A., Wurtman, R. J., Hammarström-Wiklund, B., Munro, H. N., and Davidson, C. S. (1978): Diurnal variations in plasma insulin concentrations in normal and cirrhotic subjects: Effect of dietary protein. *J. Neural Transm.* [*Suppl.*], 14:133–142.

74. Hagenfeldt, L., and Wahren, J. (1980): Experimental studies on the metabolic effects of branched chain amino acids. In: *Parenteral and Enteral Nutrition, Symposia,* edited by J. Wahren, pp. 88–92. European Society of Parenteral and Enteral Nutrition, Stockholm.

75. Fischer, J. E., Rosen, H. M., Ebeid, A. M., James, J. H., Keane, J. M., and Soeters, P. B. (1976): The effect of normalization of plasma amino acids on hepatic encephalopathy in man. *Surgery*, 80:77–82.

76. Lowenstein, J. M., and Goodman, M. N. (1978): The purine nucleotide cycle in skeletal muscle. *Fed. Proc.*, 37:2308–2312.

77. Goodlad, G. A. J. (1964): Protein metabolism and tumor growth. In: *Mammalian Protein Metabolism, Vol. II.,* edited by H. N. Munro and J. B. Allison, pp. 415–444. Academic Press, New York.

78. Munro, H. N. (1977): Tumor-host competition for nutrients in the cancer patient. *J. Am. Diet. Assoc.*, 71:380–384.

79. Lundholm, K., Edstrom, S., Karlberg, I., Ekman, L., and Scherstén, T. (1980): Relationship of food intake, body composition, and tumor growth to host metabolism in nongrowing mice with sarcoma. *Cancer Res.*, 40:2516–2522.

80. Sherman, C. D., Morton, J. J., and Mider, G. B. (1950): Potential sources of tumor nitrogen. *Cancer Res.*, 10:374.

81. Clark, C. M., and Goodlad, G. A. J. (1971): Depletion of proteins of phasic and tonic muscles in tumor-bearing rats. *Eur. J. Cancer*, 7:3–10.

82. Lundholm, K., Holm, G., and Scherstén, T. (1978): Insulin resistance in patients with cancer. *Cancer Res.*, 38:4665–4670.

83. Goodlad, G. A. J., and Clark, C. M. (1980): Leucine metabolism in skeletal muscle of the tumor-bearing rat. *Eur. J. Cancer*, 16:1153–1162.

84. Clark, C. M., and Goodlad, G. A. J. (1975): Muscle protein biosynthesis in the tumour-bearing rat. A defect in a post-initiation stage of translation. *Biochim. Biophys. Acta*, 378:230–240.

85. Lundholm, K., Bylund, A. C., Holm, J., and Scherstén, T. (1976): Skeletal muscle metabolism in patients with malignant tumor. *Eur. J. Cancer*, 12:465–473.

86. Goodlad, G. A. J., Tee, M. K., and Clark, C. M. (1981): Leucine oxidation and protein degradation in the extensor digitorum longus and soleus of the tumor-bearing host. (*personal communication*).

87. Schaur, R. J., Semmelrock, H. J., Schreimayer, W., Tillian, H. M., and Schauenstein, E. (1980): Tumor host relations. V. Nitrogen metabolism in Yoshida sarcoma-bearing rats. Reduction of growth rate and increase of survival time by administration of physiological doses of branched-chain amino acids. *J. Cancer Res. Clin. Oncol.*, 97:285–293.

88. Waterhouse, C., Jeanpetre, N., and Keilson, J. (1972): Gluconeogenesis from alanine in patients with progressive malignant disease. *Cancer Res.*, 39:1968–1972.

89. Clarke, E. F., Lewis, A. M., and Waterhouse, C. (1978): Peripheral amino acid levels in patients with cancer. *Cancer*, 42:2909–2913.

90. Munro, H. N. (1978): Nutrition and muscle protein metabolism. *Fed. Proc.*, 37:2281–2282.

91. Munro, H. N., and Gray, J. A. M. (1969): The nucleic acid content of skeletal muscle and liver in mammals of different body size. *Comp. Biochem. Physiol.*, 28:897–905.

92. Bergman, E. N., and Heitmann, R. N. (1978): Metabolism of amino acids by the gut, liver, kidneys, and peripheral tissues. *Fed. Proc.*, 37:1228–1232.

93. Morgan, E. H. (1974): Transferrin and transferrin iron. In: *Iron in Biochemistry and Medicine,* edited by A. Jacobs and M. Worwood, pp. 29–71. Academic Press, New York.

94. Waldmann, T. A., Morell, A. G., Wochner, D., Strober, W., and Sternlieb, I. (1967): Measurement of gastrointestinal protein loss using ceruloplasmin labeled with copper. *J. Clin. Invest.*, 46:10–20.

95. Crim, M. C., and Munro, H. N. (1977): Protein and amino acid requirements and metabolism in relation to defined formula diets. In: *Defined Formula Diets for Medical Purposes,* edited by M. E. Shils, pp. 5–15. American Medical Association, Chicago.

The Liver: Biology and Pathobiology, edited by
I. Arias, H. Popper, D. Schachter, and D. A. Shafritz.
Raven Press, New York © 1982.

Chapter 41

Hepatic Encephalopathy

T. E. Duffy and F. Plum

Impaired brain function is a consistent feature of severe liver disease and occurs with two forms of hepatic insufficiency. Fulminant acute hepatic failure causes a rapidly developing delirium progressing through the stages of delirium, stupor, coma, and often death. Chronic cirrhosis with portal-systemic shunting of blood produces a more insidiously evolving, relapsing encephalopathy characterized by disturbances of mentation, episodic stupor, and abnormalities in motor systems indicative of pyramidal and extrapyramidal dysfunction arising at the level of the cerebral hemispheres. The precise cause of these neurologic abnormalities is unknown, nor is it known whether acute and chronic hepatic encephalopathy share a common pathogenesis. Early diagnosis and treatment of hepatic encephalopathy is crucial and can substantially reduce the mortality and morbidity of patients with hepatic failure; early in its course, the neurological disorder is usually not associated with irreversible neuropathological changes.

CLINICAL SYNDROMES AND PRECIPITATING CAUSES OF HEPATIC ENCEPHALOPATHY

Hepatic insufficiency results in several relatively distinct neurologic disorders, the characteristics of

which depend on the acuteness or chronicity of the liver problem and the anatomy of the affected neurologic structure (Table 1). Disorders of cognition and arousal and, subsequently, motor function dominate the clinical picture of hepatic stupor and coma, conditions that occur either acutely, gradually, or episodically in the presence of advanced and worsening liver disease. Chronic hepatocerebral degeneration is an uncommon, fluctuating neurologic disorder characterized by retention of alertness but changing moods, intellectual deterioration, tremor, and varying combinations of cerebellar, extrapyramidal, and pyramidal motor dysfunction. The condition affects a small number of patients with chronic portacaval shunting and reflects the unusual neuropathologic development of areas of spongy degeneration in the brain. Wilson's disease, a disorder of copper metabolism, produces both hepatic cirrhosis and degeneration in the brain involving the corpus striatum and cerebral cortex. Whether the liver and brain abnormalities arise entirely independently or at least partly as cause and effect has not been satisfactorily settled. Hepatic myelopathy is a rare syndrome of spinal cord dysfunction leading to a spastic paresis. The cord lesion is marked by demyelination and tends to be progressive, despite treatment. It is not specifically associated with

TABLE 1. *Neurological complications and accompaniments of severe liver disease*

Hepatic encephalopathy

  Hepatic stupor or coma
    Acute (acute inflammation or necrosis due to hepatitis, hepatotoxic agents, Reye's syndrome)
    Subacute or chronic, progressive (advancing hepatitis or cirrhosis)
    Episodic or recurrent portal-systemic encephalopathy (portal bypass plus protein load)

  Chronic progressive cerebral degeneration
    Spongiform, with cirrhosis
    Wilson's disease

Hepatic myelopathy

Hepatic peripheral neuropathy

hepatic encephalopathy. Hepatic peripheral neuropathy due to segmental demyelination of the nerve sheath has been described in patients with chronic liver disease. The condition rarely produces symptoms, except when accompanied by other manifestations of nutritional insufficiency. For a more extensive discussion and bibliography of the changes in chronic hepatocerebral degeneration, hepatic myelopathy, hepatic peripheral neuropathy, and Wilson's disease, the reader may wish to consult Plum and Hindfelt (1).

The balance of this section discusses the commonly encountered syndromes of hepatic stupor and coma that accompany fulminant acute liver failure or acute worsening of chronic liver failure. As indicated in Table 2, roughly five grades of hepatic encephalopathy can be established in order of severity. Such grading is

TABLE 2. *Grades of severity in hepatic encephalopathy*[a]

Grade	Signs
1	Mild mental impairment, hypocapnic hyperventilation
2	Lethargy, confusion, asterixis, hypocapnia
3	Arousable stupor, pupillary and oculocephalic reflexes present, diffuse muscle paratonia, increased stretch reflexes, extensor plantar responses frequent, hypocapnic hyperventilation
4	Unarousable coma, pupillary and oculocephalic reflexes present, motor hypertonus, often decerebrate and extensor plantar responses, hypocapnic hyperventilation present
5	Unarousable coma, pupillary and/or oculocephalic reflexes absent, motor tone flaccid, stretch reflexes suppressed, may have metabolic or even respiratory acidosis

[a] Within any grade, all signs may not be present; to estimate prognosis, grading should be based on the single worst-level sign. Muscle flaccidity is only a grade 5 sign if preceded during the earlier course of coma by hypertonus.

crucial for identifying the severity of disease and comparing patients, imperative steps in arriving at a prognosis or determining the potential effects of therapy.

Either the acute or subacute progressive form of hapatic coma includes, in varying proportions, abnormalities in the following:

Changes in personality and mentation
Altered levels of consciousness
Abnormalities in motor function, including hyperventilation, tremor, asterixis, paratonic rigidity, hyperactive deep tendon reflexes, and, in advanced stages, extensor plantar responses and decerebrate postural responses
Characteristic neuroophthalmologic signs, including intact pupils, the emergence of brisk oculocephalic reflexes, and, sometimes, the transient development of tonic abnormal conjugate deviations of the eyes.

These symptoms and their evolution in hepatic coma somewhat resemble those encountered with several other metabolic encephalopathies, particularly the disorders produced by global hypoxia-ischemia and hypoglycemia (2). Close attention to the characteristic combination of hyperventilation, motor signs, and eye signs, however, almost always leads to the accurate clinical diagnosis of hepatic coma, even when systemic or laboratory signs of hepatic failure are not prominent.

ENCEPHALOPATHY WITH ACUTE OR FULMINANT HEPATIC FAILURE

The onset can be abrupt or insidious. In many patients, neurologic abnormalities appear and worsen markedly within a matter of no more than a few hours, especially in the presence of the sudden development or worsening of either acute or chronic liver disease. The symptoms and signs tend to be similar with either state of liver failure, and different causes of the liver failure do not confer any distinctive neurologic symptoms. What differences exist between the neurological abnormalities in fulminating or acute hepatic failure and those encountered with gradually progressive liver insufficiency lie in the rate of progression of the neurologic syndrome and the pattern of early mental changes. Sometimes, especially in explosively developing acute liver disease or in the advent of sudden gastrointestinal (GI) bleeding in a subject with extensive portacaval shunting, the neurologic disorder can precede by hours or a day the development of other clinical or laboratory evidence of hepatic insufficiency.

Symptoms of extreme restlessness, agitation, hallucinatory delirium or mania are generally confined to patients with fulminant, rapidly worsening hepatic failure. Characteristically, such psychological hyperactivity gives way to a reduced state of arousal within a matter of hours. If patients with fulminating hepatic failure, owing to acute liver disease, develop verbal unresponsiveness or unarousable coma within

24 hr, few survive. The clinical picture in severe hepatic coma in which pupillary responses and oculovestibular responses are briskly present and accompanied by bilateral abnormal motor signs, sometimes including decerebrate rigidity, is characteristic of severe metabolic brain disease. We have observed little or nothing in these patients to suggest that acute transtentorial herniation accounted for the signs of brainstem dysfunction as they first evolved. Accordingly, we suspect that autopsy reports of severe brain edema in fulminant hepatic failure reflect agonal events in patients receiving terminal life support rather than an important pathogenetic factor in the patient's death.

ENCEPHALOPATHY WITH GRADUALLY PROGRESSING OR RELAPSING HEPATIC INSUFFICIENCY

Signs and Symptoms

Patients with these forms of hepatic encephalopathy develop generally similar clinical abnormalities, although these may be modified by, respectively, differences in the rate of worsening of the liver disease, whether or not certain precipitating factors are present, and the degree to which symptoms relate themselves to abnormalities induced by portacaval shunting. Some fluctuation in neurologic signs and symptoms is almost a rule in patients with chronic progressive liver disease but is particularly characteristic in those with relapsing portal-systemic encephalopathy (PSE).

Early mental and behavioral changes in progressive liver disease or PSE include a dull, flat apathy combined with a carelessness in personal appearance and an impairment of such simple skilled movements as dressing, feeding, or writing. The abnormalities slide insidiously into a state of confusion and memory impairment that, if unreversed, eventually reaches mental unresponsiveness and finally unarousable coma.

The earliest motor warning of neurologic impairment usually consists of a fine lateral tremor of the outstretched hands accompanied or shortly followed by asterixis. The latter movement consists of irregular, coarse, quick flexion-extension movements affecting mainly the hands but extending in severe cases to involve the tongue or feet. At this stage, most patients show hyperactive facial reflexes; those with intact peripheral nerves have brisk deep tendon reflexes. Among mentally obtunded patients, skeletal muscle tone is increased, and extensor plantar responses are common. As coma deepens, decerebrate postural responses often appear. Further progression leads to skeletal muscle paralysis and flaccidity, a state that often heralds grade 5 coma. Hyperventilation with respiratory rates of 20 to 26 producing a respiratory alkalosis in the blood is the rule in all stages of hepatic encephalopathy up to grade 5; indeed, the diagnosis can hardly be made in the absence of the respiratory changes. In our experience, convulsions are uncommon in hepatic coma, except in patients withdrawing from drugs or alcohol or, less often, in those with acute water intoxication.

Neuroophthalmologic abnormalities are prominent in hepatic encephalopathy. Pupillary response to light remains intact until the terminal stages of the disorder, but disturbances in ocular motor control emerge once stupor supervenes and can take several forms. Reflecting the removal of forebrain influences on brainstem oculovestibular reflexes, patients with hepatic stupor or coma show brisk conjugate, contraversive ocular movements when one quickly turns the head from side to side or in flexion or extension. More bizarre ocular abnormalities are sometimes observed in patients in coma with an acute relapse of PSE where tonic downward or upward deviation may appear and last for several hours before spontaneously subsiding. Dysconjugate eye movements have been described rarely in such patients; such ocular dissociations, however, are more characteristic of structural than of metabolic disease of the brainstem.

The above mental, motor, and ophthalmologic abnormalities represent functional and potentially reversible depression of the brain in hepatic encephalopathy. We have observed them to appear, disappear, and reappear in various combinations in patients with PSE, especially in association with recurrent episodes of meat intoxication or GI bleeding. Even in the same patient, the combination of signs can vary from attack to attack. If signs of neurologic depression proceed beyond the above into grade 5 encephalopathy, few patients survive. Fixed pupils, flaccid skeletal muscles with areflexia, absent oculocephalic responses, or the disappearance of hyperventilation each and all imply dangerously worsening brainstem dysfunction and, usually, an irreversibly deep stage of hepatic coma.

Clinical Course

The above-described signs and symptoms of incipient or progressive brainstem dysfunction with liver disease array themselves in roughly similar patterns in patients with either progressive liver failure or with the episodic encephalopathy that accompanies relatively fixed advanced cirrhosis accompanied by a large portacaval shunt. The main difference between the two lies in the time course.

With progressive hepatic failure, the clinical course of encephalopathy, although sometimes fluctuating moderately, gradually worsens; few such patients return to a state of well-being or full mental alertness once neurologic deterioration begins. Seldom do such subacute slow courses start with an abrupt onset, and often motor abnormalities attain a less florid expression than with PSE, even in preterminal stages. One sometimes observes an exception to this principle in patients with advanced alcoholic cirrhosis who intermittently relapse during acute alcoholic bouts, each of which may produce a prolonged near-fatal neurologic illness that gradually subsides in the idealized surroundings and nutrition of the hospital.

Patients with chronic atrophic cirrhosis, by contrast with those suffering from progressive liver disease, often make remarkable recoveries from even very deep hepatic coma as long as brainstem reflexes are preserved. Among 51 patients studied by Levy et al. (3) with unarousable hepatic coma secondary mainly to cirrhosis, 35% made a good recovery to the point of self independence. Half those showing intact oculo-vestibular responses recovered, but no patient made a good recovery once that reflex disappeared. Even half of the 14 patients showing decerebrate responses to noxious stimuli recovered, four after having shown the abnormality for a full week.

Precipitating Factors

Many conditions have been incriminated as precipitants to hepatic encephalopathy in patients with chronic liver disease. Leaving aside the causes for progressive inflammation-fibrosis of the liver, the most frequent factors include a return to alcoholism, development of nutritional failure, use of sedative or opiate drugs, development of severe hypokalemia or hyponatremia, loss of large fluid volumes by sudden diureses or paracentesis, and the advent of severe systemic infection or bodily trauma. Patients with chronic cirrhosis and portacaval shunting in addition to the above are susceptible to nitrogenous loads suddenly delivered to the intestine by GI bleeding, ingestion of a large protein meal, ingestion of ammonium salts, or the taking of acetazolamide.

CEREBRAL OXIDATIVE METABOLISM AND BLOOD FLOW

The overall cerebral metabolic rate for oxygen ($CMRO_2$) is depressed in patients with hepatic encephalopathy, and the magnitude of the change tends to parallel the severity of the neurological dysfunction (4–6). The ratio of cerebral oxygen consumption to glucose utilization also appears to be abnormally low in such patients (7), suggesting that a greater than normal fraction of cerebral glucose metabolism is diverted toward nonoxidative pathways. Cerebral blood flow declines in patients with hepatic encephalopathy (5), but the reduced cerebral metabolic activity may not be entirely responsible for this effect. Patients with severe liver failure generally hyperventilate, lowering the arterial carbon dioxide tension. The results of animal studies suggest that cerebral autoregulatory mechanisms may be impaired in such individuals as well.

Stanley and Cherniak (8) observed that the cerebral hyperemic response to systemic hypoxia was diminished in goats with carbon tetrachloride-induced liver damage, and that a much milder degree of systemic hypoxia was required to reduce cerebral oxygen consumption in the liver-damaged animals compared to normal goats. Furthermore, Trewby et al. (9) found that mild arterial hypotension caused a fall in cerebral blood flow in pigs with acute liver failure secondary to total devascularization of the liver. In normal pigs, a similar maneuver was fully compensated for by adjustment of cerebral vascular resistance, so that cerebral blood flow remained unchanged. It is widely recognized that a variety of insults (hypoxia, hypoglycemia, infections, sedative drugs) that are well tolerated by patients who are free of liver disease may precipitate neurological depression or coma in patients with cirrhosis and chronic portal-systemic shunting (10). Impaired cerebral autoregulation may contribute to this increased cerebral "sensitivity" of individuals with liver disease to mild metabolic disturbances.

ACID-BASE BALANCE

Acid-base disturbances occur commonly in patients with liver disease. The most consistent abnormality is respiratory alkalosis (5,11), which often gives way, in terminal stages of the disease, to a metabolic acidosis (12). Alpha-keto acids (pyruvate, α-ketoglutarate) and lactate are increased three- to fivefold in the blood of patients with hepatic coma (13). The changes in these organic acids parallel, and may be secondary to, the respiratory alkalosis (14). They may also reflect an increased release of the acids from tissue as a consequence of impairment of their cellular oxidation. The respiratory alkalosis is thought to be compensatory, acting to protect rather than impair brain function; if the alkalosis is corrected by the administration of 5% carbon dioxide or acetazolamide, patients deteriorate clinically, and their cerebral oxygen consumption declines (5). No adequate explanation has been advanced to account for the hyperventilation accompanying liver cirrhosis, although hyperammonemia has been implicated as contributing to the abnormality either by directly stimulating the respiratory centers (15,16) or by lowering intracellular pH in brain (17). Ammonium salts will induce hyperventilation when administered to animals (18,19); voluntary hyperventilation in patients with liver disease leads to an increase in the arterial ammonia concentration (20) which, in turn, may provide a further stimulus for hyperventilation.

ELECTROENCEPHALOGRAPHIC FINDINGS

Reduction of mean dominant frequency and reactivity are the principal changes seen in the electroencephalograms (EEGs) of patients with hepatic coma. Some of these abnormalities can precede clinically obvious neurological impairment (21). The abnormally slow activity begins in the frontal area with short, bilaterally synchronous bursts that lengthen and become more widely distributed as the patient becomes less responsive (22,23). In addition, the appearance of synchronous 4 to 5 Hz triphasic wave forms consisting of a high-amplitude positive deflection preceded and followed by a low-amplitude negative deflection is a distinctive feature of the precomatose stage (23). In terminal hepatic coma, bilaterally symmetrical, high-amplitude 2 to 3 Hz activity predominates. Although the EEG changes are consistent and indicative of severe cerebral impairment, they are not diagnostic of hepatic coma and occur in other metabolic disorders, including CO_2 intoxication, hypoglycemia, or vitamin B_{12} deficiency (24), and as a consequence of hyperammonemia (25). Hawkes et al. (26) attempted to improve the diagnosis of latent hepatic encephalopathy on the basis of EEG criteria by subjecting cirrhotics and patients free of liver disease to EEG-provocative tests, including the administration of ammonia, morphine, neomycin, or a high-protein diet. No test was found to be wholly satisfactory in predicting that the abnormal EEG was due to hepatic failure. Since such measures entail a risk of precipitating encephalopathy, there is little advantage to their use.

NEUROPATHOLOGICAL FINDINGS

The neuropathological features of hepatic coma vary with the type of liver disease and its duration. The brains of patients who die in acute hepatic coma caused by fulminant hepatic failure or Reye's disease are often swollen and show signs of terminal transtentorial or medullary herniation (27–31). The mechanism of the swelling and its relation to the symptoms is not clear. No evidence exists in human studies to know how much of the increased brain volume may be due to increased blood volume, extracellular edema, or intracellular edema. Most patients dying of fulminant hepatic failure have received extensive terminal efforts at resuscitation, which add to the difficulties in judging just when during the illness the observed cerebral edema occurred. In hepatectomized rats dying in coma, Livingstone et al. (32) found increased brain water content and swelling of astrocytes and perivascular astrocytic processes in the brain. When studied during their terminal phase, the animals showed an increased permeability of the blood-brain barrier to inulin, sucrose, and trypan blue dye. Few specific cellular changes have been reported in patients with acute hepatic coma. In children with Reye's disease, pleomorphic changes, including expansion of the mitochondrial matrix, have been observed in neuronal (and liver) mitochondria, but these are thought to be fully reversible (33). Evidence of severe neuronal necrosis is more rare and has been attributed to ischemic injury secondary to the cerebral edema (30).

Chronic progressive liver disease accompanied by portal-systemic shunting of blood produces a more distinctive neuropathologic picture, typified by glial abnormalities (34,35). The most striking change is an increase in the number and size of the protoplasmic astrocytes in the cerebral cortex, thalamus, and lenticular, dentate, and pontine nuclei (Alzheimer type II change) (Fig. 1). The astrocytic nuclei are enlarged and lobulated, and the nucleoli are prominent. At the ultrastructural level, the astrocytic cytoplasm looks watery and is of a low electron density; there appears to be an accumulation of glycogen and lipofuscin granules in the cell bodies (36–38). In the more protracted cases of chronic hepatocerebral degeneration, neuronal loss may be severe; the changes mainly distribute themselves in a pseudolaminar pattern along the deeper layers of the cerebral cortices and in a "spongy" pattern of degeneration in the cerebellar cortex, most prominently in the depths of sulci (Fig. 1). The astrocytic abnormalities occur to some degree in all patients with chronic liver failure; however, they are not specific to patients with neurological symptoms and may be to some degree reversible (39,40). Similar astrocytic changes occur in the brains of children dying with hyperammonemia secondary to genetic disorders affecting the Krebs-Henseleit cycle (41). Furthermore, morphological abnormalities that are virtually identical to the human Alzheimer astrocytic changes can be produced in experimental animals by the construction of a portacaval shunt (42–44) and other measures that acutely (45) or chronically (46,47) raise the brain ammonia concentration. Several workers have suggested that the morphological changes in the astrocytes signified increased metabolic activity in these cells, possibly related to the cerebral detoxification of ammonia (48).

PATHOGENESIS OF HEPATIC ENCEPHALOPATHY

The pathogenesis of hepatic coma is unknown. The disorder is usually classified as metabolic because the neurological symptoms accompanying both acute and chronic liver failure are potentially fully reversible with appropriate treatment and, except in cases of chronic hepatocerebral degeneration, are not associated with extensive morphological damage to neurons. Because the liver is the body's principal organ of chemi-

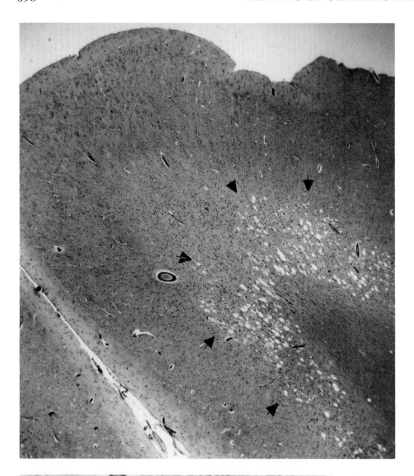

FIG. 1a. Morphological changes in the brain in chronic portal systemic encephalopathy. Lower power enlargement of parasaggital gyrus from frontal lobe showing laminar spongiform degeneration (*arrows*) involving the deep cortical layer and adjacent white matter. H&E stain.

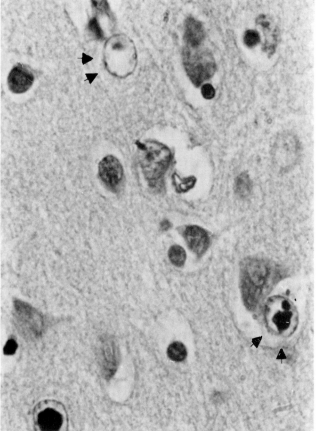

FIG. 1b. Oil immersion showing Alzheimer type 2 astrocytes. *Arrows above,* typical watery-appearing astrocytic nucleus with eccentric nucleolus; *arrows below right,* similarly enlarged astrocyte containing a PAS-positive glycogen inclusion body.

cal homeostasis, hepatic encephalopathy could result from failure of the diseased liver to (a) release nutrients and cofactors essential for normal brain metabolism and function, or (b) remove circulating neurotoxins which may then accumulate in the brain.

The brain requires constant and adequate supplies of glucose for oxidative energy production, and the liver is essential for the normal regulation of the plasma glucose concentration. This control is exerted by hepatic synthesis of glucose from noncarbohydrate precursors (gluconeogenesis), by the synthesis, storage, and release of glycogen, and by termination of the action of circulating insulin. Hypoglycemia is a frequent complication of acute liver failure (49) but occurs only rarely in patients with chronic liver disease. Early work by Geiger and co-workers (50,51) revealed that the electrical activity of an isolated, perfused cat brain preparation could be prolonged if a liver were included in the perfusion circuit. Similar results were obtained by adding to the blood perfusing the brain either liver extract or the pyrimidine nucleosides cytidine and uridine, agents that are normally synthesized and elaborated by the liver. These findings implied that substances (possibly uridine and cytidine) "essential" to brain function may be deficient in the blood of patients with liver failure. The administration of uridine and cytidine does not appear to benefit patients with hepatic encephalopathy (52), however, and no other protective substance has been found to be lacking in such individuals.

Much evidence supports the view that hepatic coma is caused by the abnormal accumulation of neurotoxins in the brain. Lascelles (53) observed that ultrafiltrates of plasma from patients with hepatic coma inhibit the respiration of rat brain-cortex slices *in vitro*, and Brennan and Plum (54) found that the infusion of cerebrospinal fluid from patients with hepatic coma into the cerebral ventricular system of rats and cats caused behavioral depression and slowing of the EEG; CSF from control subjects had no such effect. A number of known and suspected toxins are increased in the plasma and CSF of patients with hepatic encephalopathy, and measures that "cleanse" the plasma (charcoal hemoperfusion, polyacrylonitrile membrane hemodialysis) often improve consciousness in patients with acute hepatic failure (55,56). Many toxic factors have been implicated as contributing to the symptoms of hepatic encephalopathy, but the strongest arguments can be advanced for ammonia, mercaptans, short-chain fatty acids, and aromatic amine analogues of central neurotransmitters.

AMMONIA

Abnormal ammonia metabolism has been advanced as a cause of hepatic encephalopathy since the late 19th century when Eck (57) discovered that cerebral symptoms could be induced in dogs with portacaval shunts by feeding them meat. Evidence now implicates ammonia as a major contributing cause of such meat intoxication:

1. Ammonia is highly neurotoxic. The acute administration of ammonium salts to experimental animals will produce convulsions, coma, and death (58,59), and ammonia infusions into patients with chronic liver disease and portal-systemic shunting can evoke a reaction that is indistinguishable clinically from impending hepatic coma (60–62).

2. The concentration of ammonia is usually elevated in the blood and cerebrospinal fluid (CSF) of patients with hepatic encephalopathy (63). Ansley et al. (64) found that among eight conventional tests and 20 measures of nitrogen metabolism (including plasma levels of 16 amino acids) performed in 73 patients with cirrhosis, the fasting venous ammonia concentration alone correctly identified *a posteriori* 15 of the 17 patients with a history of encephalopathy and 55 of the 56 who had not experienced this complication. An individual patient's fluctuating neurological status does not always correlate with the arterial blood ammonia level (13,60,65,66)[1], but data obtained in animals with experimentally-induced liver failure suggest that blood ammonia concentrations may not accurately reflect brain ammonia concentrations in patients with liver disease, particularly when samples are obtained following an ammonia load. Thus, Navazio et al. (67) found that blood ammonia concentrations that caused a slight rise in brain ammonia in normal rats but no neurological symptoms produced higher brain ammonia concentrations and signs of hyperactivity in rats with carbon tetrachloride-induced liver damage. Ehrlich et al. (68) subsequently found that a dose of ammonium acetate, adjusted to produce comparably elevated blood ammonia concentrations in control rats and animals with portacaval shunts, caused 50 to 100% higher concentrations of ammonia in the brains of the shunted animals. Increased permeability of the blood-brain barrier to ammonia-ammonium ion may contribute to the greater accumulation of ammonia in brain in experimental liver failure (68). Whatever the explanation, the implication of the findings for patients with liver disease is that a small ammonia load, as in a protein meal, may only transiently and moderately elevate the blood ammonia concentration but may

---

[1] Venous blood ammonia determinations are a poor guide to the concentration of ammonia reaching the brain via the arterial circulation. One reason for the unreliability is that skeletal muscle possesses glutamine synthetase activity and will take up ammonia from arterial blood, converting it to glutamine. As a result, blood drawn from veins that drain skeletal muscle vasculature (e.g., the antecubital veins) may contain a significantly lower concentration of ammonia than that present in the arterial blood.

raise the brain ammonia concentration to a level high enough to cause neurological symptoms.

3. Hyperammonemia accompanies the comas of Reye's disease (69,70), inherited disorders caused by a deficiency of one or more of the enzymes of the Krebs-Henseleit cycle (41,71), and transient acute hyperammonemic encephalopathy of unknown cause in the preterm infant (72,73). Moderate to severe encephalopathy in association with hyperammonemia also occurs as a complication of (a) glutaminase-asparaginase therapy for acute lymphocytic leukemia (74), (b) ureterosigmoidostomy for the treatment of bladder cancer (75), and (c) valproic acid therapy for the management of minor motor seizures (76,77). The hyperammonemia in the latter three conditions is thought to arise from extensive hydrolysis of circulating glutamine, bacterial ureolysis in the colon with subsequent absorption of the ammonia from the urine, and direct hepatotoxicity, respectively.

4. Chronic hyperammonemia in animals, achieved either by the infusion of ammonium salts (47), administration of jack-bean urease (46), or construction of a portacaval shunt (43), leads to the development of Alzheimer astrocytic changes and other neuropathologic abnormalities that are strikingly similar to those found in the brains of patients who die in hepatic coma.

Ammonia is constantly being generated in brain by the deamination of amino acids, neurotransmitter amines, purines, and other nitrogenous substrates, and by the deamidation of glutamine. The concentration of ammonia in brain is higher than that in blood or CSF (68,78) and appears to be closely linked to the level of neural activity. Brain ammonia increases during afferent stimulation (79) and generalized seizures (80,81) and declines during sleep (82) and anesthesia (80). The immediate precursors of brain ammonia production are uncertain, but deamination of glutamate via the glutamic dehydrogenase reaction (83) and deamination of aspartate via the reactions of the purine nucleotide cycle (84) are thought to be major contributors.

Ammonia is also taken up by the brain from the blood. Direct measurements of arterial and cerebral venous concentration differences for ammonia indicate that the brain extracts a small fraction (as much as 11%) of the ammonia present in arterial blood (4,5). This finding is supported by radio scanning measurements obtained in healthy volunteers and patients with moderate to severe liver disease following the systemic administration of doses of ^{13}N-ammonia (Fig. 2) (85). Because the concentration of ammonia in hepatic portal vein blood is normally five to 10 times greater than that in mixed venous blood, the GI tract is thought to contribute most of the circulating blood ammonia (86). This ammonia originates from the action of bacterial proteases, ureases, and amine oxidases on the contents of the colon (87) and from the

hydrolysis of glutamine in the large and small intestines (88,89). The ammonia is absorbed into the intestinal venous blood and transported via the hepatic portal vein to the liver where, normally, it is largely metabolized to urea by the enzymes of the Krebs-Henseleit cycle. Liver disease interferes with this detoxification process (a) by reducing the capacity of the liver to synthesize urea, and (b) by impairing venous drainage from the intestines so that the ammonia-laden portal blood bypasses the liver to enter into the systemic circulation. In patients with liver failure and portal-systemic shunting, the burden of maintaining ammonia homeostasis shifts to other organs, notably, skeletal muscle. The ammonia taken up by muscle is converted to glutamine, which, in turn, is released from muscle in increased amounts in such patients

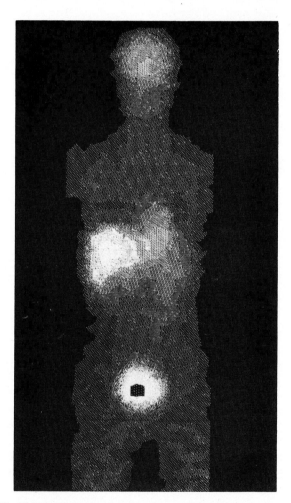

FIG. 2. Whole-body distribution of ^{13}N activity following intravenous administration of ^{13}N-ammonia to a normal individual. The brain, liver, and urinary bladder are well demarcated in this two-dimensional scan; additional activity is concentrated in the region of the heart and left kidney. The "recycled" dark area within the bladder image represents the area of highest radioactivity in this scan. Of the total observed ^{13}N activity, approximately 7% accumulated in the brain and >50% accumulated in skeletal muscle. (From ref. 85.)

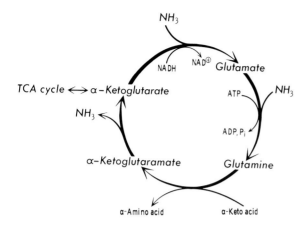

FIG. 3. Pathway of ammonia metabolism in brain. Reductive amination of α-ketoglutarate and energy-dependent amidation of glutamate are the major routes of ammonia removal in brain. Although conversion of glutamine to α-ketoglutaramate and subsequent hydrolysis of α-ketoglutaramate to α-ketoglutarate does occur in brain, the flux through this portion of the cycle is thought to be low in normal individuals. In patients with hepatic encephalopathy, increased concentrations of glutamine and certain α-keto acids (e.g., phenylpyruvate) in brain tissue may promote glutamine transamination leading to α-ketoglutaramate formation. (Modified from ref. 109.)

(90,91). Muscle wasting secondary to nutritional impairment may be an important factor that reduces the capacity of patients with liver disease to detoxify systemic ammonia (85).

Ammonia is a weak base (pK_a = 9.14) (92); at physiologic pH, approximately 99% of arterial blood ammonia exists in the ionized form (NH_4^+). Transport of ammonia from blood to brain is diffusion limited, which appears to be due mainly to the low permeability of the blood-brain barrier to ammonium ion (93–96). Lockwood et al. (85) observed that cerebral uptake of ^{13}N-ammonia in normal individuals and patients with liver disease was linearly related to the arterial blood ammonia concentration over a fivefold range; this implies that ammonia uptake into the human brain also occurs by nonfacilitated diffusion. The uptake of ammonia by the brain is a complex function of arterial pH (increasing pH increases ammonia uptake by increasing the concentration of ammonia base) (93,96,97), cerebral blood flow (94,96), blood-brain barrier permeability (96), and, possibly, the activities of the enzymes involved in cerebral ammonia metabolism (98). The pH dependency of cerebral ammonia uptake is the basis of treatments designed to counteract the blood alkalosis that accompanies hepatic coma (5) and thereby reduce the entry of ammonia into brain. Such measures, however, are unlikely to be effective; despite the low permeability of ammonium ion, its high concentration in plasma results in significant uptake of NH_4^+ by brain, even under normal circumstances (96).

The brain lacks biologically important activity of the urea cycle enzymes carbamoyl phosphate synthetase and ornithine transcarbamylase (99) and, therefore, cannot synthesize urea from precursor ammonia. Accordingly, brain metabolizes ammonia mainly through two reactions (Fig. 3): (a) reductive amination of α-ketoglutarate to form glutamate, and (b) ATP-dependent amidation of glutamate to form glutamine (100). Glutamine is continually generated in brain and released into cerebral venous blood (101–103). Under conditions of acute or chronic hyperammonemia, the concentration of glutamine rises in brain (104–106) and CSF (107–109) (Fig. 4) and appears in increased quantities in cerebral venous blood (103). Glutamine, even in high concentration, is not directly toxic to the brain (110). If the synthesis of glutamine is prevented in experimental rodents by pretreatment with the glutamine synthetase inhibitor methionine sulfoximine, the animals will survive a lethal injection of ammonium salts (111,112). The mechanism by which methionine sulfoximine protects the animals against acute ammonia intoxication has not been elucidated, but it could reflect inhibition of the synthesis of toxic metabolites of glutamine in the brain.

α-Ketoglutaramate, the transaminated metabolite of glutamine, is normally present in low concentrations in brain tissue and CSF, but its concentration may be increased 10- to 50-fold in the CSF of patients with hepatic coma (Fig. 4) (109). Pharmacologic doses of α-ketoglutaramate infused into the cerebral ventricles depress the behavior of rats (109), but it seems unlikely that the compound contributes to the symptoms of hepatic encephalopathy at the concentrations usually observed in the CSF of patients. Nevertheless, the concentration of α-ketoglutaramate in the spinal fluid provides a useful diagnostic indicator of hepatic encephalopathy and is more specific in this regard than CSF ammonia or glutamine levels alone.

Studies with nitrogen- and carbon-labeled precursors have revealed that the metabolism of ammonia-glutamate-glutamine is compartmented in brain (95, 113–115). Berl et al. (113) infused ^{15}N-ammonia in high concentrations into the carotid arteries of cats and observed a relative incorporation of label into brain metabolites of the order: glutamate < α-amino group of glutamine < amide group of glutamine. Because glutamate is the only known precursor of glutamine, Berl et al. (113) suggested that cerebral glutamine was synthesized in a small, metabolically active pool of glutamate that did not exchange readily with the bulk of brain glutamate (large pool).

Subsequent work in rats obtained at physiologic concentrations of ^{13}N-ammonia in blood (95) confirmed the existence of two pools of cerebral ammonia metabolism and further showed that (a) the incorporation of ^{13}N-ammonia into brain glutamate is only about 0.3% of that incorporated into the amide group glutamine (i.e., the glutamine synthetase reaction predominates over the glutamate dehydrogenase reaction in the metabolism of blood-borne ammonia), and (b) the incorporation of blood-borne ammonia into glutamine in brain is exceedingly rapid ($t_{1/2} \leq 3$ sec). Since little precursor glutamate was synthesized from ammonia in the small brain pool, whereas the synthesis of glutamine was rapid, Cooper et al. (95) suggested that the glutamate formed within this pool may arise by transamination of small-pool α-ketoglutarate with amino acids that are taken up by the brain from the blood. Such a mechanism may contribute to the reported effectiveness of certain enriched amino acid mixtures in the treatment of patients with hepatic encephalopathy (see below).

The astrocytes are the most likely candidates for the cells comprising the small pool of ammonia/glutamate metabolism (115). Morphologically, foot processes of astrocytes surround brain capillaries and thus constitute an integral part of the physiologic-metabolic blood-brain barrier. Distally, astrocytes abut onto neurons. The astrocytes are implicated in cerebral ammonia metabolism because they appear to contain most if not all the brain glutamine synthetase activity (116,117), and astrocytic pathology is one of the hallmarks of hyperammonemic encephalopathy in animals and man (43,47). The inactivation of transmitter glutamate, following its release from neurons and uptake into astrocytes, appears to be an important

physiological function of astrocytic glutamine synthetase (118).

The exact mechanism by which ammonia causes coma is unknown, although at both the cellular and molecular levels, high concentrations of ammonia interfere with processes that are essential to normal brain physiology and function. The acute infusion of ammonium salts into animals increases cerebral blood flow and intracranial pressure; these effects are thought to be secondary to a direct action of ammonia on cerebral resistance vessels causing vasomotor paralysis and loss of autoregulation (119,120). Ammonium ion can replace potassium ion to stimulate the membrane Na^+,K^+-activated ATPase (121); acute hyperammonemia has been shown to increase ATPase activity in the cerebral cortex, cerebellum, and brainstem of mice (122). An increase in the extracellular concentration of ammonium ions will bring about neuronal depolarization by promoting the extrusion of K^+ from neural tissue (123,124) and will block the active extrusion of Cl^- from neurons, thereby causing a shift of the inhibitory postsynaptic reversal potential toward the resting membrane potential and promoting central disinhibition (125,126). Iles and Jack (127) observed that the threshold for inhibition of the chloride pump in cat spinal motoneurons occurred at an extracellular ammonia concentration of approximately 0.1 mM, with a maximal effect (i.e., complete abolition of inhibitory hyperpolarization) at a concentration of

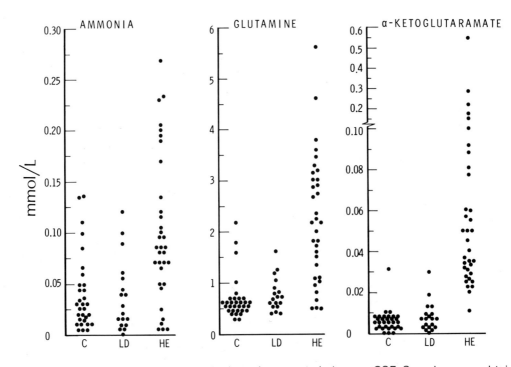

FIG. 4. Concentrations of ammonia, glutamine, and α-ketoglutaramate in human CSF. Samples were obtained by routine diagnostic lumbar puncture. Control subjects had a variety of neurological disorders but had normal liver function. Patients with hepatic encephalopathy had moderate to severe neurological dysfunction. C, control, no liver disease; LD, liver disease, no encephalopathy; HE, hepatic encephalopathy. (From ref. 233.)

0.8 mM. Since the CSF ammonia concentration often exceeds 0.1 mM in patients with hepatic encephalopathy (Fig. 4), ammonia-mediated inhibition of the chloride pump may be responsible for some of the behavioral and electroencephalographic abnormalities seen in such individuals.

Acute and chronic hyperammonemia also interfere with cerebral energy metabolism. Ammonia deinhibits phosphofructokinase, the rate-limiting enzyme of the glycolytic pathway (128), and thereby stimulates glucose utilization in brain (19,104,129). On the other hand, high concentrations of ammonia inhibit cerebral respiration *in vitro* (129,130) and reduce the amount of ^{14}C incorporated into brain glutamate, aspartate, and γ-aminobutyrate in animals injected with [U-^{14}C]glucose (131).

An early hypothesis to account for the coma of liver disease was that reductive amination of α-ketoglutarate by ammonia (via the glutamate dehydrogenase reaction) could deplete cerebral tissue concentrations of this important tricarboxylic acid cycle intermediate and thus inhibit oxidative energy production (132). Direct measurements of α-ketoglutarate, however, do not support this theory. In animals subjected to acute ammonia intoxication, the concentration of α-ketoglutarate in brain is either normal (104,133,134) or increased (78,135), presumably as a consequence in part of ammonia-mediated inhibition of α-ketoglutarate oxidation (129). Furthermore, in hyperammonemic patients with liver failure, the plasma α-ketoglutarate concentration is usually elevated, and there appears to be a net efflux of this α-keto acid from their brains (13). Schenker and co-workers (136) first noted that coma-producing acute ammonia intoxication in rats lowered phosphocreatine and ATP concentrations in the brainstem, whereas cortical concentrations of these high-energy phosphates remained unaltered. The greater sensitivity of the brainstem to ammonia-mediated abnormalities of energy metabolism is supported by results of others (78,134) and may partly reflect the lower activity of glutamine synthetase available to detoxify the ammonia in this area of the brain (137).

Ammonia-induced stupor and coma in rats with a chronic portacaval shunt are accompanied by several abnormalities of cerebral intermediary and energy metabolism. When such animals are given a small ammonia challenge, the cerebral metabolic rate for oxygen declines (103), the lactate/pyruvate ratio of brain tissue rises, and the concentrations of phosphocreatine and ATP fall (78). In addition, the concentrations of the excitatory amino acids, glutamate and aspartate, decrease, glutamine and asparagine levels increase, and the cytoplasmic redox potential (NAD$^+$/NADH) shifts toward a more reduced state (78). A failure to oxidize cytoplasmically-generated NADH may underlie some of these abnormalities. Although NADH does

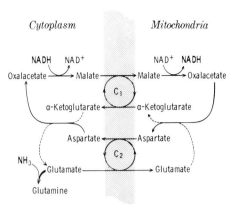

FIG. 5. Interference by ammonia in the transport of reduced equivalents from cytoplasm to mitochondria via the malate-aspartate shuttle. C_1 and C_2, membrane carriers for malate-α-ketoglutarate and glutamate-aspartate transport, respectively. According to this theory, the regeneration of oxaloacetate in the cytoplasm is dependent on the availability of cytoplasmic aspartate which, in turn, is dependent on the rate of glutamate-coupled efflux of aspartate from the mitochondria. Ammonia may interfere with the shuttle by promoting the synthesis of glutamine from cytoplasmic glutamate, thereby reducing the pool of glutamate available for exchange with aspartate. Glutamine synthetase of brain is predominantly extramitochondrial and occurs almost exclusively within astrocytes; ammonia-mediated inhibition of the malate-aspartate shuttle may be confined to this glial cell type. (From ref. 78.)

not cross the mitochondrial membrane readily, net transfer of NADH from cytoplasm to mitochondrion does occur, probably via a carrier system that transports reduced equivalents in lieu of NADH. Purified brain mitochondria have been shown to oxidize NADH only when all the cytoplasmic components of the malate-aspartate shuttle system are present in the medium (138), suggesting that this system may be responsible for regulating intracellular hydrogen transport. Because the carrier-mediated entry of glutamate into the mitochondria is an important regulator of the activity of the malate-aspartate shuttle and the affinity of the mitochondrial carrier protein for glutamate is low (139), ammonia could inhibit the shuttle by depleting the concentration of glutamate in the cytoplasmic compartment by promoting its conversion into glutamine (Fig. 5). Such a block could eventually lead to cerebral energy failure by depriving the mitochondria of oxidizable substrate (NADH). As noted previously, glutamine synthetase of brain appears to be exclusively astrocytic, so that ammonia-mediated inhibition of the malate-asparate shuttle may be confined to the astrocytes (small pool of ammonia metabolism); and may contribute to the astrocytic pathology that typifies chronic hyperammonemic encephalopathies.

AMINO ACID ABNORMALITIES

Abnormal concentrations of amino acids in plasma, CSF, and brain are a consistent finding in patients with acute hepatic failure and chronic portal-systemic encephalopathy. Among the most prominent changes in plasma are increased concentrations of methionine, phenylalanine, tyrosine, and unbound tryptophan, and decreased concentrations of the branched chain neutral amino acids, leucine, isoleucine, and valine (106, 140–143). The reasons for this altered pattern are still incompletely understood, but two factors are thought to contribute: (a) protein catabolism in muscle is increased, perhaps secondary to hyperinsulinism (144) and an elevated glucagon/insulin ratio in plasma (145); and (b) because the aromatic amino acids are degraded mainly in the liver, the capacity to metabolize them is reduced in liver disease. The branched chain neutral amino acids are metabolized mainly in skeletal muscle; muscle uptake of the branched chain amino acids is believed to be increased in cirrhotic patients (141). Elevated brain and CSF concentrations of the aromatic amino acids are probably secondary to increased plasma concentrations of the unbound amino acids (146,147), although the activity of the saturable carrier system that transports these amino acids across the blood-brain barrier may also be enhanced (148,149).

The amino acid abnormalities in the brains of patients with severe liver disease could be either the cause or consequence of abnormal protein synthesis in brain. Brun et al. (150) measured the postmortem concentrations of soluble proteins in the brains of 6 patients who died with liver failure and 6 who died lacking any evidence of liver disease or neurological dysfunction. Hepatic coma was found to be associated with a marked reduction of soluble brain proteins, particularly in areas of gray matter. Such abnormalities may be related to the chronic hyperammonemia that accompanies the disease. Hyperammonemia secondary to methionine sulfoximine administration (151) has been shown to decrease the incorporation of ^{14}C-leucine and ^{14}C-phenylalanine into proteins of the developing rat brain. Wasterlain et al. (152) found that 8 weeks after the construction of a portacaval shunt in adult rats, the incorporation of ^{14}C-lysine into protein was reduced to 50% of control in the forebrain, cerebellum, and brainstem. In the study of Wasterlain et al. (152), an acute superimposed ammonia load, sufficient to cause stupor and slowing of the EEG, depressed protein synthesis in the shunted animals by an additional 15% in all brain regions examined.

Because the aromatic amino acids compete at the blood-brain barrier for the same carrier-mediated transport system as do the branched chain neutral amino acids (153), high plasma concentrations of the aromatic amino acids could limit the cerebral uptake of essential branched chain neutral amino acids in patients with hepatic encephalopathy. Fischer and col-

leagues (154) found that the molar concentration ratio [(leucine + isoleucine + valine)/(phenylalanine + tyrosine)] in plasma correlated inversely with the severity of neurological impairment in a group of 11 patients with hepatic encephalopathy. They suggested that a cerebral imbalance of aromatic and branched chain neutral amino acids reflected by a decreased plasma [(leucine + isoleucine + valine)/(tyrosine + phenylalanine)] ratio may precipitate encephalopathy, possibly by promoting the synthesis of toxic aromatic amines. These authors have advocated the use of specially formulated amino acid mixtures, rich in branch chain neutral amino acids and low in aromatic amino acids, in order to normalize the plasma amino acid profile of patients with hepatic encephalopathy. The regimen was found to improve the survival of dogs with surgically induced portacaval shunts (155) and the neurological status of some patients with hepatic encephalopathy (154,156). Others have confirmed the effectiveness of hyperalimentation with amino acid mixtures high in branched chain amino acids but low in aromatic amino acids as adjunctive therapy for patients with hepatic encephalopathy (157,158), and Maddrey et al. (159) have reported that the administration of the α-keto acid analogues of the branched chain neutral amino acids is equally effective for this purpose. Nevertheless, it seems unlikely that an imbalance between branched chain and aromatic amino acids in either plasma or brain causes the encephalopathy. In this regard, Morgan et al. (160), in a large series of patients with liver disease of varying etiology and severity, observed that a reduction of the plasma [(valine + leucine + isoleucine)/(phenylalanine + tyrosine)] ratio was secondary to liver disease but was independent of the presence of hepatic encephalopathy. Furthermore, Ono et al. (161) found that whereas the [(valine + leucine + isoleucine)/(phenylalanine + tyrosine)] ratios in plasma and CSF were lower in cirrhotic patients compared to control subjects who were free of liver disease, these ratios were not different between cirrhotic patients who were stable and those who developed hepatic encephalopathy. In their study, only tryptophan of the amino acids measured (including methionine, phenylalanine, tyrosine, leucine, isoleucine, and valine) was significantly elevated in the CSF of cirrhotic patients with evidence of encephalopathy, compared to patients who did not experience this complication.

No satisfactory explanation for the neurological improvement of patients with hepatic encephalopathy given infusions of amino acids enriched with branched chain neutral amino acids has been advanced. Fischer and colleagues (154,155) have reasoned that by competing with the cerebral uptake of the aromatic amino acids, increased plasma concentrations of the branched chain amino acids may impede the synthesis of "false" neurotransmitter amines in brain. We suggest, as an alternative mechanism, that the branched chain amino acids, by transaminating with small-pool α-ketoglutarate, reduce the neurotoxicity of ammonia by promoting the synthesis of glutamate in the small (astrocytic) pool of cerebral ammonia metabolism (Fig. 6). Brain possesses branched chain aminotransferase activity (162) and brain slices incubated with L-[1-^{14}C]-leucine rapidly liberate $^{14}CO_2$ (163), a process that involves a transamination reaction (presumably with α-ketoglutarate) as the obligatory first step (164). Leucine is thought to be a precursor of small-pool glutamate because at early times following the injection of L-[4,5-^{3}H]leucine into normal rats or rats with 3-week portacaval shunts, the ^{3}H-glutamine/^{3}H-glutamate ratios in the animals' brains are consistently greater than 1.0 (165). Increasing the synthesis of glutamate in the astrocytic compartment would have at least two beneficial effects with respect to cerebral ammonia intoxication: (a) incorporation of ammonia into glutamine would be stimulated owing to increased availability of precursor glutamate, and (b) inhibition of the malate-aspartate shuttle caused by ammonia-mediated depletion of cytosolic glutamate would be relieved. In this connection, it is noteworthy that although high-dose valine administration tends to raise plasma ammonia levels (166), it was found to be associated with lower postmortem ammonia concentrations in the brains of cirrhotic patients dying after hepatic coma compared to similar patients who did not receive valine (167).

NEUROTRANSMITTER CHANGES

Several investigators have suggested that abnormal neurotransmitter function may contribute to the neurological complications of liver failure. Presently, however, no direct evidence supports the speculation. The concentration of tryptophan in brain, which, as noted previously, is elevated in association with severe liver disease, is a major determinant of brain serotonin synthesis (168,169). Not surprisingly, therefore, the concentrations of serotonin and 5-hydroxyindole acetic acid (5-HIAA), the major metabolite of serotonin, have both been found to be increased in the brain (especially in the brainstem) of rats with portacaval shunts (170,171), as well as in the brains and CSF (5-HIAA only) of patients with acute and chronic hepatic encephalopathy (172,173). The observation that the administration of branched chain amino acids to rats with portacaval shunts reduces the concentrations of tryptophan, serotonin, and 5-HIAA in the animals' brains (171) suggests that an imbalance of plasma aromatic and branched chain amino acids

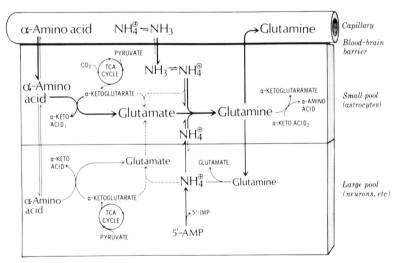

FIG. 6. Mechanism by which blood-borne amino acids may facilitate detoxification of ammonia in brain. Blood-borne and endogenously generated brain ammonia are depicted as reacting with glutamate in the small (astrocytic) pool to form glutamine, which, in turn, may diffuse into cerebral venous blood (and CSF) or into the large (neuronal) pool. Glutamate synthesis in the small pool is thought to arise mainly by transamination of small-pool α-ketoglutarate with blood-borne amino acids (95). Increased plasma and brain concentrations of the amino acids that are preferentially metabolized by transamination (e.g., branched chain amino acids) may stimulate the synthesis of glutamate in the small pool and thereby promote the incorporation of ammonia into glutamine. Depending on the nature of the transaminating amino acid (phenylalanine will also react, giving rise to phenylpyruvate), the α-keto acid formed may be further oxidized and partially replenish the carbons lost from the small pool as glutamine (branched chain α-keto acids), or it may transaminate with glutamine (phenylpyruvate) and promote the synthesis of the potential toxin α-ketoglutaramate. *Thick arrows,* processes thought to be favored. The glutaminase, glutamine transaminase, and adenylate deaminase reactions are represented in the brain compartment in which they are likely to be most active; however, all three reactions probably occur to some extent in both compartments. 5'-AMP, adenosine 5'-monophosphate; 5'-IMP, inosine 5'-monophosphate; P_i, inorganic orthophosphate.

contributes to the raised levels of brain indoles. Questions of whether and how an accumulation of serotonin in brain might cause coma are unanswereed at present, although displacement of other natural neurotransmitter amines from their presynaptic storage depots or postsynaptic receptors (i.e., false neurotransmitter hypothesis) has been advocated (174).

FALSE NEUROTRANSMITTERS

The hypothesis that inappropriate or "false" neurotransmitters may be involved in the production of hepatic coma (175) is attractive. Such false transmitters originally were suggested to be amines that were stored or released at nerve endings but had different or lesser effects at the target cell compared to the natural neurotransmitter. The concept has since been modified to include any molecule that may accumulate in nerve endings and mimic the metabolism and function of a natural neurotransmitter (176). The aromatic amines, octopamine, tyramine, and β-phenylethanolamine, have been proposed as false adrenergic neurotransmitters in hepatic coma (176), with the strongest evidence implicating the norepinephrine analog, octopamine. All three amines exhibit weak sympathetic activity and can displace norepinephrine and dopamine from their storage granules at nerve terminals (177). Patients with hepatic coma excrete tyramine and octopamine in urine in increased amounts (178), and there is a good correlation between the serum octopamine concentration and the degree of neurological disability in such individuals (179,180). Studies by Fischer and colleagues (178,181,182) have shown that the concentrations of octopamine and β-phenylethanolamine are increased in brain and CSF in animal models of liver failure, and that the brain concentrations of octopamine and β-phenylethanolamine rise prior to the increases in blood levels. This implies that the amines were being synthesized in the central nervous system (CNS) since they do not readily penetrate the blood-brain barrier. An additional factor, cited in support of the false neurotransmitter hypothesis (178), is that the administration of L-DOPA will lighten the coma of some patients with hepatic failure (175,183). It has been suggested that release of octopamine and other accumulated false neurotransmitters in brain (presumably secondary to increased synthesis of brain dopamine and norepinephrine) may be one beneficial effect of such therapy (181). Since L-DOPA may produce arousal in patients with reduced consciousness of several different causes, however, it is difficult to attribute its occasional effect in hepatic encephalopathy to disease-specific mechanisms.

Recent data from several laboratories mitigate against a disturbance of cerebral catecholamines as the primary cause of hepatic encephalopathy. Cuilleret et al. (184) found that brain dopamine and norepinephrine concentrations were similar in postmortem tissues obtained from cirrhotic patients with and without encephalopathy and from control subjects who were free of liver disease. The authors also found that octopamine levels were higher in control subjects than in patients with hepatic encephalopathy. Zieve and Olsen (185) infused octopamine into the cerebroventricular system of rats in amounts sufficient to raise brain octopamine concentrations more than 20,000-fold and reduce brain norepinephrine and dopamine levels by 86 and 92%, respectively. The treatment had no discernible effect on the alertness or activity of the animals. Other studies suggest that the beneficial effect of L-DOPA therapy may be unrelated to cerebral catecholamine metabolism. Thus, Zieve et al. (186) observed that a sufficient dosage of L-DOPA could prevent experimental hyperammonemic coma in rats, and that the presence or absence of coma correlated with the brain ammonia concentration but not with the brain dopamine concentration. These investigators further noted that the protective effect of L-DOPA was associated with an increase in the renal excretion of ammonia and suggested that the beneficial effects of L-DOPA in some patients with hepatic encephalopathy may be the result of a peripheral action of dopamine on renal function rather than a CNS action.

ACETYLCHOLINE

No firm data suggest that cholinergic function is altered in patients with hepatic coma. Ammonia inhibits the synthesis of acetylcholine *in vitro* (187), and several groups have reported decreased concentrations of acetylcholine in animals with ammonia-induced convulsions. It is uncertain from these studies, however, whether the transmitter change was caused by the hyperammonemia or was merely secondary to the convulsions. Parker et al. (188) reported that acute ammonia-induced coma had little effect upon acetylcholine concentrations in the brains of unoperated rats or rats with 1-week portacaval shunts. However, when the shunted rats were gavage-fed an ammoniated resin and developed stupor and coma over several days, a 14 to 39% reduction of acetylcholine content in the cerebral cortex, striatum, and brainstem was observed.

In attempting to account for the difference in response between animals acutely and semichronically intoxicated with ammonia, Parker et al. (188) speculated that the accumulation of ammonia over the longer period may have depleted some key cerebral acetylcholine precursor pool, but they dismissed the changes of acetylcholine as a likely cause of the coma. No studies of the effect of liver failure on the rate of turnover of acetylcholine in brain have been reported. It is now well established, however, that decreased acetylcholine turnover occurs in other metabolic encephalopathies (e.g., hypoxia, hypoglycemia) in which the cerebral concentration of acetylcholine remains unchanged (189,190). Since the turnover of the neurotransmitter more accurately reflects the activity of a neural system than does the tissue concentration of the transmitter, failure to demonstrate altered brain levels of acetylcholine in hyperammonemic encephalopathy does not rule out a possible involvement of central cholinergic mechanisms in the development of the neurologic symptoms of liver failure.

MERCAPTANS

Oral administration to patients with cirrhosis and chronic portal-systemic shunting of the sulfur-containing amino acid methionine can precipitate encephalopathy at constant plasma ammonia concentrations (191). Because the encephalopathy can be prevented or delayed by prior sterilization of the gut and fails to develop when the amino acid is given intravenously, bacterial degradation of methionine to mercaptans is thought to be responsible for the neurotoxicity (191,192). Methyl mercaptan, ethyl mercaptan, and dimethyl sulfide are excreted in increased quantities in the breath of patients with severe decompensated cirrhosis (192), and the concentration of methyl mercaptan has been shown to increase in their plasma (193) and urine (194).

Mercaptans are highly neurotoxic (195). Methyl mercaptan, the most toxic of the three mercaptans normally detectable in the breath, will cause coma in rats at a plasma concentration of 0.5 μM (196). Its toxicity is enhanced in the presence of moderately elevated plasma concentrations of ammonia or free fatty acids that, by themselves, will not cause coma (197). Since the plasma concentration of methyl mercaptan can exceed 0.5 μM in patients with hepatic encephalopathy (193), this substance acting alone or synergistically with other toxins may contribute to the neurologic abnormalities of the disorder. How the mercaptans produce their toxicity is still unclear. At much higher concentrations than those normally seen clinically, methyl mercaptan has been found to inhibit brain Na^+,K^+-activated ATPase (198); but whether or not this effect is relevant to the neurotoxicity of the compound is unknown.

FREE FATTY ACIDS

Plasma free fatty acid levels are substantially elevated in patients with chronic or fulminant hepatic failure (including Reye disease), and the increased concentrations of the short-chain fatty acids in particular have been linked to the production of encephalopathy in these disorders (199–202). Short-chain fatty acids are generated in the intestinal tract by bacterial metabolism of the intestinal lipid contents and by the incomplete β-oxidation of long-chain fatty acids by the diseased liver (203). Infusion of short-chain fatty acids into animals induces a reversible state of coma (204) accompanied by electroencephalographic changes that resemble those seen in human hepatic coma (205,206). Interestingly, short-chain fatty acids can interfere with systemic urea production (207) and will potentiate the neurotoxicity of ammonia in experimental animals (197).

The mechanism by which elevated concentrations of free fatty acids exert their neurotoxicity is poorly understood. Free fatty acids inhibit respiration and incorporation of $^{32}P_i$ into ATP of rat brain-cortex slices incubated *in vitro* (208). The coma resulting from infusions of short-chain fatty acids into animals is not the result of cerebral energy failure or decreased energy utilization in the cortex or brainstem, however, because these are normal at the onset of coma (209). Dahl (210) has shown that short-chain fatty acids inhibit the membrane Na^+,K^+-activated ATPase. Accordingly, the fatty acids may interfere with the movement of cations across neural membranes and thereby impair normal impulse propagation. In support of this view, Pettegrew and Minshew (211) have reported that the addition of octanoate to suspensions of whole blood *in vitro* alters erythrocyte membrane permeability as well as erythrocyte membrane-associated ATPase activity. Increased plasma concentrations of free fatty acids may also contribute to the neurotoxicity of tryptophan by reducing the amount of circulating tryptophan that is bound to albumin (212). In this regard, Mays (201) observed that the plasma concentration of free fatty acids per gram of serum albumin was increased as much as 10-fold in patients with hepatic coma compared to control subjects.

Difficulties with the fatty acid hypothesis of hepatic coma are: (a) concentrations of short-chain fatty acids required to cause coma in animals exceed those found in the plasma of patients with hepatic failure by at least an order of magnitude (209); and (b) the correlation of increased plasma free fatty acid levels with the encephalopathy is less than compelling (213). Furthermore, Wilcox et al. (214) observed that although the plasma concentrations of the long-chain fatty acids were increased in patients with liver disease, the concentrations were similar in severe cirrhotics with or without coma and did not correlate with the blood ammonia levels. The latter finding suggests that at least the long-chain fatty acids do not have a measurable influence on systemic ammonia metabolism in man.

TREATMENT OF HEPATIC ENCEPHALOPATHY

The proven beneficial aspects of care for the patient with hepatic encephalopathy are preventing complications, treating symptoms, and initiating measures to reduce ammonia absorption from the intestine. A number of other biochemical regimens have been advocated for treatment based on theories of toxicity or insufficiency of various amino acids, the possible deficiency of metabolic intermediates or nutritional stuffs critical to brain metabolism, or of derangements of putative neurotransmitter systems. Except for the antihyperammonemia regimens, however, none of the biochemically based proposals have met wide or independently verified success (215); their discussion is beyond the scope of this chapter.

GENERAL MEASURES

The immediate and probably most important aspect of the care of patients with hepatic encephalopathy consists of giving scrupulous attention to general medical problems. These patients are unduly sensitive to the depressant effects of sedatives and hypnotics, which must be avoided except in the rare instance of uncontrollable mania. In the latter instance, low doses of benzodiazepines, such as diazepam (2 mg), may be given repeatedly in doses sufficient to keep the patient from injuring himself or others but not to induce sleep. For patients with reduced states of consciousness, depression of behavior almost always is accompanied by impairment of autonomic reflexes and perhaps lowered systemic immunity as well. Pulmonary congestion, infection, hypoxemia, acid-base and electrolyte perturbations, renal failure, and bleeding must be searched for and corrected promptly. Patients with constipation or GI bleeding should have the gut cleansed with cathartics or enemas; recent evidence suggests that lactose enemas may be the mode of choice (see below).

Protein balance must be adjusted carefully. Authorities recommend stopping protein intake when hepatic encephalopathy appears or worsens. Most patients with chronic liver disease, however, are protein and muscle depleted, and the muscle wasting reduces their systemic capacity to detoxify ammonia (85). Accordingly, protein intake should be restarted as promptly as possible when the neurologic condition has stabilized, at which point every effort should be made gradually to increase the intake to at least 0.5 g/kg body weight (24).

Certain measures deserve particular attention. Large, abrupt reductions of fluid volume by paracentesis or too rigid diuresis threaten to worsen hepatic encephalopathy and should be avoided. As noted earlier, acetazolamide is particularly dangerous and depresses brain metabolism directly (5,216) and by increasing the ammonia concentration in renal effluent blood (217). Hyponatremia, common in hepatic encephalopathy, is a mechanism that potentially contrib-

utes to brain edema in the coma of fulminant hepatic failure. In addition, human and experimental evidence indicates that sudden corrections or overcorrections of hyponatremia, such as may accompany lactulose therapy, may precipitate central pontine myelinolysis (218), a neurological complication known to have an increased incidence in chronic portal-systemic encephalopathy. Patients with fulminant hepatic failure should not be overhydrated because of the risk of potentially fatal cerebral edema in this condition; patients with chronic cirrhosis and either portal-systemic encephalopathy or merely gradual hepatic failure and encephalopathy tend to be hypovolemic. The latter state must be corrected cautiously, because cirrhotic patients characteristically have high circulating antidiuretic hormone levels. Accurate titration between volume needs and osmolal risks requires close attention.

Malnutrition can induce increasing hepatic insufficiency and is a particular problem where alcohol ingestion provides calories but no vitamins. Wernicke's disease due to thiamin deficiency produces lethargy, drowsiness and confusion that inexperienced observers may initially mistake for impending hepatic encephalopathy. More often, nutritional encephalopathy accompanies hepatic failure. Accordingly, generous doses of oral or parenteral vitamins should be supplied.

Whenever possible, lumbar puncture should be avoided in patients with hepatic failure. A lumbar puncture is decisive only in diagnosing meningitis, a disease that heralds itself with such strong clinical implications that the purpose of a spinal tap should almost always be to answer "what kind?" rather than "is it present?" Lumbar punctures in patients with severe liver disease sometimes are followed by lumbar subdural hematomas, and the trauma can exert a nonspecific adverse effect on the clinical course.

SPECIFIC TREATMENT OF ENCEPHALOPATHY

Protein Intake

Patients with acutely worsening encephalopathy should stop all protein intake. Where portal-systemic encephalopathy has been precipitated by heavy protein feeding or GI bleeding, lactose enemas should be carried out to remove the nitrogenous substrate. Afebrile patients lying quietly in bed require little more than 600 to 800 kilocalories per day to meet their energy requirements. For a few days, this demand can be met readily by giving 10 to 20% glucose infusions without producing fluid overload. Hypertonic glucose, however, potentially creates an osmotic diuresis, and its administration should be accompanied by appropriate sodium, potassium, and, occasionally, magnesium replacement. If constipation persists, lactose enemas should be continued. Strong cathartics risk producing sudden fluid and electrolyte losses and are best avoided.

Oral Lactulose

Lactulose, a keto analog of lactose, reaches the colon largely unhydrolyzed and is metabolized there by intestinal bacteria mainly into lactic and acetic acids. Except for occasionally inducing diarrhea, the drug is nontoxic and can be regarded as the treatment of choice for patients with chronic hepatic encephalopathy (219). The low pH stimulates the growth of nonurease-containing lactobacilli and suppresses bacteroides, biologic phenomena that led Ingelfinger in 1965 (220) to suggest that the agent might reduce intestinal ammonia production and have value in treating hepatic encephalopathy. Bircher et al. (221) acted on the suggestion and several subsequent studies, some well controlled (222–224), confirmed that oral lactulose feeding lowers blood ammonia levels and improves the neurologic status of patients with PSE. Beneficial effects of lactulose have been less notable in coma associated with fulminant hepatic failure, perhaps because hyperammonemia is less consistently the major pathogenetic agent in this syndrome.

Lactulose appears to exert its beneficial action by several mechanisms, not all of which are completely understood. The increased osmolarity and decreased pH of the colon contents stimulate bowel emptying. Colon bacterial counts indicate that the decline in number of ammonia forming organisms is less rapid than either the fall of blood ammonia levels or clinical improvement following administration of the agent (225). Lactulose acidifies the intestinal contents, which may retard ammonia transfer into portal blood (222, 226). More recent studies, obtained with an *in vitro* fecal incubation system (227), suggest that lactulose provides the colonic bacteria with a fermentable substrate and reduces the ammonia content of the stool, either by promoting bacterial assimilation of the ammonia or by sparing bacterial deamination of exogenous and endogenous nitrogenous precursors. Other possible chemical effects of the agent have not been extensively explored (215).

Lactulose usually is given orally in syrup form with meals in doses of 70 to 100 g/day, the lower dose being employed if diarrhea results. For patients unable to take the agent by mouth, lactulose (or the less expensive lactose) enemas appear to be equally effective and presumably work via mechanisms similar to those that follow the oral administration of lactulose (224).

Neomycin

In oral doses up to 2 g daily, this antibiotic has been used effectively to reduce intestinal ammonia absorption and improve PSE. It is poorly absorbed and lowers the number of ureolytic and proteolytic bacteria in the gut. If kept at doses of less than 2 g/day, the potential complications of producing kidney and labyrinthine damage or inducing intestinal staphylococcal infections can be avoided or minimized. Many centers give neomycin and lactulose together to treat acute hepatic encephalopathy since individual therapeutic responses can differ unpredictably between the two drugs. Double-blind studies indicate, however, that the nontoxic lactulose is at least as effective therapeutically as neomycin when the two are compared directly (215).

L-DOPA and Bromocriptine

Parkes et al. reported in 1970 (228) that the dopamine precursor, L-DOPA temporarily improved the arousal and EEGs of some patients with hepatic encephalopathy. Several other workers reported similar neurologic improvement in small numbers of patients. Subsequently, Morgan et al. (229) reported encouraging neurologic improvement in patients with PSE treated with bromocriptine, a specific dopamine receptor agonist. Response to these agents by patients with hepatic encephalopathy has been inconsistent and temporary in our hands. In addition, controlled studies of their effects in unselected patients with PSE have not confirmed their usefulness (230,231). Both L-DOPA and bromocriptine can have an arousal effect on patients with stupor or coma resulting from several different causes, both metabolic and structural (232). We suspect that whatever arousal effect these drugs exert in hepatic encephalopathy results from nonspecific stimulation of the brain rather than any direct effect on primary mechanisms producing cerebral insufficiency.

Other Measures

As noted earlier, patients dying of fulminant hepatic failure tend to show severe brain swelling and, sometimes, acute transtentorial herniation. The cause of this presumed edema is not known, nor has any specific treatment been reported that is successful in reducing the high mortality of patients in coma from fulminating hepatic failure. Beyond keeping such patients moderately dehydrated, well oxygenated, and as free as possible of complications, little further can be done once a stage of deep unarousability is reached. Osmotic agents, steroids, passive hyperventilation, or drainage of the cerebral ventricles all have been tried, but without notable success.

ACKNOWLEDGMENT

The studies by the authors cited in this chapter were assisted by NIH grants NS03346 and AM16739.

REFERENCES

1. Plum, F., and Hindfelt, B. (1976): The neurological complications of liver disease. In: *Handbook of Neurology, Metabolic and Deficiency Diseases of the Nervous System*, edited by P. J. Vincken and G. W. Bruyn, vol. 27, pp. 349–377. North-Holland, Amsterdam.

2. Plum, F., and Posner J. B. (1981): *The Diagnosis of Stupor and Coma*, third edition. F. A. Davis, Philadelphia.

3. Levy, D. E., Bates, D., Caronna, J. J., Cartlidge, N. E. F., Knill-Jones, R. P., Singer, B. H., Shaw, D. A., and Plum, F. (1981): Prognosis in nontraumatic coma. *Ann. Intern. Med.*, 94:293–301.

4. Fazekas, J. F., Ticktin, H. E., Ehrmantraut, W. R., and Alman, R. W. (1956): Cerebral metabolism in hepatic insufficiency. *Am. J. Med.*, 21:843–849.

5. Posner, J. B., and Plum, F. (1960): The toxic effects of carbon dioxide and acetazolamide in hepatic encephalopathy. *J. Clin. Invest.*, 39:1246–1258.

6. Maiolo, A. T., Bianchi Porro, G., Galli, C., Sessa, M., and Polli, E. E. (1971): Brain energy metabolism in hepatic coma. *Exp. Biol. Med.*, 4:52–70.

7. James, I. M., Nashat, S., Sampson, D., Williams, H. S., and Garassini, M. (1969): Effect of induced metabolic alkalosis in hepatic encephalopathy. *Lancet*, 2:1106–1108.

8. Stanley, N. N., and Cherniak, N. S. (1976): Effect of liver failure on the cerebral circulatory and metabolic responses to hypoxia in the goat. *Clin. Sci. Mol. Med.*, 50:15–23.

9. Trewby, P. N., Hanid, M. A., Mackenzie, R. L., Mellon, P. J., and Williams, R. (1978): Effects of cerebral edema and arterial hypotension on cerebral blood flow in an animal model of hepatic failure. *Gut*, 19:999–1005.

10. Breen, K. J., and Schenker, S. (1972): Hepatic coma: Present concepts of pathogenesis and therapy. In: *Progress in Liver Diseases*, edited by H. Popper and F. Schaffner, vol. 4, pp. 301–332. Grune & Stratton, New York.

11. Vanamee, P., Poppell, J. W., Glicksman, A. S., Randall, H. T., and Roberts, K. E. (1956): Respiratory alkalosis in hepatic coma. *Arch. Int. Med.*, 97:762–767.

12. Prytz, H., and Thomsen, A. C. (1976): Acid-base status in liver cirrhosis. Disturbances in stable, terminal, and porta-caval shunted patients. *Scand. J. Gastroenterol.*, 11:249–256.

13. Dastur, D. K., Seshadri, R., and Talageri, V. R. (1963): Liver-brain relationships in hepatic coma. *Arch. Int. Med.*, 112:899–916.

14. Zieve, L. (1966): Pathogenesis of hepatic coma. *Arch. Int. Med.*, 118:211–223.

15. Schwab, M., and Dammaschke, H. (1962): Atmung, Säure-Basen-Gleichgewicht und Ammoniak/Ammonium in Blut und Liquor cerebrospinalis bei Lebercirrhose. *Klin. Wochenschr.*, 40:184–199.

16. Karetzky, M. S., and Mithoefer, J. C. (1967): The cause of hyperventilation and arterial hypoxia in patients with cirrhosis of the liver. *Am. J. Med. Sci.*, 254:797–804.

17. Bittar, E. E. (1964): An approach to cirrhosis of the liver. In: *Cell pH*, pp. 85–96. Butterworths, London.

18. Roberts, K. E., Thompson, F. G., III, Poppell, J. W., and Vanamee, P. (1956): Respiratory alkalosis accompanying ammonium toxicity. *J. Appl. Physiol.*, 9:367–370.

19. James, I. M., MacDonnell, L., and Xanalatos, C. (1974): Effect of ammonium salts on brain metabolism. *J. Neurol. Neurosurg. Psychiatry*, 37:948–953.

20. Berry, J. N., Owen, E. E., Flanagan, J. F., and Tyor, M. P. (1960): The effect of acute hyperventilation on the blood ammonia concentration of patients with liver disease. *J. Lab. Clin. Med.*, 55:849–854.

21. Laidlaw, J., and Read, A. E. (1963): The E.E.G. in hepatic encephalopathy. *Clin. Sci.*, 24:109–120.

22. Foley, J. M., Watson, C. W., and Adams, R. D. (1950): Significance of the electroencephalographic changes in hepatic coma. *Trans. Am. Neurol. Assoc.*, 75:161–165.

23. Bickford, R. G., and Butt, H. R. (1955): Hepatic coma: The electroencephalographic pattern. *J. Clin. Invest.*, 34:790–799.

24. Sherlock, S. (1981): *Diseases of the Liver and Biliary System*, sixth edition. Blackwell, Oxford.

25. Poser, C. M. (1958): Electroencephalographic changes and hyperammonemia. *Electroencephalogr. Clin. Neurophysiol.*, 10:51–62.

26. Hawkes, C. H., Brunt, P. W., Prescott, R. J., and Horn, D. B. (1973): EEG-provocative tests in the diagnosis of hepatic encephalopathy. *Electroencephalogr. Clin. Neurophysiol.*, 34:163–169.

27. Pirola, R. C., Ham, J. M., and Elmslie, R. G. (1969): Management of hepatic coma complicating viral hepatitis. *Gut*, 10:898–903.

28. Ware, A. J., D'Agostino, A. N., and Combes, B. (1971): Cerebral edema: A major complication of massive hepatic necrosis. *Gastroenterology*, 61:877–884.

29. Gazzard, B. G., Portmann, B., Murray-Lyon, I. M., and Williams, R. (1975): Causes of death in fulminant hepatic failure and relationship to quantitative histological assessment of parenchymal damage. *Q. J. Med.*, 44:615–626.

30. Partin, J. S., McAdams, A. J., Partin, J. C., Schubert, W. K., and McLaurin, R. L. (1978): Brain ultrastructure in Reye's disease. II. Acute injury and recovery processes in three children. *J. Neuropathol. Exp. Neurol.*, 37:796–819.

31. Hoyumpa, A. M., Jr., Desmond, P. V., Avant, G. R., Roberts, R. K., and Schenker, S. (1979): Hepatic encephalopathy. *Gastroenterology*, 76:184–195.

32. Livingstone, A. S., Potvin, M., Goresky, C. A., Finlayson, M. H., and Hinchey, E. J. (1977): Changes in the blood-brain barrier in hepatic coma after hepatectomy in the rat. *Gastroenterology*, 73:697–704.

33. Partin, J. C., Partin, J. S., Schubert, W. K., and McLaurin, R. L. (1975): Brain ultrastructure in Reye's syndrome (encephalopathy and fatty alteration of the viscera). *J. Neuropathol. Exp. Neurol.*, 34:425–444.

34. von Hösslin, C., and Alzheimer, A. (1912): Ein Beitrag zur Klinik und pathologischen Anatomie der Westphal-Strumpellschen Pseudosklerose. *Z. Gesamte Neurol. Psychiatr.*, 8:183–209.

35. Adams, R. D., and Foley, J. M. (1953): The neurological disorder associated with liver disease. In: *Metabolic and Toxic Diseases of the Nervous System*, edited by H. H. Merritt and C. C. Hare, vol. 32, pp. 198–237. Williams & Wilkins, Baltimore.

36. Victor, M., Adams, R. D., and Cole, M. (1965): The acquired (non-Wilsonian) type of chronic hepatocerebral degeneration. *Medicine*, 44:345–396.

37. Martinez, A. (1968): Electron microscopy in human hepatic encephalopathy. *Acta Neuropathol.*, 11:82–86.

38. Horita, N., Matsushita, M., Ishii, T., Oyanagi, S., and Sakamoto, K. (1981): Ultrastructure of Alzheimer type II glia in hepatocerebral disease. *Neuropathol. Appl. Neurobiol.*, 7:97–102.

39. Cavanagh, J. B., and Kyu, M. H. (1971): Type II Alzheimer change experimentally produced in astrocytes in the rat. *J. Neurol. Sci.*, 12:63–75.

40. Norenberg, M. D. (1977): A light and electron microscopic study of experimental portal-systemic (ammonia) encephalopathy. Progression and reversal of the disorder. *Lab. Invest.*, 36:618–627.

41. Bruton, C. J., Corsellis, J. A. N., and Russell, A. (1970): Hereditary hyperammonemia. *Brain*, 93:423–434.

42. Kline, D. G., Crook, J. N., and Nance, F. C. (1971): Eck fistula encephalopathy: Long-term studies in primates. *Ann. Surg.*, 173:97–103.

43. Cavanagh, J. B. (1974): Liver bypass and the glia. *Res. Publ. Assoc. Nerv. Ment. Dis.*, 53:13–35.

44. Taylor, P., Schoene, W. C., Reid, W. A., Jr., and von Lichtenberg, F. (1979): Quantitative changes in astrocytes after portacaval shunting. *Arch. Pathol. Lab. Med.*, 103:82–85.

45. Gutierrez, J. A., and Norenberg, M. D. (1975): Alzheimer II astrocytosis following methionine sulfoximine. *Arch. Neurol.*, 32:123–126.

46. Gibson, G. E., Zimber, A., Krook, L., Richardson, E. P., Jr., and Visek, W. J. (1974): Brain histology and behavior of mice injected with urease. *J. Neuropathol. Exp. Neurol.*, 33:201–211.

47. Cole, M., Rutherford, R. B., and Smith, F. O. (1972): Experimental ammonia encephalopathy in the primate. *Arch. Neurol.*, 26:130–136.

48. Zamora, A. J., Cavanagh, J. B., and Kyu, M. H. (1973): Ultrastructural responses of the astrocytes to portocaval anastomosis in the rat. *J. Neurol. Sci.*, 18:25–45.

49. Saunders, S. J., Hickman, R., MacDonald, R., and Terblauche, J. (1972): The treatment of acute liver failure. In: *Progress in Liver Diseases, Vol. 4*, edited by H. Popper and F. Schaffner, pp. 333–344. Grune & Stratton, New York.

50. Geiger, A., Magnes, J., Taylor, R. M., and Veralli, M. (1954): Effect of blood constituents on uptake of glucose and on metabolic rate of the brain in perfusion experiments. *Am. J. Physiol.*, 177:138–149.

51. Geiger, A., and Yamasaki, S. (1956): Cytidine and uridine requirement of the brain. *J. Neurochem.*, 1:93–100.

52. Shafer, W. H., and Isselbacher, K. J. (1961): Uridine metabolism in chronic liver disease. *Gastroenterology*, 40:782–784.

53. Lascelles, P. T. (1971): Oxygen electrode studies of rat brain respiration in hepatic coma. *Exp. Biol. Med.*, 4:104–106.

54. Brennan, R. W., and Plum, F. (1971): A cerebrospinal fluid transfer model for hepatic and uremic encephalopathy. *Trans. Am. Neurol. Assoc.*, 96:210–211.

55. Gazzard, B., Weston, M. J., Murray-Lyon, I. M., Flax, H., Record, C. O., Portman, B., Langley, P. G., Dunlop, E. H., Mellon, P. J., Ward, M. B., and Williams, R. (1974): Charcoal hemoperfusion in the treatment of fulminant hepatic failure. *Lancet*, 1:1301–1307.

56. Silk, D. B. A., Trewby, P. N., Chase, R. A., Mellon, P. J., Hand, M. A., Davies, M., Langley, P. G., Wheller, P. G., and Williams, R. (1977): Treatment of fulminant hepatic failure by polyacrilonitrile membrane hemodialysis. *Lancet*, 2:1–3.

57. Eck, N. V. (1877): Ligature of the portal vein. *Med. J. St. Petersburg*, 130:1–2. [Translated by Child, C. G. (1953): Eck fistula. *Surg. Gynecol. Obstet.*, 96:375–376.]

58. Torda, C. (1953): Ammonium ion content and electrical activity of the brain during the preconvulsive and convulsive phases induced by various convulsants. *J. Pharmacol. Exp. Ther.*, 107:197–203.

59. Hindfelt, B., and Siesjö, B. K. (1971): Cerebral effects of acute ammonia intoxication. I. The influence on intracellular and extracellular acid-base parameters. *Scand. J. Clin. Lab. Invest.*, 28:353–364.

60. Phillips, G. B., Schwartz, R., Gabuzda, G. J., Jr., and Davidson, C. S. (1952): The syndrome of impending hepatic coma in patients with cirrhosis of the liver given certain nitrogenous substances. *N. Engl. J. Med.*, 247:239–248.

61. McDermott, W. V., Jr., and Adams, R. D. (1954): Episodic stupor associated with an Eck fistula in the human with particular reference to the metabolism of ammonia. *J. Clin. Invest.*, 33:1–9.

62. Seegmiller, J. E., Schwartz, R., and Davidson, C. S. (1954): The plasma "ammonia" and glutamine content in patients with hepatic coma. *J. Clin. Invest.*, 33:984–988.

63. Plum, F. (1971): The CSF in hepatic encephalopathy. *Exp. Biol. Med.*, 4:34–41.

64. Ansley, J. D., Isaacs, J. W., Rikkers, L. F. Kutner, M. H., Nordlinger, B. M., and Rudman, D. (1978): Quantitative tests of nitrogen metabolism in cirrhosis: Relation to other manifestations of liver disease. *Gastroenterology*, 75:570–579.

65. Phear, E. A., Sherlock, S., and Summerskill, W. H. J. (1955): Blood-ammonium levels in liver disease and "hepatic coma." *Lancet*, 1:836–840.

66. Sullivan, J. F., Linder, H., Holdener, P., and Ortmeyer, D. (1961): Blood ammonia in cerebral dysfunction. *Am. J. Med.*, 30:893–898.

67. Navazio, F., Gerritsen, T., and Wright, G. J. (1961): Relationship of ammonia intoxication to convulsions and coma in rats. *J. Neurochem.*, 8:146–151.

68. Ehrlich, M., Plum, F., and Duffy, T. E. (1980): Blood and brain ammonia concentrations after portacaval anastomosis. Effects of acute ammonia loading. *J. Neurochem.*, 34:1538–1542.

69. Huttenlocher, P. R., Schwartz, A. D., and Klatskin, G. (1969): Reye's syndrome: Ammonia intoxication as a possible factor in the encephalopathy. *Pediatrics*, 43:443–454.

70. Glasgow, A. M., Cotton, R. B., and Dhiensiri, K. (1972): Reye's syndrome. I. Blood ammonia and consideration of the nonhistologic diagnosis. *Am. J. Dis. Child.*, 124:827–836.

71. Batshaw, M., Brusilow, S., and Walser, M. (1975): Treatment of carbamyl phosphate synthetase deficiency with keto analogues of essential amino acids. *N. Engl. J. Med.*, 292:1085–1090.

72. Ballard, R. A., Vinocur, B., Reynolds, J. W., Wennberg, R. P., Merritt, A., Sweetman, L., and Nyhan, W. L. (1978): Transient hyperammonemia of the preterm infant. *N. Engl. J. Med.*, 299:920–925.

73. Ellison, P. H., and Cowger, M. L. (1981): Transient hyperammonemia in the preterm infant: Neurologic aspects. *Neurology*, 31:767–770.

74. Holcenberg, J. S., Camitta, B. M., Borella, L. D., and Ring, B. J. (1979): Phase I study of succinylated *Acinetobacter* L-glutaminase-L-asparaginase. *Cancer Treat. Rep.*, 63:1025–1030.

75. Mortensen, E., Lyng, G., and Juhl, E. (1972): Ammonia-induced coma after ureterosigmoidostomy. *Lancet*, 1:1024.

76. Coulter, D. L., and Allen, R. J. (1980): Secondary hyperammonemia: A possible mechanism for valproate encephalopathy. *Lancet*, 1:1310–1311.

77. Rawat, S., Borkowski, W. J., and Swick, H. M. (1981): Valproic acid and secondary hyperammonemia. *Neurology*, 31:1173–1174.

78. Hindfelt, B., Plum, F., and Duffy, T. E. (1977): Effect of acute ammonia intoxication on cerebral metabolism in rats with portacaval shunts. *J. Clin. Invest.*, 59:386–396.

79. Tsukada, Y., Takagaki, G., Sugimoto, S., and Hirano, S. (1958): Changes in the ammonia and glutamine content of the rat brain induced by electric shock. *J. Neurochem.*, 2:295–303.

80. Richter, D., and Dawson, R. M. C. (1948): The ammonia and glutamine content of the brain. *J. Biol. Chem.*, 176:1199–1210.

81. Howse, D. C., and Duffy, T. E. (1975): Control of the redox state of the pyridine nucleotides in the rat cerebral cortex. Effect of electroshock-induced seizures. *J. Neurochem.*, 24:935–940.

82. Vladimirova, E. A. (1954): Ammonia formation in rat cerebral hemispheres induced by conditioned stimuli. *Daklady Akad. Nauk. (USSR)*, 95:905–908.

83. Weil-Malherbe, H. (1975): Further studies on ammonia formation in brain slices: The effect of hadacidin. *Neuropharmacology*, 14:175–180.

84. Schultz, V., and Lowenstein, J. M. (1978): The purine nucleotide cycle. Studies of ammonia production and interconversions of adenine and hypoxanthine nucleotides and nucleosides by rat brain *in situ*. *J. Biol. Chem.*, 253:1938–1943.

85. Lockwood, A. H., McDonald, J. M., Reiman, R. E., Gelbard, A. S., Laughlin, J. S., Duffy, T. E., and Plum, F. (1979): The dynamics of ammonia metabolism in man. *J. Clin. Invest.*, 63:449–460.

86. McDermott, W. V., Jr. (1957): Metabolism and toxicity of ammonia. *N. Engl. J. Med.*, 257:1076–1081.

87. Summerskill, W. H. J., and Wolpert, E. (1970): Ammonia metabolism in the gut. *Am. J. Clin. Nutr.*, 23:633–639.

88. Windmueller, H. G., and Spaeth, A. E. (1974): Uptake and metabolism of plasma glutamine by the small intestine. *J. Biol. Chem.*, 249:5070–5079.

89. Weber, F. L., Jr., and Veach, G. L. (1979): The importance of the small intestine in gut ammonia production in the fasting dog. *Gastroenterology*, 77:235–240.

90. Bessman, S. P., and Bradley, J. E. (1955): Uptake of ammonia by muscle. Its implications in ammoniagenic coma. *N. Engl. J. Med.*, 253:1143–1147.

91. Ganda, O. P., and Ruderman, N. B. (1976): Muscle nitrogen metabolism in chronic hepatic insufficiency. *Metabolism*, 25:427–435.

92. Bromberg, P. A., Robin, E. D., and Forkner, C. E., Jr. (1960): The existence of ammonia in blood *in vivo* with observations on the significance of the NH_4^+-NH_3 system. *J. Clin. Invest.*, 39:332–341.

93. Carter, C. C., Lifton, J. F., and Welch, M. J. (1973): Organ uptake and blood pH and concentration effects of ammonia in dogs determined with ammonia labeled with 10 minute half-lived nitrogen 13. *Neurology,* 23:204–213.

94. Phelps, M. E., Hoffman, E. J., and Raybaud, C. (1977): Factors which affect cerebral uptake and retention of $^{13}NH_3$. *Stroke,* 8:694–702.

95. Cooper, A. J. L., McDonald, J. M., Gelbard, A. S., Gledhill, R. F., and Duffy, T. E. (1979): The metabolic fate of ^{13}N-labeled ammonia in rat brain. *J. Biol. Chem.,* 254:4982–4992.

96. Raichle, M. E., and Larson, K. B. (1981): The significance of the NH_3-NH_4^+ equilibrium on the passage of ^{13}N-ammonia from blood to brain. *Circ. Res.,* 48:913–937.

97. Stabenau, J. R., Warren, K. S., and Rall, D. P. (1959): The role of pH gradient in the distribution of ammonia between blood and cerebrospinal fluid, brain and muscle. *J. Clin. Invest.,* 38:373–383.

98. Lockwood, A. H., Campbell, J. A., and Finn, R. D. (1980): Brain ammonia uptake correlations with enzyme activities. *Neurology,* 30:406.

99. Jones, M. E., Anderson, A. D., Anderson, C., and Hodes, S. (1961): Citrulline synthesis in rat tissues. *Arch. Biochem. Biophys.,* 95:499–507.

100. Weil-Malherbe, H. (1962): Ammonia metabolism in the brain. In: *Neurochemistry,* second edition, edited by K. A. C. Elliott, I. H. Page, and J. H. Quastel, pp. 321–330. Charles C Thomas, Springfield, Illinois.

101. Hills, A. G., Reid, E. L., and Kerr, W. D. (1972): Circulatory transport of L-glutamine in fasted mammals: Cellular sources of urine ammonia. *Am. J. Physiol.,* 223:1470–1476.

102. Abdul-Ghani, A.-S., Marton, M., and Dobkin, J. (1978): Studies on the transport of glutamine *in vivo* between the brain and blood in the resting state and during afferent electrical stimulation. *J. Neurochem.,* 31:541–546.

103. Gjedde, A., Lockwood, A. H., Duffy, T. E., and Plum, F. (1978): Cerebral blood flow and metabolism in chronically hyperammonemic rats: Effect of an acute ammonia challenge. *Ann. Neurol.,* 3:325–330.

104. Hawkins, R. A., Miller, A. L., Nielsen, R. C., and Veech, R. L. (1973): The acute action of ammonia on rat brain metabolism *in vivo*. *Biochem. J.,* 134:1001–1008.

105. Williams, A. H., Kyu, M. H., Fenton, J. C. B., and Cavanagh, J. B. (1972): The glutamate and glutamine content of rat brain after portocaval anastomosis. *J. Neurochem.,* 19:1073–1077.

106. Record, C. O., Buxton, B., Chase, R. A., Curzon, G., Murray-Lyon, I. M., and Williams, R. (1976): Plasma and brain amino acids in fulminant hepatic failure and their relationship to hepatic encephalopathy. *Eur. J. Clin. Invest.,* 6:387–394.

107. Gilon, E., Szeinberg, A., Tauman, G., and Bodonyi, E. (1959): Glutamine estimation in cerebrospinal fluid in cases of liver cirrhosis and hepatic coma. *J. Lab. Clin. Med.,* 53:714–719.

108. Steigmann, F., Kazemi, F., Dubin, A., and Kissane, J. (1963): Cerebrospinal fluid glutamine in the diagnosis of hepatic coma. *Am. J. Gastroenterol.,* 40:378–386.

109. Duffy, T. E., Vergara, F., and Plum, F. (1974): α-Ketoglutaramate in hepatic encephalopathy. *Res. Publ. Assoc. Nerv. Ment. Dis.,* 53:39–51.

110. Bradford, H. F., and McIlwain, H. (1966): Ionic basis for the depolarization of cerebral tissues by excitatory amino acids. *J. Neurochem.,* 13:1163–1177.

111. Warren, K. S., and Schenker, S. (1964): Effect of an inhibitor of glutamine synthesis (methionine sulfoximine) on ammonia toxicity and metabolism. *J. Lab. Clin. Med.,* 64:442–449.

112. Hindfelt, B., and Plum, F. (1975): L-Methionine DL-sulphoximine and acute ammonia toxicity. *J. Pharm. Pharmacol.,* 27:456–458.

113. Berl, S., Takagaki, G., Clarke, D. D., and Waelsch, H. (1962): Metabolic compartments *in vivo*. Ammonia and glutamic acid metabolism in brain and liver. *J. Biol. Chem.,* 237:2562–2569.

114. Berl, S., and Clarke, D. D. (1969): Compartmentation of amino acid metabolism. In: *Handbook of Neurochemistry,* edited by A. Lajtha, vol. 2, pp. 447–472. Plenum, New York.

115. Balázs, R., Machiyama, Y., Hammond, B. J., Julian, T., and Richter, D. (1970): The operation of the γ-aminobutyrate

116. Martinez-Hernandez, A., Bell, K. P., and Norenberg, M. D. (1976): Glutamine synthetase: Glial localization in brain. *Science,* 195:1356–1358.

117. Norenberg, M. D., and Martinez-Hernandez, A. (1979): Fine structural localization of glutamine synthetase in astrocytes of rat brain. *Brain Res.,* 161:303–310.

118. Hertz, L. (1979): Functional interactions between neurons and astrocytes I. Turnover and metabolism of putative amino acid transmitters. *Prog. Neurobiol.,* 13:277–323.

119. Altenau, L. L., and Kindt, G. W. (1977): Cerebral vasomotor paralysis produced by ammonia intoxication. *Acta Neurol. Scand. (Suppl. 56),* 64:346–347.

120. Andersson, K.-E., Brandt, L., Hindfelt, B., and Ljunggren, B. (1981): Cerebrovascular effects of ammonia in vitro. *Acta Physiol. Scand.,* 113:349–353.

121. Skou, J. C. (1960): Further investigations on a Mg^{++} + Na^+-activated adenosintriphosphatase, possibly related to the active, linked transport of Na^+ and K^+ across the nerve membrane. *Biochim. Biophys. Acta,* 42:6–23.

122. Sadasivudu, B., Rao, T. I., and Murthy, C. R. (1977): Acute metabolic effects of ammonia in mouse brain. *Neurochem. Res.,* 2:639–655.

123. Binstock, L., and Lecar, H. (1969): Ammonium ion currents in the squid giant axon. *J. Gen. Physiol.,* 53:342–361.

124. Benjamin, A. M., Okamoto, K., and Quastel, J. H. (1978): Effects of ammonium ions on spontaneous action potentials and on contents of sodium, potassium, ammonium and chloride ions in brain *in vitro*. *J. Neurochem.,* 30:131–143.

125. Lux, H. D. (1971): Ammonium and chloride extrusion: Hyperpolarizing synaptic inhibition in cat spinal motoneurons. *Science,* 173:555–557.

126. Raabe, W., and Gumnit, R. J. (1975): Disinhibition in cat motor cortex by ammonia. *J. Neurophysiol.,* 38:347–355.

127. Iles, J. F., and Jack, J. J. B. (1980): Ammonia: Assessment of its action on postsynaptic inhibition as a cause of convulsions. *Brain,* 103:555–578.

128. Lowry, O. H., and Passonneau, J. V. (1966): Kinetic evidence for multiple binding sites on phosphofructokinase. *J. Biol. Chem.,* 241:2268–2279.

129. McKhann, G. M., and Tower, D. B. (1961): Ammonia toxicity and cerebral oxidative metabolism. *Am. J. Physiol.,* 200:420–424.

130. Baraona, E., Salinas, A., Navia, E., and Orrego, H. (1965): Alterations of ammonia metabolism in the cerebral cortex of rats with hepatic damage induced by carbon tetrachloride. *Clin. Sci.,* 28:201–208.

131. Prior, R. L., and Visek, W. J. (1972): Effects of urea hydrolysis on tissue metabolite concentrations in rats. *Am. J. Physiol.,* 223:1143–1149.

132. Bessman, S. P., and Bessman, A. N. (1955): The cerebral and peripheral uptake of ammonia in liver disease with an hypothesis for the mechanism of hepatic coma. *J. Clin. Invest.,* 34:622–628.

133. Shorey, J., McCandless, D. W., and Schenker, S. (1967): Cerebral α-ketoglutarate in ammonia intoxication. *Gastroenterology,* 53:706–711.

134. Hindfelt, B., and Siesjö, B. K. (1971): Cerebral effects of acute ammonia intoxication. II. The effect upon energy metabolism. *Scand. J. Clin. Lab. Invest.,* 28:365–374.

135. Vergara, F., Duffy, T. E., and Plum, F. (1973): α-Ketoglutaramate, a neurotoxic agent in hepatic coma. *Trans. Assoc. Am. Physicians,* 86:255–262.

136. Schenker, S., McCandless, D. W., Brophy, E., and Lewis, M. S. (1967): Studies on the intracerebral toxicity of ammonia. *J. Clin. Invest.,* 46:838–848.

137. Vogel, W. H., Heginbothom, S. D., and Boehme, D. H. (1975): Glutamic acid decarboxylase, glutamine synthetase and glutamic acid dehydrogenase in various areas of human brain. *Brain Res.,* 88:131–135.

138. Dennis, S. C., and Clark, J. B. (1978): The regulation of glutamate metabolism by tricarboxylic acid-cycle activity in rat brain mitochondria. *Biochem. J.,* 172:155–162.

bypath of the tricarboxylic acid cycle in brain tissue *in vitro*. *Biochem. J.,* 116:445–467.

139. Williamson, J. R., Safer, B., LaNoue, K. F., Smith, C. M., and Walajtys, E. (1973): Mitochondrial-cytosolic interactions in cardiac tissue: Role of the malate-aspartate cycle in the removal of glycolytic NADH from the cytosol. In: *Rate Control of Biological Processes*, edited by D. D. Davies, pp. 241–281. Cambridge University Press, New York.

140. Walshe, J. M. (1953): Disturbances of amino acid metabolism following liver injury: A study by means of paper chromatography. *Q. J. Med.*, 22:483–505.

141. Iob, V., Coon, W. W., and Sloan, M. (1966): Altered clearance of free amino acids from plasma of patients with cirrhosis of the liver. *J. Surg. Res.*, 6:233–239.

142. Sherwin, R., Joshi, P., Hendler, R., Felig, P., and Conn, H. O. (1974): Hyperglucagonemia in Laennec's cirrhosis. The role of portal-systemic shunting. *N. Engl. J. Med.*, 290:239–242.

143. Rosen, H. M., Yoshimura, N., Hodgman, J. M., and Fischer, J. E. (1977): Plasma amino acid patterns in hepatic encephalopathy of differing etiology. *Gastroenterology*, 72: 483–487.

144. Munro, H. N., Fernstrom, J. D., and Wurtman, R. J. (1975): Insulin, plasma amino acid imbalance, and hepatic coma. *Lancet*, 1:722–724.

145. Soeters, P. B., and Fischer, J. E. (1976): Insulin, glucagon, aminoacid imbalance, and hepatic encephalopathy. *Lancet*, 2:880–882.

146. Mans, A. M., Saunders, S. J., Kirsch, R. E., and Biebuyck, J. F. (1979): Correlation of plasma and brain amino acid and putative neurotransmitter alterations during acute hepatic coma in the rat. *J. Neurochem.*, 32:285–292.

147. Huet, P.-M., Pomier-Layrargues, G., Duguay, L., and du Souich, P. (1981): Blood-brain transport of tryptophan and phenylalanine: Effect of portacaval shunt in dogs. *Am. J. Physiol.*, 241:G163–G169.

148. James, J. H., Escourrou, J., and Fischer, J. E. (1978): Blood-brain neutral amino acid transport activity is increased after portacaval anastomosis. *Science*, 200:1395–1397.

149. Zanchin, G., Rigotti, P., Dussini, N., Vassanelli, P., and Battistin, L. (1979): Cerebral amino acid levels and uptake in rats after portocaval anastomosis: II. Regional studies *in vivo*. *J. Neurosci. Res.*, 4:301–310.

150. Brun, A., Dawiskiba, S., Hindfelt, B., and Olsson, J.-E. (1977): Brain proteins in hepatic encephalopathy. *Acta Neurol. Scand.*, 55:213–225.

151. Sellinger, O. Z., Azcurra J. M., Ohlsson, W. G., Kohl, H. H., and Zand, R. (1972): Neurochemical correlates of drug-induced seizures: Selective inhibition of cerebral protein synthesis by methionine sulfoximine. *Fed. Proc.*, 31:160–165.

152. Wasterlain, C. G., Lockwood, A. H., and Conn, M. (1978): Chronic inhibition of brain protein synthesis after portacaval shunting. A possible pathogenic mechanism in chronic hepatic encephalopathy in the rat. *Neurology*, 28:224–228.

153. Oldendorf, W. H. (1971): Brain uptake of radiolabeled amino acids, amines, and hexoses after arterial injection. *Am. J. Physiol.*, 221:1629–1639.

154. Fischer, J. E., Rosen, H. M., Ebeid, A. M., James, J. H., Keane, J. M., and Soeters, P. B. (1976): The effect of normalization of plasma amino acids on hepatic encephalopathy in man. *Surgery*, 80:77–91.

155. Fischer, J. E., Funovics, J. M., Aguirre, A., James, J. H., Keane, J. M., Wesdorp, R. I. C., Yoshimura, N., and Westman, T. (1975): The role of plasma amino acids in hepatic encephalopathy. *Surgery*, 78:276–290.

156. Freund, H., Yoshimura, N., and Fischer, J. E. (1979): Chronic hepatic encephalopathy. Long-term therapy with a branched-chain amino-acid-enriched elemental diet. *JAMA*, 242: 347–349.

157. Okada, A., Kamata, S., Kim, C. W., and Kawashima, Y. (1981): Treatment of hepatic encephalopathy with BCAA-rich amino acid mixture. In: *Metabolism and Clinical Implications of Branched Chain Amino and Ketoacids*, edited by M. Walser and J. R. Williamson, pp. 447–452. Elsevier, New York.

158. Rakette, S., Fischer, M., Reimann, H.-J., and von Sommoggy, S. (1981): Effects of special amino acid solutions in patients with liver cirrhosis and hepatic encephalopathy. In: *Metabo-*

lism and Clinical Implications of Branched Chain Amino and Ketoacids, edited by M. Walser and J. R. Williamson, pp. 419–425. Elsevier, New York.

159. Maddrey, W. C., Weber, F. L., Coulter, A. W., Chura, C. M., Chapanis, N. P., and Walser, M. (1976): Effects of keto analogues of essential amino acids in portal-systemic encephalopathy. *Gastroenterology*, 71:190–195.

160. Morgan, M. Y., Milson, J. P., and Sherlock, S. (1978): Plasma ratio of valine, leucine and isoleucine to phenylalanine and tyrosine in liver disease. *Gut*, 19:1068–1073.

161. Ono, J., Hutson, D. G., Dombro, R. S., Levi, J. U., Livingstone, A., and Zeppa, R. (1978): Tryptophan and hepatic coma. *Gastroenterology*, 74:196–200.

162. Benuck, M., Stern, F., and Lajtha, A. (1972): Regional and subcellular distribution of aminotransferases in rat brain. *J. Neurochem.*, 19:949–957.

163. Chaplin, E. R., Goldberg, A. L., and Diamond, I. (1976): Leucine oxidation in brain slices and nerve endings. *J. Neurochem.*, 26:701–707.

164. Meister, A. (1965): *Biochemistry of the Amino Acids*, 2nd Edition, Volume II, pp. 729–757. Academic Press, New York.

165. Cremer, J. E., Heath, D. F., Patel, A. J., Balázs, R., and Cavanagh, J. B. (1975): An experimental model of CNS changes associated with chronic liver disease: Portocaval anastomosis in the rat. In: *Metabolic Compartmentation and Neurotransmission. Relation to Brain Structure and Function*, edited by S. Berl, D. D. Clarke, and D. Schneider, pp. 461–478. Plenum, New York.

166. Rudman, D., Galambos, J. T., Smith, R. B., III, Salam, A. A., and Warren, W. D. (1973): Comparison of the effect of various amino acids upon the blood ammonia concentration of patients with liver disease. *Am. J. Clin. Nutr.*, 26:916–925.

167. Weiser, M., Riederer, P., and Kleinberger, G. (1978): Human cerebral free amino acids in hepatic coma. *J. Neural Transm. (Suppl. 14)*, 95–102.

168. Fernstrom, J. D., and Wurtman, R. J. (1972): Brain serotonin content: Physiological regulation by plasma neutral amino acids. *Science*, 178:414–416.

169. Friedman, P. A., Kappelman, A. H., and Kaufman, S. (1972): Partial purification and characterization of tryptophan hydroxylase from rabbit hindbrain. *J. Biol. Chem.*, 247:4165–4173.

170. Curzon, G., Kantamaneni, B. D., Fernando, J. C., Woods, M. S., and Cavanagh, J. B. (1975): Effects of chronic portocaval anastomosis on brain tryptophan, tyrosine and 5-hydroxytryptamine. *J. Neurochem.*, 24:1065–1070.

171. Cummings, M. G., Soeters, P. B., James, J. H., Keane, J. M., and Fischer, J. E. (1976): Regional brain indoleamine metabolism following chronic portacaval anastomosis in the rat. *J. Neurochem.*, 27:501–509.

172. Knell, A. J., Davidson, A. R., Williams, R., Kantamaneni, B. D., and Curzon, G. (1974): Dopamine and serotonin metabolism in hepatic encephalopathy. *Br. Med. J.*, 1:549–551.

173. Jellinger, K., and Riederer, P. (1977): Brain monoamines in metabolic (endotoxic) coma: A preliminary biochemical study in human postmortem material. *J. Neural Transm.*, 41:275–286.

174. Baldessarini, R. J., and Fischer, J. E. (1973): Serotonin metabolism in rat brain after surgical diversion of the portal venous circulation. *Nature (New Biol.)*, 245:25–27.

175. Fischer, J. E., and Baldessarini, R. J. (1971): False neurotransmitters and hepatic failure. *Lancet*, 2:75–80.

176. Baldessarini, R. J., and Fischer, J. E. (1978): Trace amines and alternative neurotransmitters in the central nervous system. *Biochem. Pharmacol.*, 27:621–626.

177. Cohn, R. A., Kopin, I. J., Creveling, C. R., Musacchio, J. M., Fischer, J. E., Crout, J. R., and Gill, J. R., Jr. (1966): False neurochemical transmitters. *Ann. Intern. Med.*, 65:347–362.

178. Fischer, J. E. (1974): False neurotransmitters and hepatic coma. *Res. Publ. Assoc. Nerv. Ment. Dis.*, 53:53–71.

179. Lam, K. C., Tall, A. R., Goldstein, G. B., and Mistilis, S. P. (1973): Role of a false neurotransmitter, octopamine, in the pathogenesis of hepatic and renal encephalopathy. *Scand. J. Gastroenterol.*, 8:465–472.

180. Manghani, K. K., Lunzer, M. R., Billing, B. H., and Sherlock, S. (1975): Urinary and serum octopamine in patients with portal-systemic encephalopathy. *Lancet*, 2:943–946.

181. James, J. H., Hodgman, J. M., Funovics, J. M., and Fischer, J. E. (1976): Alterations in brain octopamine and brain tyrosine following portacaval anastomosis in rats. *J. Neurochem.*, 27:223–227.

182. Smith, A. R., Rossi-Fanelli, F., Ziparo, V., James, J. H., Perelle, B. A., and Fischer, J. E. (1978): Alterations in plasma and CSF amino acids, amines and metabolites in hepatic coma. *Ann. Surg.*, 187:343–350.

183. Lunzer, M., James, I. M., Weinman, J., and Sherlock, S. (1974): Treatment of chronic hepatic encephalopathy with levodopa. *Gut*, 15:555–561.

184. Cuilleret, G., Pomier-Layrargues, G., Pons, F., Cadilhac, J., and Michel, H. (1980): Changes in brain catecholamine levels in human cirrhotic hepatic encephalopathy. *Gut*, 21:565–569.

185. Zieve, L., and Olsen, R. L. (1977): Can hepatic coma be caused by a reduction of brain noradrenaline or dopamine? *Gut*, 18:688–691.

186. Zieve, L., Doizaki, W. M., and Derr, R. F. (1979): Reversal of ammonia coma in rats by L-dopa: A peripheral effect. *Gut*, 20:28–32.

187. Braganca, B. M., Falkner, P., and Quastel, J. H. (1953): Effects of inhibitors of glutamine synthesis on the inhibition of acetylcholine synthesis in brain slices by ammonium ions. *Biochim. Biophys. Acta*, 10:83–88.

188. Parker, T. H., Roberts, P. K., Vorhees, C. V., Schmidt, D. E., and Schenker, S. (1977): The effect of acute and subacute ammonia intoxication on regional cerebral acetylcholine levels in rats. *Biochem. Med.*, 18:235–244.

189. Gibson, G. E., and Blass, J. P. (1976): Impaired synthesis of acetylcholine in brain accompanying mild hypoxia and hypoglycemia. *J. Neurochem.*, 27:37–42.

190. Gibson, G. E., and Duffy, T. E. (1981): Impaired synthesis of acetylcholine by mild hypoxic hypoxia or nitrous oxide. *J. Neurochem.*, 36:28–33.

191. Phear, E. A., Ruebner, B., Sherlock, S., and Summerskill, W. H. J. (1956): Methionine toxicity in liver disease and its prevention by chlortetracycline. *Clin. Sci.*, 15:93–117.

192. Chen, S., Zieve, L., and Mahadevan, V. (1970): Mercaptans and dimethyl sulfide in the breath of patients with cirrhosis of the liver. *J. Lab. Clin. Med.*, 75:628–635.

193. McClain, C. J., Zieve, L., Doizaki, W., Gilberstadt, S., and Onstad, G. (1978): Mercaptans in portal systemic encephalopathy due to alcoholic liver disease. *Gastroenterology*, 74:1065.

194. Challenger, F., and Walshe, J. M. (1955): Methyl mercaptan in relation to fetor hepaticus. *Biochem. J.*, 59:372–375.

195. Ljunggren, G., and Norberg, B. (1943): On the effect and toxicity of dimethyl sulfide, dimethyl disulfide and methyl mercaptan. *Acta Physiol. Scand.*, 5:248–255.

196. Zieve, L., Doizaki, W. M., and Zieve, F. J. (1974): Synergism between mercaptans and ammonia or fatty acids in the production of coma: A possible role for mercaptans in the pathogenesis of hepatic coma. *J. Lab. Clin. Med.*, 83:16–28.

197. Zieve, F. J., Zieve, L., Doizaki, W. M., and Gilsdorf, R. B. (1974): Synergism between ammonia and fatty acids in the production of coma: Implications for hepatic coma. *J. Pharmacol. Exp. Ther.*, 191:10–16.

198. Quarfoth, G., Ahmed, K., Foster, D., and Zieve, L. (1976): Action of methanethiol on membrane (Na$^+$,K$^+$)-ATPase of rat brain. *Biochem. Pharmacol.*, 25:1039–1044.

199. Muto, Y. (1966): Clinical study on the relationship of short chain fatty acids and hepatic encephalopathy. *Jpn. J. Gastroenterol.*, 63:19–32.

200. Mortiaux, A., and Dawson, A. M. (1961): Plasma free fatty acid in liver disease. *Gut*, 2:304–309.

201. Mays, E. T. (1972): Encephalopathy and fatty acid toxicity. *Surg. Forum*, 23:352–354.

202. Trauner, D. A., Nyhan, W. L., and Sweetman, L. (1975): Short-chain organic acidemia and Reye's syndrome. *Neurology*, 25:296–298.

203. Rabinowitz, J. L., Staeffen, J., Blanquet, P., Vincent, J. D., Terme, R., Series, C., and Meyerson, R. M. (1978): Sources of serum [^{14}C]-octanoate in cirrhosis of the liver and hepatic encephalopathy. *J. Lab. Clin. Med.*, 91:223–227.

204. Samson, F. E., Jr., Dahl, N., and Dahl, D. R. (1956): A study on the narcotic actions of the short chain fatty acids. *J. Clin. Invest.*, 35:1291–1298.

205. White, R. P., and Samson, F. E. (1956): Effects of fatty acid anions on the electroencephalograms of unanesthetized rabbits. *Am. J. Physiol.*, 186:271–274.

206. Teychenne, P. F., Walters, I., Claveria, L. E., Calne, D. B., Price, J., MacGillivary, B. B., and Gompertz, D. (1976): The encephalopathic action of five-carbon-atom fatty acids in the rabbit. *Clin. Sci. Mol. Med.*, 50:463–472.

207. Derr, R. F., and Zieve, L. (1976): Effect of fatty acids on the disposition of ammonia. *J. Pharmacol. Exp. Ther.*, 197:675–680.

208. Ahmed, K., and Scholefield, P. G. (1961): Studies on fatty acid oxidation. The effects of fatty acids on metabolism of rat-brain cortex *in vitro*. *Biochem. J.*, 81:45–53.

209. Walker, C. O., McCandless, D. W., McGarry, J. D., and Schenker, S. (1970): Cerebral energy metabolism in short-chain fatty acid-induced coma. *J. Lab. Clin. Med.*, 76:569–583.

210. Dahl, D. R. (1968): Short chain fatty acid inhibition of rat brain Na-K adenosine triphosphatase. *J. Neurochem.*, 15:815–820.

211. Pettegrew, J. W., and Minshew, N. J. (1981): Effects of short-chain fatty acids on cellular membranes and energy metabolism: A nuclear magnetic resonance study. *Neurology*, 31:143.

212. Curzon, G., Kantamaneni, B. D., Winch, J., Rojas-Bueno, A., Murray-Lyon, I. M., and Williams, R. (1973): Plasma and brain tryptophan changes in experimental acute hepatic failure. *J. Neurochem.*, 21:137–145.

213. Morgan, M. H., Bolton, C. H., Morris, J. S., and Read, A. E. (1974): Medium chain triglycerides and hepatic encephalopathy. *Gut*, 15:180–184.

214. Wilcox, H. G., Dunn, G. D., and Schenker, S. (1978): Plasma long chain fatty acids and esterified lipids in cirrhosis and hepatic encephalopathy. *Am. J. Med. Sci.*, 276:293–303.

215. Weber, F. L. (1981): Therapy of portal-systemic encephalopathy: The practical and the promising. *Gastroenterology*, 81:174–181.

216. Laux, B. E., and Raichle, M. E. (1978): The effects of acetazolamide on cerebral blood flow and oxygen utilization in the Rhesus monkey. *J. Clin. Invest.*, 62:585–592.

217. Gabuzda, G. J. (1967): Ammonium metabolism and hepatic coma. *Gastroenterology*, 53:806–810.

218. Norenberg, M. D., Leslie, K. O., and Robertson, A. S. (1982): Association between rise in serum sodium and central pontine myelinolysis. *Ann. Neurol.*, 11:128–135.

219. Conn, H. O., and Lieberthal, M. M. (1979): *The Hepatic Coma Syndromes and Lactulose*. Williams & Wilkins, Baltimore.

220. Ingelfinger, F. J. (1964–1965): Editorial comment. In: *Year Book of Medicine*, edited by P. B. Beeson, C. Muschenheim, W. B. Castle, T. R. Harrison, F. J. Ingelfinger, and P. K. Bondy, pp. 591–592. Year Book Medical Publishers, Chicago.

221. Bircher, J., Müller, J., Guggenheim, P., and Haemmerli, U.P. (1966): Treatment of chronic portal-systemic encephalopathy with lactulose. *Lancet*, 1:890–893.

222. Elkington, S. G., Floch, M. H., and Conn, H. O. (1969): Lactulose in the treatment of chronic portal-systemic encephalopathy. A double-blind clinical trial. *N. Engl. J. Med.*, 281:408–412.

223. Atterbury, C. E., Maddrey, W. C., and Conn, H. O. (1978): Neomycin, sorbital and lactulose in the treatment of acute portal-systemic encephalopathy. A double blind controlled trial. *Am. J. Dig. Dis.*, 23:398–406.

224. Uribe, M., Berthier, J. M., Lewis, H., Mata, J. M., Sierra, J. G., García-Ramos, G., Acosta, J. R., and Dehesa, M. (1981): Lactose enemas plus placebo tablets vs neomycin tablets plus starch enemas in acute portal systemic encephalopathy. A double-blind randomized controlled study. *Gastroenterology*, 81:101–106.

225. Bircher, J., Haemmerli, U. P., Scollo-Lavizzari, G., and Hoffmann, K. (1971): Treatment of chronic portal-systemic encephalopathy with lactulose. *Am. J. Med.*, 51:148–159.

226. Price, J. B., Jr., Sawada, M., and Voorhees, A. B., Jr. (1970): Clinical significance of intraluminal pH in intestinal ammonia transport. *Am. J. Surg.*, 119:595–598.

227. Vince, A., Killingley, M., and Wrong, O. M. (1978): Effect of lactulose on ammonia production in a fecal incubation system. *Gastroenterology*, 74:544–549.

228. Parkes, J. D., Sharpstone, P., and Williams, R. (1970) Levodopa in hepatic coma. *Lancet*, 2:1341–1343.

229. Morgan, M. Y., Jakobvitz, A. W., James, I. M., and Sherlock, S. (1980): Successful use of bromocriptine in the treatment of chronic hepatic encephalopathy. *Gastroenterology*, 78:663–670.

230. Michel, H., Solere, M., Granier, P., Cauvet, G., Bali, J. P., Pons, F., and Bellet-Hermann, H. (1980): Treatment of cirrhotic hepatic encephalopathy with L-dopa. A controlled trial. *Gastroenterology*, 79:207–211.

231. Uribe, M., Farca, A., Márquez, M. A., García-Ramos, G., and Guevara, L. (1979): Treatment of chronic portal systemic encephalopathy with bromocriptine. A double-blind controlled trial. *Gastroenterology*, 76:1347–1351.

232. Ross, E. D., and Stewart, R. M. (1981): Akinetic mutism secondary to hypothalamic damage: Successful treatment with dopamine agonists. *Neurology*, 31:61.

233. Duffy, T. E., and Plum, F. (1981): Seizures, coma, and major metabolic encephalopathies. In: *Basic Neurochemistry*, 3rd edition, edited by G. I. Siegel, R. W. Albers, B. W. Agranoff, and R. Katzman, pp. 693–718. Little, Brown, Boston.

The Liver: Biology and Pathobiology, edited by
I. Arias, H. Popper, D. Schachter, and D. A. Shafritz.
Raven Press, New York © 1982.

Chapter 42

Endocrine Function

David H. van Thiel

A major function of the liver is to regulate intermediary metabolism. As such, the liver acts as a governor, directing on a moment to moment basis the rate and direction of metabolic activity as determined by the body's needs. Changes in the body's requirements that necessitate alteration in a particular metabolic pathway are signaled to the liver as any of a number of hormonal messages. To fulfill this complex function, the liver must be able to recognize individual hormonal signals (i.e., have hormone receptors) and respond to such signals (i.e., affect specific postreceptor responses) in a meaningful way.

In addition, the liver may be intimately involved in the actual fulfillment of secreted polypeptide hormone action. An example is that of growth hormone, which is secreted by the anterior pituitary. Once secreted, growth hormone induces the liver to produce a variety of "growth factors" (somatomedins), which are ultimately responsible for the biological effects of the hormone at peripheral tissues (1). An example of how critically important such hepatic function is in the ultimate manifestation of polypeptide hormone action is

the Loran dwarf (2). Such dwarfs clinically appear growth hormone deficient; however, their plasma growth hormone levels are elevated consistently. Because the livers of Loran dwarfs fail to produce somatomedins in response to growth hormone, they appear growth hormone deficient, despite growth hormone sufficiency.

Finally, in its role as an excretory organ, the liver converts lipid-soluble hydrophobic hormones into more water-soluble, hydroxylated, sulfated, or glucuronidated moieties. These generally inactive compounds are either excreted directly into bile or indirectly into plasma for final excretion into urine via the kidneys. A review of the general organization of endocrine systems is necessary in order to appreciate the effects of liver disease on the various hormonal systems.

ORGANIZATION OF ENDOCRINE SYSTEMS

At the cellular level and in all *in vitro* systems that evaluate the effect of hormones on cells, essentially all actions of hormones are viewed as occurring in an open or linear system (e.g., a system in which a cause and effect relationship exists). In such idealized systems, the hormone acts on the cell to produce a specific effect, but the cell does not act in turn upon the original stimulus (Fig. 1A). This situation does not occur *in vivo*, as it has been shown repetitively that endocrine systems are organized as closed loop systems (Fig. 1B). In such systems, the end organ or cell is capable of modifying the stimulus. Relevant to the latter observation is the recognition that in addition to classic negative feedback loops, it is possible to have positive feed-forward loops (Figs. 2A and B). In general, feed-foward loops are unstable and tend to run out of control; however, they always exist as subcomponents of larger negative feedback loops. An example of such a feed-forward loop is the release of gastric inhibitory peptide (GIP) in response to glucose loads within the duodenal lumen. (3). As a result of GIP release, insulin secretion by pancreatic β-cells is activated prior to the actual absorption of the glucose load, thereby ultimately enhancing hepatic glucose uptake. Another advantage of a feed-forward loop may be its role in coordinating activities along divergent pathways (Fig. 2B). Thus, by activating a particular step late in a sequence, the concentrations of intermediates between the initial and final step can be maintained at stable levels, despite an overall net flux through the system. Two examples of such systems are glycogenolysis and the coagulation cascade. Both systems are characterized by near total inactivity at rest but can be mobilized rapidly because of feed-forward signals.

MECHANISM OF ACTION OF HORMONES

The mechanism of action of hormones in tissues is the same whether the tissue is a generally accepted hormone-dependent target tissue or a tissue more generally considered hormone independent, such as the liver. Lipid-soluble hormones, such as iodothyronines, steroids, and vitamin D derivatives, readily transverse the lipid bilayer that makes up the plasma membrane of cells (4). Their specific receptors are intracellular; the primary site of this action is on the nucleus. Target tissues for these hormones contain high affinity (10^{-9} to 10^{-10} M), low capacity, intracellular binding proteins or receptors. Upon entering the cell by passive diffusion, the hormones associate with their cytosolic receptors, inducing a conversion of the receptor to a biochemically functional form (Fig. 3A). The transformed or activated hormone-receptor complex is translocated to the nucleus, where it binds to chromatin and, in some way, alleviates restriction on synthesis of messenger RNA that is characteristic of the hormone in hormone-dependent tissue. Enhancement of RNA synthesis in response to the action of lipophilic hormones on target tissues is thought to be the major effect of these hormones on the cell (4–7).

Physiologic doses of steroid hormone cause the disappearance of about half the total number of cytosolic receptors (7). This initial depletion induced by the interaction of specific steroid hormones with their receptors appears to stimulate new receptor synthesis and replenishment of the extranuclear receptor pool (7). Such receptor synthesis is evident within a few hours and may continue for 18 to 24 hr.

In contrast to lipophilic steroidal hormones, hydrophilic polypeptide hormones and catecholamines do not traverse the lipid bilayer of the plasma membrane of cells to exert their effects (8). Instead, the biologic activities of these hormones depend on binding to specific cell surface receptors found on the responsive cell (Fig. 3B). Such receptors have two major functions (9): (a) they recognize the specific hormone from all other materials to which the cell is exposed; and (b)

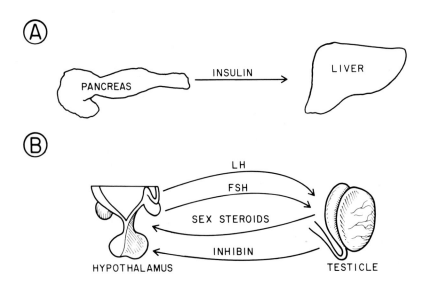

FIG. 1. Organization of endocrine systems. **A:** Idealized system in which insulin released from the pancreas as a result of any stimulus acts on the liver. The liver does not affect pancreatic insulin secretion. **B:** Classic closed loop system of negative feedback inhibition. The hypothalamus and pituitary release gonadotropins (FSH and LH) which stimulate the testes. The testes respond by releasing sex steroids and inhibin, which subsequently suppress gonadotropin release.

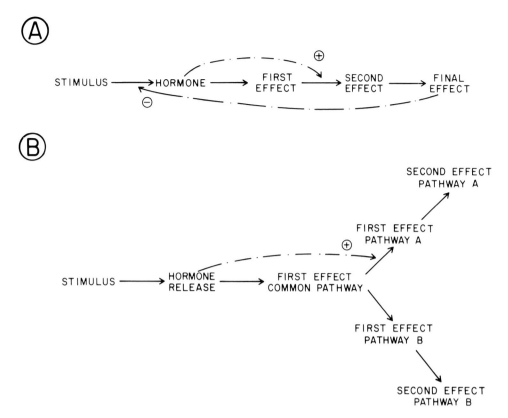

FIG. 2. Organization of endocrine systems. **A:** Schematic representation of a feedforward loop in which the hormone released as a result of a stimulus produces an effect but also activates a second step further down the response chain. Note that this feedfoward (positive) loop is enclosed by a feedback inhibitory loop (negative) from the final effect back to the interaction of the stimulus with the gland which precedes hormone release. **B:** Schematic representation of a feedforward loop that not only activates the first common pathway effect but also selectively activates pathway A.

after combining with the hormone, they initiate a series of biochemical events by which the hormonal signal is expressed by the cell. Ideally, each hydrophilic hormone should have its own unique receptor. Among the polypeptide hormones, however, there are families of hormones that have structural similarities. Not unexpectedly, structural overlap exists also in the receptors for these hormones. Thus a given polypeptide hormone has high affinity (10^{-9} M) for its own receptors but may retain some moderate affinity (10^{-7} or 10^{-8}) for receptors of structurally related hormones. Under normal circumstances, the extent of binding of one polypeptide hormone to receptors of another structurally related polypeptide hormone is so slight that fluctuations of hormone concentrations within the physiologic range cause little or no biologic effect secondary to nonspecific binding to related receptors. Under pathologic circumstances, as when the concentration of a particular hormone is elevated, disease can occur from effects mediated through binding to cross-reacting receptors (10). This type of mechanism might underlie some of the unexplained phenomena relating to changes in hormone metabolism that occur in patients with liver disease.

The cell surface receptors for these hydrophilic hormones are not static proteins; like all proteins of the cell, they are synthesized and degraded continuously. Any physiologic change of the cell, including growth, differentiation, and differences in the cell cycle, may result in a major change in their concentration (11). In addition, high concentrations of specific hormone over a period of time can act on the cell to reduce the concentration of its own receptor (12). Withdrawal of hormone can increase receptor concentations on the surface of responsive cells (13).

THE LIVER AS AN AMPLIFIER OR MODIFIER OF HORMONE ACTION

There is increasing evidence to suggest that hormones (sterols and iodothyronines) secreted by one organ (the gonads, adrenals, or thyroid) undergo metabolic transformation in plasma and other organs, particularly the liver. Transformation may lead to quantitative increase or decrease in biologic activity (e.g., the conversion of T_4 to T_3) or to qualitative change in biologic activity (e.g., the conversion of androgens to estrogens). In contrast to sterols and iodothyronines, it is generally held that polypeptide hormones do not ex-

A.) HYDROPHOBIC HORMONES (steroids and iodothyronines)

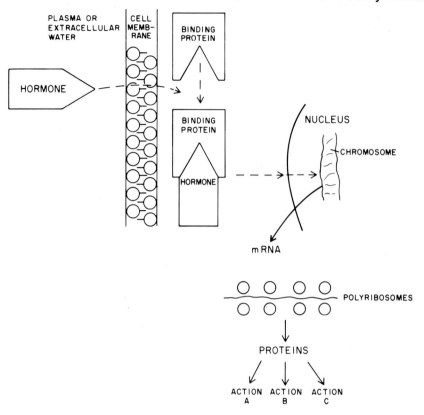

B.) HYDROPHILIC HORMONES (polypeptides and catecholamines)

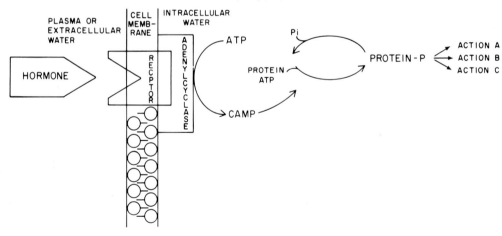

FIG. 3. Mechanism of action of hormones with receptors. **A:** Hydrophobic hormones interact with cytosolic receptors after traversing the cell membrane. The receptor-hormone complex in turn initiates hormonal action within the cell. **B:** Hydrophilic hormones are unable to traverse cell membranes and therefore interact with receptors on the cell surface which activate membrane bound enzyme systems to initiate hormone action.

hibit chemical modification following secretion. It should be noted that, at present, this possibility cannot be ruled out. It is clear that multiple forms of several specific types of polypeptide hormones exist [e.g., the various gastrins (G14, G17, and G34) and the various glucagons (2, 3.5, 9, and 160,000 dalton moieties)] (14–16).

ENERGY METABOLISM

Carbohydrate Metabolism

The liver plays a major role in the regulation of carbohydrate metabolism. It receives the majority of ingested carbohydrate via the portal circulation and plays a crucial role in glucose homeostasis. By dampening sudden surges in the concentration of fuels occurring as a consequence of eating, the liver prevents excess fluctuations in systemic osmolarity. It also must conserve, store, and convert ingested calories into suitable storage fuels.

The main source of calories ingested by man is carbohydrate, principally glucose, fructose, and galactose. Quantitatively, glucose and fructose are the most important. Even after ingestion of large amounts of glucose, there is relatively little fluctuation in the plasma glucose concentration. All ingested glucose passes through the liver via the portal vein before reaching the peripheral circulation. It has been assumed that much of this glucose is sequestered and metabolized by the liver, and only a small fraction reaches the peripheral circulation (Fig. 4).

The liver is unique in that it contains the enzyme glucokinase, which is required for phosphorylation of glucose. Glucokinase has a K_m for glucose of about 10 mM and is not inhibited by glucose-6-phosphate (17). Because the transport process for glucose across the cell membrane is very rapid, the intracellular glucose concentration in the liver closely reflects the plasma concentration. Any increase in the plasma glucose level stimulates glucose phosphorylation by the liver (17). The activity of glucokinase within the liver varies with the dietary state.

Normally, the liver does not remove glucose from portal venous blood when the blood sugar falls below 120 mg/dl (18). Above this level, however, glucose rapidly enters the hepatocyte and is converted to glucose-6-phosphate by glucokinase. Felig (19) has shown that after the oral ingestion of 100 g glucose, only 40 g appear in the hepatic vein over the next 3 hr. At the same time, hepatic glucose production decreases from the expected 25 g to zero. These studies suggest a net uptake of 85% or a real uptake of 40% of the administered glucose load. In contrast, if glucose is slowly infused directly into the portal vein, at levels such that portal venous plasma glucose remains below 120 mg/dl, no uptake can be demonstrated.

Man is an intermittent feeder; he not only uses glucose immediately following ingestion of a meal but also requires glucose to be continually available, even in the fasting state (Fig. 5). Thus the major function of the liver in glucose homeostasis is to prevent blood glucose levels from falling during fasting. Principally as a result of normal hepatic function, the blood glucose level in normal man fluctuates only minimally (less than 10% from the mean level).

Two main processes for the production of glucose exist in the normal individual: glycogenolysis, which occurs principally in the liver, and gluconeogenesis, which occurs in liver and kidney.

Glycogenolysis

In short-term starvation, certain tissues have an obligatory requirement for glucose. These include the central nervous system, peripheral nerve cells, red blood corpuscles, and white blood cells. Their glucose requirement amounts to about 160 g/day (20). Only the liver and, to a lesser extent, the kidney contain the key enzyme glucose-6-phosphatase, which allows glucose to be formed and released into the circulation for use by tissues that require glucose during fasting. After an overnight fast, approximately 75% of released glucose is derived from glycogenolysis (20–22). Another 25% comes from gluconeogenesis. Because the liver contains only 70 to 80 g glycogen, glucose production as a consequence of glycogenolysis declines rapidly after 18 to 24 hr of fasting. As starvation continues, the total body glucose requirement falls because of the adaptation of the brain to ketone body utilization (22). Thus after 5 to 6 weeks of fasting, only 40 g/day glucose is

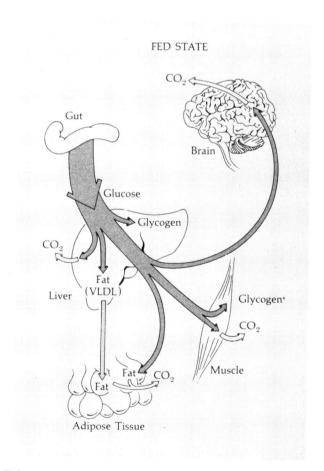

FIG. 4. Glucose metabolism in the fed state. Glucose is absorbed from the gut. Some small fraction is used within the liver for the immediate hepatic energy needs and for fat and glycogen storage. The rest is utilized by muscle, brain, and other tissues.

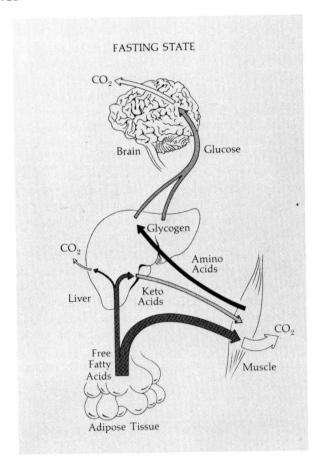

FASTING STATE

FIG. 5. Energy metabolism in the fasting state. Glucose is formed from amino acids released from muscles and from hepatic glycogen. The bulk of the energy requirement is satisfied as a result of lipolysis and fat oxidation.

required, approximating one-quarter of that required during the acute fasting state; about half of this new daily requirement is produced by the kidney (23).

The enzyme that controls the rate of glycogenolysis is glycogen phosphorylase. Two forms exist in the liver: (a) an active form, phosphorylase A, and (b) a considerably less active form, phosphorylase B. Both are interconvertible via specific enzyme-catalyzed reactions. The properties of the enzymes involved in glycogenolysis suggest that a decrease in the ADP/AMP ratio in the liver stimulates glycogenolysis and also inhibits gluconeogenesis.

Gluconeogenesis

Substate availability appears to be the limiting factor in gluconeogenesis (24). The precursors are lactate, pyruvate, glucogenic amino acids (mainly alanine), and glycerol. Quantitatively, lactate is the most important. Total lactate turnover is approximately 140 g/day, more than half of which is derived from glucose metabolism by extrahepatic tissues and muscle glycogen (25). Amino acids contribute only 6 to 12% of the

total of glucose production after an overnight fast compared to a much greater proportion with prolonged fasting (26).

During prolonged fasting, alanine and glutamine account for more than 50% of the amino acids released by muscle (27). Released glutamine is taken up mainly by gut and kidney, whereas alanine is taken up principally by the liver. In the liver, alanine undergoes transamination with oxaloacetate forming pyruvate and aspartate. The latter participates in the urea cycle yielding urea, while pyruvate passes through the gluconeogenic pathway terminating in glucose production. The key regulatory steps in gluconeogenesis are those most likely to be affected by hepatic disease: pyruvate carboxylase, phosphoenol pyruvate carboxykinase, and fructose-1,6-diphosphotase (28).

As stated previously, the liver is the major organ responsible for the regulation of carbohydrate metabolism and is an important target for insulin action. It is also important in insulin degradation. Insulin is secreted directly into the portal venous system. The rate of insulin secretion is influenced by many factors other than blood glucose such as amino acids, gut hormones, and stress. Because the liver is exquisitely sensitive to small changes in insulin levels (29), a twofold rise in portal venous insulin concentration is sufficient to inhibit hepatic glucose production completely. This fine control is aided by the fact that the liver is exposed to much higher insulin concentrations than are peripheral tissues. Most available evidence suggests that approximately 50% of insulin secreted by the pancreas is degraded on its first passage through the liver (30–32).

Hepatic cirrhosis is consistently associated with elevated peripheral venous immunoreactive insulin levels (33). This is true under fasting circumstances and in response to normal meals, oral or intravenous glucose, amino acid, or tolbutamide administration (34).

In normal man, the importance of the liver in the metabolism of glucagon is uncertain (35,36). Total plasma immunoreactive glucagon is composed of at least four fractions (15,16). The 3,500 dalton component is the biologically active form of the hormone. The 9,000 dalton moiety may be a precursor of the biologically active form but is biologically inactive. The significance of the 2,000 dalton and the 160,000 dalton fractions is as yet unknown. The liver is thought to metabolize selectively the biologically active 3,500 dalton glucagon molecule with a percent extraction of 81 ± 5% (36).

In fasting man, most of the changes in carbohydrate metabolism can be explained by changes in circulating hormone levels superimposed upon endogenous regulatory mechanisms. Thus as blood glucose concentration falls, insulin secretion decreases, and glucagon secretion increases (37). As fasting continues, the effects of insulin on amino acid transport and synthesis within peripheral tissues decrease, and the effects of glucocorticoids begin to predominate. Thus increasing levels of amino acids, particularly alanine, are released into the circulation (Fig. 5).

As a result of increased glucagon levels, the hepatic extraction of amino acids is enhanced. Glucagon increases the rate of gluconeogenesis at three specific locations (38–40): (a) transport of alanine and some other amino acids across the cell membrane into the liver, (b) conversion of phosphoenol to pyruvate, and (c) conversion of fructose triphosphate to fructose-6-phosphate.

The breakdown of skeletal muscle protein during starvation does not result in release of amino acids in proportion to the amino acid composition of the protein (39). Alanine and glutamine are released to a greater extent (50 to 60% of the total) than the other amino acids. It has been suggested that alanine released from muscle is derived from pyruvate which is produced from glucose via glycolysis. Pyruvate is transaminated, and the alanine produced is released into the bloodstream. Because the alanine released by the muscle is transported to the liver to be reconverted into glucose via gluconeogenesis and is then available to muscle as glucose, this cycle of substrate reutilization has been termed the glucose-alanine cycle (Fig. 6). The process does not permit net synthesis of glucose, since the carbons of the alanine are derived originally from glucose. The major function of this process may be to transfer ammonia from muscle to liver in the nontoxic form of alanine.

Carbohydrate Metabolism in Liver Disease

Fasting hypoglycemia is surprisingly rare in liver disease for two reasons (38–41). First, the liver has a large reserve capacity, such that normal glucose homeostasis can be maintained with as little as 20% of the normal parenchymal mass. Second, the kidney is capable of gluconeogenesis. This organ can take over a significant proportion of glucose production in individuals with hepatic disease. Hypoglycemia, when it does occur, generally is found in acute fulminant hepatic disease, such as occurs in fulminant viral hepatitis or in association with toxic liver injury secondary to drug overdose with agents such as acetaminophen (39). It can also occur, albeit rarely, in association with primary hepatic carcinoma.

In chronic liver disease, mild hypoglycemia after an overnight fast is occasionally seen; but rarely does it approach significant hypoglycemia (<40 mg/dl). The possible causes of hepatogenic hypoglycemia include impaired glycogen synthesis and breakdown as well as impaired gluconeogenesis. A common defect in many forms of liver disease is a defect in the ability to store glycogen. It has been shown that after an overnight fast, only about one-third of the total glucose production is derived from glycogen in cirrhotic patients, while 70 to 80% comes from glycogen in normal subjects (40). Similarly it has been shown that a 25% decrease in hepatic glucose production occurs in cirrhotic subjects after an overnight fast (41). Felig et al. (42) found a decreased glycemic response to glucagon in

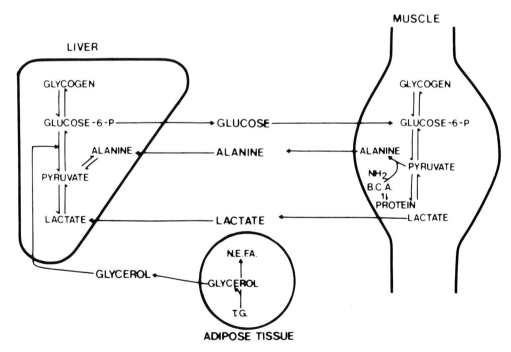

FIG. 6. The glucose alanine cycle. Alanine produced in muscle, as a result of protein breakdown, is released and deaminated in the liver to form pyruvate. Glucose is formed from pyruvate and is released to be metabolized by muscle, where it is reconverted to pyruvate and alanine, respectively, completing the cycle.

patients with viral hepatitis; Yeung and Wang (43) reported the same result in patients with postnecrotic cirrhosis.

Glucose intolerance is more common in subjects with liver disease, particularly cirrhosis, than in the normal population (44–46). Moreover, such intolerance is more apparent in response to an oral than an intravenous load. This difference in response to routes of administration is probably due to portal systemic shunting of glucose. Peripheral insulin levels are usually increased in hyperglycemia individuals with advanced liver disease, suggesting insulin resistance (45,46). However, the precise mechanisms responsible for impaired glucose tolerance in patients with liver disease are as yet unresolved.

Marco and colleagues (47) reported mean fasting plasma glucagon levels to be threefold elevated in cirrhotic patients with portal caval shunts and twice increased in patients with liver disease without shunting as compared to normal. Similarly, Sherwin and co-workers (48) reported elevated plasma immunoreactive glucagon concentrations if portal systemic shunting was present. Elevated plasma glucagon concentrations are seen also in subjects with chronic portal venous block in the absence of liver disease, such as occurs with portal vein thrombosis. The primacy of portal venous shunting in the production of hyperglucagonemia seen in liver disease suggests that diminished hepatic breakdown rather than hypersecretion is the major factor. The elevated glucagon levels in individuals with cirrhosis do not fall normally in reponse to glucose and show abnormal increases after alanine or arginine stimulation (49).

If a large portion of secreted glucagon is bypassing the liver as a result of portosystemic shunts in subjects with liver disease, important consequences might be expected. Fasting blood levels of gluconeogenic precursors are frequently elevated in individuals with liver disease and in acute viral hepatitis (50). For example, 50% of patients have elevated fasting venous lactate levels; furthermore, in mild to moderate acetaminophen poisoning, fasting lactate levels are universally increased (39). A similar situation exists in chronic liver disease, especially of the alcoholic variety (51). Fasting concentrations of glycerol are raised in about 50% of patients with liver disease. These biochemical findings may be a result of hyperglucagonemia.

One of the clinical consequences of the diminished capacity for gluconeogenesis present in individuals with liver disease is the ability to develop lactic acidosis (52–54). Thus in most patients with lactic acidosis, 60% have demonstrable evidence of hepatic disease, usually in association with circulatory failure (53). Particularly liable to lactic acidosis are patients who are treated with phenformin, ethanol, fructose, or sorbitol (54).

Lipid Metabolism

The major lipids carried in plasma are cholesterol, cholesterol esters, phospholipids, and triglycerides. Cholesterol is a precursor of bile acids and the steroid hormones and is present in all mammalian plasma membranes. With the exception of a carbocyl group at C3 and a double bond between C5 and C6, it is a fully satuated, nonpolar, water-insoluble hydrocarbon and thus is suitable to its role as a structural component of membranes. With the exception of a carboxyl group at than free cholesterol. Phospholipids, the other major constituent of biologic membranes, contain one or more phosphoric acid groups and another polar group, such as choline, ethanolamine, or sphingosine. The most abundant phospholipid in plasma and in membranes is lecithin or phosphatidylcholine. Triglycerides consistent of glycerol esterified with three fatty acids. These water-insoluble lipids occur in plasma as part of a variety of lipid protein complexes, the lipoproteins. Lipoproteins can be separated using the ultracentrifuge on the basis of their density into β- or low density lipoproteins (LDL), α- or high density lipoproteins (HDL), and pre-β-or very low density lipoproteins (VLDL) (55). A fourth class of lipoproteins, the chylomicrons, float readily in plasma and remain at the origin during electrophoresis. The protein components of the individual lipoproteins are called apoliproteins.

All lipoprotein fractions, with the exception of LDL_2, contain more than one type of apolipoprotein (56–58). Apo B is the principal apolipoprotein of LDL_2. There are at least three different types of apo C, which are the major apolipoproteins of VLDL and chylomicra. Apo C-1 is an activator of lecithin cholesterol acyltransferase (LCAT) (59). Apo C-2 is necessary for the activation of extrahepatic lipoprotein lipase (60). Apo C-3 has phospholipid binding properties and may be an inhibitor of lipoprotein lipase (61). The major apoproteins of HDL are apo A-1 and apo A-2 (62). Apo E is present in VLDL and apo D is a minor constituent of HDL.

Only the intestine and liver can synthesize and secrete plasma lipoproteins. Chylomicra are produced in the mucosal cells of the small intestine but only during dietary fat absorption. VLDL are produced in the liver and intestine. In contrast, HDL are made only in the liver; evidence suggests, however, that they may also arise as a result of intestinal production. LDL are produced mainly within the plasma as a result of the metabolism of VLDL (63). VLDL production by the liver is increased when the liver is presented with a large energy load, either as preformed fatty acid or as carbohydrate, which is converted rapidly to triglyceride (64,65).

Little is known about the factors regulating the production of HDL. HDL levels are higher in premenopausal women than in men and are increased by estrogens and reduced by androgens (62). They are decreased with high carbohydrate diets and increased as a result of alcohol intake (66).

LDL are produced in plasma as a consequence of the intravascular metabolism of VLDL. Some investigators (67) believe that LDL can also be produced *de novo* by the liver.

Two enzymes play key roles in the metabolism of plasma lipoproteins: lipoprotein lipase and, to a lesser degree, LCAT. LCAT is synthesized by the liver and probably also by the gut (68). It is secreted into the plasma, where it catalyzes the transfer of a long chain fatty acid from the β position of lecithin to the three β-hydroxy position of free cholesterol, thus forming a cholesterol ester and lysolecithin. Lipoprotein lipases are bound to the capillary walls of various tissues by a heparin-like substance which also acts as an activator (69,70). These enzymes are barely detectable in normal human plasma but are released into the circulation following the intravenous injection of heparin. They can be measured as postheparin lipolytic activity. The activity of lipoprotein lipase is influenced by a number of hormones; it is increased by insulin and decreased by glucagon, ACTH, and thyroid-stimulating hormone (TSH) (70).

Lipid Metabolism in Liver Disease

Because the liver plays a key role in the production and metabolism of plasma lipids and lipoproteins, it is not unexpected that alterations in the plasma content of such lipids and lipoproteins occur with liver disease. In patients with obstructive jaundice, there is more lipid than usual in the LDL fraction, principally as a result of a fall in LCAT activity (71,72). An absence of α lipoprotein (HDL) also is found in the plasma of patients with obstructive jaundice (73).

Frederickson et al. (74) have shown that cholesterol synthesis is increased in obstructive jaundice, which may explain the associated hypercholesterolemia. The best explanation for the hyperlipidemia of obstructive jaundice is the regurgitation of lecithin from the obstructed biliary tree into the blood (75). When plasma lipid levels reach very high levels with chronic obstructive jaundice, cutaneous xanthelasma may appear. They may be scattered or be distributed in the palmar creases around the eyes and over the elbows, buttocks, and knees (areas commonly subject to pressure or trauma).

Patients with liver disease have abnormal red cells, which contain more cholesterol or more cholesterol and phospholipid than those obtained from normal individuals (72). This results in an expansion of their surface area without a corresponding change in their volume. As a result, there is a change in their shape, and target cells develop as lecithin and free cholesterol accumulate. In acute viral hepatitis, α and β lipoproteins disappear (76,77).

PITUITARY HORMONES THAT AFFECT ENERGY BALANCE

Growth Hormone

The normal turnover of a growth hormone in plasma is rapid; its disappearance time (T½) is 19 min (78). Its secretion is pulsatile and its control complex, being affected by stress, nonesterifed fatty acids, amino acids, glucose, and adrenergic stimulation (79). Evidence suggests a negative feedback as a result of hepatic somatomedin production or by growth hormone itself (80).

The liver and kidneys are the major sites of growth hormone degradation (78). Basal growth hormone concentrations are elevated and show a paradoxical rise after glucose loading in various forms of liver disease, particularly cirrhosis (81–86). It is still uncertain whether or not the elevated levels are the result of increased secretion or diminished catabolism (82,83). Owens and co-workers (78) have shown a diminished metabolic clearance of growth hormone in individuals with cirrhosis. These results have been confirmed by Cameron et al. (81). Moreover, Taylor and his colleagues (82) have shown that the liver is responsible for 90% of the metabolic clearance of growth hormone under normal circumstances. Thus the accumulated evidence for delayed growth hormone clearance by the liver in individuals with liver disease suggests that such clearance reduction is responsible for the elevation in basal growth hormone levels seen in these patients. Alterations in the hypothalamic-pituitary control of growth hormone is suggested also in such individuals; abnormal responses to intravenous thyrotropin releasing hormone (TRH) have been reported (84,85). Altered dopaminergic function in such individuals may be responsible, at least in part, for these changes in growth hormone secretion.

Most if not all actions of growth hormone are secondary to production of a group of small peptides called the somatomedins (87). Somatomedin activity falls after hepatectomy and rises as the liver regenerates (88). Isolated rat liver perfusion experiments have demonstrated an increase in somatomedin activity when growth hormone is added (89,90). Wu and his colleagues (91) reported that nine of 10 cirrhotic subjects show low somatomedin activity, which correlates well with the degree of their liver disease. Moreover, elevated basal growth hormone levels were found in seven subjects, all of whom had decreased somatomedin activity. The decreased somatomedin levels probably result from liver damage. Abnormal estrogen metabolism also may contribute; estrogen administration decreases the somatomedin response to exogenous growth hormone in both animals and man (92–94).

Prolactin

Prolactin circulates freely in plasma in forms of differing molecular size (95). The major form is termed little prolactin (23,000 daltons) and is thought to represent the monomeric form of the hormone. Big prolactin (56,000 daltons) and the largest form, termed the void volume fraction (when eluted on Sephadex G-100), are thought to represent polymeric forms. Prolactin binds to hepatic tissue specifically. Such binding is enhanced by estrogens, is greater in females than in males, and is increased in pregnant as compared to nonpregnant women (96,97).

Prolactin has many functions, including a lactogenic effect acting in concert with estrogens, an antigonadotropic action at high doses, and an enhancing effect on luteinizing hormone (LH) binding to the gonad at normal prolactin levels (98). The specific functions of prolactin, with the exception of its lactogenic function during pregnancy, are poorly understood. Normal basal prolactin levels, greater in women than men, generally are <30 ng/ml.

In patients with advanced liver disease, particularly those with cirrhosis who are encephalopathic, prolactin levels are increased moderately. Such increases tend to mirror the level of encephalopathy (99). Such increases presumably reflect the effect of disordered neurotransmitter function. Serotonin, gamma-aminobutyric acid (GABA), arginine, and a variety of antidopaminergic agents are known to induce prolactin secretion. It is not surprising, therefore, that prolactin cell hyperplasia and adenoma have been reported to occur with greater frequency in cirrhotic individuals than in normals (100). Consistent with such reports are the clinical findings suggestive of adenoma, which include abnormal prolactin secretory responses to TRH, chlorpromazine, and sleep, in some men with advanced alcoholic liver disease (101).

TSH

TSH levels in individuals with liver disease generally have been reported to be only minimally increased or normal unless primary thyroid disease also coexists (102–105). Thus plasma TSH levels average 1.45 μU/ml in such patients, a figure not different from that for normals. TSH clearance is rapid (50.7 ml/min) in normal individuals. Free T_4 is more important than free T_3 in determining TSH levels (106). Despite a reduction in T_3 levels in individuals with advanced liver disease, basal TSH levels are usually within normal limits (102–105). Despite such apparent normal basal

levels, when the plasma TSH levels of individuals with advanced alcoholic liver disease are compared critically to those of age- and sex-matched individuals without liver disease, a statistical (although probably physiologically unimportant) increase is found (102–105). Relevant to this observation, TSH responses to various manipulations of thyroid function (both enhancement and suppression) are normal when assessed in individuals with liver disease (102).

ACTH

ACTH circulates unbound in plasma and distributes in a volume equal to that of the plasma volume. The plasma half-life of ACTH averages 8 min and ranges from 3 to 10 min in normal individuals (107,108). Plasma levels show a diurnal variation, with morning levels being greater than afternoon levels, and range from 100 to 10 pg/ml during the course of the day.

Regardless of the etiology, normal ACTH levels are reported in most individuals with liver disease. Changes in ACTH secretion seen in patients with liver disease reflect primary changes in adrenal cortical secretion. Exceptions exist; it has been reported that 10% of alcoholics (most of whom had cirrhosis) have inadequate ACTH responses to stress. Similarly, both low and paradoxically normal as well as increased ACTH levels have been reported in individuals manifesting the syndrome of alcohol-associated pseudo-Cushing (109–115). Most of these subjects have had advanced liver disease (e.g., alcoholic hepatitis or alcoholic hepatitis and cirrhosis).

OTHER PITUITARY HORMONES

Melanocyte-Stimulating Hormone, β-Lipotropin, Endorphins, and Enkephalins in Liver Disease

Essentially no information exists relevant to the levels and physiology of these substances in patients with liver disease. Increased β-melanocyte-stimulating hormone (β-MSH) levels may contribute to the hyperpigmentation that occurs in individuals with advanced liver disease, particularly those with portal hypertension and those who have undergone surgical portocaval shunting. It is interesting to speculate what role the endorphins and smaller enkephalins may play in the pathophysiology of hepatic encephalopathy. Although the total number of naturally occurring opioid peptides is still uncertain, there are two well-characterized pentapeptides, methionine-enkephalin and leucine-enkephalin. The most important long chain opioid peptide is β-endorphin, which consists of amino acid residues 61-91 of β-lipotropin (Fig. 7). In the brain, β-endorphin is found in the hypothalamus,

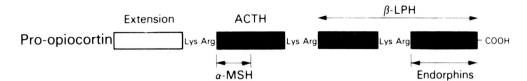

FIG. 7. Schematic representation of the component parts of pro-opiocortin, which consists of ACTH, α-MSH, β-lipotropin (β-LPH), and β-endorphin.

midbrain, medulla, and pons, with little or no activity in the striatum, cortex, cerebellum, and spinal cord (116). These same areas are those that manifest abnormal function in hepatic encephalopathy (117). In contrast, the enkephalins are located in areas separate from the endorphin system, being widely distributed throughout the central and peripherial nervous system (118). However, the locations in the central nervous system containing the greatest number of enkephalin binding sites are also the hypothalamus, amygdala, thalamus, and periventricular and periaquaductal grey areas. Thus they are the same areas that demonstrate the greatest enkephalin immunoreactivity (119,120) and the sites most disturbed in patients with hepatic encephalopathy (117).

Using the electron microscope and immunocytochemistry, methionine-enkephalin has been found in the perikarya and dendrites of catecholaminergic neurons (119). Moreover, enkephalin immunoreactive nerve terminals form a dense network around sympathetic ganglia and chromaffin cells contained within the adrenal medulla (120,121).

Enkephalins are readily degraded by aminopeptidases, carboxypeptidase, and enkephalinase. Their measurement in plasma, therefore, is difficult and fraught with methodologic problems (122–125). Similarly, plasma β-endorphin levels in normal men and women are near the detection limits of most radioimmunoassay systems (4 to 12 fmoles/ml). The role of opioid peptides in cerebrospinal fluid (CSF) is as yet uncertain (125–129). Levels in the CSF of individuals with hepatic encephalopathy have not yet been reported.

Although there is a great deal of information concerning the biosynthesis of β-endorphin from corticotropin-β-lipotropin precursor (a polypeptide containing 265 amino acids) and the more immediate opiocorticotropin (a polypeptide containing 134 amino acids) which also contains the ACTH sequence (amino acids 1-39), β-lipotropin (amino acids 42-134), there is little information available concerning the origin of the enkephalins (Fig. 7). However, it is generally believed that methionine-enkephalin is not derived from β-endorphin. It is also unlikely that enkephalins are produced in neurons that have no opioid activity (130–134). ³H-Tyrosine has been incorporated into methionine- and leucine-enkephalins (135,136).

Opioid peptides do not readily penetrate the blood-brain barrier. The resistance provided to their passage is uneven, however, and the hypothalamus appears to be an area that is particularly leaky. Thus parenteral administration of opioid peptides has a greater effect on the hypothalamus and therefore on endocrine function than in other parts of the central nervous system. Considerable evidence has accumulated documenting enkephalin release of prolactin and growth hormone. Moreover, the release of both can be shown to be inhibited by opiate antagonists (137–141). Such prolactin and growth hormone release is probably attributable to inhibition of dopaminergic inhibitory mechanisms which occur within the mediobasal hypothalamus rather than at the pituitary. Increased enkephalin activity in such brain areas of encephalopathic patients might account for the increased prolactin and growth hormone levels commonly seen in cirrhotic subjects. Moreover, the same mechanism also may account for the "normal" LH levels seen in most alcoholic cirrhotic men despite severe gonadal failure (142–144).

Clearly, the study of endogenous opioids in subjects with liver disease with and without encephalopathy would be a fruitful area of future clinical investigation.

Gonadotropins

The two gonadotropins, follicle-stimulating hormone (FSH) and LH, share a common α chain with each other and with thyrotropin. Each, however, has a unique β-chain that is responsible for its particular biologic function. Both distribute in a volume equivalent to 1.5 the plasma volume and circulate unbound in plasma. Because the metabolic clearance rate of LH (25 ml/min) is greater than that of FSH (13.5 ml/min), its levels fluctuate more markedly than those of FSH. Neither is metabolized to any degree by the liver; moreover, neither has a recognized hepatic function. Therefore, liver disease affects their regulation only indirectly by altering gonadotropin releasing factor (GRF) clearance and/or that of sex steroids. Thus changes in the plasma levels of gonadotropins in liver disease primarily reflect associated disease either in the gonads (as occurs in alcoholic liver disease) or in the hypothalamic pituitary unit (as occurs in both alcoholic liver disease and hemochomatosis).

Antidiuretic Hormone

The maintenance of volume and osmolarity of body fluids requires an intact thirst system to control intake and also a system that allows for regulation of water losses. Antidiuretic hormone (ADH) or vasopressin accomplish this function by acting on the kidneys Vasopressin secretion is responsive to both volume and osmolar signals. The osmoregulatory system is more sensitive than the volume regulatory system; however, a 1 or 2% change in osmolarity alters vasopressin secretion dramatically, whereas a 7 to 10% volume depletion is required to alter ADH secretion.

Alcohol, in addition to being a potent and commonplace hepatotoxin, is also a powerful inhibitor of ADH secretion (145). Diphenylhydantoin is also an inhibitor of ADH release (146). Other potent stimulators of ADH secretion or action that occur commonly in patients with liver disease, regardless of etiology, include nicotine and chlorpropamide (147,148).

Vasopressin circulates unbound in plasma and distributes in a volume nearly equal to that of plasma. It is degraded by both the kidney and the liver; circulating levels range from undetectable with overhydration to 20 μU/ml with severe dehydration.

Many factors affect the renal action of ADH. Urea, the end product of protein metabolism, plays an important role in the renal concentrating process (149). A decrease in urea formation by the liver impairs renal concentrating capacity by limiting the hypertonicity achievable by the renal medullary interstitium (149, 150). Similarly, sodium restriction, which is prescribed commonly in individuals with liver disease, reduces the ultimate ability of the kidney to concentrate urine (151). Diuretics, by virtue of their actions on tubular sodium or chloride reabsorption, also affect water reabsorption. The thiazides, which act principally on the cortical diluting segment, affect maximal free water clearance; the potent loop diuretics, such as furosemide and ethacrynic acid, impair free water reabsorption as well as free water clearance (152).

It is generally held that the reduction in total peripheral resistance that occurs in decompensated cirrhosis allows for a reduction in the effective intravascular volume, which in turn leads to enhanced aldosterone and ADH secretion; this ultimately enhances salt and water retention, respectively.

THE LIVER AND ITS INTERACTION WITH VARIOUS ENDOCRINE SYSTEMS

Hypothalamic-Pituitary-Gonadal Axis

The normal hypothalamic-pituitary-gonadal axis consists of three separate organs, the hypothalamus, pituitary, and gonads. Each is separated from the others but functions in response to endocrine signals from the other two in a classic endocrine regulatory manner utilizing negative feedback inhibition.

The hypothalamus consists of neuronal nuclei which receive afferent signals from a wide variety of sites, including the cerebral cortex. It discharges peptidergic signals into the hypophyseal portal circulation, which regulates pituitary function. It also contains sex steroid receptors that allow it to recognize and respond to alterations in gonadal function manifested by the circulating levels of androgens and estrogens. Luteinizing hormone releasing factor (LHRF) is the principal hypothalamic factor involved in regulating pituitary gonadotropin production and secretion (both FSH and LH). When sex steroid levels (either testosterone in the male or estradiol in the female) are reduced, hypothalamic sex steroid receptors are unoccupied and hypothalamic release of LHRF is enhanced. When sex steroid levels are normal or increased, sex steroid receptors in the hypothalamus are occupied, and the release of LHRF is inhibited.

In response to LHRF, gonadotrophs in the pituitary gland release the two gonadotropins FSH and LH. FSH is a trophic factor for the reproductive compartment of the gonads; LH is a trophic factor affecting growth and development of the endocrine cells within the gonads.

In humans, the binding of sex steroids in the circulation occurs primarily to sex steroid binding globulin, which binds steroids with high affinity but low capacity. Binding is believed to determine the concentration of free sex steroid, particularly testosterone (approximately 1% of the total), in the circulation (153). Binding of sex steroids to serum protein is not required for their actions to be manifest. Specifically, the sex steroids are soluble enough in plasma to circulate at concentrations at which they are fully active. Considerable evidence suggests that the metabolic disposition of androgens is influenced by the presence of sex hormone binding globulin. Thus the metabolic clearance rate of a given androgen can be shown to be related inversely to the affinity of the androgen for sex hormone binding globulin (154). Moreover, sex hormone binding globulin may provide a reservoir of bound hormone that effectively dampens wide oscillations in the free hormone concentration.

The principal steroidal androgens present in the blood of males are testosterone, dihydrotestosterone, and androstanediol. Other androgenic steroids secreted by endocrine tissues include androstenedione and dehydroepiandrosterone. The Leydig cells, the testicular interstitial tissue, represent the major source of testicular androgens.

Testosterone, the principal androgen found in plasma, is secreted in episodic bursts throughout the day; thus multiple peaks can be observed if frequent blood sampling is performed. Normal plasma testosterone levels in men range between 3.0 and 12.0 ng/ml, with a mean value of 6 to 7 ng/ml. Testosterone and dihydrotestosterone are metabolized to a variety of different 17-ketosteroids (155), which are then conjugated with glucuronic acid and sulfate and ultimately excreted in urine. Of the total urinary 17-ketosteroids in man, testicular secretion accounts for only 30%. Moreover, urinary excretion of testosterone is not directly proportional to testosterone production rates. Finally, only traces of testosterone metabolites are found in bile and feces.

Small amounts of estrogen are produced by the normal testes. Most plasma estrogen present in men arises as a result of peripheral conversion of weak adrenal androgens (Fig. 8) (156). Estradiol in blood, like testosterone, is bound to sex hormone binding globulin but with less affinity. Estrogens, like androgens, are metabolized largely in the liver and conjugated with glucuronic acid or sulfuric acid and finally excreted in bile and urine.

In addition to being an endocrine organ, the testes also function as a reproductive organ. Spermatogenesis is closely regulated by FSH. Testosterone is also necessary for normal spermatogenesis. It is likely that the close approximation of Leydig cells to the seminiferous tubules allows for a high local concentration of androgen to reach the developing spermatogonia, thereby stimulating spermatogenesis (157).

In the female, estradiol production varies during the menstrual cycle, ranging between 250 and 500 μg/24 hr. The plasma level is lower in the follicular (60 to 100 pg/ml) than in the luteal (300 to 700 pg/ml) phase. The

production rate of estrone is approximately 40 μg/24 hr; most of this arises as a result of peripheral conversion from androstenedione, which is secreted from both the ovaries and the adrenal glands (Fig. 8). In normal, lean, premenopausal women, the conversion of androstenedione to estrone is on the order of 1 to 1.5% (158,159).

Following menopause, ovarian secretion of androstenedione falls to negligible amounts, while the adrenals continue to secrete 1.0 to 1.5 mg/day androstenedione. The rate at which androstenedione is converted to estrone increases after menopause to levels of 2 to 3%, such that about 40 μg/day estrone is produced, maintaining plasma levels near those prior to the menopause (160).

In both men and women, a number of conditions increase the production of estrone, including hyperthyroidism, aging, hepatic disease, and obesity (161–166). In each of these conditions, the increased production of estrone is the result of an increased conversion of androstenedione to estrone. Despite extensive study, the principal site of this conversion is uncertain.

The observed alterations that occur in the functioning of the hypothalamic-pituitary-gonadal axis of individuals with liver disease vary depending on the etiology of the disease (142,167). In individuals with alcoholic liver disease, primary gonadal failure appears to be the major finding. In such individuals, hypogonadism characterized by loss of gonadal reproductive and endocrine function is obvious. Alcoholic men frequently have small testes containing greatly reduced numbers of germ cells (168–170) (Fig. 9). Not surprisingly, ejaculates obtained from such men are frequently azoospermic or contain reduced numbers of spermatozoa or an increased number of bizarre and/or immature germ cells (143,171).

Plasma testosterone levels are reduced in 50% of alcoholic men (143). (Fig. 10). In contrast to the total plasma testosterone level, which is normal in 50%, free testosterone levels are reduced almost universally as a consequence of the eightfold increase in the plasma sex hormone binding globulin concentration in such men (143,172) (Fig. 11). Plasma gonadotropins are within the normal range or are moderately increased; considering the degree of reproductive and endocrine failure present, these levels are inappropriately low (142–144). Moreover, the LH responses of alcoholic men to the provocative stimulus LHRF are reduced in most (173). Therefore, evidence for combined hypothalamic-pituitary-gonadal dysfunction occurs in the majority (144,173).

In addition to manifesting evidence for hypothalamic-pituitary-gonadal dysfunction, alcoholic men commonly appear feminized. Feminization is manifest by a female escutcheon body habitus, palmar

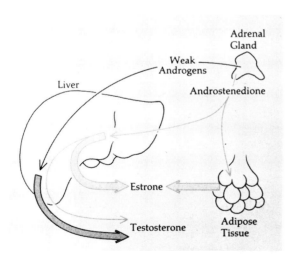

FIG. 8. Schematic representation of the biotransformation of weak adrenal androgens to estrone and to a lesser extent estradiol by the liver and adipose tissues. The testosterone formed from such weak adrenal androgens for the most part is conjugated with glucuronide and excreted either in bile or urine.

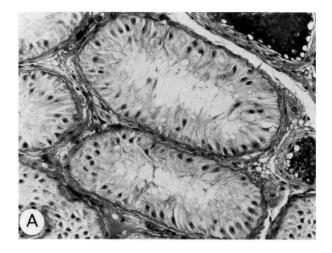

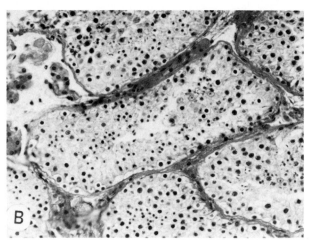

FIG. 9. Testicular histology. **A:** Alcoholic. **B:** Normal control. Both are shown at 200×.

erythema, spider angiomata, and gynecomastia. In addition, the patients are biochemically feminized, as manifested by increased levels of sex hormone binding globulin, estrogen-sensitive neurophysin, prolactin, growth hormone, TSH, and estrone, all of which are presumed to be estrogenic responses (172,174,175).

Alcoholic individuals with liver disease are more likely to be feminized than those without liver disease; as a result, the presence of liver disease per se has been advanced as the immediate cause of the feminization (174). Alcoholic males with Laennec cirrhosis convert androstenedione to estrone and estradiol at a greater rate than do men without such disease (166). Portal systemic shunts are associated with increased plasma estrone levels (176). Presumably, shunts allow estrogens excreted into the bile to be reabsorbed and bypass the liver and hepatic reexcretion. Quantitatively more important is reabsorption of weak androgens, such as androstenedione, which are excreted initially into bile and then into the bowel. Upon being reabsorbed in patients with portal systemic shunts, they escape hepatic reexcretion. Once reabsorbed,

weak androgens are converted to and act as estrogens (principally estrogen) at estrogen-responsive tissues without ever having circulated in the plasma as estrogens (174–176). The absolute amount of estrogen receptor in hepatic tissue is increased in liver obtained from alcohol-fed animals as compared to that of isocaloric controls (177–179). This permits the hepatic cells of alcohol-fed rats and presumably men to experience relatively more estrogen for any given ambient estrogen level (177–179).

In contrast to the male, the chronic alcoholic female is not superfeminized but shows severe gonadal failure commonly manifested by oligoamenorrhea, loss of secondary sex characteristics, such as breast and pelvic fat accumulation, and infertility (142,174,180). Histologic studies of ovaries obtained at autopsy from chronic alcoholic women who died of cirrhosis while still in their reproductive years (20 to 40 years of age) show a paucity of developing follicles and few or no corpora lutea (100).

In contrast to the considerable information available evaluating the hypothalamic-pituitary-gonadal function in individuals with alcohol-induced Laennec cirrhosis, few data are available concerning hypothalamic-pituitary function in individuals with postnecrotic or viral-induced liver disease (142,167). In a recent evaluation of the hypothalamic-pituitary-gonadal axis of adult hemophiliac males with advanced liver disease of presumed viral etiology, testosterone levels were not reduced when compared with those of age-matched controls (167). In addition, sperm concentrations were not reduced, and ejaculates collected from such men were no different than those obtained from age-matched controls without liver disease.

In hemochromatosis, gonadal failure characterized by a high prevalence of reduced libido, impotence, reduction in sexual body hair, and a reduction of testicular size has been reported in male patients (181–184). In about one-half of the reported studies, LH levels were reduced, suggesting secondary hypogonadism. In many others, however, LH levels have been increased, suggesting primary gonadal failure. These variable results are not unexpected if one recalls that, at autopsy, iron deposition is common in both the hypothalamus and pituitary and is occasionally seen in the testes of men dying with hemochromatosis. Feminization is less common in males with hemochromatosis than in those with alcohol-induced liver disease, presumably because portal systemic shunting is less severe and/or the hypogonadism appears so much later in life that feminization does not become manifest except in unusual circumstances.

Probably because hemochromatosis is unusual in women, except in those well beyond menopause, no data are available evaluating hypothalamic-pituitary-gonadal function in such women.

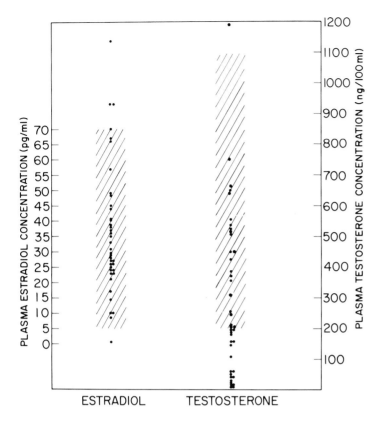

FIG. 10. Plasma sex steroids in men with alcoholic liver disease. *Cross-hatched areas,* range of values for age-matched nonalcoholic controls.

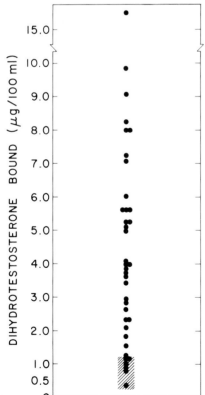

FIG. 11. Plasma sex steroid binding capacity of men with alcoholic liver disease. The binding capacity has been determined by displacing endogenous sex steroids with dihydrostestosterone. *Shaded area,* range of values observed for age-matched nonalcoholic controls.

Few studies evaluating hypothalamic-pituitary-gonadal function have been performed in subjects with Wilson disease (142). Similarly, few autopsy data specifically evaluating the hypothalamus, pituitary, and/or gonads obtained from individuals dying with Wilson disease are available. Those patients studied show no evidence of hypothalamic-pituitary-gonadal disease until they had such advanced hepatocellular disease that it proved lethal despite appropriate therapy. It is of interest to note that copper stimulates secretion of all known anterior pituitary hormones except prolactin (185).

As is the case with Wilson disease, hypothalamic-pituitary-gonadal function, when evaluated in individuals with advanced biliary cirrhosis, either primary or secondary to extrahepatic bile duct obstruction or cystic fibrosis, has been found to be universally normal (142). This also may be due to enhanced copper levels at hypothalamic-pituitary sites (185). Because the major site for copper excretion is the biliary system, disease of the biliary system is associated with tissue accumulation of copper.

Adrenal Gland

Cortisol is the major glucocorticoid secreted by the adrenal cortex in man; its $T_{1/2}$ is approximately 70 min (186). Plasma levels range from 5 to 35 mg/dl. Under normal conditions, a diurnal variation exists, with highest levels occurring in the morning and lower levels present in the afternoon and evening (187). Ninety-five percent of the plasma cortisol is bound to protein, principally cortisol binding globulin (CBG) and to a lesser extent albumin (188). Cortisol is degraded principally by the liver as a result of A-ring reduction to tetrahydrocortisone and subsequent conjugation with glucuronic acid, which is followed by urinary excretion (186). In patients with liver disease, there is a decreased cortisol clearance (186,189–192). In hepatic failure, 20-α reduction is favored over A-ring reduction. Consequently, tetrahydrocortisol formation is decreased, and 20-$\propto$ cortalone is increased.

In most cases of liver disease, particularly those with significant portal hypertension, plasma levels of CBG are increased, as are, consequently, total cortisol levels. In contrast, free cortisol levels are usually normal, and measurement of urinary free cortisol levels clearly differentiates between those with adrenal disease and those with liver-associated alterations in CBG levels as a cause of elevated plasma cortisol levels.

Clinical evidence of cortisol excess (i.e., striae, obesity, facial mooning, and acne) is common in patients with idiopathic chronic active hepatitis (192). Such patients often have other forms of endocrine disease commonly associated with the HLA B8 and DW 3 antigens, such as Hashimoto thyroiditis, autoimmune gonadal (particularly ovarian) failure, and adrenal insufficiency.

Aldosterone is the major mineralocorticoid produced by the human adrenal gland. With the exception of the unusual syndrome of primary hyperaldosteronism, hyperaldosteronism is usually a secondary phenomenon occurring in response to excessive and prolonged adrenal stimulation by angiotensin II produced as a result of hyperreninemia (193). In such situations, the aldosterone hypersecretion is appropriate for the degree of activation of the renin-angiotensin system. In decompensated hepatic disease states, characterized as having an inadequate effective plasma volume, renal hyperreninemia develops, and angiotensin II levels increase with the resultant hypersecretion of aldosterone. Aldosterone hypersecretion results in enhanced salt and water retention, ascites formation, and ultimately anasarca. Spironolactone therapy in such individuals is quite effective but often requires high doses (400 to 800 mg/day).

Recent recognition of a pseudo-Cushing syndrome in alcoholic patients, many of whom have liver disease, has rekindled interest in the effects of liver disease and alcohol per se on the hypothalamic-pituitary-adrenal axis (109–115). The mechanisms responsible and the specific site for this stimulation, however, have not been determined fully. Recent data suggest a possible adrenal as well as pituitary site for such stimulation (194–196). Compounding such observa-

tions, however, is the additional observation that up to 25% of chronic alcoholic subjects have inadequate ACTH response to insulin-induced hypoglycemia (195,196). It should be remembered, however, that both syndromes (pseudo-Cushing and ACTH deficiency) are likely to result from alcohol ingestion per se rather than from the associated liver disease.

Hypothalamic-Pituitary-Thyroidal Axis

In normal subjects, the thyroid produces 78 μg/day thyroxine, of which 16 μg are either conjugated and excreted in bile or undergo oxidative deamination (197,198). The remaining 62 μg are deiodinated to either triiodothyrinine (T_3), accounting for 23 μg/day or reverse T_3 (RT_3), 29 μg/day. RT_3 is generally considered to be biologically inactive. On the molar basis, T_3 is several times more potent than T_4 (199). Therefore, peripheral conversion of T_4 to T_3 may be considered a form of hormone activation. Because the liver is the major organ responsible for the peripheral conversion of T_4 to T_3 (199), it has a major role in thyroid hormone metabolism and is involved in its conjugation, biliary excretion, oxidative deamination, and peripheral deiodination. T_4-5'-deiodinase is a particulate enzyme which is dependent in part on the presence of various cytosolic components (200). Hepatic T_4-5'-deiodinase is inhibited *in vitro* by a variety of drugs, such as propylthiouracil, ioponoic acid and other cholecystographic contrast agents, propanalol, and salicylates (201–205). Its activity is decreased in liver by starvation, hypothyroidism, glucocorticoid administration, diabetes mellitus, and uremia (203–205) because of decreased enzyme activity and decreased cofactor availability (204,205). Another factor determining hepatic T_4 conversion to T_3 is T_4 uptake by the liver, which reflects the capacity of hepatic cytosolic proteins to bind T_4 (205).

The majority of patients with liver disease are clinically euthyroid, as manifested by indirect measures of thyroid hormone function, such as Achilles tendon reflex time and indices of myocardial contractility. However, some patients with acute alcohol-related liver disease may have increased thyroidal radioactive iodine uptake and clearance, particularly if studied early on admission to hospital (206). Thyroidal iodine uptake returns to normal during hospitalization without any specific thyroid therapy and can be suppressed appropriately with T_3. Accelerated thyroidal uptake of ^{131}I has been reported to occur also in hepatobiliary giardiasis (207).

Serum total and free T_4 levels are normal or slightly increased in most subjects with advanced liver disease (208–212). In an occasional patient, however, the total

T_4 level may be considerably increased or decreased, occurring in association with alteration in thyroxin binding protein levels. Estimation of the free thyroxin index, which is calculated from the serum thyroxin and thyroid hormone binding globulin level, is normal in such subjects.

Nomura and colleagues (210) reported that a reduced T_4 to T_3 conversion is common in cirrhotic patients. In their studies, these patients had a T_4 to T_3 conversion one-half that found in normal subjects. In addition, the authors noted that reduced conversion of T_4 to T_3 returns to normal with convalescence and improved hepatic function.

Estimation of TSH concentrations is a sensitive index of thyroid function, particularly hypothyroidism. In four recent reports (209,210,212–215), TSH levels have been elevated to twice normal (but within the normal range) in individuals with chronic liver disease. In contrast to the responses of individuals with true hypothyroidism, peak TSH responses to TRH are usually normal in individuals with advanced liver disease (209, 210,212). This has been construed as suggesting that liver disease, particularly alcoholic liver disease, is associated with an abnormality of pituitary secretion of TSH, independent of the thyroid (212).

Finally, it should be noted that both chronic active hepatitis and primary biliary cirrhosis often are associated with an autoimmune thyroiditis of the Hashimoto variety (214,215).

Calcium Metabolism

The level of ionized calcium in the plasma is maintained within the narrow normal range by the integrated actions of parathormone, vitamin D, and calcitonin (216). Parathyroid hormone affects the movement of calcium in three ways: (a) by increasing intestinal calcium absorption, (b) by increasing renal tubular reabsorption of calcium, and (c) by increasing bone reabsorption. The active metabolite of vitamin D, 1,25-dihydroxycholecalciferol, like parathormone, increases intestinal absorption and bone reabsorption of calcium (217). Together, these two hormones function to increase the serum level. Conversely, calcitonin inhibits reabsorption of calcium from bone and therefore tends to lower serum calcium (218). The rates of secretion of parathormone, 1,25-dihydroxycholecalciferol, and calcitonin are controlled by the plasma level of ionized calcium. Hypocalcemia stimulates the production of parathormone and 1,25-dihydroxycholecalciferol, while hypercalcemia diminishes their production but enhances the secretion of calcitonin. In addition, calcitonin stimulates while parathormone inhibits 1-hydroxylation of 25-hydroxycholecalciferol to 1,25-dihydroxycholecalciferol within the kidney.

The most important aspect of vitamin D chemistry is

that it is a steroid, albeit a secosteroid, in which the B-ring of the steroid nucleus is replaced by a 5,7-diene bridge (219). Cholecalciferol, or vitamin D_3, the form that is produced in the skin by ultraviolet radiation, is the most important form of vitamin D. A second and important nutritional form of vitamin D is that of vitamin D_2, or ergocalciferol.

The absorption of vitamin D requires bile salts. Once absorbed, vitamin D is transported via lymphatics to the bloodstream, where it binds to vitamin D transport globulin (220–223); this transport protein is an α_1-globulin (221–223). Vitamin D transport globulin is responsible for transporting all the vitamin D moieties and is found in huge excess relative to the total amount of the vitamin and its various metabolites present in plasma.

Cholecalciferol characteristically accumulates rapidly in the liver from plasma. Vitamin D metabolites do not accumulate in the liver, indicating that this phenomenon is specific for the cholecalciferol molecule itself (224–226). In the liver, cholecalciferol undergoes its first metabolic activation, being converted to 25-hydroxycholecalciferol (227,228). This compound is the major circulating form of vitamin D, being present in plasma at levels of 20 to 30 ng/ml. This is in contrast to the circulating level of the parent cholecalciferol, which is about 1 ng/ml.

The 25-hydroxylation of cholecalciferol occurs in the endoplasmic reticulum and/or microsomal fractions and requires the presence of NADPH, molecular oxygen, magnesium, and a cytoplasmic factor (229). 25-Hydroxycholecalciferol is transferred to the kidney, where it undergoes its next obligatory reaction prior to becoming functionally active in the form of 1,25-dihydroxycholecalciferol (224–226). 25-Hydroxycholecalciferol can undergo a variety of other metabolic conversions in the kidney, intestine, and cartilage where there exists another enzyme system, namely, 25-hydroxy-D-24-R-hydrolase (224). This enzyme is absent in vitamin D deficiency and is induced by vitamin D. The 24-R-hydrolase requires that the substrate contain the 25-hydroxyl function and is apparently mitochondrial in location (230,231). It acts not only on 25-hydroxycholecalciferol but also on 1,25-dihydroxycholecalciferol to produce the corresponding 24-R-hydrolylated metabolite. The 24-R-hydrolylated forms of vitamin D are almost as active as the precursor 25-hydroxy forms (232). It has been suggested that 24,25-dihydroxycholecalciferol plays an important role in the mineralization of bone (233). Vitamin D compounds are excreted primarily in the bile, ultimately resulting in their excretion with the feces. There is an enterohepatic circulation of 25-hydroxycholecalciferol (234–238).

The biologic activity of 1,25-dihydroxycholecalciferol is 10 times of that of cholecalciferol, while

25-hydroxycholecalciferol is approximately three times more active than cholecalciferol (239). 24,25-Dihydroxycholecalciferol is about twice as active as cholecalciferol. The major function of vitamin D in the form of 1,25-dihydroxycholecalciferol is to elevate plasma calcium and phosphorus concentrations to supersaturating levels in order to support normal mineralization of newly forming bone. It does this principally by elevating the plasma calcium concentration by stimulating the active absorption of calcium by the small intestine (224–226).

In addition, 1,25-dihydroxycholecalciferol also stimulates the active absorption of phosphate (226,240, 241); evidence also suggests that it stimulates renal absorption of calcium in the distal renal tubules (242, 243) and functions with parathormone to mobilize calcium and phosphate from bone (244). The regulation of vitamin D 25-hydrolase in the liver is of limited capacity, as large circulating levels of 25-hydroxycholecalciferol can be produced by the administration of large doses of vitamin D (228,245).

The major site of regulation of vitamin D metabolism is at the level of the renal 25-hydroxycholecalciferol 1-α-hydrolylase and the 25-hydroxycholecalciferol, 24-R-hydrolylase. Under circumstances of vitamin D deficiency, together with its characteristic secondary hyperparathyroidism, high levels of 25-hydroxy-D 1-α-hydrolylase and virtually no measurable 25-hydroxycholeciferol 24-R-hydrolylase is found (246). Administration of vitamin D brings about the suppression of 1-α-hydrolylase and a stimulation of the 24-R-hydrolylase (247). The specific stimulant is 1,25-dihydroxycholecalciferol, which seems to induce the 24-R-hydrolylase and at the same time suppresses the 1-hydrolylase. Calcium affects vitamin D levels as follows: Hypocalcemia, when sensed by the parathyroid glands, results in the secretion of parathromone. Parathromone in turn stimulates 25-hydroxycholecalciferol α-hydrolylase and suppresses the 24-R-hydrolylase. The resultant 1,25-hydroxycholecalciferol then stimulates the mobilization of calcium in the small intestine, bone, and distal tubules.

Besides regulation by calcium and parathyroid hormone, it is clear that plasma phosphate also plays an important role in the regulation of 1,25-hydroxycholecalciferol metabolism (248). Under hypophosphatemic conditions, 1,25-dihydroxycholecalciferol accumulates in the plasma; under conditions of hyperphosphatemia, 24-R-25-hydroxycholecalciferol accumulates. Because vitamin D oxidative metabolites have certain structural similarities to steroid hormones, it was recognized early that vitamin D steroids might also be subject to increased hepatic microsomal metabolism, which occurs in anticonvulsant-treated patients. In both man and animals, chronic anticonvulsant therapy results in a marked reduction in the

serum half-life of cholecalciferol and 25-hydroxycholecalciferol, with an associated increase in the appearance of more polar products, which are not active as vitamin D (249–253). Additionally, the coadministration of phenobarbital further increases the hepatic microsomal uptake and metabolism of vitamin D. It also enhances the biliary excretion of vitamin D metabolites and accelerates the *in vitro* microsomal conversion of vitamin D and 25-hydroxycholecalciferol to inactive polar metabolites.

A variety of cholestalic diseases and syndromes, most notably primary biliary cirrhosis and biliary atresia, are complicated by metabolic bone disease (254–258). Because 25-hydroxycholecalciferol, the major circulating form of vitamin D, is synthesized mainly or exclusively in the liver, several groups (256,257,259) have measured serum 25-hydroxycholecalciferol concentrations in patients with primary biliary cirrhosis. The 25-hydroxycholecalciferol concentrations in these patients have been found to be low when compared to those in various control groups. The lower serum 25-hydroxycholecalciferol concentrations are associated with skeletal demineralization (257). The bone lesion that occurs most commonly in primary biliary cirrhosis has been characterized histologically and appears to consist of two lesions: osteomalacia combined with osteoporosis. The most common finding on bone biopsy, however, is osteomalacia (257).

Investigation of the pathogenesis of these bone lesions has aroused considerable controversy. Workers in Chicago (257) studying a small group of patients with advanced primary biliary cirrhosis found that neither oral nor parenteral vitamin D increased the serum 25-hydroxycholecalciferol concentrations or prevented further skeletal demineralization. In contrast, oral 25-hydroxycholecalciferol increased serum 25-hydroxycholecalciferol concentrations in all patients tested and stabilized the bone mineral content in most. Thus, while noting that bone disease in primary biliary cirrhosis is undoubtably multifactorial, Rosenberg et al. (260) have suggested that a low serum 25-hydroxycholecalciferol concentration in these patients might be of pathogenic significance. It is important to note that bile duct ligation in rats is associated with a reduction in the hepatic vitamin D 25-hydrolylase activity, whereas hepatic vitamin D uptake and 25-hydroxycholecalciferol released from liver remain normal (261).

Biliary atresia is the most important cause of osteomalacia in children with hepatic biliary disease. Kobayashi et al. (258) found radiographic evidence of rickets in 23 or 39 children with uncorrected extrahepatic biliary atresia. Daum et al. (262) reported that these patients have low serum 25-hydroxycholecalciferol concentrations and that oral 25-hydroxycholecalciferol therapy heals or prevents rickets in these children.

Low 25-hydroxycholecalciferol concentrations are reported in other types of cirrhosis, particularly alcoholic cirrhosis (263). In one series of patients with severe advanced alcoholic cirrhosis, low serum 25-hydroxycholecalciferol concentrations were found in 44% and were restored to normal by modest doses of oral vitamin D (264). Although subtle defects in 25-hydrolylation could not be excluded, the low serum 25-hydroxycholecalciferol concentrations in these patients was believed to be due to a combination of factors, including malabsorption, poor dietary intake, and lack of sunlight exposure, or a direct effect of alcohol on vitamin D metabolism.

Adrenal Medullary Function

Little was known of the metabolic fate of catecholamines until it was shown that 3-methoxy,4-hydroxymandelic acid (VMA) is a urinary metabolite or norepinephrine (265). Monoamine oxidase (MOA) deaminates epinephrine, and the deaminated product is O-methylated and excreted (266). Axelrod et al. (267) demonstrated that O-methylated derivatives of the catecholamines could be formed in vitro by liver homogenates and are present in free and conjugated form. Catechol-O-methyltransferase, the enzyme responsible for the O-methylation of catecholamines, has been pufiried partially. Although it is present in almost all tissues, it is found in highest concentrations in the liver and kidneys (268). Deamination of catecholamines by MAO results in the formation of aldehydes, which are oxidized further to the corresponding acids, which in turn are reduced to alcohol (glycol) derivatives (269,270).

Normal levels of norepinephrine in plasma are in the range of 0.2 to 0.4 ng/ml and of epinephrine 0.02 to 0.4 ng/ml. Because of the rapid turnover rates of plasma catecholamines, their levels are rapidly responsive to changes in the rate of their entry into circulation. The observation that dopamine-β-hydroxylase is released along with norepinephrine has allowed investigators to examine factors that stimulate the sympathetic nervous system by assaying dopamine-β-hydroxylase in plasma (271).

Mobilization of glucose from glycogen stores and the formation of glucose from short chain fatty acids and amino acids is stimulated by catecholamines. The formation and release of fatty acids from triglyceride stores in adipose tissue is increased also as a result of catecholamine stimulation (272). It is generally believed that the local metabolic effect of catecholamines is to substrate for immediate local consumption. Glycogenolysis in heart and skeletal muscle and glycerol release from adipose tissue are all catecholamine-stimulated activities (272). Of greater importance for overall energy metabolism, however, catecholamines stimulate the mobilization of major fuel stores in the liver, adipose tissue, and muscle for the production of readily usable substrates required for the immediate energy needs of rapidly metabolizing tissues (Fig. 12).

The predominant biochemical effect of catecholamine stimulation within a tissue is the activation of previously synthesized enzymes and the inactivation of others. Thus glycogen phosphorylase, triglyceride lipase, and glucose-6-phosphatase are activated by catecholamines, while glycogen synthetase is inactivated (272). Such a system of enzyme regulation by catecholamines provides for the prompt responses to acute environmental demands, while de novo enzyme synthesis would require considerably more time. As a result, gluconeogenesis from lactate and endogenous amino acids is accelerated (273,274). Similarly, catecholamines accelerate ketogenesis by exerting a direct effect on the liver, thereby promoting ketone production while inhibiting hepatic triglyceride release (274).

Insulin antagonizes most of the metabolic changes that occur as a result of the action of catecholamines, while glucagon potentiates their action by increasing glycogenolysis, gluconeogenesis, and ketogenesis. Thus the ability of catecholamines to suppress insulin and stimulate glucagon provides the proper hormonal environment in which the full expression of catecholamines effects on hepatic metabolism can be manifested.

Catecholamines greatly influence hepatic blood flow. Stimulation of splanchnic sympathetics or the infusion of epinephrine and norepinephrine into either hepatic artery or the portal vein reduces hepatic blood flow by 50% (275). Recently, glucagon has been shown to inhibit this vasoconstrictive action of norepinephrine (276). Thus the increased secretion of glucagon stimulated by catecholamines may serve not only to promote catecholamine effects on hepatic metabolism but also to prevent, to some extent, the decrease in hepatic blood flow associated with increased catecholamine activity.

The nonspecificity of the enzymes involved in the formation of norepinephrine and the ability of the neurosecretory vesicles to store and release compounds similar in structure to that of norepinephrine results in the accumulation of compounds that release the physiologic transmitter when appropriate precursors or amines are available. Such false neurotransmitters are generally less potent than norepinephrine (277). The disturbance of hepatic encephalopathy must involve derangements in neurotransmission. It is yet to be determined whether these changes in neurotransmission occur primarily as a result of alterations in

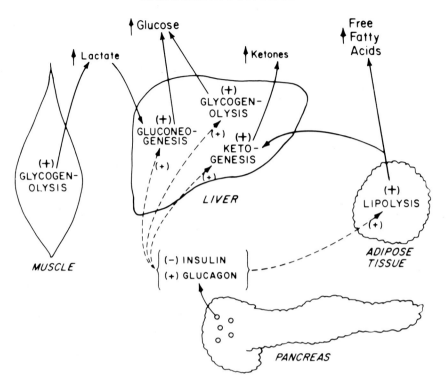

FIG. 12. Effects of catecholamines on the generation of usable substrates from stored fuels as a result of catecholamine modulation of insulin and glucagon action. (+), Stimulation, (−), inhibition.

energy or alterations in synthesis and/or metabolism of neurotransmitters.

Ammonia has traditionally been the leading candidate as the putative toxin responsible for hepatic encephalopathy (278). Such a hypothesis is an extension of the observation that meat intoxication has been recognized for nearly 100 years in animals with hepatic damage following Eck fistula. Moreover, the recognition that ammonia intoxication in such animals mimics spontaneous hepatic encephalopathy has served to fuel the argument. It was initially thought that ammonia blocked energy production utilized in the synthesis of glutamine (279). This hypothesis is no longer tenable, as it has been shown that brain glutamine is derived from the synthesis of ammonia via glutamic acid rather than 2-oxoglutarate (280). Ammonia has been thought to act as a toxin by increasing the brain levels of the inhibitory neurotransmitter GABA (281). In addition, ammonia has been shown to inhibit acetylcholine synthesis. Recent neurophysiologic evidence suggests that ammonia cannot be the sole toxin in hepatic encephalopathy, as the site of ammonia toxicity has been localized to the cortex and perhaps the amygdala. In contrast, the reticular activating system, which is severely involved in hepatic encephalopathy, is not affected by ammonia (282). Moreover, the striking elevations of trytophan and serotonin levels, alterations in brain phenylalanine, tyrosine, and derivative amines, and alterations in

metabolism of dopamine and serotonins seen in hepatic encephalopathy are not inducible with ammonia intoxication (283–288).

The recognition that butyrate, valerate, and octonoate are increased in the blood and CSF of patients with hepatic encephalopathy has suggested that short chain fatty acids might contribute to the pathogenesis of hepatic encephalopathy (289,290). Such a hypothesis is supported by the observation that intraperitoneal injection of butyrate, valerate, and octonoate can produce coma in experimental animals (291). It should be noted, however, that the clinical status of encephalopathy in patients with cirrhosis correlates poorly with the circulating levels of any of the short chain fatty acids (291). Zieve et al. (292) have proposed that a synergism exists between ammonia and fatty acids in the pathogenesis of encephalopathy. More recently, the concept of false neurotransmitters in the pathogenesis of hepatic encephalopathy has evolved (286,293,294). It is proposed that false neurotransmitters might accumulate under toxic or pharmacologic conditions or in response to the accumulation of their precursors in patients with advanced liver disease. Such substances are taken up by the central and peripheral nervous systems.

The blood-brain barrier selectively allows neurotransmitter precursor amino acids to enter the central nervous system but excludes the others. It operates on a series of competitive principles, however, by which decreased plasma concentrations of certain amino acids may result in increased uptake of others (295). With the failure of hepatic function, both the peripheral and central nervous systems can be found to accept amino acids normally excluded or incorrect amounts of neurotransmitter precursors which might lead to altered neurotransmitter synthesis.

In patients and animals with encephalopathy, derangements in plasma levels of many of the common dietary amino acids are well established (296–305). The pattern consists of increased phenylalanine, tyrosine, free but not total tryptophan, methionine, histidine, glutamate, and aspartate, together with decreased or normal levels of the branched chain amino acids, leucine, isoleucine, and valine. Presumably because of the increased plasma-free tryptophan level serotonin, an inhibitor transmitter derived from tryptophan, is greatly increased (286,306).

Since the initial neurotransmitter hypothesis was proposed, the finding of octopamine in the brain and blood of experimental animals and the blood and urine of patients with hepatic encephalopathy has been reported (307–309). It is important to note that phenylalanine and other amines capable of acting as false neurotransmitters have been found to be increased in the brains of experimental animals with hepatic encephalopathy (310). It should also be noted, however, that octopamine introduced into the CSF of animals at concentrations well above those seen clinically in hepatic encephalopathy does not produce coma in animals (311). Elevated glutamine concentrations are found consistently in the brain and CSF of man and animals with hepatic coma (313). In contrast, levels of the inhibitory neurotransmitter GABA usually are found to be normal (312–314).

Much remains to be learned about hepatic encephalopathy. The same admonition pertains to the interactions of the liver, hepatic disease, and endocrine systems. Hopefully this chapter will serve as a starting point for those interested in expanding knowledge of such interrelationships and as a source of information for clinicians faced with caring for patients with liver disease who also manifest evidence of endocrine dysfunction.

REFERENCES

1. Van Wyk, J. J., and Hintz, R. G. (1979): Peptide growth factors. In: *Endocrinology, Vol. 3*, edited by L. J. DeGroot, G. F. Cahill, Jr., W. D. Odell, L. Martini, J. T. Potts, Jr., D. H. Nelson, E. Steinberger, and A. L. Winegrad, pp. 1767–1775. Grune & Stratton, New York.
2. Laron Z. (1974): Syndrome of familial dwarfism and high plasma immunoreactive growth hormone. *Isr. J. Med. Sci.*, 10:1247.
3. Dupre, J., Ross, S. A., Watson, D., and Brown, J. C. (1973): Stimulation of insulin secretion by gastric inhibitory polypeptide in man. *J. Clin. Endocrinol. Metab.*, 37:826.
4. Jensen, E. V., Mohla, S., Gorell, T. A., and DeSombre, E. R. (1974): The role of estrophilin in estrogen action. *Vitam. Horm.*, 32:89.
5. Gorski, J., and Gannon F. (1976): Current models of steroid hormone QP801 V5V837 action: A critique. *Annu. Rev. Physiol.*, 38:425.
6. O'Malley, B. W., and Schrader, W. T. (1976): The receptors of steroid hormones. *Sci. Am.*, 234:32.
7. Jensen, E. V., and DeSombre, E. R. (1979): Steroid sex hormone receptors and action. In: *Endocrinology, Vol. 3*, edited by L. J. DeGroot, G. F. Cahill, Jr., W. D. Odell, L. Martini, J. T. Potts, Jr., D. H. Nelson, E. Steinberger, and A. L. Winegrad, pp. 2055–2061. Grune & Stratton, New York.
8. Roth, J. (1973): Peptide hormone binding to receptors: A review of direct studies in vitro. *Metabolism*, 22:1059.
9. Pastan, I., Roth, J., and Macchia, V. (1966): Binding of hormone to tissue: The first step in polypeptide hormone action. *Proc. Natl. Acad. Sci. USA*, 56:1801.
10. Van Thiel, D. H. (1981): Disorders of the hypothalamic-pituitary-gonadal axis in patients with liver disease. In: *Hepatology*, edited by D. Zakim and T. D. Boyer. Saunders, Philadelphia (*in press*).
11. Schimke, R. T. (1975): Turnover of membrane proteins in animal cells. In: *Methods in Membrane Biology, Vol. 3*, edited by E. D. Korn, pp. 201–236. Plenum, New York.
12. Gavin, J. R., Roth, J., Neville, D. M., Jr., DeMeyts, P., and Buell, D. N. (1974): Insulin dependent regulation of insulin receptor concentrations. *Proc. Natl. Acad. Sci. USA*, 71:84.
13. Davidson, M. B., and Kaplan, S. A. (1977): Increased insulin binding by hepatic plasma membranes from diabetic rats. *J. Clin. Invest.*, 59:22.
14. Rehfeld, J. F., and Stadil, F. (1973): Gel filtration studies on immunoreactive gastrin in serum from Zollinger-Ellison patients. *Gut*, 14:369.
15. Marks, V. (1972): Glucagon. *Clin. Endocrinol. Metab.*, 1:829.
16. Valverde, I. (1968): Demonstration and characterization of a second fraction of glucagon like immunoreactivity in jejunal extracts. *Am J. Med. Sci.*, 225:415.
17. Issekutz, B. (1977): Studies on hepatic glucose cycles in normal and methyl prednisolone treated dogs. *Metabolism*, 26:157.
18. Combes, B., Adams, R. H., Strickland, W., and Madison, L. L. (1961): The physiological significance of the secretion of endogenous insulin into portal circulation. *J. Clin. Invest.*, 40:1706.
19. Felig, P. (1976): The liver in glucose homeostasis in normal man and in diabetes. In: *Diabetes: Its Physiological and Biochemical Basis*, edited by J. Vallence-Owen, pp. 53–123. MIP Press, Lancaster.
20. Cahill, G. F., and Owen, O. E. (1968): Some observations on carbohydrate metabolism in man. In: *Carbohydrate Metabolism and Its Disorders*, edited by F. Dirkens, P. J. Randle, and W. J. Whelon, pp. 447–522. Academic Press, New York.
21. Felig, P. (1973): The glucose alanine cycle. *Metabolism*, 22:179.
22. Owen, O. E., Morgan, A. P., Kemp, H. G., Sullivan, J. N., Herrera, M. G., and Cahill, G. F. (1967): Brain metabolism during fasting. *J. Clin. Invest.*, 46:1589.
23. Owen, O. E., Felig, P., Morgan, A. P., Wahren, J., and Cahill, G. F. (1969): Liver and kidney metabolism during prolonged fasting. *J. Clin. Invest.*, 48:574.
24. Dietze, G., Wicklmayr, M., Hepp, K. D., Bogner, W., Mehnert, H., Czempiel, H., and Henftling, H. G. (1976): On gluconeogenesis of human liver: Accelerated hepatic glucose formation by increased percursor supply. *Diabetologia*, 12:555.
25. Kreisberg, R. A. (1972): Glucose-lactate interrelations in men. *N. Engl. J. Med.*, 287:132.
26. Sugden, M. C., Sharples, C., and Rundle, P. J. (1976): Carcass glycogen as a potential source of glucose during short term starvation. *Biochem. J.*, 160:817.
27. Felig, P., Pozefsky, T., Marliss, E., and Cahill, G. F. (1970): Alanine: Key role in gluconeogenesis. *Science*, 167:1003.
28. Alberti, K. H. M. M., and Johnston, D. G. (1979): Carbohy-

drate metabolism in liver disease. In: *Liver and Biliary Disease*, edited by R. Wright, K. G. M. M. Alberti, S. Korran, and G. H. Mullward-Sadler, p. 46. Saunders, Philadelphia.

29. Felig, P., and Wahren, J. (1971): Influence of endogenous insulin secretion on sphanchnic glucose and amino acid balance in man. *J. Clin. Invest.*, 50:1702.

30. Camu, F. (1975): Hepatic balances of glucose and insulin in response to physiological increases of endogenous insulin during glucose infusions in dogs. *Eur. J. Clin. Invest.*, 5:101.

31. Kaden, M., Harding, P., and Field, J. B. (1973): Effect of intraduodenal glucose administration on hepatic extraction of insulin in the anesthetized dog. *J. Clin. Invest.*, 52:2016.

32. Kanazawa, Y., Kuzuya, T., Ide, T., and Kosaka, K. (1966): Plasma insulin responses to glucose in femoral, hepatic and pancreatic veins in dogs. *Am. J. Physiol.*, 211:442.

33. Johnston, D. G., and Alberti, K. G. M. M. (1976): Carbohydrate metabolism in liver disease. *Clin. Endocrinol. Metab.*, 5:675.

34. Greco, A. V., Fedeli, G., Ghirlanda, G., Manna, R., and Patrono, C. (1974): Behavior of pancreatic glucagon, insulin and HGH in liver cirrhosis after arginine and IV glucose. *Acta Diabetol. Lat.*, 11:330.

35. Felig, P., Gusberg, R., Hendler, R., Grump, F. E., and Kinney, J. M. (1974): Concentrations of glucagon and the insulin: Glucagon ratio in the portal and peripheral circulation. *Proc. Soc. Exp. Biol. Med.*, 147:88.

36. Jaspan, J. B., Huen, A. H. J., Morley, C. G., Moossa, A. E., and Rubenstein, A. H. (1977): The role of the liver in glucagon metabolism. *J. Clin. Invest.*, 60:421.

37. Unger, R. H. (1971): Glucagon and the insulin glucagon ratio in diabetes and other catabolic illnesses. *Diabetes*, 20:834.

38. Samols, E., and Holdsworth, D. (1968): Disturbances in carbohydrate metabolism: Liver disease. In: *Carbohydrate Metabolism and Its Disorders, Vol. 2*, edited by F. Dickins, P. J. Rundle, and W. J. Whelan, pp. 289–336. Academic Press, New York.

39. Record, C. V., Chase, R. A., Alberti, K. G. M. M., and Williams, R. (1975): Disturbances in glucose metabolism in patients with liver damage due to paracetamol overdose. *Clin. Sci. Mol. Med.*, 49:473.

40. Owen, O. E., Patel, M. S., Block, B. S. B., Kremlen, T. H., Reichle, F. A., and Mozzoli, M. A. (1976): Gluconeogenesis in normal, cirrhotic and diabetic humans. In: *Gluconeogenesis: Its Regulations in Mammalism Species*, edited by R. W. Hanson and M. A. Mehlman, pp. 533–558. Wiley, New York.

41. Meyers, J. D. (1950): Net splanchnic glucose production in normal man and in various disease states. *J. Clin. Invest.*, 29:1421.

42. Felig, P., Brown, W. V., Levine, R. A., and Klatskin, G. (1970): Glucose homeostasis in viral hepatitis. *N. Engl. J. Med.*, 283:1436.

43. Yeung, R. T. T., and Wang, C. C. L. (1974): A study of carbohydrate metabolism in post-necrotic cirrhosis of the liver. *Gut*, 15:907.

44. Megyesi, C., Samols, E., and Marks, V. (1967): Glucose tolerance and diabetes in chronic liver disease. *Lancet*, ii:1051.

45. Johnston, D. G., Alberti, K. G. M. M., Faber, O. K., Binder, C., and Wright, R. (1977): Hyperinsulinism of hepatic cirrhosis: Diminished degradation or hypersecretion. *Lancet*, i:10.

46. Johnston, D. G., Alberti, K. G. M. M., Wright, R., Smith-Liang, G., Stewart, A. M., Sherlock, S., Faber, O., and Binder, C. (1978): C peptide and insulin in liver disease. *Diabetes* [*Suppl.*], 27:201.

47. Marco, J., Diego, J., Villaneuva, M. L., Diza-Fierros, M., Valverde, I., and Segovia, J. M. (1973): Elevated plasma glucagon levels in cirrhosis of the liver. *N. Engl. J. Med.*, 289:1107.

48. Sherwin, R. S., Joshi, P., Hendler, P., Felig, P., and Conn, H. O. (1974): Hyperglucagonemia in Laennec's cirrhosis, the role of portal systemic shunting. *N. Engl. J. Med.*, 290:239.

49. Grecco, A. V., Crucitti, F., Ghirlanda, G., Manna, R., Altomonte, L., Rebuzzi, A., and Bertoli, A. (1981): Insulin and glucagon concentrations in portal and peripheral veins in hepatic cirrhosis. *Diabetologia* (*in press*).

50. Leevy, C. M., Thomson, P., and Baker, H. (1970): Vitamins and liver injury. *Am. J. Clin. Nutr.*, 23:453.

51. Alberti, K. G. M. M. (1974): In: *Some Metabolic Aspects of Liver Disease*, edited by S. C. Truelove and J. Trowell, pp. 341–359. Blackwell, Oxford.

52. Connor, H., Woods, H. F., Murray, J. D., and Ledingham, J. G. G. (1978): The kinetics of elimination of a sodium l-lactate load in man: The effect of liver disease. *Clin. Sci. Mol. Med.*, 54:33.

53. Mulhausen, R., Eichenholz, A., and Blumentals, A. (1967): Acid base disturbances in patients with cirrhosis of the liver. *Medicine*, 46:185.

54. Cohen, R. D. (1976): Disorders of lactic acid metabolism. *Clin. Endocrinol. Metab.*, 5:613.

55. Lindgren, F. T., and Jensen, L. C. (1972): The isolation and quantitative analysis of serum lipoproteins. In: *Blood Lipids and Lipoproteins*, edited by G. J. Nelson, p. 181. Wiley, New York.

56. Alaupovic, P. (1972): Studies on the composition and structure of plasma lipoproteins. *Biochem. Biophys. Acta*, 260:689.

57. Fredrickson, D. S., Lux, S. E., and Herbert, P. N. (1972): The apolipoproteins. *Adv. Exp. Med. Biol.*, 26:25.

58. Morrisett, J. D., Jackson, R. L., and Gotto, A. M. (1975): Lipoproteins: Structure and function. *Annu. Rev. Biochem.*, 44:183.

59. Marcel, Y. L., and Vezina, C. (1973): Lecithin cholesterol acyltransferase of human plasma: Role of chylomicrons, very low and high density lipoproteins in the reaction. *J. Biol. Chem.*, 248:8254.

60. Havel, R. J., Fielding, C. J., and Olivercrona, T. (1973): Cofactor activity of protein components of human VLDL in the hydrolysis of triglycerides by lipoprotein lipase from different sources. *Biochemistry*, 12:1828.

61. Brown, V. W., and Baginsky, M. C. (1972): Inhibition of lipoprotein lipase by an apoprotein of human VLDL. *Biochem. Biophys. Res. Commun.*, 46:375.

62. Schonfeld, G. (1979): Hormonal control of lipoproteins metabolism. In: *Endocrinology, Vol. 3*, edited by L. J. DeGroot, G. F. Cahill, Jr., W. D. Odell, L. Martini, J. T. Potts, Jr., D. H. Nelson, E. Steinberger, and A. L. Winegrad, pp. 1855–1882. Grune & Stratton, New York.

63. Eisenberg, S., Bilheimer, D. W., and Luy, R. I. (1973): On the metabolic conversion of human plasma very low density lipoprotein to low density lipoprotein. *Biochem. Biophys. Acta*, 326:361.

64. Schonfeld, G., and Pfleger, B. (1971): Overproduction of very low density lipoproteins by liver of genetically obese rats. *Am. J. Physiol.*, 220:1178.

65. Quarfordt, S. H., Frank, A., and Shames, D. M. (1970): Very low density lipoprotein triglyceride transport in type IV hyperlipoproteinemia and the effects of carbohydrate rich diets. *J. Clin. Invest.*, 49:2281.

66. Johansson, B. G., and Medhus, A. (1974): Increase in plasma α lipoproteins in chronic alcoholics after acute abuse. *Acta Med. Scand.*, 195:273.

67. Soutar, A. K., Myant, N. B., and Thompson, G. R. (1977): Simultaneous measurements of apolipoprotein B turnover in very low and low density lipoproteins in familial hypercholesterolemia. *Atherosclerosis*, 28:247.

68. Clark, S. B., and Norum, K. R. (1977): The lecithin cholesterol acyltransferase activity of rat intestinal lymph. *J. Lipid Res.*, 18:293.

69. Korn, E. D. (1955): Clearing factor, α heparin-activated lipoprotein lipase. *J. Biol. Chem.*, 215:1.

70. Robinson, D. S., and Wing, D. R. (1971): Studies on tissue clearing factor lipase related to its role in the removal of lipoprotein triglyceride from the plasma. In: *Plasma Lipoproteins*, edited by R. M. S. Smellie, pp. 123–135. Academic Press, New York.

71. Calandra, S., Marin, M. J., and McIntyre, N. (1971): Plasma lecithin cholesterol acyltransferase activity in liver disease. *Eur. J. Clin. Invest.*, 1:352.

72. Gjone, E., and Norum, K. R. (1970): Plasma lecithin cholesterol acyltransferase and erythocyte lipids in liver disease. *Acta Med. Scand.*, 187:153.

73. Gofman, J. W., Delalla, O., Glazier, F., Freeman, N. K., Lindgren, F. T., Nichols, A. V., Strisower, B., and Tamplin, A. R. (1954): The serum lipoprotein transport system in health, metabolic disorders, atherosclerosis and coronary heart disease. *Plasma,* 2:413.

74. Fredrickson, D. S., Loud, A. V., Hinkelman, B. T., Schneider, H. S., and Frantz, I. D., Jr. (1954): The effect of ligation of the common bile duct on cholesterol synthesis in the rat. *J. Exp. Med.,* 99:43.

75. Quarfordt, S. H., Oedschlaeger, H., Krighaum, W. R., Jakoi, L., and Davis, R. (1973): Effect of biliary obstruction on canine plasma and biliary lipids. *Lipids,* 8:522.

76. Gjone, E., Blomhoff, J. P., and Wiencke, I. (1971): Plasma lecithin cholesterol acyltransferase activity in acute hepatitis. *Scand. J. Gastroenterol.,* 6:161.

77. Seidel, D., Greten, H., Geisen, H. P., Wengler, H., and Wieland, H. (1972): Further aspects on the characterization of high and very low density lipoproteins in patients with liver disease. *Eur. J. Clin. Invest.,* 2:359.

78. Owens, D., Srivastava, M. C., Tompkins, C. V., Nabarro, J. D. N., and Sonksen, P. H. (1973): Studies on the metabolic clearance rate, apparent volume of distribution space and plasma half disappearance time of unlabelled human growth hormone in normal subjects and in patients with liver disease, renal disease, thyroid disease and diabetes mellitus. *Eur. J. Clin. Invest.,* 3:284.

79. Root, A. W. (1976): Clinical studies of human growth hormone. *Pharmacol. Ther.,* 1:15.

80. Muller, E. E., Sawano, S., and Arimura, A. (1967): Mechanism of action of growth hormone in altering its own secretion rate: comparison with action of dexamethasone. *Acta Endocrinol. (Copenh.),* 56:499.

81. Cameran, D. P., Berger, H. G., Catt, K. J., Gordon, E., and McWatts, J. (1972): Metabolic clearance of human growth hormone in patients with hepatic and renal failure and in the isolated perfused pig liver. *Metabolism,* 21:895.

82. Taylor, A. L., Upman, R. L., Salam, A., and Mintz, D. H. (1972): Hepatic clearance of human growth hormone. *J. Clin. Endocrinol.,* 34:395.

83. Pimstone, B. L., LeRoith, D., Epstein, S., and Kronheim, S. (1975): Disappearance rates of plasma growth hormone after intravenous somatostatin in renal and liver disease. *J. Clin. Endocrinol. Metab.,* 41:392.

84. Van Thiel, D. H., Gavaler, J. S., Wight, C., Smith, I. I., Jr., and Abuid, J. (1978): Thyrotropin releasing hormone (TRH) induced growth hormone responses in alcoholic men. *Gastroenterology,* 75:66.

85. Zanoboni, A., and Zanoboni-Muciaccia, W. (1977): Elevated basal growth hormone levels and growth hormone responses to TRH in alcoholic patients with cirrhosis. *J. Clin. Endocrinol. Metab.,* 45:576.

86. Panerai, A. E., Salemo, P., and Menneschi, M. (1977): Growth hormone and prolactin responses to thyrotropin releasing hormone in patients with severe liver disease. *J. Clin. Endocrinol. Metab.,* 45:134.

87. Merimee, T. J. (1979): Growth hormone: Secretion and action. In: *Endocrinology, Vol. 1,* edited by L. J. DeGroot, G. F. Cahill, Jr., W. D. Odell, L. Martini, J. T. Potts, Jr., D. H. Nelson, E. Steinberger, and A. L. Winegrad, pp. 123–132. Grune & Stratton, New York.

88. Uthne, K., and Uthne, T. (1972): Influence of liver resection and regeneration on somatomedin activity in sera from normal and hypophysectomized rats. *Acta Endocrinol.,* 71:255.

89. McConaghky, P. (1972): The production of sulphation factor by rat liver. *J. Endocrinol.,* 52:1.

90. McConaghky, P., and Sledge, C. B. (1970): Production of sulfation factor by perfused liver. *Nature,* 225:1249.

91. Wu, A., Grant, D. B., Hambley, J., and Levi, A. J. (1974): Reduced somatomedin activity in patients with chronic liver disease. *Clin. Sci. Mol. Med.,* 47:359.

92. Philips, L. S., Herington, A. C., and Daughaday, W. H. (1975): Steroid hormone effects on somatomedin. *Endocrinology,* 97:780.

93. Wiedemann, E., and Schwartz, E. (1972): Suppression of growth hormone dependent human serum sulfation factor by estrogen. *J. Clin. Endocrinol. Metab.,* 34:51.

94. Wiedemann, E., Schwartz, E., and Frantz, A. G. (1976): Acute and chronic estrogen effects upon serum somatomedin activity, growth hormone and prolactin in man. *J. Clin. Endocrinol. Metab.,* 42:942.

95. Suhh, K., and Frantz, A. G. (1974): Size heterogeneity of human prolactin in plasma and pituitary extracts. *J. Clin. Endocrinol. Metab.,* 39:928.

96. Posner, H. J., Kelly, P. A., and Friesen, H. G. (1974): Induction of a lactogenic receptor in rat liver: influence of estrogen and the pituitary. *Proc. Natl. Acad. Sci. USA,* 71:2407.

97. Aragona, C., Bohnet, H. G., and Friesen, H. G. (1976): Prolactin binding sites in male rat liver following castration. *Endocrinology,* 99:1017.

98. Nicoll, C. S. (1974): Physiological actions in prolactin. In: *Handbook of Physiology Vol. IV, Part 12,* edited by R. O. Greep, p. 253. Williams & Wilkins, Baltimore.

99. McClain, C. J., Kromhout, J. P., and Van Thiel, D. H. (1981): Serum prolactin concentrations in portal systemic encephalopathy. *Dig. Dis. Sci. (in press).*

100. Jung, Y., and Russfield, A. B. (1972): Prolactin cells in the hypophysis of cirrhotic patients. *Arch. Pathol.,* 94:265.

101. Van Thiel, D. H., McClain, C. J., Elson, M. K., McMillan, M. J., and Lester, R. (1978): Evidence for autonomous secretion of prolactin in some alcoholic men with cirrhosis and gynecomastia. *Metabolism,* 27:1178–1184.

102. Chopra, I. J., Solomon, D. H., Chopra, U., Young, R. T., and Chua Teco, G. N. (1974): Alterations in circulating thyroid hormone and thyrotropin in hepatic cirrhosis. *J. Clin. Endocrinol. Metab.,* 39:501.

103. Cuttelod, S., LeMarchiand-Berand, T., Magnenet, P., Perret, C., Poli, S., and Vanotti, A. (1974): Effect of age and role of kidneys and liver in thyrotropin turnover in man. *Metabolism,* 23:101.

104. Nomura, S., Pittman, C. S., Chambers, J. B., Buck, M. W., and Shimizu, T. (1975): Reduced peripheral conversion of thyroxine to triiodothyronine in patients with hepatic cirrhosis. *J. Clin. Invest.,* 56:643.

105. Van Thiel, D. H., Smith, W. I., Jr., Wight, C., and Abuid, J. (1979): Elevated basal and abnormal thyrotropin-releasing hormone-induced thyroid-stimulating hormone secretion in chronic alcoholic men with liver disease. *Alc. Clin. Exp. Res.,* 3:302–308.

106. Silva, J. E., and Larson, P. R. (1978): Contributions of plasma T_3 and local T_4 to T_3 monodeiodination to nuclear T_3 receptor saturation in pituitary, liver and kidney of hypothyroid rats. *J. Clin. Invest.,* 61:1247.

107. Krieger, D. T., and Allen, W. (1975): Relationship of bioassayable and immunoassayable plasma ACTH and cortisol concentrations in normal subjects and in patients with Cushing's disease. *J. Clin. Endocrinol. Metab.,* 40:675.

108. Gallagher, T. F., Yoshida, K., and Raffmarg, J. D. (1973): ACTH and cortisol secretory patterns in man. *J. Clin. Endocrinol. Metab.,* 36:1058.

109. Smals, A. G., Kloppenborg, P. W., Njo, K. T. et al. (1976): Alcohol-induced Cushingoid syndrome. *Br. Med. J.,* ii:1298.

110. Paton, A. (1976): Alcohol-induced Cushingoid syndrome. *Br. Med. J.,* ii:1298.

111. Rees, L. H., Besser, G. M., Jeffcoate, W. J. et al. (1977): Alcohol-induced pseudo-Cushing's syndrome. *Lancet,* i:726–728.

112. Frajria, R., and Angeli, A. (1977): Alcohol-induced pseudo-Cushing's syndrome. *Lancet,* i:1050–1051.

113. Smals, A., and Kloppenborg, P. (1977): Alcohol-induced pseudo-Cushing's syndrome. *Lancet,* i:1369.

114. Smals, A. G., Nijo, K. T., Knoben, J. M. et al. (1977): Alcohol-induced Cushingoid syndrome. *J. R. Coll. Physicians Lond.,* 12:36–41.

115. Binkiewiez, A., Robinson, M. J., and Senior, B. (1978): Pseudo-Cushing's syndrome caused by alcohol in breast milk. *J. Pediatr.,* 93:965.

116. Rossier, J., Vargo, T. M., Minick, S., Ling, N., Bloom, F. E., and Guillemin, R. (1977): Regional dissociation of β endorphin

and enkephalin content in rat brain and pituitary. *Proc. Natl. Acad. Sci. USA*, 74:15162.

117. Lockwood, A. H., McDonald, J. M., and Reiman, R. E. (1979): The dynamics of ammonia metabolism in man: effects of liver disease and hyperammonia. *J. Clin. Invest.*, 63:449.

118. Watson, S. J., Akil, H., Richard, C. W., and Barchos, J. D. (1978): Evidence for two separate opiate peptide neural pathways. *Nature*, 275:226.

119. Pickel, V. M., Joh, T. H., Reis, D. J., Leeman, S. E., and Miller, R. J. (1979): Electron microscopic localization of substance P and enkephalin in axon terminals related to dendrites of catecholaminergic neurons. *Brain Res.*, 160–387.

120. Schultzburg, M., Hökfelt, T., Terenius, L., Elfvin, L. G., Lundberg, J. M., Brandt, J., Elde, R., and Goldstein, M. (1979): Enkephalin immunoreactive nerve terminals and cell bodies in sympathetic ganglia of the guinea pig and rat. *Neuroscience*, 4:249.

121. Schultzburg, M., Lundberg, J. M., Hökfelt, T., Terenius, L., Brandt, J., Elde, R., and Goldstein, M. (1978): Enkephalin like immunoreactivity in gland cells and nerve terminals of the adrenal medulla. *Neuroscience*, 3:1169.

122. Hambrook, J. M., Morgan, B. A., Ronce, M. J., and Smith, C. F. C. (1976): Mode of deactivation of the enkephalins by rat and human plasma and rat brain homogenates. *Nature*, 262:782.

123. Maefroy, B., Swerts, J. P., Gayon, A., Rogues, B. P., and Schwartz, J. C. (1978): High affinity enkephalin degrading peptidase in brain is increased after morphine. *Nature*, 276:523.

124. Gayon, A., Rogues, B. P., Guyon, F., Foucault, A., Perdrisot, R., Swerts, J. P., and Schwartz, J. C. (1979): Enkephalin degradation in mouse brain studied by a new HPLC method. *Life Sci.*, 25:1605.

125. Akil, H., Watson, S. J., Sullivan, S., and Barchas, J. D. (1978): Enkephalin like material in normal CSF: measurement and levels. *Life Sci.*, 23:121.

126. Almay, B. L. G., Johansson, F., von Knorring, L., Terenius, C., and Wahlstrom, A. (1978): Endorphins in chronic pain. I. Differences in CSF endorphin levels between organic and psycogenic pain syndromes. *Pain*, 5:153.

127. von Knorring, L., Almay, B. G. L., Johansson, F., and Terenius, L. (1978): Pain perception and endorphin levels in cerebrospinal fluid. *Pain*, 5:359.

128. Shorr, J., Foley, K., and Spector, S. (1978): Presence of a non-peptide morphine like compound in human cerebrospinal fluid. *Life Sci.*, 23:2057.

129. Sarne, Y., Azov, R., and Weissman, B. A. (1978): A stable enkephalin like immunoreactive substance in human CSF. *Brain Res.*, 151:399.

130. Heller, J. M., Pearson, J., and Simon, E. J. (1973): Distribution of stereospecific binding of the potent narcotic analgesic etorphine in the human brain: predominance in the limbic system. *Res. Commun. Chem. Pathol. Pharmacol.*, 6:1052.

131. Kuhor, M. J., Pert, C. B., and Snyder, S. H. (1973): Regional distribution of opiate receptor binding in monkey and human brain. *Nature*, 245:447.

132. Lewis, R. V., Stein, S., Gerber, L. D., Rubenstein, M., and Udenfriend, S. (1979): High molecular weight opioid containing proteins in striatum. *Proc. Natl. Acad. Sci. USA*, 75:4021.

133. Beaumont, A., Dell, A., Hughes, J., Malfray, B., and Morris, H. R. (1980): Studies on possible precursors for the enkephalins. In: *Endogenous and Exogenous Opiate Agonists and Antagonists*, edited by E. L. Way, p. 209. Pergamon Press, New York.

134. McKnight, A. T., Sosa, R. P., Corbett, A. D., and Kosterlitz, H. W. (1980): Enkephalin precursors from guinea pig myenteric plexus. In: *Endogenous and Exogenous Opiate Agonists and Antagonists*, edited by E. L. Way, p. 213. Pergamon Press, New York.

135. Sosa, R. P., McKnight, A. T., Hughes, J., and Kosterlitz, H. W. (1977): Incorporation of labeled amino acids into enkephalins. *FEBS Lett.*, 84:195.

136. McKnight, A. T., Hughes, J., and Kosterlitz, H. W. (1979): Synthesis of enkephalins by guinea pig striatum in vitro. *Proc. R. Soc. Lond. [Biol.]*, 205:199.

137. Cusan, L., Dupont, A., Kledzik, G. S., Labrie, F., Coy, D. H., and Schally, A. V. (1977): Potent prolactin and growth hormone releasing activity of male analogues of met-enkephalin. *Nature*, 268:544.

138. Rivier, C., Vale, W., Ling, N., Brown, M., and Guillemin, R. (1977): Stimulation in vivo of the secretion of prolactin and growth hormone by β endorphin. *Endocrinology*, 100:238.

139. Shaar, C. J., Frederickson, R. C. A., Dininger, N. B., and Jackson, L. (1977): Enkephalin analogues and naloxone modulate the release of growth hormone and prolactin—evidence for regulation by an endogenous opioid peptide in brain. *Life Sci.*, 21:853.

140. Cicero, T. J., Schainker, B. A., and Meyer, E. R. (1979): Endogenous opioids participate in the regulation of the hypothalamic-pituitary-luteinizing hormone axis and testosterone's negative feedback control of luteinizing hormone. *Endocrinology*, 104:1286.

141. Meyers, B. M., and Baum, M. J. (1979): Facilitation by opiate antagonists of sexual performance in the male rat. *Pharmacol. Biochem. Behav.*, 10:615.

142. Van Thiel, D. H., and Lester, R. (1980): Hypothalamic-pituitary-gonadal function in liver disease. *Viewpoints Dig. Dis.*, 12:13–16.

143. Van Thiel, D. H., Lester, R., and Sherins, R. J. (1974): Hypogonadism in alcoholic liver disease: Evidence for a double defect. *Gastroenterology*, 67:1188–1199.

144. Van Thiel, D. H., and Lester, R. (1976): Alcoholism: Its effect on hypothalamic pituitary gonadal function. *Gastroenterology*, 71:318–327.

145. Kleeman, C. R., Rubini, M. E., Lambin, E., and Epstein, F. H. (1954): Studies in alcohol diuresis. II. The evaluation of ethyl alcohol in inhibition of the neurohypophysis. *J. Clin. Invest.*, 34:448.

146. Fichman, M. P., and Bethune, J. E. (1968): The role of adrenocorticoids in the inappropriate antidiuretic hormone syndrome. *Ann. Int. Med.*, 68:806.

147. Cadnapaphornchai, P., Boykin, J. L., Berl, T., MacDonald, K., and Schrier, R. W. (1974): Mechanism of effect of nicotine on renal water excretion. *Am. J. Physiol.*, 227:1216.

148. Moses, A. M., Numann, P., and Miller, M. (1973): Mechanisms of chloropropamide induced antidiuresis in man: Evidence for release of ADH and enhancement of peripheral action. *Metabolism*, 22:59.

149. Levinsky, N. G., and Berliner, R. W. (1959): The role of urea in the urine concentrating mechanism. *J. Clin. Invest.*, 38:741.

150. Epstein, F. H., Kleeman, C. R., Pursel, S., and Hendrick, A. (1957): The effect of feeding protein and urea on the renal concentrating process. *J. Clin. Invest.*, 36:635.

151. Goldsmith, C., Beasly, H. K., Wholley, P. J., Rector, F. C., and Seldin, D. W. (1961): Effect of salt deprivation on urinary concentrating mechanism in dog. *J. Clin. Invest.*, 40:2043.

152. Suki, W. N., Eknoyan, G., and Martinez-Maldonaldo, M. (1973): Tubular sites and mechanisms of diuretic action. *Annu. Rev. Pharmacol.*, 13:91.

153. Pearlman, W., and Crepy, O. (1967): Steroid-protein interaction with particular reference to testosterone binding by human serum. *J. Biol. Chem.*, 242:182.

154. Lipsett, M. B. (1979): In: *Hirsutism in Endocrinology, Vol. 3*, edited by L. J. DeGroot, G. F. Cahill, Jr., W. D. Odell, L. Martini, J. T. Potts, Jr., D. H, Nelson, E. Steinberger, and A. L. Winegrad, p. 1453. Grune & Stratton, New York.

155. Horton, R. (1979): Testicular steroid secretions, transport and metabolism. In: *Endocrinology, Vol. 3*, edited by L. J. DeGroot, G. F. Cahill, Jr., W. D. Odell, L. Martini, J. T. Potts, Jr., D. H. Nelson, E. Steinberger, and A. L. Winegrad, pp. 1521–1525. Grune & Stratton, New York.

156. Kelch, R., Jenner, M., Weinstein, R., Kaplan, S. L., and Grumbach, M. M. (1972): Estradiol and testosterone in the male. *J. Clin. Invest.*, 51:824.

157. Steinberger, E. (1975): Hormonal regulations of the seminiferous tubule function. In: *Hormonal Regulation of Spermatogenesis*, edited by F. S. French, V. Hansson, E. M. Ritgenand, and S. N. Nayfek, p. 337. Pleneum Press, New York.

158. MacDonald, P. L., Roubaut, R. P., and Siiteri, P. K. (1967):

Plasma precursors of estrogen: Extent of conversion of plasma Δ^4 androstenedione to estrone in normal males and nonpregnant normal, castrate and adrenalectomized females. *J. Clin. Endocrinol. Metab.,* 27:1103.

159. Longcope, C., Kato, T., and Horton, R. (1969): Conversion of blood androgens to estrogens in normal adult men and women. *J. Clin. Invest.,* 48:2191.

160. Grodin, J. M., Siiteri, P. K., and MacDonald, P. C. (1973): Source of estrogen production in the postmenopausal woman. *J. Clin. Endocrinol. Metab.,* 36:207.

161. Southren, A. L., Olivo, J., and Gordon, G. G. (1974): The conversion of androgens to estrogens in hyperthyroidism. *J. Clin. Endocrinol. Metab.,* 38:207.

162. Bolt, H. M., and Gobel, P. (1972): Formation of estrogens from androgens by human subcutaneous adipose tissue in vitro. *Human Metab. Res.,* 4:312.

163. Schindler, A. E., Ebert, A., and Frederick, E. (1972): Conversion of androstenedione to estrone by human fat tissue. *J. Clin. Endocrinol. Metab.,* 35:627.

164. Nimrod, A., and Ryan, K. J. (1975): Aromatization of androgens by human abdominal and breast fat tissue. *J. Clin. Endocrinol. Metab.,* 40:367.

165. MacDonald, P. C., Edman, C. D., and Hemsell, D. L. (1978): Effect of obesity on conversion of plasma andostenedione to estrone in postmenopausal women with and without endometrial cancer. *Am. J. Obstet. Gynecol.,* 130:4489.

166. Gordon, G. G., Olivo, J., and Rafii, F. (1975): Conversion of androgens to estrogens in cirrhosis of the liver. *J. Clin. Endocrinol. Metab.,* 40:1018.

167. Van Thiel, D. H., Gavaler, J. S., Spero, J. A., Egler, K. M., Wight, C., Sanghvi, A., Hasiba, U., and Lewis, J. H. (1981): Patterns of hypothalamic-pituitary-gonadal dysfunction in men with liver disease due to differing etiologies. *Hepatology (in press).*

168. Rather, L. J. (1947): Hepatic cirrhosis and testicular atrophy. *Arch. Intern. Med.,* 80:397–405.

169. Bennett, H. S., Boggenstoss, A. H., and Butt, H. R. (1970): The testes, breast and prostate of men who die of cirrhosis of the liver. *Am. J. Clin. Pathol.,* 20:814–819.

170. Morrione, T. (1944): The effect of estrogen on the testes in hepatic insufficiency. *Arch. Pathol.,* 37:39–47.

171. Van Thiel, D. H., Gavaler, J. S., Smith, W. I., Jr., and Rabin, B. S. (1977): Testicular and spermatozoal autoantibody in chronic alcoholic males with gonadal failure. *Clin. Immunol. Immunopathol.,* 8:311–317.

172. Van Thiel, D. H., Gavaler, J. S., Lester, R., Loriaux, D. L., and Braunstein, G. D. (1975): Plasma estrone, prolactin, neurophysin and sex steroid binding globulin in chronic alcoholic men. *Metabolism,* 24:1015–1019.

173. Van Thiel, D. H., Lester, R., and Vaitukaitis, J. (1978): Evidence for a defect in pituitary secretion of luteinizing hormone in chronic alcoholic men. *J. Clin. Endocrinol. Metab.,* 47:499–507.

174. Van Thiel, D. H., and Lester, R. (1979): Hypothalamic-pituitary-gonadal dysfunction in patients with alcoholic liver disease. In: *Problems in Liver Disease,* edited by C. S. Davidson, pp. 289–298. Stratton Intercontinental, New York.

175. Van Thiel, D. H. (1979): Feminization of chronic alcoholic men: A formulation. *Yale J. Biol. Med.,* 52:219–225.

176. Van Thiel, D. H., Gavaler, J. S., Slone, F. L., Cobb, C. F., Smither, W. I., Jr., Bron, K. M., and Lester, R. (1980): Is feminization in alcoholic men due in part to portal hypertension: A rat model. *Gastroenterology,* 78:81–91.

177. Eagon, P. K., Porter, L. E., Gavaler, J. S., Egler, K. M., and Van Thiel, D. H. (1981): Effect of ethanol feeding upon levels of a male-specific hepatic estrogen binding protein: A possible mechanism for feminization. *Alc. Clin. Exp. Res. (in press).*

178. Eagon, P. K., and Zdunek, J. R., Van Thiel, D. H., Singletary, B. K., Egler, K. M., Gavaler, J. S., and Porter, L. E. (1981): Alcohol-induced changes in hepatic estrogen binding proteins: A mechanism explaining feminization in alcoholics. *Arch. Biochem. Biophys. (in press).*

179. Lester, R., Eagon, P. K., and Van Thiel, D. H. (1979): Feminization of the alcoholic: The estrogen/testosterone ration (E/T). (Editorial.) *Gastroenterology,* 76:415–417.

180. Van Thiel, D. H., and Lester, R. (1979): The effect of chronic alcohol abuse on sexual function. *Clin. Endocrinol. Metab.,* 8:499–510.

181. Stocks, A. E., and Powell, L. W. (1972): Pituitary function in idiopathic haemochromatosis and cirrhosis of the liver. *Lancet,* 1:298–300.

182. Simon, M., Franchimont, P., Murie, N., Ferrand, B., Van Lauwenberge, H., and Bourel, M. (1979): Study of somatotropic and gonadotropic pituitary function in idiopathic haemochromatosis (31 cases). *Eur. J. Clin. Invest.,* 2:384–389.

183. Walsh, C. H., Wright, A. D., Williams, J. W., and Holder, G. (1976): A study of pituitary function in patients with idiopathic hemochromatosis. *J. Clin. Endocrinol. Metab.,* 43:866–872.

184. Bezuoda, W. R., Bothwell, T. H., Vander Walt, L. A., Kronheim, S., and Pimstone, B. L. (1977): An investigation into gonadal dysfunction in patients with idiopathic haemochromatosis. *Clin. Endocrinol.,* 6:377–385.

185. La Bella, F., Dulor, R., and Vivian, S. (1973): Releasing or inhibiting activity of metal ions present in hypothalamic extracts. *Biochem. Biophys. Res. Commun.,* 52:786–794.

186. Peterson, R. E., Wyngarden, J. B., and Guerra, S. L. (1955): The physiological disposition and metabolic fate of hydrocortisone in man. *J. Clin. Invest.,* 34:1779.

187. Westzman, E. D., Fukushima, D., and Nogeine, C. (1971): Twenty-four hour pattern of the episodic secretion of cortisol in normal subjects. *J. Clin. Endocrinol. Metab.,* 33:14.

188. West, C. D., and Meikle, A. W. (1979): Laboratory tests for the diagnosis of Cushing's syndrome and adrenal insufficiency and factors affecting these tests. In: *Endocrinology, Vol. 2,* edited by L. J. Degroot, G. F. Cahill, Jr., W. D. Odell, L. Martini, J. T. Potts, Jr., D. H. Nelson, E. Steinberger, and A. L. Winegrad, p. 1159. Grune & Stratton, New York.

189. Peterson, R. E. (1960): Adrenocortical steroid metabolism and adrenal cortical function in liver disease. *J. Clin. Invest.,* 39:320.

190. Zumoff, B., Bradlow, H. L., and Gallagher, T. F. (1967): Cortisol metabolism in cirrhosis. *J. Clin. Invest.,* 46:1735.

191. Tucci, J. R., Albocete, R. A., and Martin, M. M. (1966): Effect of liver disease upon steroid circadian rhythms in man. *Gastroenterology,* 50:634.

192. McCann, V. J., and Fullon, T. T. (1975): Cortisol metabolism in chronic liver disease. *J. Clin. Endocrinol. Metab.,* 40:1038.

193. Melby, J. C. (1979): Diagnosis and treatment of hyperaldosteronism and hypoaldosteronism. In: *Endocrinology, Vol. 3,* edited by L. J. Degroot, G. F. Cahill, Jr., W. D. Odell, L. Martini, J. T. Potts, Jr., D. H. Nelson, E. Steinberger, and A. L. Winegrad, pp. 1225–1234. Grune & Stratton, New York.

194. Cobb, C. F., Van Thiel, D. H., Gavaler, J. S., and Lester, R. (1981): Effects of ethanol and acetaldehyde on the rat adrenal. *Metabolism (in press).*

195. Merry, J., and Marks, V. (1973): Hypothalamic-pituitary-adrenal function in chronic alcoholics. In: *Alcohol Intoxication and Withdrawal: Experimental Studies. Advances in Experimental Medicine and Biology,* edited by M. M. Gross, p. 167. Plenum, New York.

196. Wright, J. (1978): Endocrine effects of alcohol. *Clin. Endocrinol. Metab.,* 7:351–367.

197. Pittman, C. S. (1979): Hormone metabolism. In: *Endocrinology, Vol. 3,* edited by L. J. DeGroot, G. F. Cahill, Jr., W. D. Odell, L. Martini, J. T. Potts, Jr., D. H. Nelson, E. Steinberger, and A. L. Winegrad, p. 365. Grune & Stratton, New York.

198. Galton, V. A., and Nisula, B. C. (1972): The enterohepatic circulation of thyroxine. *J. Endocrinol.,* 54:187.

199. Visser, T. (1978): Tentative review of recent in vitro observations of the enzymatic deiodination of iodothyronines and its possible physiological implications. *Mol. Cell. Endocrinol.,* 10:241.

200. Kaplan, M. M., and Utiger, R. D. (1978): Iodothyronine metabolism in rat liver homogenate. *J. Clin. Invest.,* 61:459.

201. Van Noorden, C. J. F., Wiersinga, W. M., and Touber, J. L. (1979): Propranolol inhibits that in vitro conversion of

thyroxine into triiodothyronine by isolated rat liver parenchymal cells. *Horm. Metab. Res.*, 11:366.

202. Chopra, I. J., Solomon, D. H., and Chua-Teco, G. H. (1980): Inhibition of hepatic outer ring monodiiodinations of thyroxine and 3,3',5'-triiodothyronine by sodium salicylate. *Endocrinology*, 106:1728.

203. Balsam, A., and Ingbar, S. H. (1978): The influences of fasting, diabetes, and several pharmacological agents on the pathways of thyroxine metabolism in rat liver. *J. Clin. Invest.*, 62:415.

204. Kaplan, M. M. (1979): Subcellular alterations causing reduced hepatic thyroxine 5'-monodiiodinase activity in fasted rats. *Endocrinology*, 104:58.

205. Jennings, A. S., Ferguson, D. C., and Utiger, R. D. (1979): Regulation of the conversion of thyroxine to triiodothyronine in the perfused rat liver. *J. Clin. Invest.*, 64:1614.

206. Shipley, R. A., and Chudzik, E. B. (1957): Thyroidal uptake and plasma clearance of I^{131} and I^{125} in cirrhosis of the liver. *J. Clin. Endocrinol. Metab.*, 17:1229.

207. Lepyanko, A. G. (1970): Functional state of the thyroid gland in patients with lambliasis with predominant involvement of the hepatobiliary system. *Klin. Med. (Mosk.).*, 48:83.

208. Carter, J. N., Eastman, C. J., Corcoran, J. M., and Lazarus, L. (1974): Effect of severe chronic illness on thyroid function. *Lancet*, ii:971.

209. Inada, M., and Sterling, K. (1967): Thyroxine turnover and transport in Laennec's cirrhosis of the liver. *J. Clin. Invest.*, 46:1275.

210. Nomura, S., Pittman, C. S., Cambers, J. B., Berk, M. W., and Shimizu, T. (1975): Reduced peripheral conversion of thyroxine to triiodothyronine in patients with hepatic cirrhosis. *J. Clin. Invest.*, 56:643.

211. Sheridan, P., Chapman, C., and Losowsky, M. S. (1978): Interpretation of laboratory tests of thyroid function in chronic active hepatitis. *Clin. Chim. Acta*, 86:73.

212. Van Thiel, D. H., Smith, W. I., Jr., Wight, C., and Abuid, J. (1979): Elevated basal and abnormal thyrotropin-releasing hormone-induced thyroid-stimulating hormone secretion in chronic alcoholic men with liver disease. *Alc. Clin. Exp. Res.*, 3:302–308.

213. Cutlelod, S., Le Marchord-Beaud, T., Magnenat, P., Perret, G., Poli, S., and Vanotti, A. (1974): Effect of age and role of kidneys and liver on thyrotropin turnover in man. *Metabolism*, 23:101.

214. Pokroy, N., Epstein, S., Hendricks, S., and Pimstone, B. (1974): Thyrotropin response to intravenous thyrothyrotropin releasing hormone in patients with hepatic and renal disease. *Horm. Metab. Res.*, 6:132.

215. Doniack, D., Roitt, M., Walker, J. G., and Sherlock, S. (1966): Tissue antibodies in primary biliary cirrhosis, active lupoid hepatitis, cryptogenic cirrhosis and other liver diseases and their clinical implications. *Clin. Exp. Immunol.*, 1:237.

216. Rasmussen, H. (1972): The cellular basin of mammalian calcium homeostasis. *Clin. Endocrinol. Metab.*, 1:3.

217. Kodicek, E. (1972): Recent advances in vitamin D metabolism. *Clin. Endocrinol. Metab.*, 1:305.

218. Hirsch, P. F., and Munson, P. L. (1969): Thyrocacitonin. *Physiol. Rev.*, 49:458.

219. DeLuca, H. P. (1980): Vitamin D: Revisited 1980. *Clin. Endocrinol. Metab.*, 9:3.

220. Botham, K., Ghazarian, J. G., Kream, B. E., and DeLuca, H. F. (1970): Isolation of a potent inhibition of 25 hydroxyvitamin D$_3$-1-hydroxylase from rat serum. *Biochemistry*, 15:2130.

221. Bouillon, R., Van Baselen, H., Rombauts, W., and De Moor, P. (1976): The purification and characterization of the human serum binding protein for the 25 hydroxycholecalciferal. *Eur. J. Biochem.*, 66:285.

222. Haddad, J. G., and Walgate, J. (1976): 25-Hydroxyvitamin D transport in human plasma. *J. Biol. Chem.*, 251:4803.

223. Imawari, M., Kida, K., and Goodman, D. S. (1976): The transport of vitamin D and its 25 hydroxymetabolite in human plasma. *J. Clin. Invest.*, 58:514.

224. DeLuca, H. F., and Schroes, H. K. (1976): Metabolism and mechanism of action of vitamin D. *Ann. Rev. Biochem.*, 45:631.

225. DeLuca, H. F. (1978): Vitamin D. In: *The Fat Soluble Vitamin, Vol. II. Handbook of Lipid Research,* edited by H. F. DeLuca, p. 69. Plenum, New York.

226. DeLuca, H. F. (1979): Vitamin D: Metabolism and function. In: *Monographs on Endocrinology, Vol. 13,* edited by F. Gross, M. M. Grumbach, A. Labhart, M. B. Lipsett, T. Mann, L. T. Samuels, and J. Zander, p. 979. Springer, New York.

227. Horsting, M., and DeLuca, H. F. (1969): In vitro production of 25-hydroxycholecalciferal. *Biochim. Biophys. Res. Commun.* 36:251.

228. Blunt, J. W., DeLuca, H. F., and Schroes, H. K. (1978): 25-Hydroxycholecalciferal, a biologically active metabolite of vitamin D$_3$. *Biochemistry*, 7:3317.

229. Bhattachargya, M. H., and DeLuca, H. F. (1974): The regulation of calciferal-25-hydroxylase in the chick. *Biochem. Biophys. Res. Commun.*, 59:734.

230. Madlak, T. C., Schnoes, H. K., and DeLuca, H. F. (1977): Mechanism of 25-hydroxyvitamin D$_3$ 24 hydroxylation. *Biochemistry*, 16:2142.

231. Tanaka, Y., DeLuca, H. F., Akaiwa, A., Morisaki, M., and Ikekama, N. (1976): Synthesis of 24S, 24R hydroxy (24-^{3}H) vitamin D$_3$ and their metabolism in rachitic rats. *Arch. Biochem. Biophys.*, 177:615.

232. Tanaka, Y., DeLuca, H. F., Ikekawa, N., Morisaki, M., and Koizumi, N. (1975): Determination of stereochemical configuration of the 24 hydroxyl group of 24,25-dehyroxyvitamin D$_3$. *Arch. Biochem. Biophys.*, 170:620.

233. Goodwin, D., Noff, D., and Edelstein, S. (1978): 24,25-Dehydroxyvitamin D is a metabolite of vitamin D essential for bone formation. *Nature*, 276:517.

234. Arnaud, S. B., Allen, B., Lenardon, A., and Wong, L. (1979): Enterohepatic recycling of 25 hydroxyvitamin D in the monkey. *Gastroenterology*, 77:A2.

235. Arnaud, S. B., Goldsmith, R. S., Lambert, P. W., and Go, V. L. W. (1975): 25-Hydroxyvitamin D$_3$ evidence of an entrohepatic circulation in man. *Proc. Soc. Exp. Biol. Med.*, 149:570.

236. Kumar, R., Nagubandi, S., Mattox, V. R., and Londowski, J. M. (1980): Enterohepatic physiology of 1,25-dihydroxyvitamin D$_3$. *J. Clin. Invest.*, 65:277.

237. Kumar, R., Nagubandi, S., and Landowski, J. M. (1980): Enterohepatic physiology of 24,25-dihydroxyvitamin D$_3$. *J. Lab. Clin. Med.*, 95:278.

238. Wiesner, R. H., Kumar, R., Sieman, E., and Go, V. L. W. (1980): Enterohepatic physiology of 1,25-dihydroxyvitamin D$_3$ metabolites in normal man. *J. Lab. Clin. Med.*, 96:1094.

239. Tanaka, Y., Frank, H., and DeLuca, H. P. (1973): Biological activity of 1,25-dihydroxyvitamin D$_3$ in the rat. *Endocrinology*, 92:417.

240. DeLuca, H. P. (1974): Vitamin D: The vitamin and the hormone. *Fed. Proc.*, 33:2211.

241. Kodicek, E. (1974): The study of vitamin D from vitamin to hormone. *Lancet*, i:325.

242. Steele, T. H., Engh, J. E., Tanaka, Y., Lorenc, R. S., Dudgeon, K. L., and DeLuca, H. F. (1975): Phosphotemic action of 1,25-dihydroxyvitamin D$_3$. *Am. J. Physiol.*, 229:489.

243. Sutton, R. A. L., Harris, C. A., Wong, N. L. M., and Dirks, J. (1977): Effects of vitamin D on renal tubular calcium transport. In: *Vitamin D: Biochemical, Clinical, and Clinical Aspects Related to Calcium Metabolism,* edited by A. W. Norman, K. Schaefer, J. W. Coburn, and H. F. DeLuca, p. 451. Walter de Gruyter, Berlin.

244. Raiz, L. G. (1980): Direct effects of vitamin D and its metabolites on skeletal tissue. *Clin. Endocrinol. Metab.*, 9:27.

245. Haddud, J. G., and Stamp, T. C. B. (1974): Circulating 25-hydroxyvitamin D in man. *Am. J. Med.*, 57:57.

246. Boyle, I. T., Gray, R. W., and DeLuca, H. F. (1971): Regulation by calcium of in vivo synthesis of 1,25-dihydroxycholecalciferol. *Proc. Natl. Acad. Sci. USA*, 68:2131.

247. Tanaka, Y., Lorenc, R. S., and DeLuca, H. F. (1975): The role of 1,25-dehydroxyvitamin D$_3$ and parathyroid hormone in the regulation of chick renal 25-hydroxyvitamin D$_3$-24-hydroxylase. *Arch. Biochem. Biophys.*, 171:521.

248. Tanaka, Y., and DeLuca, H. F. (1973): The control of 25-

hydroxyvitamin D metabolism by inorganic phosphate. *Arch. Biochem. Biophys.*, 154:566.

249. Hahn, T. J., Birge, S. J., Scharp, C. R., and Avioli, L. V. (1972): Phenobarbital-induced alterations in vitamin D metabolism. *J. Clin. Invest.*, 51:741.

250. Silver, J., Neale, G., and Thompson, G. R. (1974): Effect of phenobarbitone treatment on vitamin D metabolism in mammals. *Clin. Sci. Mol. Med.*, 46:433.

251. Hahn, T. J., Hendin, B. A., Scharp, C. R., and Haddud, J. G., Jr. (1972): Effect of chronic anticonvulsant therapy on serum 25-hydroxycalciferol levels in adults. *N. Engl. J. Med.*, 287:900.

252. Gascon-Barre, M., and Cote, M. G. (1978): Effects of phenobarbital and diphenylhydantoin on acute vitamin D toxicity in the rat. *Toxicol. Appl. Pharmacol.*, 43:125.

253. Norman, A. W., Bayless, J. D., and Tsai, H. C. (1975): Biological effects of short term phenobarbital treatment on the response to vitamin D and its metabolites in the chick. *Biochem. Pharmacol.*, 25:161.

254. Ahrens, E. H., Payne, M. A., and Byer, P. B. (1950): Primary biliary cirrhosis. *Medicine*, 29:299.

255. Atkinson, M., Nordin, B. E. C., and Sherlock, J. (1956): Malabsorption and bone disease in prolonged obstructive jaundice. *Q. J. Med.*, 25:299.

256. Long, R. G., Skinner, R. K., Wills, M. R., and Sherlock, S. (1976): Serum 25-hydroxyvitamin D in intoxicated parenchymal and cholestatic liver disease. *Lancet*, ii:650.

257. Wagonfeld, J. B., Nemchansky, B. A., Bolt, M., Vancher Horst, J., Boyo, J. L., and Rösenberg, I. H. (1976): Comparison of vitamin D and 25 hydroxyvitamin D in the therapy of primary biliary cirrhosis. *Lancet*, ii:391.

258. Kobayashi, A., Kawai, S., Utsonomiya, T., and Ohbe, Y. (1974): Bone disease in infants and children with hepatobiliary disease. *Arch. Dis. Child.*, 49:641.

259. Avioli, L. V., and Haddud, J. G. (1973): Vitamin D current concepts. *Metabolism*, 22:507.

260. Rosenberg, I. H., Boyer, J. L., Bolt, M., and Wagonfeld, J. B. (1976): Vitamin D in primary biliary cirrhosis. *Lancet*, ii:796.

261. Bolt, M., Sitrin, M., Farus, M. J., and Rosenberg, I. H. (1977): Hepatic 25-hydroxylase: Inhibition by bile duct ligation or bile salts in vivo. *Clin. Res.*, 25:606A.

262. Daum, F., Rosen, J. F., Roginsky, M., Cohen, M. I., and Fineberg, L. (1976): 25-Hydroxycholecalciferol in the management of rickets with extrahepatic biliaryatresia. *J. Pediatr.*, 88:1041.

263. Hepner, G. W., Roginsky, M., and Moo, M. F. (1976): Abnormal vitamin D metabolism in patients with cirrhosis. *Am. J. Dig. Dis.*, 21:527.

264. Posner, D. B., Russell, R. M., Abgood, S., Connor, J. B., Davis, C., Martin, L., Pruce, M. A., Tomlinson, S., and Ribot, C. A. (1975): Studies of vitamin D deficiency in man. *Q. J. Med.*, 64:575.

265. Armstrong, M. D., McMillan, A., and Jhaw, K. N. F. (1957): 3-Hethoxy-4-hydroxy-d-mandelic acid, a urinary metabolite of norepinephrine. *Biochem. Biophys. Acta*, 25:422.

266. Blaschko, H., Richter, D., and Shlossman, H. J. (1937): Inactivation of adrenaline. *J. Physiol.*, 90:1.

267. Axelrod, J., Senoh, S., and Witkop, B. B. (1958): O-methylation of catechol amines in vivo. *J. Biol. Chem.*, 233:697.

268. Axelrod, J., and Tomchick, R. (1958): Enzymatic O-methylation of norepinephrine and other catechols. *J. Biol. Chem.*, 233:702.

269. Kopin, I. J., Axelrod, J., and Gordon, E. K. (1961): The metabolic fate of H^3 epinephrine is C^{14} metanephrine in the rat. *J. Biol. Chem.*, 236:2109.

270. LaBrosse, E. H., Axelrod, J., Kopin, I. J., and Kety, S. S. (1961): Metabolism of 7-H^3-epinephrine-d-bitartrate in normal young men. *J. Clin. Invest.*, 40:253.

271. Weinshilbaum, R. M., and Axelrod, J. (1971): Serum dopamine-β-hydroxylase activity. *Circ. Res.*, 28:307.

272. Young, J. B., and Landsberg, L. (1977): Catecholamines and intermediary metabolism. *Clin. Endocrinol. Metab.*, 6:599.

273. Kneer, N. M., Bosch, A. L., Clark, M. G., and Lardy, H. A. (1974): Glucose inhibition of epinephrine stimulation of hepatic gluconeogenesis by blockade of the α-receptor function. *Proc. Natl. Acad. Sci. USA*, 71:4523.

274. Himms-Hagen, J. (1972): Effects of catecholamines on metabolism. In: *Catecholamines. Handbook of Experimental Pharmacology, XXXIII*, edited by H. Blaschko and E. Muschall, p. 363. Springer Verlag, Berlin.

275. Hirsch, L. J., Ayake, T., and Glick, G. (1976): Direct effects of various catecholamines on liver circulation in dogs. *Am. J. Physiol.*, 230:1394.

276. Richardson, P. D. I., and Withrington, P. G. (1976): The inhibition by glucagon of the vasoconstrictor actions of norepinephrine, angiotensin and vasopressin on the hepatic arterial vascular bed of the dog. *Br. J. Pharmacol.*, 57:93.

277. Muschall, E. (1972): Adrenergic false transmitters. In: *Catecholamines. Handbook of Experimental Pharmacology, XXXIII*, edited by H. Blaschko and E. Muschall, p. 618. Springer-Verlag, Berlin.

278. Schenker, S., Breen, K. J., and Hoyumpa, A. A. (1974): Hepatic encephalopathy: Current status. *Gastroenterology*, 66:121.

279. Bessman, S. P., and Bessman, A. W. (1955): The cerebral and peripheral uptake of ammonia in liver disease with a hypothesis for the mechanism of hepatic coma. *J. Clin. Invest.*, 34:622.

280. Shorey, J., McCandless, D. W., and Schenker, S. (1967): Cerebral alpha ketogluterate in ammonia intoxication. *Gastroenterology*, 53:706.

281. Goetchus, J. S., and Webster, L. T. (1965): α-Aminobutyrate and hepatic coma. *J. Lab. Clin. Med.*, 65:257.

282. Holm, E. (1975): *Ammoniak und Hepatische Enzephalopathie*. Gustav Fischer Verlag, Stuttgart.

283. Baldessarini, R. J., and Fischer, J. E. (1973): Serotonin metabolism in rat brain after surgical diversion of the portal venous circulation. *Nature*, 254:272.

284. Cummings, M. G., Soeters, P. B., James, J. H., Keane, J. M., and Fischer, J. E. (1976): Regional brain indoleamine metabolism following chronic portocaval anastomasis in the rat. *J. Neurochem.*, 27:501.

285. Fischer, J. E. (1974): False neurotransmitters and hepatic coma. *Res. Publ. Assoc. Res. Nerv. Ment. Dis.*, 53:53.

286. Knott, P. J., and Curzon, G. (1974): Effect of increased rat brain tryptophan on 5-hydroxytryptamine and 5-hydroxyindolyl acetic acid in the hypothalamus and other brain regions. *J. Neurochem.*, 22:1065.

287. Fischer, J. E. (1976): Nonaminoacids: Nontoxic or antitoxic. *Gastroenterology*, 71:329.

288. Knell, A. J., Davidson, A. R., Williams, R., Kentamaneni, B. D., and Gurzon, G. (1974): Dopamine and serotonin metabolism in hepatic encephalopathy. *Br. Med. J.*, ii:549.

289. Chen, S., Mahadevan, V., and Zieve, L. (1970): Volatile fatty acids in the breath of patients with cirrhosis of the liver. *J. Lab. Clin. Med.*, 75:622.

290. Takahaski, Y. (1963): Serum lipids in liver disease, liver disease and the relationship of serum lipids and hepatic coma. *Jpn. J. Gastroenterol.*, 60:571.

291. Walker, C. O., McCandless, D. W., McCarry, J. D., and Schenker, S. (1970): Cerebral metabolism in short chain fatty acid induced coma. *J. Lab. Clin. Med.*, 76:569.

292. Zieve, F. G., Zieve, L., Doizaki, W. M., and Gilsdorf, R. B. (1974): Synergism between ammonia and fatty acids in the production of coma. *J. Pharmacol. Exp. Ther.*, 191:10.

293. Fischer, J. E., and Baldessarini, R. J. (1971): False neurotransmitters and hepatic failure. *Lancet*, ii:75.

294. Fischer, J. E., and Baldessarini, R. J. (1976): Pathogenesis and therapy of hepatic coma. In: *Progress in Liver Disease*, edited by H. Popper and F. Schaffer, p. 363. Grune & Stratton, New York.

295. Oldendorf, W. K. (1971): Brain uptake of radiolabelled amino acids, amines and hexoses after arterial injection. *Am. J. Physiol.*, 221:1629.

296. Aguirre, A., Yoshimura, M., Westman, T., and Fischer, J. E. (1974): Plasma amino acids in dogs with two experimental forms of liver damage. *J. Surg. Res.*, 16:339.

297. Bollman, J. R., Glock, E. V., Gindley, J. H., Brickford, R. G., and Lichtenheld, F. R. (1957): Coma with increased amino acids of brain in dogs with Eck's fistula. *Arch. Surg.*, 75:405.

298. Fischer, J. E., Yoshimura, N., James, J. H., Cummings, M. G., Abel, R. M., and Diendoefer, F. (1974): Plasma amino acids in patients with hepatic encephalopathy. Effects of amino acid infusions. *Am. J. Surg.,* 127:40.

299. Iber, F. L., Rosen, H., Levenson, S. M., and Chalmers, T. C. (1957): The plasma amino acids in patients with liver failure. *J. Lab. Clin. Med.,* 50:417.

300. Iob, V., Coon, W. W., and Sloan, M. (1966): Altered clearance of free amino acids from plasma of patients with cirrhosis of the liver. *J. Surg. Res.,* 6:233.

301. Iob, V., Mattson, W. J., Jr., Sloan, M., Coon, W. W., Turcotte, J. G., and Child, C. G., III (1970): Alterations in plasma free amino acids in dogs with hepatic insufficiency. *Surg. Gynecol. Obstet.,* 130:794.

302. Mattson, W. J., Jr., Job, V., Sloan, M., Coon, W. W., Turcotte, J. G., and Child, C. G., III (1970): Alterations of individual free amino acids in brain during acute hepatic coma. *Surg. Gynecol. Obstet.,* 130:263.

303. Richmond, J., and Girdwood, R. H. (1962): Observations on amino acid absorption. *Clin. Sci.,* 22:301.

304. Svec, M. H., and Freeman, S. (1949): Effect of impaired hepatic circulation on plasma free amino acids of dogs. *Am. J. Physiol.,* 159:357.

305. Wu, C. J., Gollman, G., and Butt, H. R. (1955): Changes in free amino acids in plasma during hepatic coma. *J. Clin. Invest.,* 34:845.

306. Cummings, M. G., James, J. H., Soeters, P. B., Keane, J. M., Foster, J., and Fischer, J. R. (1976): Regional brain study of indoleamine metabolism in the rat in acute hepatic failure. *J. Neurochem.,* 27:741.

307. Lam, K. C., Tall, A. R., Goldstein, G. B., and Mistillis, S. P. (1973): Role of a false neurotransmitter octopamine in the pathogenesis of hepatic and renal encephalopathy. *Scand. J. Gastroenterol.,* 8:465.

308. Manghani, K. K., Lunzer, M. R., Billing, B. H., and Sherlock, S. (1975): Urinary and serum octopamine in patients with portal systemic encephalopathy. *Lancet,* ii:943.

309. Rossi-Fanelli, F., Cargiano, C., Attili, A., Angelico, M., Casano, A., Capocaccia, L., Strom, L., and Crito, C. (1976): Octopamine plasma levels and hepatic encephalopathy; a reappraisal of the problem. *Clin. Chem. Acta,* 67:255.

310. Rossi-Fanelli, F., Smith, A. R., Cangiano, C., Bazzi, A., James, J. H., Kay, L. A., Perlle, B. A., Capococcira, L., and Fischer, J. E. (1981): Simultaneous determination of phenylethanolamine and octopamine in plasma and cerebrospinal fluid. In: *Biochemistry of Phenylethylamines,* edited by A. Moosmain. Raven Press, New York.

311. Zieve, L., and Olsen, R. L. (1977): Can hepatic coma be caused by a reduction of brain noradrenaline or dopamine. *Gut,* 18:688–691.

312. Beebuyck, J., Funovics, J., Dedrick, D. F., Scherer, Y. D., and Fischer, J. E. (1975): Neurochemistry of hepatic coma. Alterations in putative neurotransmitter amino acids. In: *Artificial Liver Support,* edited by R. Williams and I. M. Murray-Lyon, pp. 51–60. Pitman, London.

313. Gebor, E., Szeinberg, A., Tauman, G., and Bodonige, E. (1959): Glutamine estimation in cerebrospinal fluid in cases of liver cirrhosis and hepatic coma. *J. Lab. Clin. Med.,* 53:714.

314. Houpani, B. T., Hamlin, E. M., and Reynolds, T. B. (1971): Cerebrospinal fluid glutamine as a measure of hepatic encephalopathy. *Arch. Int. Med.,* 127:1033.

The Liver: Biology and Pathobiology, edited by
I. Arias, H. Popper, D. Schachter, and D. A. Shafritz.
Raven Press, New York © 1982.

Chapter 43

The Kidney in Liver Disease

Murray Epstein

> When the liver is full of fluid and this overflows into the peritoneal cavity, so that the belly becomes full of water, death follows.
>
> *Hippocrates, ca. 400 B.C.* (1)

The interrelationship of liver disease and simultaneous kidney dysfunction has been appreciated for thousands of years. More than 2,400 years ago, Hippocrates recorded the association of ascites and liver disease (1). During the subsequent two millennia, the scope of liver-kidney interrelationships has been amplified and extended; currently, such interrelationships are voluminous and exceedingly complex. Table 1 comprises a proposed framework for considering those conditions that involve both the liver and the kidney, and in which relationships have been reasonably well defined. Basically, three major categories of disease states subtend such interrelationships: (a) disorders involving both the liver and the kidney directly, (b) primary disorders of the kidney with secondary hepatic involvement, and (c) primary disorders of the liver with secondary renal dysfunction.

This chapter does not consider the entire spectrum of diseases that simultaneously involve both the liver and kidney. Consideration is given only to derangements of renal function that secondarily complicate primary disorders of the liver. Table 2 summarizes some of the alterations in renal function and electrolyte metabolism that frequently accompany liver disease. These complications are diverse and comprise a wide continuum, varying from complications with little clinical significance to others that are serious and require therapeutic intervention.

Providing an overview of such a large and complex subject has made it necessary to select the information presented and to establish rather arbitrary priorities concerning which areas receive more detailed discussion. In the present review, emphasis is placed on abnormalities of renal sodium and water handling and the syndromes of acute renal failure (ATN) and the hepatorenal syndrome (HRS) which often supervene in patients with severe liver disease. In addition, immune-complex glomerulonephritides, which complicate liver disease, are reviewed.

To facilitate consideration of these varying syndromes, this chapter focuses on the clinical and biochemical derangements peculiar to each and how these relate to the specifics of diagnosis and management. Although each is discussed separately for clarity, it should be remembered that they often do not occur clinically as separate entities but rather in a mixed or overlapping form. As an example, it is common for a patient with renal sodium retention to manifest simultaneously dilutional hyponatremia with water retention.

RENAL SODIUM HANDLING

One of the most frequent and florid renal complications of liver disease is the impairment of renal sodium

TABLE 1. *Abnormalities affecting the liver and the kidney simultaneously*

1. Disorders involving both the liver and kidney directly
2. Primary disorder of the kidney with secondary hepatic involvement
3. Primary disorders of the liver with secondary renal dysfunction
   a. Extrahepatic biliary obstruction with secondary impairment of renal function
   b. Parenchymal liver disease with secondary renal dysfunction

handling. Recently, several reviews (2–4) and editorials (5,6) have attempted to bring this complex medical problem into clearer focus. This body of literature has characterized many of the important features of the syndrome, but the pathogenesis and rational management remain controversial.

As noted elsewhere (3), there is a paucity of information in man on aberrations of sodium homeostasis in hepatic conditions other than cirrhosis. Discussion of the pathogenesis of renal sodium retention, therefore, is restricted to the cirrhotic population.

Clinical Features

Patients with Laennec cirrhosis manifest a remarkable capacity for sodium retention; indeed, they frequently excrete urine virtually free of sodium (7–11). Extracellular fluid accumulates excessively and eventually becomes evident as clinically detectable ascites and edema. Cirrhotic patients who are unable to excrete sodium continue to gain weight and accumulate ascites and edema as long as dietary sodium content exceeds maximal urinary sodium excretion. If access to sodium is not curtailed, the relentless retention of sodium may lead to accumulation of vast amounts of

TABLE 2. *Renal abnormalities in liver disease*

Parenchymal liver disease with secondary impairment of renal function
  Deranged renal sodium handling
  Impaired renal water excretion
  Impaired renal concentrating ability
  HRS
  ATN
  Glomerulopathies
    Cirrhosis
    Acute viral hepatitis
    Chronic viral hepatitis
  Impaired renal acidification
Extrahepatic biliary obstruction with secondary impairment of renal function
  Acute renal failure

ascites (on occasion up to 25 liters). Weight gain and ascites formation promptly cease when sodium intake is limited to approximate maximal sodium excretion.

The abnormality of renal sodium handling in cirrhosis is not fixed; cirrhotic patients may undergo a spontaneous diuresis followed by a return to avid salt retention (12,13). Although many patients who are maintained on a sodium-restricted diet demonstrate a spontaneous diuresis, there is inadequate information about the incidence with which this occurs.

In this regard, the report of Bosch et al. (14) is of interest. These observers reported that 35 of 124 hospitalized patients with cirrhosis and ascites underwent a spontaneous diuresis in response to bedrest and dietary sodium restriction. Since all patients with liver disease and ascites in the area served by the hospital were hospitalized during the period of the report, the figure of 28% reported by these authors may be representative of the frequency with which spontaneous diuresis occurs.

The primary renal excretory abnormality causing fluid retention is a disturbance of *sodium* rather than of water excretion. Many sodium-retaining patients with ascites and edema can excrete urine of low osmolality when given excessive amounts of water without sodium (13,15,16); when sodium is administered, however, it is not excreted.

Etiology of Hepatic Disease as a Determinant of Renal Sodium Retention

In contrast to the findings in patients with Laennec cirrhosis in whom renal sodium retention is common, patients with primary biliary cirrhosis (PBC) do not manifest this abnormality. Chaimovitz et al. (17) recently assessed the natriuretic and diuretic responses to extracellular fluid volume expansion (ECVE) in five patients with PBC. Despite conspicuous evidence of portal hypertension, ascites and edema were absent; the natriuretic and diuretic responses exceeded those observed in healthy normal volunteers and in edema-free patients with Laennec cirrhosis. The authors suggest that a common mechanism may underlie the augmented natriuretic response to volume in PBC patients and the rarity of fluid retention (17).

Fulminant Hepatic Failure

Limited data are available on fulminant hepatic failure, and an association with sodium retention has been suggested (18). Detailed observations in this patient population are required.

Pathogenesis

The pathogenetic events leading to sodium retention in cirrhosis are complex and controversial. The following discussion considers some of the afferent and efferent alterations that contribute to sodium retention.

Afferent events constitute the signal(s) for sodium retention, and efferent events mediate the antinatriuresis. Two major concepts of afferent events that have received recent attention include (a) diminished "effective" blood volume, and (b) the "overflow" theory of ascites formation.

Role of Diminished Effective Volume

Traditionally, it has been proposed that ascites formation in cirrhotic patients begins when a critical imbalance of Starling forces in the hepatic sinusoids and splanchnic capillaries causes lymph formation which exceeds the capacity of the thoracic duct to return lymph to the general circulation (19). Consequently, excess lymph accumulates in the peritoneal space as ascites, with subsequent contraction of circulating plasma volume. As ascites develops, there is a progressive redistribution of plasma volume. Although

total plasma volume may be increased in this setting, the physiologic circumstance mimics a reduction in plasma volume (a reduced effective plasma volume).

Although an imbalance of Starling forces in the hepatosplanchnic microcirculation may contribute to the relative decrease in effective blood volume, this is not the sole mechanism. An additional determinant is total peripheral resistance, which is significantly diminished in most patients with cirrhosis who retain sodium and water. The decrease in peripheral vascular resistance is partially related to anatomic arteriovenous shunts, but another undefined vasodilator (either produced by or not inactivated by the diseased liver) plays a role. Thus, despite an increase in total plasma volume, the relative fullness of the arteriovenous tree is diminished. Several hemodynamic events act in concert to diminish effective volume, thereby activating the mechanisms of sodium retention (Fig. 1). It should be emphasized that the traditional formulation suggests that renal retention of sodium is a secondary rather than a primary event.

In this context, the term "effective" plasma volume refers to that part of the total circulating volume that is effective in stimulating volume receptors. The concept is somewhat elusive since the actual volume receptors remain incompletely defined. Diminished effective

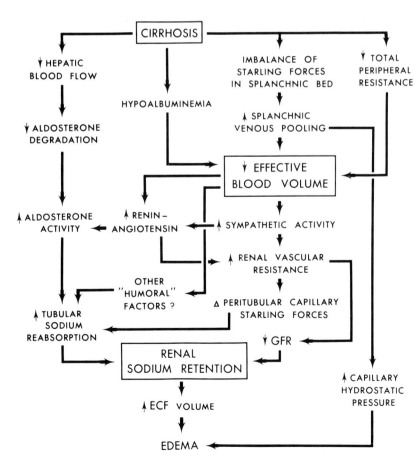

FIG. 1. Schematic representation of the major pathophysiologic mechanisms leading to renal sodium retention in cirrhosis. An imbalance of Starling forces in the hepatosplanchnic microcirculation favors sequestration of fluid within the splanchnic bed. Concomitantly, total peripheral resistance is diminished significantly, with a resultant decrease in the relative fullness of the arteriovenous tree. Thus, several hemodynamic events act in concert to diminish effective volume, thereby promoting renal sodium retention through a number of hormonal, hemodynamic, and neural mechanisms.

volume may reflect subtle alterations in systemic hemodynamic factors, such as decreased filling of the arterial tree or diminished central blood volume, or both. Since the stimulus is unknown and the afferent receptors are incompletely elucidated, alterations in effective volume must be defined in a functional manner, as exemplified by the kinetic response to volume expansive maneuvers, such as the infusion of exogenous expanders (20–22) or head-out water immersion (23,24).

"Overflow" Theory

An alternative hypothesis has been proposed. Lieberman and associates (25,26) proposed the overflow theory for ascites formation. This suggests that the primary event is inappropriate retention of excessive sodium by the kidneys with a resultant expansion of plasma volume. In the setting of abnormal Starling forces (both portal venous hypertension and reduction in plasma colloid osmotic pressure) in the portal venous bed and hepatic sinusoids, the expanded plasma volume is sequestered preferentially in the peritoneal space with ascites formation. According to this formulation, renal sodium retention and plasma volume expansion precede rather than follow the formation of ascites.

Since promulgation of the overflow theory of ascites formation, controversy has centered on which of the two hypotheses is correct (5,27). The demonstration that plasma volume is increased in cirrhosis with ascites but not during spontaneous diuresis has been cited as evidence to support the overflow hypothesis. This hypothesis has received additional support from a series of elegant investigations performed by Levy et al. (27) on dogs with experimental portal cirrhosis. The authors succeeded in developing a canine model for cirrhosis by the feeding of dimethylnitrosamine and demonstrated that renal sodium retention is an initial event which precedes ascites formation.

These investigators (27) attempted to test this hypothesis further by studying dogs with experimental cirrhosis before and after insertion of a peritoneovenous shunt, thereby preventing the reformation of ascites. In essence, the authors sought to study a model in which the liver remains damaged but where vascular underfilling, because of fluid leaving the circulation, cannot occur. It was demonstrated that increasing oral sodium intake in these dogs resulted in development of anasarca and weight gain but not ascites. Since the cirrhotic animals retained sodium in the absence of peritoneal sequestration of fluid, the authors interpreted their data as supporting the overflow theory of ascites formation.

Although these observations are collectively consistent with the overflow theory of ascites formation, certain considerations temper such an interpretation. The canine model utilized to support the overflow theory has many similarities with cirrhotic man, but differences may confound extrapolation of these findings to man. A case in point is the difference in glomerular filtration rate (GFR). In light of the postulated decrease in effective volume in cirrhosis, one would anticipate a resultant diminution in GFR. Most sodium-retaining cirrhotic patients manifest a modest and reversible decrement in GFR (2,5). In contrast, the dimethylnitrosamine dog model is not associated with such decrements.

The available evidence favors a prominent role for diminished effective volume in mediating avid sodium retention in many cirrhotic patients. Diminished effective volume and overflow may not be mutually exclusive. Virtually all available clinical studies of deranged sodium homeostasis were performed at a time when decompensation was well established; little information is available during the incipient stage of sodium retention. The two ostensibly differing formulations may be reconciled by viewing the pathogenesis of abnormal sodium retention in cirrhosis as a complex clinical constellation in which differing forces participate to varying degrees as the derangement in sodium homeostasis evolves. Thus, a primary defect in renal sodium handling may assume a more prominent role in the early stages of cirrhosis, and diminished effective volume may constitute the major determinant of sodium retention in many patients once the derangement is established.

Effectors of Renal Sodium Retention

Initial attempts to explain the abnormalities of renal sodium handling focused on the decrement in GFR that occurs frequently in patients with advanced liver disease (2,28). A number of observations indicate that decreased GFR cannot constitute the major determinant of abnormalities in renal sodium handling; many observers have reported derangements in renal sodium handling, despite preserved GFR. Furthermore, avid sodium reabsorption occurs despite supranormal GFR (13,29).

Whereas evidence demonstrates that the renal sodium retention accompanying cirrhosis is attributable primarily to enhanced tubular reabsorption rather than to alterations in the filtered load of sodium, the precise nephron sites which are operative remain controversial. Most evidence suggests that the avid reabsorption of filtrate along the proximal tubule is responsible in large part for sodium retention in cirrhosis (20,21,30). Several investigators have emphasized the importance of excessive sodium reabsorption at more distal sites (29).

The mediators of enhanced tubular reabsorption of sodium in cirrhosis and their relative participation in avid sodium retention have not been elucidated completely. Several mechanism(s) have been suggested: (a) hyperaldosteronism, (b) alterations in intrarenal blood flow distribution, (c) alterations in the endogenous release of renal prostaglandins, (d) an increase in sympathetic nervous system activity, (e) changes in the kallikrein-kinin system, and (f) the possible role of a humoral natriuretic factor. These mechanism(s) and their inter-relationships are summarized schematically in Fig. 2.

Role of Hyperaldosteronism

Cirrhosis frequently is associated with increased levels of aldosterone in urine and plasma (31–33). The elevation of plasma aldosterone is attributable to increased adrenal secretion and decreased metabolic degradation of the hormone (34). The rate of hepatic degradation is related directly to hepatic blood flow, which is markedly decreased in patients with decompensated cirrhosis.

The etiologic relationship between hyperaldosteronism and sodium retention is uncertain. The traditional view held that aldosterone is a major determinant of sodium retention. Evidence demonstrates dissociation between sodium excretion and plasma aldosterone in several experimental conditions (32,35), thereby challenging the predominance of elevated plasma aldosterone levels in mediating sodium retention in cirrhosis. Unfortunately, none of these studies

assesses kinetically the responses of plasma aldosterone and renal sodium excretion to acute volume manipulation. Epstein and co-workers (23,24) investigated the role of aldosterone in mediating the abnormal renal sodium handling in cirrhosis by performing studies utilizing a newly developed investigative tool, the model of head-out water immersion. Water immersion results in prompt and sustained increase in central blood volume comparable to the infusion of 2 liters isotonic saline (36–38). In contrast to saline, the volume expansive effect of immersion is promptly reversible, rendering it a less hazardous maneuver in edematous patients (37–39).

Immersion studies during chronic spironolactone administration permitted further elucidation of the relative contribution of aldosterone to sodium retention (24). Spironolactone administration without immersion resulted in only a modest increase in sodium excretion. In contrast, there was a marked increase when immersion was performed during chronic spironolactone administration, thereby indicating that the major contribution to natriuresis is enhanced distal delivery of filtrate (24). More compelling evidence mitigating against a predominant role for aldosterone in prompting the antinatriuresis of cirrhosis is derived from recent immersion studies kinetically assessing the relationship of plasma aldosterone responsiveness to renal sodium handling (23). Despite suppression in plasma aldosterone to comparable nadir levels in 16 cirrhotic patients, half the patients manifested absent or blunted natriuretic responses during immersion. This demonstration of a dissociation between the suppression of circulating aldosterone and the absence of nat-

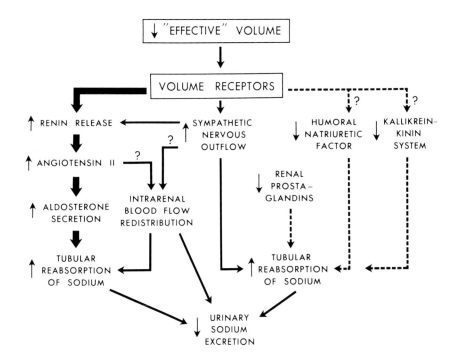

FIG. 2. Schematic drawing of possible hormonal mechanisms whereby a diminished effective volume results in sodium retention. *Heavy arrows,* pathways for which evidence is available; *dashed lines,* proposed pathways, the existence of which remains to be established. (Reproduced with permission of the American Gastroenterological Association, Inc.; from ref. 3.)

riuresis lends strong support to the interpretation that aldosterone is not the primary determinant of impaired sodium excretion in cirrhosis.

Role of Renal Prostaglandins and Renal Sodium Handling

The possibility that prostaglandins participate in mediating the sodium retention of cirrhosis must be considered. Since recent studies suggest the possibility that alterations in prostaglandin release may constitute a determinant of the natriuretic response to extracellular fluid volume expansion (39a), alterations in renal prostaglandin synthesis may contribute to derangements in renal sodium handling. Several studies demonstrate that the administration of inhibitors of prostaglandin synthetase to patients with decompensated cirrhosis results in profound decrements of renal hemodynamics, GFR, and sodium excretion (40,41). These provocative observations suggest a possible role for renal prostaglandins as determinants of the abnormal sodium retention in cirrhosis.

Kallikrein-Kinin System

Increasing evidence has suggested that bradykinin and other kinins synthesized in the kidney may participate in modulation of intrarenal blood flow and renal sodium handling (42–44). Since recent studies have demonstrated depressed levels of plasma prekallikrein in patients with chronic alcoholic liver disease (45,46), diminished kinin formation may contribute to abnormal renal sodium handling in advanced liver disease.

Role of Humoral Natriuretic Factor

Several lines of evidence suggest that a circulating natriuretic factor may constitute a component part of the biologic control system regulating sodium excretion in man (47,48). Since this natriuretic factor functions in uremia, and its role in the regulation of sodium excretion in normal physiologic states has been postulated, deficiencies of this hormone could mediate, at least in part, sodium retention in cirrhosis (Fig. 2). Implicit in this concept is the hypothesis that sodium retention results from a failure to elaborate natriuretic hormone when extracellular fluid volume increases in response to renal sodium retention.

Several preliminary observations utilizing bioassay systems, including isolated frog skin and hydrated rats, are consistent with such a formulation (49). Additional studies are warranted to assess the role of a natriuretic factor in the pathogenesis of sodium retention in cirrhosis.

Sympathetic Nervous System Activity

An increase in sympathetic nervous system activity may also contribute to the sodium retention in cirrhosis. Considerable evidence indicates that alterations in central blood volume are perceived by cardiopulmonary receptors with resultant changes in renal sympathetic activity (50). Furthermore, recent studies have demonstrated that an increase in sympathetic tone promotes an antinatriuresis by altering intrarenal hemodynamics and by a direct tubular effect (51,52).

Although these theoretical considerations suggest a role for the sympathetic nervous system in the sodium retention of cirrhosis, no data available bear directly on this possibility.

Possible Role of Estrogens

In the search for additional sodium-retaining factors in cirrhosis, it has been suggested that an impaired hepatic inactivation of estrogens, with a resultant increase in circulating estrogen, participates in mediating the sodium retention. Estrogens exert a moderate sodium-retaining effect in man, independent of their ability to stimulate aldosterone (53). Furthermore, evidence indicates that these hormones are normally inactivated by the liver (54).

The male alcoholic patient frequently manifests stigmata of feminization, including gynecomastia, testicular atrophy, decreased libido and potency, and spider angiomata (55,56). Several studies have demonstrated elevated urinary estrogen levels in cirrhosis (55–57). Studies utilizing radioimmunoassay techniques confirm the elevated estradiol levels in cirrhosis (58,59), although this is not a universal finding (60).

The presence of elevated estradiol levels per se does not establish an etiologic role for elevated estrogen activity in the antinatriuresis of cirrhosis. The observations of Preedy and Aitken (61) are of interest in this regard. These investigators assessed the effect of daily administration of 10 mg estradiol benzoate on sodium and water balance. Cirrhotic patients with ascites and edema manifested significant retention of sodium and water, as compared to normal control subjects. In contrast, the resultant retention of sodium and water in cirrhotic patients without ascites was less marked, although it exceeded that manifested by normal control subjects given estradiol. Additional studies are necessary to assess the role of elevated estradiol levels in cirrhotic patients in mediating sodium retention.

RENAL WATER HANDLING IN CIRRHOSIS

Clinical Features

The impairment of renal diluting capacity occurs frequently in cirrhosis (16). Hyponatremia, the expression of this impaired capacity to excrete water, is a commonly encountered clinical problem in cirrhotic patients. A critical review of the available data suggests that it is difficult to correlate the capacity of water diuresis with specific clinical features. Although the majority of compensated (without clinical evidence of ascites and/or edema) patients excrete water normally, decompensated (presence of ascites and/or edema) patients manifest widely varying responses to oral water loading. Furthermore, prospective studies indicate that the transition from compensation to decompensation, or vice versa, is not necessarily accompanied by concomitant changes in renal water handling.

Pathogenesis

The mechanism(s) responsible for the impairment in water diuresis in cirrhosis are not fully established. Two principal mechanisms have been proposed, including enhanced antidiuretic hormone (ADH) activity and decreased delivery of filtrate to the diluting segments of the nephron.

Increased Activity of ADH

Several lines of evidence suggest that the impairment in water excretion is attributable to increased levels of ADH, with a resultant increased back diffusion of free water in the collecting tubule. Most of the experimental evidence supporting a role for vasopressin has been indirect, involving an assessment of the responses to the administration of agents that either alter ADH release or interfere with its peripheral actions. Thus the ingestion of alcohol increased urine flow and decreased urine osmolality in severely decompensated cirrhotic patients with normal GFR (62). More recently, the administration of demeclocycline, a tetracycline derivative that appears to antagonize the peripheral action of ADH, has been shown to enhance free water generation in patients with cirrhosis and ascites (63).

The question as to whether levels of ADH are elevated in advanced liver disease remains unanswered. Despite the development of sensitive and specific radioimmunoassays for ADH, published observations of ADH levels in cirrhosis are preliminary and incomplete. The available reports suggest that decompensated cirrhosis is associated with a wide spectrum of ADH levels varying from normal to elevated values (64). The possible mechanisms for increased vasopressin levels in cirrhosis are multiple. It has been proposed that enhanced vasopressin activity may be mediated by known nonosmotic stimuli, including a decrease in peripheral resistance and arterial pressure (16). Alternatively, abnormalities in the metabolic clearance of vasopressin may contribute to the increase in the vasopressin activity (65).

Decreased Delivery of Filtrate to the Diluting Segments of the Nephron

Theoretical considerations suggest that a decreased delivery of the filtrate to the diluting segments of the nephron contribute to the impaired water excretion in cirrhotic patients. Many decompensated cirrhotic patients manifest a decrease in GFR (2). Furthermore, evidence suggests avid reabsorption of filtrate along the proximal tubule (30,20). Collectively, these events should impose a quantitative limitation to maximal urine flow and free water generation in such patients. The demonstration that free water generation is improved in some cirrhotic patients following expansion with infusions of hypotonic saline, isotonic mannitol, or saline and albumin (20,62,21) supports a role for increasing distal delivery of filtrate in the enhancement of water excretion. Decreased delivery of filtrate probably contributes to the impaired water excretion in most patients with liver disease.

MANAGEMENT OF ASCITES AND EDEMA IN LIVER DISEASE

Ascites is associated with unwanted side effects in patients with liver disease (66,67). Clearly, the accumulation of marked ascites is associated with significant discomfort. Some observers have proposed a causal relationship between ascites and the subsequent development of complications of cirrhosis, including variceal bleeding and spontaneous bacterial peritonitis (67). While ascites may indeed be the "... root of much evil" (66), the decision to relieve ascites with diuretic agents is not clear cut; several studies (68,69) suggest that diuretic therapy in the cirrhotic patient may be associated with a substantial risk of adverse effects.

A Rational Approach to Management

Since sodium is retained as long as access to sodium is not curtailed, the initial goal of any treatment program should be an attempt to obtain spontaneous diuresis by consistent and scrupulous adherence to a well-balanced diet with rigid dietary sodium restriction (250 mg/day). It should be emphasized that the sodium intake prescribed for cardiac patients (1,200 to 1,500 mg/day) is not sufficiently restrictive for the cirrhotic patient who continues to gain weight on such a regimen. When the response to dietary management is inadequate, or when the imposition of rigid dietary sodium restriction is not feasible due to cost or unpalatability of the diet, the use of diuretic agents may be considered.

Since the attributes and efficacy of the varying diuretic agents have been reviewed in detail elsewhere (69a,70), therapeutic considerations unique to the cirrhotic patient are emphasized. When diuretics are used, the therapeutic aim is a slow and gradual diuresis not exceeding the capacity for mobilization of ascitic fluid. Shear et al. (71) have demonstrated that ascites absorption averages about 300 to 500 ml/day during spontaneous diuresis; its upper limits are 700 to 900 ml/day. Thus, any diuresis that exceeds 900 ml/day (in the ascitic patient without edema) must be mobilized at the expense of the plasma compartment with resultant volume contraction.

SYNDROMES OF ACUTE AZOTEMIA

Acute renal failure (ATN) frequently complicates the course of patients with hepatic and biliary disease. While acute azotemia may often represent reversible volume contraction or classic ATN, cirrhotic patients may also develop a unique form of renal failure for which a specific cause cannot be elucidated: the "hepatorenal syndrome" (HRS). This section reviews the spectrum of acute azotemic syndromes, initially discussing HRS and subsequently ATN in the setting of hepatic and biliary disease.

THE HEPATORENAL SYNDROME

Progressive oliguric renal failure commonly complicates the course of advanced hepatic disease (72). Although this condition has been designated by many names, including functional renal failure and the renal failure of cirrhosis, the more appealing albeit less specific term HRS is the most commonly used. For the purpose of this discussion, HRS is defined as unexplained renal failure occurring in patients with liver disease in the absence of clinical, laboratory, or anatomic evidence of other known causes of renal failure.

Clinical Features

A review of the clinical features of HRS reveals marked variability regarding both the clinical presentation and course (72). HRS usually occurs in cirrhotic patients who are alcoholic, although cirrhosis is not a *sine qua non* for development of HRS. HRS may complicate other liver diseases, including acute hepatitis, fulminant hepatic failure, and hepatic malignancy (73–75). Numerous reports emphasize the development of renal failure following events that reduce effective blood volume, including abdominal paracentesis, vigorous diuretic therapy, and gastrointestinal bleeding, although it can occur in the absence of an apparent precipitating event. In this context, several careful observers have noted that HRS patients sel-

dom arrive in the hospital with preexisting renal failure (72); rather, HRS seems to develop in the hospital, raising questions as to whether events in the hospital precipitate this syndrome.

Virtually all HRS patients have ascites, which is often tense; clinical stigmata of portal hypertension are usually present. The degree of jaundice is extremely variable, and occasionally renal failure may develop at a time when the serum bilirubin concentration is decreasing. The majority of patients have a modest decrease in systemic blood pressure, but significant hypotension occurs usually as a terminal event. The serum creatinine characteristically increased before the BUN in the series reported by Shear and co-workers (76), whereas the opposite was true in the Mayo Clinic series (77). These data emphasize the great variability in HRS, both within and between series of patients. The majority of patients die within 3 weeks of onset of azotemia (78), although rare patients have survived for several months with mild azotemia.

HRS patients manifest a characteristic urine excretory pattern, voiding urine that is practically sodium free and retaining the capacity to concentrate urine to a modest degree. The biochemical characteristics of the urine in such patients is indistinguishable from that seen in hypovolemia, underscoring the importance of considering hypovolemia in any diagnostic evaluation of azotemia in liver disease.

Pathogenesis

A substantial body of evidence lends strong support to the concept that the renal failure in HRS is functional in nature. Despite the severe derangement of renal function, pathologic abnormalities are minimal and inconsistent (72). Furthermore, tubular functional integrity is maintained during the renal failure, as manifested by a relatively unimpaired sodium reabsorptive capacity and concentrating ability. Finally, more direct evidence is derived from the demonstration that kidneys transplanted from patients with HRS are capable of resuming normal function in the recipient (79).

Despite extensive study, the precise pathogenesis of HRS remains obscure. Many studies utilizing diverse hemodynamic techniques have documented a significant reduction in renal perfusion (80–82). Since a similar reduction of renal perfusion is compatible with urine volumes exceeding 1 liter in many patients with chronic renal failure (83), it is unlikely that a reduction in mean blood flow per se is responsible for the encountered oliguria.

Our laboratory applied the ^{133}Xe washout technique and selective renal arteriography to the study of HRS and demonstrated a significant reduction in calculated mean blood flow and preferential reduction in cortical perfusion (80). In addition, cirrhotic patients manifested marked vasomotor instability characterized not only by variability between serial xenon washout studies but also by instability within a single curve (80). This phenomenon has not been encountered in renal failure of other etiologies. In addition, Epstein and co-workers (80) performed simultaneous renal arteriography to delineate further the nature of the hemodynamic abnormalities. Selective renal arteriograms disclosed marked beading and tortuosity of the interlobar and proximal arcuate arteries and an absence of distinct cortical nephrograms and vascular filling of the cortical vessels (Fig. 3, left). Postmortem angiography performed on the kidneys of five patients studied during life disclosed a striking normalization of the vascular abnormalities with reversal of all the vascular abnormalities in the kidneys (Fig. 3, right). The peripheral vasculature filled completely, and the previously irregular vessels became smooth and regular. These findings provide additional evidence for the functional basis of the renal failure, operating through active renal vasoconstriction.

Although renal hypoperfusion with preferential renal cortical ischemia has been shown to underlie the renal failure of HRS, the factors responsible for sustaining reduction in cortical perfusion and suppression of filtration in HRS have not been elucidated. Several major hypotheses have been implicated or suggested, including: (a) alterations of the renin-angiotensin system, (b) an increase in sympathetic nervous system activity, (c) alterations in the endogenous release of renal prostaglandins, (d) changes in the kallikrein-kinin system, (e) increased levels of vasoactive intestinal peptide, and (f) endotoxemia. These proposed mechanisms and their interrelationships are summarized schematically in Fig. 4.

Role of Effective Volume

Examination of the proposed pathogenetic schema in Fig. 4 ascribes an important role to a diminished effective volume in the pathogenesis of HRS (84). Thus a diminution of effective volume constitutes the linchpin activating many of the hormonal and neural mechanisms that mediate the diminished renal perfusion of HRS. It is appropriate, therefore, to consider

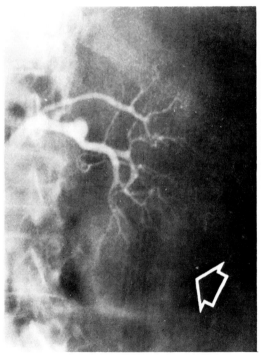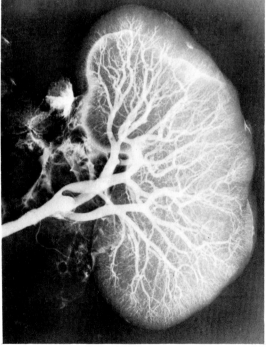

FIG. 3. Left: Selective renal arteriogram carried out in a patient with oliguric renal failure and cirrhosis (T.L.) Note the extreme abnormality of the intrarenal vessels, including the primary branches off the main renal artery and the interlobar arteries. The arcuate and cortical arterial system is not recognizable, nor is a distinct cortical nephrogram present. *Arrow,* edge of the kidney. (Reproduced with permission from ref. 80.) **Right:** Angiogram carried out postmortem on the same kidney with the intraarterial injection of micropaque in gelatin as the contrast agent. Note filling of the renal arterial system throughout the vascular bed to the periphery of the cortex. The vascular attenuation and tortuosity are no longer present. The vessels were also histologically normal. (Reproduced from ref. 80.)

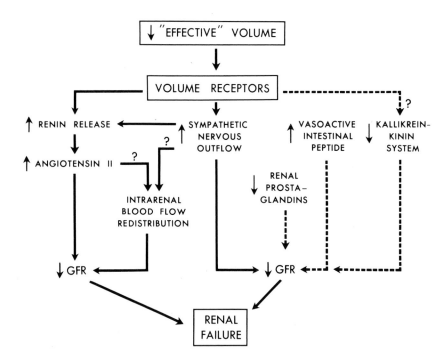

FIG. 4. Schematic representation of possible mechanisms whereby a diminished effective volume might modulate a number of hormonal effectors, eventuating in renal failure. *Solid arrows,* pathways for which evidence is available; *dashed arrows,* proposed pathways, the existence of which remains to be established. (Modified from ref. 28.)

briefly the evidence for such a postulate. Several studies, which mitigate against such a possibility (22,85), have attempted to assess the etiologic role of blood volume alterations and have focused on determination of total blood volume and plasma volume. While many investigators have observed an increase in plasma volume in cirrhotic patients with ascites (26,85) and in patients with HRS (72), the relevance of such observations to a critical assessment of the postulate that effective volume is diminished is questionable.

Pequignot and associates (86) determined blood volume in a series of 137 patients with cirrhosis and ascites, 74 of whom were azotemic. Although mean blood volume was not diminished in absolute terms in the azotemic group, mean blood volume in this group was significantly less than that observed in the group of 63 comparable patients with cirrhosis and ascites but without azotemia. Furthermore, the authors determined blood volume in 18 of the patients before and after the onset of azotemia. Mean blood volume was significantly less during the azotemic phase than during the period before azotemia ensued. Taken together, these observations suggest that blood volumes which are deemed "normal" in absolute terms when compared to control subjects may be hypovolemic for cirrhotic patients with hyperdynamic circulation, extensive collateral vasculature, and portal hypertension.

Renin-Angiotensin System

Several lines of evidence suggest a role for the renin-angiotensin axis in sustaining the vasoconstric-

tion in HRS (87). Patients with decompensated cirrhosis frequently manifest marked elevations of plasma renin levels. An examination of the relationship between renal function and plasma renin levels has disclosed that cirrhotic patients with impaired renal function manifested the most profound elevations in plasma renin levels (88) (Fig. 5). Although the elevation of plasma renin is attributable in part to decreased hepatic inactivation of renin, the major determinant is increased renin secretion by the kidney (89) (Fig. 6). The elevation of plasma renin often occurs despite presumed failure of hepatic synthesis of the alpha-2 globulin renin substrate (89).

There are at least two alternative explanations for the increased renin secretion in cirrhosis. First, renal hypoperfusion may be the primary event, with a resultant activation of the renin-angiotensin system. Alternatively, activation of the renin-angiotensin system (perhaps in response to a diminished effective blood volume) may constitute the primary event. Regardless of mechanism(s), activation of the renin-angiotensin system has profound implications for renal function. In light of experimental evidence that angiotensin plays an important role in the control of the renal circulation (87), it is tempting to speculate that enhanced angiotensin levels contribute to renal vasoconstriction and reduction in filtration rate of renal failure in cirrhosis (Fig. 6).

An additional mechanism whereby perturbations in the renin-angiotensin system may mediate the renal failure of liver disease has been proposed. Berkowitz (90) postulated that renin substrate depletion per se may be the principal etiologic factor for the hemodynamic abnormalities that accompany HRS. Ob-

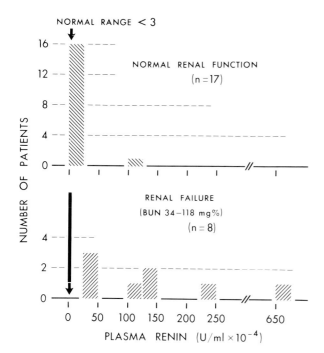

FIG. 5. Relationship between renal function and plasma renin levels in 24 patients with cirrhosis and ascites. The range for normal subjects (0 to 3.5×10^{-4} Goldblatt units/ml) on dietary sodium restriction is depicted by the solid arrow to the left of the lower panel; 17 patients had normal renal function (*upper panel*), whereas seven had azotemia with BUNs ranging from 34 to 118 mg/dl (*lower panel*). In contrast to the normal or modestly elevated plasma renin levels in cirrhotic patients with normal GFRs, most patients with azotemia manifested profound elevations in plasma renin levels markedly exceeding the values of the nonazotemic group. (Based on data from ref. 88.)

servations following hepatic transplantation (91) and during the infusion of renin substrate-rich fresh frozen plasma into patients with HRS (90) raised the possibility that a rise in renin substrate may precede transient improvements in renal function. Additional studies are needed to establish the significance of these provocative preliminary observations.

Role of Renal Prostaglandins

The possibility that prostaglandins participate in mediating the renal failure of cirrhosis must be considered. Attempts to investigate the role of renal prostaglandins in mediating the sodium retention in cirrhosis include administration of exogenous prostaglandins and alteration of endogenous production of prostaglandins by inhibition of prostaglandin synthesis. Initially, the problem was approached by examining the renal hemodynamic response to the administration of exogenous prostaglandins (92). Unfortunately, the relevance of such studies in cirrhotic man is tenuous; recent studies suggest that any action of prostaglandins on the kidney must be as a local tissue hormone (93). Thus, any evaluation of the physiologic role of prostaglandins on renal function necessitates an experimental design in which the endogenous production of lipids is altered.

Several investigators have demonstrated that the administration of inhibitors of prostaglandin synthetase (both indomethacin and ibuprofen) results in significant decrements in GFR and renal plasma flow (ERPF) in patients with alcoholic liver disease (40,41).

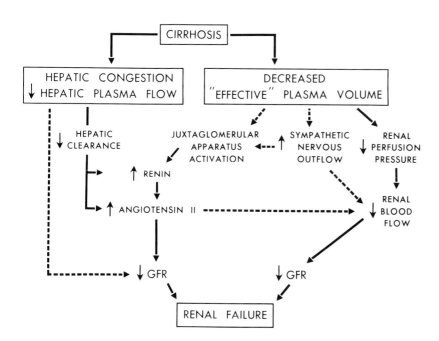

FIG. 6. Schematic drawing of probable mechanisms whereby the renin-angiotensin system and the sympathetic nervous system interact to produce renal failure. Both a diminished effective volume and impaired hepatic clearance of renin-angiotensin result in a marked enhancement of circulating PRA with a resultant decrease in GFR. An increase in sympathetic nervous system activity (possibly attributable to decreased effective volume) decreases GFR both by diminishing renal perfusion and by activating the renin-angiotensin system. (Reproduced with permission from Epstein, ref. 28.)

The decrement in renal hemodynamics varied directly with the degree of sodium retention; i.e., the patients with the most avid sodium retention manifested the largest decrements in GFR (41).

The above findings are not isolated observations. As noted recently (6), one may conceive of renal prostaglandins as constituting critical modulators of renal function during conditions or disease states involving volume contraction. The demonstration that synthetase inhibition affected renal function only in decompensated (presence of ascites and/or edema) and not in compensated cirrhotic subjects, and that the effects of synthetase inhibition varies as a function of the degree of renal sodium avidity, is consistent with this formulation.

As the above-cited studies examined the effect of inhibiting endogenous production of renal prostaglandins, it would be of interest to assess the effect of augmenting endogenous prostaglandins on renal functional alterations. Our recent demonstration that head-out water immersion constitutes a unique means of augmenting urinary prostaglandin excretion, and presumably renal prostaglandin synthesis (39a), prompted an examination of the relationship of immersion-induced changes in prostaglandin and renal function. Immersion of cirrhotic patients was associated with prompt and marked increments in prostaglandin excretion (*unpublished observations*). The demonstration that the majority of these patients manifest increments in GFR is consistent with the interpretation that augmentation of renal prostaglandin synthesis may constitute a determinant of renal hemodynamics in decompensated cirrhosis. Additional studies are necessary to characterize further the role of prostaglandins as determinants of the renal failure of cirrhosis.

Kallikrein-Kinin System

The interdependence of prostaglandins and other vasoactive hormonal systems dictates that consideration should be given to the possible pathogenetic role of these hormonal systems, and the kallikrein-kinin system in particular. That the latter system may be involved in mediating sodium retention of liver disease is suggested by several preliminary reports of abnormalities of the plasma kallikrein system (45,46). Wong (45) measured plasma prekallikrein levels in patients with HRS. Undetectable levels were found in many such patients, raising the possibility that the decrease in prekallikrein levels results in diminished kinin formation. Since bradykinin has been suggested to be a physiologic renal vasodilator, failure of bradykinin

formation may contribute to the renal cortical vasoconstriction encountered in HRS.

Endotoxins

Systemic endotoxemia may participate in the pathogenesis of the renal failure of cirrhosis. It has been hypothesized that enteric endotoxin is liberated into the systemic circulation through naturally or surgically created portasystemic shunts, thus bypassing the hepatic Kupffer cells, the major site of endotoxin removal (95). Recent studies have measured endotoxin by the limulus lysate technique and reported that endotoxin is present in the portal and systemic circulation of many cirrhotic patients, particularly those with ascites. Since several investigators have demonstrated a high frequency of positive limulus assays in cirrhotic patients with renal failure but not in the absence of renal failure (94), endotoxins may contribute to the pathogenesis of the renal failure. This hypothesis awaits additional study and confirmation.

ACUTE RENAL FAILURE (ATN)

Although much attention has been directed to HRS, it should be borne in mind that cirrhotic patients are not less vulnerable than noncirrhotic patients to the development of ATN. A review of several published series shows that, among liver disease patients in whom renal failure developed, the etiology of renal failure was more commonly ATN than HRS (76). The increased frequency of ATN may relate to the hypotension, bleeding dyscrasias, infection, and multiple metabolic disorders that complicate the clinical course.

Finally, the association between obstructive jaundice and ATN merits comment. More than 15 years ago, Dawson noted that, in patients undergoing surgery for the relief of obstructive jaundice, the incidence of ATN was many times greater than that encountered in a comparable group of nonjaundiced patients (95). It was further noted that the greater the degree of jaundice, the greater the risk of ATN. The demonstration that the risk of ATN is higher in the most deeply jaundiced patients prompted an investigation of the mechanism(s) in the Gunn rat (a species unable to conjugate bilirubin) (96). These studies suggest that circulating conjugated bilirubin may be responsible for the increased proclivity of jaundiced animals to develop renal failure. It should be noted, however, that there is a lack of unanimity of opinion regarding the uniqueness of the association of biliary tract disease and ATN (97).

Diuretic-Induced Azotemia

As noted earlier, cirrhotic patients who are treated with diuretics frequently develop azotemia. Although there are many reasons to believe that this complication develops as a consequence of overly vigorous therapy in which negative fluid balance is attained, which exceeds the maximal rate at which ascites can be mobilized, isolated observations raise the possibility that this phenomenon may be more complex. It has been proposed that mechanisms other than volume depletion per se may be causative. These speculations require confirmation.

Treatment of HRS

The management of HRS has been discouraging in view of the absence of any effective treatment modality. Since knowledge about its pathogenesis is incomplete, therapy is supportive. The initial step in management is not to equate decreased renal function with HRS, but rather to search for and treat correctable causes of azotemia, such as volume contraction, cardiac decompensation, and urinary tract obstruction.

Once correctable causes of renal functional impairment are excluded, the mainstay of therapy is careful restriction of sodium and fluid intake. While a number of specific therapeutic measures have been attempted, none has proved to be of practical value. Attempts at volume expansion with different exogenous expanders and exchange transfusion have not resulted in significant improvement in the outcome (72,98). Dialysis has not been effective in managing HRS (99).

Recently, there has been enthusiasm for the use of the peritoneovenous shunt (LeVeen shunt) in the management of HRS (100). Since the underlying abnormality is thought to be maldistribution of ECF with a resultant diminished effective blood volume, attention has focused on developing procedures to replenish the central compartment at a time when ascites is decreasing. Earlier attempts at autogenous reinfusion of ascites proved too cumbersome a technique to constitute a useful form of therapy. In 1974, Le Veen and associates developed a one-way valve activated by a pressure gradient which facilitates continuous P-V shunting of ascitic fluid. Since then, a number of reports have suggested reversal of HRS following P-V shunting (100,101). Unfortunately, most reports have been anecdotal, with insufficient details to allow critical assessment (102). Furthermore, there is increasing awareness that P-V shunting is attended by many complications (102,103). Controlled prospective studies are currently underway to delineate the possible role of this therapeutic modality in the treatment of HRS.

GLOMERULAR CHANGES IN LIVER DISEASE

Glomerular changes occur primarily in patients with cirrhosis and acute and chronic viral hepatitis.

Cirrhosis

Glomerular changes are common in patients with cirrhosis of the liver (104). On a histopathologic basis, it is possible to distinguish two types of glomerular abnormalities: forms with and without proliferation.

The changes without proliferation are characterized by sclerosis and increase in mesangial matrix. Electron microscopy reveals electron-dense deposits that are mainly mesangial but frequently extend into the subendothelial stage. It has been suggested that IgA constitutes the main immunoglobulin in the deposits, often accompanied by IgG and/or IgM. Although these glomerular changes are usually not associated with urinary abnormalities, some patients have proteinuria or microscopic hematuria or both.

Glomerular changes with proliferation are characterized by slight mesangial hypercellularity, endo- and extracapillary proliferation, and mesangial interposition, giving a pattern similar to that of membranoproliferative glomerulonephritis. IgA is the major immunoglobulin in the deposits. The cases with endocapillary proliferation present with a clinical picture similar to that of acute glomerulonephritis. Patients with membranoproliferative glomerulonephritis may have no urinary abnormalities or may present with proteinuria and microscopic hematuria.

The pathogenesis of these glomerular changes and their relationship to the underlying hepatic disease is unsettled. While it is possible for glomerulonephritis unrelated to hepatic disease to develop in a patient with cirrhosis, the available evidence suggests that the glomerular changes are related to the liver disease per se. Because the major immunoglobulin in the glomerular deposits in cirrhotic patients is IgA, which is uncommon in acute glomerulonephritis, the majority of cases of proliferative glomerulonephritis encountered in cirrhotic patients may be related to the presence of hepatic disease.

Viral Hepatitis

Renal morphologic and functional alterations occur in patients with acute and chronic viral hepatitis (106). In the majority of patients with acute viral hepatitis, renal function is only mildly impaired. The most common findings include a modest degree of proteinuria, hematuria, and mild reduction in GFR. Renal biopsies in patients with acute viral hepatitis reveal mild proliferative glomerulonephritis (105). Immunofluorescence shows IgG, IgM, IgA, and complement as discrete nodular deposits with electron-dense deposits primarily near the mesangial areas on electron microscopy. Although follow-up information in most of these patients is limited, preliminary indications suggest that most patients with acute viral hepatitis manifest a return to normal renal function with respect to GFR and proteinuria (106).

In contrast to acute viral hepatitis, more severe impairment of renal function occurs in patients with persistent HB$_s$Ag antigenemia associated with chronic active hepatitis (105). The characteristic glomerular lesion in such cases with progressive deterioration of renal function has been a membranoproliferative or epimembranous glomerulonephritis. Clinically, these patients have proteinuria, nephrotic syndrome, or renal failure. The glomerulonephritides associated with with HB$_s$Ag hepatitis are due to an immune complex-mediated glomerulonephritis, which is initiated by deposition of HB$_s$Ag in the glomerular basement membrane or, more likely, by circulating immune complexes formed by the binding of HB$_s$Ag to specific antibodies in the serum and subsequent deposition in the glomerular basement membrane. The prognosis of glomerulonephritis in patients with persistent HB$_s$Ag remains to be delineated (106).

REFERENCES

1. Hippocrates. Cited in Atkinson, M. (1956): Ascites in liver disease. *Postgrad. Med. J.*, 32:482–485.
2. Epstein, M. (1978): Renal sodium handling in cirrhosis. In: *The Kidney in Liver Disease*, edited by M. Epstein, pp. 35–53. Elsevier, New York.
3. Epstein, M. (1979): Deranged sodium homeostasis in cirrhosis. *Gastroenterology*, 76:622–635.
4. Levy, M. (1978): The kidney in liver disease. In: *Sodium and Water Homeostasis*, edited by B. M. Brenner and J. H. Stein, pp. 73–116. Churchill Livingstone, New York.
5. Epstein, M. (1979): Renal sodium handling in cirrhosis: A reappraisal. *Nephron*, 23:211–217.
6. Epstein, M. (1980): Determinants of abnormal renal sodium handling in cirrhosis: A reappraisal. *Scand. J. Clin. Lab. Invest.*, 40:689–694.
7. Barnardo, D. E., Summerskill, W. H. J., Strong, C. B., and Baldus, W. P. (1970): Renal function, renin activity and endogenous vasoactive substances in cirrhosis. *Am. J. Dig. Dis.*, 15:419–425.
8. Eisenmenger, W. J., Blondheim, S. H., Bongiovanni, A. M., and Kunkel, H. G. (1950): Electrolyte studies on patients with cirrhosis of the liver. *J. Clin. Invest.*, 29:1491–1499.
9. Faloon, W. W., Eckhardt, R. D., Cooper, A. M., and Davidson, C. S. (1949): The effect of human serum albumin, mercurial diuretics and a low sodium diet on sodium excretion in patients with cirrhosis of the liver. *J. Clin. Invest.*, 28:595–602.
10. Jones, R. A., McDonald, G. O., and Last, J. H. (1952): Reversal of diurnal variation in renal function in cases of cirrhosis with ascites. *J. Clin. Invest.*, 31:326–334.
11. Papper, S., and Rosenbaum, J. D. (1952): Abnormalities in the excretion of water and sodium in "compensated" cirrhosis of the liver. *J. Lab. Clin. Med.*, 40:523–530.
12. Gabuzda, G. J. (1970): Cirrhosis, ascites, and edema. Clinical course related to management. *Gastroenterology*, 58:546–553.
13. Klingler, E. L., Jr., Vaamonde, C. A., Vaamonde, L. S., Lancestremere, R. G., Morosi, H. J., Frisch, E., and Papper, S. (1970): Renal function changes in cirrhosis of the liver. *Arch. Intern. Med.*, 125:1010–1015.
14. Bosch, J., Arroyo, V., Rodes, J., Bruguera, M., and Teres, J. (1974): Compensanea espontanea de la ascitis en la cirrosis hepatica. *Rev. Clin. Esp.*, 133:441–446.
15. Papper, S., and Saxon, L. (1959): The diuretic response to administered water in patients with liver disease. II. Laennec's cirrhosis of the liver. *Arch. Intern. Med.*, 103:750–757.
16. Vaamonde, C. A. (1978): Renal water handling in liver disease. In: *The Kidney in Liver Disease*, edited by M. Epstein, pp. 67–89. Elsevier, New York.
17. Chaimovitz, C., Rochman, J., Eidelman, S., and Better, O. S. (1977): Exaggerated natriuretic response to volume expansion in patients with primary biliary cirrhosis. *Am. J. Med. Sci.*, 274:173–178.
18. Wilkinson, S. P., Arroyo, V., Moodie, H. E., Blendis, L. M., and Williams, R. (1974): Renal failure and site of abnormal renal retention of sodium in fulminant hepatic failure. *Gut*, 15:343.
19. Witte, M. H., Witte, C. L., and Dumont, A. E. (1971): Progress in liver disease: Physiological factors involved in the causation of cirrhotic ascites. *Gastroenterology*, 61:742–750.
20. Schedl, H. P., and Bartter, F. C. (1960): An explanation for and experimental correction of the abnormal water diuresis in cirrhosis. *J. Clin. Invest.*, 39:248–261.
21. Vlahcevic, Z. R., Adam, N. F., Jick, H., Moore, E. W., and Chalmers, T. C. (1965): Renal effects of acute expansion on plasma volume in cirrhosis. *N. Engl. J. Med.*, 272:387–391.
22. Yamahiro, H. S., and Reynolds, T. B. (1961): Effects of ascitic fluid infusion on sodium excretion. *Gastroenterology*, 40:497–503.
23. Epstein, M., Levinson, R., Sancho, J., Haber, E., and Re, R. (1977): Characterization of the renin-aldosterone system in decompensated cirrhosis. *Circ. Res.*, 41:818–829.
24. Epstein, M., Pins, D. S., Schneider, N., and Levinson, R. (1976): Determinants of deranged sodium and water homeostasis in decompensated cirrhosis. *J. Lab. Clin. Med.*, 87:822–839.
25. Lieberman, F. L., Denison, E. K., and Reynolds, T. B. (1970): The relationship of plasma volume, portal hypertension, ascites and renal sodium retention in cirrhosis: The overflow theory of ascites formation. *Ann. NY Acad. Sci.*, 170:202–212.
26. Lieberman, F. L., Ito, S., and Reynolds, T. B. (1969): Effective plasma volume in cirrhosis with ascites. Evidence that a decreased value does not account for renal sodium retention, a spontaneous reduction in glomerular filtration rate (GFR) and a fall in GFR during drug-induced diuresis. *J. Clin. Invest.*, 48:975–981.
27. Levy, M., Wexler, M. J., and McCaffrey, C. (1979): Sodium retention in dogs with experimental cirrhosis following removal of ascites by continuous peritoneovenous shunting. *J. Lab. Clin. Med.*, 94:933–946.
28. Epstein, M. (1982): The kidney in liver disease. In: *Textbook of Nephrology*, edited by S. G. Massry and R. B. Glassock. Elsevier, New York (*in press*).
29. Chaimovitz, C., Szylman, P., Alroy, G., and Better, O. S. (1972): Mechanism of increased renal tubular sodium reabsorption in cirrhosis. *Am. J. Med.*, 52:198–202.
30. Chiandussi, L., Bartoli, E., and Arras, S. (1978): Reabsorption

of sodium in the proximal renal tubule in cirrhosis of the liver. *Gut*, 19:497–503.

31. Coppage, W. S., Jr., Island, D. P., Cooner, A. E., and Liddle, G. W. (1962): The metabolism of aldosterone in normal subjects and in patients with hepatic cirrhosis. *J. Clin. Invest.*, 41:1672–1680.

32. Rosoff, L., Jr., Zia, P., Reynolds, T., and Horton, R. (1975): Studies of renin and aldosterone in cirrhotic patients with ascites. *Gastroenterology*, 69:698–705.

33. Vecsei, P., Dusterdieck, G., Jahnecke, J., Lommer, D., and Wolff, H. P. D. (1969): Secretion and turnover of aldosterone in various pathological states. *Clin. Sci.*, 36:241–256,

34. Saruta, R., Saito, I., Nakamura, R., and Oka, M. (1978): Regulation of aldosterone in cirrhosis of the liver. In: *The Kidney in Liver Disease*, edited by M. Epstein, pp. 271–282. Elsevier, New York.

35. Chonko, A. M., Bay, W. H., Stein, J. H., and Ferris, T. F. (1977): The role of renin and aldosterone in the salt retention of edema. *Am. J. Med.*, 63:881–889.

36. Epstein, M. (1976): Cardiovascular and renal effects of head-out water immersion in man. Application of the model in the assessment of volume homeostasis. *Circ. Res.*, 39:619–628.

37. Epstein, M. (1978): Renal effects of head-out water immersion in man: Implications for an understanding of volume homeostasis. *Physiol. Rev.*, 58:529–581.

38. Levinson, R., Epstein, M., Sackner, M. A., and Begin, R. (1977): Comparison of the effects of water immersion and saline infusion on central hemodynamics in man. *Clin. Sci. Mol. Med.*, 52:343–350.

39. Epstein, J., Pins, D. S., Arrington, R., DeNunzio, A. G., and Engstrom, R. (1975): Comparison of water immersion and saline infusion as a means of inducing volume expansion in man. *J. Appl. Physiol.*, 39:66–70.

39a. Epstein, M., Lifschitz, M., Hoffman, D. S., and Stein, J. (1979): Relationship between renal prostaglandin E and renal sodium handling during water immersion in normal man. *Circ. Res.*, 45:71–80.

40. Boyer, T. D., Zia, P., and Reynolds, T. B. (1979): Effect of indomethacin and prostaglandin A₁ on renal function and plasma activity in alcoholic liver disease. *Gastroenterology*, 77:215–222.

41. Zipser, R. D., Hoefs, J. C., Speckart, P. F., Zia, P. K., and Horton, R. (1979): Prostaglandins: Modulators of renal function and pressor resistance in chronic liver disease. *J. Clin. Endocrinol. Metab.*, 48:895–900.

42. Nasjletti, A., Colina-Chourio, J., and McGiff, J. C. (1975): Disappearance of bradykinin in the renal circulation of dogs: Effects of kininase inhibition. *Circ. Res.*, 37:59–65.

43. Stein, J. H., Congbalay, R. C., Karsh, D. L., Osgood, R. W., and Ferris, T. F. (1972): The effect of bradykinin on proximal tubular sodium reabsorption in the dog: Evidence for functional nephron heterogeneity. *J. Clin. Invest.*, 51:1709–1721.

44. Stein, J. H., Ferris, R. F., Huprich, J. E., Smith, T. C., and Osgood, R. W. (1971): Effect of renal vasodilation on the distribution of cortical blood flow in the kidney of the dog. *J. Clin. Invest.*, 50:1429–1438.

45. Wong, P. Y. (1978): The kallikrein-kinin and related vasoactive systems in cirrhosis of the liver. In: *The Kidney in Liver Disease*, edited by M. Epstein, pp. 299-310. Elsevier, New York.

46. Wong, P. Y., Colman, R. W., Talamo, R. C., and Babior, B. M. (1972): Kallikrein-bradykinin system in chronic alcoholic liver disease. *Ann. Intern. Med.*, 77:205–209.

47. Bricker, N. S. (1978): Extracellular fluid volume regulation: On the evidence for a biologic control system. In: *The Kidney in Liver Disease*, edited by M. Epstein, pp. 19–30. Elsevier, New York.

48. DeWardener, H. E. (1977): Natriuretic hormone. *Clin. Sci. Mol. Ved.*, 53:1–8.

49. Kramer, H. J. (1976): Natriuretic activity in plasma following extracellular volume expansion. In: *Central Nervous Control of Na⁺ Balance—Relations to the Renin-Angiotensin System*, edited by W. Kaufmann and D. K. Krause, pp. 126–133. George Thieme Verlag, Stuttgart.

50. Thames, M. D. (1977): Neural control of renal function: Contribution of cardiopulmonary baroreceptors to the control of the kidney. *Fed. Proc.*, 37:1209–1213.

51. DiBona, G. F. (1977): Neurogenic regulation of renal tubular sodium reabsorption. *Am. J. Physiol.*, 233:F73–F81.

52. Stein, J. H., Boonjarern, S., Wilson, C. B., and Ferris, T. F. (1973): Alterations in intrarenal blood flow distribution. Methods of measurement and relationship to sodium balance. *Circ. Res.*, 32,33:61–72.

53. Christy, N. P., and Shaver, J. C. (1974): Estrogens and the kidney. *Kidney Int.*, 6:366–376.

54. Pearlman, W. H. (1948): The chemistry and metabolism of the estrogens. In: *The Hormones, Vol. I*, edited by G. Pincus and K. V. Thimann, pp. 351–405. Academic Press, New York.

55. Lloyd, C. W., and Williams, R. H. (1948): Endocrine changes associated with Laennec's cirrhosis of the liver. *Am. J. Med.*, 4:315–327.

56. Rupp, J., Cantarow, A., Rakoff, A. E., and Paschkis, K. E. (1952): Hormone excretion in liver disease and in gynecomastia. *J. Clin. Endocrinol. Metab.*, 11:688–699.

57. Dohan, F. C., Richardson, E. M., Bluemle, L. W., Jr., and Gyorgy, P. (1952): Hormone excretion in liver disease. *J. Clin. Invest.*, 31:481–498.

58. Chopra, I. J., Tulchinsky, D., and Greenway, F. L. (1973): Estrogen-androgen imbalance in hepatic cirrhosis. Studies in 13 male patients. *Ann. Intern. Med.*, 79:198–203.

59. Kley, H. K., Nieschlag, E., Wiegelmann, W., Solbach, H. G., and Kruskemper, H. L. (1975): Steroid hormones and their binding in plasma of male patients with fatty liver, chronic hepatitis and liver cirrhosis. *Acta Endocrinol.*, 78:275–285.

60. Galvao-Teles, A., Burke, C. W., Anderson, D. C., Marshall, J. C., Corker, C. S., Brown, R. L., and Clark, M. L. (1973): Biologically active androgens and oestradiol in men with chronic liver disease. *Lancet*, 1:173–177.

61. Preedy, J. R. K., and Aitken, E. H. (1956): The effect of estrogen on water and electrolyte metabolism. II. Hepatic disease. *J. Clin. Invest.*, 35:430–442.

62. Strauss, M. B., Birchard, W. H., and Saxon, L. (1956): Correction of impaired water excretion in cirrhosis of the liver by alcohol ingestion or expansion of extracellular fluid volume: The role of the antidiuretic hormone. *Trans. Assoc. Am. Physicians*, 69:222–228.

63. DeTroyer, A., Pilloy, W., Broeckaert, I., and Demanet, J. D. (1976): Demeclocycline treatment of water retention in cirrhosis. *Ann. Intern. Med.*, 85:336–337.

64. Padfield, P. L., and Morton, J. J. (1974): Application of a sensitive radioimmunoassay for plasma arginine vasopressin to pathological conditions in man. *Clin. Sci. Mol. Med.*, 47:16P–17P.

65. Skowsky, R., Riestra, J., Martinez, I., Swan, L., and Kikuchi, T. (1976): Arginine vasopressin (AVP) kinetics in hepatic cirrhosis. *Clin. Res.*, 24:101A.

66. Conn, H. O. (1977): Diuresis of ascites: Fraught with or free from hazard. *Gastroenterology*, 73:619–621.

67. Conn, H. O., and Fessel, J. M. (1971): Spontaneous bacterial peritonitis in cirrhosis. Variations on a theme. *Medicine*, 50:161–197.

68. Naranjo, C. A., Pontigo, E., Valdenegro, C., Gonzalez, G., Ruiz, I., and Busto, U. (1979): Furosemide-induced adverse reactions in cirrhosis of the liver. *Clin. Pharm. Ther.*, 25:154–160.

69. Sherlock, S. (1970): Ascites formation in cirrhosis and its management. *Scand. J. Gastroenterol. [Suppl.].* 7:9–15.

69a. Linas, S. L., Anderson, R. J., Miller, P. D., and Schrier, R. W. (1978): Rational use of diuretics in cirrhosis. In: *The Kidney in Liver Disease*, edited by M. Epstein, pp. 313–323. Elsevier, New York.

70. Burg, M. B. (1976): Mechanisms of action of diuretic drugs. In: *The Kidney*, edited by B. M. Brenner and F. C. Rectors, pp. 737–762. Saunders, Philadelphia.

71. Shear, L., Ching, S., and Gabuzda, G. J. (1970): Compartmentalization of ascites and edema in patients with hepatic cirrhosis. *N. Engl. J. Med.*, 282:1391–1396.

72. Papper, S. (1978): Renal failure in cirrhosis (the hepatorenal

syndrome). In: *The Kidney in Liver Disease*, edited by M. Epstein, pp. 91-112. Elsevier, New York.

73. Epstein, M., Oster, J. R., and DeVelasco, R. E. (1976): Hepatorenal syndrome following hemihepatectomy. *Clin. Nephrol.*, 5:128–133.

74. Ritt, D. J., Whelan, G., Werner, D. J., Eigenbrodt, E. H., Schenker, S., and Combes, B. (1969): Acute hepatic necrosis with stupor or coma. *Medicine*, 48:151–172.

75. Vesin, P., Roberti, A., and Viguie, R. R. (1965): Defaillance renale fonctionnelle terminale chez des malades atteints de cancer due foie, primitif ou secondaire. *Sem. Hop. Paris*, 26:1216–1220.

76. Shear, L., Kleinerman, J., and Gabuzda, G. J. (1965): Renal failure in patients with cirrhosis of the liver. I. Clinical and pathologic characteristics. *Am. J. Med.*, 39:184–198.

77. Baldus, W. P., Feichter, R. N., and Summerskill, W. H. J. (1964): The kidney in cirrhosis I. Clinical and biochemical features of azotemia in hepatic failure. *Ann. Intern. Med.*, 60:353–365.

78. Goldstein, H., and Boyle, J. D. (1965): Spontaneous recovery from the hepatorenal syndrome. Report of four cases. *N. Engl. J. Med.*, 272:895–898.

79. Koppel, M. H., Coburn, J. W., Mims, M. M., Goldstein, H., Boyle, J. D., and Rubini, M. E. (1969): Transplantation of cadaveric kidneys from patients with hepatorenal syndrome. Evidence for the functional nature of renal failure in advanced liver disease. *N. Engl. J. Med.*, 280:1367–1371.

80. Epstein, M., Berk, D. P., Hollenberg, N. K., Adams, D. F., Chalmers, T. C., Abrams, H. L., and Merrill, J. P. (1970): Renal failure in the patient with cirrhosis. The role of active vasoconstriction. *Am. J. Med.*, 49:175–185.

81. Kew, M. C., Varma, R. R., Williams, H. S., Brunt, P. W., Hourigan, K. J., and Sherlock, S. (1971): Renal and intrarenal blood flow in cirrhosis of the liver. *Lancet*, 2:504–510, 1971.

82. Schroeder, E. T., Shear, L., Sancetta, S. M., and Gabuzda, G. J. (1967): Renal failure in patients with cirrhosis of the liver. III. Evaluation of intrarenal blood flow by para-amino-hippurate extraction and response to angiotensin. *Am. J. Med.*, 43:887–896.

83. Hollenberg, N. K., Epstein, M., Basch, R. I., Oken, D. E., and Merrill, J. P. (1968): Acute oliguric renal failure in man: Evidence for preferential renal cortical ischemia. *Medicine*, 47:455–474.

84. Papper, S., and Vaamonde, C. A. (1968): Renal failure in cirrhosis. Role of plasma volume. *Ann. Intern. Med.*, 68:958–959.

85. McCloy, R. M., Baldus, W. P., Tauxe, W. N., and Summerskill, W. H. J. (1967): Plasma volume and renal circulatory function in cirrhosis. *Ann. Intern. Med.*, 66:307–311.

86. Pequignot, E., Viallet, A., Combrisson, A., and Caroli, J. (1962): L'hypovolemie relative des cirrhotiques hyperazotemiques, circonstance d'apparition. In: *Aktuelle Probleme der Hepatologie: Ultrastruktur Steroidstoffwechsel, Durchblutung, Liber und Niere*, edited by G. A. Martinin and S. Sherlock, pp. 110–118. George Thieme Verlag, Stuttgart.

87. Hollenberg, N. K. (1978): Renin, angiotensin, and the kidney: Assessment with angiotensin antagonists. In: *The Kidney in Liver Disease*, edited by M. Epstein, pp. 187–205. Elsevier, New York.

88. Schroeder, E. T., Eich, R. H., Smulyan, H., Gould, A. B., and Gabuzda, G. J. (1970): Plasma renin level in hepatic cirrhosis. *Am. J. Med.*, 49:186–191.

89. Saruta, T., Kondo, K., Saito, I., and Nakamura, R. (1978): Characterization of the components of the renin-angiotensin system in cirrhosis of the liver. In: *The Kidney in Liver Disease*, edited by M. Epstein, pp. 207–233. Elsevier, New York.

90. Berkowitz, H. D. (1978): Renin substrate in the hepatorenal syndrome. In: *The Kidney in Liver Disease*, edited by M. Epstein, pp. 251–270. Elsevier, New York.

91. Iwatsuki, S., Popovtzer, M. M., Corman, J. L., Ishikawa, M., Putnam, C. W., Katz, F. H., and Starzl, T. E. (1973): Recovery from hepatorenal syndrome after orthotopic liver transplantation. *N. Engl. J. Med.*, 289:1155–1159.

92. Arieff, A. I., and Chidsey, C. A. (1974): Renal function in cirrhosis and the effects of prostaglandin A_1. *Am. J. Med.*, 56:695–703.

93. McGiff, J. C., and Itskovitz, H. D. (1973): Prostaglandins and the kidney. *Circ. Res.*, 33:479–488.

94. Wilkinson, S. P., Smith, I. K., and Williams, R. (1978): Renal failure in liver disease: Role of endotoxins and renin-angiotensin system. In: *The Kidney in Liver Disease*, edited by M. Epstein, pp. 113–120. Elsevier, New York.

95. Dawson, J. L. (1965): The incidence of postoperative renal failure in obstructive jaundice. *Br. J. Surg.*, 52:663–665.

96. Baum, M., Stirling, G. A., and Dawson, J. L. (1969): Further study into obstructive jaundice and ischaemic renal damage. *Br. Med. J.*, 2:229–231.

97. Bismuth, H., Kuntziger, H., and Corlette, M. B. (1975): Cholangitis with acute renal failure. *Ann. Surg.*, 181:881–887.

98. Horisawa, M., and Reynolds, T. B. (1976): Exchange transfusion in hepatorenal syndrome with liver disease. *Arch. Intern. Med.*, 136:1135–1137.

99. Perez, G. O., and Oster, J. R. (1978): A critical review of the role of dialysis in the treatment of liver disease. In: *The Kidney in Liver Disease*, edited by M. Epstein, pp. 325–336. Elsevier, New York.

100. Kinney, M. J., Wapnick, S., Ahmed, N., Ip, M., Grosberg, S., and LeVeen, H. H. (1978): Cirrhosis, ascites, and impaired renal function: Treatment with the LeVeen-type chronic peritoneal-venous shunt. In: *The Kidney in Liver Disease*, edited by M. Epstein, pp. 349–364. Elsevier, New York.

101. Pladson, T. R., and Parrish, R. M. (1977): Hepatorenal syndrome: Recovery after peritoneovenous shunt. *Arch. Intern. Med.*, 137:1248–1249.

102. Epstein, M. (1980): The LeVeen shunt for ascites and hepatorenal syndrome. *N. Engl. J. Med.*, 302:628–630.

103. Greig, P. D., Langer, B., Blendis, L. M., Taylor, B. R., and Glynn, M. F. X. (1980): Complications after peritoneovenous shunting for ascites. *Am. J. Surg.*, 139:125–131.

104. Berger, J., Yaneva, H., and Nabarra, B. (1977): Glomerular changes in patients with cirrhosis of the liver. In: *Advances in Nephrology, Vol. 7*, edited by J. Hamburger, J. Crosnier, J. P. Grunfeld, and M. Maxwell pp. 3–14. Year Book Medical, Chicago.

105. Eknoyan, G., Gyorkey, F., Dichoso, C., Martinez-Maldonado, M., Suki, W. N., and Gyorkey, P. (1972): Renal morphological and immunological changes associated with acute viral hepatitis. *Kidney Int.*, 1:413–419.

106. Eknoyan, G. (1982): Glomerular abnormalities in liver disease. In: *The Kidney in Liver Disease*, 2nd ed., edited by M. Epstein, Elsevier, New York (*in press*).

The Liver: Biology and Pathobiology, edited by
I. Arias, H. Popper, D. Schachter, and D. A. Schafritz.
Raven Press, New York © 1982.

Chapter 44

Blood Coagulation

Robert W. Colman and Ronald N. Rubin

The liver plays several vital roles in the coagulation system. Hepatocytes are responsible for the synthesis of 11 proteins critical to the hemostatic mechanism. As illustrated in Table 1, these proteins include coagulation factors (fibrinogen, prothrombin, factors V, VII, IX, and XII, prekallikrein, and high molecular weight kininogen), critical inhibitor proteins (antithrombin III), and fibrinolytic proteins (plasminogen). Recent evidence suggests that the liver may have a role in factor VIII synthesis by producing the low molecular weight procoagulant portion (VIII:C)(1).

In addition to these synthetic functions, the liver, as an organ of the reticuloendothelial system, is a major clearance and catabolic organ for coagulation proteins. Many activated coagulant serine proteases, as well as plasminogen activators of the fibrinolytic system, are cleared and/or metabolized by the liver (2). The need for this clearance function is dramatically demonstrated, for example, by experience with the use of concentrates of vitamin K-related factors in the treatment of patients with hepatic failure complicated by hemorrhage. Such concentrates, which contain small amounts of activated clotting proteins (probably IXa and Xa), have been used successfully to "bypass" the factor VIII requirement in hemophiliac patients with antibodies to VIII (3). When given to cirrhotic patients, however, these same activated proteins are not cleared from the circulation, resulting in profound thrombotic diathesis, clinically manifested as major venous thrombosis and disseminated intravascular coagulation (4,5).

The liver may indirectly influence platelet count and function and thus impair primary hemostasis. Vascular changes in the liver which result in hypertension in the portal system eventually result in increased pressure and pooling in the spleen. Normally, 30% of the body platelet pool is sequestered in the spleen (6). Although these platelets are in equilibrium with and eventually are made available to the remainder of the total body pool, human spleens cannot contract to release such platelets rapidly to the general circulation. The sequestered platelets, therefore, are unavailable for immediate hemostatic functions. If the portal system is expanded and the spleen enlarged, common events in liver disease, the sequestered platelet pool increases. Massively enlarged spleens may sequester up to 90% of the body's platelets and result in thrombocytopenia and enhanced predisposition to hemorrhage (7,8). This situation exists in the patient with advanced cirrhosis, portal hypertension, and splenomegaly in which steady-state peripheral platelet count is 50 to 75,000 but total body platelet/megakarocyte mass as measured with radioisotopes is normal (7,8).

METHODS OF STUDY

Investigators have utilized several major techniques to define the role of the liver in regulation and/or synthesis of clotting proteins. A commonly employed method involves studying human subjects with severe hepatic damage (either acute, as with certain mushroom poisonings, or chronic, as in severe Laennec cirrhosis) and recording the effects of such damage on coagulation protein levels (9,10). Diminished levels imply a role for hepatic synthesis but do not rule out

TABLE 1. *Coagulation proteins and the liver*

Factor	Function	Molecular weight	Biologic half-life	Effects of hepatic disease
Fibrinogen (I)	Thrombin clottable protein	340,000	4 days	Significant reserve depressed only when liver failure severe; Dysfibrinogen variants in hepatoma and advanced cirrhosis
Prothrombin (II)	Precursor of thrombin	65,000	2–3 days	Vitamin K-dependent post-translational modification; synthesis decreased in liver disease
Factor V	Cofactor in common pathway to enhance prothrombin activation by factor Xa	290,000	1.5 days	Similar to fibrinogen, significant depression requires severe liver disease
Factor VII	Reacts with tissue thromboplastin to activate X (extrinsic pathway)	63,000	6 hr	Vitamin K-dependent post-translational modification; synthesis decreased in liver disease
Factor VIII	Cofactor in intrinsic pathway to enhance activation of factor X by factor IXa	180,000	8–12 hr	Small procoagulant portion may be synthesized in liver; traditionally a "nonhepatic" clotting protein
Factor IX	Contact phase of intrinsic coagulation pathway	50,000	24 hr	Vitamin K-dependent post-translational modification; synthesis decreased in liver disease
Factor X	In common pathway reaction with V, Ca^{2+}, and phospholipid, it activates prothrombin	60,000	3–4 days	Vitamin K-dependent post-translational modification; synthesis decreased in liver disease
Factor XI	Contact phase of intrinsic coagulation	160,000	4–5 days	Depressed in liver disease but less so than vitamin K group
Factor XII	Contact phase of intrinsic coagulation	80,000	4 days	Depressed in liver disease but less so than vitamin K group
Prekallikrein	Contact phase of intrinsic coagulation	88,000	3 days	Depressed in moderate liver disease (30%) and markedly in severe liver disease (0–12%)
High molecular weight kininogen	Cofactor of contact phase intrinsic coagulation	120,000	?	Depressed in liver disease but less so than vitamin K group
Factor XIII	Cross links and stabilizes fibrin clot	320,000	4 days	Decreased in liver disease

enhanced catabolism. This approach is further applied in animals whose livers are damaged experimentally by drugs or removed surgically; the effects on specific protein levels are noted (11–13). Turnover studies using radiolabeled proteins are also employed (14). Finally, elegant demonstrations involve the *in vitro* incubation of hepatocytes in culture or of liver slices and subsequent assay of the supernatant media for specific coagulation-related proteins (15,16) or treatment of the cells with immunofluorescent stains specific for clotting proteins (17).

The remainder of this chapter is devoted to the discussion of the role of the liver in the metabolism of specific clotting proteins. Where appropriate, illustrative clinical examples are referred to. Omitted are the vitamin K-dependent factors, II, VII, IX, and X, since vitamin K biotransformations are discussed in detail elsewhere in this volume.

Coagulation Proteins

Fibrinogen

Of the coagulation proteins synthesized by the liver, fibrinogen has been the object of most study because of its abundance and importance. Fbrinogen is a dimer composed of three chains (α_2, β_2, γ_2) with total molecular weight of 340,000 (18). The complete amino acid sequence of all three chains has been delineated. In normal plasma, about 15% of fibrinogen exists in a lower molecular weight but still clottable form, probably due to *in vivo* fibrinolysis. Nevertheless, most of its degradation is not related to consumption either by coagulation or fibrinolysis, since the half-life of 4 days is unaffected by either heparin anticoagulation or inhibition of fibrinolysis by epsilon-amino-caproic acid (19). It is likely that fibrinogen catabolism is intracellular, possibly in vascular endothelial cells. It has been shown that fibrinogen is synthesized in the liver using immunofluorescent staining techniques (17). Such evidence favors the hepatocyte rather than the Kupffer cell as the cell of origin (17), although this is not universally accepted (20). Experimental evidence suggests that fibrinogen synthesis may be controlled by feedback related not to circulating fibrinogen levels but to circulating levels of fibrinogen-fibrin degradation products (21,22).

In mild or moderate liver disease, the fibrinogen synthetic capacity is well maintained. Thus in certain early inflammatory or neoplastic diseases of the liver, fibrinogen behaves as an acute phase protein, and considerably elevated levels are found. For example, in early or moderate liver disease due to metastatic cancer, it is the rule rather than the exception to find the fibrinogen in excess of 500 mg% (23). Similarly, normal or elevated levels are seen in mild hepatitis (2). This behavior must be considered when one tries to interpret a "normal" fibrinogen level in such subjects. As hepatocyte function progressively deteriorates, fibrinogen levels in the 100 to 150 mg% range are observed, while in patients with fulminant hepatitis, fibrinogen concentrations in plasma may be less than 100 mg%. The lowest levels are indicative of severe and massive compromise of hepatocyte mass and are ominous prognostically (24).

Altered fibrinogen, a dysfibrinogen which is antigenically similar to fibrinogen but cannot function properly, has been described in the plasma of patients with hepatoma (25) and in patients with severe Laennec cirrhosis (26). The abnormality is a manifestation of a posttranslational defect in the fibrinogen molecule, specifically, an increase in sialic acid content, which renders the molecule less functional in its ability to form a clot (26). This finding is seen in advanced cases of cirrhosis and is a poor prognostic sign (26). This abnormality is detected by prolonged thrombin time in the face of clottable fibrinogen measurements in excess of 100 mg%, where a normal thrombin time is expected. Normal amounts of fibrinogen antigen are found.

Factor V

Factor V is similar to fibrinogen. Its molecular weight is in the 290,000 range, and its half-life is approximately 1.5 days. Both immunofluorescent staining techniques and isolated liver slice perfusion have demonstrated that the hepatocyte is the source of factor V (15,27). Its synthesis is clearly decreased in hepatocellular disease and, like fibrinogen, is much less sensitive than the vitamin K-dependent factors as a marker for cellular damage (26).

Factor VIII

Factor VIII is a large molecule with a molecular weight of more than 2 million and a plasma half-life in the range of 10 to 18 h. It is composed of a large subunit containing the VIII-related antigenic site and the von Willebrand factor responsible for platelet adhesiveness and a smaller subunit with factor VIII procoagulant activity. The VIII-related antigen (von Willebrand factor) appears to be synthesized by vascular endothelial cells (28). Evidence has been presented that the procoagulant fraction may be made in the liver (29). When trying to differentiate liver disease from consumptive coagulopathies, simultaneous measurements are often performed of factor VIII along with a protein synthesized in the liver but not usually consumed in coagulation, such as factor VII. If VIII alone is depressed, consumptive coagulopathy is often diagnosed. Although some investigations (30) indicate that this approach reliably distinguishes consumptive coagulopathy from liver disease, the great intrinsic variability in plasma VIII levels (increased with stress, oral contraceptives, fever) coupled with the data suggesting some hepatic role in factor VIII metabolism suggests caution in interpreting such studies.

Factors XI and XII, Prekallikrein, and High Molecular Weight Kininogen

These factors in the contact phase of intrinsic coagulation are synthesized in the liver (31). Data suggest that levels of these proteins are depressed in liver diseases; with the exception of prekallikrein, these changes are less sensitive than those of the vitamin K factors. Prekallikrein can be reduced to levels of 30% of normal in the presence of a normal prothrombin time (32).

Factor XIII

Factor XIII catalyzes the formation of covalent crosslinks between α- and γ-chains of fibrin, rendering the clot more stable and resistant to plasmin degradation. Evidence exists for its hepatic synthesis, but there are too few studies available to characterize its behavior in liver disease.

Inhibitors

Plasma contains five proteins that inhibit activated coagulation proteins. Table 2 lists the proteins, their molecular weight, concentration in plasma, and variation in liver disease. The bulk of the inhibitory activity resides in antithrombin III (At III), which accounts for 75% of plasma inhibitory activity against serine pro-

TABLE 2. *Inhibitors of blood coagulation*

Inhibitor	Function	Molecular weight	Grams per liter	Changes in liver
AT III	Major inhibitor of factors IXa, Xa, and thrombin provides 75% of plasma inhibition of serine proteases	62,000	0.29	Depressed in severe hepatocellular liver disease (cirrhosis); does not behave as acute phase protein
α-2-Antiplasmin	Major inhibitor of plasmin	67,000	0.07	Decreased in hepatic cirrhosis; level correlated with liver synthetic function
Cl inhibitor	Major inhibitor of factor XII and kallikrein	105,000	0.18	Deficiency results in angioneurotic edema syndrome; rarely decreased in liver disease although synthesized in liver
α-1-Antitrypsin	Major inhibitor of tissue proteases; Inhibits factor XIa	55,000	2.5	Deficiency results in cirrhosis and liver damage; acute phase reactant; mild elevation in liver disease
α-2-Macroglobulin	Secondary inhibition for many serine proteases	725,000	2.5	Mild elevation in cirrhosis

tease activity (33). The subsequent discussion centers on this protein, which is an α-2-globulin of molecular weight 62,000 daltons. Evidence for hepatic synthesis includes lowered levels in severe hepatic disease (34), although studies with liver tissue slices have yet to be reported. Its steady-state concentration in plasma is in the range of 0.22 to 0.37 g/liter. Like other inhibitor proteins, and unlike most coagulation proteins, this concentration is tightly controlled by undetermined mechanisms. Thus, unlike fibrinogen, for example, elevated levels of AT III are rarely encountered. AT III does not behave as an acute phase protein (34,35). The level is decreased in disseminated intravascular coagulation (35) and in congenital deficiency (36). The latter group manifests a significant thrombotic diathesis (36).

Table 3 demonstrates the profound depression of AT III in patients with parenchymal liver disease (Laennec cirrhosis and alcoholic hepatitis). There is a rough correlation between depression of AT III and elevation of the prothrombin time in such patients. Of interest is the fact that patients with metastatic liver disease do not have depressed AT III levels. This finding cannot be explained on the basis of an elevation of an acute phase reactant secondary to neoplastic disease coupled with hepatic metastases and decreased hepatic synthetic capacity (34). Thus AT III synthesis appears to be affected only be general insults to the liver affecting essentially all the hepatocytes (as in cirrhosis), while metastatic deposits, which are likely to spare hepatocyte function in many areas, do not significantly affect AT III synthesis.

α 2-Plasmin Inhibitor

α-2-Plasmin inhibitor (α-2-PI), a recently identified plasma protein, physiologically is the most important inhibitor of plasmin (37–39). The reaction between plasmin and α-2-PI is very rapid and results in the formation of a 1:1 stoichiometric inactive complex. The α-2-PI inhibits fibrin clot dissolution in three ways: (a) in plasma, it inhibits plasmin; (b) in the fibrin network, it interferes with plasminogen binding (40); and (c) it is incorporated in the clot by factor XIIIa, rendering the fibrin relatively resistant to fibrinolysis (41). Congenital deficiency results in severe hemorrhagic state following trauma (42). The concentration of α-2-PI is decreased in hepatic cirrhosis, and the level is correlated with liver synthetic function (43). The decrease provides another mechanism for the increased fibrinolytic activity found in cirrhosis.

Cl-Inhibitor

C1 inhibitor inhibits kallikrein, plasmin, and complement via formation of 1:1 stoichometric inactive complexes (46). Congenital deficiency results in hereditary angioedema (47) but no hemostatic disturbance. Im-

TABLE 3. *Antithrombin III levels in hepatic disease states*[a]

Patient group	AT III level	
	Functional (%)	Immunological (mg %)
Normal (N = 75)	100 ± 18	25 ± 7
Laennec cirrhosis and alcoholic hepatitis (N = 21)	32 ± 20	7 ± 2.9
Cancer with hepatic metastasis (N = 51)	106 ± 22	25.7 ± 8.4
Cancer without hepatic mestastasis	101 ± 20	24.7 ± 7

[a] From ref. 34.

munofluorescent studies suggest that the liver is the site of synthesis (48). No decrease in C1 inhibitor has been documented in liver disease. Its role is probably the regulation of the activity of Hageman factor-dependent pathways.

α-1-Antitrypsin

Although α-1-antitrypsin is the most abundant proteolytic enzyme inhibitor, its role in hemostasis appears minor. Congenital deficiency results in proteolytic destruction of lung tissue without thrombotic or hemorrhagic tendency. Inhibition of thrombin and plasmin are slow, and the role of factor XIa inhibition is unknown. Liver disease is associated with increased levels of α-1-antitrypsin.

α-2-Macroglobulin

α-2-Macroglobulin binds a variety of proteases, including kallikrein, plasmin, and thrombin (49). A part of the proteolytic activity may still be expressed after binding. While not an acute phase reactant, it rises in liver disease. Congenital deficiency (50) has been detected in an asymptomatic individual.

Impaired Hepatic Clearance

In addition to the impaired synthetic functions of liver disease and their consequences for coagulation and fibrinolysis, hepatic clearance and metabolic functions also are impaired and have a significant influence on hemostasis.

One such function involves the clearance of activated coagulation proteins. The half-life in the circulation of factor Xa is 3 to 4 min rather than 3 to 4 days for the zymogen factor X (51). Survival of factor Xa in experimental animals however, is prolonged when the liver is excluded from the circulation (51); thus when coagulation is activated, the activated proteases persist, predisposing to disseminated intravascular coagulation. A similar situation occurs with plasminogen activators and plasmin removal from the circulation. In severe liver disease, activation of the fibrinolytic system may be attributable to impaired clearance of these substances (52–54). Such activation clearly occurs in lower animals, such as the rat, in which plasmin is taken up by the liver and excreted in the bile (54). In man, "primary fibrinolysis" has been reported in a variety of liver diseases (52–54); however, whether all such reported instances were fibrinolysis is controversial, since other etiologies for abnormal fibrinogen catabolism, such as dysfibrinogenemia (25,26), and disseminated intravascular coagulation (53,54), are probably far more common. Primary fibrinogenolysis due to impaired clearance of

plasmin and plasminogen activators probably occurs only rarely because of severe liver disease, most likely in the setting of liver transplantation and fulminant acute liver necrosis.

A more common hemostatic defect related to impaired hepatic clearance involves fibrinogen/fibrin degradation products (FDP). It is well known that elevations of FDP are common in moderate to severe liver disease (24,53,54). The genesis of such FDP is controversial and has been the subject of reviews (55). These FDP have been attributed to low-grade disseminated intravascular coagulation in hepatic disease (24,56), to increased catabolism of an abnormal fibrinogen synthesized in liver disease (26,53), to increased catabolism and absorption of extravascular fibrinogen in ascites (53), and, finally, as described previously, to the presence of primary fibrinolysis itself. Regardless of their genesis, the FDP are cleared in part by the reticuloendothelial system of the liver (57). Serious liver diseases, therefore, result in increases of FDP to detectable and biologically active levels. Once in the circulation in significant titers, the FDP exert specific activities on the coagulation system. These include antithrombin activity with prolongation of the thrombin time (58), interference with normal fibrinogen polymerization (59), and antiplatelet properties that induce abnormal platelet function with a prolonged bleeding time (60). All these phenomenon have been reported in liver diseases ranging from Laennec cirrhosis to chronic active hepatitis (53,56). As expected, the FDP, elevated as a result of impaired hepatic clearance functions, often aggravated the already compromised coagulation function in these patients.

Hemostatic Testing in Liver Disease

Traditionally, assessment of the coagulation system has been utilized in the study of hepatic disease. As has been described in this chapter and elsewhere in this text, the intimate dependence of the coagulation system on hepatic synthetic and metabolic pathways makes such testing logical. Problems arise in interpretation, however, because of the extremely complex interplay between synthesis and catabolism of coagulation proteases and coagulation inhibitors, all of which are influenced by liver function. Thus the use of specific clotting assays to help define a specific liver disease or its prognosis is limited. The most sensitive and valuable set of tests remains the prothrombin time and the partial thromboplastin time, especially when measured after vitamin K therapy. Hepatic damage significant enough to impair hepatic synthetic function will result in abnormalities in these tests. The prognostic significance depends on whether or not the insult to the liver is reversible. Other investigators have reported prognostic significance when specific clotting factors, such as V (24) and VII (61), are very low; but most studies have involved a small number of patients, and not all investigators agree with these findings. In addition, the platelet count in such patients may be useful since the incidence of hypersplenism is quite high.

Management of Hemostatic Failure in Liver Disease

A patient with liver disease may manifest any of a number of coagulation abnormalities during the course of the disease, ranging from decreased platelets, decreased coagulation function, and enhanced fibrinolysis due to impaired clearance of plasminogen activators. Specific therapy depends on specific diagnosis. Before implementing treatment, therefore, it may be necessary to go beyond the routine screening tests of prothrombin time, partial thromboplastin time, and platelet count. In the instance of hepatic failure complicated by hemorrhage, additional studies, such as fibrinogen, FDP, and platelet function, may be needed. The following therapeutic approaches have been used in this group of patients: (a) platelet concentrates, (b) fresh plasma, (c) prothrombin complex concentrates, and (d) heparin. Since there is always a possibility of vitamin K deficiency, a course of parenteral vitamin K should be given.

Platelet concentrates should not be withheld from a bleeding patient with thrombocytopenia less than 75,000, regardless of the presumed or proven etiology. However, such transfusions often do not result in significant increments or clinical effects, since the transfused platelets equilibrate between the spleen and peripheral blood in the same ratio as existed prior to transfusion. Thus massive transfusions may be needed to effect marginal platelet increments in the peripheral blood.

In theory, fresh frozen plasma is optimal for patients with hepatocellular disease. It contains adequate amounts of prothrombin complex proteins and, in addition, contains the labile proteins V and VIII, which are lost in bank blood (62). The limiting factor, however, is the volume required to replace the factors. For 50% of clotting activity, for example, between 1 and 2 liters are required (8). Since several of the proteins, notably factor VII, have short half-lives, frequent therapy is required to retain hemostatic levels. Many patients with liver failure, already overloaded with salt and water, tolerate such volumes very poorly (63). For acute problems, however, fresh frozen plasma may be used with reasonably acceptable results.

Prothrombin complex concentrates are obtained from barium salt eluates of plasma or ion exchange chromatography and are extremely potent sources of the vitamin K-dependent factors II, VII, IX, and X. Other factors which are synthesized in the liver but are not vitamin K-dependent, such as factor V, are not supplied by this material. These complexes, therefore, may not completely correct hepatic failure in patients requiring surgery or with severe bleeding, as reported by several investigators (63–65). Several strong contraindications have prevented more widespread use of prothrombin complex concentrates. It has been reported that up to 30% of recipients may contract hepatitis (66,67). Such a complication can be disastrous in a patient with existing severe hepatic disease. Another frequently reported complication is thrombosis and even disseminated intravascular coagulation in patients with hepatic failure given such concentrates (68,69). Such thrombotic complications are caused by the presence of activated clotting proteins, especially Xa and IXa, which cannot be metabolized and cleared adequately by the diseased liver (69,70). Recently, attempts to obviate this problem have included modified concentrates which contain heparin and less of the measurable activated factors and/or addition of fresh frozen plasma to elevate AT III levels which will complex the activated proteins (63). Although some investigators use such concentrates, many avoid their use in patients with significant liver failure.

Heparin has been shown to increase fibrinogen half-life in patients with cirrhosis (71). Disseminated intravascular coagulation does complicate certain liver diseases, and improvement in hemostatic functions in patients given heparin has been reported (71–73). The use of this anticoagulant in liver disease is controversial; we rarely use heparin in hepatic patients with hemostatic disorders. Similarly, although a fibrinolytic inhibitor, such as epsilon-amino-caproic acid has been used to treat the proposed fibrinolytic state in certain liver patients (2,8), its utility remains to be established by further studies.

ACKNOWLEDGMENTS

This work was partially supported by SCOR grant HC-14217 and by research grant HL-24365 from the National Institutes of Health.

REFERENCES

1. Shaw, E., Giddings, J. C., Peake, I. R., and Bloom, A. L. (1979): Synthesis of procoagulant factor VIII, factor VIII related antigen and other coagulation factors by the isolated perfused rat liver. *Br. J. Haematol.,* 41:585.
2. Roberts, H. R., and Cedarbaum, A. I. (1972): The liver and blood coagulation. Physiology and pathology. *Gastroenterology,* 63:297.

3. Sonoda, T., Solomon, A., Krauss, S., Cruz, P., and Levin, J. (1976): Use of prothrombin complexes concentrates in the treatment of a hemophiliac patient with an inhibitor of factor VIII. *Blood*, 47:983.

4. Blatt, P. M., Lundblad, R. L., Kingdon, H. S., McLean, G., and Roberts, H. R. (1974): Thrombogenic materials in prothrombin complex concentrates. *Ann. Int. Med.*, 81:766.

5. Rubin, R. N. (1977): Disseminated intravascular coagulation. *Transfusion*, 17:198.

6. Aster, R. H. (1966): Pooling of platelets in the spleen: Role in the pathogenesis of "hypersplenic" thrombocytopenia. *J. Clin. Invest.*, 45:645.

7. Harker, L. A., and Finch, C. A. (1969): Thrombokinetics in man. *J. Clin. Invest.*, 48:963.

8. Penny, R., Rosenberg, M. C., and Firkin, B. G. (1966): The splenic platelet pool. *Blood*, 27:1.

9. Smith, H. P., Warner, E., and Brinkhous, K. M. (1937): Prothrombin deficiency and the bleeding tendency in liver injury. *J. Exp. Med.*, 66:801.

10. Rapaport, S. I., Ames, S., Mikkelson, S., and Goodman, J. R. (1960): Plasma clotting factors in chronic hepatocellular disease. *N. Engl. J. Med.*, 263–278.

11. Andrus, W.D.E.W., Lord, J. W., Jr., and Moore, R. A. (1939): The effect of hepatectomy on the plasma prothrombin and the utilization of vitamin K. *Surgery*, 6:899.

12. Zucker, M. B., Siegal, M., Cliffton, E. E., Bellville, J. W., Howland, W. S., and Grossi, C. E. (1957): The effect of hepatic lobectomy on some blood clotting factors and on fibrinolysis. *Ann. Surg.*, 146:772.

13. Mann, F. D., Shonyo, E. S., and Mann, F. C. (1951): Effects of removal of the liver on blood coagulation. *Am J. Physiol.* 164:111.

14. Hawker, R. J., and Hawker, L. M. (1976): A rapidly produced I^{125} labelled autogenous fibrinogen: In vitro properties and preliminary metabolic studies in man. *J. Clin. Pathol.* 29:495.

15. Olson, J. P., Miller, L. L., and Troup, S. B. (1966): Synthesis of clotting factors by isolated perfused rat livers. *J. Clin. Invest.*, 45:690.

16. Kazmier, F. J., Spiffell, J. A., Bowie, E. J. W., Thompson, J. H., and Owen, C. A. (1968): Release of vitamin K dependent coagulation factors by isolated perfused rat liver. *Am. J. Physiol.*, 214:919.

17. Foreman, W. B., and Barnhart, M. I., (1964): Cellular site for fibrinogen synthesis. *JAMA*, 187:128.

18. Doolittle, R. F. (1975): Fibrinogen and fibrin. In: *The Plasma Proteins*, p. 109. Academic Press, New York.

19. Collen, D., Tygat, N., Claez, H., and Piessous, R: (1972): Metabolism and distribution of fibrinogen. I. Fibrinogen turnover in physiological conditions in humans. *Br. J. Haematol.*, 22:681.

20. Hamashima, Y., Harter, J., and Loons, A. (1964): The localization of albumin and fibrinogen in human liver cells. *J. Cell Biol.*, 20:271.

21. Barnhart, M. I., Cress, D. C., Nooman, S. M., and Forman, W. B. (1970): Influence of fibrinolytic products on hepatic release and synthesis of fibrinogen. *Thromb. Diath. Haemorrh.* [*Suppl.*], 39:143.

22. Kessler, C. M., and Bell, W. R. (1980): Stimulation of fibrinogen synthesis: A possible functional role of fibrinogen degradation. *Blood*, 55:40.

23. Keis, M. K., Posch, J. J., and Rubin, R. N. (1980): Hemostatic function in cancer patients. *Cancer*, 46:831–837.

24. Dymock, I. W., Tucher, J. S., Woolf, I. L., Poller, L., and Thompson, J. M. (1975): Coagulation studies as a prognostic index in acute liver failure. *Br. J. Haematol.*, 29:385.

25. Gralnick, H. R., Givelbar, H., and Abrams, E. (1978): Dysfibrinogenemia associated with hepatoma. *N. Engl. J. Med.*, 299:221.

26. Martinez, J., Palarcarl, J. E., and Kwasniak, D. (1978): Abnormal sialic acid content of the dysfibrinogenemia associated with liver disease. *J. Clin. Invest*, 61:535.

27. Barnhart, M. I., Ferar, J., and Aoki, H. (1963): Demonstration of globulin in bovine hepatocytes. *Fed. Proc.*, 22:164.

28. Jaffe, E. A., Hoyer, L. W., and Nachman, R. L. (1973): Synthesis of antihemophiliac factor antigen by cultured endothelial cells. *J. Clin. Invest.*, 52:2757.

29. Owen, C. A., Jr., Bowie, E. J. W., and Fass, D. N. (1979): Generation of factor VII coagulant activity by isolated, perfused neonatal pig livers and adult rat livers. *Br. J. Haematol.*, 43:307.

30. Corrigan, J. J., Jr., Bennett, B. B., and Buflee, B. (1973): The value of factor VIII levels in acquired hypofibrinogenemia. *Am. J. Clin. Pathol.*, 60:897.

30a. Colman, R. W., Robboy, S. J., and Minna, J. D. (1979): Disseminated intravascular coagulation: A reappraisal. *Ann. Rev. Med.*, 30:355.

31. Wong, P. Y., Talamo, R. C., and Williams, G. H. (1981): Kallikrein-kinin and renin angiotensin systems in functional renal failure in cirrhosis of the liver. (*In press.*)

32. Wong, P. Y., Colman, R. W., Talamo, R. L., and Babior, B. M. (1972): Kallikrein bradykinin system in chronic alcoholic liver disease. *Ann. Intern. Med.*, 77:205.

33. Rosenberg, R. R. (1975): Actions and interactions of antithrombin and heparin. *N. Engl. J. Med.*, 292:146.

34. Rubin, R. N., Posch, J. J., and Kies, M. K. (1980): Measurements of antithrombin III in solid tumor patients with and without hepatic metastases. *Thromb. Res.*, 18:353–360.

35. Bick, R. L., Dukes, M. L., Wilson, W. L., and Follete I.F. (1977): Antithrombin III (AT III) as a diagnostic aid in disseminated intravascular coagulation. *Thromb. Res.*, 10:721.

36. Von Kaulla, E., and Von Kaulla, K. M. (1972): Deficiency of anti-thrombin III activity associated with hereditary thrombosis tendency. *J. Med.*, 3:349.

37. Moroi, M., and Aoki, N. (1976): Isolation and characterization α2 plasmin inhibitor from human plasma. A novel proteinase inhibitor which inhibits activator induced clot lysis. *J. Biol. Chem.*, 251:5956.

38. Collen, D. (1976): Identification and some properties of a new fast reacting plasmin inhibitor in human plasma. *Eur. J. Biochem.*, 69:209.

39. Mullertz, S., and Qemmensen, I. (1976): The primary inhibitor of plasmin in human plasma. *Biochem. J.*, 159:545.

40. Aoki, N., Moroi M., and Tachiya, K. (1978): Effects of α2 plasmin inhibitor on fibrin lysis. Its comparison with α2 macroglobulin. *Thromb. Haemostas.*, 39:22.

41. Sahata, Y., and Aoki, N. (1980): Cross-linking of α2 plasmin inhibitor to fibrin by fibrin stabilizing factor. *J. Clin. Invest.*, 65:290.

42. Harpel, P. C. (1976): CI inactivator. In: *Methods in Enzymology*, *Vol. 45*, edited by L. Lorand, p. 751. Academic Press, New York.

43. Aoki, N., and Yamanaka, T. (1978): The α2-plasmin inhibitor levels in liver diseases. *Clin. Chem. Acta*, 84:99.

44. Harpel, P. C., Mosesson, M. W., and Cooper, N. R. (1975): Studies on the structure and function of α2-monoglobulin and CI-inactivator. In: *Proteases and Biological Controls*, edited by E. Reich, D. B. Rifkin, and E. Shaw, p. 387. Cold Spring Harbor Laboratory, New York.

45. Heck, L. W., and Kaplan, A. P. (1974): Substrates of Hageman factor. I. Isolation and characterization of human factor XI (PTA) and inhibition of the activated enzyme by α1-antitrypsin. *J. Exp. Med.*, 140:1615.

46. Harpel, P. C., and Cooper, N. R. (1975): Studies on human plasma CI inactivation-enzyme interactions. I. Mechanisms of interaction with CI, plasmin and trypsin. *J. Clin. Invest.*, 55:593.

47. Donaldson, V. H., and Evans, R. R. (1963): A biochemical abnormality in hereditary angioneurotic edema. Absence of serum inhibitor of C′ l-esterase. *Am. J. Med.*, 35:37.

48. Johnson, A. M., Alper, C. A., Rosen, F. S., and Craig, J. M. (1971): CI inhibitor: Evidence for decreased hepatic synthesis in hereditary angioneurotic edema. *Science*, 173:553.

49. Harpel, P. C., and Rosenberg, R. D. (1979): α2-Macroglobulin deficiency. *Scand. J. Haematol.*, 23:443.

50. Bergquist, D., and Nilsson, I. M. Hereditary α2-macroglobulin deficiency. *Scand. J. Haemetol.*, 23:433.

51. Deykin, D. (1966): The role of the liver in serum-induced hyper-coaguability. *J. Clin. Invest.*, 45:256.
52. Fletcher, A. P., Biederman, O., Moore, D., Alkjaersig, N., and Sherry, S. (1964): Abnormal plasminogen-plasma system activity (fibrinolysis) in patients with hepatic cirrhosis: Its cause and consequences. *J. Clin. Invest.*, 43:681.
53. Bloom, A. (1975): Intravascular coagulation and the liver. *Br. J. Haematol.*, 30:1.
54. Owen, C. A., Jr., and Bowie, E. J. W. (1974): Chronic intravascular coagulation. *Thromb. Diath. Haemorrh.*, 33:107.
55. Straub, P. W. (1974): A case against heparin therapy of intravascular coagulation. *Thromb. Diath. Haemorrh.*, 33:107.
56. Clark, R. D., Gazzard, B. G., Lewis, M. L., Flute, P. T., and Williams, R. (1975): Fibrinogen metabolism in acute hepatitis and active chronic hepatitis. *Br. J. Haematol.*, 30:95.
57. Heene, D. L. (1977): Disseminated intravascular coagulation: Evaluation of therapeutic approaches. *Semin. Thromb. Hemostas.* 4:291.
58. Marder, V. J., and Shulman, N. E. (1969): High molecular weight derivatives. Human fibrinogen produced by plasmin. II. Mechanisms of their anticoagulant activity. *J. Biol. Chem.*, 244:2120.
59. Marder, V. J., and Budzynski, A. Z. (1974): Fibrinogen and its derivatives, hereditary and acquired abnormalities. *Schweiz. Med. Wochenschr.*, 104:1338.
60. Cronberg. S. (1975): Effect of fibrinolysis on adhesion and aggregation of human platelets. *Thromb. Diath. Haemorrh.*, 14:202.
61. Green, G., Poller, L., Thomson, I., and Dymocl, I. W. (1976): Factor VII as a marker of hepatocellular synthetic function in liver disease. *J. Clin. Pathol.* 29:271.
62. Goldstein, R., Bunker, J. P., and McGovern, J. J. (1964): The effect of storage of whole blood and anticoagulants upon certain coagulation factors. *Ann. NY Acad. Sci.*, 115:422.
63. Mannucci, P. M., Franchi, F., and Diognardi, N. (1976): Correction of abnormal coagulation in chronic liver disease by combined use of fresh-frozen plasma and prothrombin complex concentrations in liver disease. *Lancet*, 2:542.
64. Green, G., Dymoch, I. W., Pollen, L., and Thromson, J. M. (1975): Use of factor VII rich prothrombin complex concentrates in liver disease. *Lancet*, 1:1311.
65. Gazzard, B. G., Henderson, J. M., and Williams, R. (1975): The use of fresh frozen plasma or a concentrate of factor IX as replacement of therapy before liver biopsy. *Gut*, 16:621.
66. Wyke, R. J., Tsraquaye, K. N., Thorton, A., White, Y., Portman, B., Das, P. K., Zuckerman, A., and Williams, R. (1979): Transmission of non A non B hepatitis to chimpanzees by factor IX concentrates after fatal complications in patients with chronic liver disease. *Lancet*, 1:520.
67. Grammens, G. L., and Breckinridge, R. T. (1974): Complications of Christmas factor (factor IX) concentrates. *Ann. Intern. Med.*, 80:666.
68. Marassi, A., DiCarlo, V., Manzullo, V., and Manucci, P. M. (1978): Thromboembolism following prothrombin complex concentrates and major surgery in severe liver disease. *Thromb. Haemostas.*, 39:787.
69. Blatt, P. M., Lundblag, R. L., Kingdon, H. S., and Roberts, H. K. (1972): Thrombogenic materials in prothrombin complex concentrates. *Ann. Intern. Med.*, 81:766.
70. Hultin, M. B. (1979): Activated clotting factors in factor IX concentrates. *Blood*, 54:1028.
71. Coleman, M., Finlayson, M., Bettigole, R. I., Sadula, D., Cohn, M., and Pasmantier, M. (1975): Fibrinogen survival in cirrhosis: Improvement by low dise heparin. *Ann. Intern. Med.*, 83:73–78.
72. Rake, M. O., Flute, P. T., Shilkin, K. B., Lewis, M. L., Winch, J., and Williams, R. (1971): Early and intensive therapy of intravascular coagulation in acute liver failure. *Lancet*, 2:1215.
73. Tytgat, G. M., Collen, D., and Verstaete, M. (1971): Metabolism of fibrinogen in cirrhosis of the liver. *J. Clin. Invest.*, 50:1690.

Pathobiologic Analysis of Major Disease Mechanisms

The Liver: Biology and Pathobiology, edited by
I. Arias, H. Popper, D. Schachter, and D. A. Shafritz.
Raven Press, New York © 1982.

Chapter 45

Hepatocellular Degeneration and Death

Hans Popper

The mechanism of death of hepatocytes, a key phenomenon in virtually all hepatic diseases, is still poorly understood. The exception is rapid interruption of cellular respiration, as in cyanide poisoning, when cell death is not expressed in any morphologic, even ultrastructural, alteration, and the vital appearance is fixed in the specimen. Otherwise, most forms of hepatocellular death are step-like processes (1), which are recognized in light microscopic and fine structural lesions. Earlier steps may be more specific for the etiologic factor; later steps involve a common terminal pathway. An understanding of these different steps provides an opportunity for therapeutic intervention even after the initial events have occurred (2). Investigation of hepatocellular death, therefore, is one of the most promising and challenging tasks of basic research in hepatology.

These considerations call for definitions. Cell death is the state of equilibrium precluding any vital function; the cells have either disintegrated or appear as remnants or debris. Necrosis represents a step-like process leading to an irreversible state (3,4). Hepatocellular degeneration is the precursor lesion preceding but not necessarily leading to necrosis and death.

In the definition of degeneration, the separation from a physiologic response, part of which is adaptation to an altered milieu, is difficult. Environmental and endogenous factors perturb the normal equilibrium, including imbalance of metabolites or accumulation of xenobiotics, to which the cell responds by genetically determined reactions (5). Only if a status unfavorable to the cell or organism results, degeneration or injury can be assumed. Steatosis is an example of an unfavorable state, although it need not be associated with measurable dysfunction. The irreversible step that terminates in necrosis (the point of no return) (6), is difficult to identify. Thus hepatocellular injury and death are discussed as (a) morphologic expressions, with emphasis on human lesions, (b) mechanisms, mainly explored in experimental animals, (c) target structures, and (d) briefly, human diseases with acute hepatic failure.

MORPHOLOGIC EXPRESSIONS OF HEPATOCYTIC INJURY AND DEATH

Three forms of cell death are recognized. One, only recently described, is apoptosis, which is postulated to be the normal turnover of cells, including hepatocytes, and represents a physiologic process. The name was coined in analogy to mitosis and implies a "falling off" of cells (7,8). The cytoplasm in scattered cells condenses and, simultaneously, nuclear alterations occur. After budding of cytoplasmic portions, small cell fragments form, which characteristically contain parts of the nucleus and in which cytoplasmic organelles appear preserved. These apoptotic bodies usually are too small to be recognized by light microscopy. The exceptions are larger acidophilic round bodies, which, despite their rarity, are considered to be the light microscopic hallmark of apoptosis. Apoptotic fragments are taken up by phagocytosis by neighboring, epithelial and mesenchymal cells, including macrophages, and are digested by lysosomes without release of bioactive substances which lead to the characteristic inflammation of other forms of necrosis. This silent, or nonreactive, disappearance of single cells found in normal cell turnover is conspicuously accentuated during resorption of the tail of the tadpole, in involution of endocrine organs, in tumors after chemotherapy, after radiation, and in experimentally induced lymphocytotoxicity (9). The claim has been made that the periportal disappearance of hepatocytes in chronic active hepatitis results from apoptosis (10), which would separate the inflammatory reaction in the disease from hepatocellular necrosis, a concept that is not yet fully accepted. Further studies are required to identify the role of apoptosis in liver disease.

The second form of cell death is cytolysis, which usually involves groups of cells (11). Release of bioactive substances results in inflammation with accumulation of specialized and active mesenchymal cells and eventual fibroplasia. Since the disintegration of the cell is usually rapid, morphologic visualization by static morphologic techniques is difficult and requires cinematographic techniques, which have only barely been applied to hepatocytes *in vivo*. The only recognizable expression is cell blisters, which appear on electron microscopy to rupture; but artifacts cannot be excluded. In common histologic usage, focal cytolytic necrosis is recognized by accumulation of reactive inflammatory cells replacing lost hepatocytes, with macrophages that contain PAS-positive granules participating to varying degrees. The recent recognition of lymphocytotoxicity and secretion of bioactive agents by macrophages (12) makes morphologic separation of the scavenger action of inflammatory cells from their contribution to cell death difficult.

Morphologically better defined is the third form, "coagulative" necrosis, as exemplified by contiguous remnants of cells, as occurs in hypoxia or by the acidophilic body. Conventionally, the latter is considered to result from water loss caused by presumed membrane changes. The organelles are preserved in a dark lyophilized cell, which is expelled from the liver cell plate and lies in the tissue spaces, with or without pycnotic nuclei (13). Its subsequent uptake by macrophages indicates cell death. Although apoptosis may also result in the formation of acidophilic bodies, their association with "dark" hepatocytes with reduced water content in the surrounding parenchyma supports the coagulative necrotic nature of the cells.

By light microscopy, it is difficult to recognize hepatocellular degeneration because of fixation and processing vagaries, which obscure subtle changes. The functional deficit in nonfatal acute hepatitis of any etiology is reflected in variations in size and staining qualities of cytoplasm and nuclei of neighboring hepatocytes, independent of necrosis (14,15). These alterations are reflected in the transmission electron microscope by various changes in hepatocytic organelles, such as shattering of the rough endoplasmic reticulum, loss of attachment and disappearance of polysomes, variations in mitochondria, alterations of microvilli of the sinusoidal cell membrane, and increased endocytosis (16,17). Several histochemical alterations (for instance, loss of glucose-6-phosphatase and oxidative enzymes) support the electron microscopic findings. However, the heterogeneity of the enzyme distribution and the functional capacity of hepatocytes throughout the lobule or acinus must be taken into consideration (18,19) in interpreting degenerative processes.

Enzymes that reflect oxidative energy metabolism, gluconeogenesis, and transferases, including glucuronidation (20), are located preferentially around the portal tracts; glycolysis, lipogenesis, and oxidative biotransformation predominantly occur around the hepatic vein tributaries. To what degree gradients in oxygen and hormone concentrations or variations in innervation are responsible for these features is not established. Bile acids are secreted almost entirely by hepatocytes around the portal tracts (21). Necrosis and degeneration of hepatocytes in one zone result in compensatory takeover of the function by another zone (22), all of which complicates the histochemical interpretation. These variations also determine localization of lesions in the acinus of Rappaport (18), which distinguishes the oxygen-rich zone 1 around the portal tracts, the intermediate zone, and the relatively oxygen-poor zone around the hepatic vein tributaries. Necrosis induced by metabolites of many toxic agents [e.g., carbon tetrachloride (CCl_4) and acetaminophen] occurs in zone 3, primarily because of the preferential localization of biotransformation, coupled with protection by the conjugating activity preferentially localized in zone 1. Immunohistochemical variations in visualized proteins, such as albumin, fibrinogen, or alpha$_1$-antitrypsin, and sometimes of nondefined proteinic cytoplasmic inclusions (23), are usually an expression of impaired secretion of the proteins (24). Autophagy by lysosomes of cytoplasmic components is a normal turnover of organelles. It is increased in any type of nonspecific stress (25); and in focal cytoplasmic degeneration, injured portions of the parenchyma are digested by an energy-dependent process (26).

Morphologic expression and functional evaluation of degeneration are vaguer than that of necrosis. Focal necrosis need not cause a significant functional deficit if the function of surrounding hepatocytes is not altered. In most liver diseases, therefore, the number and status of viable hepatocytes determine the functional deficit (27). Viability need not be reflected in the morphologic appearance. This is illustrated in an experimental counterpart of fulminant hepatic failure, which develops in rabbits a few days after receiving galactosamine intravenously (28). The animals die in coma, with biochemical evidence of fulminant hepatic failure. The hepatocytes, however, are almost all present, although they show degeneration with karyorrhexis and acidophilic bodies; silver impregnation shows a fully preserved lobular architecture.

Zone 3 necrosis is produced more frequently by circulatory and toxic factors. Periportal zone 1 necrosis is associated with hepatitis resulting from immunologic attack, prolonged cholestasis, and, occasionally, circulatory and toxic factors; the latter occur mainly in experimental animals, as produced by allyl alcohol, for example.

Necrosis of hepatocytes causes hepatic failure when massive and submassive necrosis remove hepatocytes from a large portion of the liver, as occurs in viral hepatitis and some drug-induced lesions (29). This is in keeping with observations in animals and man that a large portion of the liver can be excised without causing hepatic failure or significant functional deficiency as detected by conventional hepatic tests (30). Even with extensive necrosis, the remaining viable hepatocytes determine the functional deficit and explain the difficulty in distinguishing morphologically patients with acute hepatic failure. Reversibility to normal function of viable hepatocytes cannot be recognized morphologically, which explains the difficulty in evaluating the degree of hepatic insufficiency and the prognosis of severe chronic active or alcoholic hepatitis, when most hepatocytes are altered but present. Quantitative parameters of the functional hepatic mass, measured, for instance, by galactose clearance (31), are neither practical nor informative. Examination of biopsy specimens of patients in acute hepatic failure does not provide a reliable criterion. In the few cases in which such biopsies have been obtained, morphometrically determined loss of hepatocytic volume (i.e., reduction in the volume fraction of preserved hepatocytes from 85 to 95% to less than 28 to 35% of total liver) and decreasing glycogen content have been considered unfavorable signs regarding prognosis (32,33). The regenerative potential of the hepatocytes may not be the key factor in survival (162).

Hepatic failure in man is more often determined by the function of remaining viable hepatocytes than by the loss of hepatocytes. This is particularly exemplified by cases of hepatic failure associated with diffuse steatosis.

A third cause of human hepatic failure, besides dysfunction and necrosis of hepatocytes, is hepatic circulatory insufficiency, which is characteristic of cirrhosis (35). The hepatic parenchyma suffers from insufficient perfusion by blood, which bypasses the lobular parenchyma through extrahepatic collaterals and intrahepatic anastomoses between afferent and efferent blood vessels. This shunting deprives the organism of function by the liver, independent of functional status of hepatocytes.

MECHANISM OF HEPATOCYTIC DEATH

Most processes associated with hepatocellular necrosis have been studied in experimental animals. Apoptosis, in contrast to the other forms of cell death, is not accompanied by the processes discussed below. For example, apoptosis is not preceded by loss of cellular energy (reflected in reduction of high-energy nucleotides) or by changes in plasma membrane permeability, nor is it associated with inflammation related to release of irritating bioactive substances in the step-like process of the common forms of necrosis. Regeneration, which is stimulated by necrosis (either by deficit of functional tissue or by release of growth-stimulating factors) is not induced by apoptosis.

In the complex mechanism of hepatocellular degeneration leading to cell death, all cell constituents are eventually altered; it is difficult, therefore, to distinguish primary from secondary events. In an excellent review that provides much information and detailed literature on the problems, Farber (36) emphasizes that cell death does not simply result from "interference with one or more of its metabolic functions" but requires a specific disarrangement, still to be established, which is a potential target of therapeutic intervention. In the processes listed below, an attempt is made to distinguish those causing necrosis from those that do not.

Hypoxia

In experimental animals, limitation of oxygen supply is readily reproducible, and degree and duration can be quantitated. It reduces the NAD/NADH and ATP/ADP ratios and leads to disintegration of polysomes with reduction of ribosomes, loss of effectiveness of transfer RNA (37–39), and alterations of intercellular gap junctions (40). Degradation of phospholipids, including those of the plasma membrane, is accelerated (41); in this respect, chlorpromazine has a stabilizing effect (42). Cytosolic factors have been incriminated in reducing protein synthesis (37). Hypoxia, however, is also a secondary effect in many processes leading to necrosis, in part explained by interference with circulation, which has been well delineated for many experimental conditions (43). For example, in early acetaminophen intoxication, hepatocellular alterations are associated with centrolobular congestion from hepatocellular swelling and detached sinusoidal cells (44). Hypoxia may be the most frequent cause of cell death in human disease.

The mechanism has been explored more extensively in tissues other than the liver (4,45), but the principles can be extrapolated to the hepatocytes. Five stages are postulated (4). Basically, decrease in ATP with increase of ADP stimulates glycolysis. Glycogen is rapidly depleted, and lactate accumulates, decreasing cellular pH, which is also favored by an increase in phosphates. The decrease in ATP interferes with the action of the ion pumps, which leads to swelling of the cell and its organelles and to disturbed ion equilibrium with leakage of potassium and influx of sodium. The ion shift and loss of high energy reduce protein synthesis. Cellular enzymes leak into the plasma, particularly lactate dehydrogenase, aspartate aminotransferase, and glutamic dehydrogenase. The elevated serum activity of these enzymes, reflecting leakage from still viable hepatocytes, is the basis of the common hepatic tests. In hypoxic conditions, such as cardiac failure, the serum activities are particularly high. Cell water, however, may be increased or decreased, explaining the simultaneous presence of hydropic and "dark" hepatocytes. The mitochondrial changes are complex (46) and vary from initial shrinkage and condensation to subsequent enlargement. These changes depend on progressive deterioration of mitochondrial respiration, which is associated with altered permeability of the inner mitochondrial membrane and with ion shifts. Activated mitochondrial phospholipases attack mitochondrial membrane phospholipids. Acidosis favors release of lysosomal hydrolases; their importance in cell degeneration and death, however, may be less than in postmortal autolysis (47).

The irreversible step at which homeostasis cannot restore viability is characterized by denaturation and dislocation of cell macromolecules, lysosomal digestion of cell components, and excess cellular calcium. Clumping of cell proteins is recognized by light microscopy, which also shows eosinophilia, which may result from unfolding of proteins. Nuclear chromatin is clumped, phospholipids form myelin whorls, and other lipids aggregate in "fat phanerosis." Digestive action increases free amino acids and acid-soluble phosphorus and decreases specific stainability of DNA and RNA. The electric resistance of the cell membrane is decreased; increased uptake of vital dyes and release of chromium characterize necrotic cells. Terminal events, best studied in the readily controllable effects of hypoxia, probably are identical for all types of cell death.

Relative hypoxia has also been considered a cause of characteristic zone 3 hepatocytic injury in active alcoholic liver disease because of its control by propylthiouracil (48), which is said to decrease a hypermetabolic state and suppresses liver lesions induced by hypoxia on high protein diets (49). The effect of the drug, at least in acetaminophen intoxications, however, has also been ascribed to actions other than suppressing thyroid function, for instance, to increase hepatocellular glutathione content and glucuronidation (50).

Trapping of Essential Cofactors

Ethionine depletes adenosine triphosphatase (51,52) and galactosamine uridine triphosphate (53). Phosphate is trapped by deoxygalactose, which results in hepatocytic injury but not necrosis (54); the lesion is aggravated by inhibition of uridilate biosynthesis (55). Reduction in cellular adenosylmethionine by ethionine interferes with many cell functions, including respiration, ionic equilibrium, and synthesis of RNA and proteins, but the hepatocyte does not become necrotic. In contrast, galactosamine, which induces similar changes, produces dose- and time-dependent necrosis, which is prevented by uridine. This develops in living adult animals and in perfused rat liver (56) and isolated hepatocytes (57,58). Reduction in UTP, UDP, and UDPG to less than 15% of control values inhibits biosynthesis of membrane glycoproteins, which is considered to be the lethal event (59). Although other factors enter in galactosamine toxicity, this metabolic event, which is ameliorated by uridine even during the course of intoxication, suffices to produce cell death. The tolerance of young animals, regenerating liver, and hepatoma cells to galactosamine may also be explained by metabolic conditions, such as prolonged lifespan of the membrane glycoproteins (60).

Interaction of Chemicals With Phospholipids and Macromolecules

Metabolism of Agents

The reaction of chemicals with macromolecules requires their entrance into hepatocytes, except for direct action on the cell membrane. The majority of hepatotoxic agents enter hepatocytes as lipid-soluble compounds, which undergo biotransformation mainly in the smooth endoplasmic reticulum but also in the nuclear membrane and mitochondria to a bioactive metabolite which interacts with macromolecules. These hepatotoxins also include environmental agents, some of which are metabolized without necessarily being injurious to the hepatocytes, although many may be stored in the fat tissue for a long time.

The stepwise transformation is accomplished mainly

by monooxygenases of the cytochrome P-450 type, often along different pathways, as with water-soluble dimethylnitrosamine (61), and may result in free radicals, such as chlorine, e.g., in CCl₄ intoxication, hydroxylates, epoxides, superoxides, and oxygen. Some of the observations on macrophages regarding oxygen toxicity (163) may also apply to the hepatocyte. Most bioactive metabolites undergo further change, such as enzymatic hydration of epoxides, conjugation with glucuronic acid, and binding to glutathione by transferases, but also trapping by antioxidants, as with vitamin E. The toxic effect depends on the amount and lifespan of the bioactive metabolite. Usually the initial, mainly oxidative phase I reactions (62) produce more toxic and carcinogenic compounds; the subsequent phase II reactions usually detoxify. Exceptions to this rule include phase II without phase I reactions, detoxification by monooxygenases, and increased toxicity from phase II reactions.

The importance of this complex biotransformation system lies in the different distribution of both types of reactions in the hepatic acinus, which favors zone 3 necrosis, but also in the influence of many factors on both types of reactions. These factors include the genetic determination of enzyme activities, now well demonstrated for acetylation (63) and oxidative metabolism (64), and inhibition or increase in the enzymatic reaction by other chemicals. The latter process, designated "induction," may result from either enhanced synthesis or reduced breakdown of the enzymes. For instance, phenobarbital, which increases cytochrome P-450 activity, or polychlorinated biphenyls, which increase both cytochrome P-450 and P-448 activities, enhance hepatocellular necrosis caused by other agents or induce necrosis otherwise not present (65,66). Human examples are hepatic adverse drug reactions, for example, toxicity following isoniazid, which is aggravated by rifampicin (67). Different metabolites of the same drug may produce different reactions; halothane may be transformed by a reductive pathway requiring cytochrome P-450 to a metabolite which produces hepatocellular necrosis in animals, particularly if they are treated with polychlorinated biphenyls or phenobarbital and exposed to hypoxia (160,161). This rapidly disappearing lesion may be the counterpart to the mild hepatotoxic and self-limited reaction that frequently follows halothane anesthesia in man. In contrast, an oxidative pathway of halothane (68), which apparently requires cytochrome P-448, may lead to metabolites that induce, in rare instances, a severe and dangerous reaction explained by hapten formation (69).

Many hepatotoxic agents and most common environmental factors may modulate biotransformation, usually by aggravating the injury but sometimes by protecting against it. The latter is reflected in protection by preadministration of toxic agents in small "inducing" doses or in very large doses, which block metabolism (70). Smoking (71) and ethanol (72) have been incriminated; the latter is exemplified by more severe human response to acetaminophen in alcoholics (73). Dietary variations influence biotransformation by altering enzymatic activity, acting on phospholipids in the endoplasmic reticulum membrane in which the enzymes are located and by determining the available hepatic concentration of glutathione. Low protein diets reduce cytochrome P-450 and are protective in CCl₄ intoxication (74). The influence of these factors on the amount and lifespan of the bioactive metabolite creates unpredictable effects of drugs in animals and man. In general, inducing agents and undernutrition appear to accentuate drug toxicity.

Interaction with Phospholipids

Phospholipids are the backbone of cellular and organelle membranes, and their fatty acid composition can be altered by nutritional variations, in their physical state (viscosity) by chemicals [e.g., assumed for porphyrin-inducing agents (75)], and especially by destructive peroxidation. Free radicals attack the unsaturated bonds of the fatty acids, which initiates a chain reaction by additional cleavage. Breakdown of the membranes leads to dislocation and dysfunction of membrane proteins and enzymes. This process was first demonstrated in CCl₄ intoxication (76,164) and is measured by formation of malonic dialdehydes, dienes, and ethanes. The destruction of microsomal membrane enzymes, such as cytochrome P-450 and glucose-6-phosphatase, is fully accounted for by lipid peroxidation (77). Free radicals probably affect the plasma membrane (36,77) and may cause its destruction. To what degree cell death by lipid peroxidation applies to intoxications other than CCl₄ is not established. The concept holds true for free radicals from ionizing radiation and, particularly when superoxide and singlet oxygen are formed, following exposure to acetaminophen (65) or paraquat (78). It applies to various halogenated hydrocarbons (79), but whether it plays a role in hepatocellular necrosis from nitrosamines (61) or after iron overload (80) is not established.

A significant application of the free radical concept is the protective action of antioxidants, including alpha-tocopherol, glutathione, other sulfhydryl compounds, free radical scavengers, such as diethyldithiocarbamates (2), and a large number of other agents with mainly antioxidative activity. Not only binding to glutathione, but also the activity of glutathione peroxidase, a selenium-containing enzyme, may be involved. Glutathione and other antioxidants not only bind free radicals, they also act on other metabolites, e.g., epoxides, in part by transferases. Protection, therefore, is not specific. In human intoxication, e.g., with acetaminophen, hepatic glutathione concentration is the limiting factor, and its repletion by cysteamine or N-acetyl cysteine prevents hepatocellular necrosis and death (81).

Interaction with Proteins

Covalent binding of metabolites to proteins has been considered to be necrogenic (82), mainly on the basis of parallelism between the extent of binding and hepatocellular necrosis; it has not been established as a critical event. The problem is the specific nature of the protein bound and the chance that the chemical or its metabolite contacts a functional protein, in view of the many others present in the cell. Nevertheless, covalent binding should alter the tertiary structure of the protein and change its lifespan and enzymatic activity. Reduction of cytochrome P-450 system by metals and porphyria-inducing agents (83) does not produce hepatocellular necrosis, nor does otherwise conspicuous reduction of cytochrome P-450. Inhibition of hepatocellular protein synthesis for many hours by inhibitors of protein synthesis, such as cycloheximide (84) or puromycin (85), produces steatosis and not hepatic necrosis. Indeed, cycloheximide protects against liver cell injury from 2-acetylaminofluorene and 3-methyl-4-diaminoazobenzene (86), CCl_4 (87), and galactosamine (88). Besides impaired formation of toxic metabolites, lethal enzymes are incriminated, but this matter is not resolved (36).

Interaction with RNA

Necrogenic mushroom poisons of the amatoxin variety, such as amanitine, inhibit RNA polymerase, which forms messenger RNA (89). Aflatoxin binds to DNA and interferes with RNA polymerase (90,91), but it is not established whether these actions are necrogenic. RNA synthesis is inhibited by many agents, not all of which produce hepatocellular necrosis.

Interaction with DNA

Many agents bind to DNA, and demonstration of the adduct is an important aspect in carcinogenesis. Alkylation is well established for nitrosamines (92,93), but it is not clear whether this DNA alteration results in necrosis, particularly since it does not seem to inhibit replication (94). Actinomycin binds to DNA but does not produce necrosis. This lack of necrogenic effect may be explained by the long lifespan of the hepatocyte and may account for the tolerance of the human liver to most cancer chemotherapeutic agents that affect macromolecular synthesis (95).

Evaluation

This abbreviated review of the possible effects of chemical agents and their metabolites does not permit explanation of the role of most agents in hepatocellular necrosis. There is no doubt that the mechanisms have many similarities and differences (96). This ignorance contrasts with the better appreciated mechanism of hypoxic necrosis. Pharmacologic manipulation of the necrogenic effect clarifies these ambiguities only slightly. Some agents, such as chlorpromazine, probably have multiple effects, one of which may be simply to reduce body temperature (97). The beneficial effect of the antioxidant diethyldithiocarbamate in many intoxications (2), including galactosamine hepatitis (98), suggests common pathways, as do the claimed effects of flavonoids in protecting against acute CCl_4 and galactosamine intoxications (165). Even more complex is the explanation of acute necrotizing liver injury in man. The human liver, however, seems to be protected against some effects of environmental agents that produce hepatocellular necrosis in experimental animals (99).

Action of Agents on the Cell Membrane

Water-soluble agents enter the cell frequently by interaction with its membrane, often by binding to receptors or through energy-dependent transport, which is coupled to hydrolysis of ATP, facilitated by the ion pump, or involves hydrophilic channels (either ion-coupled or with the help of carrier proteins). The penetration of toxins into the cell has been studied in models other than hepatocytes (100). The relatively few studies on hepatocytes include abrin and ricin (101) and diphtheria toxin (102), which, after binding to glycoprotein receptors, enter the hepatocytes where they block protein synthesis within the cytoplasm (101). These agents do not produce necrosis of hepatocytes except in tissue culture, although they cause necrosis of Kupffer cells *in vivo*. Metals, particularly mercury, are toxic to hepatocytes by interaction with the plasma membrane, as has been demonstrated for parachloromercurobenzene sulfonate (100). An alteration of plasma membrane sulfhydryl groups is postulated. The toxin of Clostridium perfringens, a phospholipase A, attacks the plasma membrane with subsequent release of lipids in man (4).

The most interesting aspect of receptors and transport mechanisms in toxic injury is the tolerance of hepatocytes to toxins if these receptors are missing or blocked. An example is phalloidin, which acts only on hepatocytes because of their specific receptors or transport mechanisms (103). Young animals and regenerating livers are unaffected by phalloidin, presumably because of the absence of receptors (104). Various hepatocellular toxins, such as diethylnitrosamine

(105), decrease phalloidin sensitivity, and phalloidin decreases galactosamine toxicity (106). The claim is also made that protection by some flavonoids against phalloidin injury also involves blocking of the receptor mechanism. The same may hold true for the tolerance of transformed hepatocytes to toxins. Blocking of receptors or transport mechanisms may represent an important avenue to avoid toxicity.

Other aspects are ultrastructural cell membrane alterations from toxic agents, such as acetaminophen (44), or increased microvilli in the intercellular space, which is an indication of regeneration (107) and precedes necrosis from ethinylestradiol.

Immunologic Hepatocellular Injury

Only a few viruses act on liver cells by direct cytopathic reaction, for example, the various herpes viruses in man and murine and canine hepatitis virus. There is no convincing evidence for a cytopathic action in human viral hepatitis, although a cytopathic component has not been excluded for hepatitis A virus, because of its relation to cytopathic enteroviruses, and for the hepatitis non-A/non-B virus. Otherwise, in human viral hepatitis, immunologic reactions are incriminated in hepatocellular degeneration and necrosis. A direct action of antibodies is not considered. An effect of immune complexes on the liver has been suggested but is not fully accepted, whereas it is for extrahepatic locations (108). A cytotoxic effect of activated complement is suggested by its binding to hepatocytic plasma membranes of galactosamine-treated rats (109); necrosis fails to develop in complement-deficient animals. The main effect is a cell-dependent toxicity. Experimental evidence suggests that lymphocytes with exposed galactose on their surface after neuraminidase treatment attach to hepatocytes with potential subsequent cell injury (110,111). In viral hepatitis B, lymphocytotoxic action is directed against viral antigens, and acute viral hepatitis B has been considered to result from elimination of hepatocytes carrying these antigens on or near their cell membrane (112). Chronic active hepatitis may result from incomplete elimination, because of an immune defect, of hepatocytes carrying the antigen. The carrier state and possibly chronic persistent hepatitis may be caused by persistence of hepatocytes which carry excess surface antigen in their endoplasmic reticulum.

These hepatocytes may persist because they are tolerant to immunologic attack. There are, however, other potential membrane antigens for cell-mediated attack, including so-called liver-specific lipoproteins (LSP), a group of antigens, not all of which are liver-specific (113). They are also a target in hepatitis B and in many other liver diseases. Antibodies to liver antigens occur in many conditions, including experimental injury (114), but their pathogenetic role is still not established. Of greater specificity is another liver membrane antigen, to which antibodies are found characteristically in autoimmune hepatitis (113) and in primary biliary cirrhosis. Many other immune markers, like antibodies to actin or intermediate fibrils (so-called smooth muscle antibodies), mitochondria, ribosomes, and nucleoproteins play no pathogenetic role in liver disease. In some forms of drug-induced liver injury, however, metabolites may act as haptens, which may become a membrane-localized target of cell-mediated immunologic attack, which histologically is reflected in a picture resembling viral hepatitis. This has been suggested for severe, potentially fatal, halothane hepatitis, where a specific antibody, and cellular immune reaction, have been demonstrated (69). Both manifestations of toxic and immunologic injury of nonpredictable or idiosyncratic nature may occur together (115).

The mechanism of lymphocytotoxicity in the liver is still not clear (116). There is evidence for (a) an antibody-dependent lymphocytotoxicity mainly by killer lymphocytes with FC receptors (ADCC), and (b) an action of T-lymphocytes with allogenic restriction to HLA-determined antigens in the cell membrane, antigens which, however, are not common in hepatocytes; so far, natural killer cells with direct action on virus and tumor cells are not incriminated. Macrophages may be cytotoxic. However, the classification of cytotoxic lymphocytes and immune regulation by helper or suppressor T-cells and humoral factors are still problematic.

Defect of Protective Effect of Sinusoidal Cells

The sinusoidal cells, including endothelial cells, macrophages (Kupffer cells), and fat-storing cells, normally form a protective barrier. The receptors of macrophages differ from those of hepatocytes, and thus they preferentially take up toxins. The best studied model is the action of the toxin of frog hepatitis virus, which proliferates only in cold-blooded animals (117). The toxin damages mammalian sinusoidal cells, initially Kupffer cells, and subsequently endothelial cells, permitting subsequent injury of hepatocytes which take up material that they normally exclude, such as carbon and herpes virus (118), or become sensitive to endotoxins. A clinical application of this principle is the effect of endotoxins (119), which are considered important pathogenetic factors in extrahepatic manifestations of chronic liver disease, but are now given significance in hepatocellular injury after endotoxin has altered Kupffer cells (120). Whether endotoxins are important in alcoholic liver injury by this mechanism (121) is not established. In galactosamine hepatitis, hepatocellular injury is, at least in part, produced by complement which is activated by endotoxins (109). The *in vivo* importance of this effect, supplemental to the metabolic injury demonstrated in isolated hepatocytes or in perfused liver, is not clear, but galactosamine does sensitize the liver to the lethal effects of endotoxin (122).

Chronic Liver Cell Injuries

Almost all the mechanisms discussed may lead to chronic liver dysfunction without necessarily proceeding to cell death, which may occur at any time during continued exposure to a noxious regimen. In chronic exposure, the process is modified by two types of adaptive changes. The first concerns disappearance of the original injury, despite continuation of the noxious regimen, for which an unexplained metabolic adaptation is responsible. Induction of microsomal and mitochondrial enzymes, which increase the handling of xenobiotics, is one possibility. Other adaptive changes include alterations of lysosomes (sometimes associated with pigment deposition), cellular hypertrophy, fatty metamorphosis, changes in transcription and replication, cell surface adaptation with variations of transport into the cells, and adaptation in intracellular storage and transport (123). Late phenomena responsible for cell death are fibroplasia, which encircles hepatocytes, and cirrhosis, which interferes with parenchymal perfusion and is more frequently the cause of death in man than in experimental animals. However, the multitude of processes makes analysis of specific mechanisms particularly difficult in chronic liver injury.

TARGET STRUCTURES

The effect on hepatocyte organelles has been discussed. The following list of targets supplements this information and states to what degree injury of an organelle initiates hepatocellular necrosis.

Mitochondria

Mitochondrial injury is an important effect of hypoxia and acute and prolonged exposure to ethanol, in which functional and structural alterations have been well studied. The basic lesion is a defect in energy transduction associated with nucleotide deficiency, mainly in the inner mitochondrial membrane (124,125). There is no evidence that mitochondrial injury initiates hepatocellular necrosis in alcoholic liver injury, however, probably because the large number of mitochondria in each hepatocyte maintains cell function even if many mitochondria are malfunctioning. The same holds true for experimental conditions in which mitochondrial injury is observed and for human

diseases in which mitochondrial morphologic changes are frequent, such as Wilson disease (126). However, early effects of mitochondrial dysfunction cannot always be excluded (166).

Lysosomes

Release of lysosomal hydralases is not a common cause of hepatocellular death but is important in postmortal autolysis, which is particularly effective in the liver, in view of its large number of lysosomes. Swelling of lysosomes, for instance, following administration of triton, does not produce cell death (127). Hepatic fibrosis accompanies some lysosomal storage diseases and may also follow deficient lysosomal storage of metals. Cell death from iron overload has been hypothetically related to faulty iron storage in lysosomes, causing release of acid hydralases (80). Transfer to the cytoplasm of copper from lysosomes has been incriminated in hepatocytic injury in Wilson disease (126). Thus a challenge of the protective function of lysosomes may cause hepatocytic necrosis.

Cytoskeleton

In view of the importance of the cytoskeleton in maintaining cell shape and integrity, its injury deserves consideration. Phalloidin prevents the depolymerization of actin. Actin filaments aggregate along the cell membrane particularly near the tight junction, which reduces cell tonus, as reflected in blisters of hepatocytes in cultures and in invaginations of cells *in situ* due to intravital hemodynamic pressure (103,128). Cytochalasin binds to the growing ends of the actin filament and prevents polymerization (129). Phalloidin and cytochalasin cause functional and structural changes of hepatocytes, including cholestasis, which also results from the action of sex steroids and chlorpromazine metabolites on these structures. Necrosis, however, is not a necessary consequence; in human intoxications with *Amanita phalloides*, amotoxins, not phalloidin, are responsible for liver injury (89).

Although microtubules play an important role in lipid and protein secretion on the sinusoidal and possibly also on the canalicular surface, inhibition of secretion by the tubulin poisons cholchicine and conavalin A does not cause cell death. Ethanol and acetaldehyde have been incriminated in inhibition of protein secretion by hepatocytes by impairing the tubulin system (130). This causes the characteristic hydropic changes in hepatocytes in alcoholic liver injury which may proceed to necrosis (131). Injury of the tubulin system is also considered to cause accumulation of intermediate fibrils, which are, at least partly, the hyalin of Mallory (132). Other tubulin-injuring agents, such as griseofulvin, favor accumulation of hyalin in experimental animals, which also has been produced by dimethyl nitrosamine (133). It is questionable, however, whether deposition of hyalin causes cell death, since it may disappear from viable hepatocytes (132). Excessive copper deposition in the terminal stages of Indian childhood cirrhosis may cause death of hepatocytes, which is associated with abundant hyalin; copper also has an antitubulin effect (134). In prolonged cholestasis, similar hydropic swelling and deposition of copper and hyalin occur; the detergent action of excess intracellular bile acid seems to be responsible. However, bile acids also act on other cellular structures. They destroy cytochrome P-450 by detergent action. Dihydroxy and conjugated bile acids are more effective than are trihydroxy and unconjugated bile acids (135). Hepatocytes become necrotic in prolonged cholestasis, although the primary target of the detergent action remains to be established.

Nucleus

Nuclear changes are characteristic of all types of hepatocellular degeneration and necrosis. Only rarely are cytoplasmic changes preceded by morphologically recognizable nuclear lesions, including segregation, degradation, and fragmentation of structural components. An exception is thioacetamide, which causes nuclear enlargement (136), which differs in structural characteristics from that occurring in rats on deficient diets (137).

Cell Membrane

Injury of the hepatocyte plasma membrane is the best established cause of hepatocellular necrosis and may represent the terminal event in many mechanisms. Current evidence incriminates a disturbance in calcium homeostasis as the crucial irreversible event in cell membrane injury. In older studies by Judah et al. (74), protection by drugs against hepatocytic necrosis was explained by inhibition of ion movements and prevention of toxin-induced disturbance of the semipermeable property of the cell membrane. Lethal intracellular concentrations of calcium are reflected in high total liver calcium (138,139). Extensive studies by Farber (36) have clarified these observations, including the protective effect of phenothiazines noted in various models of hepatocellular necrosis (42,58,140,141).

In galactosamine (58) and phalloidin (142) intoxications, a correlation between early plasma membrane injury and elevation of intracellular calcium was established. Failure of cellular calcium homeostasis may be related to calcium pumps in the endoplasmic reticulum and mitochondria, not necessarily in the cell membrane, but different from $Na^+K^+ATPase$ (143). This failure results in excess lethal calcium influx through the plasma membrane (36). A role of the calcium-binding protein calmodulin (144) is possible. The death of primary cultures of adult rat hepatocytes exposed to a large number of hepatotoxins uniformly depends on extracellular calcium concentrations (145). This suggests that disruption of integrity of the cell membrane by different mechanisms may be followed by excess entry of calcium as a common final step in cell death. However, the preceding steps of disruption of the cell membrane remain to be explained in the different models.

HUMAN DISEASES ASSOCIATED WITH ACUTE HEPATIC FAILURE

Hepatic failure as a result of hepatocytic death or faulty function of persisting cells may develop in many chronic conditions, especially in cirrhosis and chronic hepatitis of any etiology. The list of potential causes is long and not informative. In contrast, enumeration of the causes of acute hepatic failure (defined by occurrence within 2 months after onset of the disease) supplements the preceding discussion. In Western countries, viral hepatitis is the most frequent cause, although the incidence has recently declined for unknown reasons. Hepatitis B is the most common type, and the risk to patients is highest (1.3% in the U.S. in 1977), particularly after transfusion of blood or blood products (3.33% in 1977). Hepatitis A, now well identified immunologically, causes massive necrosis in a lower incidence and has a lower risk. The incidence seems to be higher in hepatitis non-A/non-B, but the risk has not been established (146). The survival rate following grade 4 coma from massive hepatic necrosis in viral hepatitis is estimated at about 15%; therapy with corticosteroids or hyperimmune globulin (in hepatitis B) were not effective and possibly detrimental. Younger age and, possibly, male sex increase the survival rate, which may explain the better prognosis in drug addicts. Other virus infections, such as infectious mononucleosis, cytomegalovirus disease, and several forms of herpes are rare causes of acute hepatic failure. In exotic viral disease, exemplified by Lassa fever and Marburg green-monkey disease, death is caused by systemic or extrahepatic alterations, despite distinct hepatic lesions (147). In most intoxication, the survival rate is higher than in viral hepatitis, which is probably explained by the limited time of exposure, removal of the responsible agent by hemodialysis or similar procedures, and counteraction of the toxic effect by specific pharmacologic agents, particularly with acetaminophen (81). In contrast, survival is the lowest in intoxications in which immunologic reactions combine with direct toxicity, as in severe halothane hepatitis.

There are several examples of acute hepatic failure in the absence of significant hepatocellular necrosis. Besides the rare instances of generalized dysfunction of viable hepatocytes, diffuse steatosis may be the morphologic substrate. One example is Reye syndrome (148), which occurs in adults (149,150) as well as in children. The disease is triggered by viral infections; in some cases, a genetic defect in ornithine transcarbamylase activity may predispose. A mitochondrial defect identified by functional and morphologic investigations seems to be generalized (151,152). The clinical manifestations sometimes progress to death, while the hepatic changes regress or disappear. Aflatoxin as etiologic factor is still not excluded (153). Another example is pernicious steatosis of pregnancy, characterized by microvesicular fat, limited necrosis, and mild cholestasis. A peculiar toxicity of fatty acids has been postulated (154), as well as alteration in mitochondrial urea cycle enzymes, similar to Reye syndrome (155). Histologic and clinical manifestations are similar in the potentially fatal steatosis previously encountered after intravenous administration of large doses of tetracycline in the presence of impaired renal function; pregnancy adds to the risk (156). This form of microvesicular steatosis is explained, at least in part, by inhibition of hepatic lipoprotein secretion. Finally, in young women abusing alcohol, a huge fatty liver without significant necrosis may lead to fatal hepatic failure by unknown mechanisms (157).

Severe congestive failure, including that from acute obstruction of hepatic veins (Budd-Chiari syndrome), may cause acute hepatic failure in rare instances (158). In contrast, severe cholestasis does not cause hepatocellular necrosis to an extent which explains similarity in manifestations of acute hepatic failure. As in other conditions with hepatic complications of extrahepatic diseases, gram-negative septicemia and endotoxemia cause similar manifestations.

Clinically, the deficit of hepatic function in fulminant hepatic failure is often not the ultimate cause of death. Extrahepatic sequelae, such as cardiac, circulatory, renal, and pulmonary failure, gastrointestinal hemorrhage, septicemia, brain edema, and, of course, hepatic coma, are the causes of death. These complications constitute the factors in survival (159).

OUTLOOK

The main processes in hepatocellular death are (a) loss of homeostasis with ion shifts and consequent variations in volume of cell compartments, and (b) failing energy supply, particularly associated with mi-

tochondrial alterations and cell membrane change. Inhibition of macromolecular synthesis is only of terminal significance. As a rule, many factors are involved. Although more questions have been raised than answered in this review, possibilities of therapeutic strategies gradually arise. In addition to antidotes in specific intoxications and modulation of immunologic attacks, they include (a) amelioration of the hypoxic component in many injuries, (b) increase of factors, including glutathione and other antioxidants, which trap toxic metabolites, (c) modulation of hepatocellular transport mechanisms, mainly plasma membrane receptors, preventing the entrance of toxins, (d) strengthening of the barrier of the sinusoidal cell lining, and (e) protection of the plasma membrane by restoration of altered proteins by stimulating biosynthesis or reducing degradation, particularly to prevent calcium influx. The beneficial effect of various agents of different chemical nature, such as chlorpromazine, antihistaminics, diethyldithiocarbamate, cycloheximide, and some flavonoids, in different types of intoxications suggests protection from common injurious, possibly endogenous, factors. Replacement of liver function by transplantation and artificial devices is still in infancy.

ACKNOWLEDGMENT

This work was supported in part by National Institute of Environmental Health Sciences grant 2 P30 E500928 06.

REFERENCES

1. Farber, E. (1971): Biochemical pathology. *Ann. Rev. Pharmacol.*, 11:71–96.
2. Ying, T. S., Sarma, D. S. R., and Farber, E. (1980): The sequential analysis of liver cell necrosis. *Am. J. Pathol.*, 99:159–174.
3. Majno, G., Lagattuta, M., and Thompson, E. T. (1960): Cellular death and necrosis: Chemical, physical and morphologic changes in rat liver. *Virchows Arch. [Pathol. Anat.]*, 333:421–465.
4. Trump, B. F., Laiho, K. A., Mergner, W. J., and Arstila, A. U. (1974): Studies on the subcellular pathophysiology of acute lethal cell injury. *Beitr. Pathol.*, 152:243–271.
5. Cameron, R., Murray, R. K., and Farber, E. (1979): Some patterns of response of liver to environmental agents. *Ann. NY Acad. Sci.*, 329:39–47.
6. Van Lancker, J. L. (1976): *Molecular and Cellular Mechanisms in Disease*, 2, pp. 627–629. Springer-Verlag, Berlin.
7. Kerr, J. F. R., and Searle, J. (1980): Apoptosis: Its nature and kinetic role. In: *Radiation Biology in Cancer Research*, edited by R. E. Meyn and H. R. Withers, pp. 367–384. Raven Press, New York.
8. Wyllie, A. H., Kerr, J. F. R., and Currie, A. R. (1980): Cell death: The significance of apoptosis. *Int. Rev. Cytol.*, 68:(in press).
9. Don, M. M., Ablett, G., Bishop, C. J., Bundesen, P. G., Donald, K. J., Searle, J., and Kerr, J. F. R. (1977): Death of cells by apoptosis following attachment of specifically allergized lymphocytes *in vitro*. *Aust. J. Exp. Biol. Med. Sci.*, 55:407–417.

10. Kerr, J. F. R., Cooksley, W. G. E., Searle, J., Halliday, J. W., Halliday, W. J., Holder, L., Roberts, I., Burnett, W., and Powell, L. W. (1979): The nature of piecemeal necrosis in chronic active hepatitis. *Lancet*, 2:827–828.

11. Cossell, L. (1966): Electronenmikroskopische Befunde beim intravitalen Untergang von Leberepithelzellen (Beitrag zur Kenntnis von Kolliquations- und Koagulationsnekrose). *Beitr. Pathol. Anat.*, 133:156–185.

12. Unanue, E. R. (1976): Secretory function of mononuclear phagocytes. A review. *Am. J. Pathol.*, 83:396–426.

13. Klion, F. M., and Schaffner, F. (1966): The ultrastructure of acidophilic "Councilman-like" bodies in the liver. *Am. J. Pathol.*, 48:755–767.

14. Popper, H., Steigmann, F., and Szanto, P. B. (1949): Quantitative correlation of morphologic liver changes and clinical tests. *Am. J. Clin. Pathol.*, 19:710–724.

15. Popper, H., Dienstag, J. L., Feinstone, S. M., Alter, H. J., and Purcell, R. H. (1981): Lessons from the pathology of viral hepatitis in chimpanzees. In: *Virus and the Liver*, edited by L. Bianchi, W. Gerok, K. Sickinger, and G. A. Stalder. MTP Press, Lancaster (*in press*).

16. Miyai, K. (1979): Ultrastructural basis for toxic liver injury. In: *Toxic Injury of the Liver, Part A*, edited by E. Farber and M. M. Fisher, pp. 59–154. Marcel Dekker, New York.

17. Trump, B. F., Kim, K. M., Jones, R. T., and Valigorsky, J. M. (1976): Pathology of organelles in the human hepatic parenchymal cell. In: *Progress in Liver Diseases, Volume V*, edited by H. Popper and F. Schaffner, pp. 51–68. Grune & Stratton, New York.

18. Rappaport, A. M. (1980): Hepatic blood flow: Morphologic aspects and physiologic regulation. In: *Liver and Biliary Tract Physiology I. International Review of Physiology, Vol. 21*, edited by N. B. Javitt, pp. 1–63. University Park Press, Baltimore.

19. Jungermann, K., and Sasse, D. (1978): Heterogeneity of liver parenchymal cells. *TIBS*, September:198–202.

20. Branch, R. A., Desmond, P. V., James, R., and Schenker, S. (1980): Periportal localization of glucuronidation in the rat. *Gastroenterology*, 79:1006.

21. Jones, A. L., Hradek, G. T., Renston, R. H., Wong, K. Y., Karlaganis, G., and Paumgartner, G. (1980): Autoradiographic evidence for hepatic lobular concentration gradient of bile acid derivative. *Am. J. Physiol.*, 238:G233–G237.

22. Gumucio, J. J., Katz, M. E., Miller, D. L., Balabaud, C. P., Greenfield, J. M., and Wagner, R. M. (1979): Bile salt transport after selective damage to acinar zone 3 hepatocytes by bromobenzene in the rat. *Toxicol. Appl. Pharmacol.*, 50:77–85.

23. Pfeiffer, U., and Klinge, O. (1974): Intracisternal hyalin in hepatocytes of human liver biopsies. *Virchows Arch. [Cell Pathol.]*, 16:141–155.

24. Feldman, G. (1979): Morphologic aspects of hepatic synthesis and secretion of plasma proteins. In: *Progress in Liver Diseases, Vol. VI*, edited by H. Popper and F. Schaffner, pp. 23–41. Grune & Stratton, New York.

25. Salas, M., Tuchweber, B., and Kourounakis, P. (1980): Liver ultrastructure during acute stress. *Pathol. Res. Pract.*, 167:217–233.

26. Shelbourne, J. D., Arstila, A. U., and Trump, B. F. (1973): Studies on cellular autophagocytosis. Cyclic AMP- and dibutyryl cyclic AMP-stimulated autophagy in rat liver. *Am. J. Pathol.*, 72:521–540.

27. Popper, H. (1971): The problem of hepatitis. *Am. J. Gastroenterol.*, 55:335–346.

28. Blitzer, B. L., Waggoner, J. G., Jones, E. A., Gralnick, H. R., Towne, D., Butler, J., Weise, V., Kopin, I. J., Walters, I., Teychenne, P. F., Goodman, D., and Berk, P. D. (1978): A model of fulminant hepatic failure in the rabbit. *Gastroenterology*, 74:664–671.

29. Popper, H. (1976): Pathogenesis of hepatic failure. *Kidney Int.*, 10:S225–S228.

30. Sekas, G., and Cook, R. T. (1979): The evaluation of liver function after partial hepatectomy in the rat: Serum changes. *Br. J. Exp. Pathol.*, 60:447–452.

31. Ramsøe, K., Andreason, B., and Ranek, L. (1980): Functioning liver mass in uncomplicated and fulminant acute hepatitis. *Scand. J. Gastroenterol.*, 15:65–72.

32. Gazzard, B. G., Portmann, B., Murray-Lyon, I. M., and Williams, R. (1975): Causes of death in fulminant hepatic failure and relationship to quantitative histological assessment of parenchymal damage. *Q. J. Med.*, 44:615–626.

33. Scotto, J., Opolon, P., Eteve, J., Vergoz, D., Thomas, M., and Caroli, J. (1973): Liver biopsy and prognosis in acute liver failure. *Gut*, 14:927–933.

34. Testas, P., Benichou, J., Benhamou, M., Trivin, F., Vieillefond, A., Ghika, I., Jan, D., and Ollier, A. (1975): L'insuffisance hépatocellulaire expérimentale aiguë grave avec coma. *Med. Chir. Dig. [Suppl.]*, 2:21–23.

35. Popper, H. (1977): Pathologic aspects of cirrhosis. A review. *Am. J. Pathol.*, 87:228–274.

36. Farber, J. L. (1979): Reactions of the liver to injury. Necrosis. In: *Toxic Injury of the Liver, Part A*, edited by E. Farber and M. M. Fisher, pp. 215–241. Marcel Dekker, New York.

37. Cajone, F., Schiaffonati, L., and Bernelli-Zazzera, A. (1976): Protein synthesis in liver injury. Soluble factors of protein synthesis in the cytosol from ischemic rat liver. *Lab. Invest.*, 34:387–393.

38. Chien, K. R., and Farber, J. L. (1977): Microsomal membrane dysfunction in ischemic rat liver cells. *Arch. Biochem. Biophys.*, 180:191–198.

39. Ferrero, M. E., Orsi, R., and Bernelli-Zazzera, A. (1980): Cell repair after liver injury. Membranes of the endoplasmic reticulum, ribosomes, and amino acids in post-ischemic livers. *Exp. Mol. Pathol.*, 32:32–42.

40. Peracchia, C. (1977): Gap junctions. Structural changes after uncoupling procedures. *J. Cell Biol.*, 72:628–641.

41. Chien, K. R., Abrams, J., Serroni, A., Martin, J. T., and Farber, J. L. (1978): Accelerated phospholipid degradation and associated membrane dysfunction in irreversible, ischemic liver cell injury. *J. Biol. Chem.*, 253:4809–4817.

42. Chien, K. R., Abrams, J., Pfau, R. G., and Farber, J. L. (1977): Prevention by chlorpromazine of ischemic liver cell death. *Am. J. Pathol.*, 88:539–558.

43. Rappaport, A. M. (1979): Physioanatomical basis of toxic liver injury. In: *Toxic Injury of the Liver, Part A*, edited by E. Farber and M. M. Fisher, pp. 1–57. Marcel Dekker, New York.

44. Walker, R. M., Racz, W. J., and McElligott, T. F. (1980): Acetaminophen-induced hepatotoxicity in mice. *Lab. Invest.*, 42:181–189.

45. Vogt, M. T., and Farber, E. (1968): On the molecular pathology of ischemic renal death. *Am. J. Pathol.*, 53:1–26.

46. Mergner, W. J., Marzella, L., Mergner, C., Kahng, M. W., Smith, M. W., and Trump, B. F. (1977): Studies on the pathogenesis of ischemic cell injury. VII. Proton gradient and respiration of renal tissue cubes, renal mitochondrial and submitochondrial particles following ischemic cell injury. *Beitr. Pathol.*, 161:230–243.

47. Riede, U. N., Lobinger, A., Grünholz, D., Steimer, R., and Sandritter, W. (1976): Einfluss einer einstuendigen Autolyse auf die quantitative Zytoarchitektur der Rattenleberzelle (Eine ultrastrukturell-morphometrische Studie). *Beitr. Pathol.*, 157:391–411.

48. Orrego, H., Kalant, H., Israel, Y., Blake, J., Medline, A., Rankin, J. G., Armstrong, A., and Kapur, B. (1979): Effect of short-term therapy with propylthiouracil in patients with alcoholic liver disease. *Gastroenterology*, 76:105–115.

49. Orrego, H., Israel, Y., Carmichael, F. J., Khanna, J. M., Phillips, M. H., and Kalant, H. (1978): Effect of dietary proteins and amino acids on liver damage induced by hypoxia. *Lab. Invest.*, 38:633–639.

50. Linsheer, W. G., Raheja, K. L., Cho, C., and Smith, N. J. (1980): Mechanisms of the protective effect of propylthiouracil against acetaminophen (Tylenol) toxicity in the rat. *Gastroenterology*, 78:100–107.

51. Farber, E. (1959): Studies on the chemical pathology of lesions produced by ethionine. *Arch. Pathol.*, 67:1–8.

52. Okazaki, K., Shull, K. H., and Farber, E. (1968): Effects of

ethionine on adenosine triphosphate levels and ionic composition of liver cell nuclei. *J. Biol. Chem.*, 243:4661–4666.

53. Decker, K., and Keppler, D. (1972): Galactosamine-induced liver injury. In: *Progress in Liver Diseases, Vol. IV*, edited by H. Popper and F. Schaffner, pp. 183–199. Grune & Stratton, New York.

54. Lattke, H., Koch, H. K., Lesch, R., and Keppler, D. O. R. (1979): Consequences of recurrent phosphate trapping induced by repeated injections of 2-deoxy-D-galactose. Biochemical and morphological studies in rats. *Virchows Arch. [Cell Pathol.]*, 30:297–312.

55. Decker, K., Keppler, D., Rudiger, J., and Domschke, W. (1971): Cell damage by trapping of biosynthetic intermediates. The role of uracil nucleotides in experimental hepatitis. *Hoppe Seylers Z. Physiol. Chem.*, 352:412–418.

56. Rasenack, J., Koch, H. K., Nowack, J., Lesch, R., and Decker, K. (1980): Hepatotoxicity of D-galactosamine in the isolated perfused rat liver. *Exp. Mol. Pathol.*, 32:264–275.

57. Hofmann, F., Wilkening, J., Nowack, J., and Decker, K. (1976): Response of isolated rat hepatocytes to D-galactosamine and uridine. *Hoppe Seylers Z. Physiol. Chem.*, 357:427–433.

58. Schanne, F. A. X., Pfau, R. G., and Farber, J. L. (1980): Galactosamine-induced cell death in primary cultures of rat hepatocytes. *Am. J. Pathol.*, 100:25–38.

59. Bachmann, W., Harms, W., Hasses, R., Henninger, H., and Reutter, W. (1977): Studies on rat liver plasma membrane altered protein and phospholipid metabolism after injection of D-galactosamine. *Biochem. J.*, 166:455–462.

60. Reutter, W., Bauer, C., Bachmann, W., and Lesch, R. (1975): The galactosamine refractory regenerating rat liver. In: *Liver Regeneration After Experimental Injury*, edited by R. Lesch and W. Reutter, pp. 259–268. Stratton Intercontinental, New York.

61. Godoy, H. M., Diaz Gomez, M. I., and Castro, J. A. (1980): Relationship between dimethylnitrosamine metabolism or activation and its ability to induce liver necrosis in rats. *J. Natl. Cancer Inst.*, 64:533–538.

62. Jollow, D., Kocsis, J., and Snyder, R. (editors) (1977): *Biological Reactive Intermediates. Formation, Toxicity and Inactivation.* Plenum Press, New York.

63. Zysset, T., Bircher, J., and Preisig, R. (1980): Acetylator status. In: *Drug Reactions and the Liver*, edited by M. Davis and R. Williams (*in press*).

64. Smith, R. L. (1980): In: *Drug Reactions and the Liver*, edited by M. Davis and R. Williams (*in press*).

65. Mitchell, J. R., Nelson, S., Thorgeirsson, S. S., McMurtry, R. J., and Dybing, E. (1976): Metabolic activation: Biochemical basis for many drug-induced liver injuries. In: *Progress in Liver Diseases, Vol. V*, edited by H. Popper and F. Schaffner, pp. 259–279. Grune & Stratton, New York.

66. Reynolds, E. S., Treinen Moslen, M., Szabo, S., Jaeger, R. J., and Murphy, S. D. (1975): Hepatotoxicity of vinyl chloride and 1,1-dichloroethylene. *Am. J. Pathol.*, 81:219–236.

67. Miguet, J. P., Mavier, D., Soussy, C. J., and Dhumeaux, D. (1977): Induction of hepatic microsomal enzymes after brief administration of rifampicin in man. *Gastroenterology*, 72:924–926.

68. Cohen, E. N., Trudell, J. R., Edmunds, H. N., and Watson, E. (1975): Urinary metabolites of halothane in man. *Anesthesiology*, 43:392–401.

69. Vergani, D., Mieli-Vergani, G., Alberti, A., Neuberger, J., Eddleston, A. L. W. F., Davis, M., and Williams, R. (1980): Antibodies to the surface of halothane-altered rabbit hepatocytes in patients with severe halothane-associated hepatitis. *N. Engl. J. Med.*, 303:66–71.

70. Flaks, B., and Nicholl, J. W. (1975): Modification of toxic liver injury in the rat. II. Protective effect of cycloheximide on ethionine-induced damage and autoprotective effects of high doses of ethionine, 3'-methyl-4-dimethylaminoazobenzene, and 2-acetylaminofluorene. *Toxicol. Appl. Pharmacol.*, 32:603–620.

71. Cooksley, W. G. E., Farrell, G. C., Cash, G. A., and Powell, L. W. (1979): The interaction of cigarette smoking and chronic

drug ingestion on human drug metabolism. *Clin. Exp. Pharmacol. Physiol.*, 6:527–533.

72. Boobis, A. R., Brodie, M. J., Bulpitt, C. J., and Davies, D. S. (1979): Environmental factors affecting monooxygenase activity of microsomal fractions of human liver biopsies. *Br. J. Pharmacol.*, 66:426P–427P.

73. Licht, H., Seeff, L. B., and Zimmerman, H. J. (1980): Apparent potentiation of acetaminophen hepatotoxicity by alcohol. *Ann. Intern. Med.*, 92:511.

74. Judah, J. D., McLean, A. E. M., and McLean, A. E. (1970): Biochemical mechanisms of liver injury. *Am. J. Med.*, 49:609–616.

75. Nelson, I. R., Chaykowski, F. T., Singer, M. A., and Marks, G. S. (1979): A possible association between membrane-fluidizing properties and porphyrin-inducing activity of drugs. *Biochem. Pharmacol.*, 28:3589–3593.

76. Recknagel, R. O., and Glende, E. A., Jr. (1973): Carbon tetrachloride hepatotoxicity: An example of lethal cleavage. *Crit. Rev. Toxicol.*, 2:263–297.

77. Rodgers, M., Glende, E. A., Jr., and Recknagel, R. O. (1977): Prelytic damage of red cells in filtrates from peroxidizing microsomes. *Science*, 196:1221–1222.

78. Burk, R. F., Lawrence, R. A., and Lane, J. M. (1980): Liver necrosis and lipid peroxidation in the rat as the result of paraquat and diquat administration. Effect of selenium deficiency. *J. Clin. Invest.*, 65:1024–1031.

79. Reynolds, E. S., and Treinen Moslen, M. (1979): Environmental liver injury: Halogenated hydrocarbons. In: *Toxic Injury of the Liver, Part B*, edited by E. Farber and M. M. Fisher, pp. 541–596. Marcel Dekker, New York.

80. Seldon, C., Seymour, C. A., and Peter, T. J. (1980): Activities of some free-radical scavenging enzymes and glutathione concentrations in human and rat liver and their relationship to the pathogenesis of tissue damage in iron overload. *Clin. Sci.*, 58:211–219.

81. Black, M. (1980): Acetaminophen hepatotoxicity. *Gastroenterology*, 78:382–392.

82. Gillette, J. R., Mitchell, J. R., and Brodie, B. B. (1974): Biochemical mechanisms of drug toxicity. *Ann. Rev. Pharmacol.*, 14:271–288.

83. Maines, M. D., and Kappas, A. (1977): Metals as regulators of heme metabolism. *Science*, 198:1215–1221.

84. Verbin, R. S., Lognecker, D. S., Tang, H., and Farber, E. (1971): Some observations on the acute histopathologic effects of cycloheximide in vivo. *Am. J. Pathol.*, 62:111–126.

85. Robinson, D. S., and Seakins, A. (1962): The development in the rat of fatty livers associated with reduced plasma-lipoprotein synthesis. *Biochem. Biophys. Acta*, 62:163–165.

86. Flaks, B., and Basley, W. A. (1980): Acute and persistent ultrastructural changes in rat liver after a single dose of 2-acetylaminofluorene: Effect of co-administration of cycloheximide. *J. Pathol.*, 131:1–20.

87. Lieberman, M. W. (1972): DNA metabolism, cell death, and cancer chemotherapy. In: *The Pathology of Transcription and Translation*, edited by E. Farber, pp. 37–53. Marcel Dekker, New York.

88. Koff, R. S., and Connelly, L. J. D. (1976): Modification of the hepatotoxicity of D-galactosamine in the rat by cycloheximide. *Proc. Soc. Exp. Biol. Med.*, 151:519–522.

89. Faulstich, H. (1979): New aspects of Amanita poisoning. *Klin. Wochenschr.*, 57:1143–1152.

90. Butler, W. H. (1970): Liver injury induced by aflatoxin. In: *Progress in Liver Diseases, Vol. III*, edited by H. Popper and F. Schaffner, pp. 408–418. Grune & Stratton, New York.

91. Garyican, L., Cajone, F., and Rees, K. R. (1973): The mechanism of action of aflatoxin B_1 on protein synthesis. Observations on malignant viral transformed and untransformed cells in culture. *Chem. Biol. Interact.*, 7:39–50.

92. Craddock, V. M., and Magee, P. N. (1963): Reaction of the carcinogen dimethylnitrosamine with nucleic acids in vivo. *Biochem. J.*, 89:32–37.

93. Pegg, A. E., (1977): Alkylation of rat liver DNA by dimethylnitrosamine: Effect of dosage on O^6-methylguanine levels. *J. Natl. Cancer Inst.*, 58:681–687.

94. Abanobi, S. E., Columbano, A., Mulivor, R. A., Rajalakshmi, S., and Sarma, D. S. R. (1980): In vivo replication of hepatic deoxyribonucleic acid of rats treated with dimethylnitrosamine: Presence of dimethylnitrosamine-induced O⁶-methylguanine, N⁷-methylguanine, and N³-methyladenine in the replicated hybrid deoxyribonucleic acid. *Biochemistry,* 19: 19:1382–1387.

95. Menard, D. B., Gisselbrecht, C., Marty, M., Reyes, F., and Dhumeaux, D. (1980): Antineoplastic agents and the liver. *Gastroenterology,* 78:142–164.

96. D'Acosta, J. A., Castro, J. A., De Castro, C. R., Diaz Gomez, M. I., De Ferreyra, E. C., and De Fenos, O. M. (1975): Mechanism of dimethylnitrosamine and carbon tetrachloride-induced liver necrosis: Similarities and differences. *Toxicol. Appl. Pharmacol.,* 32:474–471.

97. Marzi, A., De Toranzo, E. G. D., and Castro, J. A. (1980): Mechanism of chlorpromazine prevention of carbon tetrachloride-induced liver necrosis. *Toxicol. Appl. Pharmacol.,* 82–88.

98. Homann, J., Gerhardt, H., Kratz, F., Matthes, K., and Hopf, F. (1980): Kurative Wirkung von Diäthyldithiocarbamat (Dithiocarb) auf die Galaktosaminhepatitis der Ratte. *Hepatogastroenterology [Suppl.],* 279.

99. Popper, H., Gerber, M. A., Schaffner, F., and Selikoff, I. J. (1979): Environmental hepatic injury in man. In: *Progress in Liver Diseases, Vol. VI,* edited by H. Popper and F. Schaffner, pp. 605–638. Grune & Stratton, New York.

100. Pritchard, J. B. (1979): Toxic substances and cell membrane function. *Fed. Proc.,* 38:2220–2225.

101. Olsnes, S. (1978): Binding, entry, and action of abrin, ricin, and modeccin. In: *Transport of Macromolecules in Cellular Systems,* edited by S. C. Silverstein, pp. 103–116. Dahlem Konferenzen, Berlin.

102. Boquet, P., Silverman, M. S., Pappenheimer, A. M., Jr., and Vernon, W. B. (1976): Binding of triton X-100 to diphtheria toxin, cross-reacting material 45, and their fragments. *Proc. Natl. Acad. Sci. USA,* 73:449–453.

103. Frimmer, M. (1979): Phalloidin, ein leberspezifisches Pilzgift. *Biol. in unserer Zeit,* 9:147–152.

104. Ziegler, K., Petzinger, E., Grundmann, E., and Frimmer, M. (1979): Decreased sensitivity of isolated hepatocytes from baby rats, from regenerating and from poisoning livers to phalloidin. *Naunyn Schmiedebergs Arch. Pharmacol.,* 306:295–300.

105. Ziegler, K., Petzinger, E., and Frimmer, M. (1980): Decreased phalloidin response, phallotoxin uptake and bile acid transport in hepatocytes prepared from Wistar rats treated chronically with diethylnitrosamine. *Naunyn Schmiedebergs Arch. Pharmacol.,* 310:245–247.

106. Agostini, B., Wieland, T., and Lesch, R. (1977): Decreased phalloidin toxicity in rats pretreated with D-galactosamine. *Naturwissenschaften,* 64:649.

107. Cole, F. M., and Sweeney, G. D. (1970): Changes in rat hepatocyte plasma membranes caused by synthetic estrogens. *Lab. Invest.,* 42:225–230.

108. Nowoslawski, A. (1979): Hepatitis B virus-induced immune complex disease. In: *Progress in Liver Diseases, Vol. VI,* edited by H. Popper and F. Schaffner, pp. 393–406. Grune & Stratton, New York.

109. Liehr, H., Grün, P., Seelig, H.-P., Seelig, R., Reutter, W., and Heine, W.-D. (1978): On the pathogenesis of galactosamine hepatitis. Indications of extrahepatocellular mechanisms responsible for liver cell death. *Virchows Arch. [Cell Pathol.],* 26:331–344.

110. Kolb-Bachofen, V., and Kolb, H. (1979): Autoimmune reactions against liver cells by syngeneic neuraminidase-treated lymphocytes. *J. Immunol.,* 123:2830–2834.

111. Novogrodsky, A., and Ashwell, G. (1977): Lymphocyte mitogenesis induced by a mammalian liver protein that specifically binds desialylated glycoproteins. *Proc. Natl. Acad. Sci. USA,* 74:676–678.

112. Bianchi, L., and Gudat, F. (1979): Immunopathology of hepatitis B. In: *Progress in Liver Diseases, Vol. VI,* edited by H. Popper and F. Schaffner, pp. 371–392. Grune & Stratton, New York.

113. Meyer zum Büschenfelde, K.-H., Hüttenroth, T. H., Arnold, W., and Hopf, U. (1979): Immunologic liver injury: The role of hepatitis B viral antigens and liver membrane antigens as targets. In: *Progress in Liver Diseases, Vol. VI,* edited by H. Popper and F. Schaffner, pp. 407–424. Grune & Stratton, New York.

114. Smith, C. I., Cooksley, W. G. E., and Powell, L. W. (1980): Cell mediated immunity to liver antigen in toxic liver injury. II. Role in pathogenesis of liver damage. *Clin. Exp. Immunol.,* 3:1–8.

115. Popper, H., and Geller, S. A. (1981): Pathogenetic considerations in the histologic diagnosis of drug induced liver injury. In: *Progress in Surgical Pathology, Vol. III,* edited by C. M. Fenoglio and M. Wolff, pp. 223–246. Masson, New York (*in press*).

116. Eddleston, A. L. W. F., Weber, J. C. P., and Williams, R. (editors) (1979): *Immune Reactions in Liver Disease.* Pitman Medical, Kent.

117. Bingen, A., and Kirn, A. (1977): Hepatocellular necrosis during frog virus 3-induced hepatitis of mice: An electron microscopic study. *Exp. Mol. Pathol.,* 27:68–80.

118. Kirn, A., Gendrault, J. L., Bingen, A., Gut, J. P., and Steffan, A. M. (1980): Alterations in communication between the hepatocytes produced by frog virus 3. In: *Communications of Liver Cells,* edited by H. Popper, L. Bianchi, and F. Gudat, pp. 195–203. MTP Press, Lancaster.

119. Ramadori, G., and Hopf, U. (1979): Die klinische Bedeutung von Endotoxin. *Inn. Med.,* 99:108.

120. Ruiter, D. J., Warnaar, S. O., Wisse, E., Brouwer, A., van der Heide, D., Hummel, M., Mauw, B. J., van der Meulen, J., and van der Ploeg, J. C. M. (1980): Some cell biologic and pathologic aspects of the interaction of endotoxin with the liver. In: *The Reticuloendothelial System (RES) and the Pathogenesis of Liver Disease,* edited by H. Liehr, pp. 267–277. Elsevier, Amsterdam.

121. Nolan, J. P., and Leibowitz, A. I. (1980): Influence of alcohol on Kupffer cell function and possible significance in liver injury. In: *The Reticuloendothelial System (RES) and the Pathogenesis of Liver Disease,* edited by H. Liehr. pp. 125–148. Elsevier, Amsterdam.

122. Galanos, C., Freudenberg, M. A., and Reutter, W. (1979): Galactosamine-induced sensitization to the lethal effects of endotoxin. *Proc. Natl. Acad. Sci. USA,* 76:5939–5943.

123. Artila, A. U., Hirsimäki, P., and Trump, B. F. (1974): Studies on the subcellular pathophysiology of sublethal chronic cell injury. *Beitr. Pathol.,* 152:211–242.

124. Thayer, W. S., and Rubin, E. (1979): Effects of chronic ethanol intoxication on oxidative phosphorylation in rat liver submitochondrial particles. *J. Biol. Chem.,* 254:7717–7723.

125. Rottenberg, H., Robertson, D. E., and Rubin, E. (1980): The effect of ethanol on the temperature dependence of respiration and ATPase activities of rat liver mitochondria. *Lab. Invest.,* 42:318–326.

126. Sternlieb, I. (1972): Evolution of the hepatic lesion in Wilson's disease (hepatolenticular degeneration). In: *Progress in Liver Diseases, Vol. IV,* edited by H. Popper and F. Schaffner, pp. 511–525. Grune & Stratton, New York.

127. Trout, J. J., and Viles, J. M. (1979): Cellular changes associated with triton WR-1339 accumulation in rat hepatocytes. II. Lysosomal triton WR-1339 accumulation. *Exp. Mol. Pathol.,* 31:81–90.

128. Virtanen, I., and Miettinen, A. (1980): The role of actin in the surface integrity of cultured rat liver parenchymal cells. *Cell Biol. Int. Rep.,* 4:29–36.

129. Grumet, M., Flanagan, M. D., Lin, D. C., and Lin, S. (1979): Inhibition of nuclei-induced actin polymerization by cytochalasins. *J. Cell Biol.,* 83:316a.

130. Baraona, E., Leo, M. A., Borowsky, S. A., and Lieber, C. S. (1977): Pathogenesis of alcohol-induced accumulation of protein in the liver. *J. Clin. Invest.,* 60:546–554.

131. Lieber, C. S. (1980): Alcohol, protein metabolism and liver injury. *Gastroenterology,* 79:373–390.

132. Denk, H., Franke, W. W., Kerjaschki, K., and Eckerstorfer, R. (1979): Mallory bodies in experimental animals and man. *Int. Rev. Exp. Pathol.,* 20:78–121.

133. Borenfreund, E., Higgins, P. J., and Peterson, E. (1980): Intermediate-sized filaments in cultured rat liver tumor cells with Mallory body-like cytoplasm abnormalities. *J. Natl. Cancer Inst.,* 64:323–333.

134. Popper, H., Goldfischer, S., Sternlieb, I., Nayak, C. N., and Madhavan, T. V. (1979): Cytoplasmic copper and its toxic effects. Studies in Indian childhood cirrhosis. *Lancet,* 1:1205–1208.

135. Popper, H., Schaffner, F., and Denk, H. (1976): Molecular pathology of cholestasis. In: *The Hepatobiliary System. Fundamental and Pathological Mechanisms,* edited by W. Taylor, pp. 605–629. Plenum Press, New York.

136. Svoboda, D., Racela, A., and Higginson, J. (1967): Variations in ultrastructural nuclear changes in hepatocarcinogenesis. *Biochem. Pharmacol.,* 16:651–657.

137. Lutzeler, J., Verney, E., and Sidransky, H. (1979): Nuclear-cytoplasmic transport of RNA in liver of rats fed a deficient diet. *Exp. Mol. Pathol.,* 31:261–268.

138. Kröner, H., and Planker, M. (1977): The significance of intracellular calcium in rat liver cell damage by carbon tetrachloride. *Beitr. Pathol.,* 160:245–259.

139. Reynolds, E. (1963): Liver parenchymal cell injury. *J. Cell Biol.,* 19:139–157.

140. Gallagher, C. H., Gupta, D. N., Judah, J. D., and Reese, K. R. (1956): Biochemical changes in liver in acute thioacetamide intoxication. *J. Pathol.,* 72:193–201.

141. Vaino, T., Judah, J. D., and Bjotvedt, G. (1964): Mechanism of cellular damage by virus: A study of antihistamine drugs. I. Murine hepatitis and liver explant cultures. *Exp. Mol. Pathol.,* 1:15–25.

142. Kane, A. B., Young, E. E., Schanne, F. A. X., and Farber, J. L. (1980): Calcium dependence of phalloidin-induced liver cell death. *Proc. Natl. Acad. Sci. USA,* 77:1177–1180.

143. Itzitsu, K., and Smuckler, E. A. (1978): Effects of carbon tetrachloride on rat liver plasmalemmal calcium adenosine triphosphatase. *Am. J. Pathol.,* 90:145–158.

144. Cheung, W. Y. (1979): Calmodulin plays a pivotal role in cellular regulation. *Science,* 207:19–27.

145. Schanne, F. A. X., Kane, A. B., Young, E. E., and Farber, J. L. (1979): Calcium dependence of toxic cell death: A final common pathway. *Science,* 296:700–702.

146. Mathiesen, L. R., Skinoj, P., Nielsen, J. O., Purcell, R. H., Wong, D., and Ranek, L. (1980): Hepatitis type A, B, and non-A non-B in fulminant hepatitis. *Gut,* 21:72–77.

147. Zuckerman, A. J., and Simpson, D. I. H. (1979): Exotic virus infections of the liver. In: *Progress in Liver Diseases, Vol. VI,* edited by H. Popper and F. Schaffner, pp. 425–438. Grune & Stratton, New York.

148. Crocker, J. F. S. (editor) (1979): *Reye's Syndrome II (Proceedings of the International Conference on Reye's Syndrome, Halifax, Nova Scotia, Canada).* Grune & Stratton, New York.

149. Atkins, J. N., and Haponik, E. F. (1979): Reye's syndrome in the adult patient. *Am. J. Med.,* 67:672–678.

150. Varma, R. R., Reidel, D. R., Komorowski, R. A., Harrington, G. J., and Nowak, T. V. (1979): Reye's syndrome in non-pediatric age groups. *JAMA,* 242:1373–1375.

151. Brown, T., Hug, G., Lansky, L., Bove, K., Schave, A., Ryan, H., Brown, H., Schubert, W. K., Partin, J. C., and Lloyd-Still, J. (1976): Transiently reduced activity of carbamyl phosphate synthetase and ornithine transcarbamylase in liver of children with Reye's syndrome. *N. Engl. J. Med.,* 294:861–867.

152. Snodgrass, P. J., and DeLong, G. R. (1976): Urea-cycle enzyme deficiencies and an increased nitrogen load producing hyperammonemia in Reye's syndrome. *N. Engl. J. Med.,* 294:855–860.

153. Thurlow, P. M., Desai, R. K., Newberne, P. M., and Brown, H. (1980): Aflatoxin B_1 acute effects on three hepatic urea cycle enzymes using semiautomated methods: A model for Reye's syndrome. *Toxicol. Appl. Pharmacol.,* 53:293–298.

154. Eisele, J. W., Barker, E. A., and Smuckler, E. A. (1975): Lipid content in the liver of fatty metamorphosis of pregnancy. *Am. J. Pathol.,* 81:545–560.

155. Weber, F. L., Jr., Snodgrass, P. J., Powell, D. E., Rao, P., Huffman, S. L., and Bradley, P. G. (1979): Abnormalities of hepatic mitochondrial urea-cycle enzyme activities and hepatic ultrastructure in acute fatty liver of pregnancy. *J. Lab. Clin Med.,* 94:27–41.

156. Lewis, M., Schenker, S., and Combes, B. (1967): Studies on the pathogenesis of tetracycline-induced fatty liver. *Am. J. Dig. Dis.,* 12:429–438.

157. Popper, H., and Szanto, P. B. (1957): Fatty liver with hepatic failure in alcoholics. *J. Mt. Sinai Hosp.,* 24:1121–1131.

158. Nouel, O., Henrion, J., Bernau, J., Degott, C., Rueff, B., and Benhamou, J.-P. (1980): Fulminant hepatic failure due to transient circulatory failure in patients with chronic heart disease. *Dig. Dis. Sci.,* 25:59.

159. Berk, P. D., and Popper, H. (1978): Fulminant hepatic failure: Annotated abstracts of a workshop held at the National Institutes of Health, Bethesda, MD, 7-9, February, 1977. *Am. J. Gastroenterol.,* 69:349–400.

160. Cousins, M. J., Sharp, J. H., Gourlay, G. K., Adams, J. F., Haynes, W. D., and Whitehead, R. (1979): Hepatotoxicity and halothane metabolism in an animal model with application for human toxicity. *Anaesth. Intens. Care,* 7:9–24.

161. Sipes, I. G., and Brown, B. R. (1976): An animal model of hepatotoxicity associated with halothane anesthesia. *Anesthesiology,* 45:622–628.

162. Milandri, M., Gaub, J., and Ranek, L. (1980): Evidence for liver cell proliferation during fatal acute liver failure. *Gut,* 21:423–427.

163. Klebanoff, S. J. (1980): Oxygen metabolism and the toxic properties of phagocytes. *Ann. Int. Med.,* 93:480–489.

164. Willis, R. J. (1980): Possible role of endogenous toxigenic lipids in the carbon tetrachloride poisoned hepatocyte. *Federation Proc.,* 39:3134–3137.

165. Perrissoud, D., and Weibel, I. (1980): Protective effect of (+)cyanidanol-3 in acute liver injury induced by galactosamine or carbon tetrachloride in the rat. *Naunyn-Schmiedeberg's Arch. Pharmacol.,* 312:285–291.

166. Reynolds, E. S., Treinen Moslen, M., Boor, P. J., and Jaeger, R. J. (1980): 1,1-dichloroethylene hepatotoxicity. Time course of GSH changes and biochemical aberrations. *Am. J. Pathol.,* 101:331–344.

The Liver: Biology and Pathobiology, edited by
I. Arias, H. Popper, D. Schachter, and D. A. Shafritz.
Raven Press, New York © 1982.

Chapter 46

Cholestasis

Juerg Reichen and Francis R. Simon

The physiologist, biochemist, morphologist, and clinician each views cholestasis from a different vantage point. The term was originally coined to indicate stagnation of bilirubin in the biliary passages and hepatocytes as viewed under the light microscope (1). In contrast to the previous use of "obstructive jaundice," the term cholestasis indicated that defects in secretion of bile could be due not only to mechanical obstruction but to abnormalities at the level of the liver cell. This morphologic definition was expanded with the development of electron microscopes. These studies showed that in both extra- and intrahepatic cholestasis, biliary canaliculi were decreased in number, and their microvilli were either distorted or absent. Canaliculi frequently were greatly dilated and contained electron-dense amorphous material (2). Subsequent studies demonstrated alterations of the canalicular cytoplasm (3), in particular the cytoskeletal elements, such as microfilaments (4,5). A new dimension to the morphologic examination of the liver was added with the use of scanning electron microscopy, which gives great magnification yet provides a three-dimensional view of the liver cell. These studies confirmed and extended previous transmission electron microscopic studies showing that the lumina of canaliculi are widened and often are either entirely devoid or contain blunted, edematous-appearing microvilli (6,7). Thus morphologists were the first to describe cholestasis and characterize the process. However, the morphologic appearance of intra- and

extrahepatic cholestasis was similar, suggesting that the abnormalities observed may have been secondary; moreover, forms of intrahepatic cholestasis without any classic morphologic changes have been observed (8,9).

Not all authors agreed with this morphologic definition; its usefulness was justified, however, by its association with biochemical changes in the serum. Characteristically, substances normally secreted into bile, such as bilirubin, bile acids, and cholesterol, are elevated in the serum. In addition, enzymes and proteins found in bile, such as alkaline phosphatase, 5'-nucleotidase, gamma-glutamyltranspeptidase, leucine aminopeptidase, and immunoglobulin A, generally are increased in the serum of patients with cholestasis. The increase in serum activities of alkaline phosphatase, gamma-glutamyltranspeptidase, and leucine aminopeptidase may not reflect reduced biliary secretion as originally believed; elevation of alkaline phosphatase in serum may be due to increased hepatic production (10,11) rather than regurgitation; hepatic clearance of IgA in man apparently is unrelated to transport across the hepatocyte, in contrast to findings in the rat (12).

Because the morphologic definition did not meet the requirements needed to explain the apparent functional impairment in bile flow, a more physiologically oriented definition was suggested, which required only that bile flow be decreased (13). Although determination of bile flow is not a practical measurement in humans, it potentially provides an undisputable, direct quantitative measurement of bile secretion. This functional definition emphasizes the obvious importance of understanding the multiple and complex steps involved in bile secretion, which include at least secretion of bile salts, other organic anions, electrolytes, and water (14–16). In addition to hepatocellular excretion, there is indirect evidence for paracellular movement of water, electrolytes, and small organic molecules (14–16). The biliary epithelium plays a poorly defined role in the bidirectional flux of biliary constitutents. Decreased bile flow may result from abnormalities in the flux of water and bile constituents at several levels. Generally, cholestasis refers only to these disorders associated with abnormalities at the canalicular level.

Biliary secretion has been divided into three major components, referred to as (a) bile salt-dependent bile flow, (b) a second canalicular fraction independent of bile flow, and (c) ductular in origin, mainly driven by bicarbonate secretion under control of gastrointestinal hormones, predominantly secretin (16). Most disorders of bile secretion fall into abnormalities of one or both of the two hepatocellular components. However, genetic disorders involving selective abnormalities in biliary secretion of organic anions other than bile salts may have normal bile flow but nevertheless present clinically with jaundice. The most common disorder of this type is the Dubin-Johnson syndrome (17). It has been suggested, therefore, that the term "bile secretory failure" be substituted for cholestasis, since neither bile plugs nor decreased bile flow is present in these conditions (13). These genetic disorders and the subclinical abnormalities seen with administration of sex steroid hormones (18) and selective hormonal deficiencies (19) emphasize both the possibility of selective abnormalities and the large functional hepatic reserve which may hide major abnormalities in bile secretion before they can be detected by currently available clinical tests (20).

The term cholestasis may refer to various abnormalities of the bile secretory process, depending on one's orientation, morphologic or physiologic. With the newer developments in imaging of the biliary secretory apparatus, clinicians and physiologists may be able to think of cholestasis in terms of selective and subclinical disorders of bile secretion manifested by quantitative abnormalities in bile flow and/or organic anion secretion.

HISTORIC EVOLUTION OF BASIC CONCEPTS OF PATHOGENESIS OF CHOLESTASIS

Emphasis on the pathogenesis of cholestasis has changed from one of a mechanical process in the biliary tree to alterations at the hepatocyte-canalicular

membrane level. Cholestasis due to obstruction of bile ducts has been known since Galen of Permagon (quoted in ref. 21). Most of the early theories regarding pathogenesis of jaundice indicated that the mechanism involved either obstruction to bile flow or its regurgitation either from the ducts or between liver cells. Virchow (2) attributed viral hepatitis ("catarrhal jaundice") to duodenitis and a mucus plug in the papilla of Vater, while Naunyn and Minkowsky (2) postulated regurgitation of bile through the hepatocyte. Eppinger described bile canalicular rupture and possibly paracellular regurgitation (quoted in ref. 2). This latter concept was accepted by Rich (22) as part of his classification of jaundice. Emphasis on mechanical factors as pathogenetic for cholestasis is seen as late as 1946 with the description of cholangiolitic hepatitis as the cause of jaundice without large duct obstruction as observed in hepatitis and induced by drugs (23). Later, the association of a large number of drugs causing jaundice (24) and the application of the electron microscope to liver tissue from patients with cholestasis shifted the emphasis to the hepatocyte, with particular attention to the canalicular network, referred to as the bile secretory apparatus (25).

The search for the pathogenesis of cholestasis has changed focus from the bile ducts to the hepatocytes. Using primarily animal models of cholestasis, a number of intracellular and membrane organelles have been implicated in its pathogenesis. Of the steps involved in bile formation, most have been shown to be abnormal, including the endoplasmic reticulum, liver surface membranes, intracellular energy stores, cytoskeleton, and altered permeability of the tight junction.

SUBCELLAR MECHANISMS OF CHOLESTASIS

The first unifying concept for the pathogenesis of cholestasis was that postulating a hypoactive hypertrophic smooth endoplasmic reticulum (26). Clearly, in experimental bile duct ligation, mixed function oxidase is reduced, but correction of the apparent abnormalities with drugs and dissociation of cholestasis with abnormalities in drug metabolism have suggested that the observed abnormalities are secondary to cholestasis, rather than its cause (27,28). Histochemical as well as electron microscopic abnormalities have suggested that alterations in canalicular membranes may be involved in the pathogenesis of cholestasis (29). This hypothesis was supported by direct measurements of enzyme activities *in vitro* (9) and the demonstration that plasma membrane lipid composition and thereby fluidity may be changed (30,31). It is still unclear whether such changes are the primary event rather than secondary to cholestasis and whether similar abnormalities occur in humans. Although abnormal mitochondria are seen by electron microscopy (32), only severe depletion of ATP and hypoxemia cause decreased bile flow and organic anion secretion (33,34), suggesting that insufficient energy supplies are not likely to be an important event in cholestasis.

Malfunction of other intracellular organelles may be involved in cholestasis. Recent data suggest that lysosomes fuse with the canalicular membrane and export enzymes; in ethinyl estradiol-induced cholestasis, however, this process was not affected (35). Quantitative electron microscopic studies have demonstrated an increase in pericanalicular vesicles in bile acid-infused animals, suggesting a possible role of the Golgi apparatus in cholestasis; no definitive evidence is currently available (36).

A number of investigators have provided indirect evidence from physiologic and morphologic studies for a possible role of cytoskeletal elements in regulating bile flow (4). Certain drugs, such as cytochalasin B, phalloidin (37,38), and norethandrolone (5), may cause cholestasis by interfering with microfilament function.

Despite the emphasis in recent years on intracellular events in the pathogenesis of cholestasis, morphologic and physiologic studies of bile using sucrose and mannitol support the early ideas that regurgitation may be an important factor. As in other epithelial tissues (39), much of the water and cations secreted into bile may actually reach the canaliculus via the paracellular shunt pathway through what had previously been interpreted to be the tight junction. Several drugs, as well as extrahepatic obstruction, have been shown to increase the permeability of this pathway providing for back diffusion (regurgitation) of secreted substances. Whether this pathway is quantitatively important, and whether this event is primary rather than secondary to cholestasis of many types, is unknown at this time.

The proliferation of drugs that cause cholestasis has led to a renewed interest in the mechanisms of intrahepatic cholestasis. Examination of their effects in experimental animals is inspired by their potential usefulness to increase our understanding of normal transport phenomena and by their potential for our future understanding of the pathogenesis of cholestasis.

POTENTIAL MECHANISM OF CHOLESTASIS

Permeability Changes in the Biliary Tree

Altered permeability could occur at the level of the canalicular part of the hepatocytic membrane or at the level of the junctional complex. This has led to the regurgitation theory, first documented for the cholestasis induced by estrone in rats (40). Increased permeability has also been documented in cholestasis induced by ethinyl estradiol (41) taurolithocholate (42),

chlorpromazine (43), phalloidin (37,38), and bile duct ligation (44,45). Permeability can be assessed only indirectly, usually by determining the clearance of high molecular weight substances, such as inulin or sucrose (40). Other approaches have included measurement of the biliary recovery of retrogradely injected marker substances (41) or electron microscopic demonstration of peroxidase (45). Neither of these techniques identifies the level at which such permeability changes occur or allows for quantitation of these changes.

Altered Permeability of the Canalicular Membrane

Taurolithocholate administration leads to characteristic alterations in membrane appearance (6,46−48), which are associated with an increase in cholesterol content of the membrane (49). Increased permeability to inulin is prevented by coinfusion of taurocholate, which also prevents the membrane alterations usually induced by taurolithocholate (47). Based on these studies, Layden and Boyer (47) concluded that the diffusion permeability coefficient had to be increased threefold to explain the observed biliary clearances. These findings, although indirect, favor the existence of an abnormally elevated permeability at the level of the canalicular membrane or the tight junction. The markers employed in clearance studies equilibrate with bile water earlier than with cell water (15). Therefore, permeability changes may occur at the level of the tight junction rather than at the level of the canalicular membrane. On the other hand, increase in membrane cholesterol content in erythrocyte membrane inhibits transmembrane water movement (50), which led Kakis et al. (51) to postulate a decreased permeability of the canalicular membrane in lithocholate- and taurolithocholate-induced cholestasis; membrane cholesterol content is increased in both. These authors, however, provided no measure of permeability to support their hypothesis.

Another cholestatic model in which alteration of the permeability characteristics of the canalicular membrane must be considered is that induced by ethinyl estradiol (41). This model is characterized by an increase in the cholesterol ester content of the membrane (30). Triton WR 1339 reverses cholestasis and the increased cholesterol ester incorporation into the membrane (31), but this has not yet been correlated with alterations in permeability.

Altered Permeability of the Junctional Complex

The existence of a paracellular pathway for fluid transport has been documented morphologically by Layden et al. (52), the quantitative significance of which remains to be determined. An increased permeability of the tight junction to peroxidase was first described after bile duct ligation by Metz et al. (45). Bile duct ligation leads to a characteristic morphologic alteration of the tight junction, consisting of a decrease in the number of strands visualized by the freeze-fracture technique, disruption of strands, and a loss of their parallel orientation (45,53,54). Similar findings have recently been described in human extrahepatic cholestasis (55). Whether such changes are responsible for increased junctional permeability is unclear.

Microfilaments are enriched in the perijunctional area (56) and may be a regulator of the permeability of the tight junction. Phalloidin, which prevents depolymerization of actin, leads to cholestasis characterized by increased permeability to sucrose (37,38) and to permeation of ionic lanthanum into the junctional complex (38). Similar to other models of cholestasis, phalloidin leads to an extensive rearrangement of junctional strands (38,57). Whether cytochalasin B, another cholestatic microfilament inhibitor (4), leads to similar permeability changes is unknown.

Atypical Bile Salts

Taurolithocholate leads to a characteristic cholestatic syndrome in the rat (46) and hamster (58). Similar effects have been observed with unconjugated lithocholate (59) and, to a lesser extent, with 3-β-hydroxy-5-cholenoic acid (46,59). It has been suggested that atypical bile salts may be pathogenetic in some forms of cholestatic syndromes in humans (60–62). These potentially hepatotoxic bile salts are detoxified to a significant extent by sulfation (63) and glucuronidation (64) in cholestasis; such esters are readily excreted by the kidney (65–69). To which extent increased formation of monohydroxy bile salts (62,66,70) or 6-α-hydroxylation (68,71) represent changes specific for cholestasis is unclear. It is known that the fetal liver produces increased amounts of 3-α-hydroxy-5-cholenoic acid and performs unusual hydroxylation, such as at positions 1 and 6; coplanar (allo) bile salts also are found in meconium (72). In certain inborn errors of bile salt metabolism (73,74) and in Byler's disease (60,75,76), atypical bile salts may be the initiating event. In most forms of cholestasis, however, the presence of such atypical bile salts represents regression of bile salt metabolism to a fetal pattern (67,72). Although the pathogenetic role of atypical bile acids in human disease remains to be established, the study of their effects in animal models has enhanced our understanding of potential mechanisms of cholestasis.

Taurolithocholate

Taurolithocholate, a conjugated monohydroxy bile salt, leads to a dose-dependent, reversible cholestasis, affecting both bile salt excretion (46,58) and the bile salt-independent fraction (66,77). Besides the usual morphologic features of cholestasis, such as loss of microvilli and canalicular dilatation, taurolithocholate administration leads to a characteristic alteration of the canalicular plasma membrane with disruption of the membrane, evagination of the cytoplasm, and, finally, a peculiar lamellar transformation of the canalicular membrane (6,46,78). Intracanalicular precipitates of amorphous, lipid-soluble material were initially thought to be taurolithocholate crystals (46) but later were shown by cytochemical methods to be cholesterol (79).

Different hypotheses have been proposed to explain taurolithocholate-induced cholestasis. Mechanical obstruction by crystalline precipitation (46) probably is only a contributing factor. The finding that bile salt-independent fraction of bile is severely affected (58) led to investigation of the effect of taurolithocholate on membrane Na^+,K^+-ATPase activity. While this enzyme is markedly reduced after bolus injection of taurolithocholate (77), prolonged infusion of this bile salt does not affect enzyme activity, although it does lead to a similar degree of bile flow inhibition (49). Bile salt secretion is moderately decreased after infusion (46,51) but slightly increased after bolus injection (77). The decreased secretion rate could be due to inhibition of bile salt uptake, as described in isolated hepatocytes (80); nevertheless, this phenomenon is insufficient to explain the degree of cholestasis observed after taurolithocholate infusion.

In contrast to lithocholate, taurolithocholate is not incorporated into hepatocellular plasma membranes (49); however, it increased membrane cholesterol content twofold (49). Such a dramatic change, albeit less than that observed after administration of the unconjugated analog, may be expected to change membrane properties. If the observed increase in permeability of the biliary tree to sucrose (47), contrary to theoretical expectation (50), is attributable to such changes in membrane composition remains to be established. Decreased bile flow (46), changes in membrane morphology (46,74) and composition (49), and permeability of the biliary tree (74) are prevented by concomitant administration of taurocholate (46,74), cholate (81), or taurochenodeoxycholate (46). This protective effect seems to be related to detergent properties of these bile salts, since the nonmicelle-forming bile salt dehydrocholate only partially prevents cholestasis, morphologic alterations, and changes in permeability (47). The protective effect has been ascribed to complex formation between taurolithocholate and the other bile salts (81).

Lithocholate

While taurolithocholate immediately decreases bile flow, lithocholate-induced cholestasis is preceded by a choleretic phase (49). The morphologic changes induced by the unconjugated bile salt are similar to those observed after administration of the taurine conjugate (48). In addition, loss of particulate material on the canalicular surface membrane has been observed in scanning electron microscopy (59). Lithocholate leads to a six- to sevenfold increase in cholesterol content of canalicular-enriched membrane fractions, as compared to a twofold increase induced by taurolithocholate (49). These changes are associated with a marked decrease in Na^+,K^+-ATPase activity and other membrane enzymes (49). It is tempting to speculate that the loss of particulate matter in the membrane (59) is related to the loss of enzymatic activity. Like taurolithocholate, lithocholate-induced cholestasis is prevented by simultaneous cholate infusion, which prevents both the morphologic (48) and biochemical (81) sequelae.

Monohydroxy Bile Salt Sulfate Esters

Sulfation was believed to be a protective mechanism for hepatotoxic bile salts (65,69,82); it has been demonstrated recently that this is not necessarily true. While taurolithocholate sulfate appeared readily in bile and did not affect bile flow, lithocholate sulfate—appearing in bile somewhat delayed and mostly as taurine conjugate—led to a transient 20% decrease in bile flow; neither bile salt affected the morphologic appearance of the canalicular membrane. Glycolithocholate sulfate, by contrast, reduced bile flow in a dose-dependent fashion to a much greater extent than did lithocholate sulfate. This was associated with the appearance of membrane-bound vacuoles but not with any of the changes characteristic for the nonsulfated monohydroxy bile salts (83a). Therefore, glycolithocholate appears to produce cholestasis by a mechanism different from that responsible for lithocholate or taurolithocholate-induced cholestasis. Since no precipitates were seen, it is unlikely that this effect is related to the poor solubility of this compound.

3-β-Hydroxy-5-Cholenoic Acid

3-β-Hydroxy-5-cholenoic acid has been described in meconium (72) and also has been found in cholestasis. It leads to changes similar to those induced by lithocholate, but to a lesser extent (46,49). Its cholestatic effect is prevented by coadministration of cholate or chenodeoxycholate (46,48). Although its cholestatic mechanism has not yet been investigated, given the similarities with taurolithocholate and lithocholate, it is probable that it exerts cholestatic effects in a manner similar to that of the saturated monohydroxy bile salts.

Allo Bile Salts

3-β-Hydroxy-5-α-cholanic acid and its sulfate ester have recently been shown to produce reversible, dose-dependent cholestasis with marked reduction in bile salt and lipid secretion. They were about four times as potent as their β-analogs. The canaliculi showed loss of microvilli, dilatation, and ectoplasmic evagination, as well as intracanalicular precipitates, but no lamellar transformation (83).

Physiologic Bile Salts

Taurocholate leads to cholestasis in the *in situ* perfused rat liver at rates exceeding its excretory transport maximum (84). Similar findings were reported in the whole animal for taurocholate as well as the dihydroxy bile salts taurodeoxycholate and chenodeoxycholate (85). In the latter study, the cholestatic potency (DC > CDC > C) corresponded to hemolytic potency (86) and to damaging properties in isolated hepatocellular plasma membranes (87). The levels of bile salts achieved in these studies (84,85) are far above those encountered in cholestatic conditions; the effects, therefore, may represent direct toxic effects of intracellular accumulation of bile salts, since the uptake capacity exceeds the secretory capacity about sixfold (88). Whether similar effects are responsible for cholestasis induced by other organic anions (89–92) remains to be established.

Alteration of Liver Surface Membrane Composition

Most of the studies reported below were performed with membrane fractions purportedly enriched in bile canalicular domains. As pointed out elsewhere in this volume, all such fractions seem to be contaminated to some extent with lateral and even sinusoidal membrane components. These reservations notwithstanding, studies on membrane composition have dramatically increased our understanding of potential pathogenetic mechanism of cholestasis. While it has to be assumed that the changes to be described are not specific for the canalicular domain, further progress can be expected once we are able to separate reliably canalicular from lateral and sinusoidal membrane domains.

Alterations in Total Membrane Protein Content

Bile salts remove protein from liver plasma membrane *in vitro*; this is paralleled by a loss of surface membrane activity (87); a similar effect does not occur *in vivo* (93). Among the many models of cholestasis studied, there is only one report of decreased membrane protein recovery, i.e., acute bolus administration of taurolithocholate (77). If the same agent is given as a constant infusion, recovery of membrane protein is not affected (49). The latter authors reported a dramatic increase of cholesterol content in canalicular-enriched plasma membrane fraction. One would anticipate that such a change would affect the behavior of plasma membranes in the isopycnic centrifugation employed for their isolation. It must be noted that balance sheet data of protein and enzyme recoveries in different cell fractions in cholestasis have not been presented. Correlation of such data with morphometric analysis of canalicular membrane surface density is needed to estimate reliably whether a loss of canalicular proteins and their presumptive function in bile formation is a possible cause for cholestasis.

Alterations in Membrane Lipid Content

Bile salt secretion is one of the major determinants of biliary lipid secretion. The source of biliary phospholipids and the mechanisms whereby canalicular membranes are protected from the detergent actions of bile salts have only partially been elucidated. A potentially protective mechanism is the particular phospholipid composition of canalicular membranes. They are reported to have a high (18 to 25%) sphingomyelin content, and phospholipid solubilization by bile salts is selective and diphasic; from plasma membranes other than the canalicular domain, it is nonspecific and monophasic (94). Similarly, erythrocytes with a high sphingomyelin/phosphatidyl choline ratio are better protected from bile salt-induced hemolysis (86). *In vivo*, other mechanisms, such as local protection by rapid turnover of membrane phospholipids, may be operative. The detergent bile salt taurocholate increases membrane phospholipid content, while the nondetergent dehydrocholate does not affect biliary lipid secretion and membrane lipid composition (95). Total phospholipid content is not altered by ethinyl estradiol (9,30,96), lithocholate (49), or bile duct ligation (9). In contrast, taurolithocholate significantly increases phospholipid in noncanalicular plasma membranes but not in canalicular-enriched liver plasma membrane fractions (49). The significance of the latter finding is unclear. A promising approach may be the study of the individual phospholipid composition in different models of cholestasis.

Changes in membrane cholesterol content in nonhepatic plasma membranes are known to influence Na^+,K^+-ATPase activity (97) and water permeability (50). Total cholesterol content is not affected in ethinyl estradiol-induced cholestasis (9,30), but cholesterol esters are significantly increased by this drug (30). The increase in cholesterol ester content is associated with increased membrane microviscosity and decreased Na^+,K^+-ATPase activity (30). All these changes are reversible by administration of the detergent Triton WR 1339 (31).

While ethinyl estradiol increases cholesterol ester alone, lithocholate and taurolithocholate led to a six- and twofold increase, respectively, in total membrane cholesterol (49). The effect of these cholestatic bile salts on the distribution of free versus esterified cholesterol has not yet been investigated. Only lithocholate-induced increase in cholesterol was associated with a decrease in membrane Na^+,K^+-ATPase activity, while taurolithocholate did not affect the activity of this enzyme (49). These authors attributed this differential effect to the lack of incorporation of taurolithocholate into membranes, while lithocholate is incorporated into membranes up to 400 nmoles/mg protein. Cholesterol could be demonstrated on the membrane and in canaliculi by cytochemical methods after taurolithocholate administration (79). This accumulation of cholesterol is inhibited by simultaneous administration of the micelle-forming cholate, but not by the nonmicelle-forming dehydrocholate (81). The effects of coinfusion of taurolithocholate and cholate and dehydrocholate on bile flow are somewhat at variance: cholate completely abolishes the cholestatic effect of taurolithocholate, while coinfusion of taurolitho- and dehydrocholate leads to an intermediate response in bile flow (47). This protective effect has been ascribed to formation of complexes between the two bile salts; but evidence for this is lacking (47,81).

It is evident that our understanding of the influence of membrane lipid composition is scanty. Whereas, in other membranes, regulation of membrane enzyme activity by lipids as well as regulation of physical characteristics has reached a sophisticated level (50,97), little is known about the influence of lipid composition of the different domains of the hepatocellular surface membrane or its permeability. Influences of such alterations on permeability of the tight junction remain to be elucidated.

Alterations of Individual Membrane Enzymes

Various enzymes have been investigated in different models of cholestasis, either because of their presumed role in bile formation or because they are used as marker enzymes for cholestasis in clinical medicine.

Na^+K^+-ATPase.

Na^+K^+-ATPase, the biochemical equivalent of the sodium pump, is correlated to bile flow in several conditions (19,98). At one time, it was thought to regulate bile salt-independent bile flow, but the weaknesses of this hypothesis have recently been discussed (14,16). The enzyme is located predominantly at the basolateral portion of the hepatocellular surface membrane and could not be demonstrated histochemically at the canalicular portion (99).

Na^+K^+-ATPase is inhibited by ethinyl estradiol (30,98). This has been attributed to an increased rigidity of the membrane secondary to increased cholesterol ester incorporation into the membrane (30); the number of enzyme sites is not altered in this model of cholestasis (31).

In chlorpromazine-induced cholestasis, Na^+K^+-ATPase activity also is inhibited (100). Since ultraviolet treatment as well as adminsitration of H_2O_2 together with peroxidase *in vitro* enhances toxicity, the semiquinone has been implicated as the main inhibiting agent (100). This inhibition has been studied *in vitro*, where it was established that the inhibition is dose dependent, reversible, and caused by a decrease in V_{max}, while K_m is not altered (101). The most potent metabolites in this study were 7,8-dihydroxy- and dioxochlorpromazine. Chlorpromazine sulfate was about half as potent as chlorpromazine and 7-hydroxychlorpromazine (101), while the sulfate ester was inactive in the former study (100).

The effects of bile salts on Na^+K^+-ATPase *in vitro* have been described in the paragraph on bile salt metabolism. The effect of tauro- and lithocholate cholestasis on Na^+,K^+-ATPase is controversial. After continuous infusion of these bile salts, a decrease induced by lithocholate but not by its taurine conjugate was described (49,51). This effect was only discernible in so-called canalicular-enriched plasma membrane fractions, not in presumably sinusoidal plasma membranes. In contrast, if taurolithocholate is given in a similar dose as an intravenous bolus, enzyme activity is decreased (77). Taurolithocholate inhibits Na^+,K^+-ATPase as well as other bile salts *in vitro* (102,103). Phenobarbital pretreatment, which elevates NaK-ATPase activity by inducing enzyme synthesis (104), is unable to prevent the lithocholate-induced decrease in canalicular NaK-ATPase activity (51).

Similar to the findings reported with lithocholic acid, bile duct ligation decreased NaK-ATPase activity in a light plasma membrane fraction, which contained bile canaliculi, while a heavy fraction presumably composed of sinusoidal domain was not affected (105). In the unobstructed segment of the liver after selective biliary obstruction, enzyme activity is compensatorily increased (93). These effects on NaK-ATPase activity by different cholestatic agents cannot be explained by a unifying concept. Although there are clear indications that bile formation and enzyme activity are correlated under different experimental conditions (19, 98), there are several instances where a divergent behavior can be observed (102,105). A better understanding of the role of Na^+K^+-ATPase in the pathogenesis of cholestasis will require simultaneous measurement

of enzyme activity, bile salt transport, permeability of liver plasma membrane, and the tight junction in different situations of choleresis and cholestasis.

Mg^{2+}ATPase.

The role of Mg^{2+}-ATPase is even less understood than that of Na^+K^+-ATPase. Histochemically, it is localized predominantly at the canalicular surface of the hepatocyte (99) and is thought to be an integral membrane enzyme (106). Microfilaments are known to have Mg^{2+}-ATPase activity, but to what extent the pericanalicular web and microfilaments attached to membrane preparations contribute to Mg^{2+}-ATPase activity measured in any membrane preparation is not known. Although present in ductular epithelium, its activity is much higher in hepatocellular plasma membrane fractions (56). All bile salts, except dehydrocholate, inhibit Mg^{2+}-ATPase *in vitro* (102,103). The effect of different models of cholestasis on Mg^{2+}-ATPase in plasma membrane fractions is controversial. Bile duct ligation seems to decrease enzyme activity (9). Chlorpromazine has been described to decrease (107) as well as to increase (100) enzyme activity. The reason for this discrepancy is unclear. Similarly, in ethinyl estradiol-induced cholestasis, conflicting results have been reported: decrease (9), no change (98), or increases (31,96) have been reported.

An interesting model with respect to Mg^{2+}-ATPase is the cholestasis induced by cytochalasin B, a presumed inhibitor of microfilaments. Parallel to a loss of microfilaments, enzyme activity is lost after application of cytochalasin B (108), suggesting a relationship between Mg^{2+}-ATPase and microfilaments. This hypothesis awaits confirmation by use of a more specific microfilament toxin, such as phalloidin.

Alkaline Phosphatase.

As a marker enzyme for cholestasis in clinical medicine, alkaline phosphatase has been thoroughly investigated, although its function is unknown. Most of the data have been gathered in bile duct ligation as a model of cholestasis. It is evident that the well-known increase in alkaline phosphatase activity in serum is paralleled by an increase in enzyme activity in the liver (9–11,103).

Alkaline phosphatase occurs in hepatocellular and ductular epithelial cells, the former being more stimulated after bile duct ligation (109). The time course of alkaline phosphatase increase after bile duct ligation has been carefully studied by De Vos et al. (110), who found that staining was most intense in type I and types III–IV canaliculi, which increase after bile duct ligation, while type II canaliculi decrease in number. The increase in alkaline phosphatase activity reaches its peak 24 hr after bile duct ligation, while ductular proliferation increased up to 7 days (111). This dissociation suggests that the increase seen in whole liver is predominantly due to an increase in hepatocellular alkaline phosphatase; this could be further investigated by making use of the different electrophoretic behaviors and the differences in heat stability of the hepatocellular and ductular isoenzymes (109).

The stimulus for increased alkaline phosphatase synthesis is unknown, but the finding that bile salts stimulate its synthesis specifically in cultured hepatocytes raises the possibility that bile salt elevation in cholestasis may be the messenger (112). The stimulation *in vitro* is cycloheximide sensitive and not related to the detergent property of bile salts (112). *In vivo* administration of dehydrocholate but not taurocholate increased alkaline phosphatase activity (95). While there seems to be a differential effect on Na^+K^+- and Mg^{2+}-ATPase on cholestatic liver plasma membranes of different densities, this is not true for alkaline phosphatase, which is elevated in both light (canaliculi containing) and heavy liver plasma membranes (105). Furthermore, alkaline phosphatase seems to be universally elevated in extra- and intrahepatic cholestasis (9,113).

Other Marker Enzymes of Cholestasis.

Other enzymes that have been studied as marker enzymes of cholestasis include 5'-nucleotidase, leucine naphthylamidase, phosphodiesterases, and gamma-glutamyltranspeptidase. They are all thought to be surface membrane enzymes which are embedded to different degrees into the membrane (87,114). Their time course after bile duct ligation is different (111), and their response to different cholestatic toxins may also be variable (9,31,96,107). Since these enzymes are not thought to be involved in the formation of bile, little can be gained from their study in different forms of cholestasis. However, the described alterations emphasize the potentially important role of alterations of specific membrane proteins in the pathogenesis of cholestasis.

Abnormal Endoplasmic Reticulum

Hypoactivity of the smooth endoplasmic reticulum with consequent reduction in bile acid hydroxylation has been postulated as a mechanism of cholestasis (26). There is no doubt that cholestasis affects the activity of a variety of enzymes of the endoplasmic reticulum (28,115,116). Most of these changes seem to be related to decreased protein synthesis (28) and, therefore, are the sequelae rather than the cause of cholestasis. Alteration of drug-metabolizing enzymes may lead to altered pathways of drug metabolism with the formation of toxic (cholestatic) compounds under certain conditions. Such a mechanism occurs in chlorpromazine cholestasis, where inhibition of the microsomal enzyme system acclerates toxicity (115).

The Cytosol

The only study investigating cytosolic function in cholestasis reported a decrease in the anion-binding protein ligandin after ethinyl estradiol administration (117). The mechanism for this decrease is unclear but could compound decreased anion transport.

Lysosomes

Lysosomal protein transport is not affected by ethinyl estradiol-induced cholestasis (35). Other forms of cholestasis have not yet been investigated with respect to lysosomal function.

Pump Failure

Bile Salt Transport

Bile salt transport is impaired in ethinyl estradiol-induced cholestasis (118), after bile duct ligation (119), and by androgenic steroids (120) and chlorpromazine (121). Estrogens and androgenic steroids interfere with bile salt uptake into isolated hepatocytes (120). Whether canalicular excretion is also affected remains to be established. A carrier thought to be responsible for bile salt transport has been tentatively identified (122), but ethinyl estradiol-induced cholestasis is the only model where bile salt carriers have been measured. Ethinyl estradiol decreases bile salt transport maximum into bile (30,118) but does not affect the number of bile salt carriers (31). In contrast, following administration of cycloheximide, an inhibitor of protein synthesis, bile salt and sulfobromophthalein (BSP) transport maxima (T_m) are progressively decreased over 24 hr. The decrease in bile salt T_m is associated with a similar change in the number of bile salt binding sites (31). These studies suggest that these binding sites represent the putative bile salt carrier. The lack of an effect of estrogens on the number of bile salt carriers suggests that, at least in this model, bile salt transport is not affected by direct interference with the number or character of bile salt carriers, but by the lipid environment and/or the driving forces for bile salt transport. This driving force has not been identified but could be related to Na^+,K^+-ATPase. Clearly, studies are needed which investigate bile salt uptake and excretion in conjunction with measurements of the binding characteristics of the bile salt carrier, its lipid environment, and Na^+,K^+-ATPase.

Other Pumps

The role of Na+,K+-ATPase in the generation of the so-called bile salt-independent fraction (BSIF) of bile is controversial. Since the driving force for BSIF is unknown, no marker exists for the pump(s) responsible for its generation and its possible impairment in cholestasis. A number of candidates have been suggested, among them bicarbonate (123), chloride (14), and other anions (124), but their role in cholestasis remains to be defined.

Decreased Substrate

It is well established that hypothermia, anoxia, and depletors of energy-rich substrates lead to cholestasis (for references, see ref. 16). These are unphysiologic manipulations; at present, there is no evidence that interference with generation of energy-rich substrates is a major pathogenetic force in the development of cholestasis.

Abnormal Membrane Fluidity

Increased rigidity of the membrane due an increase in cholesterol esters has been demonstrated for ethinyl estradiol cholestasis (30); this is reversible by treatment with Triton WR 1339 (30). Altered fluidity is known to affect permeability characteristics of membranes (50) as well as activity of enzymes, such as Na+,K+-ATPase (97). The only other model of cholestasis where fluidity has been investigated is that induced by chlorpromazine and its metabolites. They are incorporated into the membrane and increase rigidity (101). More work is needed in this area; although changes in lipid composition leading to altered microviscosity could explain most of the phenomena described in cholestasis, identification of the pumps responsible for ion transport and correlation of their activity to the lipid environment of the membrane are needed to evaluate fully the contribution of fluidity to the pathogenesis of cholestasis.

Alterations of the Cytoskeleton

Microfilaments

A role for microfilaments in bile formation was postulated based on the observation that administration of cytochalasin B leads to cholestasis (4). Cytochalasin B administration causes dilatation of canaliculi and a loss of microvilli (4), a feature encountered in several other forms of cholestasis. Cytochalasin B detaches microfilaments from the plasma membrane (108). It has been speculated that microfilament inhibition by cytochalasin B leads to cholestasis by loss of canalicular tone (4), but evidence for this hypothesis is lacking. Recently, contractile movement presumably generated by microfilaments has been demonstrated in canaliculi. Another potential contributing factor is inhibition of bile salt transport induced by cytochalasin B administration (125). While cytochalasin B acts by detaching microfilaments from their insertion into the plasma membrane, phalloidin shifts the equilibrium from unpolymerized G actin to the filamentous F actin (126). Phalloidin also leads to cholestasis characterized by increased permeability to sucrose (37,126). Phalloidin cholestasis is characterized morphologically by an increase in filamentous actin around the canaliculi and the tight junction (37). Such changes also are seen in different forms of human cholestasis (3,127a). Other forms of cholestasis where interference with the function of microfilaments has been postulated include chlorpromazine- (126) and norethandrolone- (5) induced cholestasis.

Intermediate Filaments

The physiologic role of intermediate filaments is unclear. The only potential involvement of this structure stems from the observation of Mallory bodies, which presumably are composed of intermediate filaments, in griseofulvin-induced cholestasis (113).

Microtubules

The role of microtubules in cholestasis has yet to be elucidated. Colchicine, an inhibitor of tubulin polymerization, does not affect basal bile flow but decreases bile salt excretion and thereby reduces the bile salt-dependent fraction of bile flow (127). If administered together with phalloidin, it decreases bile flow in a synergistic fashion (127). These studies suggest that microtubule alterations interfere with bile salt transport, as demonstrated in isolated hepatocytes (125). Therefore, microtubules may be required for the formation of bile. Whether inhibition of microtubules contributes to the development of cholestasis remains to be established.

Canalicular Precipitates

Precipitation of taurolithocholate within the canaliculi was initially thought to be responsible for taurolithocholate-induced cholestasis (46). Indeed crystals can clearly be seen obliterating the canalicular lumen soon after administration of this bile salt (46,48). These crystals have been demonstrated to be composed at least in part of cholesterol (79). Whether this mechanism contributes to monohydroxy bile salt cholestasis is doubtful. Another model of cholestasis where such a mechanism has been invoked is chlorpromazine-induced cholestasis. Chlorpromazine interferes with the formation of bile salt micelles, but this effect is prevented by the addition of phosphatidylcholine (128).

Hepatic Blood Flow and Lobular Gradient

Over physiologic ranges, blood flow presumably does not affect bile secretion (16). In the perfused rat liver, decrease in perfusion leads to centralization of blood flow and a decrease in bile salt-independent bile formation, while bile salt secretion is not affected (129). Distribution of perfusion does not play a significant role in cholestasis.

The role of specialization of hepatocytes in the generation of bile has received attention only lately. Studies making use of selective central or portal toxins have revealed that portal and central hepatocytes have about the same capacity to extract and excrete bile salts, while the generation of bile salt-independent bile flow seems to be a function of central hepatocytes (130). Such a lobular gradient had been demonstrated earlier by scanning electron microscopy (42). The implication of the lobular gradient for the generation of hepatocellular bile flow and its role in cholestasis are far reaching; however, it is too early to speculate about their role in the pathogenesis of cholestasis.

CHOLESTASIS IN CLINICAL PRACTICE

Chief clinical manifestations of intrahepatic as well as extrahepatic cholestasis include jaundice, pruritus, and elevations of bile salts, bilirubin, alkaline phosphatase, and related enzymes in serum. In the future, when measurements of serum bile acids will be a routine clinical laboratory test, their elevation will be a *sine qua non* for the diagnosis of cholestasis. However, the large reserve capacity for hepatic excretory function reflects abnormalities by elevated serum indicators only when more than 80% of its functional capacity is impaired. Therefore, a noninvasive quantitative measurement of bile flow is needed to detect subclinical cases of cholestasis.

The main clinical manifestations and most of the histologic characteristics of intrahepatic ("medical") and extrahepatic ("surgical") cholestasis are similar. For centuries, clinicians have argued the characteristic features that distinguish one process from the other. Today, it is usually possible, after careful evaluation of clinical, serologic, and histologic features, to draw accurate conclusions about the pathogenesis of cholestasis by utilizing newer imaging techniques, such as ultrasound, radionuclide imaging, percutaneous transhepatic cholangiography, and endoscopic retrograde cholangiography, to achieve an accurate anatomical di-

agnosis preoperatively. Thus it is possible to separate extra- from intrahepatic cholestasis.

On the other hand, intrahepatic cholestasis has multiple causes (Table 1). With the exceptions of the Dubin-Johnson syndrome and estrogen-induced cholestasis, the specific hepatic processes that are altered are unknown. Because of the availability of an animal model for Dubin-Johnson syndrome (mutant Corriedale sheep), this disorder has been shown to result from an abnormality in biliary secretion of organic anions other than bile salts (131). Similarly, administration of ethinyl estradiol to rats produces abnormalties in biliary secretion similar to those found in women taking contraceptive steroids (104). These studies suggest that estrogens decrease all canalicular transport functions through changes in the membrane lipid composition. Idiopathic cholestasis of pregnancy is the most common inherited type of cholestasis; it is particularly prevalent in Chile and in the Scandinavian countries (132,133). The syndrome may present as a spectrum ranging from "pruritus gravidarum" to cholestatic jaundice anytime during pregnancy but usually during the last trimester. All cholestatic features disappear rapidly after delivery. Susceptible individuals have a constitutional abnormality either in

TABLE 1. *Causes of intrahepatic cholestasis*

Familial
   Classic cholestasis
      Idiopathic cholestasis of pregnancy
      Benign recurrent cholestasis
      Familial intrahepatic cholestasis
   Selective cholestasis
      Dubin-Johnson syndrome
      Rotor syndrome
Drugs (1,131)
   Canalicular: Estrogenic and oral anabolic steroids
   Hepatocanalicular
      Drugs: phenothiazines, erythromycins, others
      Chemicals: 4-4'-diaminodiphenylmethane (99)
Developmental
   Neonatal
Secondary causes
   Indirect involvement
      Postoperative (139)
      Endotoxin (79)
      Total parenteral nutrition (14)
      Hodgkin disease
      Sickle cell crisis
      Stauffer syndrome (32)
      Hypophysectomy (17)
      Erythropoietic protoporphyria (86)
   Direct involvement
      Intrahepatic biliary atresia
      Cholangiocarcinoma
      Caroli disease
      Viral hepatitis
      Alcoholic hepatitis/steatosis
      Primary biliary cirrhosis
      Pericholangitis

estrogen metabolism or, more likely, in hepatic secretory function. Idiopathic cholestasis of pregnancy is a benign disorder which may predispose to gallstones; more frequently, however, it confuses the physician when it is not considered in the differential diagnosis of cholestasis.

Familial benign recurrent intrahepatic cholestasis may be confused with cholestasis of pregnancy because it can be provoked by estrogens and pregnancy. Generally, however, its clinical onset is independent of drugs, pregnancy, or other known factors associated with cholestasis (134). The underlying defect in these patients is unknown, although it has been suggested to be a primary defect in bile salt transport. Indocyanine green but not cholylglycine transport is abnormal in this syndrome. There is no known therapy to prevent attacks.

Familial intrahepatic cholestasis is a confusing group of syndromes (135), including arteriohepatic dysplasia (or Alagille syndrome), Byler syndrome, the THCA syndrome, and Norwegian cholestasis. The pathogenesis and long-term prognosis in each of these entities are clearly different. Clinical presentation is usually in the neonatal period. Patients with Byler syndrome and THCA syndrome progressively deteriorate to death at an early age, while the others have a wide variability in clinical expression. Although these are rare causes of cholestasis, careful investigation of such genetic causes may provide a better understanding of the bile secretory process and the pathogenesis of cholestasis.

Dubin-Johnson and Rotor syndromes are rare disorders characterized by chronic, nonhemolytic, conjugated hyberbilirubinemia with normal bile salt levels. Histology is normal, with the exception of an excess of melanin-like hepatocellular pigment in Dubin-Johnson syndrome (136). Although the clinical presentation is similar, Dubin-Johnson and Rotor syndromes differ in several important characteristics. In the former but not the latter coproporphyrin I excretion is increased, and the biliary T_m for BSP is virtually zero, while BSP storage is normal. These observations suggest that only Dubin-Johnson represents an example of selective bile secretory failure for organic anions other than bile salts, while Rotor syndrome represents a defect of hepatic uptake of such compounds.

Drugs are the most common cause of intrahepatic cholestasis (137). In most cases the mechanism(s) for drug-induced cholestasis is unknown primarily because of the low incidence of cholestasis associated with the majority of therapeutic agents (24). A major exception is ethinyl estradiol, where a wealth of information has accumulated from studies in rats that indicate that estrogens may produce cholestasis by either or both of two possible mechanisms: (a) increased permeability, presumably via the paracellular pathway

(40), or (b) alterations in membrane lipid fluidity (30,104). The observation that clinical evidence of cholestasis (normal values for serum bilirubin, bile salts, and alkaline phosphatase) is usually absent may be related to the capacity of this drug to decrease bile flow while only mildly affecting excretion of organic anions. Estrogens produce clinically apparent cholestasis only in susceptible individuals.

The mechanism for cholestasis associated with oral androgen administration is less clear. Similar to effects of estrogens, androgen effects are dose- and time-dependent and reversible; in both situations, liver histology is unremarkable. Since bile flow is not reduced with androgen administration, at least in the rat, its mechanism of action is probably different from that described for estrogens.

Many other drugs may produce cholestasis; except for chlorpromazine, however, the mechanisms are unclear. Frequently, immune mechanisms have been invoked, but expermental support for such an etiology is scant. A prime example of this is chlorpromazine-associated cholestasis, which long was thought to be an allergic reaction. Recently, abnormalities of the cytoskeleton, Na^+,K^+-ATPase, membrane fluidity, and micelle formation have been demonstrated. As we learn more about mechanisms of cell injury and the genetics of drug metabolism, many therapeutic agents will be found to cause cholestasis at specific subcellular sites in susceptible individuals.

Physiologic hyperbilirubinemia is well characterized in man. Similarly, it appears that the bile acid secretory pathway is also immature at birth. In normal neonates, serum bile acid levels are elevated for several months after birth (138). These studies suggest that normal neonates may have impairment of biliary secretion, even when physiologic jaundice is not present.

Many processes may affect the biliary excretory system and produce cholestasis. These causes have been arbitrarily divided into either direct or indirect causes (Table 1). In almost all these situations, the mechanism of cholestasis is unknown.

CONCLUSION

The presumed driving forces for bile flow generation have been discussed in an earlier chapter and are schematized in Figure 1. Hypothetically, impairment of bile salt-dependent bile flow could result from abnormalities in (a) uptake, related either to a decreased number of carriers or to an altered sodium gradient; (b) translocation across the hepatocyte, presumably involving the cytoskeleton; (c) canalicular excretion; (d) changes in membrane fluidity; and (e) paracellular regurgitation. It is hoped that in the future we will be able to organize cholestatic syndromes into such a

Lobular Gradient   **Hepatocyte**   **Surface Membrane**

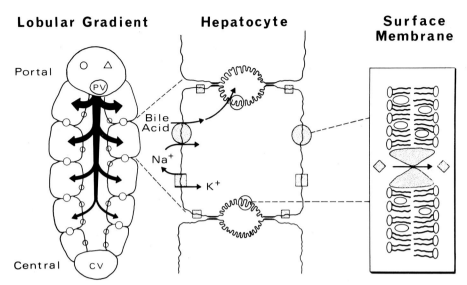

FIG. 1. Schematic representation of bile acid transport in the liver. Delivery of bile acids to hepatocytes depends on a lobular gradient where their concentration is greater at the portal zone I area. Uptake into the hepatocyte requires a putative bile acid "carrier," which is apparently embedded in the surface membrane lipid bilayer. Active uptake is driven by the sodium gradient generated by Na$^+$K$^+$-APTase. Translocation across the hepatocyte is directed toward the canalicular membrane, where another carrier (*open circle*) is proposed to be present and is responsible for biliary secretion.

physiologic framework. A tentative classification of agents that may affect these specific steps is given in Table 2. In many cases, one agent has been shown to interfere with different steps in the formation of bile. In addition, many of these agents are used in dosages greatly exceeding concentrations achieved in humans; therefore, the resemblance of these cholestatic syndromes in animals to that in humans is often poor.

Our concepts regarding the pathogenesis of intrahepatic cholestasis have gradually evolved over the past century in a remarkable fashion. A lesion, which was initially believed to result from regurgitation, moved from the biliary ducts to the paracellular junctions. A lesion orginally described in morphologic terms is now

TABLE 2. *Steps in formation of hepatocellular bile which may be affected in intrahepatic cholestasis*

Site and abnormality	Agents	References
Sinusoidal uptake		
Decreased number of carriers	Not described	
Decreased driving forces	Chlorpromazine	100
	Porphyrins	140
	Estrogens	30,31,98
	Endotoxin	133a
	Taurolithocholate	77
Decreased bile salt delivery	Ileal resection, bile duct drainage	
Competitive inhibition	Various drugs	80,120
Cellular translocation		
Microtubules	Colchicine	125,127
Microfilaments	Cytochalasin B	108,125
	Norethandrolone	5
	Phalloidin	4,37,38,57
Excretion		
Decreased carriers	Cycloheximide	104
Membrane fluidity		
	Ethinyl estradiol	30
	Tauro- and lithocholate	35
	Chlorpromazine	101
Paracellular regurgitation		
	Ethinyl estradiol	40,41
	Phalloidin	4,37,57
	Bile duct ligation	44,45,54
	Taurocholate	43,47

characterized by physiologic and biochemical parameters. A lesion initially believed to be unique to humans has now been reproduced in experimental animals. Although our understanding of the mechanisms involved in the elaboration of bile have greatly improved, definition of specific steps is still vague. In the future, it will be necessary to characterize the specific bile salt carrier, its relation to the sodium pump, and the translocation of bile salts across the hepatocyte before we can precisely define the pathogenesis of cholestasis and devise specific therapeutic agents.

REFERENCES

1. Popper, H., and Szanto, P. B. (1956): Intrahepatic cholestasis (cholangiolitis). *Gastroenterology,* 31:683–700.
2. Popper, H., and Schaffner, F. (1970): Pathophysiology of cholestasis. *Human Pathol.,* 1:1–24.
3. Badaruddin, R. H., Waldrop, F. S., and Puchtler, H. (1976): Alterations of the myoid pericanalicular layer in liver. *Arch. Pathol. Lab. Med.,* 100:616–619.
4. Phillips, M. J., Oda, M., Mak, E., Fisher, M. M., and Jeejeebhoy, K. N. (1975): Microfilament dysfunction as a possible cause of intrahepatic cholestasis. *Gastroenterology,* 69:48–58.
5. Phillips, M. J. Oda, M., and Fumatsu, K. (1978): Evidence for microfilament involvement in norethandrolone-induced intrahepatic cholestasis. *Am. J. Pathol.,* 93:729–739.
6. Layden, T. J., and Boyer, J. L. (1975): Scanning electron microscopy of the rat liver. Studies of the effect of taurolithocholate and other models of cholestasis. *Gastroenterology,* 69:724–738.
7. Vial, J. D., Simon, F. R., and Mackinnon, A. M. (1976): Effect of bile duct ligation on the ultrastructural morphology of hepatocytes. *Gastroenterology,* 70:85–92.
8. Kleiner, G. J., Kresch, L., and Arias, I. M. (1965): Studies on hepatic excretory function. II. The effect of norethynodrel and mestranol on bromsulphalein sodium metabolism in women of child-bearing age. *N. Engl. J. Med.,* 273:420–423.
9. Simon, F. R., and Arias, I. M. (1973): Alteration of bile canalicular enzymes in cholestasis. A possible cause of bile secretory failure. *J. Clin. Invest.,* 52:765–775.
10. Kaplan, M. M., and Righetti, A. (1970): Induction of rat liver alkaline phosphatase: The mechanism of the serum elevation in bile duct obstruction. *J. Clin. Invest.,* 49:508–516.
11. Kaplan, M. H. (1972): Alkaline phosphatase. *Gastroenterology,* 62:452–468.
12. Nagura, H., Smith, P. D., Nakane, P. K., and Brown, W. R. (1981): IgA in human bile and liver. *J. Immunol.,* 126:587–595.
13. Javitt, N. B., and Arias, I. M. (1967): Intrahepatic cholestasis: A functional approach to pathogenesis. *Gastroenterology,* 53:171–175.
14. Boyer, J. L. (1980): New concepts of mechanisms of hepatocyte bile formation. *Physiol. Rev.,* 60:303–326.
15. Forker, E. L. (1977): Mechanisms of hepatic bile formation. *Annu. Rev. Physiol.,* 39:323–347.
16. Reichen, J., and Paumgartner, G. (1979): The excretory function of the liver. In: *Physiology of the Liver. International Reviews of Physiology,* edited by N.B. Javitt, pp. 103–150. University Park Press, Baltimore.
17. Cohen, L., Lewis, C., and Arias, I. M. (1972): Pregnancy, oral contraceptives, and chronic familial jaundice with predominantly conjugated hyperbilirubinemia (Dubin-Johnson syndrome). *Gastroenterology,* 62:1182-1190.
18. Adlercreutz, H., and Terhunen, R. (1970): Some aspects of the interactions between natural and synthetic female sex hormones and the liver. *Am. J. Med.,* 49:630–648.
19. Layden, T. J., and Boyer, J. L. (1976): The effect of thyroid hormone on bile salt-independent bile flow and Na$^+$,K$^+$-

20. Arias, I. M. (1963): Studies on a plant acid (icterogenin) and certain anabolic steroids on the hepatic metabolism of bilirubin and sulfobromophthalein (BSP). *Ann. N.Y. Acad. Sci.,* 104:1014–1025.
21. Popper, H. (1981): Cholestasis: the future of a past and present riddle. *Hepatology,* 1:187–191.
22. Rich, A. R. (1930): The pathogenesis of the forms of jaundice. *Bull. Johns Hopkins Hosp.,* 47:338–377.
23. Watson, C. J., and Hofbauer, F. W. (1946): Problem of prolonged hepatitis with particular reference to cholangiolitic type and to development of cholangiolitic cirrhosis of the liver. *Ann. Int. Med.,* 25:195–227.
24. Plaa, G. L., and Priestly, B. G. (1977): Intrahepatic cholestasis induced by drugs and chemicals. *Pharmacol. Rev.,* 28:207–273.
25. Popper, H., and Schaffner, F. (1963): Fine structural changes of the liver. *Ann. Int. Med.,* 59:674–691.
26. Schaffner, F., and Popper, H. (1969): Cholestasis is the result of hypoactive hypertrophic smooth endoplasmatic reticulum in the hepatocyte. *Lancet,* 2:355–359.
27. Drew, R., and Priestley, B. G. (1978): Failure of hypoactive hypertrophic smooth endoplasmatic reticulum to produce cholestasis in rats. *Toxicol. Appl. Pharmacol.,* 45:191–199.
28. Mackinnon, M., Sutherland, E., and Simon, F. R. (1977): Effects of ethinyl estradiol on hepatic microsomal proteins and the turnover of cytochrome P-450. *J. Lab. Clin. Med.,* 90:1096–1106.
29. Goldfisher, S., Arias, I. M., Essner, E., and Novikoff, A. B. (1962): Cytochemical and electron microscopic studies of rat liver with reduced capacity to transport conjugated bilirubin. *J. Exp. Med.,* 115:467–475.
30. Davis, R. A., Kern, F., Showalter, R., Sutherland, E., Sinensky, M., and Simon, F. R. (1978): Alterations of hepatic Na$^+$,K$^+$-ATPase and bile flow by estrogen: Effects on liver surface membrane lipid structure and function. *Proc. Natl. Acad. Sci. USA,* 75:4130–4134.
31. Simon, F. R., Gonzalez, M., Sutherland, E. Accatino, L., and Davis, R. A. (1980): Reversal of ethinyl estradiol-induced bile secretory failure with Triton WR-1339. *J. Clin. Invest.,* 65:851–860.
32. Carruthers, J. S., and Steiner, J. W. (1962): Experimental extrahepatic biliary obstruction: Fine structural changes of liver cell mitochondria. *Gastroenterology,* 42:419–430.
33. Shorey, J., Schenker, S., and Combes, B. (1969): Effect of acute hypoxia on hepatic excretory function. *Am. J. Physiol.,* 216:1441–1452.
34. Slater, T. F., and Eakins, M. N. (1976): Biochemical studies on bile secretion. In: *The Hepatobiliary System,* edited by W. Taylor, pp 61–78. Plenum, New York.
35. Lopez del Pino, V. H., and LaRusso, N. F. (1981): Dissociation of bile flow and biliary lipid secretion from biliary lysosomal enzyme output in experimental cholestasis. *J. Lipid Res.,* 22:229–244.
36. Jones, A. L., Schmucker, D. L., Mooney, J. S., Adler, R. D., and Ockner, R. (1978): A quantitative analysis of hepatic ultrastructure in rats during enhanced bile secretion. *Anat. Rec.,* 192:277–288.
37. Dubin, M., Maurice, M., Feldmann, G., and Erlinger, S. (1978): Phalloidin-induced cholestasis in the rat: Relation to changes in microfilaments. *Gastroenterology,* 75:450–455.
38. Elias, E., Hruban, Z., Wade, J. B., and Boyer, J. L. (1980): Phalloidin-induced cholestasis: A microfilament-mediated change in junctional complex permeability. *Proc. Natl. Acad. Sci. USA,* 77:2229–2233.
39. Schultz, S. G. (1977): The role of paracellular pathways in isotonic fluid transport. *Yale J. Biol. Med.,* 50:99–113.
40. Forker, E. L. (1969): The effect of estrogen on bile formation in the rat. *J. Clin. Invest.,* 48:654–663.
41. Peterson, R. E., and Fujimoto, J. M. (1977): Increased biliary tree permeability produced in rats by hepatoactive agents. *J. Pharmacol. Exp. Ther.,* 202:732–739.
42. Layden, T. J., and Boyer, J. L. (1978): Influence of bile acids in bile canalicular membrane morphology and the lobular gradient in canalicular size. *Lab. Invest.,* 39:110–119.

ATPase activity in liver plasma membranes enriched in bile canaliculi. *J. Clin. Invest.,* 57:1009–1018.

43. Strasberg, S. M., Kay, R. M., Ilson, R. G., Petrunka, C. N., and Paloheimo, J. E. (1979): Taurolithocholic acid and chlorpromazine cholestasis in the Rhesus monkey. *Can. J. Physiol. Pharmacol.,* 57:1138–1147.

44. Jakab, F., Donath, T., and Szabo, G. (1976): The escape of bile from the intrahepatic biliary tree in acute bile stasis. *Z. Mikrosk. Anat. Forsch.,* 90:200–205.

45. Metz, J., Aoki, A., Merlo, M., and Forssman, W. G. (1977): Morphological alterations and functional changes of interhepatocellular junctions induced by bile duct ligation. *Cell Tissue Res.* 182:299–310.

46. Javitt, N. B., and Emerman, S. (1968): Effect of sodium taurolithocholate on bile flow and bile acid excretion. *J. Clin. Invest.,* 47:1002–1014.

47. Layden, T. J., and Boyer, J. L. (1977): Taurolithocholate-induced cholestasis: Taurocholate, but not dehydrocholate, reverses cholestasis and bile canalicular membrane injury. *Gastroenterology,* 73:120–128.

48. Miyai, K., Mayr, W. W., and Richardson, A. L. (1975): Acute cholestasis induced by lithocholic acid in the rat. A freeze-fracture replica and thin section study. *Lab. Invest.,* 32:527–535.

49. Kakis, G., and Yousef, I. M. (1978): Pathogenesis of lithocholate- and taurolithocholate-induced intrahepatic cholestasis in rats. *Gastroenterology,* 75:595–607.

50. Cooper, R. A., Leslie, M. H., Fishcoff, S., Shinitzky, M., and Shattil, S. J. (1978): Factors influencing the lipid composition and fluidity of red cell membranes in vitro: Production of red cell possessing more than two cholesterols per phospholipid. *Biochemistry,* 17:327–331.

51. Kakis, G., Phillips, M. J., and Yousef, I. M. (1980): The respective role of membrane cholesterol and of sodium potassium adenosine triphosphatase in the pathogenesis of lithocholate-induced cholestasis. *Lab. Invest.,* 43:73–81.

52. Layden, T. J., Elias, E., and Boyer, J. L. (1978): Bile formation in the rat. The role of the paracellular shunt pathway. *J. Clin. Invest.,* 62:1375–1385.

53. De Vos, R., and Desmet, V. J. (1978): Morphologic changes of the junctional complex of the hepatocytes in rat liver after bile duct ligation. *Br. J. Exp. Pathol.,* 59:220–227.

54. Metz, J., and Bressler, D. (1979): Reformation of gap and tight junctions in regenerating rat liver after cholestasis. *Cell Tissue Res.,* 199:257–270.

55. Robenek, H., Herwig, J., and Themann, H. (1980): The morphologic characteristics of intercellular junctions between normal human liver cells and cells from patients with extrahepatic cholestasis. *Am. J. Pathol.,* 100:93–114.

56. Oda, M., and Phillips, M. J. (1975): Electron microscopic cytochemical characterization of bile canaliculi and bile ducts in vitro. *Virchows Archiv.* [Cell Pathol.], 18:109–118.

57. Montesano, R., Gabbiani, G., Perrelet, A., and Orci, L. (1976): In vivo induction of tight junction proliferation in rat liver. *J. Cell Biol.,* 68:793–798.

58. King, J. E., and Schoenfield, L. J. (1971): Cholestasis induced by sodium taurolithocholate in isolated hamster liver. *J. Clin. Invest.,* 50:2305–2312.

59. Miyai, K., Richardson, A. L., Mayr, W., and Javitt, N. B. (1977): Subcellular pathology of rat liver in cholestasis and choleresis induced by bile salts. 1. Effects of lithocholic, 3-hydroxy-5-cholenoic, cholic and dehydrocholic acids. *Lab. Invest.,* 36:249–258.

60. De Vos, R., De Wolf-Peters, C., Desmet, V., Eggermont, E., and Van Acker, K. (1975): Progressive intrahepatic cholestasis (Byler's disease): Case report. *Gut,* 16:943–950.

61. Jenner, R. E., and Howard, E. R. (1975): Unsaturated monohydroxy bile acids as a cause of idiopathic obstructive cholangiopathy. *Lancet,* 2:1073–1075.

62. Murphy, G. M., Jansen, F. H., and Billing, B. H. (1972): Unsaturated monohydroxy bile acids in cholestatic liver disease. *Biochem. J.,* 129:491–494.

63. Palmer, R. H. (1967): The formation of bile acid sulfates: A new pathway of bile acid metabolism in human. *Proc. Natl. Acad. Sci. USA,* 58:1047–1050.

64. Back, P., Spaczynski, K., and Gerok, W. (1974): Bile salt glucuronides in urine. *Hoppe Seylers Z. Physiol. Chem.,* 335:749–752.

65. Galeazzi, R., and Javitt, N. B. (1977): Bile acid excretion: The alternate pathway in the hamster. *J. Clin. Invest.,* 60:693–701.

66. Makino, I., Sjovall, J., Norman, A., and Strandvik, B. (1971): Excretion of 3-beta-hydroxy-5-cholenic and 3-alpha-hydroxy-5-alpha-cholanoic acids in urine of infants with biliary atresia. *FEBS Lett.* 15:161–164.

67. Stiehl, A., Becker, M., Czygan, P., Froehling, W., Kommerell, B., Rotthauwe, H. W., and Senn, M. (1980): Bile acids and their sulphated and glucuronidated derivatives in bile, plasma and urine of children with intrahepatic cholestasis: effects of phenobarbital treatment. *Eur. J. Clin. Invest.,* 10:307–316.

68. Summerfield, J. A., Billing, B. H., and Shackleton, C. H. L. (1976): Identification of bile acids in the serum and urine in cholestasis. Evidence for 6-alpha-hydroxylation of bile acids in man. *Biochem. J.,* 154:507–516.

69. Summerfield, J. A., Cullen, J., Barnes, S., and Billing, B. H., (1977): Evidence for renal control of urinary excretion of bile acids and bile acid sulfates in the cholestatic syndrome. *Clin. Sci. Mol. Med.,* 52:51–65.

70. Mitropoulos, K. A., and Myant, N. B. (1967): The formation of lithocholic acid, chenodeoxycholic acid and alpha- and beta-muricholic acid from cholesterol incubated with rat liver mitochondria. *Biochem. J.,* 103:472–479.

71. Alme, B., Bremmelgard, A., Sjoevall, J., and Thomassen, P. (1977): Analysis of metabolic profiles of bile acids in urine using a lipophilic anion exchanger and computerized gas-liquid chromatography–mass spectrometry. *J. Lipid Res.,* 18:339–361.

72. Back, P., and Walter, K. (1980): Developmental pattern of bile acid metabolism as revealed by bile acid analysis of meconium. *Gastroenterology,* 78:671–676.

73. Eyssen, H., Parmentier, G., Compernolle, F., Boon, J., and Eggermont, E. (1972): Trihydroxycoprostanic acid in the duodenal fluid of two children with intrahepatic bile duct anomalies. *Biochim. Biophys. Acta,* 273:212–221.

74. Hanson, R. F., Isenberg, J. N., Williams, G. C., Hackey, D., Klein, P. D., and Sharp, H. L. (1975): The metabolism of 3α, 7α, 12α-trihydroxy-P-cholestan-26-oic acid in two siblings with cholestasis due to intrahepatic bile duct anomalies. An apparent inborn error of cholic acid synthesis. *J. Clin. Invest.,* 56:577–587.

75. Linarelli, L. G., Williams, C. N., and Phillips, M. J. (1972): Byler's disease: Fatal intrahepatic cholestasis. *J. Pediatr.,* 81:484–492.

76. Williams, C. N., Kaye, R., Baker, L., Hurwitz, R., and Senior, J. R. (1972): Progressive familial cholestatic cirrhosis and bile acid metabolism. *J. Pediatr.,* 81:493–500.

77. Reichen, J., and Paumgartner, G. (1979): Inhibition of hepatic Na$^+$,K$^+$-adenosinetriphosphatase in taurolithocholate-induced cholestasis in the rat. *Experientia,* 35:1186–1188.

78. Priestley, B. G., Cote, M. G., and Plaa, G. L. (1971): Biochemical and morphological parameters of taurolithocholate cholestasis. *Can. J. Physiol. Pharmacol.,* 49:1078–1091.

79. Bonvicini, F., Gautier, A., Gardiol, D., and Borel, G. A. (1978): Cholesterol in acute cholestasis induced by taurolithocholic acid. *Lab. Invest.,* 38:487–495.

80. Schwenk, M., Schwarz, L. R., and Greim, H. (1977): Taurolithocholate inhibits taurocholate uptake by isolated hepatocytes at low concentrations. *Naunyn Schmiedebergs Arch. Pharmacol.,* 298:175–179.

81. Kakis, G., and Yousef, I. M. (1980): Mechanism of cholic acid protection in lithocholate-induced intrahepatic cholestasis in rats. *Gastroenterology,* 78:1402–1411.

82. Makino, I. (1973): Sulphated bile acid in urine of patients with hepatobiliary disease. *Lipids,* 8:47–49.

83. Vonk, R. J., Tuchweber, B., Masse, D., Perea, A., Audet, M., Roy, D. D., and Yousef, I. M. (1981): Intrahepatic cholestasis induced by allo monohydroxy bile acids in the rat. *Gastroenterology,* 80:242–249.

83a. Yousef, I. M., Tuchweber, R., Vonk, R. J., Masse, D., Audet, M., and Roy, C. C. (1981): Lithocholate cholestasis—sulfated glycolithocholate-induced intrahepatic cholestasis in rats. *Gastroenterology,* 80:233–241.

84. Herz, R., Paumgartner, G., and Preisig, R. (1976): Inhibition of bile formation in high doses of taurocholate in the perfused rat liver. *Scand. J. Gastroenterol.,* 11:741–746.

85. Drew, R., and Priestley, B. G. (1978): Choleretic and cholestatic effects of infused bile salt in the rat. *Experientia,* 35: 809–811.

86. Coleman, R., Lowe, P. J., and Billington, D. (1980): Membrane lipid composition and susceptibility to bile salt damage. *Biochim. Biophys. Acta,* 599:294–300.

87. Vyvoda, O. S., Coleman, R., and Holdsworth, G. (1977): Effects of different bile salts upon the composition and morphology of a liver plasma membrane preparation. Deoxycholate is more membrane damaging than cholate and its conjugates. *Biochim. Biophys. Acta,* 465:68–76.

88. Reichen, J., and Paumgartner, G. (1976): Uptake of bile acids by the perfused rat liver. *Am. J. Physiol.,* 231:734–742.

89. De Lamirande, E., and Plaa, G. L. (1979): Dose and time relationships in manganese-bilirubin cholestasis. *Toxicol. Appl. Pharmacol.,* 49:257–263.

90. Dhumeaux, D., Erlinger, S., Benhamou, J. P., and Fauvert, R. (1970): Effects of Rose Bengal on bile secretion in the rabbit: inhibition of a bile salt independent fraction. *Gut,* 11:134–140.

91. Horak, W., Grabner, G., and Paumgartner, G. (1973): Inhibition of bile salt-independent bile formation by indocyanine green. *Gastroenterology,* 64:1005–1012.

92. Witzleben, C. L. (1972): Physiologic and morphologic natural history of a model of intrahepatic cholestasis (manganese-bilirubin overload). *Am. J. Pathol.,* 66:577–588.

93. Wannagat, F. J., Adler, R. D., and Ockner, R. K. (1978): Bile acid-induced increase in bile acid-independent flow and plasma membrane Na$^+$,K$^+$ATPase activity in rat liver. *J. Clin. Invest.,* 61:297–307.

94. Yousef, I. M., and Fisher, M. M. (1976): In vitro effect of free bile acids on the bile canalicular membrane phospholipids in the rat. *Can. J. Biochem.,* 54:1040–1046.

95. Nemchausky, B. A., Layden, T. J., and Boyer, J. L. (1977): Effects of chronic choleretic infusions of bile acids on the membrane of the bile canaliculus. A biochemical and morphological study. *Lab. Invest.,* 36:259–267.

96. Keeffe, E. B., Scharschmidt, B. F., Blankenship, N. M., and Ockner, R. K. (1979): Studies of relationships among bile flow, liver plasma membrane Na$^+$,K$^+$-ATPase, and membrane microviscosity in the rat. *J. Clin. Invest.,* 64:1590–1598.

97. Kimmelberg, H. K., and Paphadjopoulos, D. (1974): Effects of phospholipid acyl chain fluidity, phase transitions and cholesterol on Na$^+$-K$^+$-stimulated adenosine triphosphatase. *J. Biol. Chem.,* 249:1071–1080.

98. Reichen, J., and Paumgartner, G. (1977): Relationship between bile flow and Na$^+$,K$^+$-adenosine triphosphatase in liver plasma membranes enriched in bile canaliculi. *J. Clin. Invest.,* 60:429–434.

99. Blitzer, B. L., and Boyer, J. L. (1978): Cytochemical localization of Na$^+$,K$^+$-ATPase in the rat hepatocyte. *J. Clin. Invest.,* 62:1104–1108.

100. Samuels, A. M., and Carey, M. C. (1978): Effects of chlorpromazine hydrochloride and its metabolites on Mg^{2+}- and Na$^+$,K$^+$-ATPase activities of canalicular enriched rat liver plasma membranes. *Gastroenterology,* 74:1183–1190.

101. Keeffe, E. B., Blankenship, N. M., and Scharschmidt, B. F. (1980): Alteration of rat liver plasma membrane fluidity and ATPase activity by chlorpromazine hydrochloride and its metabolites. *Gastroenterology,* 79:222–231.

102. Meijer, D. K. F., Vonk, R. J., and Weitering, J. G. (1978): The influence of various bile salts and some cholephilic dyes on Na$^+$,K$^+$- and Mg^{2+}-activated ATPase of rat liver in relation to cholestatic effects. *Toxicol. Appl. Pharmacol.,* 43:597–612.

103. Scharschmidt, B. F., Keeffe, E. B., Vessey, D. A., Blankenship, N. M., and Ockner, R. K. (1981): In vitro effect of bile salts on rat liver plasma membrane fluidity and ATPase activity. *Hepatology,* 1:137–145.

104. Simon, F. R., Sutherland, E., Accatino, L., Vial, J., and Mills, D. (1977): Studies on drug-induced cholestasis: effect of ethinyl estradiol on hepatic bile acid receptors and NaK-ATPase. In: *Bile Acid Metabolism in Health and Disease,* edited by G. Paumgartner and A. Stiehl, pp. 133–143. MTP Press, Lancaster, England.

105. Toda, G., Kako, M., Oka, H., Oda, T., and Ikeda, Y. (1978): Uneven distribution of enzymatic alterations on the liver cell surface in experimental extrahepatic cholestasis of rat. *Exp. Mol. Pathol.,* 28:10–24.

105. Miner, P. B., Sutherland, E., and Simon, F. R. (1980): Regulation of hepatic sodium plus potassium-activated adenosine triphosphatase activity by glucocorticoids in the rat. *Gastroenterology,* 79:212–221.

106. Evans, W. H., Kremmer, T., and Culvenor, J. G. (1976): Role of membranes in bile formation. Comparison of the composition of bile and a liver bile-canalicular plasma membrane subfraction. *Biochem. J.,* 154:589–595.

107. Tavaloni, N., Reed, J. S., Hruban, Z., and Boyer, J. L. (1979): Effect of chlorpromazine on hepatic perfusion and bile secretory function in the isolated perfused rat liver. *J. Lab. Clin. Med.,* 94:726–741.

108. Oda, M., and Phillips, M. J. (1977): Bile canalicular membrane pathology in cytochalasin B induced cholestasis. *Lab. Invest.,* 37:350–356.

109. Wootton, A. M., Neale, G., and Moss, D. W. (1975): Some properties of alkaline phosphatases in parenchymal and biliary tract cells separated from rat liver. *Clin. Chim. Acta,* 61:183–190.

110. De Vos, R., De Wolf-Peters, C., Desmet, C., Bianchi, L., and Rohr, H. P. (1975): Significance of liver canalicular changes after experimental bile duct ligation. *Exp. Mol. Pathol.,* 23:12–34.

111. Kaplan, M. M., Kanel, G. C., and Singer, J. A. (1979): Enzyme changes and morphometric analysis of bile ducts in experimental bile duct obstruction. *Clin. Chim. Acta,* 99:113–119.

112. Hatoff, D. E., and Hardison, W. G. M. (1979): Induced synthesis of alkaline phosphatase by bile acids in rat liver cell culture. *Gastroenterology,* 77:1062–1067.

113. Yokoo, H., Craig, R. M., Harwood, T. R., and Cochrane, C. (1979): Griseofulvin-induced cholestasis in Swiss albino mice. *Gastroenterology,* 77:1082–1087.

114. Billington, D., Evans, C. E., Godfrey, P. P., and Coleman, R. (1980): Effects of bile salts on the plasma membranes of isolated hepatocytes. *Biochem. J.,* 188:321–327.

115. Tavaloni, N., and Boyer, J. L. (1980): Relationship between hepatic metabolism of chlorpromazine and cholestatic effects in the isolated perfused rat liver. *J. Pharmacol. Exp. Ther.,* 214:269–274.

116. Tsyrlov, I. B., Polyakova, N. E., Gromova, O. A., Rivkind, N. B., and Lyakhovich, V. V. (1979): Cholestasis as an in vivo model for analysis of the induction of liver microsomal monooxygenases by sodium phenobarbital and 3-methylcholanthrene. *Biochem. Pharmacol.,* 28:1473–1478.

117. Reyes, H., Levi, A. J., Gatmaitan, Z., and Arias, I. M. (1972): Studies on Y and Z, two hepatic cytoplasmic organic anion-binding proteins: Effect of drugs, chemicals, hormones and cholestasis. *J. Clin. Invest.,* 50:2242–2252.

118. Gumucio, J. J., and Valdivieso, V. D. (1971): Studies on the mechanism of ethinylestradiol impairment of bile flow and bile salt excretion in the rat. *Gastroenterology,* 61:339–344.

119. Accatino L., Contreras, A., Fernandez, S., and Quintana, C. (1979): The effect of complete biliary obstruction on bile flow and bile acid excretion: Postcholestatic choleresis in the rat. *J. Lab. Clin. Med.,* 93:706–717.

120. Schwarz, L. R., Schwenk, M., Pfaff, E., and Greim, H. (1977): Cholestatic steroid hormones inhibit taurocholate uptake into isolated rat hepatocytes. *Biochem. Pharmacol.,* 26: 2433–2437.

121. Ros, E., Small, D. M., and Carey, M. C. (1979): Effects of chlorpromazine hydrochloride on bile salt synthesis, bile formation and biliary lipid secretion in the rhesus monkey: a model for chlorpromazine-induced cholestasis. *Eur. J. Clin. Invest.,* 9:29–41.

122. Accatino, L., and Simon, F. R. (1976): Identification and

characterization of a bile acid receptor in isolated liver surface membranes. *J. Clin. Invest.*, 57:496–508.

123. Hardison, W. G. M., and Wood, C. A. (1978): Importance of bicarbonate in bile salt independent fraction of bileflow. *Am. J. Physiol.*, 235:E158–E164.

124. Klos, C., Paumgartner, G., and Reichen, J. (1979): Cation-anion gap and choleretic properties in rat bile. *Am. J. Physiol.*, 236:E434–E440.

125. Reichen, J., Berman, M. D., and Berk, P. D. (1981): The role of microfilaments and of microtubules in taurocholate uptake by isolated rat liver cells. *Biochim. Biophys. Acta*, 643:126–133.

126. Elias, E., and Boyer, J. L. (1979): Chlorpromazine and its metabolites alter polymerization and gelation of actin. *Science*, 206:1404–1406.

127. Dubin, M., Maurice, M., Feldman, G., and Erlinger, S. (1980): Influence of colchicine and phalloidin on bile secretion and hepatic ultrastructure in the rat. *Gastroenterology, 79:* 646–654.

127a. Adler, M., Chung, K. W., and Schaffner, F. (1980): Pericanalicular hepatocytes and bile ductular microfilaments in cholestasis in man. *Am. J. Pathol.*, 98:603–616.

128. Carey, M. C., Hirom, P. C., and Small, D. M. (1976): A study of the physicochemical interactions between biliary lipids and chlorpromazine hydrochloride. *Biochem. J.*, 153:519–531.

129. Tavaloni, N., Reed, J. S., and Boyer, J. L. (1978): Hemodynamic effects on determinants of bile secretion in isolated rat liver. *Am. J. Physiol.*, 234:E584–592.

130. Gumucio, J. J., Balabaud, C., Miller, D. L., DeMason, L. F., Appleman, H. D., Stoecker, T. J., and Franzblau, D. R. (1978): Bile secretion and liver cell heterogeneity in the rat. *J. Lab. Clin. Med.*, 91:350–362.

131. Alpert, S., Mosher, M., Shanske, A., and Arias, I. M. (1969): Multiplicity of hepatic excretory mechanisms for organic anions. *J. Gen. Physiol.*, 53:238–247.

132. Haemmerli, U. P., and Wyss, H. I. (1967): Recurrent intrahepatic cholestasis of pregnancy. *Medicine,* 46:299–321.

133. Reyes, H., Gonzalez, M. C., Ribolta, J., Abento, H., Matus, C., Schramm, G., Katz, R., and Medina, E. (1978): Prevalence of intrahepatic cholestasis in Chile. *Ann. Int. Med.*, 88:487–493.

133a. Utili, R., Abernathy, C. O., and Zimmerman, H. J. (1977): Studies on the effect of *Escherichia coli* endotoxin on canalicular bile formation in the isolated perfused rat liver. *J. Lab. Clin. Med.*, 89:471–482.

134. De Pagter, A. G. F., Van Berge-Hennegouwen, G. P., ten Bokkel, A., and Brandt, K. H. (1976): Familial benign recurrent intrahepatic cholestasis. Interrelation with intrahepatic cholestasis of pregnancy and from oral contraceptives. *Gastroenterology, 71:202–207.

135. Riely, C. A. (1979): Familial intrahepatic cholestasis: an update. *Yale J. Biol. Med.*, 52:89–98.

136. Dubin, I. N. (1958): Chronic idiopathic jaundice: A review of fifty cases. *Am. J. Med.*, 24:268–292.

137. Zimmerman, H. J. (1979): Intrahepatic cholestasis. *Arch. Int. Med.*, 139:1038–1045.

138. Sucky, F. J., Balistreri, W. F., Heubi, J. E., Searcy, J. E., and Levin, R. S. (1981): Physiologic cholestasis: Elevation of the primary serum bile acid concentrations in normal infants. *Gastroenterology, 80:1037–1041.

139. Bloomer, J. R., Phillips, M. J., Davidson, D. C., and Klatskin, G. L. (1975): Hepatic disease in erythropoietic porphyria. *Am. J. Med.*, 58:869–882.

140. Avner, D. L., Lee, R. G., and Berenson, M. M. (1981): Protoporphyrin-induced cholestasis in the isolated in-situ perfused rat liver. *J. Clin. Invest.*, 67:385–394.

The Liver: Biology and Pathobiology, edited by
I. Arias, H. Popper, D. Schachter, and D. A. Shafritz.
Raven Press, New York © 1982.

Chapter 47

Fibrogenesis

Marcos Rojkind

Cirrhosis of the liver is one of the major causes of death worldwide. In the eastern hemisphere, hepatosplenic schistosomiasis is the most prevalent form of chronic liver disease (1). In the western hemisphere, alcohol may be responsible for at least 60% of total deaths attributable to liver cirrhosis (2,3). In Mexico and the United States, liver cirrhosis is the third cause of death for men between 30 and 60 years of age, and the incidence of the disease is increasing. In Mexico, approximately 30,000 people die every year from complications of liver cirrhosis (2).

The important cultural and socioeconomic problems associated with the consumption of alcohol or with the mode of transmission of schistosomiasis have made it difficult to establish proper programs for prevention of related liver disease. It has been suggested that a better understanding of the pathophysiology of liver cirrhosis could provide clues as to how to modify the course of the disease, prevent scar formation, and facilitate regeneration of undamaged liver cells (4).

Fibrosis is only one component of liver cirrhosis. Since many complications of the disease are associated with the increase in liver connective tissue, this chapter deals primarily with alterations in composition and metabolism of liver collagens. The relationship of changes resulting from the etiologic agent(s) that result in a fibrogenic response is analyzed. Modifications in collagen synthesis, deposition, and degradation are presented, with a brief analysis of the regulatory mechanisms. Alterations in glycosaminoglycans

are not analyzed; a complete reevaluation of this field is currently needed. The chemistry of collagen is discussed elsewhere in this volume, and reviews of liver fibrosis and collagen metabolism in the liver have been published (5–7).

LIVER COLLAGENS

Genetic Types and Changes in Distribution

Liver contains collagen types I, III, IV, and V. The total amount of liver collagen is 5.5 ± 1.6 mg/g fresh tissue (8). For a normal liver weighing approximately 1,500 g, total collagen content is 8.25 g. In terminal cases of liver cirrhosis, collagen content is increased above 30 mg/g. Since the size of the liver can be as small as 500 g, the net collagen content of an end-stage cirrhotic liver is approximately 15.0 g. These findings indicate that, although the size of the liver decreases threefold, the amount of liver collagen doubles. However, changes in the distribution of different collagen types, with the concomitant distortion of liver architecture, may be more important than the actual increase in collagen content. Thus the main alteration is a change in the ratio of parenchyma (cells) to stroma (extracellular matrix) (9).

All collagen types are increased in the liver of cirrhotic persons (8,10,11). Depending on the total amount of collagen present, the ratios of the different genetic types vary. In liver containing less than 20 mg collagen/g fresh tissue, all collagens are proportionally increased, and the ratio of type I to type III collagen is 1, a value similar to that found in normal liver. In liver with more than 20 mg/g, however, type I collagen is predominant, and the ratio of type I to type III increases (>2.0). Analysis of liver collagen types in cirrhosis produced by different etiologic agents has shown that the alterations are independent of the agent that produced cirrhosis. The final scar in the liver is similar to scars formed in the skin.

Immunocytochemical studies with antibodies against different collagens in the liver have shown that all antibodies react strongly with the dense collagen deposits of portal triads, terminal venule areas, and fibrous septa (12–15). The sinusoidal lining of the hepatocytes strongly stain with antitype IV and type V collagens but not as intensely with antitype III. No staining with antitype I collagen was detected in the central portions of the regenerative nodules. The projections of septa to the centrolobular regions stain with antibodies to collagens I, III, IV, and V (12–15).

GLYCOPROTEINS ASSOCIATED WITH COLLAGEN

The extracellular matrix of the liver contains several glycoproteins, two of which have been characterized. Fibronectin is associated with collagen and with the cellular plasma membrane of fibroblasts (16). Laminin is a component of some but not all basement membranes (14,17).

In cirrhosis, the amounts of fibronectin and laminin are increased. These data are based on immunocytochemical studies, however, and not on quantitative determinations (14). Fibronectin and laminin antibodies stain the connective tissue of portal triads and septa. Although fibronectin also stains some fibrilar structures of the intercellular matrix, laminin antibodies do not stain these structures. In many areas, laminin antibodies were localized in the parenchyma, where they encircle single cells or liver cell islands. This localization is different from that observed with antitype IV collagen antibodies (14).

According to the distribution of liver collagen in cirrhosis (12–15) collagenization of the space of Disse (18), thickening of the sinusoidal lining with a concomitant diminution of the sinusoidal caliber, and/or rigidity of the fibrosed wall may be responsible for the increase in portal pressure observed in this disease.

The changes in collagen content and distribution can explain some complications of chronic liver disease. The extracellular matrix closely interacts with the plasma membrane of hepatocytes and, in many cells, plays an important role in development and cell differentiation (19). It is possible that changes in collagen

(8,10–15), glycoproteins (14), and glycosaminoglycans (20,21) not only change the physical properties of the tissue but also modify the microenvironment. This may lead to a change in the phenotypic expression of liver cells. Another factor may be distortion of the lobular architecture. Hepatocytes in the normal liver lobule are heterogeneous with respect to their enzymatic content and intermediary metabolism (22). Since hepatocytes are genotypically similar, the phenotypic differences may be related to oxygen, hormonal, and metabolite gradients generated from the portal vein to the terminal venule areas (zones 1, 2, and 3 of the acinus) (23). Following formation of regenerative nodules and shunting of blood, the organization of liver plates is distorted, and hepatocyte function is altered.

Metabolic Changes Associated with Liver Fibrogenesis

Proline Metabolism

It has long been emphasized that proline is biosynthetically derived from glutamate. Experiments performed with liver slices from normal animals showed that a small amount of proline was derived from glutamic acid (24). In liver slices from cirrhotic animals, this amount was increased, but not sufficiently to explain the large increase in the liver proline pool (24). Therefore, the biosynthesis of proline from arginine and ornithine was explored in chick embryos during active biosynthesis of collagen (25), in liver of cirrhotic individuals (26), and animals (27). In all cases thus far studied, most if not all proline was derived from arginine and ornithine. This pathway (Fig. 1) is important; arginine, an essential amino acid, is used for the biosynthesis of proline and glutamate. Glutamate can readily be made available from many other sources, including glucose.

Ornithine has three possible metabolic pathways. One is formation of urea, which is a self-generating cycle, in which ornithine is not consumed. Another pathway is decarboxylation of ornithine via ornithine decarboxylase (28) to produce putrescine; this participates in the synthesis of polyamines, which are involved in RNA metabolism. Finally, ornithine may form proline, which is chiefly used for collagen biosynthesis or as fuel in mitochondria after oxidation by proline oxidase (29).

In CCl_4-induced liver cirrhosis, in addition to increased formation of proline from ornithine, liver proline oxidase is inhibited (29). Furthermore, alcohol inhibits hormonal induction of ornithine decarboxylase (30) providing additional ornithine for proline biosynthesis in alcoholic patients.

Although it has been suggested that the proline pool plays an important role in regulation of collagen syn-

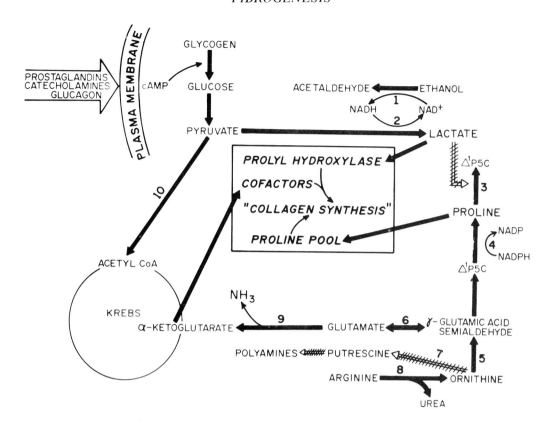

FIG. 1. Potential interrelationships between intermediary metabolism and liver fibrogenesis. Several factors, such as prostaglandins, catecholamines, and glucagon, stimulate liver adenyl cyclase and increase the concentration of cAMP. Liver glycogen is degraded to glucose, which eventually produces pyruvate. Under normal conditions, pyruvate enters the Krebs cycle, **10.** In the presence of liver damage produced by ethanol, metabolism to acetalhyde generates NADH, **1,** which favors formation of lactic acid from pyruvate, **2.** Lactic acid inhibits degradation of proline, **3,** and thereby increases the concentration of proline.

After liver injury, proline production from arginine, **8,** and ornithine, **5,** is increased. Alcohol inhibits formation of polyamines from ornithine, **7,** and facilitates the use of ornithine for proline biosynthesis. Although it has been suggested that glutamic acid is the precursor of proline, **6,** there is more evidence to suggest that radiolabeled ornithine generates both radiolabeled proline and glutamic acid. Whether glutamic acid is formed from glutamic acid semialdehyde or from Δ^1pyrroline-5-carboxylic acid (Δ^1P5C) is not known. Glutamic acid can produce α-ketoglutarate, **9.** As illustrated in the center box, lactate stimulates the activity of prolyl hydroxylase. The increased production of proline and inhibition of its degradation contributes to an increased proline pool in the liver and blood (alcoholic patients). α-Ketoglutarate, the cosubstrate of prolyl hydroxylase, facilitates the hydroxylation of prolyl residues in collagen. These factors and others which may stimulate collagen production by different cell populations link intermediary metabolism with liver fibrogenesis. *Black arrows,* metabolic pathways; *light arrows with cross lines,* inhibition of proline oxidation by lactic acid and inhibition of polyamine formation by alcohol. The enzymes involved in the metabolic pathways listed are: **1,** alcohol dehydrogenase; **2,** lactic dehydrogenase; **3,** proline oxidase; **4,** Δ^1P5C reductase; **5,** ornithine transaminase; **6,** glutamate kinase and dehydrogenase; **7,** ornithine decarboxylase; **8,** arginase; **9,** glutamic acid dehydrogenase; and **10,** pyruvate dehydrogenase.

thesis (24,31), proline alone is not responsible for increased collagen synthesis. The increased proline pool is needed for more efficient incorporation of the amino acid into collagen. In several animal models of cirrhosis and in human cirrhosis, proline is limiting (6,31). With increasing concentrations of proline in the incubation medium, there is increased incorporation of proline into collagen, reaching constant rates of synthesis at proline concentrations of 0.48 mM (29,32).

In alcoholic liver disease, in addition to an elevation in liver proline, there is also an increase in serum proline (33,34). Alcoholic patients with liver disease have hyperlactacidemia (35,36), which inhibits proline

oxidase activity (37). Thus hyperlactacidemia and inhibition of ornithine decarboxylase in the cirrhotic liver may be responsible for an increase in serum proline. We cannot exclude alterations in the transport of proline secondary to changes in membrane composition or lactacidemia per se.

Changes in Liver tRNA

In several systems that produce specific proteins as major biosynthetic products of a particular cell, their tRNA content and free amino acid pool closely resemble the amino acid composition of the specific protein synthesized (38). In tissues that produce collagen, there are some tRNA species in relatively larger concentrations than are found in the normal liver. A specific tRNA glycine may be selectively used for collagen biosynthesis (39,40).

Analysis of tRNA species in normal and cirrhotic rat liver has been presented (31,41). *In vivo*, tRNA amino acylation in cirrhotic liver is increased, and approximately 75% of tRNA appears to be amino acylated. In normal liver, only 25% of tRNA is amino acylated in preparation for protein synthesis (31,41). In addition to these findings, changes in the isoacceptor species of proline tRNA have been detected in liver of rats with cirrhosis induced with CCl_4 (41,31).

Enzymes Involved in Posttranslational Modifications of Collagen

All the enzymes involved in posttranslational modifications of collagen are elevated in the liver of animals or patients with cirrhosis (6); general properties of these enzymes are shown in Table 1. Alterations in individual steps of collagen synthesis observed in cirrhosis are summarized in Table 2.

Prolyl hydroxylase (42,43) and galactosylhydroxylysyl glucosyl transferase (44) are increased in liver and sera of patients with cirrhosis. Lysyl oxidase is elevated in liver of CCl_4-treated animals (45) but has not been investigated in human liver.

In liver fibrosis, no information is available with respect to the dolychol system, which is required for attachment of sugars to the procollagen peptide region, or regarding procollagen peptidases, which are involved in the cleavage of procollagen extensions. (For a recent review, see ref. 46.)

CELLS INVOLVED IN COLLAGEN SYNTHESIS

Several cell types are capable of producing different genetic types of collagen *in vitro* (47). Whether the same cells produce the same genetic types *in vivo* remains to be established. That different cells possess the necessary elements to produce collagen makes them potentially important in the general response of parenchymatous tissues to injury. In the liver, hepatocytes, fat-storing cells, fibroblasts, and endothelial cells could contribute to the production of collagen. Since the distribution of collagen types is not homogeneous throughout the liver (see Chapter 32), different cells may participate in the production of different genetic types of collagen. Recently, it was demonstrated that hepatocyte clones in culture produce

types I and III collagens and the trimer of $\alpha 1$ (I) collagen (48). Furthermore, primary cultures of rat hepatocytes contain most of the activity of collagen prolyl hydroxylase present in the intact liver (49).

CONNECTIONS BETWEEN LIVER INJURY AND LIVER FIBROGENESIS

Several factors are capable of modifying the synthesis of collagen and/or collagenase produced by several cells in culture. Nondialyzable materials released by lymphocytes or macrophages stimulate the proliferation of diploid guinea pig fibroblasts (50,51). Granulomas obtained from mice liver with experimental schistosomiasis produce a fibroblast-stimulating activity (52). Human mononuclear cells produce factors that either increase collagen accumulation (53) or selectively inhibit collagen synthesis when added to monolayer cultures of human skin fibroblasts (54). Lectin-stimulated monocytes increase production of the inhibitory factors (54). Liver from animals injured with CCl_4 produces factors that stimulate collagen synthesis and enhance the activity of collagen prolyl hydroxylase (55).

With respect to collagen degradation, it has been shown that proteases stimulate the production and release of collagenase and plasminogen activator by fibroblasts (56). Lymphokines (57,58), colchicine (59), and cytochalasin B (59,60) induce the production of proteases that activate the release of collagenase; serum contains factors that inhibit the release of such proteases (56) or block the activity of collagenase by direct combination with the enzyme. Tissues also contain peptides that inhibit collagenase activity (61).

The nature of the factors produced or the mediators involved is not known. Prostaglandins and cAMP may participate as either mediators or effectors. Prostaglandins stimulate collagen synthesis in some systems (62) and inhibit collagen deposition in others (63). The latter reaction is secondary to an increment in intracellular degradation of collagen (64). The interrelationships between prostaglandins and cAMP in the fibrotic process are not known; however, liver plasma membrane adenylate cyclase activity and cellular cAMP are stimulated by prostaglandins (65), and both are elevated in liver of rats made cirrhotic with CCl_4 (66).

Elevations of liver cAMP, if also present in alcoholic persons, may have important implications in the pathophysiology of liver fibrosis (see Fig. 1). cAMP promotes glycogen degradation. Excess pyruvate derived from glucose is transformed into lactic acid by the increased concentrations of NADH produced during the metabolism of alcohol by alcohol dehydrogenase. Lactate can inhibit proline oxidase (37), promote the elevation of liver proline (6), stimulate collagen syn-

TABLE 1. *Liver fibrogenesis* [a]

Known steps in collagen biosynthesis	Studied events in liver fibrogenesis
Transcription	Gene selection: All collagen types (I, III, IV, V) are increased.
Translation	
mRNA	?
tRNA	Functional tRNA is increased, total tRNA is normal. There are changes in the isoacceptor species of prolyl tRNA.
Amino acid pools	Several amino acids are increased. The increase in proline is proportional to total liver collagen content. Collagen synthesis is dependent on proline concentration and is saturable at 0.48 mM proline. Proline oxidase activity is inhibited. Proline is derived chiefly from ornithine and arginine.
Intracellular posttranslational modifications	
Hydroxylation of proline and lysine residues	The activities of prolyl and lysyl hydroxylases are increased prior to an increase in liver collagen content. Serum immunoreactive prolyl hydroxylase closely follows changes in liver enzyme.
Glycosylation of hydroxylysine	Galactosylhydroxylysyl glucosyl transferase.
Glycosylation of noncollagenous extensions of procollagen	Requires dolichol phosphate intermediates. Inhibited by tunicamycin.
Disulfide bonding and helix formation	Occurs only after complete hydroxylation and glycosylation of collagen chains.
Transcellular movement of collagen	At physiologic temperature, only completed and triple helical collagen chains are secreted. Microtubules are involved in transcellular movement.
Extracellular posttranslational modifications	
Conversion of procollagen to collagen	At least two different enzymes are needed. No information about these enzymes is available in liver fibrosis.
Fiber formation	Occurs only if the procollagen peptides have been cleaved. The peptides may be found in serum. Type III procollagen may exist as such in the liver. Correlation of procollagen peptide levels in serum with liver cell necrosis and inflammation.
Oxidation of lysine and hydroxylysine residues to aldehydes	Lysyl oxidase is increased and follows liver fibrogenesis.
Formation of intramolecular and intermolecular crosslinks	Spontaneous reactions (?). Collagen crosslinks may slow down collagen degradation by tissue collagenase.
Association with other macromolecules	Noncollagenous glycoproteins (fibronectin) are increased and may inhibit binding of collagenase to collagen. Changes in microenvironment may modify phenotypic expression of liver cells.
Degradation	Collagenase activity is increased or normal and cleaves only newly synthesized collagen. There is no binding of collagenase to liver collagen fibers.

[a] Modified from ref. 83.

thesis, and activate collagen prolyl hydroxylase (67). Whether these mechanisms are specific for alcohol liver injury or are mediated through the same mechanisms as in other chronic liver diseases remains to be determined.

Lysosomal enzymes, which are released after cell injury or produced by inflammatory cells, may promote the production of collagenase, which mediates remodeling of damaged liver. Factors produced by platelets or other cells, including inflammatory cells can stimulate cell proliferation and collagen biosynthesis. The same factors may also stimulate collagen biosynthesis by nonfibroblastic cells. Subsequently, when repair has been completed, inhibitory factors reduce collagen synthesis to normal values. In chronic liver diseases, however, while the injurious agent persists, only the first part of the process is activated, and collagen synthesis and liver fibrogenesis continue. In the reversible stage of the disease, cessation of liver injury allows the inhibitory factors to arrest the fibrogenic response. Nevertheless, if the mechanisms that control the aforementioned reactions are modified or destroyed, liver fibrosis can become irreversible.

TABLE 2. Some properties of enzymes involved in posttranslational modification of collagen[a]

Enzyme	Substrate	General information
4-Prolylhydroxylase	Prolyl residues in α-chains. Second proline in the triplet glycine-proline-proline.	Active enzyme: tetramer of 240,000 daltons. Monomers of 60,000 and 64,000 daltons inactive. Cofactors: O_2, Fe^{2+}, α-ketoglutarate, ascorbate. Inhibitors: N_2, chelating agents, corticosteroids. Not active with triple helical collagen.
3-Prolylhydroxylase	Prolyl residues in α-chains. First proline in the triplet glycine-proline-proline.	Same requirements as 4-prolylhydroxylase; MW 160,000 daltons.
Lysylhydroxylase	Lysyl residues in α-chains.	Two forms: 200,000 and 500,000 daltons. Same requirements as the prolylhydroxylases.
Collagen galactosyltransferase	Hydroxylysyl residues in α-chains.	MW 200,000 and 450,000 daltons. Requires MN^{2+}. Transfers galactose from UDP-galactose. Decreased activity with triple helical collagen. Inactive with free hydroxylysine.
Collagen glucosyltransferase	Galactosylhydroxylysyl residues in α-chains.	MW 55,000 daltons. Requires Mn^{2+}. Transfers glucose from UDP-glucose. Decreased activity with triple helical collagen. Active with free galactosylhydroxylysine.
Sugar transferases	Asparagine residues in noncollagenous extensions of pro-α-chains.	Dolichol phosphate intermediates; it is inhibited by tunicamycin.
Procollagen peptidase	Intact procollagen.	MW 70,000 daltons. Requires Ca^{2+}. Purified enzyme cleaves only N-terminal propeptides; there must be other peptidases for the C-terminal propeptides.
Lysyl oxidase	Some lysyl and/or hydroxylysyl residues in triple helical collagen.	MW 62,000 daltons. Requires Cu. Inhibited by copper chelators, β-aminopropionitrile and other lathyrogens, and high concentrations of penicillamine.

[a] Modified from ref. 6.

COLLAGEN SYNTHESIS AND DEPOSITION

Increased collagen content in the diseased liver is a result of an imbalance between collagen synthesis and deposition, and collagen degradation. In all types of cirrhosis thus far analyzed, collagen synthesis is increased *in vitro* (6,26). Furthermore, this increase correlates with the amount of collagen present in the liver, which suggests that most fibrous tissue is produced by active deposition. Collapse of the preexisting parenchyma may also play a role in liver fibrosis.

Collagen degradation has been investigated in CCl_4-induced liver cirrhosis and in murine schistosomiasis. In the former, normal or increased collagenase activity is detected at early stages of the disease (68); subsequently, collagenase activity decreases (69). Using immunofluorescent antibodies against collagenase, the enzyme was localized bound to collagen in the extracellular space (70). The enzyme has a wide distribution; almost every section that contains collagen fibers also contains collagenase. In early stages of liver cirrhosis, antibodies to collagenase localize on the outer parts of collagen bundles; in late stages of the

disease, no localization of collagenase is observed (71). In contrast to the results of immunochemical studies, direct measurements of collagen degradation *in vivo* reveal active collagen turnover (M. Rojkind, M. A. Giambrone, J. Cordero, and C. Soto, *unpublished results*). However, the rates of degradation of individual collagen types *in vivo* are unknown.

In murine schistosomiasis, collagen synthesis and collagenase activity *in vitro* increase during the first 8 weeks postinfection (72). Subsequently, both decrease to almost normal levels. Maximal collagen deposition in the liver is attained at 8 weeks and continues up to 11 weeks. As judged from these results, the increase in collagen synthesis surpasses the extent of collagen degradation, which results in net collagen accumulation (72).

If the net increase in liver collagen content is due to active fibrogenesis, several important questions arise in relation to liver cirrhosis and fibrosis:

(a) Will withdrawal of the toxic agent or elimination of biologic agents that produce liver fibrosis arrest liver fibrogenesis? Owing to the lack of nonagressive methods to explore liver fibrogenesis in human liver disease, this question has been explored mainly in CCl_4-induced liver fibrosis in rats. Discontinuation of CCl_4 administration to rats previously treated for 7 or more weeks to produce cirrhosis is accompanied by a return to normal of the pool of liver proline (29), inhibition of mitochondrial proline oxidase activity (29), and increased incorporation of radiolabeled proline into collagen hydroxyproline (29,73). Furthermore, liver collagenase activity determined *in vitro* doubled (74). In man, we have indirect evidence of a ''better course of the disease'' in some patients who stop drinking alcohol (75) and in patients with Wilson disease (76) or PBC (77) in whom liver copper levels are reduced following treatment with penicillamine. However, no direct measurements of liver collagen synthesis have been performed.

(b) If the etiologic agent that produced liver cirrhosis is eliminated, can the liver remove excess collagen and reverse the disease, or is the disease self-perpetuating? Two recent reviews analyzed animal models (69) and patients (6,69) in whom complete histologic reversibility of liver fibrosis was documented. Whether potential reversibility exists in all types of human liver cirrhosis has yet to be determined. In some patients, however, cirrhosis of the liver appears to be reversible.

(c) If a self-perpetuating mechanism(s) begins at a specific time during evolution of liver cirrhosis, can we modify the mechanism(s) or enhance removal of liver collagen? Several attempts have been made to develop a pharmacologic therapy of liver fibrogenesis. The rationale consists in using chemicals that inhibit collagen synthesis and deposition and/or enhance collagen degradation. This ''magic bullet'' is not available, although encouraging results have been obtained using colchicine in the treatment of animal (78) and human (79,80) liver cirrhosis.

Thus far, we have considered excess collagen deposition as the primary event in liver cirrhosis. No attention has been paid to damage produced to the hepatocyte. It is important to determine whether at any stage of the disease the damage produced to hepatocytes is reversible. If we succeed in removing excess liver collagen, will remaining hepatocytes be able to function normally? This question has not been answered because no effective therapy for liver fibrosis currently exists.

NONAGGRESSIVE PARAMETERS OF LIVER FIBROGENESIS

Despite several claims that enzymes involved in posttranslational modifications of collagen may be used as markers of liver fibrogenesis (42–44), evidence of their reliability in routine analysis of human samples is lacking. Prolyl hydroxylase and galac-

tosylhydroxylysyl glucosyl transferase activities have been determined in serum and liver in cirrhotic patients (42–44). The results, compared with those obtained in patients with liver disease without fibrosis, suggest that serum prolyl hydroxylase activity does not always reflect liver fibrogenesis. Serum immunoreactive prolyl hydroxylase values reflect changes in enzyme activity in the liver and may serve as a marker. The enzyme is elevated in patients with PBC, alcoholic liver cirrhosis, acute hepatitis, cancer with liver metastasis, and some nonhepatic tumors, even in the absence of liver metastasis. In acute hepatitis, serum immunoreactive prolyl hydroxylase decreases rapidly with time (42). Serum galactosylhydroxylysyl glucosyl transferase correlates with serum prolyl hydroxylase immunoreactive protein levels and is increased in the same diseases (44). Although these enzymes are increased in the serum of cirrhotic patients, they are also increased in other diseases unrelated to liver cirrhosis.

Sensitive immunoassays have been developed to quantitate the immunoreactive procollagen type III peptide in biologic fluids (81), as well as other connective tissue proteins (82). In the serum of patients with alcoholic liver disease, procollagen peptide is increased two- to 20-fold as compared to control values. The peptide is also elevated in many patients with acute or chronic active hepatitis. Although the peptide is also elevated in patients with other nonhepatic diseases, the increases are smaller.

In patients with alcoholic liver cirrhosis, procollagen peptide levels correlate with the degree of inflammation and necrosis observed in liver biopsies. A similar correlation was reported for increased serum proline values in patients with alcoholic liver disease (34).

Further prospective studies of larger populations of patients with chronic liver diseases who were followed for prolonged periods will eventually determine whether these parameters are useful markers of liver fibrogenesis. Perhaps they may select patients with acute liver damage who are more sensitive to the injurious agent; these constitute the 30% population of alcoholics who eventually develop liver cirrhosis (3).

TREATMENT OF LIVER FIBROSIS

Several chemicals are currently being used in attempts to arrest liver fibrosis. A recent review summarized the available agents and their mechanism of action (83). Except for colchicine in several forms of liver cirrhosis (79) (alcoholic, cryptogenic, and posthepatitic) and penicillamine in PBC (77), the results are discouraging. These two drugs are far from ideal. More research is needed to produce nontoxic compounds with tissue or cellular specificity which reach the target organ and inhibit fibrogenesis.

ACKNOWLEDGMENTS

I wish to thank my students for helping me check references and particularly Mr. Javier Cordero for proofreading the manuscript, and Mrs. Josefina Quiroga for typing the manuscript. The author's original work was supported in part by Grant AM 17702, and subcontracts 612-1671 and 612-1749 with the Liver Research Center, Albert Einstein College of Medicine, New York, and Grants 1576 and 63(2)0136 from CONACyT-México.

REFERENCES

1. Warren, K. S. (1978): Hepatosplenic schistosomiasis: A great neglected disease of the liver. *Gut,* 19:572–577.
2. Dajer, F., Guevara, L., Arosamena, L., Suárez, G. I., and Kershenobich, D. (1978): Consideraciones sobre la epidemiología de la cirrosis hepática alcóholica en México. *Rev. Invest. Clin.,* 30:13–28.
3. Galambos, J. T. (editor) (1979): Epidemiology. In: *Cirrhosis. Major Problems in Internal Medicine. Vol. XVII,* pp. 91–127, Saunders, Philadelphia.
4. Rojkind, M., and Kershenobich, D. (1975): Regulation of collagen synthesis in liver cirrhosis. Inhibition of fibrogenesis in rats and humans. In: *Collagen Metabolism in the Liver,* edited by H. Popper and K. Becker, pp. 129–138. Stratton Intercontinental, New York.
5. Popper, H., and Piez, K. A. (1978): Collagen metabolism in the liver. *Dig. Dis.,* 23:641–659.
6. Rojkind, M., and Dunn, M. A. (1979): Hepatic fibrosis. *Gastroenterology,* 76:849–863.
7. Stern, R. (1979): Experimental aspects of hepatic fibrosis. In: *Progress in Liver Diseases, Vol. VI,* edited by H. Popper and F. Schaffner, pp. 173–185. Stratton Intercontinental, New York.
8. Rojkind, M., Giambrone, M. A., and Biempica, L. (1979): Collagen types in normal and cirrhotic liver. *Gastroenterology,* 76:710–719.
9. Pérez-Tamayo, R. (1965): Some aspects of connective tissue of the liver. In: *Progress in Liver Disease,* edited by H. Popper and F. Schaffner, pp. 192–210. Grune & Stratton, New York.
10. Rojkind, M., and Martínez-Palomo, A. (1976): Increase in type I and type III collagens in human alcoholic liver cirrhosis. *Proc. Natl. Acad. Sci. USA,* 73:539–543.
11. Seyer, J. M., Hutcheson, E. T., and Kang, A. H. (1977): Collagen polymorphism in normal and cirrhotic human liver. *J. Clin. Invest.,* 59:241–248.
12. Biempica, L., Morecki, R., Wu, C. H., Giambrone, M. A., and Rojkind, M. (1980): Immunocytochemical localization of type B collagen. A component of basement membrane in human liver. *Am. J. Pathol.,* 98:591–602.
13. Gay, S., Fietzek, P. P., Remberger, K., Eder, M., and Kühn, K. (1975): Liver cirrhosis. Immunofluorescence and biochemical studies demonstrate two types of collagen. *Klin. Wochenschr.,* 53:205–208.
14. Hahn, E., Wick, G., Pencev, D., and Timpl, R. (1980): Distribution of basement membrane proteins in normal and fibrotic human liver: Collagen type IV, laminin and fibronectin. *Gut,* 21:63–71.
15. Remberger, K., Gay, S., and Fietzek, P. P. (1975): Immunohistochemische untersuchen zur kollagencharakterisierung in libercirrhosen. *Virchows Arch. (Cell Pathol.),* 367:231–240.
16. Pearlstein, E., Gold, L. I., and García-Pardo, A. (1980): Fibronectin: A review of its structure and biological activity. *Mol. Cell. Biochem.,* 29:103–128.
17. Timpl, R., Rohde, H., Gehron-Robey, P., Rennard, S. I., Foidart, J. M., and Martin, G. R. (1979): Laminin—A glycoprotein from basement membranes. *J. Biol. Chem.,* 254: 9933–9937.
18. Orrego, H., Medline, A., Blendis, L. M., Rankin, J. G., and Kreaden, D. A. (1979): Collagenization of the Disse space in alcoholic liver disease. *Gut,* 20:673–679.
19. Reid, L. M., and Rojkind, M. (1979): New techniques for culturing differentiated cells: Reconstituted basement membrane rafts. *Methods Enzymol.,* 58:263–278.
20. Galambos, J. T, Hollingsworth, M. A., Falek, A., and Warren, W. D. (1977): The rate of synthesis of glycosaminoglycans and collagen by fibroblasts cultured from adult human liver biopsies. *J. Clin. Invest.,* 60:107–114.
21. Koizumi, T., Nakamura, N., and Abe, H. (1967): Changes in acid mucopolysaccharide in the liver in hepatic fibrosis. *Biochim. Biophys. Acta,* 148:749–756.
22. Jungermann, K., and Sasse, D. (1978): Heterogeneity of liver parenchymal cells. *TIBS,* 3:198–202.
23. Rappaport, A. M., (1976): The microcirculatory acinar concept of normal and pathological hepatic structure. *Beitr. Pathol.,* 157:215–243.
24. Rojkind, M., and Díaz De León, L. (1970): Collagen biosynthesis in cirrhotic rat liver slices. A regulatory mechanism. *Biochim. Biophys. Acta,* 217:512–522.
25. Zinker, S., and Rojkind, M. (1972): Collagen biosynthesis in the chick embryo. I. The source of free proline and collagen hydroxyproline. *Connect. Tissue Res.,* 1:275–281.
26. Dunn, M. A., Kamel, R., Kamel, I. A., Biempica, L., Kholy, A., Hait, P. K., Rojkind, M., Warren, K. S., and Mahmoud, A. F. (1979): Liver collagen synthesis in Schistosomiasis mansoni. *Gastroenterology,* 76:978–982.
27. Dunn, M. A., Rojkind, M., Hiat, P. K., and Warren, K. S. (1978): Conversion of arginine to proline in murine Schistosomiasis. *Gastroenterology,* 75:1010–1015.
28. Russell, D. H. (1980): Ornithine decarboxylase as a biological and pharmacological tool. *Pharmacology,* 20:117–129.
29. Ehrinpreis, M. N., Giambrone, M. A., and Rojkind, M. (1980): Liver proline oxidase activity and collagen synthesis in rats with cirrhosis induced by carbon tetrachloride. *Biochim. Biophys. Acta,* 629:184–193.
30. Lumeng, L. (1979): Hormonal control of ornithine decarboxylase in isolated liver cells and the effect of ethanol oxidation. *Biochem. Biophys. Acta,* 587:556–566.
31. Díaz de León, L., Ehrinpreis, M. N., Kershenobich, D., and Rojkind, M. (1979): Liver injury and liver fibrogenesis. In: *Metabolic Effects of Alcohol,* edited by P. Avogaro, C. R. Sirtori, and E. Tremoli, pp. 269–280. Elsevier, New York.
32. Dunn, M. A., Rojkind, M., Warren, K. S., Hait, P. K., Rifas, L., and Seifter, S. (1977): Liver collagen synthesis in murine schistosomiasis. *J. Clin. Invest.,* 59:666–674.
33. Cerra, F. B., Caprioli, J., Siegel, J. H., McMenamy, R. R., and Border, J. R. (1979): Proline metabolism in sepsis, cirrhosis and general surgery. The peripheral energy deficit. *Ann. Surg.,* 190:577–586.
34. Mata, J. M., Villarreal, E., Kershenobich, D., and Rojkind, M. (1975): Serum free proline and free hydroxyproline in patients with chronic liver disease. *Gastroenterology,* 68:1265–1269.
35. Kershenobich, D., García-Tsao, G., and Rojkind, M. (1979): Relationship between serum lactic acid and serum proline in alcoholic liver cirrhosis. *Gastroenterology,* 77:A–22.
36. Lieber, C. S., Jones, D. P., Losowsky, M. S., and Davidson, C. S. (1962): Interrelation of uric acid and ethanol metabolism in man. *J. Clin. Invest.,* 41:1863–1970.
37. Kowaloff, E. M., Phang, J. M., Granger, A. S., and Downing, S. J. (1977): Regulation of proline oxidase activity by lactate. *Proc. Natl. Acad. Sci. USA,* 74:5368–5371.
38. Rojkind, M., Zinker, S., and Díaz de León, L. (1972): Collagen biosynthesis: A regulatory mechanism. In: *Molecular Basis of Biological Activity,* edited by K. Gaede, B. L. Horecker, and W. J. Whelan, pp. 275–293. Academic Press, New York.
39. Carpousis, A., Christner, P., and Rosenbloom, J. (1977): Preferential usage of glycyl-tRNA isoaccepting species in collagen synthesis. *J. Biol. Chem.,* 252:2447–2449.
40. Carpousis, A., Christner, P., and Rosenbloom, J. (1977): Preferential usage of tRNA isoaccepting species in collagen synthesis. *J. Biol. Chem.,* 252:8023–8026.
41. Díaz de León, L. (1975): *Regulación de la Biosíntesis de Col-*

ágena en la Cirrosis Experimental: Cambios en la Poza de Aminoacidos Libres y en la Población del tRNA. Doctoral dissertation, Cinvestav, Mexico.

42. Kuutti-Savolainen, E-R., Risteli, J., Miettinen, T. A., and Kivirikko, K. I. (1979): Collagen biosynthesis enzymes in serum and hepatic tissue in liver disease. I. Prolyl hydroxylase. *Eur. J. Clin. Invest.*, 9:89–95.

43. Mann, S. W., Fuller, G. C., Rodil, J. V., and Vidins, E. I. (1979): Hepatic prolyl hydroxylase and collagen synthesis in patients with alcoholic liver disease. *Gut* 20:825–832.

44. Kuutti-Savolainen, E. R., Anttinen, H., Miettinen, T. A., and Kivirikko, K. I. (1979): Collagen biosynthesis enzymes in serum and hepatic tissue in liver disease. II. Galactosylhydroxylysyl glucosyltransferase. *Eur. J. Clin. Invest.*, 9:97–101.

45. Siegel, R. C., Chen, K. H., Greenspan, J. S., and Aguiar, J. M. (1978): Biochemical and immunochemical study of lysyl oxidase in experimental hepatic fibrosis in the rat. *Proc. Natl. Acad. Sci. USA*, 75:2945–2949.

46. Minor, R. R. (1980): Collagen metabolism: A comparison of diseases of collagen and diseases affecting collagen. *Am. J. Pathol.*, 98:226–280.

47. Bornstein, P., and Sage, H. (1980): Structurally distinct collagen types. *Ann. Rev. Biochem.*, 49:957–1003.

48. Hata, R., Ninomiya, Y., Nagai, Y., and Tsukada, Y. (1980): Biosynthesis of interstitial types of collagen by albumin-producing rat parenchymal cell (hepatocyte) clones in culture. *Biochemistry*, 19:169–176.

49. Guzelian, P. S., and Diegelmann, R. F. (1979): Localization of collagen prolyl hydroxylase to the hepatocyte. *Exp. Cell Res.*, 123:269–279.

50. Leibovich, S. J., and Ross, R. (1976): A macrophage-dependent factor that stimulates the proliferation of fibroblasts *in vitro*. *Am. J. Pathol.*, 84:501–514.

51. Wahl, S. M., Wahl, L. M., and McCarthy, J. B. (1978): Lymphocyte mediated activation of fibroblast proliferation and collagen production. *J. Immunol.*, 121:942–946.

52. Wyler, D. J., Wahl, S. M., and Wahl, L. M. (1978): Hepatic fibrosis in schistosomiasis: Egg granulomas secrete fibroblast stimulating factor *in vitro*. *Science*, 202:438–440.

53. Johnson, R. L., and Ziff, M. (1976): Lymphokine stimulation of collagen accumulation. *J. Clin. Invest.*, 58:240–252.

54. Jiménez, S. A., McArthur, W., and Rosenbloom, J. (1979): Inhibition of collagen synthesis by mononuclear cell supernates. *J. Exp. Med.*, 150:1421–1431.

55. McGee, J. O'D., O'Hare, R. P., and Patrick, R. S. (1973): Stimulation of collagen biosynthetic pathway by factors isolated from experimentally injured liver. *Nature*, 243:121–123.

56. Werb, Z., and Aggeler, J. (1978): Proteases induce secretion of collagenase and plasminogen activator by fibroblasts. *Proc. Natl. Acad. Sci. USA*, 75:1839–1843.

57. Dayer, J. M., Russell, R. G. G., and Krane, S. M. (1977): Collagenase production by rheumatoid synovial cells: Stimulation by a human lymphocyte factor. *Science*, 195:181–183.

58. Vasalli, J-D., and Reich, M. (1977): Macrophage plasminogen activator: Induction by products of activated lymphocyte cells. *J. Exp. Med.*, 145:429–437.

59. Gordon, S., and Werb, Z. (1976): Secretion of macrophage neutral proteinase is enhanced by colchicine. *Proc. Natl. Acad. Sci. USA*, 73:872–876.

60. Harris, E. D., Reynolds, J. J., and Werb, Z. (1975): Cytochalasin B increases collagenase production by cells *in vitro*. *Nature*, 257:243–244.

61. Harper, E. (1980): Collagenases. *Ann. Rev. Biochem.*, 49: 1063–1078.

62. Blumenkrantz, N., and Søndergaard, J. (1972): Effect of prostaglandins E_1 and F_{1a} on biosynthesis of collagen. *Nature* 239:246.

63. Baum, B. J., Moss, J., Bruel, S. D., and Crystal, R. G. (1978): Association in normal human fibroblasts of elevated levels of adenosine 3':5'-monophosphate with a selective decrease in collagen production. *J. Biol. Chem.*, 253:3391–3394.

64. Baum, B. J., Moss, J., Breul, S. D., and Crystal, R. G. (1980): Effect of cyclic AMP on the intracellular degradation of newly synthesized collagen. *J. Biol. Chem.*, 255:2843–2847.

65. Okamura, N., and Terayama, H. (1977): Prostaglandin receptor-adenylate cyclase system in plasma membranes of rat liver and ascites hepatomas, and the effect of GTP upon it. *Biochim. Biophys. Acta*, 465:54–67.

66. Mourelle, M., Rojkind, M., and Rubalcava, B. (1981): Colchicine improves the alterations in the liver adenylate cyclase system of cirrhotic rats. *Toxicology* (*in press*).

67. Cardinale, G. J., and Undenfriend, S. (1974): Prolyl hydroxylase. *Adv. Enzymol.*, 41:245–300.

68. Okazaki, I., and Maruyama, K. (1974): Collagenase activity in experimental hepatic fibrosis. *Nature*, 252:49–50.

69. Pérez-Tamayo, R. (1979): Cirrhosis of the liver. A reversible disease? *Pathol. Ann.*, 14:183–213.

70. Montfort, I., and Pérez-Tamayo, R. (1975): The distribution of collagenase in normal rat tissues. *J. Histochem. Cytochem.*, 23:910–920.

71. Montfort, I., and Pérez-Tamayo, R. (1978): Collagenase in experimental carbon tetrachloride cirrhosis of the liver. *Am. J. Pathol.*, 92:411–418.

72. Takahashi, S., Dunn, M. A., and Seifter, S. (1980): Liver collagenase in murine schistosomiasis. *Gastroenterology*, 78: 1425–1431.

73. Galligani, L., Lonati-Galligani, M., and Fuller, G. (1979): Collagen metabolism in the liver of normal and carbon tetrachloride-treated rats. *Biomedicine*, 31:199–201.

74. Rojkind, M., Takahashi, S., and Giambrone, M. A. (1978): Collagenase and reversible hepatic fibrosis in the rat. *Gastroenterology*, 75:984.

75. Soterakis, J., Resnick, R. H., and Iber, F. L. (1973): Effect of alcohol abstinence on survival in cirrhotic portal hypertension. *Lancet*, 2:65–67.

76. Sternlieb, I. (1980): Copper and the liver. *Gastroenterology*, 78:1615–1628.

77. Epstein, O., De-Villiers, D., Jains, S., and Sherlock, S. (1979): Reduction of immune complexes and immunoglobulins induced by D-penicillamine. *N. Engl. J. Med.*, 300:274–275.

78. Rojkind, M., and Kershenobich, D. (1975): Effect of colchicine on collagen, albumin and transferrin synthesis by cirrhotic rat liver slices. *Biochim. Biophys. Acta*, 378:415–423.

79. Kershenobich, D., Uribe, M., Suárez, G. I., Mata, J. M., Pérez-Tamayo, R., and Rojkind, M. (1979): Treatment of cirrhosis with colchicine. A double-blind randomized trial. *Gastroenterology*, 77:532–536.

80. Rojkind, M., Uribe, M., and Kershenobich, D. (1973): Colchicine and the treatment of liver cirrhosis. *Lancet*, 1:38–39.

81. Rohde, H., Vargas, L., Hahn, E., Kalbfleisch, H., Bruguera, M., and Timpl, R. (1979): Radioimmunoassay for type III procollagen peptide and its application to human liver disease. *Eur. J. Clin. Invest.*, 9:451–459.

82. Rennard, S. I., Berg, R., Martin, G. R., Foidart, J. M., and Gehron-Robey, P. (1980): Enzyme-linked immunoassay (ELISA) for connective tissue components. *Anal. Biochem.*, 104:205–214.

83. Rojkind, M. (1981): Antifibrogenic therapy in liver disease. *It. J. Gastroenterology*, 12:97–103.

The Liver: Biology and Pathobiology, edited by
I. Arias, H. Popper, D. Schachter, and D. A. Shafritz.
Raven Press, New York © 1982.

Chapter 48

Neoplastic Transformation

Emmanuel Farber

The liver is a target for neoplastic transformation in experimental animals by chemicals of diverse structure (1,2), radiation (3), and at least two viruses (4). In man, several chemicals, hormones (5,6), and possibly hepatitis B virus (7,8) are incriminated.

As with other cancers, liver cancer, which results from various etiologic agents, develops slowly over decades in man and several months in small experimental animals, such as rats and mice. The development of hepatocellular carcinoma is characterized by appearance of many changes involving hepatocytes and other cell types; these morphologic alterations have been studied since the first major report in 1935 by Sasaki and Yoshida (9) of liver cancer induction with *o*-aminoazotoluene in an experimental animal. The past 10 years have seen new developments in experimental models for liver cancer, including more definitive ways to analyze sequentially the carcinogenic process in the liver at different levels of organization (10).

The subject of liver cancer in man and experimental animals has been reviewed comprehensively (10–16). This chapter presents a critical overview with emphasis on mechanisms and on major gaps in our understanding of how cancer may develop. The focus is on chemicals as etiologic agents, since almost all knowledge about liver carcinogenesis has been obtained with such carcinogenic stimuli. An attempt is made to integrate, where possible, factual data obtained at different levels of cellular organization into a biologically meaningful view of neoplastic transformation. As emphasized recently (17), distinction must be made between agents that cause disease, including cancer, and the processes that lead or relate to chronic disease. This distinction, although not absolute, is essential in attempting to reconstruct a pathogenetic mechanism of any disease or progressive biologic phenomenon.

CARCINOGENESIS AS A MULTISTEP PROCESS

Before concentrating on the liver, it is worthwhile to discuss several general aspects of carcinogenesis. As is clear for almost all organs and tissues, the development of epithelial cancer with chemicals, various types of radiation, and possibly viruses appears to consist of a process of cellular evolution from normal, through initiated, preneoplastic, and premalignant lesions to carcinoma. One regularly sees a change in a rare cell (rare event) (13) followed by expansion, amplication, or differential cell growth of the rare cells to create a second population, nodules, polyps, papillomas, and so forth (13). These are sites for a second change in a rare cell (second rare event), which subsequently are expanded to create another new population and so on until a population appears that has obviously malignant behavior. This repeating process of rare event-selection is consistent with a mutation-selection or a clonal evolution (see ref. 13 for references) concept of cancer development.

Possible alternate hypotheses to account for the rare

events must be considered until more information about mechanisms is available. For example, normal development is associated with many irreversible changes in cells and tissues, which lead to highly specialized organs and tissues. Until the nature of these changes and how they differ from mutations are understood, no conclusion concerning the role of mutation in cancer development is possible (13).

Unfortunately, even though the chemical-biochemical, histologic, and biologic evidence favors this formulation, the models available in any system for its study are poorly developed. As with any multistep process of biologic organization, each significant stage must be identified and studied separately *in vivo* and *in vitro* if we are to understand and control the process. This includes determination of relative rates of the different steps, so that rate-limiting steps can be delineated and regulated.

Models that allow such studies should have at least the following properties:

1. Testable working hypotheses of mechanisms.
2. Ability to control the induction and fate of each step.
3. Synchronization of each new cell population.
4. Quantitation of each new relevant cell population.
5. Genetic or other markers for each discrete step or cell population.
6. Ability to identify grossly and harvest each new cell population for cellular metabolic and molecular studies.

We are far from such models in any organ, but recent innovations offer optimism for their development in the liver.

How do these considerations fit with what we know about the skin, which has been studied in greatest detail regarding experimental carcinogenesis? By 1950, studies in the skin of mice and rabbits indicated that skin cancer development could be separated into at least two major stages: (a) a short, more or less irreversible step, initiation; and (b) a much more prolonged period of cancer development, promotion. Each phenomenon could be induced by different agents. With small doses and single applications, some known carcinogens could initiate the process but not stimulate further development. The latter could be effected by other types of agents that came to be known as promoters. Examples of the latter are croton oil and its component phorbol esters, phenols, and auramine. With relatively large doses, and with repeated application of the initiating carcinogen, many carcinogens can initiate and promote (18).

Research in the 1970s extended this basic principle to other tissues, including the liver, urinary bladder, kidney, and bronchial tree (12,13,19). Thus a unifying concept of carcinogenesis has developed, which includes liver cancer (13,19).

Reconciliation of the "two-stage" concept and the "multistep mutation-selection or clonal evolution" concept now seems possible. There is increasing evidence that initiated cells induced by carcinogens have not acquired measureable autonomy of growth but require an environment that creates a selection pressure (13,17,20). This is provided by promoting agents. Thus the first sequence of "rare event-selection" is environment dependent and reflects two effects: a rare initiated cell, and the selective growth of such cells, each induced by a different manipulation. Once this sequence occurs, the remaining sequences no longer depend on environmental manipulation but are self-generating (20). Thus initiation-promotion is only the first of an unknown number of sequences, the majority of which are apparently environment independent.

MODELS FOR LIVER CARCINOGENESIS

Continuous or Intermittent Chronic Exposure: Classic Models

Virtually all models studied until the past few years used relatively long periods of continuous or intermittent exposure to one or more carcinogens in food or drinking water or sometimes by parenteral administration. Such studies showed focal alterations, which include islands or foci of hepatocytes with altered histochemistry, foci and nodules of hyperplastic hepatocytes, hyperbasophilia, ductular proliferation ("oval cell proliferation"), nodules within nodules having morphologic resemblance to hepatocellular carcinoma, and a variety of cell and tissue changes around the focal areas (4,21–23). Although these studies have suggested some regular patterns of tissue changes during carcinogenesis, the relatively long exposure to carcinogens almost certainly induced an increasing number of overlapping events, which preclude analysis of their sequence. This criticism also applies to the models that induce large hyperplastic nodules by intermittent feeding of carcinogen-containing and carcinogen-free diets (24,26,31).

Model of Peraino: Initiation and Promotion

Peraino and his colleagues in 1971 reported development of a new model for the study of liver cancer (27). This model utilizes young weanling rats, in which proliferating hepatocytes are numerous. The animals are exposed to 2-acetylaminofluorene (2-AAF) [or other strong or weak carcinogens: 3'-methyl-4-dimethylaminoazobenzene (3'-Me-DAB), 2-methyl-4-dimethylaminoazobenzene (2-Me-DAB), diethylnitrosamine (DEN) (28)] in the diet for 2 to 3 weeks. After a short rest period (1 week), they are fed a diet containing 0.05% phenobarbital (PB) or polychlorinated biphenyls (PCBs) (29) for several months. Hyperplastic nodules and hepatocellular carcinomas are more numerous with than without PB. Thus the model mimics the classic skin model with the use of two different treatments: exposure to an initiating carcinogen, and a promoting environment.

These studies established that carcinogenesis in the liver resembled carcinogenesis in mouse or rabbit skin and opened up new ways to identify initiators and promoters. For example, 2-Me-DAB is an initiator but not a potent promotor, whereas DDT is an effective promoter.

Model of Scherer and Emmelot

Scherer, Emmelot, and their co-workers in 1971 (see refs. 30 and 31 for references) reported development of a new quantitative approach for the study of liver carcinogenesis. Using a single exposure to DEN [or other carcinogens, e.g., dimethylnitrosamine (DMN), 3'-Me-DAB, aflatoxin B_1 (AFB$_1$), ethionine] after partial hepatectomy (PH), they measured the number, size, and behavior patterns of microscopic islands of altered hepatocytes, which were deficient in ATPase (AP) and glucose-6-phosphatase (GP). These islands also show persistence of glycogen and increased activity of arylesterase.

Without further treatment of the animals, the islands of altered hepatocytes persist for long periods with only a small increase in size. On exposure to low levels of DEN for more than 375 days, cancer occurs. It is presumed but not yet established that cancer originates from one or more enzyme-altered islands.

The importance of this model is the introduction of quantitation of early presumptive steps in liver carcinogenesis. However, the absence of a hypothesis as to how early altered hepatocytes function as precursors for subsequent hyperplastic and neoplastic focal cell populations, the microscopic nature of the altered islands, and the relatively large ratio of number of islands to number of cancers are limitations of the model.

Model of Pitot: Combined Peraino and Scherer-Emmelot Models

Pitot and his colleagues (see refs. 32–34 for references) combined the Peraino and the Scherer-Emmelot models into a useful synthesis. Rats are subjected to PH; within 24 hr, they are given a single dose of DEN or other carcinogen. After a recovery period of 2 months, the animals are fed a diet containing 0.05% PB for a period of 6 months. Enzyme-altered islands [(decrease in ATPase (nucleotide polyphosphatase) and in GP

and increase in γ-glutamyltransferase) (γ-glutamyltranspeptidase) (GGT)], hyperplastic nodules, and hepatocellular carcinomas, are quantitated. This model, as the original Peraino model, is useful in identifying promoters, promoting environments, and initiating carcinogens.

Resistant Cell Model of Solt and Farber

Solt, Farber, and their colleagues (35) developed a model for sequential analysis of liver cancer development based on the hypothesis that initiating doses of a carcinogen produce an initiated cell which is resistant to cytotoxic effects of the carcinogen, particularly the inhibitory effect on cell proliferation. This idea was based on an early suggestion of Haddow (36) that resistance to the cytotoxic effects of a carcinogen may be important during carcinogenesis. This suggestion has been discussed by several investigators (see refs. 13, 20, 23, and 35 for references) and derived from the observation that cancer cells are relatively insensitive to cytocidal and other toxic effects of polycyclic aromatic hydrocarbons (PAH) and other carcinogens. These suggestions were integrated with the following considerations in formulating the resistant cell hypothesis: (a) many carcinogens are inhibitors of cell proliferation and/or DNA synthesis; (b) autonomous, semiautonomous, or independent growth of putative premalignant hepatocytes appears to be acquired relatively late in the carcinogenic process; and (c) new hepatocyte populations seen during liver carcinogenesis are focal and show a variety of properties that indicate resistance to cytotoxic effects of hepatotoxins and hepatocarcinogens.

In the model, adult rats are exposed briefly (single or, rarely, a few doses) to an initiating carcinogen. After recovery from any immediate toxicity, a selection procedure is imposed that is designed to measure the number of hepatocytes that proliferate in an environment that inhibits proliferation of the vast majority of normal or uninitiated hepatocytes. In the model, which is in current use as a standard, animals are fed a relatively low level of 2-AAF for 7 days to create the mitoinhibitory (mitosis inhibiting) environment and then are subjected to a stimulus for cell proliferation, such as PH or a single necrogenic dose of CCl$_4$. Regeneration of the bulk of the liver is inhibited, but isolated, widely scattered hepatocytes rapidly proliferate to form foci and visible nodules within 1 to 10 days. Liver cancer ultimately develops by 8 months; in some instances, metastasizing cancer arises within nodules. New cell populations resembling hepatocellular carcinoma arise in discrete hyperplastic nodules as nodules within nodules. The selecting environment per se has not been found to induce significant numbers of resistant cells over background in hundreds of animals. As presently conceived, the cytotoxic mitoinhibitory effects of carcinogens are exerted upon the majority of the original or uninitiated hepatocytes, while the key positive effect, induction of resistance, is induced in only a rare target cell.

PROCESS OF NEOPLASTIC TRANSFORMATION AS A SEQUENCE

Although the process of neoplastic transformation is by no means understood, major progress has been made over the past two decades in clarifying the sequence of effects and changes seen during development of liver cancer with chemicals. A summary of this sequence is presented, followed by a discussion of some of the fundamental questions and issues that are currently evident.

Sequence of Changes During Carcinogenesis

Initiation

Initiation of liver carcinogenesis consists of at least a two-step process: (a) induction of a biochemical event, an apparently reversible process, and (b) fixation of this as yet unidentified biochemical event by a round of cell proliferation.

Step 1: Induction of biochemical or molecular events by activated carcinogens. It is now almost certain that most carcinogens are not active by themselves but require metabolic conversion to one or more active derivatives. The liver is the most active and versatile organ in converting potential carcinogens to reactive products. For most known carcinogens, the reactive products are positively charged and have an affinity for sites of high electron density (37). Such electrophilic reactants are being increasingly characterized for different types of potential carcinogens. They react with many different sites in DNA, RNA, proteins, and other cellular constituents (37). The reactions with DNA have been studied most intensively (38), since it is generally accepted that perhaps one or more of these reactions are especially important for initiation of carcinogenesis. Although certain specific loci of interaction, such as 0–6 of guanine and other sites for hydrogen bonding between base pairs, have been particularly singled out as being relevant to carcinogenesis, this is based on the premise that altered base pairing is involved in the process. This assumption, although reasonable, is not essential in formulating working hypotheses for the molecular basis for initiation. For example, recent work by Columbano et al. (39) indicates that an extensive interchange occurs between parental and daughter strands of DNA during cell replication after exposure to DMN or N-methyl-N-nitrosourea (MNU). This suggested recom

bination offers alternatives to faulty single base pairing as a possible molecular basis for initiation.

The enzymology of carcinogen activation has received increasing attention in recent years. For the majority of carcinogens, including PAH, nitrosamines, aromatic amines, aflatoxins, and others, the mixed function monooxygenase systems, which are located predominantly in the endoplasmic reticulum (ER), play an important role. This system contains several cytochrome P-450s and NADPH reductase, among other components, and participates in carcinogen activation in either an alternate (e.g., 2-AAF) or sequential (e.g., PAH) pathway (22). The increasing emphasis on enzymology may clarify how the liver metabolizes carcinogens and other xenobiotic agents, including the manner in which a balance is created between activation (the genesis of more reactive molecules) and inactivation (the genesis of less reactive molecules).

This balance is now appreciated as having a key role in initiation. With any compound, the ultimate biochemical or molecular consequences are a reflection of the extent and rates of opposing reactions. Therefore, the modulation of this system can play a crucial role in determining whether or not a particular regimen will be carcinogenic or not (40). For example, PB and 3-methylcholanthrene can each prevent liver cancer induction with 3'-Me-DAB or other carcinogens when administered from the outset. Also, many drugs, foods, and xenobiotic agents modulate the development of cancer with chemicals (41) in experimental animals.

It is likely that the levels of normal cell constituents, such as glutathione and other trapping agents, and enzymes that use these substrates, may influence the availability of reactive moieties, the electrophilic reactants, for interactions with the presumed key macromolecules, such as DNA. This type of modulation is worthy of further exploration, since it may diminish the risk of initiation under certain circumstances.

Step 1A: Repair of crucial biochemical events. If exposure to a hepatocarcinogen at a nonnecrogenic dose is not followed within 2 days by one round cell replication, the pertinent or relevant biochemical lesions disappear, and initiation does not occur.

The nature of the relevant target molecules and alterations that relate to initiation are not known with certainty. Most of the available evidence, however, points to DNA as the likely target of importance, either exclusively or as part of a complex. Repair systems in liver can remove or repair many of the known DNA adducts (see ref. 38 for references). The availability of an assay for initiation in the resistant hepatocyte model of Solt and Farber makes it possible to approach this problem with more precision and celerity, since experiments can be completed in a few weeks instead of having to wait 1 to 2 years for cancer to develop.

Step 2: Genesis by cell proliferation of resistant

hepatocytes as one form of initiation. Initiation of liver cancer by chemicals appears to depend on cell proliferation within 48 hr. If cell proliferation occurs, a permanent change is induced in some hepatocytes and allows subsequent evolution to hepatocellular carcinoma. This becomes manifest in at least 3 ways: (a) appearance of cancer (see ref. 50 for references); (b) appearance or increase in the number of islands of hepatocytes with altered histochemical properties (see refs. 30 and 31 for references); or (c) appearance of hepatocytes that can be stimulated to proliferate, to form focal proliferations—at first small (foci) and than large (nodules) (see refs. 13 and 20 for references).

The mechanistic role of cell proliferation is not known. It may be related to DNA replication and/or to metabolic properties associated with different phases of the cell cycle. DNA replication in the presence of "damage" in the parental strand may induce double stranded damage and permanence. Transfer of altered DNA from parental to daughter strands by recombination, altered repair kinetics, or other possible modulations must be entertained as possibilities.

Cell proliferation can occur either by a primary mitogenic event, such as with partial hepatectomy, with a chemical mitogen, or as a secondary response to cell death. With the usual hepatocarcinogens, cell death occurs regularly; thus these chemicals have a built in cell proliferation component when given in necrogenic doses. With subnecrogenic doses, or with many nonhepatocarcinogens, a stimulus for cell proliferation must be added for initiation to occur. In a recent study (42) when hepatic necrosis was prevented by posttreatment with a protective agent, such as diethyldithiocarbomate (DEDTC) (half the molecule of disulfiram), initiation with DEN, a good hepatocarcinogen, is largely prevented, even though ethylation of DNA, RNA, and protein occurs. Initiation was restored by inducing cell proliferation without necrosis after posttreatment with DEDTC.

The implications of this study for human cancer are far reaching. With nonnecrogenic carcinogenic stimuli (many if not the majority of carcinogens), the rate-limiting step is not exposure to carcinogen but occurrence of cell damage and cell regeneration. This may be important for cancer development in many quiescent organs, such as pancreas, salivary glands, urinary bladder, thyroid, and liver. This could be one way in which hepatitis, either toxic or viral, might be synergistic with chemicals in inducing liver cancer in man.

Cancer Development

Step 3: Selective stimulation (promotion) of initiated hepatocytes to form nodules. If no selective stimulation occurs, initiated hepatocytes persist for long periods. If selective stimulation is exerted, initiated hepatocytes proliferate to form focal nodules. This can occur by various mechanisms.

Differental Inhibition.

If the promoting environment creates a stimulus for cell proliferation but inhibits normal cells from responding, only initiated cells that are resistant are able to respond. Thus focal proliferations can be rapidly or slowly generated, depending on the intensity of the selecting environment. In the Solt-Farber model, the selection pressure (promoting environment) is intense; as a result, nodules appear within 1 to 10 days. Under natural circumstances, with prolonged exposure to carcinogens, the kinetics are different, and nodules appear more slowly and are not synchronized. We visualize this to be the usual form in liver cancer in animals and man.

Differential Stimulation.

Schulte-Hermann and his colleagues (see refs. 17, 20, and 43 for references) found that with some chemicals which are mitogens for liver, such as cyproterone acetate or α-hexachlorocyclohexane, the majority of uninitiated hepatocytes lost their response after one or two cell cycles, while nodule cells continue to expand. Thus initiated hepatocytes continue to be stimulated to proliferate and generate nodules of ever-increasing size. The proliferating foci have at least two options.

Step 3A: Small foci persist. If the foci are small and remain so, they persist and show, in general, low epoxide hydratase activity (43). These foci do not seem to remodel or mature.

Step 3B: Hyperplastic nodules. If the foci show progressive growth stimulation to form larger collections of altered hepatocytes, hyperplastic nodules, remodeling, or maturation to normal-looking liver may occur. With a few hundred or a few thousand nodules per liver, the majority (90 to 95%) of nodules undergo a complex process of remodeling called neodifferentiation (13), while the minority persist and show progressive phenotypic changes. The hepatocytes in these persistent nodules show fairly uniform hypertrophy, mainly due to a large increase in their smooth ER (SER). These cells become typical "ground-glass cells" and closely resemble those seen in patients who are carriers of hepatitis B virus. The nuclei become pale, with apparent decrease of heterochromatin, and have large single nucleoli, although many of these hepatocytes are not proliferating.

The hepatocytes in hyperplastic nodules are arranged in two or more cell thick plates and have many biochemical, cytologic, physiologic, and biologic markers (35). During remodeling, they architecturally and histochemically change to resemble more closely normal, mature liver (4).

The hyperplastic nodules show no growth on transplantation, and their hepatocytes show no growth in culture. There is no evidence that these new hepatocyte populations have acquired independence or autonomy of growth and are considered by us and others to be hyperplastic, not neoplastic (13).

Thus the focal proliferations of altered hepatocytes express at least three options: when small, persistence; when large (nodules), remodeling for the majority and persistence for a few.

Step 3C: Transfer to other animals. The availability of large hyperplastic nodules with a reasonable degree of synchrony has allowed preparation and study *in vitro* of hepatocytes from nodules, and their transfer and growth (transplantation) into other animals. *In vitro,* the hepatocytes show resistance to the cytocidal effects of aflatoxin B$_1$ and other hepatotoxins (45–46). These hepatocytes have no apparent ability to grow autonomously, since they do not take in recepient syngeneic animals when injected into the portal vein. However, if an appropriate selection pressure is created in the recipient in a manner similar to that created during selection, islands of nodule hepatocytes seed and grow in the recepient liver, and some progress to lesions resembling hepatocellular carcinoma (36,45). These findings offer new approaches to the sequential analysis of liver carcinogenesis.

Steps 4, 5 . . . n: A change in a rare cell in a persistent hyperplastic nodule. Occasionally, an obvious new hepatocyte population arises in the middle of a hyperplastic nodule, creating nodules within nodules.

This new population is arranged with two or more cell thick plates. The cells are smaller than in the surrounding hyperplastic nodule and show a larger nuclear-cytoplasmic ratio. In a few hyperplastic nodules, unequivocal hepatocellular carcinoma has been seen with metastasis in the lung.

The number of rare events and new cell populations seen during cancer development is unknown, since no model is available for study of this important segment of carcinogenesis.

A tentative sequence of the early steps in development of liver cancer is outlined in Fig. 1. The rare events occur in a small number of cells in a large population at risk. They are probably clonal in nature. The selection process with options is akin to a phase of differentiation.

Hyperplastic nodules are one site of origin for hepatocellular carcinoma. Whether other sites exist is not known, since there is no model in which cancer develops without prior development of hyperplastic nodules (28). Until such a model becomes available, no conclusions can be made concerning the origin of cancer outside nodules.

Hepatocellular carcinoma might arise from oval cells (ductular cells plus ?) which undergo differentiation to hepatocytes (see ref. 13 for references). This was suggested for liver cancer induced with azo dyes, since an apparent transition between large oval cells and hepatocytes occurs with these carcinogens. Such transition has not been reported with other types of hepatocarcinogens. Development of a precise model

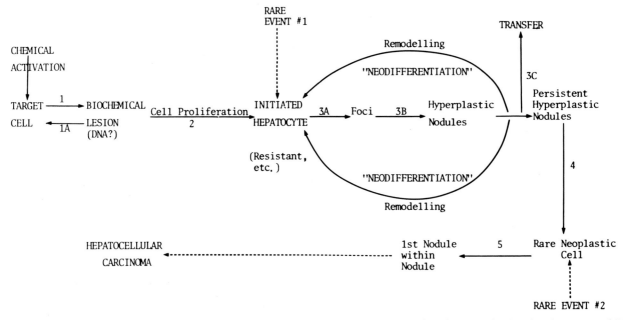

FIG. 1. Diagrammatic representation of our current concept of the sequence of early steps in the development of liver cancer with chemicals. Rare events are apparently irreversible cellular events occurring in a rare cell as discrete steps in the carcinogenic process. "Transfer" refers to the growth in the liver of putative preneoplastic hepatocytes from hyperplastic nodules on transfer by intraportal injection into a syngeneic recipient, prepared by creating an appropriate selection pressure by dietary 2-AAF plus PH or CCl$_4$.

for study of such histogenetic sequence is desirable and would offer new opportunities to explore how cancer develops with chemicals.

Fundamental Questions and Issues

As with any multistep process at any level of organization, the understanding of cancer development depends on understanding the nature and role of each major step, new cell population, and the generating and controlling forces. This requires experimental systems in which each important step can be isolated and studied *in vivo* and *in vitro*. This approach is now possible for some of the early steps but not for any subsequent ones, especially those that follow the first neoplastic change.

There is an emerging confidence that similar patterns of cancer development pertain in different tissues and with different initiating carcinogens and promoting environments (13,19). This awareness is fairly new and encourages further exploitation of the thesis that a study in depth and in detail of one system for chemical carcinogenesis will be useful in other tissues of different structure, architecture, and physiology.

Assuming the basic validity of this thesis, it is timely to focus on some fundamental issues using liver cancer as the model.

Initiation

There is abundant evidence that most chemicals that induce liver cancer in animals or man are converted into chemically reactive derivatives which can react with many different macromolecules, including DNA, and induce many more or less ''permanent'' changes in some cells at risk. Whether the mechanism of change is by mutation or unknown mechanisms that account for ''permanent'' changes in cells during normal prenatal and postnatal development remains unknown.

As with any multistep process initiated by a brief perturbation, does the carcinogen instruct the cell in a way that has direct relevance to behavior as a cancer or does it merely induce a change that favors further changes toward cancer? This is by no means only of theoretical interest, since commitment to explore novel ways to interrupt carcinogenesis depends on its resolution. There is some evidence (see ref. 13 for references) that the preneoplastic phase of cancer development may have survival value for the host and may constitute a fundamentally useful adaptive response (13,49).

What is the role of cell proliferation in the initiation process? This seems to be a fundamental requirement of carcinogenesis with DNA viruses, radiation, and chemicals *in vitro* and *in vivo* (13,50). Is it largely related to DNA replication, or are there metabolic modulations during the cell cycle which influence the metabolic fates of chemicals?

What are the functional or physiologic changes in target cells that enable a few to act as initiated cells? If an initiated cell can be stimulated to proliferate to form focal proliferations (nodules), what determines selection? Are there few or many types of initiated hepatocytes?

Is promotion in liver carcinogenesis merely the expansion of one or more types of initiated hepatocytes, or are there additional effects of a promoting environment that are necessary for evolution to cancer? If the former is valid, then it should be possible to interrupt carcinogenesis at this phase by understanding the nature of the nodules with respect to their evolution to cancer.

Since hepatocytes in persistent hyperplastic nodules have architectural and vascular patterns which differ considerably from normal, mature liver, are such changes sufficient to favor the next step in the process, rare event #2, or does the initiating carcinogen or promoting environment add additional instruction for this step?

Are persistent nodules fundamentally different from remodeling nodules, or are the differences merely a reflection of the intensity of the promoting environment, i.e., a result of a stochastic phenomenon?

Since additional exposures to a known carcinogen do not seem to be necessary for rare event #2 and the subsequent rare cell changes which result in nodules within nodules, what is the nature of these changes? Are they ''spontaneous,'' resulting from some organizational change in the nucleus or cytoplasm of the cells at risk, or are they due to background mutations (51)?

Is carcinogenesis with chemicals a multihit process in which the carcinogen imposes more than one change on the cells at risk (see ref. 30), or does the carcinogen ''instruct'' the target cell in only one respect?

A striking alteration in the hepatocytes in hyperplastic nodules is the apparent paucity of heterochromatin, i.e., condensed DNA (35). Normally, this condensation occurs during the recovery phase after cell proliferation. Is there some fundamental alteration in the mechanisms for condensation that favors rare changes in hepatocytes in nodules and in nodules within nodules? Such a lack of condensation could favor ''apparently inappropriate expression of genetic information,'' a characteristic of neoplastic hepatocytes.

Early preneoplastic hepatocyte populations have many biochemical, physiologic, and structural markers (35). Are any of these important mechanistically, or are they merely expressions of some fundamental change in cell metabolic programming?

Obviously, these are only a few of the issues in our ''understanding'' of how cancer develops. Some can be answered with current techniques and concepts;

others will probably remain elusive for some time to come. In-depth analysis of the carcinogenic process will almost certainly generate new insights into fundamental aspects of how the liver responds to environmental perturbations.

ACKNOWLEDGMENTS

The research included in this review was supported in part by research grants from the National Cancer Institute of Canada, National Cancer Institute of the National Institutes of Health (CA-21157 and CA-25094), and Medical Research Council of Canada (MA-5994).

I would like to express my sincere thanks to Miss Helene Robitaille for the assistance in the preparation of this manuscript.

REFERENCES

1. Pitot, H. C. (1970): Recent advances in the mechanism of hepatic carcinogenesis. In: *Progress in Liver Disease,* Vol. 3, edited by H. Popper and F. Schaffner, pp. 77–88. Grune & Stratton, New York.

2. Wogan, G. M. (1976): The induction of liver cell cancer with chemicals. In: *Liver Cell Cancer,* edited by H. M. Cameron, D. A. Linsell, and G. P. Warwick, pp. 121–152. Elsevier, Amsterdam.

3. Cole, L. J., and Nowell, P. C. (1965): Radiation carcinogenesis: The sequence of events. *Science,* 150:1782–1786.

4. Farber, E. (1976): The pathology of experimental liver cell cancer. In: *Liver Cell Cancer,* edited by H. M. Cameron, D. A. Linsell, and G. P. Warwick, pp. 243–277. Elsevier, Amsterdam.

5. Nunnerley, H., Laws, J. W., Davis, M., and Williams, R. (1980): Chemical and drug-induced liver tumors. In: *Induced Disease. Drug, Irradiation, Occupation,* edited by L. Preger, pp. 3–26. Grune & Stratton, New York.

6. Sherlock, S. (1980): Hepatic effects of steroid sex hormones. In: *Toxic Injury of the Liver,* edited by E. Farber and M. M. Fisher, pp. 595–627. Marcel Dekker, New York.

7. Blumberg, B. S. (1977): Australia antigen and the biology of hepatitis B. *Science,* 197:17–25.

8. Zuckerman, A. J., and Howard, C. R. (1979): *Hepatitis Viruses of Man.* Academic Press, London.

9. Sasaki, T., and Yoshida, T. (1935): Experimentalle Enzeugung des Lebercarcinoms durch Fütterung mit o-Amidozotoluol. *Virchows Arch. Path. Anat. Physiol.,* 295:175–200.

10. Emmelot, P. (editor) (1980): Developmental phases in liver carcinogenesis. *Biochim. Biophys. Acta,* 605:149–304.

11. Cameron, H. M., Linsell, D. A., and Warwick, G. P. (editors) (1976): *Liver Cell Cancer.* Elsevier, Amsterdam.

12. Farber, E., and Sporn, M. B. (editors) (1976): Early lesions and the development of epithelial cancer. *Cancer Res.,* 36:2475–2806.

13. Farber, E., and Cameron, R. (1980): The sequential analysis of cancer development. *Adv. Cancer Res.,* 31:125–226.

14. Newberne, P. M., and Butler, W. H. (editors) (1978): *Rat Hepatic Neoplasia.* MIT Press, Cambridge.

15. Okuda, K., and Peters, R. L. (editors) (1976): *Hepatocellular Carcinoma.* Wiley, New York.

16. Remmer, H., Bolt, H. M., Bannasch, P., and Popper, H. (editors) (1978): *Primary Liver Tumors.* MTP Press, Lancaster.

17. Farber, E. (1982): Sequential events in chemical carcinogenesis. In: *Cancer: A Comprehensive Treatise,* 2nd edition, edited by F. F. Becker. Plenum, New York.

18. Berenblum, I. (1975): Sequential aspects of chemical carcino-genesis in skin. In: *Cancer: A Comprehensive Treatise, Vol. I,* edited by F. F. Becker, pp. 323–344. Plenum, New York.

19. Pitot, H. C. (1979): Biological and enzymatic events in chemical carcinogenesis. *Ann. Rev. Med.,* 30:25–39.

20. Farber, E. (1980): The sequential analysis of liver cancer induction. *Biochim. Biophys. Acta,* 605:149–166.

21. Farber, E. (1963): Ethionine carcinogenesis. *Adv. Cancer Res.,* 7:383–474.

22. Farber, E. (1976): On the pathogenesis of experimental hepatocellular carcinoma. In: *Hepatocellular Carcinoma,* edited by K. Okuda and R. L. Peters, pp. 3–22. Wiley, New York.

23. Farber, E. (1978): Experimental liver carcinogenesis: A perspective. In: *Primary Liver Tumors,* edited by H. Remmer, H. M. Bolt, P. Bannasch, and H. Popper, pp. 357–375. MTP Press, Lancaster.

24. Epstein, S. M., Ito, N., Merkow, L., and Farber, E. (1967): Cellular analysis of liver carcinogenesis: The induction of large hyperplastic nodules in the liver with 2-fluorenylacetamide or ethionine and some aspects of their morphology and glycogen metabolism. *Cancer Res.,* 27:1702–1711.

25. Reuber, M. D. (1965): Development of preneoplastic and neoplastic lesions of the liver in male rats given 0.025% N-2-fluorenylacetamide. *J. Natl. Cancer Inst.,* 34:697–723.

26. Teebor, G. W., and Becker, F. F. (1971): Regression and persistence of hyperplastic nodules induced by N-2-fluorenylacetamide and their relationship to hepatocarcinogenesis. *Cancer Res.,* 31:1–3.

27. Peraino, C., Fry, R. J. M., and Grube, D. D. (1978): Drug-induced enhancement of hepatic tumorigenesis. In: *Carcinogenesis: Mechanisms of Tumor Promotion and Cocarcinogenesis, Vol. 2,* edited by T. J. Slaga, A. Sivak, and R. K. Boutwell, pp. 421–432. Raven Press, New York.

28. Weisburger, J. H., Madison, R. M., Ward, J. M., Viguera, C., and Weisburger, E. K. (1975): Modification of diethylnitrosamine liver carcinogenesis with phenobarbital but not by immunosuppression. *J. Natl. Cancer Inst.,* 54:1185–1188.

29. Nishizumi, M. (1976): Enhancement of diethylnitrosamine hepatocarcinogenesis in rats exposed to polychlorinated biphenyls or phenobarbital. *Cancer Lett.,* 2:11–16.

30. Emmelot, P., and Scherer, E. (1980): The first relevant cell stage in rat liver carcinogenesis. A quantitative approach. *Biochim. Biophys. Acta,* 605:247–304.

31. Scherer, E., Hoffmann, M., Emmelot, P., and Friedrich-Freksa, H. (1972): Quantitative study on foci of altered liver cells induced in the rat by a single dose of diethylnitrosamine and partial hepatectomy. *J. Natl. Cancer Inst.,* 49:93–106.

32. Pitot, H. C. (1979): Drugs as promoters of carcinogenesis. In: *The Induction of Drug Metabolism,* edited by R. W. Estabrook and E. Lindenlaub, pp. 471–483. Schattauer, Stuttgart.

33. Pitot, H. C., and Sirica, A. E. (1980): The stages of initiation and promotion in hepatocarcinogenesis. *Biochim. Biophys. Acta,* 605:191–215.

34. Pitot, H. C., Barsness, T., Goldsworthy, T., and Kitagowa, T. (1978): Biochemical characterization of stages of hepatocarcinogenesis after a single dose of diethylnitrosamine. *Nature,* 271:456–458.

35. Farber, E., Cameron, R. G., Laishes, B., Lin, J-C., Medline, A., Ogawa, K., and Solt, D. B. (1979): Physiological and molecular markers during carcinogenesis. In: *Carcinogens: Identification and Mechanisms of Actions,* edited by A. C. Griffin and C. R. Shaw, pp. 319–335. Raven Press, New York.

36. Haddow, A. (1938): Cellular inhibition and the origin of cancer. *Acta Union Int. Contre Cancer,* 3:342–353.

37. Miller, E. C. (1978): Some current perspectives on chemical carcinogenesis in humans and experimental animals. Presidential address. *Cancer Res.,* 38:1479–1496.

38. Rajalakshmi, S., Rao, P. M., and Sarma, D. S. R. (1982): Chemical carcinogenesis: Interactions of carcinogens with nucleic acids. In: *Cancer: A Comprehensive Treatise,* 2nd edition, edited by F. F. Becker. Plenum, New York.

39. Columbano, A., Rao, P. M., Rajalakshmi, S., and Sarma, D. S. R. (1980): Presence of dimethylnitrosamine (DMN) induced methylated products in the parental strand of the in vivo replicated,

S₁ nuclease resistant, hybrid liver DNA. *Proc. Am. Assoc. Cancer Res.*, 21:86.

40. Farber, E. (1982): The possible toxicological significance of liver hypertrophy produced by drug-metabolizing enzyme inducers. *Ciba Found. Symp.*, 76:261–274.

41. Wattenberg, L. W. (1979): Inhibitors of carcinogenesis. In: *Carcinogenesis: Identification and Mechanisms of Action*, edited by A. C. Griffin and C. R. Shaw, pp. 299–316. Raven Press, New York.

42. Ying, T. S., Sarma, D. S. R., and Farber, E. (1979): Role of liver cell necrosis in the induction of preneoplastic lesions. *Proc. Am. Assoc. Cancer Res.*, 20:14.

43. Schulte-Hermann, R. (1979): Reactions of the liver to injury adaptation. In: *Toxic Liver Injury*, edited by E. Farber and M. M. Fisher, pp. 385–444. Marcel Dekker, New York.

44. Enomoto, K., and Farber, E. (1980): Immunohistochemical study of epoxide hydratase (EH) activity in rat liver during chemical carcinogenesis. *Proc. Am. Assoc. Cancer Res.*, 21:82.

45. Laishes, B. A., and Rolfe, P. B. (1982): Quantitative assessment of liver carcinoma incidence in rats receiving intravenous injec-

tions of isogenic liver cells isolated during hepatocarcinogenesis. *Cancer Res.*, 40: (in press).

46. Laishes, B. A., Roberts, E., and Farber, E. (1978): In vitro measurement of carcinogen-resistant liver cells during hepatocarcinogenesis. *Int. J. Cancer*, 21:186–193.

47. Laishes, B. A., and Farber, E. (1978): Transfer of viable putative preneoplastic hepatocytes to the livers of syngeneic host rats. *J. Natl. Cancer Inst.*, 61:507–512.

48. Williams, G. M. (1980): The pathogenesis of rat liver cancer caused by chemical carcinogens. *Biochim. Biophys. Acta*, 605:167–189.

49. Cameron, R., Murray, R. K., Farber, E., and Sharma, R. N. (1979): Some patterns of response of liver to environmental agents. *Ann. N.Y. Acad. Sci.*, 329:39–47.

50. Craddock, V. M. (1976): Cell proliferation and experimental liver cancer. In: *Liver Cell Cancer*, edited by H. M. Cameron, D. A. Linsell, and G. P. Warwick, pp. 152–201. Elsevier, Amsterdam.

51. Burnet, F. M. (1974): *Intrinsic Mutagenesis: A Genetic Approach to Ageing*. Wiley, New York.

The Liver: Biology and Pathobiology, edited by
I. Arias, H. Popper, D. Schachter, and D. A. Shåfritz.
Raven Press, New York © 1982.

Chapter 49

The Pathophysiology of Portal Hypertension

Harold O. Conn and Roberto J. Groszmann

ANATOMY OF THE PORTAL VENOUS SYSTEM

The portal venous system can be regarded as a great river. It arises from small streams in the highlands of the spleen, pancreas, colon, small intestine, and stomach, which join in orderly fashion to form the mighty portal. After it enters the liver, the portal vein divides and redivides into progressively smaller branches to form a delta that terminates in the sinusoidal network of the liver. It is a unique venous system that exists between two capillary beds—upstream, the sinusoids of the spleen and the capillaries of the digestive tract, and downstream, the sinusoidal bed of the liver.

Anatomically, the portal vein originates in the pulp of the spleen, where splenic blood, after being screened in the splenic pulp, enters venules, which merge to form the splenic trunks, which in turn join to form the splenic vein (Fig. 1). Into this vein flow the left gastroepiploic vein, the pancreatic veins, the inferior mesenteric vein, which arises in the capillary beds of the left colon and rectum, and, finally, the left gastric (coronary) vein. The portal vein per se begins at the confluence of the splenic and the superior mesenteric veins, the latter of which arises in the capillary beds of right colon, small intestine, and pancreas. The portal vein, which is 1 to 1.4 cm in diameter and 5 to 8 cm in length, flows directly to the liver. It is joined near the liver by a few small tributaries from the

pancreas, duodenum, and biliary tree. As it enters the liver, it abruptly divides into the right and left portal veins, which rebranch until the hepatic sinusoidal network is formed. The anatomic pattern described is the classic one which sets the norm. An infinite number of anatomic variations on this theme, of little functional significance, may occur.

The microcirculation of the liver is based on the acinar structure of the hepatic parenchyma (1). Each acinus, the structural unit of the liver, is supplied with an arteriole, a portal venule, and a terminal hepatic venule (central vein) (Fig. 2). Each also has lymph vessels and nerves. The arterioles, portal venules, and biliary ductules travel together in the portal tracts as they repeatedly branch. Some of the terminal hepatic arterioles, which range from 15 to 50 μm in diameter, form dense capillary networks around bile ductules; others flow into the sinusoids, usually into zone 1 of the acinus (1). Based on studies in rats, some arterioles may terminate in acinar zones 2 and 3, often near collecting venules (2) (Fig. 3). The much larger portal venules divide into distributing portal venules, from which inlet venules supply the sinusoids at many points. The sinusoids, which are infinitely interconnected, flow into collecting venules which join to form the terminal hepatic venules. Recent studies have shown a pO$_2$ gradient from zone 1 to zone 3 which parallels the distribution of blood flow through the acinus. The endothelial lining of the sinusoids, which is thin and fenestrated, permits the rapid passage of

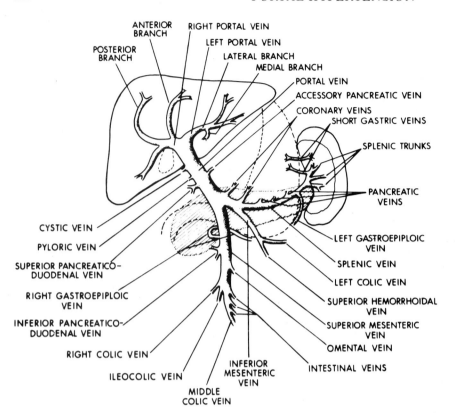

FIG. 1. Anatomy of the portal venous system. Stomach and duodenum, *dotted lines;* pancreas, *cross hatched.*

fluids and nutrients into the space of Disse. This is an extremely vulnerable site, where the deposition of collagen, for example, can both impair transport and compromise homeostatic mechanisms.

PHYSIOLOGY OF THE HEPATIC CIRCULATION

The physiology of the hepatic circulation is discussed in detail elsewhere in this volume. Those aspects that deal with portal hypertension and its consequences are discussed here.

It has long been known that a reciprocal relationship exists between the hepatic arterial and portal venous blood flows (3). Normally, the hepatic arterial flow, which amounts to 500 ml/min, joins the portal vein, which carries 1,000 ml/min, in the sinusoids and contributes to the portal venous pressure. Manometrically, the hepatic artery can be considered a tributary of the portal vein. This effect, however, is small since the arterial pressure is dissipated in the sinusoidal bed, which is relatively large and of low resistance.

A decrease in portal flow is almost invariably followed by an increase in hepatic arterial blood flow. This relationship has been explained by the mechanical effects of merging a small, rapidly flowing system with one that is large and slowly flowing. When they merge, the blood flow and pressure in the low flow portal system are increased, while the pressure and flow in the fast hepatic arterial system are propor-

tionally diminished. Therefore, reduction in portal flow is equivalent to reduction in resistance to hepatic arterial blood flow. Consequently, a decrease in portal flow induces a rapid increase in hepatic arterial blood flow (Fig. 4). This reciprocal relationship is communicated via arterioportal, presinusoidal connections between the portal and arterial systems.

As cirrhosis develops, shunts between the hepatic artery and the hepatic vein develop, which may impair normal relationships between the hepatic arterial and portal venous flows (4). The effects of reducing hepatic arterial flow on portal flow are not as clearcut, as increments, decrements, and no crements have been reported.

Alternative possibilities have been postulated by other investigators. Some suggest that the hepatic arterial response is dependent on the metabolic requirements of the liver for oxygen (5). Others postulate that the hepatic arterial blood flow varies inversely with the portal blood flow in compensatory fashion to maintain total hepatic blood flow at a constant level (6).

Streaming in the Portal Vein

Although it had long been assumed that streaming exists in the portal vein (i.e., blood derived from the splenic vein flows primarily to the left lobe of the liver and blood from the superior mesenteric vein to the right), recent observations suggest that this pattern is not significant physiologically. Isotopes injected into

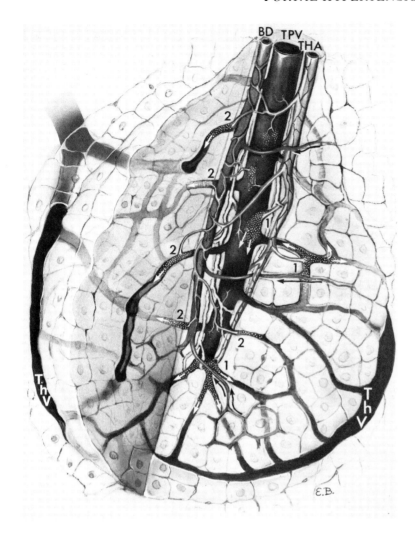

FIG. 2. Microcirculatory hepatic unit. The unit consists of the terminal portal venule (TPV) with the sinusoids branching off and forming a glomus; the terminal hepatic arteriole (THA) forms a plexus around the terminal bile ductule (BD). The arterioles empty either directly (1) or via the peribiliary plexus (2) into the TPV sinusoids. The sinusoids run along the outside of cell plates; inside are the capillaries of the hepatic secretory and excretory systems. The glomus of sinusoids is drained by at least two terminal hepatic venules (ThV). LY, lymphatics. (From ref. 1.)

the superior mesenteric artery show similar dilution curves recorded in the right and left hepatic veins (7). Injections of large amounts of radioopaque constrast material into the spleen show homogenous opacification of the portal venous system. When small amounts of contrast material are injected into the spleen, they tend to flow preferentially to the left lobe. Neoplasms arising in the domain of tributaries of either the inferior mesenteric or superior mesenteric veins tend to metastasize to the right and left lobes of the liver, respectively. Most metastases from carcinomas of either the ascending or descending colon are found in the right lobe. Since the volume of the right lobe is five to six times greater than that of the left lobe, it is not surprising that 80 to 90% of metastases are found there. Physiologically, the portal blood carries to the liver and, ultimately, to the systemic circulation, nutrients and other exogenous substances absorbed from the alimentary tract, metabolic products of unabsorbed foodstuffs, endogenous substances produced by enteric enzymes and bacteria, hormones secreted by the pancreas and gastrointestinal tract, hormonal

substances and formed elements of the blood released by the spleen, and, sometimes, bacteria that may enter portal venous blood after injury to the intestinal mucosa. Thus the liver receives first for appropriate disposition those substances which are potentially beneficial and harmful and which are ingested orally or arise in the splanchnic circulation. The liver deserves its sobriquet, "guardian of the body."

PORTAL HYPERTENSION

Portal hypertension is the abnormal state of a sustained increase of pressure in the portal venous system or portion thereof. Portal pressure is the resultant of blood flow through the portal venous system and the total resistance to blood flow through its component branches. Portal pressure levels, like arterial pressure, vary widely; unlike arterial pressure, which can be measured easily and safely, however, portal pressure can be determined only with difficulty and with some danger. It has not been studied extensively in normal

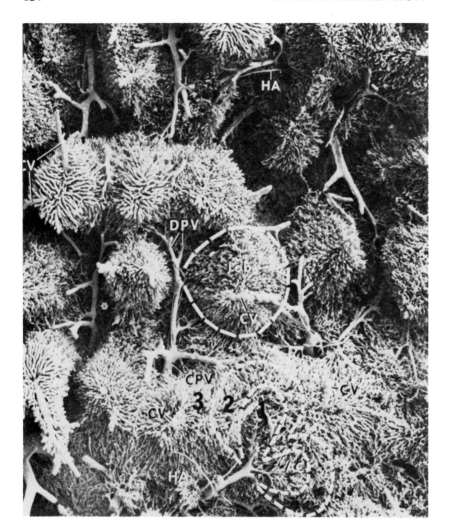

FIG. 3. Hepatic microcirculation as seen by scanning electron microscopy of corrosion cast of rat liver. Zones one (1), two (2), and three (3) of the liver acinus are denoted at the bottom of the figure. Adjacent areas contain sinusoids (Si), the arrangement of which corresponds to a lobular (Lob) parenchymal organization, conducting portal veins (CPV), distributing portal veins (DPV), collecting venules (CV), hepatic arterioles (HA), and noncasted areas in portal tracts (*). (Republished from ref. 2 with permission.)

individuals, therefore, and the definition of normal portal pressure is empiric. The normal portal pressure measured in the supine position at rest and expressed as the portal venous pressure gradient, i.e., the difference between the absolute portal venous pressure and the intraabdominal systemic venous pressure, ranges from 3 to 6 mm Hg.

The absolute level of portal pressure may be a clinically misleading value. Consequently, the portal venous pressure must be expressed in terms of a zero reference point. Determinations of portal pressure made with different methods may differ, depending primarily on the choice of the zero reference point, which may be an external, fixed measurement, such as an arbitrary distance (12 cm) above the level of the table on which the patient lies or an arbitrary estimate of the level of the right atrium (5 cm below the sternal angle), or an internal, functional pressure, such as that of the right atrium or the inferior vena cava. The use of an internal zero reference point, such as the inferior vena cava or the free (unwedged) hepatic vein, corrects for extraneous, intraabdominal effects on the portal pressure.

The increase in portal pressure is limited to that portion of the portal venous system upstream to the site of obstruction to blood flow. The method of measurement of the pressure in such a portion of the portal system is often determined by the nature and location of the lesion.

PORTAL VENOUS PRESSURE MEASUREMENTS

Portal pressure can be estimated at a variety of sites in a number of ways (Table 1). These measurements can be made directly by entering the portal venous system, or indirectly by measuring the pressure extraportally at a site that accurately reflects the portal venous pressure (PVP) (Fig. 5).

Direct Measurement of PVP

Operative PVP

Operative PVP, which was first used at the end of the 19th century for measuring the portal pressure, is

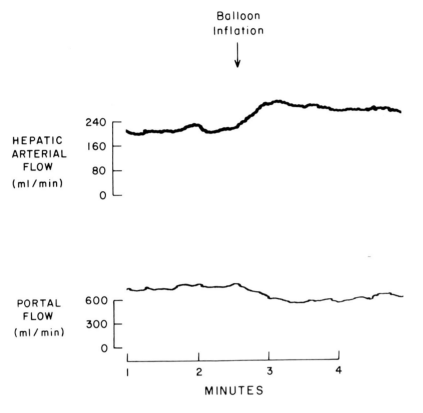

FIG. 4. Simultaneous recording of mean hepatic arterial flow and mean portal venous flow before and during reduction in portal blood flow by inflation of a balloon catheter in the superior mesenteric artery. The decrease in portal venous flow is followed promptly by an increase in hepatic arterial flow. (Reprinted from ref. 56 with permission.)

accomplished by inserting a needle into a branch of the portal vein at surgery. This technique has a number of disadvantages. Since it can be used only at surgery, it is not possible to compare pre- and postoperative pressure levels. In addition, it is difficult to determine a reliable baseline, intraabdominal venous pressure. Without this basal pressure, one cannot correct for any of the many factors that may affect PVP, such as ascites, cardiac decompensation, or inferior vena caval compression. Ascites, for example, may cause a significant increment in the PVP and intraabdominal venous pressure, which increases with the amount of ascites and the tightness of the abdomen (8) (Fig. 6). One can measure the pressure in the inferior vena cava, but this is not always possible at laparotomy without extensive dissection. Consequently, arbitrary reference levels have been used. These include the level of the operating table or the level of the right atrium. It has been determined at autopsy that the portal vein is approximately 12 cm above the post-

mortem table; consequently, 12 cm H_2O is subtracted from the gross PVP to determine the "true" PVP. This empiric estimate differs in different patients. The difference between a 100-pound woman and a 200-pound man may represent a 25% error. Although the right atrium provides a useful benchmark, it is usually taken to be 5 cm below the level of the sternal angle, another soft estimate. Both these measurements are meaningful only when the patient is supine; but surgery often is performed with the patient in other positions.

There is a variable effect of an open abdomen on the portal pressure. The wedged hepatic venous pressure (WHVP) may change unpredictably when the abdomen is opened. Unless carefully monitored, many variables, such as the type and depth of anesthesia, medications, hemodynamic status, pO_2, pCO_2, and respiration, may render operative measurements of PVP unreliable. The hepatic venous pressure gradient (see below) remains relatively constant, however. Finally, most surgeons do not use electronic transducers for these measurements. They tend to use water manometers, which measure a column of fluid that is sometimes only sluggishly responsive to changes in pressure, which frequently clot when mixed with blood and which are so cumbersome as to discourage serial measurements.

Operative Umbilical Vein Catheterization

The unbilical vein, which collapses after birth, offers an avenue into the portal venous system throughout

TABLE 1. *Methods of measuring PVP*

Direct
  Operative mesenteric venous
  Operative umbilical venous
  Percutaneous transhepatic portal venous
Indirect
  Percutaneous transsplenic pulp
  Percutaneous transhepatic parenchymal
  Percutaneous wedged hepatic venous

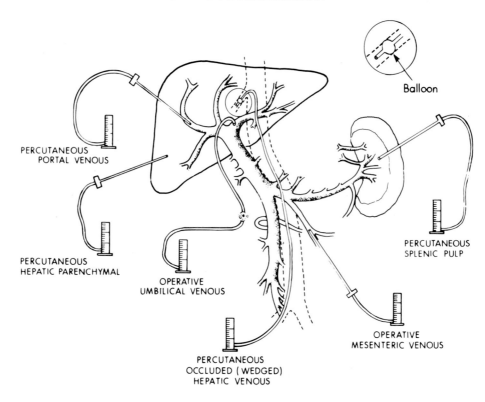

Balloon

PERCUTANEOUS
PORTAL VENOUS

PERCUTANEOUS
HEPATIC PARENCHYMAL

OPERATIVE
UMBILICAL VENOUS

PERCUTANEOUS
SPLENIC PULP

OPERATIVE
MESENTERIC VENOUS

PERCUTANEOUS
OCCLUDED (WEDGED)
HEPATIC VENOUS

FIG. 5. Sites and methods of measuring PVP.

adult life. The technique of cannulating the umbilical vein through a superficial incision in the hypogastrium was first described in 1959. When the left intrahepatic portal vein is entered in this manner, one can measure portal pressure directly, blood samples can be easily obtained, and, by manipulation of the catheter, the whole portal venous system can be visualized angiographically (9). This technique has been used for experimental purposes in man to great advantage.

Zimmon and Kessler (10) have studied the effects of stepwise increments and decrements in portal blood flow by infusing or withdrawing blood from the portal vein via an umbilical catheter. Access to the umbilical vein is not always easy, however. The umbilical vein remnant must be identified, cannulated, and dilated and the cannula passed into the portal vein. Several veins may be present, and the false ones are almost invariably entered first. The venous wall is atrophic and the residual route tortuous; perforations are common. The success rate ranges from 30 to 90%. To catheterize the vein successfully, some surgeons extend their dissections to enter the peritoneal cavity in identifying an appropriate vessel. This extension converts a minor surgical procedure to a major one that may require general anesthesia and may have important metabolic consequences. A second disadvantage of this procedure is that a reliable basal intraabdominal venous pressure is not easily available.

Percutaneous, Transhepatic PVP (Chiba Needle)

Percutaneous, transhepatic PVP, which is an outgrowth of percutaneous, transhepatic "skinny needle" cholangiography, is another method of directly measuring the PVP. In this type of portomanometry, the needle is advanced toward the confluence of the intrahepatic portal veins using a small gauge needle (external diameter, 0.7 mm; internal diameter, 0.5 mm). As the needle is withdrawn, radioopaque material is gently injected, and the position of the tip of the needle can be identified to be in the biliary, portal venous, hepatic venous, hepatic arterial, or lymphatic system fluoroscopically. The same technique is used in visualizing the biliary tree, but the target is different.

In patients with portal hypertension, this technique usually is successful because the portal veins are dilated and occupy a relatively large fraction of liver volume. In patients without portal hypertension, the portal veins may be missed.

The main disadvantage of this technique is the inability to obtain a basal, intraabdominal pressure level. The University of Southern California physicians who devised this technique agree that the baseline pressure is essential for proper interpretation and, consequently, determine it in a hepatic vein with a skinny needle. If they cannot, they perform percutaneous femoral vein catheterization to measure the inferior

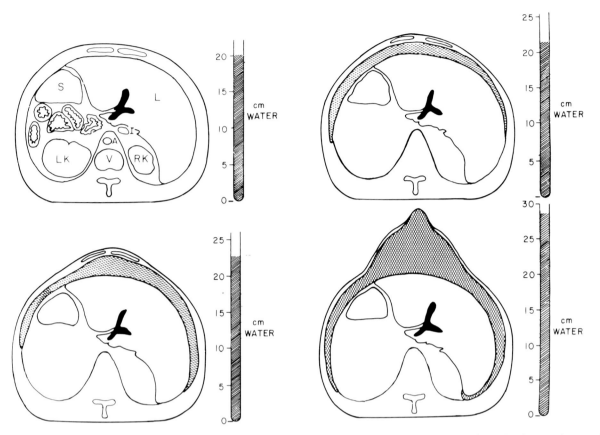

FIG. 6. Effect of increasing amounts of ascites on portal pressure. Supine cross sections of the body are shown at the level of the bifurcation of the portal vein in a cirrhotic patient. **Upper left:** No ascites. PVP is 20 cm water. **Upper right:** Small amount of ascites indicated by cross hatching. The layer of ascites 3 cm deep adds 3 cm to the portal pressure. **Lower left:** Moderate amount of ascites. In the supine position, the 6 cm of ascites adds 6 cm to the portal pressure. **Lower right:** Tight ascites. The pressure in the bulging abdomen is transmitted to the portal vein in excess of the "depth" of ascites. L, liver; S, spleen; A, aorta; LK, left kid   y; V, vertebra; RK, right kidney. The portal vein is shown in black. (Republished from ref. 51 with permission.)

vena caval pressure. This vena caval measurement can be used with any of the other methods as well, but it involves a separate procedure.

The other drawback is the small gauge of the needle, which results in sluggish responses to changes in pressure and which makes essential the use of electronic manometers. Clotting is also a problem with small needles. Boyer and associates (11) were able to measure PVP in 101 of 123 patients (82%) in this manner compared to WHVP, which was successful in 119 of the 123 patients (96%). The authors found an almost perfect correlation between WHVP and skinny needle PVP in alcoholic cirrhosis (Fig. 7). In chronic active hepatitis, they found the portal pressure to be higher than the WHVP, which they attributed to a presinusoidal obstructive component in this disease. This observation has recently been confirmed using an umbilical venous catheter measuring PVP directly.

The advantage of this method is its safety. These small gauge needles can be passed into the liver repeatedly without hazard, if no coagulopathy exists.

This percutaneous technique using a larger needle and a guide wire for the passage of a catheter has been used for portal venography and to perform therapeutic intervention in patients with bleeding varices (12). Coronary and short gastric veins have been obliterated in active bleeding and to prevent recurrent episodes of hemorrhage.

Indirect Methods

Percutaneous Splenic Pulp Pressure

It has been recognized for 30 years that portal pressure can be estimated by measuring splenic pulp pressure (13). The spleen is a vascular organ that consists of an envelope supported by a trabecular skeleton filled with blood, which drains directly into the portal venous system. A large bore needle inserted into the splenic pulp will record a pressure that is 1 or 2 mm higher than portal pressure. The pressure recorded approximates the vascular pressure in the spleen, al-

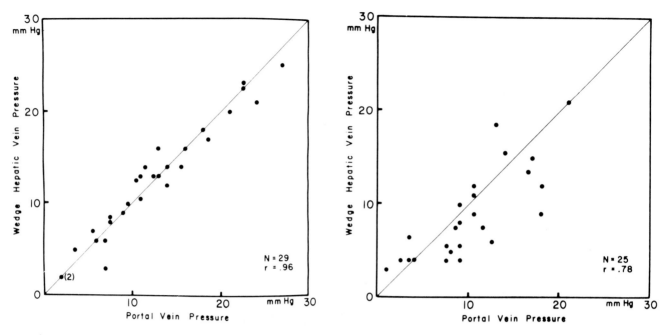

FIG. 7. Comparison of WHVP with PVP (skinny needle). **Left:** In alcoholic liver disease, an almost perfect correlation was observed. **Right:** In chronic active hepatitis, PVP was often higher than WHVP. (Republished from ref. 11 with permission.)

though the system may not respond rapidly to changes in pressure, such as those that occur with respiration.

This technique is useful in obtaining good visualization of the portal venous system, although the injection of a large bolus of contrast medium under high pressure may distort the portal venous pattern and show false retrograde flow in the inferior mesenteric or other tributary veins (14) (Fig. 8).

Splenic pulp pressure measurements do not permit an accurate internal "zero" pressure. Much more distressing is the fact that a small but significant fraction of patients (1 or 2%) have serious intraperitoneal bleeding after splenoportography. These measurements are for practical purposes a one-time technique; serial measurements cannot be made without undue risk.

At present, splenic pulp pressures are not commonly measured. They are done when other, safer measures are not possible or when other techniques have failed. Occasionally, as in splenic vein thrombosis, it is the only method other than surgery that permits measurement of the PVP upstream to the obstruction.

Percutaneous Hepatic Parenchymal Pressure

This technique is the hepatic equivalent of the splenic pulp pressure. Several groups in the mid-1960s demonstrated that a large bore needle inserted into the liver parenchyma will record the intrahepatic pressure, which reflects the PVP surprisingly closely (15,16). It has been suggested that it measures sinusoidal pres-

sure, which, of course, is not increased in presinusoidal obstruction. The intrahepatic parenchymal pressure is the resultant of a number of vectors, such as hepatic arterial, portal venous, and sinusoidal pressure, the degree of fibrosis of the liver, the amount of glycogen deposition, fatty infiltration, and inflammation, any of which may affect the measurement of portal pressure. Its reliability, however, has been questioned (17).

This technique is about as safe as a liver biopsy, a procedure that is probably too risky for pressure measurement alone. In addition, it is another of the procedures that does not permit estimation of the corrected portal pressure. This technique is rarely employed to measure PVP.

Percutaneous WHVP

The WHVP measurement of PVP is in principle the same as the wedged pulmonary arterial pressure measurement of pulmonary capillary or "left atrial" pressure (18). In either technique, a catheter is advanced until it "wedges," i.e., completely obstructs a branch vessel. The fluid in the wedged hepatic venous catheter forms a continuous column with the blood in the hepatic vein, sinusoids, and portal veins. In the normal liver, extensive intersinusoidal anastomoses dissipate some of the pressure from the wedged sinusoids, and the measured WHVP is slightly lower than the PVP (Fig. 9). A wedged hepatic venous catheter, therefore, records the pressure in the sinusoidal bed, which approximates portal pressure.

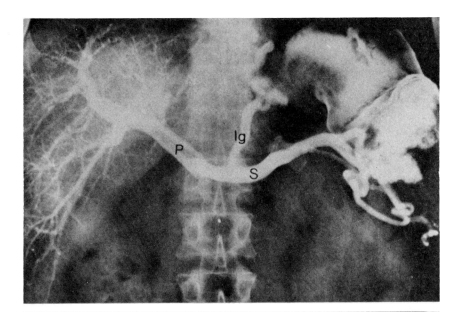

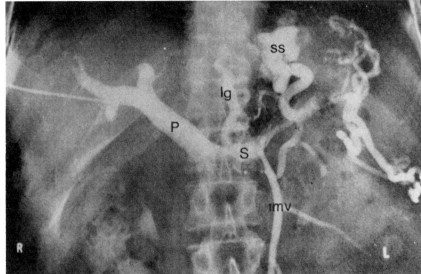

FIG. 8. Comparison between splenic and transhepatic portagram. **Top:** Splenic venogram shows patent portal system with a left gastric vessel leading to esophageal varices. Transhepatic portagram reveals a large spontaneous splenorenal shunt in addition. **Bottom:** Reprinted from ref. 14 with permission.

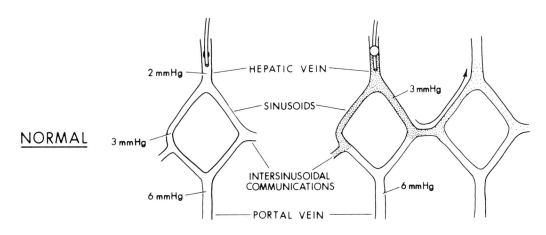

FIG. 9. No obstruction. Diagram showing presinusoidal, sinusoidal, and postsinusoidal pressure relationships during measurement of hepatic vein wedged pressure in a normal subject. With the hepatic vein unoccluded **(left)**, the pressure is highest in the portal vein and decreases as it passes through the sinusoids to the hepatic veins. With the hepatic vein occluded **(right)**, the measured pressure is lower than the PVP due to dissipation of pressure to unoccluded hepatic veins via the intersinusoidal communications (*arrow*). Pressure levels at various sites are representative.

In presinusoidal obstruction, due, for example, to portal vein thrombosis, the column of blood, which cannot be continuous with the hypertensive portion of the portal vein, terminates in the sinusoids where pressure dissipation results in a normal pressure level (Fig. 10). In posthepatitic cirrhosis, the PVP is often appreciably higher than the WHVP, indicating that a presinusoidal component of increased resistance is operative (11). In alcoholic cirrhosis, in which the site of increased resistance appears to be sinusoidal, intersinusoidal communications are diminished. Dissipation of pressure in the wedged vessels is relatively insignificant, and the WHVP virtually equals the PVP (Fig. 11). When the site of obstruction is postsinusoidal, some dissipation of pressure via intersinusoidal communications can occur; therefore, the WHVP may be theoretically lower than the PVP (Fig. 12). In posthepatic obstruction, all hepatic veins are equally obstructed, and the PVP and WHVP are equal.

The greatest virtue of this technique is that it permits measurement of an ideal reference pressure—the free hepatic venous pressure (FHVP) or the inferior vena caval pressure. Using this value, one can calculate the hepatic venous pressure gradient (HVPG) by subtracting the FHVP from the WHVP (WHVP − FHVP = HVPG). The use of a balloon catheter greatly simplifies and improves this measurement (19). With the catheter in a large hepatic vein and the balloon uninflated, one measures the FHVP; with the balloon inflated, one measures the occluded hepatic venous pressure (Fig. 13). Occluded and wedged hepatic venous pressures are almost identical. Simply by inflation and deflation, one can repeatedly measure the pressure at the same site without moving the catheter. With the balloon method, one measures the pressure in a larger segment of the liver than when the catheter itself obstructs a smaller vessel, i.e., a form of pressure averaging. These catheters, which do not obstruct flow, can be left *in situ* for long periods and can be used to monitor portal pressure clinically, e.g., during pharmacologic therapy for bleeding varices. Another advantage of the balloon catheter is that the femoral approach can be employed. With conventional catheters, it is difficult to wedge a catheter passed through the femoral vein, and the transcardiac passage of the catheter thus can be avoided.

A disadvantage of measuring portal pressure by the wedged or occluded hepatic vein technique is that the different sites of lesions that cause the portal hypertension affect the pressure measurements differently (Fig. 14). In obstruction of the portal vein, the HVPG does not approximate the PVP, and different types of cirrhosis may affect the HVPG-PVP relationship differently. When the HVPG and the PVP are both measured, however, the site of increased resistance can be unequivocally established (20). The other disadvantage is that the WHVP methods require fluoroscopic equipment for passage and positioning of the catheter. This disadvantage, which may be considered the price of medical progress, offers many additional advantages.

CLASSIFICATION OF PORTAL HYPERTENSION

A sustained increase in PVP many arise from a wide variety of different disorders and may give rise to many clinical syndromes. A unifying classification of the anatomic locations of the increased resistance to portal venous flow, which correlate closely with the hemodynamic alterations observed in these sites of increased resistance, and the types of etiologic lesions that induce them are shown in Table 2.

Prehepatic Portal Hypertension

Prehepatic portal hypertension is caused by lesions that obstruct some portion of the portal venous system

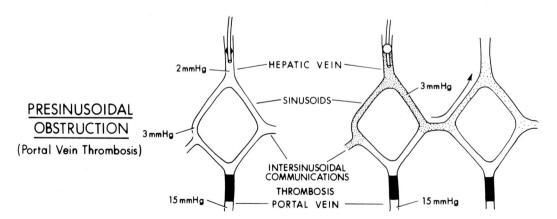

FIG. 10. Presinusoidal obstruction. In the unoccluded system **(left)**, the PVP upstream to the obstruction is higher than in the sinusoidal bed. When the hepatic vein is occluded **(right)**, the wedged or occluded hepatic venous pressure is measured, approximating the sinusoidal pressure.

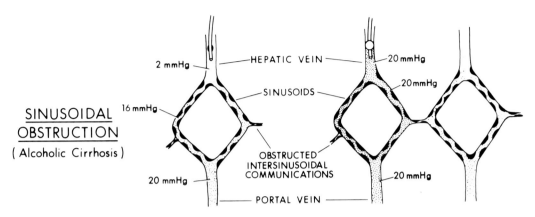

FIG. 11. Sinusoidal obstruction. In alcoholic cirrhosis, the primary site of obstruction is in the sinusoids, and the intersinusoidal communications are largely obliterated. In the unoccluded system **(left)**, the pressure progressively decreases as flow proceeds through the sinusoids. In the occluded position **(right)**, the WHVP and the PVP are equal, because obstruction of the intersinusoidal communications prevents pressure dissipation.

before it enters the liver or which contribute large amounts of exogenous blood to the portal system. Most commonly, prehepatic portal hypertension results from the thrombosis of the splenic or portal vein or branches thereof. These thromboses may follow infections, such as omphalitis or pylephlebitis, pancreatitis, tumor, trauma, or hypercoagulopathic disorders. The pressure in the portal venous system proximal to the obstruction is elevated. Measurement of percutaneous splenic pulp pressure, operative mesenteric or umbilical venous pressure, or percutaneous transhepatic PVP may be elevated according to the location of the obstruction. HVPG and percutaneous hepatic parenchymal pressure are not increased.

Arteriovenous fistulae, involving splenic mesenteric or hepatic arteries and a venous tributary of the portal venous system, may be responsible for prehepatic portal hypertension. Such fistulae are usually the sequelae of abdominal trauma, such as gunshot or stab wounds, but may follow laparotomy, percutaneous liver biopsy, angiography or cholangiography, or a

ruptured aneurysm. Rarely are they congenital, and even more rarely do they develop in association with intrahepatic malignancies. Arteriovenous fistulae usually are silent but may be accompanied by abdominal pain or by visible collateral vessels. They are often characterized by an arterial bruit, which may be systolic or continuous and which is localized to the area of the fistula. By all the techniques described, the pressure in the splenic pulp or in the portal veins is elevated; the HVPG is normal.

The increase in portal pressure with arteriovenous fistulae is not only due to the direct transmission of pressure from the artery to the vein but also results from increased blood flow into the portal system. The volume of flow depends on the size of the fistula and the resistance offered by the hepatic vasculature. Although detailed hemodynamic studies are lacking, the hemodynamic data from one well-studied patient showed reduced hepatic blood flow, which suggests that the resistance to flow, rather than the flow itself, is increased (21). Furthermore, high output cardiac

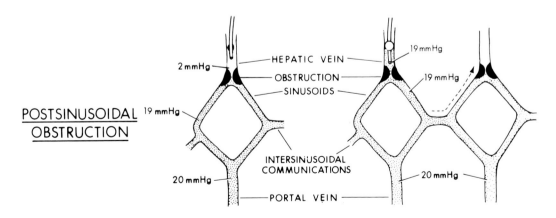

FIG. 12. Postsinusoidal obstruction. In the unoccluded system **(left),** the pressure is increased upstream to the obstruction. In the occluded system **(right),** the WHVP is slightly lower than the PVP due to some dissipation of pressure via the patent intersinusoidal communications.

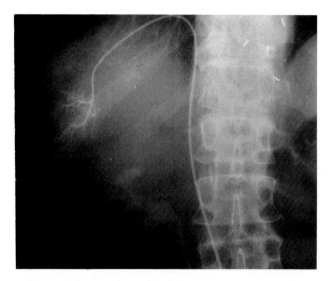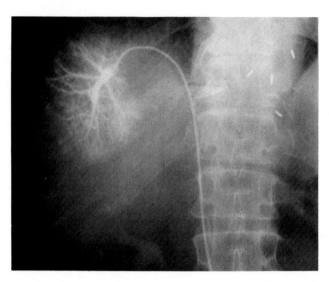

FIG. 13. Left: Radiologic demonstration of a catheter wedged in the hepatic vein. Pressure injection of contrast material into a segmental hepatic vein through a conventional, wedged catheter opacifies the sinusoids that drain into the occluded vein. **Right:** Pressure injection of contrast material through a balloon catheter occluding a lobar hepatic vein in the same patient opacifies the sinusoids of a much larger portion of the liver. Note that the "wedged" (occluded) position has been achieved without advancing the catheter nearly so far into the hepatic vein. (Reprinted from ref. 19 with permission.)

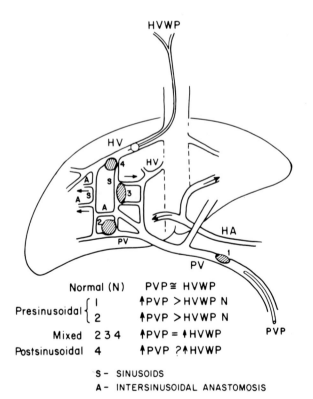

FIG. 14. Diagrammatic representation of the relationship between WHVP and PVP during blockage of the hepatic circulation at different levels. In the diagram, sinusoids (S) and intersinusoidal anastomoses (A) are represented. In the "mixed sinusoidal" form of portal hypertension (seen mainly in alcoholic cirrhosis), obstruction occurs at presinusoidal, sinusoidal, and postsinusoidal areas within the liver (sites 2, 3, and 4 in the diagram). (Reprinted with permission from ref. 57.)

failure is rare in this syndrome. It is hypothesized that hepatic vascular resistance is elevated, probably at the level of the portal venules, in an analogous fashion to that observed in the pulmonary circulation in patients with left-to-right ventricular shunts. The increased resistance in the portal venules does not occur promptly after an arteriovenous fistula develops but probably is a late manifestation. The diagnosis is best established by selective arteriography of the celiac axis and/or mesenteric arteries. Early filling of the dilated portal venous system during the arterial phase of the examination is pathognomonic of the defect (Fig. 15). This syndrome is correctable by closure of the fistula.

Occasionally, the diagnosis of prehepatic portal hypertension of unknown origin, as occurs in tropical splenomegaly, is made when there is no evidence of intrahepatic or posthepatic obstruction or fistulae (22). This disorder is characterized by splenomegaly, hypersplenism, and the development of portal-systemic collateral circulation; sometimes, bleeding from gastroesophageal varices is the first sign of the syndrome. The pathogenesis of this syndrome is not known, but it has been postulated that an enormous, progressive increase in splenic arterial flow is the primary defect, in effect acting as a massive arteriovenous fistula. An increase in intrahepatic resistance to portal flow has not been unequivocally excluded (23). Splenectomy, with or without splenorenal shunt, will correct the disorder, although if the increased flow hypothesis is right, and if intrahepatic resistance does not increase as a consequence of prolonged portal hypertension, the splenorenal shunt is unnecessary.

TABLE 2. *Classification of portal hypertension*

Prehepatic
  Venous thrombosis
    Splenic
    Portal
  Arteriovenous fistula
  Idiopathic
Intrahepatic
  Presinusoidal
    Schistosomiasis
    Nodular regeneration
    Congenital hepatic fibrosis
    Myeloproliferative disorders
    Metastatic liver disease
    Idiopathic
  Sinusoidal
    Cirrhosis
      Alcoholic
      Cryptogenic
      Other
  Postsinusoidal
    Venoocclusive disease
    Hepatic venous thrombosis
    Hepatic venous web
Posthepatic
  Venacaval obstruction
  Constrictive pericarditis
  Congestive heart failure

There are three vulnerable anatomic locations at which increased resistance can occur within the liver: (a) presinusoidal portal venules, (b) sinusoids themselves, and (c) postsinusoidal branches of the hepatic veins.

In presinusoidal intrahepatic portal hypertension, the major resistance to portal flow is localized in the portal venules. Anything that obstructs, impinges on, or otherwise narrows the intrahepatic portal venules falls into this category. Such disorders are characterized by elevated portal pressure by any of the methods that measure PVP per se, but the HVPG is not elevated. Clinically, these disorders of diminished inflow share the development of portal-systemic collaterals, often with hemorrhage from esophageal varices, but ascites is rare.

Schistosomiasis, the most common cause of portal hypertension, is the prototype of presinusoidal portal hypertension. The portal venules are obstructed by the schistosome ova. The preferred habitat in mammalian species of *Schistosoma mansoni* and *japonicum* is the portal venous system, into which the adult worms de-

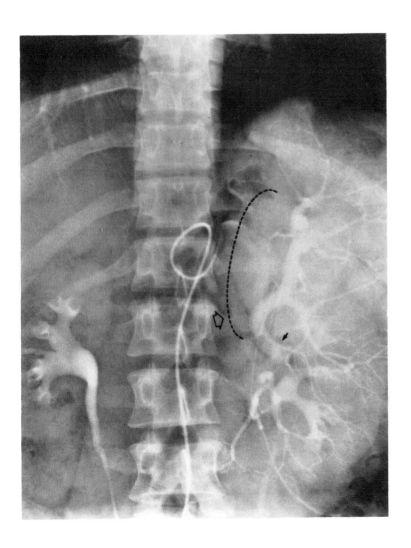

FIG. 15. Arteriovenous fistula in the portal venous system. During the arterial phase of splenic arteriography, the splenic vein (*dotted lines* and *open arrow*) is visualized by filling from the splenic artery through the arteriovenous fistula (*closed arrow*). (Reprinted from ref. 58 with permission.)

liver their eggs. The degree of portal hypertension is proportional to the oval load or the severity of the schistosomial infestation. The venooclusive effects of the ova are enhanced by the periportal granulomatous reaction to these foreign bodies. As these granulomata mature, they undergo fibrosis, which intensifies the degree of portal obstruction. As with other forms of presinusoidal portal hypertension, portal pressure is elevated, but the WHVP remains normal. The reduction in portal venous inflow is compensated for by an increment in hepatic arterial flow, which maintains the total hepatic blood flow at normal levels. During late stages of the disease, sinusoidal fibrosis and nodule formation may develop, accompanied by a rise in the HVPG, indicative of sinusoidal or postsinusoidal portal hypertension. At this stage, which may be considered the cirrhotic phase of schistosomiasis, ascites and other manifestations of hepatic outflow obstruction may appear.

Nodular regeneration of the liver is a rare disease characterized by the presence of many minute nodules scattered diffusely throughout the liver. There is little or no fibrosis. Although the cause is not known, it is postulated to be an immunopathologic disorder. This hypothesis, which is based on the concurrence of nodular regeneration with autoimmune diseases, such as Felty syndrome and scleroderma, and its appearance after renal transplantation, can be considered pathogenesis by association. The portal hypertension probably results from nodule-induced distortion of the intrahepatic portal venules. Rougier et al. (24) demonstrated a pressure gradient between the PVP and WHVP, indicative of resistance to blood flow at the presinusoidal level. The diagnosis of this disease can be established only histologically; larger, surgical biopsies are superior to needle biopsies for this purpose.

Congenital hepatic fibrosis, an autosomal recessive genetic disorder, is characterized by microscopic, intrahepatic cysts, which often communicate with the bile ducts. These cysts, which are accompanied by pericystic fibrosis, are found exclusively in the portal tracts. There they distort portal venules and biliary ducts, giving rise to portal hypertension and/or cholangitis, respectively. When the portal hypertension is severe, recurrent hemorrhage from gastroesophageal varices, which is rarely fatal, begins usually between the ages of 10 and 30.

Myeloproliferative disorders frequently infiltrate the liver, resulting in hepatomegaly and/or cholestasis. Rarely do these infiltrates induce portal hypertension by increasing portal venular resistance. When splenomegaly coexists, the increased splenic blood flow may intensify the degree of portal hypertension by increasing the portal blood flow. Although increased resistance to portal inflow is the primary defect, it cannot be excluded that the portal hypertension is solely the consequence of increased portal blood flow in patients with enormous splenomegaly.

Metastatic liver disease, a common disorder, is an uncommon cause of portal hypertension. It occasionally causes presinusoidal portal hypertension by the growth of a tumor, by tumor embolization into the portal veins, or by distortion of portal venules by tumor nodules.

Idiopathic portal hypertension, also termed hepatoportal sclerosis or noncirrhotic portal fibrosis, is a mysterious syndrome which is a diagnosis of exclusion. It is one of the frequent causes of portal hypertension in India and Japan but is uncommon in the Western world. It consists of portal hypertension in the presence of a patent extrahepatic portal venous system and in the absence of cirrhosis. Histologically, it is characterized by small amounts of portal fibrosis. Injection cast studies suggest that narrowing and destruction of intrahepatic branches of the portal vein are responsible. Microthrombosis of the portal vessels has been postulated (25). Radiologically, this disorder appears to show abrupt tapering of the intrahepatic portal vein segment just distal to the bifurcation and a paucity of middle-order portal veins and by decreased filling of small portal venules at the periphery of the liver (26). These are all subjective and controversial findings that have not been established by objective means. Hemodynamically, this disorder usually exhibits an increase in PVP but normal HVPG. We and others have occasionally observed patients with an increase in HVPG, indicative of increased resistance at the sinusoidal level or beyond. In some of these cases, a striking deposition of collagen within the space of Disse can be demonstrated electron microscopically.

Although neither its etiology nor its pathogenesis is known, arsenic toxicity, copper toxicity (in vineyard sprayers), hypervitaminosis A, and exposure to vinyl chloride have all been implicated. It has been reported recently in patients after renal transplantation (27) and may represent a spectrum of diseases caused by various etiologic agents.

Sarcoidosis, which is characterized by the predominantly periportal distribution of granulomata, tends to give rise to a predominantly presinusoidal form of portal hypertension.

In sinusoidal intrahepatic portal hypertension, the site of increased resistance to blood flow is in the sinusoids themselves. This form of portal hypertension usually is seen in various forms of cirrhosis, the prototype of which is alcoholic cirrhosis. It has long been believed that the location of the obstruction in cirrhosis was postsinusoidal, and that its mechanism was compression of hepatic venules by regenerating nodules. Recent investigations suggest that although elements of pre- and postsinusoidal obstruction are present in cirrhosis, the primary lesions are at the sinusoidal level, where the deposition of collagen in the sinusoids has been demonstrated (28) (Fig. 16). Furthermore, portal hypertension has been documented in cirrhotic patients in the absence of regenerative nodules (29).

In sinusoidal obstruction, all measurements of portal pressure, whether direct or indirect, are elevated, and the WHVP and the PVP are equal. Clinically, this type of portal hypertension is associated with the development of portal-systemic collaterals throughout the portal venous system and often with ascites, the presence or absence of which depends on the degree of obstruction of hepatic venous blood flow.

In postsinusoidal intrahepatic portal hypertension, the resistance to blood flow is in the hepatic venules. Venoocclusive disease is the prototype of this form of portal hypertension. This syndrome, which is the small vessel equivalent of the Budd-Chiari syndrome, was first described in Jamaica as a consequence of the in-

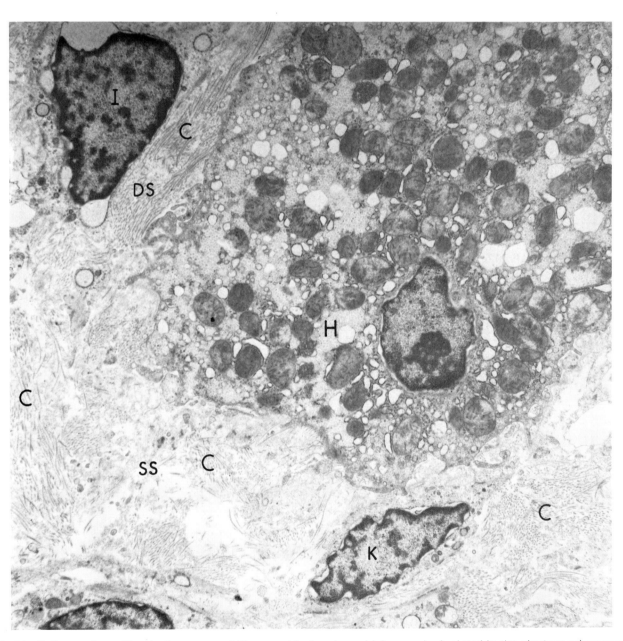

FIG. 16. Collagen deposition in the space of Disse and in the sinusoidal space is depicted in the electron micrograph. The lumen of the sinusoid is narrowed by extruded collagen. C, collagen; DS, Disse space; H, hepatocyte; I, Ito cell; K, Kuppfer cell. (Photograph kindly provided by Dr. Rosa Enriquez.)

gestion of bush tea. It has been seen wherever pyrrolizidine (senechio) alkaloids are ingested chronically (30). It can be reproduced in experimental animals by the administration of *Crotalaria fulva* or monocrotaline. It has also been seen in patients who have received 6-mercaptopurine, azothioprine, 6-thioguanine, or radiotherapy. In this disorder, the intrahepatic venules are affected by perivenular edema, fibrin deposition, and secondary scarring. Hemodynamic data are rare. Theoretically, the portal pressure is elevated and equal to the sinusoidal pressure. The major clinical manifestation of this form of hepatic outflow obstruction is ascites, although the portal-systemic collaterals develop, and hemorrhage from varices may occur.

Hepatic vein thrombosis (the Budd-Chiari syndrome) is characterized by hepatomegaly, right upper quadrant pain, and the rapid appearance of ascites, which is often intractable. Hemorrhage from esophageal varices, signs of inferior vena caval obstruction, and hypotension may appear alone or in combination as consequences of this disorder. It is relatively common in women who are taking oral contraceptives. Patients with polycythemia or other forms of hypercoagulopathy are susceptible. It may be associated with neoplasms that compress the hepatic venules and precipitate thrombosis. Pathologically, the liver is large and congested. The cut surface shows dark reddish congested areas around terminal hepatic veins (zone 3 of Rappaport) that are clearly differentiable from the peripheral, paler zones (Fig. 17). Microscopically intense sinusoidal dilatation with the disappearance and atrophy of parenchymal cells and hemorrhages around the hepatic venules are seen. When the hepatic veins are completely thrombosed, it is impossible to introduce a catheter.

Congenital hepatic venous webs, which may obstruct hepatic veins intrahepatically, mimic the Budd-Chiari syndrome, although if recognized and removed, their hosts have a more positive outcome.

Neoplasms sometimes cause compression of intrahepatic hepatic venules, although the site of obstruction may be presinusoidal and sinusoidal as well.

Posthepatic Portal Hypertension

Extrahepatic diseases that prevent the normal egress of hepatic venous blood from the liver and increase central venous pressure superimpose portal hypertension on the underlying disease. These disorders, which include obstruction of the inferior vena cava above the entry of the hepatic veins, constrictive pericarditis, and severe tricuspid insufficiency, are characterized by a Budd-Chiari-like picture. Management of the syndrome requires treatment of the primary lesion, which varies from complete correction by removal of congenital vena caval webs or by stripping of a constricting pericardium, to little relief in patients with intractable congestive heart failure.

PORTAL-SYSTEMIC COLLATERAL VESSELS

The collateral pattern that develops in response to obstruction of the portal venous system is determined by the location of the obstacle (Fig. 18). Every site of blockage has a pattern all its own. The collateral pattern is determined by the site of obstruction, the length of the obstruction, the differential in pressure between the blocked vessel and potential downstream sites of anastomosis, the nature of the tissues that must be traversed, the ability of the individual to regenerate, and the vascular anlagen that are unique for every individual.

Nature abhors an obstruction as much as a vacuum. The functional goal of collateral development is to restore the vascular right-of-way that existed before the blockage. Indeed, in this area, the wisdom expressed of the body has never been surpassed by human attempts to redirect the flow from obstructed vessels. This is not to say that solutions found in nature are

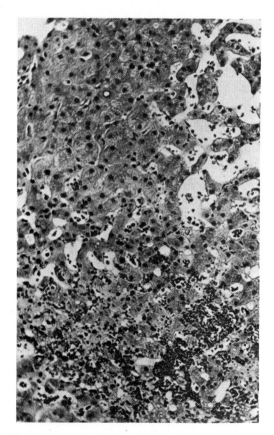

FIG. 17. Light microscopic appearance of liver in congested liver. Sinusoids are dilated, liver plates are atrophied, and red blood cells fill the central portion of the lobule.

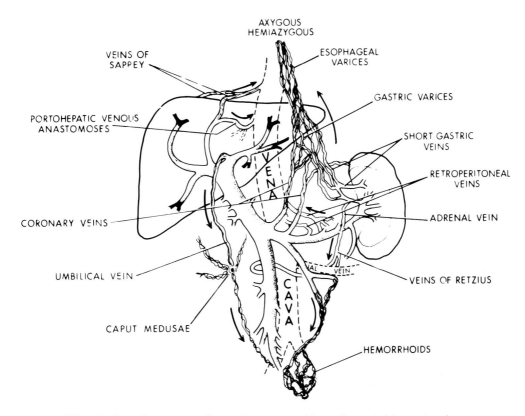

FIG. 18. Portal venous collateral patterns of hepatic portal hypertension.

perfect, or that under certain circumstances collateral circulation may not be improved by surgical intervention. Clearly, the choice of the structurally flimsy esophageal wall within the negative pressure of the tho-

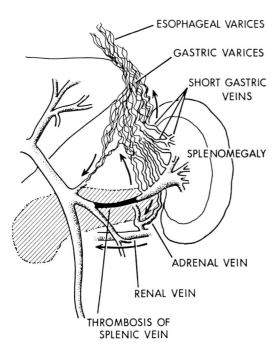

FIG. 19. Diagram of the patterns of collateral flow in splenic vein thrombosis. The pancreas is hatched.

racic cavity as a route of escape of large volumes of portal blood is neither optimal nor free of hazard. The poorly supported tortuous collateral veins, which carry blood sluggishly, develop a vicious cycle of stasis, anoxia, dilatation, and often rupture. Human attempts to find a better way are not necessarily better. Portal-systemic shunts, which divert blood flow from the varices, may divert too much blood in the process, depriving the liver of hepatotrophic portal blood, with encephalopathic consequences.

Anatomically, the farther upstream the site of the blockage, the less severe the collateral consequences. Obstruction of a splenic vein trunk, for example, stimulates little or no collateral circulation. Intrasplenic shunting redistributes the blood flow through parallel channels.

With splenic vein occlusion, localized splenic venous hypertension develops. The splenic vein proximal to the obstruction distends, the spleen becomes congested, and splenomegaly develops. The short gastric veins, the major route of splenic collaterals, rapidly enlarge and carry trapped splenic blood to the stomach and esophagus, where they become gastric and esophageal varices en route to the azygos vein (Fig. 19). The left gastroepiploic vein, which is in continuity with the branches of the left gastric vein via a rich collateral network, may drain into the left adrenal vein or newly formed splenorenal collaterals. The coronary

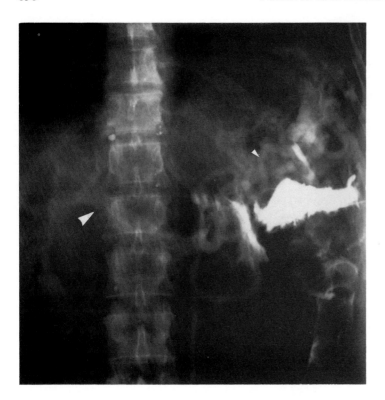

FIG. 20. Splenic vein thrombosis. A splenoportogram reveals the replacement of the splenic vein by an extensive network of collaterals (*small arrow*). The portal vein is patent (*large arrow*); it has been filled by bridging collateral veins that bypass the obstruction.

vein may carry increased amounts of blood in the physiologic direction, i.e., to the portal vein, and may help to decompress the gastroesophageal varices (Figs. 19 and 20).

When the portal vein becomes occluded, all the vessels upstream to the site of obstruction that normally form the portal vein are obstructed. The pressure in these vessels increases, the vessels distend, and collaterals develop to decompress them. All the collaterals that develop with a splenic vein obstruction develop in this situation as well. In addition, the inferior mesenteric vein is involved and results in stasis in the veins of the descending colon and the development of a hemorrhoidal variceal network (Fig. 18). The superior mesenteric flow is blocked, and stasis of the veins of the small intestine develops; exudation of splanchnic tissue fluids may occur. Ascites is uncommon but occurs occasionally. The coronary veins become dilated and carry blood to the gastroesophageal plexus with the formation of varices. The pancreatic veins become distended, the pancreas edematous, and retroperitoneal collaterals develop wherever the pancreas and mesentery contact the retroperitoneal tissues and the posterior peritoneal wall. Collaterals to the abdominal wall may become prominent. In the late stages, collaterals may develop from venae comitantes around the hepatic artery and may actually bridge the block, entering the unobstructed, intrahepatic portal vein. The unbilical vein distal to the blockage may reopen and carry blood from the abdominal wall to the left intrahepatic portal vein. A portovenogram of an obstructed portal vein can be described as collateral chaos (Fig. 21).

HEPATIC BLOOD FLOW MEASUREMENTS

Since portal pressure results from blood flow through the liver and resistance to that flow, methods to measure hepatic blood flow (HBF) and its portal venous and hepatic components are extremely important. The classic methods are presented in Table 3 and discussed in detail elsewhere in this volume.

Since the complications of portal hypertension (portal-systemic encephalopathy, hemorrhage from varices, spontaneous bacterial peritonitis) are in effect consequences of portal-systemic shunting, quantitation of such shunting is equally important. The methods used are based on the same principles used to measure blood flow. Using a modification of the indicator dilution technique, one can inject a known amount of an indicator that is not metabolized by the liver into the portal vein or hepatic artery with good mixing and calculate the HBF, which is directly proportional to the amount of hepatic blood that has diluted the indicator (31). The following formula expresses this concept:

$$\text{HBF (ml/min)} = \frac{I \times 60}{Cm \times t}$$

I is the amount of indicator injected, Cm is the mean amount of indicator collected in the hepatic vein, and t

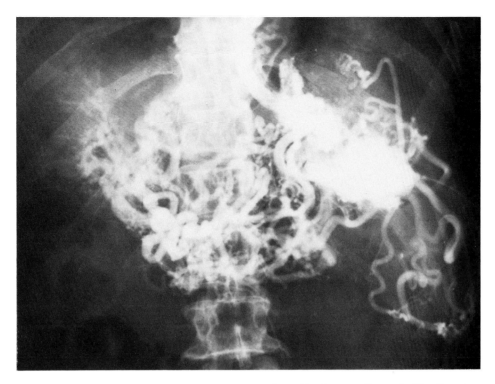

FIG. 21. Portal vein thrombosis. The portal venous system is replaced by large collaterals. The liver is partially opacified by bridging collaterals. (Kindly made available by Dr. M. Glickman.)

is the total time curve duration (seconds). If the splanchnic circulation is normal, injection of the indicator substance into either the hepatic, superior mesenteric, or splenic artery results in the same recovery of indicator in the hepatic vein (Fig. 22). The calculation of the indicator dilution curve obtained from any one of these vessels accurately reflects HBF. In the presence of either splenoportosystemic or mesoportosystemic shunting, however, some or all the dye will be lost through spontaneous splanchnosystemic shunts. By calculating the amount of indicator

TABLE 3. *Methods of measuring hepatic blood flow*

Direct
  Mechanical
    Stromuhr
    Venous outflow
    Bubble meter
    Rotameter
  Electromagnetic flowmeter
    Extravascular
    Intravascular
Indirect
  Clearance
    Single injection
    Constant infusion
  Oral-intravenous pharmacokinetic
  Indicator dilution
  Inert gas
  Distribution of cardiac output (radiolabeled
    microspheres)

recovered in the hepatic vein after each regional injection, it is possible to calculate the amount of blood flow shunted in each regional bed (32) (Fig. 23). The most accurate method for measuring regional blood flow and portal-systemic shunting is the radioactive microsphere method, which is not yet applicable to measurements in man (Fig. 24).

COMPLICATIONS OF PORTAL HYPERTENSION

Portal hypertension gives rise to a variety of clinicopathologic syndromes, such as ascites or portal-systemic encephalopathy. Each may lead to secondary complications, such as spontaneous bacterial peritonitis or hepatocerebrolenticular degeneration which may in turn give rise to tertiary complications or iatrogenic consequences (Table 4).

Treatment may illuminate critical aspects of the pathophysiology of various clinical manifestations of this protean disorder. Ideally, therapy is selected to interrupt the disease at the rate-limiting step of its pathogenic sequence using the least hazardous types of treatment. Frequently, the most desirable sites are inaccessible or invulnerable to attack by available therapy, and less logical approaches must be made. Often the therapy selected is ineffective or too toxic. Sometimes, however, therapeutic experience revises our understanding of the pathophysiology. For this

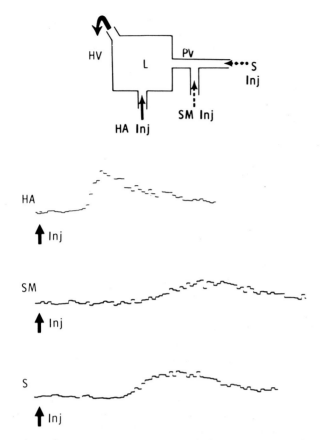

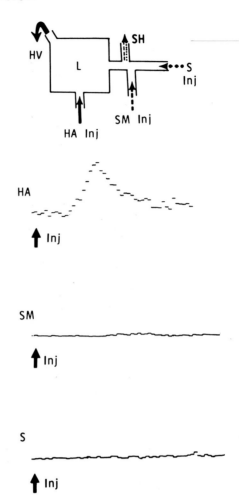

FIG. 22. Indicator dilution method of measuring blood flow through the liver (L). Recording of isotope concentration in hepatic venous (HV) blood after injection of ^{131}I-albumin into the hepatic artery (HA), superior mesenteric artery (SM), and splenic artery (S) of a normal subject. Area under each of the three curves is practically identical, thus indicating the absence of significant portal-systemic shunting. Patterns of blood flow in the portal venous (PV) and hepatic beds in the absence of shunting are shown diagrammatically. (Reprinted from ref. 32 with permission.)

FIG. 23. Portal hypertensive patient with total portal-systemic shunting. Intermediate amounts of shunting have also been observed. The absence of any radioactivity in the hepatic vein indicates that no blood from either the superior mesenteric or splenic system flows through the liver. (Symbols same as in Fig. 22.) (Reprinted from ref. 32 with permission.)

reason, a brief discussion of the pathogenesis and therapy of the major complications of portal hypertension is presented.

ASCITES

Ascites is the most important of the primary clinical complications of the portal hypertension of cirrhosis. In the most simplistic sense, ascites results from an increase in intravascular hydrostatic pressure (PVP) and a decrease in intravascular osmotic pressure (hypoalbuminemia), the two primary components of the Starling equilibrium and the major vascular and synthetic derangements of advanced cirrhosis, respectively (33).

Actually, the pathogenesis of ascites formation is far more complex. Portal hypertension sets in motion a complicated series of events. The trigger is postulated to be an as yet unidentified baroreceptor in the hepatic sinusoids which employs an unknown messenger that initiates fluid retention, the first detectable event in ascites formation. Clearly, sodium retention and the expansion of plasma volume precedes the appearance of ascitic fluid—the "overflow" hypothesis of ascites formation (34). Fluid retention is accompanied by increments in renin, angiotensin, and aldosterone production, but their role in initiating ascites formation is not known. Once the process is initiated, however, ascites increases inexorably until a new equilibrium is achieved.

Ascites has a number of clinical correlates and effects. The change in body shape may embarrass the host and profoundly affect psychosocial relationships. The physical presence of ascites may interfere with the

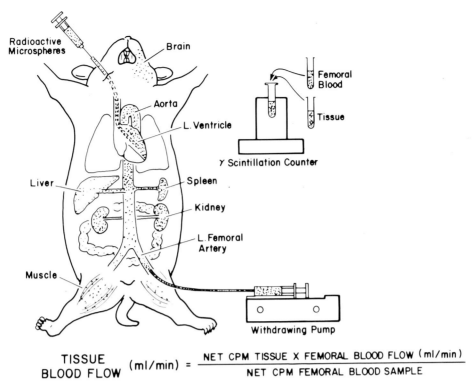

$$\text{TISSUE BLOOD FLOW (ml/min)} = \frac{\text{NET CPM TISSUE} \times \text{FEMORAL BLOOD FLOW (ml/min)}}{\text{NET CPM FEMORAL BLOOD SAMPLE}}$$

FIG. 24. Diagram of measurement of systemic and splanchnic blood flow in the rat using radioactive microspheres. While blood is withdrawn at a constant rate from the femoral artery, radioactive microspheres are injected into the left ventricle. The microspheres are distributed throughout the organs proportional to the blood flow of each organ. Blood flow is determined by comparing the radioactivity in each organ with the radioactivity in the reference blood sample. (From ref. 59.)

TABLE 4. *Consequences of portal hypertension*

Direct
  Ascites
    Bacterial peritonitis
    Abdominal hernias
      Intestinal obstruction
      Rupture
    Respiratory phenomena
      Atelectasis
      Pneumonitis
      Hypoxemia
    Inferior vena caval compression
      Peripheral edema
      Impaired venous return
    Iatrogenic
      Azotemia
      Electrolyte disturbances
  Hepatorenal syndrome
  Intestinal stasis
  Hypersplenism
Indirect
  Portal-systemic collateral network
    Neurologic
      Gastroesophageal varices
      Hemorrhoids
      Other collaterals
      Portal–systemic shunting
    Portal-systemic encephalopathy
      Impaired drug metabolism
      Altered carbohydrate metabolism
    Ulcer diathesis
    Pulmonary hypertension
    Impaired reticuloendothelial function

patient's livelihood. Surgeons may not be able to get close enough to the operating table to operate, and firemen may fall off their ladders.

Ascites may precipitate the development of all types of abdominal hernias, i.e., inguinal, umbilical, hiatal, and ventral, occasionally with morbid consequences. It raises the diaphragm, interferes with respiratory function, and sets the stage for atelectasis and pneumonitis. It may suppress appetite and aggravate an already meager nutritional state. It makes sexual congress technically difficult if that appetite persists.

In a more lethal vein, ascites increases the absolute level of portal pressure (Fig. 25) and may play a role in initiating or prolonging hemorrhage from varices. Spontaneous bacterial peritonitis never occurs in the absence of ascites. Ascites is a *sine qua non* of the hepatorenal syndrome, although it should not be considered a cause per se.

For these many reasons, patients seek medical attention. Rational therapy is based on reversing or interrupting pathogenic, precipitatory factors. Unfortunately, completely rational therapy is neither possible nor applicable in the majority of patients.

We now consider the therapy of ascites from a purely pathophysiologic point of view. In descending

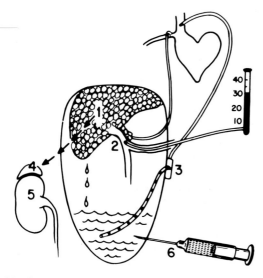

FIG. 25. A rational approach to the treatment of ascites. The numbers indicate the sites of therapy in descending order of logic. 1: Elimination of the underlying disease (venous webs). 2: Correction of the pathophysiologic abnormalities, such as portal hypertension (side-to-side portacaval shunt). 3: Enhancement of the physiologic mobilization of ascites (peritoneovenous anastomosis). 4: Inhibition of pathophysiologic mechanisms of ascites formation, such as aldosterone synthesis or renal tubular effects (spironolactone). 5: Selective intoxication of renal effects (furosemide diuresis). 6: Removal of ascites (paracentesis). (Reprinted from *Problems on Liver Diseases* with permission of C. S. Davidson and Stratton Intercontinental ref. 60.)

order of reason (Fig. 25), one would first desire to eradicate the cirrhosis. This goal has not yet been accomplished medically, although preliminary studies suggest that colchicine may have the capacity to do so (35). Orthotopic transplantation of the liver has reduced portal pressure to normal, improved hepatic synthetic function, and eliminated ascites and the hepatorenal syndrome (36). These, however, are ideas whose time has not yet come. In the noncirrhotic patient, removal of a congenital web from the hepatic vein or vena cava may completely correct the disorder.

Second, one would like to reduce portal pressure. Preliminary studies suggest that this goal may be accomplished at least transiently with propranolol (37) and can be accomplished surgically with a side-to-side portacaval anastomosis (38). This form of therapy, which must be reserved for those patients with only mild hepatic decompensation, carries a high operative mortality and frequently is followed by portal-systemic encephalopathy.

Third, one might assist the thoracic duct to enhance the transport of ascitic fluid from the peritoneal cavity to the systemic circulation. This can be accomplished by inserting a mechanical peritoneovenous shunt, such as that devised by LeVeen et al. (39), which may be

considered a man-made accessory thoracic duct. It can also be accomplished by reanastomosing the thoracic duct to the subclavian vein, in effect dilating the anatomically normal, but relatively stenotic, flow-limiting thoracosubclavian orifice (40).

Fourth, one can pharmacologically inhibit the synthesis of aldosterone and its effects on the renal tubules. It is less rational and less effective to restrict sodium intake, and it is often irrational and counterproductive to restrict water intake.

Fifth, one may pharmacologically suppress sodium reabsorption by the renal tubules by any of a number of potent diuretic drugs, which are often accompanied by azotemia and electrolyte imbalances.

Finally, and least rational, is the invasive removal of ascites. Although to treat ascites with a trochar is a direct and effective approach, it wastes protein and risks lethal infection.

Physical therapy and the order in which various forms of treatment are employed are determined by what is available rather than by what is rational. The conventional therapeutic triad has long consisted of bedrest, sodium restriction, and diuretic therapy. The role of bedrest has never been tested objectively, but it appears to be minor and should be eliminated. Salt restriction is mathematically a losing proposition, since it is rarely possible to reduce intake to levels below the renal capacity to conserve sodium. Potent diuretic therapy has rendered salt restriction archaic. Indeed, Reynolds and co-workers, in a preliminary controlled trial, have suggested that salt restriction and diuretic therapy do not increase the rate of diuresis, although they increase the rate of diuretic complications.

Since increased aldosterone secretion is an important mechanism of sodium retention, spironolactone has been found to be one of the safest and most effective diuretics. When used in progressively increasing dosage, it can induce diuresis in the majority of cirrhotic patients without inducing azotemia, hypokalemia, or other electrolyte disturbances.

It has been known for more than 20 years that spironolactone is a potent inhibitor of aldosterone at the renal tubule. More recently, it was learned that spironolactone may inhibit the synthesis of aldosterone by its action on the adrenal gland (41). Since 1963, unusual cytoplasmic inclusions have been observed in the adrenal glands of patients receiving spironolactone (Fig. 26). These "spironolactone bodies," which occur exclusively in the zona glomerulosa of the adrenal glands, appear as plasma and urinary aldosterone levels decrease. They increase in number with continuous spironolactone administration. These bodies persist in cirrhotic patients as long as spironolactone is administered but gradually disappear after it is discontinued. They appear to represent a morphologic ex-

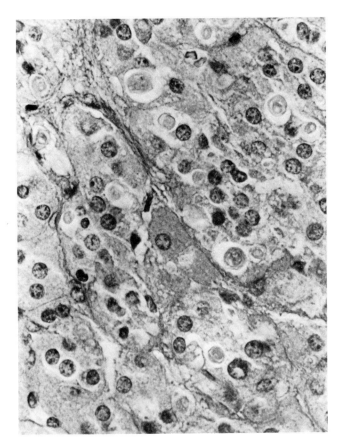

FIG. 26. Spironolactone bodies. Many of the cells of an adrenal adenoma contain pale, eosinophilic, bullseye cytoplasmic inclusions surrounded by a pale halo. (Reprinted with permission of S. S. Shrago and the American Medical Association. Originally published in 1975, *Arch. Pathol.*, 99:416.)

pression of the inhibition of aldosterone biosynthesis by spironolactone. It is reassuring that spironolactone, the safest and sanest diuretic agent for cirrhosis, happens to inhibit both the synthesis and target organ effects of the principal hormone of fluid retention.

Peritoneovenous shunts are still in the investigational stage, and their place in the treatment of ascites is not yet assured (39).

Side-to-side portacaval anastomosis, although effective, is too risky for most cirrhotic patients and must be reserved for that small fraction of ascitic patients who have both acceptable hepatic function and aggressive surgeons.

Spontaneous Bacterial Peritonitis

Spontaneous bacterial peritonitis (SBP) is a disease of ascitic patients in whom bacteria find their way into the hospitable ascitic fluid (42). This disorder usually is characterized by abdominal pain and tenderness and fever or hypothermia; it may be silent. The ascitic fluid is cloudy and contains an increased number of poly-

morphonuclear leukocytes and, usually, a single species of aerobic bacteria. Bacteremia is the most common precipitory event, although bacteria also can enter the peritoneal cavity transmurally through the intestinal wall or the avascular abdominal wall, via the lymphatics or through the Fallopian tubes.

Portal hypertension sets the stage for bacterial peritonitis in several ways. First, it is the cause of the ascites, which is an ideal bacterial culture medium. Second, it stimulates the development of portal-to-systemic collateral vessels, which act as a hole in the hepatic reticuloendothelial filter and prolong bacteremias that are normally rapidly cleared. Approximately two-thirds of episodes of SBP are caused by enteric bacteria, the most common of which are *E. coli*. Anaerobic bacteria, which make up the overwhelming majority of intestinal organisms, however, are extremely rare causes of SBP. One-third of the species arise from nonenteric sources, of which the pneumococcus is the most common. Since the majority of these infections occur more than 1 week after admission to the hospital, bacterial peritonitis is certainly a nosocomial and, probably, an iatrogenic syndrome. Medical procedures, such as infusions, transfusions, enemas, rectal examinations, angiography, catheterizations, endoscopies, biopsies, and barium contrast examinations, all of which may induce bacteremia, can initiate this disorder. In many, however, no such predisposing factor is evident. The disease is frequently fatal, either from the infection per se or with the infection serving as a contributory event. The disease may be prevented by elimination of ascites and, perhaps, by prophylaxis during potentially bacteremogenic procedures.

Hemorrhage From Gastroesophageal Varices

The most lethal of the consequences of portal hypertension is hemorrhage from esophagogastric varices. This complication occurs when the dilated, thin-walled, poorly supported collateral veins in the esophageal submucosa rupture. More than one-half the patients who bleed from varices die of the hemorrhage, aided and abetted by other problems associated with advanced cirrhosis. Another 10% die during definitive therapy. Only one-third leave the hospital alive.

Evidence indicates that the majority of hemorrhages results from the increase in portal pressure (explosion hypothesis) rather than from ulcerations of the esophageal mucosa (erosion hypothesis). In cirrhotic patients examined at esophagotomy during active variceal hemorrhage, evidence of esophageal erosions or esophagitis was uncommon (43). It has long been known that patients with corrected portal pressure levels (or hepatic venous pressure gradients of <14 mmHg) rarely bleed from varices and probably never bleed at levels below 12 mm Hg (44). Clinical observations suggest that patients with the largest varices and the highest portal pressure levels are most prone to bleed, although the degree of abnormality is not linearly related to the risk of hemorrhage. It is logical to assume that the risk rises with the pressure, although such a relationship is unproved.

Although the gradient between the wedged and free hepatic venous pressures provides a reliable prognostic and therapeutic clinical guide, it is still not clear whether the HVPG is the critical pressure measurement. Theoretically, the pressure gradient between the portal vein and the esophageal varices may be more important. The absolute PVP, which is increased by ascites and affected by other intraabdominal phenomena, is transmitted via the collateral vessels to the varices, which exist in the hypobaric thorax. The gradient may be between the head of pressure in the portal vein and the pressure within the lumen of the esophagus into which the varix bleeds. This gradient varies during respiration (Fig. 27), but is greatest in inspiration. Hemodynamic principles indicate that in a nonrigid system, the pressure gradient is decreased between compartments of different pressure by constriction of compressible communicating vessels (45).

Whether the pressure gradient or the volume of blood flow through the collateral vessels is more important in terms of hemorrhage from varices is not known. The much greater frequency of hemorrhage from esophageal varices than from gastric varices may reflect the higher portovariceal pressure gradient in the former, but other factors may be responsible for this difference.

The management of this lethal disorder is intrinsically rational. Esophageal tamponade, the most widely used form of therapy, is used to impede the flow of portal blood from the abdomen into the esophageal varices by compressing gastric collaterals against the diaphragm with an inflated gastric balloon (Fig. 28). Most such balloons also have an intraesophageal, hot-dog shaped balloon, which is designed to compress the esophageal varices against the esophageal wall. Although reasonably effective, this technique is complicated and frequently associated with serious or lethal complications (46). Other, more direct attacks on the site of hemorrhage are in active use and under intense investigation. The endoscopic injection of esophageal varices with sclerosing solutions is an old technique that is being reconsidered because of the availability of fiberoptic endoscopes and broad expertise in their use (Fig. 29). Preliminary reports of two

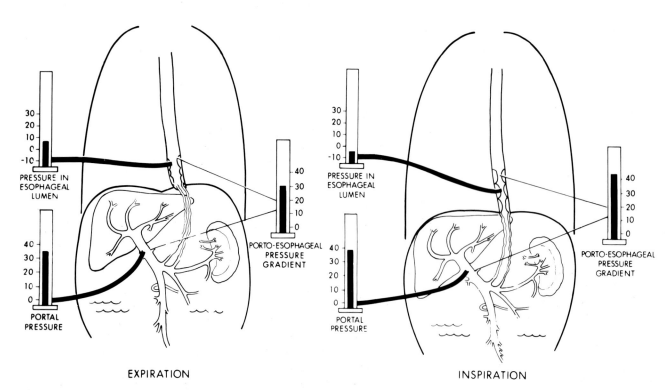

FIG. 27. The portoesophageal pressure gradient. The gradient between the PVP and the pressure in the lumen of the esophagus may be critical in initiating and perpetuating hemorrhage from esophageal varices. **Left:** Portoesophageal pressure gradient during expiration. The absolute PVP is 35 mm Hg; the esophageal pressure is +5 mm Hg; the gradient is 30 mm Hg. **Right:** Same gradient during inspiration when the portal pressure is slightly higher (38 mm Hg) than in expiration. The esophageal luminal pressure is negative, −5 mm Hg; the gradient is 43 mm Hg. The effect of respiration emphasizes the role of the negative pressure of the thorax on this pressure gradient.

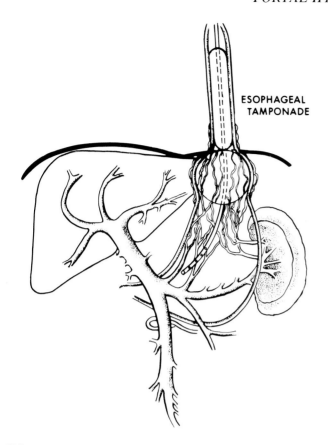

FIG. 28. Esophageal tamponade. The diagram shows an inflated Sengstaken-Blakemore tube *in situ*. The gastric balloon impedes the upward flow of gastric collateral veins. The esophageal balloon compresses mucosal varices against the esophageal wall. Distended esophageal serosal varices are shown.

ongoing controlled investigations of endoscopic sclerosis suggest that bleeding can be controlled and the frequency of hemorrhage reduced, so far without significantly decreasing mortality (47,48). Percutaneous transhepatic obliteration of the coronary veins has been performed by aggressive angiographers. Various coagulating-sclerosing-obstructing agents have been used, including buterylacrylocyanate, sodium morrhuate, gelfoam, and precoiled steel wire (49) (Fig. 29). This method requires more sophisticated, more expensive, and less available expertise, equipment, and personnel than endoscopic sclerosis. It has the advantage of affecting gastric varices, which cannot be effectively sclerosed endoscopically.

Another logical form of therapy is the use of vasoconstrictive agents, which constrict the splanchnic arteries and thereby diminish portal blood flow and portal pressure. Vasopressin, the most widely used agent, can be administered intravenously or intraarterially into the superior mesenteric artery (50). This form of therapy is often limited by the systemic effects of the agent, which decrease cardiac output and blood flow in the coronary and other venous systems. Vaso-

pressin, which stimulates the contraction of smooth muscle, may cause contraction of the esophageal wall, thus diminishing the flow of blood from serosal to mucosal varices.

The limitations of each of these forms of therapy are that hemorrhage from esophageal varices is a recurrent phenomenon, and definitive surgical portal decompression often is required. A discussion of the relative efficacy and complications of the various operations currently in use is beyond the scope of this chapter. In brief, the portacaval anastamosis is an effective procedure that prolongs survival.

Portal Systemic Encephalopathy

The pathophysiology of portal systemic encephalopathy (PSE) is determined by the portal-systemic collateral circulation that develops to compensate for the obstruction of portal blood flow. Potentially toxic materials are shunted from the portal veins directly into the systemic circulation, where they create many metabolic derangements, the most distressful of which is PSE.

The pathogenesis of PSE is unknown and is under intensive investigation. It is so metabolically diverse and involves so many metabolic abnormalities that it has been impossible to identify any one substance as *the* cause of PSE. Ammonia, a number of individual amino acids (tyrosine, phenylalanine, methionine, and tryptophan), an increased molar ratio of aromatic to branched chain amino acids, fatty acids of all chain lengths, phenols, mercaptans, and unidentified, inert neurotransmitter amines have all been touted as serious candidate toxins (51). These substances all have neurotoxic properties, are of enteric origin, and are either hepatically detoxified or compensated for.

Ammonia is the prime culprit. It was the first putative toxin and the one about which the most is known. A variety of ammonium salts induce encephalopathy in both cirrhotic patients and experimental animals. Similarly, ammonium-liberating cation exchange resins induce PSE. Infusions of amino acids, such as glycine, which are rapidly deaminated, may also cause coma in patients with liver disease. Orally ingested proteins induce encephalopathy in cirrhotic patients. All the urea cycle enzyme deficiencies, which represent five different syndromes, each of which is characterized by increased blood ammonia levels, are associated with an encephalopathic pattern similar to that of PSE. These disorders are characterized by increased blood ammonia concentrations. Nonnitrogenous forms of hepatic coma do not exhibit elevated blood ammonia levels. Successful therapy is designed to reduce the amount of ammonia that enters the systemic circulation from the alimentary canal and to increase the en-

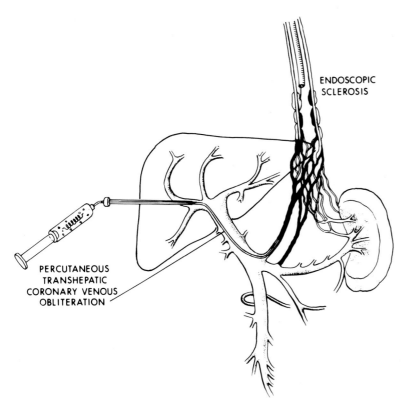

FIG. 29. Endoscopic and transhepatic obliteration of varices. *Upper right,* a varix is being injected with a flexible endoscope. The black varices have already undergone sclerosis. *Left,* a catheter passes through a percutaneous cannula, through the portal vein, and into the left gastric (coronary) vein. The black veins have already been obliterated. Within the syringe, gelfoam particles and a coil in a sclerosing solution are represented.

teric and urinary excretion of ammonia and its products.

Recent investigations of the dynamics of ammonia metabolism in normal and encephalopathic human subjects provide new understanding of the pathophysiology of this substance (52). After the intravenous injection of $^{13}NH_3$, a positron-emitting isotope with a half-life of 10 min, the ammonia, which is distributed throughout the body water, is promptly cleared from the blood and metabolized. Ammonia clearance from the blood is proportional to the arterial ammonia concentration. At equilibrium, approximately 6% of the ^{13}N is found in the blood. Approximately 7% is located in the brains of normal subjects with slightly more in the brains of cirrhotic patients. Brain uptake is linearly related to arterial ammonia concentration, which is higher in patients with cirrhosis. The ammonia taken up by brain is trapped in a compartment that constitutes approximately 20% of brain volume. It is postulated that this small ammonia pool is contained in the astrocytes, where most of the ammonia that enters the brain is incorporated into the amide nitrogen of glutamine. Glutamine synthetase, the enzyme that catalyzes this critical reaction, is an astrocytic enzyme (53). These observations are in accord with the astrocyte abnormalities observed in PSE and the histologic changes in astrocyte nuclei induced by portacaval anastomosis. Approximately 7% of the activity was found in the liver. The liver, which synthesizes urea, an excretable product, plays the most important role in ammonia homeostasis.

Skeletal muscle, which constitutes 40% of body weight, is estimated to contain 50% of the ^{13}N. By virtue of its mass, muscle is second only to the liver in the amount of ammonia removed. Skeletal muscle, like brain, contains glutamine synthetase, which can detoxify large amounts of ammonia by synthesizing glutamine. This glutamine is carried to the liver, where it is converted to urea. Clearly, the amount of ammonia that can be detoxified is directly related to the muscle mass. Just as muscle is important in the extraction of ammonia from blood, it has long been known that muscle releases ammonia into the blood during exercise. There are small increments in arterial ammonia concentration after mild physical exercise, such as walking up two flights of stairs, and larger increments after severe exercise. The incremental ammonia is liberated from adenylic acid, which accumulates in muscle during anaerobic exercise. Subsequently, ammonia is reincorporated into the purine nucleotide cycle to replenish adenosine triphosphate (54).

Scintigraphs of the head taken with a high-energy gamma rectilinear scanner show that normally, the highest ^{13}N activity is seen in the gray matter of the brain. In patients with cirrhosis, there is a redistribution in the uptake of ^{13}N, with a progressive decrease in the parietal area as encephalopathy develops. These dramatic scintiscans represent the first "photographs" of hepatic coma (52).

It has been shown recently that different portions of the bowel function differently in ammonia homeostasis

(55). The gut is actually the primary source of the ammonia in blood. In the dog, most of the ammonia is derived from the colon, in which urea is hydrolyzed by bacterial urease. A smaller amount arises from the small intestine, which takes up glutamine. The ammonia released is not solely related to bacterial activity. It must be kept in mind that ammonia can be released from the intestinal tract of germ-free animals. The substrate for ammonia liberation in germ-free animals is dietary protein or blood, but urea does not liberate ammonia in germ-free animals. The hepatic coma induced in rats by total hepatectomy develops just as rapidly in germ-free as in germy rats. Although ammonia can be derived from nonbacterial metabolism, the metabolic chaos of the liverless animal is quite different from clinical PSE and from most experimental models.

The three principal aspects of the treatment of PSE are, like the classic chemical reaction, directed at the substrate, the enzyme, and the product. Reduction in dietary protein intake and evacuation of the gastrointestinal tract are designed to reduce the ammoniagenic substrate. Antibiotic therapy, such as neomycin, effectively suppresses the bacteria and, thereby, the bacterial enzymes that degrade urea and other nitrogenous substrates. Lactulose creates an internal acid dialysis system, which dialyzes ammonia, the product of this reaction, from the body, traps it in the intestinal lumen, and excretes it in the feces. All are effective forms of therapy, and each individually can lower the blood ammonia level and restore normal cerebral function in patients with PSE.

Hypersplenism

Splenomegaly is a common physical sign of portal hypertension. Although the size of the spleen per se is not a problem, the hematocytopenic consequences of splenomegaly may be. Thrombocytopenia (<100,000/cu mm) occurs in about 20% of cirrhotic patients with esophageal varices, leukopenia (<4,000/cu mm) occurs in about 15%, and hemolytic anemia in about 10%. Hypersplenism, with suppression of one or more of the formed elements of blood, occurs in about 35%. In most instances, the cytopenia represents a numerical rather than a disease-inducing abnormality, although occasionally thrombocytopenia causes bleeding, leukopenia permits the development of bacterial infection, and hemolytic anemia requires transfusions. The presence and degree of hypersplenism tend to fluctuate over long periods of observation. After portal decompression surgery, there is often transient improvement. When clinically severe, hypersplenism may require splenectomy, which usually is permanently effective.

The pathophysiology of portal hypertension is a many-faceted story; we have just begun to develop the tools that may permit elucidation of its mysteries. Each of the clinical consequences of portal hypertension has a pathogenesis equally complex to that of portal hypertension per se. Clearly, portal hypertension will be a fertile field for the study of the basic physiology and clinical manifestations of portal hypertension for the foreseeable future.

REFERENCES

1. Rappaport, A. M. (1975): *Anatomic Considerations. Diseases of the Liver,* edited by L. M. Schiff. Lippincott, Philadelphia.
2. Kardon, R. H., and Wessel, R. G. (1980): Three-dimensional organization of the hepatic microcirculation in the rodent as observed by scanning electron microscopy of corrosion casts. *Gastroenterology,* 79:72–81.
3. Ternberg, J. L., and Butcher, H. R., Jr. (1965): Blood flow relation between artery and portal vein. *Science,* 150:1030–1031.
4. Groszmann, R. J., Kravetz, D., and Parysow, O. (1977): Intrahepatic arteriovenous shunting in cirrhosis of the liver. *Gastroenterology,* 73:201–204.
5. Cohn, R., and Kountz, S. (1963): Factors influencing control of arterial circulation in the liver of the dog. *Am. J. Physiol.,* 205:1260–1264.
6. Lautt, W. W. (1980): Control of hepatic arterial blood flow: independence from liver metabolic activity. *Am. J. Physiol.,* 239:H559–H564.
7. Groszmann, R. J., Kotelanski, B., and Cohn, J. N. (1971): Hepatic lobar distribution of splenic and mesenteric blood flow in man. *Gastroenterology,* 60:1047–1052.
8. Knauer, C. M., and Lowe, H. M. (1967): Hemodynamics in the cirrhotic patient during paracentesis. *N. Engl. J. Med.,* 276:491–496.
9. Lavoie, P., Jacob, M., Ledue, J., Legare, A., and Viallet, A. (1966): The umbilicoportal approach for the study of the splanchnic circulation: Technical radiological and hemodynamic considerations. *Can. J. Surg.,* 9:338–343.
10. Zimmon, D. S., and Kessler, R. E. (1980): Effect of portal venous blood flow diversion on portal pressure. *J. Clin. Invest.,* 65:1388–1397.
11. Boyer, T. D., Triger, D. R., Horisawa, M., Redeker, A. G., and Reynolds, T. B. (1977): Direct transhepatic measurement of portal vein pressure using a thin needle. *Gastroenterology,* 72:584–589.
12. Viamonte, M., Jr., LePage, J., Lunderquist, A., Pereiras, R., Russell, E., Viamonte, M., and Camacho, M. (1975): Selective catherization of the portal vein and its tributaries. *Radiology,* 114:456–460.
13. Panke, W. F., Bradley, E. G., Moreno, A. H., Ruzicka, F. F., and Rousselot, L. M. (1959): Techniques, hazards and usefulness of percutaneous splenic portography. *JAMA,* 169:1032–1037.
14. Smith-Laing, G., Camilo, M. E., Dick, R., and Sherlock, S. (1980): Percutaneous transhepatic portography in the assessment of portal hypertension. Clinical correlations and comparison of radiographic techniques. *Gastroenterology,* 78:197–205.
15. Orrego-Matte, H., Amenabar, E., Lara, G., Baraona, E., Palmar, R., and Messaro, F. (1964): Measurements of intrahepatic pressure as index of portal pressure. *Am. J. Med. Sci.,* 247:278–282.
16. Vennes, J. A. (1966): Intrahepatic pressure: An accurate reflection of portal pressure. *Medicine,* 45:445–452.
17. Petursson, M. K., Wenger, J., Landy, M. S., Crawley, S., and Lindsay, J. (1971): Intrahepatic pressure measurement: Some pitfalls. *Scand. J. Gastroenterol.,* 6:745–750.
18. Friedman, E. W., and Weiner, R. S. (1951): Estimation of hepatic sinusoid pressure by means of venous catheters and estimation of portal pressure by hepatic vein catheterization. *Am. J. Physiol.,* 165:527–531.
19. Groszmann, R. J., Glickman, M., Blei, A. T., Storer, E., and

Conn, H. O. (1979): Wedged and free hepatic venous pressure measured with a balloon catheter. *Gastroenterology,* 76: 254–258.

20. Groszmann, R. J., and Atterbury, C. E. (1980): Clinical applications of the measurement of portal venous pressure. *J. Clin. Gastroenterol.,* 2:379–386.

21. Donovan, A. J., Reynolds, T. B., Mikkelsen, W. P., and Peters, R. L. (1969): Systemic-portal arteriovenous fistulas: Pathological and hemodynamic observations in two patients. *Surgery,* 66:474–482.

22. Williams, R., Parronson, A., Sommers, K., and Hamilton, P. G. S. (1966): Portal hypertension in idiopathic tropical splenomegaly. *Lancet,* ii:329–333.

23. Sato, T., Woyama, K., Watomabe, K., and Kimura, S. (1969): Experimental study on the effect of increase in splenic blood flow upon the portal pressure. *J. Exp. Med.,* 98:65–74.

24. Rougier, P., Degot, T. C., Ruef, B., and Benhamou, J. P. (1978): Modular regenerative hyperplasia of the liver. Report of six cases and review of the literature. *Gastroenterology,* 75:169–172.

25. Boyer, J. L., Hales, M. R., and Klatskin, G. (1974): Idiopathic portal hypertension due to occlusion of intra-hepatic portal vein by organized thrombi. *Medicine,* 53:77–91.

26. Futagawa, S., Fukazawa, M., Horisawa, M., Musha, H., Ito, T., Sugiura, M., Kameda, H., and Okuda, K. (1980): Portographic liver changes in idiopathic non cirrhotic portal hypertension. *Am. J. Roentgenol.,* 134:917–923.

27. Natal, C., Feldman, G., Lebree, D., Degot, D., Deseamps, J. N., Rueff, B., and Benhamou, J. P. (1979): Idiopathic portal hypertension (perisinusoidal fibrosis) after renal transplantation. *Gut,* 20:531–537.

28. Edmundson, H. E., Peters, R., Frankel, H. H., and Borowsky, S. (1967): The early stage of liver injury in the alcoholic. *Medicine,* 46:119–129.

29. Reynolds, T. B., Hidemura, R., Michel, H., and Peters, R. (1969): Portal hypertension without cirrhosis in alcoholic liver disease. *Ann. Int. Med.,* 70:497–506.

30. Stillman, A. E., Huxtable, R., Consroe, P., Kohnen, P., and Smith, S. (1977): Hepatic veno-occlusive disease due to pyrrolizidine (senechio) poisoning in Arizona. *Gastroenterology,* 73:349–352.

31. Cohn, J. N., Kharti, I., Groszmann, R. J., and Kotelanski, B. (1972): Hepatic blood flow in alcoholic liver disease measured by an indicator dilution technique. *Am. J. Med.,* 53:704–714.

32. Groszmann, R. J., Kotelanski, B., and Cohn, J. N. (1972): Quantitation of portasystemic shunting from the splenic and mesenteric beds in alcoholic liver disease. *Am. J. Med.,* 53:715–722.

33. Atkinson, M., and Losowsky, M. S. (1962): Plasma colloid osmotic pressure in relation to the formation of ascites and edema in liver disease. *Clin. Sci.,* 22:383–389.

34. Levy, M. (1977): Sodium retention and ascites formation in dogs with experimental portal cirrhosis. *Am. J. Physiol.,* 233:F572–F585.

35. Kersenobich, D., Uribe, M., Suarez, G. I., Mata, J. M., Perez-Tamayo, R., and Rojkind, M. (1979): Treatment of cirrhosis with colchicine. A double-blind randomized trial. *Gastroenterology,* 77:532–536.

36. Iwatsuki, S., Popovtzer, M. M., Corman, J. L., Ishikawa, M., Putnam, C. W., Katz, F. H., and Starzl, T. E. (1973): Recovery from "hepatorenal syndome" after orthotopic transplantation. *N. Engl. J. Med.,* 289:1155–1159.

37. Lebrec, D., Poynard, T., Hillon, P., et al. (1981): Propranolol for prevention of recurrent gastrointestinal bleeding in patients with cirrhosis. *N. Engl. J. Med.,* 305:1371–1374.

38. Orloff, M. J., and Johansen, K. H. (1978): Treatment of Budd-Chiari syndrome by side-to-side portacaval shunt: Experimental and clinical results. *Am. Surg.,* 188:494–512.

39. LeVeen, H. H., Wapnick, S., Grosberg, S., and Kinney, M. J. (1976): Further experience with peritoneovenous shunt for ascites. *Ann. Surg.,* 184:574–581.

40. Dumont, A. E., and Mullholland, J. H. (1960): Flow rate and composition of thoracic duct lymph in patients with cirrhosis. *N. Engl. J. Med.,* 263:471–474.

41. Conn, J. W., and Hinerman, D. L. (1977): Spironolactone-induced inhibition of aldosterone biosynthesis in primary aldosteronism. Morphological and functional studies. *Metabolism,* 26:1293–1307.

42. Conn, H. O., and Fessel, J. M. (1971): Spontaneous bacterial peritonitis in cirrhosis. Variations on a theme. *Medicine,* 50:161–197.

43. Orloff, M. J., and Thomas, H. S. (1963): Pathogenesis of esophageal varix rupture. *Arch. Surg.,* 87:301–306.

44. Viallet, A., Marleau, D., Huet, M., Martin, F., Farley, A., Villeneuve, J-P., and Lavoie, P. (1975): Hemodynamic evaluation of patients with intrahepatic portal hypertension: Relationship between bleeding varices and the portohepatic gradient. *Gastroenterology,* 69:1297–1300.

45. Doppman, J., Rubinson, R. M., Rockoff, S. P., Vasko, J. S., Shapiro, R., and Morrow, A. G. (1966): Mechanism of obstruction of the infradiaphragmatic portion of the inferior vena cava in the presence of increased intra-abdominal pressure. *Invest. Radiol,* 1:37–53.

46. Chojkier, M., and Conn, H. O. (1980): Esophageal tamponade in the treatment of bleeding varcies. *Dig. Dis. Sci.,* 25:267–272.

47. Macdougall, B. R. D., Westaby, D., Theodossi, A., Dawson, J. L., and Williams, R. (1982): Increased long-term survival in variceal haemorrhage using injection sclerotherapy: results of a controlled trial. *Lancet,* i:124–127.

48. Terblanche, J., Northover, J. M. A., Bornmann, P., Kahn, D., Silber, W., Barbezat, G. O., Sellars, S., Campbell, J. A., and Saunders, S. J. (1979): A prospective controlled trial of scleroptherapy in the long-term management of patients after esophageal variceal bleeding. *Surg. Gynecol. Obstet.,* 148: 323–333.

49. Lunderquist, A., Borjesson, B., Owman, T., and Bengmark, S. (1978): Isobutyl 2-cyanoacrylate (Bucrylate) in obliteration of gastric coronary vein and esophageal varices. *Am. J. Roentgenol.,* 130:1–6.

50. Conn, H. O., Ramsby, G. R., Storer, E. H., Mutchnick, M. G., Joshi, P. H., Phillips, M. M., Cohen, G. A., Fields, G. N., and Petroski, D. (1975): Intraarterial vasopressin in the treatment of upper gastrointestinal hemorrhage: A prospective, controlled clinical trial. *Gastroenterology,* 68:211–221.

51. Conn, H. O., and Lieberthal, M. M. (1979): *The Hepatic Coma Syndromes and Lactulose.* Williams & Wilkins, Baltimore.

52. Lockwood, A. H., McDonald, J. M., Reiman, R. E., Gelbard, A. S., Laughlin, J. S., Duffy, T. E., and Plum, F. (1979): The dynamics of ammonia metabolism in man: Effects of liver disease and hyperammonemia. *J. Clin. Invest.,* 63:449–460.

53. Martinez-Hernandez, A., Bell, K. P., and Norenberg, M. D. (1977): Glutamine synthetase: Glial localization in brain. *Science,* 195:1356–1358.

54. Lowenstein, J. M. (1972): Ammonia production in muscle and other tissues: The purine nucleotide cycle. *Physiol. Rev.,* 52:382–414.

55. Weber, F. L., and Veach, G. L. (1979): The importance of the small intestine in gut ammonium production in the fasting dog. *Gastroenterology,* 77:235–240.

56. Groszmann, R. J., Blei, A., Storer, E., and Conn, H. O. (1978): Portal pressure reduction induced by partial mechanical obstruction of the superior mesenteric artery in the anesthetized dog. *Gastroenterology,* 74:187–192.

57. Groszmann, R. J. (1981): Portal hypertension: hemodynamic and physiopathologic aspects. In: *Enfermedades del Aparato Digestivo y de Higado,* edited by D. Cantor, and R. J. Groszmann. Salvat, Barcelona.

58. Bredfeldt, J. E., and O'Laughlin, J. C. (1980): Portal hypertension secondary to a congenital splenic arteriovenous fistula. *J. Clin. Gastro.,* 2:355–358.

59. Groszmann, R. J., Vorobioff, J., and Riley, E. (1981): The measurement of splanchnic and systemic hemodynamics in the normal and cirrhotic rat by using radioactive microspheres. In: *Hepatic Circulation in Health and Disease,* edited by W. Wyane Lautt. Raven Press, New York.

60. Taggart, G. J., and Conn, H. O. (1979): Ascites: its causes, complications and correction. In: *Problems in Liver Disease,* edited by C. S. Davison. Stratton Intercontinental Medical Book Corp., New York.

SUBJECT INDEX

Subject Index

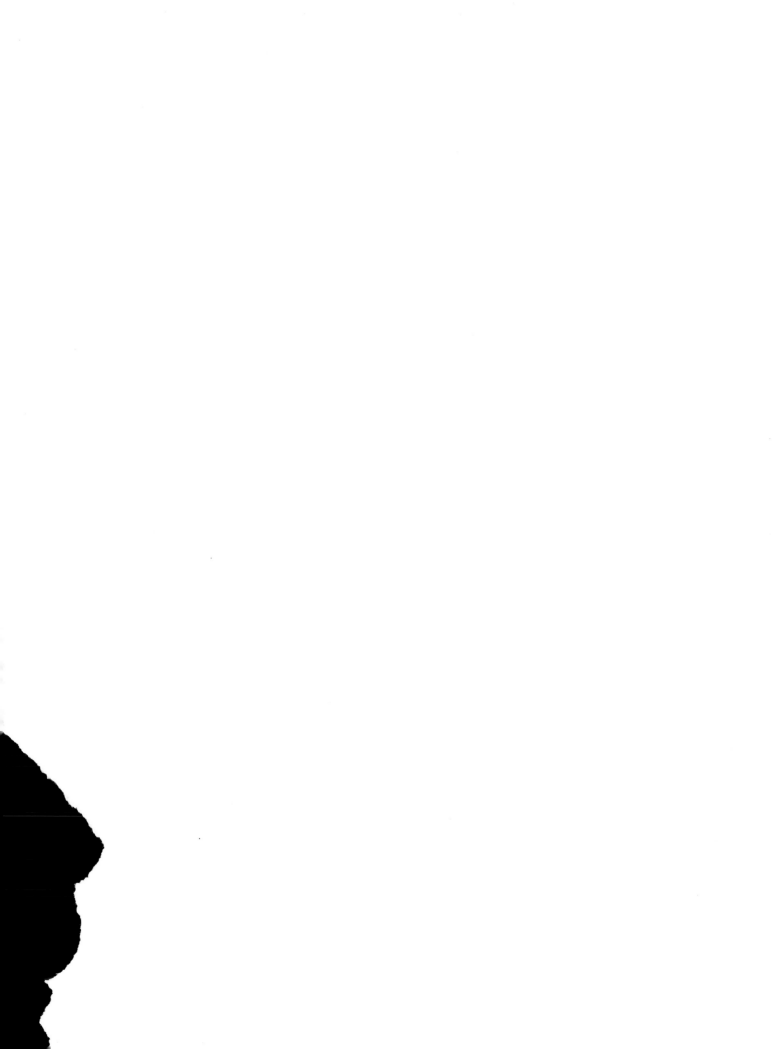